Alexander's Nursing Practice

Alexander's Nursing Practice

Hospital and Home

6TH EDITION

Edited by

Ian Peate, OBE, FRCN, EN(G) RGN, DipN(Lond), RNT B.Ed (Hons), MA, LLM

Editor in Chief, British Journal of Nursing; Consultant Editor, Journal of Paramedic Practice;
Consultant Editor, International Journal for Advancing Practice;
Visiting Professor, Northumbria University;
Visiting Professor, St Georges University of London and Kingston University London;
Professorial Fellow, Roehampton University;
Visiting Senior Clinical Fellow, University of Hertfordshire, UK

ELSEVIER

Publisher's note: Elsevier takes a neutral position with respect to territorial disputes or jurisdictional claims in its published content, including in maps and institutional affiliations.

First edition 1994
Second edition 2000
Third edition 2006
Fourth edition 2011
Fifth edition 2019

Notices

Practitioners and researchers must always rely on their own experience and knowledge in evaluating and using any information, methods, compounds or experiments described herein. Because of rapid advances in the medical sciences, in particular, independent verification of diagnoses and drug dosages should be made. To the fullest extent of the law, no responsibility is assumed by Elsevier, authors, editors or contributors for any injury and/or damage to persons or property as a matter of products liability, negligence or otherwise, or from any use or operation of any methods, products, instructions, or ideas contained in the material herein.

ISBN: 978-0-4431-1022-1

Content Strategist: Robert Edwards
Content Project Manager: Arindam Banerjee
Design: Christian Bilbow
Marketing Manager: Deborah Watkins

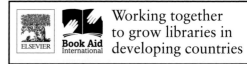

Printed in India
Last digit is the print number: 9 8 7 6 5 4 3 2 1

Contents

This text is dedicated to my brother Alan David Peate.

Contributors

Irene Anderson, MSc, BSc Hons, PG Cert HE, PG Cert Management & Leadership
Principal Lecturer
Tissue Viability
Associate Professor
Learning and Teaching
School of Health and Social Work
University of Hertfordshire
Hatfield, Hertfordshire, UK

Kim Bezzant, RN, BEd (Hons), MSc in Professional and Policy Studies (Age and Ageing)

Emma Burnett, PhD, MSc, PGCert, BN, SPQ, RGN
Head of Campus
Fatima College of Health Sciences
Institute of Applied Technology
Ajman, UAE

Trish Burton, BSc (Nursing and Human Sciences), PgCert (Practice Education)
Patient and Family Liaison Nurse
Centre for Excellence
Essex & Herts Air Ambulance
Essex, UK

Clare Butler, MSc, SFHEA, BSc, RN
Programme Lead
Advanced and Specialist Practice CPD
Oxford School of Nursing and Midwifery
Faculty of Health and Life Sciences
Oxford Brookes University
Oxford, UK

Carl Clare, MSc, BSc
Senior Lecturer Adult Nursing
University of Hertfordshire
Hatfield, Hertfordshire, UK

Elaine Crosby-Jones
Acute Oncology Lead Nurse
East Sussex Healthcare Trust
Eastbourne and Hastings, UK

Susanne Cruickshank, PhD, FHEA, MSc (Cancer), BSc, RGN
Strategic Lead for Applied Health Research
Health Services Research
The Royal Marsden NHS Foundation Trust
London, UK;
Honorary Professor
Faculty of Health Sciences and Sport
University of Stirling
Stirling, UK

Jacqui Fletcher, BSc, PG Cert, MSc, OBE
Clinical Lead Pressure Ulcers
Stop the Pressure Programme
NHS England
London, UK;
Independent Nurse Consultant
Jacqui Fletcher Limited, UK

Sue M. Green, RN, PGCert, BSc, MedSci, PhD
Professor and Deputy Head
Department for Nursing Sciences
Faculty of Health and Social Sciences
Bournemouth University
Bournemouth, Dorset, UK

Hilary Harkin, BSc (Hons) RGN
ENT Clinical Nurse Specialist
Guys and St. Thomas' NHS Foundation Trust
London, UK

Barry Hill, MSc Adv Prac, PGCAP, BSc (Hons) CCRN, DipHE/O.A. Dip, SFHEA, TEFL, NMC RN RNT/TCH V300
Associate Professor of Nursing and Critical Care
Module Leader for Critical Care Nursing
Advanced Diploma Adult Critical Care Nursing - Level 6/ Postgraduate Certificate
Adult Critical Care Nursing - Level 7
Employability Lead for Nursing, Midwifery and Health
Champion for Equality, Diversity, and Inclusion (LGBTQ+)
Northumbria University
Newcastle upon Tyne, UK

Cheryl Holman, PhD, MSc, BEd (Hons)
Associate Dean Academic Quality Assurance
Health and Social Work
University of Hertfordshire
Hatfield, UK

Lucy Victoria Jamieson, BSc (Hons) RGN
ENT Nurse
Guys and St. Thomas' NHS Foundation Trust
London, UK

Noleen Patricia Jones, BSc, Med, FHEA
Principal Lecturer (Ag)
School of Health Studies
Gibraltar Health Authority
St. Bernard's Hospital
Gibraltar

Patricia Kydd, MSc, PGCAPHE, BN, RN
Lecturer
School of Health Sciences
University of Dundee
Dundee, UK

Rachael Lear, PhD, FHEA, RN
Advanced Nurse Practitioner
Robin Hood Lane Health Centre
Sutton, UK
Research Fellow
Faculty of Medicine
Imperial College London
London, UK

Georgina Lewis, MSc (Surgical Care Practice from Edge Hill), BSc (Perioperative Care Staffordshire)
Surgical Care Practitioner (Gynae)
Gloucestershire Hospitals NHS Trust
Gloucester, UK

Vicky MacArthur, RGN, BSc (Hons), MSc, DHPE
Deputy Programme Lead Advanced and Specialist Practice
Course Lead Integrated Degree Apprenticeship Advanced
    Clinical Practitioner
Oxford Brookes University
Oxford, UK

Ruth Magowan, MSc, BSc (Hons), PG Cert, RGN, RSCN, SFHEA
Interim Head of Division
Division of Nursing and Paramedic Science
Queen Margaret University
Edinburgh, UK

Breeda McCahill, BSc, PGDip, NBSDip, RN
Burns Nurse Practitioner
Burns Clinic
Glasgow Royal Infirmary
Course Leader
Nursing and Health
University of Glasgow
Glasgow, UK

Katharine Martyn, RN, RNut
SSHS Apprenticeships
Technical Education and Flexible Learning Lead
Honorary Fellow International Academy of Nutrition Educators
Senior Fellow Higher Education Academy
Principal Lecturer Nutrition
School of Sport and Health Sciences
University of Brighton
Brighton, UK

Jane Marquesen, BSN, MPH, FHEA
Lecturer
School of Sport and Health Science
University of Brighton
Fellowship of Higher Education Academy
University of Brighton
Post Graduate Certificate of Academic Practice
University of Brighton
Brighton, UK

Johannes Mellinghoff, BSc, MSc, RN
Senior Lecturer
School of Sport and Health Sciences
University of Brighton
London, UK

Emma Menzies-Gow, BSc (Hons), MA, RNT, FHEA
Senior Lecturer
School of Sport and Health Sciences
University of Brighton
Brighton, UK

Jacqueline Metcalfe, BSc (Hons), MSc, RN
Safeguarding Learning and Improvement Lead
    (Adults, Children and LAC)
Hampshire and Isle of Wight Integrated Care Board
Southampton, Hampshire, UK

Sally Pannifex, BSc (Nursing)
Alcohol Related Liver Disease CNS
Gastro/Hepatology
St Georges Hospital NHS Foundation Trust
London, UK

Ruth Paterson, PhD, MPhil, FHEA, RN
Associate Professor
Head of Subject (Nursing)
Honorary Research Consultant NHS Lothian
School of Health and Social Care
Edinburgh Napier University
Edinburgh, UK

Jill Peters, MSc, BSc, RGN, Dip NP, PGD, NISP, CMS
Dermatology Nurse Practitioner
Dermatology Department
Ipswich Hospital
Ipswich, Suffolk, UK

Allyson Sanderson, MA, ECP, PGCE LTHE, RN
Regional Senior Nurse
HC One-The Kind Care Company
Darlington, County Durham, UK
Senior Lecturer in Adult Nursing
School of Health and Life Sciences
Teesside University
Middlesbrough, UK

Anthony Shanahan, MSc, BSc
Surgical Care Practitioner in Urology
Urology Department
Cwm Taf University Health Board
Pontyclun, Wales, UK

Julie Santy-Tomlinson, RN (Ret), PhD
Freelance Author and Editor
Hull, UK

Penelope Stanford, BSc (Hons), MSc, PhD, PGDE, RN, OND, RNT
Senior Lecturer
Chair, RCN Ophthalmic Forum
Division of Nursing
Midwifery and Social Work
University of Manchester
Greater Manchester, Manchester, UK

Martin Steggall, BSc (Hons), MSc, PhD, RN (Adult), FHEA
Pro Vice Chancellor Research and Innovation
University of South Wales
Pontypridd, UK
Honorary Clinical Nurse Specialist (Urology)
Cwm Taf University Health Board
Pontyclun, Wales, UK

Suzan Thompson, MSc, BSc (Hons), RN, DMCC, FHEA
Senior Lecturer in Paramedic Science (pre-registration)
Paramedic Section
Centre for Allied Health
St George's, University of London
London, UK

Jitka Vseteckova, PhD, D.Prof., SFHEA
Chair Carers Research Group OU
School of Health, Wellbeing and Social Care
Faculty of Wellbeing, Education and Language Studies
The Open University
Milton Keynes, UK

Susan Walker, MA, BSc (Hons)
Senior Lecturer
School of Health and Society
University of Salford
Salford, Greater Manchester, UK

Catheryne Waterhouse, MSC Nursing
Clinical Nurse Educator
Neuro Intensive Care
Royal Hallamshire Hospital
Sheffield, South Yorkshire, UK

Anthony Wheeldon, MSc Cardiorespiratory Nursing, PGDip Learning and Teaching, BSc (Hons), RN
Senior Lecturer
Adult Nursing and Primary Care
University of Hertfordshire
Hatfield, Hertfordshire, UK

Dean Whiting, RN, RNT, BN (Hons), BSc (Hons), PgCAP, PgDip, MSc, DipMSKMed, FHEA
Principal Lecturer in Advanced Clinical Practice
The School of Health and Social Work
University of Hertfordshire
Hatfield, UK

Sue Woodward, RN, MSc, PGCEA, PhD, FRCN
Senior Lecturer
Florence Nightingale Faculty of Nursing
Midwifery and Palliative Care
King's College London
London, UK

Preface

I am delighted to present the sixth edition of *Alexander's Nursing Practice: Hospital and Home*. As the provision of healthcare continues to evolve, so too must the resources that shape the education of future nurses. This latest edition reflects the most up-to-date advances in the field, ensuring that readers are equipped with the knowledge and skills that are essential for success in their ever changing and demanding profession. Since the publication of the previous edition, health and care provision has experienced profound changes, predominantly due to the COVID-19 pandemic.

I extend my sincere gratitude to the nursing community for their ongoing support and feedback, which has been instrumental in helping to shape this edition. I am confident that *Alexander's Nursing Practice: Hospital and Home* will serve as an invaluable resource for students, educators and practitioners alike, contributing to the development of competent, compassionate and forward-thinking health and care provision.

In this new edition, we have meticulously revised and expanded the content to encompass the latest developments in nursing practice, technology and healthcare policies. Our overarching aim has been to provide readers with a comprehensive resource that not only meets academic needs but also prepares them for the challenges that they will encounter in practice.

Alexander's Nursing Practice: Hospital and Home has retained its well-received format that readers have told us they find useful and user friendly. This updated edition continues to provide readers with high quality illustrations, figures and tables that can help them develop further their understanding of the complexities associated with offering people high quality nursing care. This new edition explores the latest trends, ethical considerations and cultural competencies that shape nursing practice, as nurses strive to deliver patient centred care.

The sixth edition retains the three-sections style. The three sections are progressive; assisting readers as they move from the broad approach of Section 1 to a more in-depth understanding of essential nursing issues in Section 2 and the care needs of different patient groups in Section 3. Cross-referencing between chapters helps make links and follow lines of enquiry. The dedicated web-based materials have been retained and include:

- additional evidence-based information
- critical thinking questions with outline answers
- over 250 MCQs with answers and feedback

An icon used throughout the text directs the reader to the website ⊕ for further information, figures or to critical thinking questions.

In the UK and other countries there are ageing populations. These populations present more complex health conditions and an increased proportion of the population are living with long-term conditions. As more people experience multiple diseases, the complexity of acute admissions will continue to increase. Chapters in this updated sixth edition of *Alexander's Nursing Practice* provide insight and information concerning a range of conditions, acute and long-term.

The overarching aspiration of any nurse is to protect the public (NMC, 2018) and regardless of the many radical changes occurring, and will continue to occur, this should never waiver. *Alexander's Nursing Practice* continues to emphasise this important aspect of practice throughout. Protecting the public will incorporate promoting patient safety, adhering to professional standards and instilling confidence in those we have the privilege to care for.

The provision of evidence-based care is again emphasised in this edition, equipping readers with the skills that are required to critically appraise the evidence available and integrate the latest evidence into their clinical decision-making. There is an overriding focus on holistic, patient-centred care, this remains central. Case studies and scenarios illustrate the application of nursing concepts in real-life situations, fostering a deeper understanding of patient needs.

Recognising the integral role of technology in contemporary healthcare, this edition explores the latest advances and their impact on nursing practice, from electronic health records to telehealth.

Healthcare continues to become increasingly collaborative; this edition emphasises the importance of working within interprofessional teams, preparing readers for the collaborative nature of the healthcare setting. Collaborative health care provision must have the patient at the heart of all that is done.

Critical thinking and reflective practice are integral to nursing with the potential to enhance decision-making, problem-solving, patient-centred care and the promotion of continuous learning. Reflective practice is a tool that is used for ongoing professional development, enabling nurses to assess their strengths and weaknesses, set goals for improvement and to engage in activities that enhance their skills and knowledge over time. Throughout the text, readers are encouraged to develop critical thinking skills and engage in reflective practice, fostering a mindset of lifelong learning and continuous improvement. These components contribute to the overall effectiveness, adaptability and professionalism of nurses in providing high-quality healthcare.

In England, the role of the nursing associate is now embedded. The nursing associate sits alongside existing healthcare support workers and other registered nurses to deliver hands-on care for patients. The introduction of this has created a significant shift within the nursing and care workforce and brings with it implications for how care is managed.

Practicing as a contemporary nurse and providing contemporary nursing care, navigating health and social care systems that are dynamic and ever-changing, addressing the nature and breadth of nursing and the underpinning concepts of nursing theory and practice are all issues that have to be considered. This updated and revised sixth edition of *Alexander's Nursing Practice* has been written by clinical experts and academics with a wealth and breadth of experience helps the reader lay down the foundations of practice so that the care offered to people is compassionate, of a high standard, patient-centred and above all else, is safe and effective. This edition, as was the case with previous editions, serves as a guide, laying down a robust basis for nursing practice. Its purpose is to empower nurses to deliver care that is not only compassionate and of the highest quality but also centered around the patient.

Throughout a nurse's career there is a requirement to demonstrate a commitment to lifelong learning. The Nursing and Midwifery Council (NMC) (2021) require registrants to revalidate every three years to maintain their registration. Revalidation is a process through which registered nurses demonstrate that they remain fit to practice and meet the necessary professional standards.

We wish you an enriching and successful learning experience. We trust you will enjoy reading this new edition as much as we have enjoyed updating and revising the content ensuring that it remains fit for purpose. We hope to inspire in you, confidence and competence, to subscribe to being a lifelong learner and to delve deeper, regardless of where you are in your career trajectory.

Ian Peate
London
January 2024

References

Nursing and Midwifery Council. The Code. Professional Standards of Practice and Behaviour for Nurses, Midwives and Nursing Associates; 2018. Available at: https://www.nmc.org.uk/standards/code/. Last accessed January 2024.

Nursing and Midwifery Council. Revalidation: Guidance and Information; 2021. Available at: https://www.nmc.org.uk/revalidation/. Last accessed January 2024.

Acknowledgements

I would like to acknowledge and thank those contributors, new and old, who have provided their support in making the production of this text possible. Thank you all for your total commitment and generosity.

My thanks go to my partner of over 40 years, Jussi Lahtinen. Thank you also to those staff at the Royal College of Nursing Library, London.

I am grateful to Mr Arindam Banerjee who has been so very supportive and encouraging; an absolute joy to work with.

1

On Being a Nurse

JACQUELINE METCALFE, KIM BEZZANT

CHAPTER OUTLINE

Introduction

Nurses work in a wide variety of settings: in people's homes, care homes, hospitals, general practice (GP) surgeries, hospices, factories and as lecturers in universities; indeed, nurses work anywhere where there are people. Nurses are found working in health and social care settings, working with people who may have mental health problems and those with a learning disability in the adult and child care settings. Nurses often work in multidisciplinary teams, however, they also work independently. Moreover, nurses care for people throughout their lives from birth until death.

The role of the nurse has become increasingly complex, with roles and responsibilities reflecting the various changes that are occurring in our society. Nurses are professionals in their own right and must conduct themselves in a manner which promotes trust and confidence.

In this chapter, some of the core values and principles on which all areas of nursing are based and which support nurses in this diverse landscape of nursing practice will be explored. This exploration will provide an overview of how nursing contributes to the care of adult patients with a comprehensive range of needs and vulnerabilities. In particular, there will be an exploration of the values that sustain nurses in difficult times, and to support the provision of safe and effective care and the requirement to uphold the reputation of this unique profession.

Within contemporary health and social care settings, the team has grown significantly and has become more diverse in its composition over recent years. New roles, for example, the assistant practitioner (AP) and the nursing associate (NA) (in England), have been established and care is delivered by nurses in an increasing number of different settings. Nurses are helped by support workers who now provide a large proportion of hands-on care in

many settings. As the number of NAs increase, they will be contributing to core aspects of direct patient care working closely with other team members.

All staff working in the NHS are required to uphold certain standards. The NHS is founded on a common set of principles and values for both the people for whom the NHS cares and the staff who work within the service, and these principles are set out in the NHS Constitution (Department of Health and Social Care [DHSC] 2021) (in England). All NHS bodies are required to have due consideration for this Constitution by law. The values of the NHS which underpin its activities are (DHSC 2021):

- Working together for patients
- Respect and dignity
- Commitment to quality of care
- Compassion
- Improving lives
- Everyone counts

Nurses need to be familiar with the details of the NHS Constitution as it guides professionals in practice, and upholds the human rights of both patients and staff.

Nursing as Part of a Team

All nurses must be part of the UK nursing register (Nursing and Midwifery Council [NMC] 2018). No person can practice as a nurse in the UK unless they are active on this register. A registered nurse is also known as a 'registrant'.

During a nursing career, nurses will work with colleagues from many other disciplines who are part of a wider team supporting the patients for whom they are caring. This will include individuals who are professionally registered, such as social workers, therapists and doctors, as well as those with specialist skills in mental health and different conditions and disabilities. The team also includes other people with important skills and knowledge for safe and effective care provision, such as support workers and ancillary and voluntary workers, and those who patients choose to be involved in their care, including family and friends. Nurses often have a role in coordinating care interventions from this wider team and it is important for nurses to understand the contribution and value of the roles of others to ensure that patients receive the most comprehensive and best quality care available to them.

The care team will notably now include the 'nursing associate'. NAs are skilled health and care workers who have successfully completed a programme of education and training to enable them to support registered nurses in their roles. Because of the more advanced level at which they will practice, they are, like registered nurses, accountable for their practice and are registered with NMC in the same way as registered nurses.

There are many different members of staff who make up the clinical care team. Some will be registered with the NMC, some with other professional regulators such as the General Medical Council (GMC) for doctors and the Health and Care Professions Council (HCPC) for professionals such as physiotherapists and occupational therapists. Other members will be nonregistered healthcare staff. Patients may find this plethora of staff confusing and may feel intimidated. Staff should be wearing clearly visible ID badges so patients and their families know who is who and nurses should ensure good communication with patients to support them to understand the role of each person.

Non-Registered Health and Social Care Staff

There is a variety of nonregistered staff who carry out a number of roles. They usually provide direct patient care, undertaking roles such as supporting patients to maintain their activities of living, but they may well undertake other duties such as recording observations or vital signs and helping with assessment. Support workers are central to delivering a timely, compassionate and efficient healthcare service. There are a number of job titles that refer to nonregistered staff and they can include:
- Clinical support worker
- Support worker
- Care assistant
- Midwifery care assistant
- Nursing assistant
- Healthcare assistant
- Senior healthcare assistant

Some unregistered staff can undertake other roles; they may have titles such as physiotherapy assistant, ambulance care worker, phlebotomist and electrocardiograph (ECG) assistant. Healthcare assistants/nonregistered nursing staff have their nursing tasks delegated to them and are supervised by registered professionals and supported by NAs. They are guided by protocols, performing duties that correspond to these protocols. This will be discussed later in the chapter.

There are areas of overlap that occur between the roles of registered nurses and nonregistered staff when delivering nursing care; the distinguishing feature between them concerns clinical decision-making and leadership. It is the registered nurse who makes judgements and decisions according to the clinical context and the patient's condition. Regardless of role, the focus for any healthcare and social worker has to be on putting the person being cared for at the heart of the care delivered.

Being a Nurse

Nursing is defined by an important set of core values. These values underpin and guide all nursing practice and reflect the humanity that is an indispensable and core aspect of nursing. Regardless of the specialty in which a nurse works, these values are paramount and it is the responsibility of each and every nurse to uphold them at all times. Nurses help people who face challenging and life-changing circumstances and give them support and care throughout their illnesses and difficulties. This often involves developing close and intimate relationships with people who are experiencing some of the most demanding times of their lives. Through such situations, upholding nursing values ensures that care remains focused on the patient and makes them the nurse's first and foremost priority. The maintenance of these nursing values also

ensures that nurses are always a force for good in their patients' lives. Florence Nightingale identified this as a key aim of care:

> *It may seem a strange principle to enunciate as the very first requirement in a hospital that it should do the sick no harm…*
> **FLORENCE NIGHTINGALE**

Modern nurses have been provided with further direction in their roles in a document called *Compassion in Practice*:

> *To be a nurse, a midwife or member of care staff is an extraordinary role. What we do every day has deep importance. Nurses are key to the drive to enable people to stay healthy and well for longer through promoting health and well-being, and supporting as much independence as possible. We help people to recover from illness, sometimes when they are at their most vulnerable. We support hundreds of thousands of people in living with illness. We provide care and comfort when people's lives are coming to an end. We care for everyone, from the joy at the beginning of new life to the sadness at its end. We do so in the privacy of people's homes, in the local surgery, in the community, in care homes, in hospices, and in hospitals. We support the people in our care and their families when they are at their most vulnerable. We have the clinical expertise, compassion and humanity with which to shape the culture of our health service and our care and support system (Cummings and Bennett 2012, p. 5).*

To help understand how nurses deliver care in this way, it is useful to examine in a little detail the values that guide and sustain nurses.

The Importance of Caring

Caring is core and central to the nursing profession and nursing practice. Patients know when they feel 'cared about', rather than just 'cared for' (that is, when their physical needs are met but their emotional and psychological needs are not). It is this true caring which defines nursing, drawing people to into the profession and also providing them with satisfaction in their roles. Caring is so integral to nursing that without caring nursing could not be defined as nursing. It is founded in a desire to help and support people with whatever their health needs are, including those who undergo intensive treatments for life-threatening or life-limiting disease, those rehabilitating from injury, those seeking advice and guidance to manage long-term conditions or disabilities and many who come to nurses for one episode of care and are otherwise well.

In particular, it should be remembered that nurses often have access to the minds and bodies of people when they are at their most vulnerable and fearful, and true nursing cannot be undertaken without empathy and caring. The maintenance of a caring approach is particularly important in modern nursing where nurses work in increasingly complex and busy environments. Karlsson (2020) describes that nursing is essentially a human endeavour based on the whole person (holism) and focused solely on the patient (person-centredness) adding that there is a risk that challenges such as increasing patient complexity and a lack of time mean that nursing risks becoming more technical without the essential and underpinning core of 'caring substance.' The concepts of person-centredness and holism are further explored later.

Of great importance is that excellence in nursing practice cannot be achieved without care being delivered with empathy and compassion, upholding the principles of dignity and respect for each individual who is cared for and understanding each person as a unique human being. Caring is demonstrated through communicating, both verbally and nonverbally, concern for patients and for the people who matter to them, through the way in which nurses behave when they are with patients and through the strength of the relationships that nurses form with patients.

Skilled caring responses such as active listening and well-timed and appropriate touch conveying concern and support are as important as technical interventions within nursing practice. Through building open and trusting relationships with patients, nurses are privileged to share their patients' stories, hear their hopes and fears and be present with them during their disappointments and their successes. Caring is open-minded and non-judgemental and nurses stand in the shoes of their patients to enable them to know and empathise with the unique wishes and preferences that each individual has for their health and well-being.

> *Care is our core business and that of our organisations, and the care we deliver helps the individual person and improves the health of the whole community. Caring defines us and our work. People receiving care expect it to be right for them, consistently, throughout every stage of their life (Cummings and Bennett 2012, p. 13).*

Person-Centred Care

Person-centred care is a key principle which guides nurses in their roles: It means putting the patient at the centre, as an expert of their own experience. The nurse supports the patient to be an equal partner in their care, goals and care plan. The emphasis is on 'doing with' and not 'doing to' the patient. Person-centred care has been defined as relying on a number of care practices, including:

- People's values and putting people at the centre of care
- Taking into account people's preferences and chosen needs
- Ensuring people are physically comfortable and safe
- Emotional support involving family and friends
- Making sure people have access to appropriate care that they need, when and where they need it
- Ensuring people get all the information they need, in a way that is accessible for them, to make decisions for their care and support (SCIE 2022).

To achieve person-centred care, nurses need to plan, deliver and review care with an understanding of the physical, emotional and cultural context that is important to the individual for whom they are caring.

The Health Foundation (2014) set out four key principles which underpin the provision of person-centred care:

1. Affording people dignity, compassion and respect.
2. Offering coordinated care, support or treatment.
3. Offering personalised care, support or treatment.
4. Supporting people to recognise and develop their own strengths and abilities to enable them to live independent and fulfilling lives.

Essentially, in order to achieve person-centred care, nurses need to work with individuals to identify and achieve aims that reflect what is most important to those individuals, and to do this with compassion and respect. This necessitates nurses working in close partnership with patients and the people they choose to support them, taking their lead from the patient whenever possible. The following quote refers to care in a hospital but the sentiment expressed applies equally to care in all settings:

> *A Patient is the most important Person in our Hospital. He is not an interruption to our work. He is the purpose of it. He is not an outsider in our Hospital, He is part of it. We are not doing him a favour by serving him, he is doing us a favour by giving us an opportunity to do so.*
>
> **ADAPTED FROM A QUOTATION OF MAHATMA GANDHI**

Compassionate Care

Caring requires compassion. Compassion describes an approach to caring that demonstrates characteristics such as empathy, sensitivity, kindness and warmth. When nurses focus on the activity alone rather than undertaking the activity with a compassionate attitude, the patient is likely to have a poor experience. Treating patients with compassion costs nothing and compassionate care is a core value that is central to the provision of the best standard of care. Patients feel that care is compassionate when the nurse knows them and gives them time. They feel that the nurse is standing in their shoes (Curtis 2015). Compassion is an essential component of good nursing care and can be conveyed through the smallest actions.

It could be said that compassion is nursing's most precious asset and that providing compassionate care is

> *…more than a professional requirement. Instead it is the result of an authentic bond between a nurse and a patient and the virtue that allows a nurse to enter into the pain, suffering, and adversities a patient experiences as a way of establishing a meaningful connection (Burnell 2009, p. 319).*

Care and compassion are key nursing values but there are also others identified as essential to nursing practice, and these are encapsulated in what is known as the '6 Cs'.

The 6 Cs

Professional nursing practice is underpinned by six values which are considered to be essential for the delivery of the best standard of nursing care: the '6 Cs' (NHS England 2012). Each value is of equal importance to the others.

It would seem to be self-evident that these values should be part of everyday nursing practice. However, despite nurses aspiring to uphold these values as they enter the profession, it is unfortunately sometimes found that they have difficulty in maintaining this aspiration. Nursing leaders and healthcare organisations should focus on creating climates and cultures where compassion in nursing can flourish. Nurses need to be compassionate, but within a healthcare organisation, everybody at every level has a responsibility to ensure there is a culture of compassion for both staff and those whom they care for.

The lack of a compassionate culture sadly has been seen in the findings of investigations into serious failings in care delivery such as those at Mid Staffordshire NHS Trust (Francis 2013) and in Winterbourne View care home (Flynn 2012). These investigations uncovered inadequate and abusive nursing practices and the reports still remain important today, highlighting how patients can be harmed when there is not a culture of professionalism. More recently, the Ockenden Report (2022) highlighted how poor staff behaviour and a bullying culture (within a midwifery setting) were present towards patients and within the wider team and organisation. So what affects a nurse's ability to maintain nursing values and what supports nurses in this respect? One theory suggests that a 'moral compass' supports nurses in the maintenance of their professional nursing values.

Maintaining a Moral Compass

Individuals enter the nursing profession because they want to care for people and to ensure that they provide comfort and safety to vulnerable individuals. The term 'moral compass' (Moore and Gino 2013) is used to describe an individual's sense of right and wrong together with their motivation to make sound ethical judgements and take ethical actions, and this is particularly pertinent to nursing practice. When the moral compass is pointing north it suggests sound ethical practice. However, a moral compass can be pulled from its true north by a number of influencing factors.

For example, within nursing, moral neglect may result when a nurse works in a team that is not delivering high-quality care but, in order to 'fit' into the team, the nurse accepts the prevailing standards of care and lowers their personal standard of care delivery, losing sight of the possible consequences of their actions. Or when, perhaps, a patient is considered to be 'difficult' (MacDonald 2005) or 'unpopular' (Stockwell 1984), and there is a failure to consider the uniqueness and humanity of the individual (Metcalfe 2014) by an individual nurse or a group of nurses. Organisations can also influence a nurse's moral compass through the presence of priorities which are not focused on patients first and foremost (Francis 2013). Most nurses provide excellent care every day they attend to their patients, but it is important that nurses are astute in relation to influences which may negatively impact their judgment, behaviours and actions at all times.

Having identified the importance of the maintenance key nursing values, it is useful to set this in context of the environments in which nurses work in the 21st century.

Current Challenges for Healthcare in the UK

UK healthcare provision is largely led by our NHS. The founding principle of the NHS was to provide free healthcare at the point of delivery for all UK citizens irrespective of their age, ethnicity, gender or socio-economic standing. Despite the NHS being over 70 years old, this principle remains its driving philosophy. However, our modern world is very different from the one in which the NHS was created and we need to acknowledge the challenges for nurses working in a modern NHS with a richly diverse patient population and an increasing focus on efficiency.

Government decisions about priorities for allocation of resources are central to how patients and healthcare workers experience healthcare. These decisions can present challenges to nurses who are required to provide care regardless of the impact on their day-to-day roles. However, despite these challenges, the fundamental need for nurses to uphold nursing values and to provide holistic and person-centred care has not changed since the inception of nursing as a profession over a century ago and is clearly spelled out in the Nursing and Midwifery Code set out by the UK nursing regulator, the NMC (2018). The primary role of the NMC is to protect the public. In order to ensure this, the NMC's Code contains the standards that nurses, midwives and NAs must uphold to practise effectively. When nurses, NAs and midwives join the professional register of the NMC, they are signing up to upholding the standards of the profession.

Ensuring Professionalism and the NMC Code

The NMC exists to protect the public. It has a statutory role in regulating nurses and midwives in the four countries of the UK. It sets standards of education, training, conduct and performance so that nurses and midwives can deliver high-quality healthcare throughout their careers. All nurses, midwives and NAs in the UK are regulated by the NMC and students nurses and trainee NAs are also required to adhere to guidance and regulations produced by the NMC. The NMC sets standards for professional conduct which must be upheld; that is, they are not negotiable or discretionary. Nurses, NAs and student nurses must be familiar with their duties under the Code and ensure that if they are not clear

what the Code requires of them in any given situation they discuss this with other nursing colleagues to gain clarity. The Code also upholds the principles of the Human Rights Act (HM Government 1998), the Care Act (HM Government 2014) and the NHS Constitution (DHSC 2021).

The Code also makes clear that responsibility for those receiving care lies not only with the nurse who provides hands-on care in a clinical setting, but also with those nurses who are working in policy, education and management roles and other roles where they hold their nursing registration with the NMC.

The upholding of nursing values is a central and core theme of professional practice as it acts to foster the trust and confidence of patients and the public. The Code is composed of a succession of statements which, when taken together, indicate what good nursing practice looks like. The interests of patients and service users are put first; their care must be safe and effective and trust through professionalism is promoted throughout the standards. The Code (NMC 2018) sets out four core categories of standards of conduct and behaviour to be upheld by the nursing profession. This includes four key areas:

- **Prioritise people** – this means putting people who need nursing services first and ensuring their care and safety needs are met whilst upholding their dignity. Patients should be cared for in a respectful manner without any discriminatory attitudes or behaviours.
- **Practise effectively** – this means that nurses must assess care needs and provide evidenced-based care in a timely manner. Communication must be good and clear and accurate records must be maintained. Nurses must share their knowledge and skills and be open to any feedback, and reflect on this to improve their nursing practice.
- **Preserve safety** – nurses must ensure that patient or public safety is not compromised. They must work within the limits of their competence and raise any concerns about patient or public safety. They must also take the necessary actions to deal with any concerns where appropriate.
- **Promote professionalism and trust** – every nurse must uphold the standards of the profession at all times and have a strong personal commitment to these. Each nurse is expected to be a model of integrity and show leadership in practice so that others can learn from them and aspire to be like them.

Clear and transparent processes exist to enable the NMC to investigate nurses and midwives who fall short of their standards. They also maintain a register of nurses and midwives who are permitted to practice in the UK. The NMC assumes the same responsibilities for NAs and is responsible for their professional regulation.

If a nurse fails to comply with the Code, they may bring their fitness to practice into question. Following regulatory procedures by the NMC, a nurse may only be able to practice with certain conditions attached to their professional registration and in serious cases the nurse may be removed from the professional register. At all times the nurse is personally accountable for their actions or omissions.

Nurses are also expected to display integrity in their behaviour and practice. Integrity means that nurses must do the right thing regardless of any adverse personal consequences. It is clear, however, that this can be difficult and there have been times when nurses have not shown integrity. This was noted in the inquiry into the failings at Mid Staffordshire NHS Trust (Francis 2013), but it should not be assumed that this is a rare incidence and nurses must always be aware of this key professional responsibility.

In a report that followed on from the Mid Staffordshire inquiry, Sir Robert Francis made recommendations aimed at creating an honest and open culture in the NHS, with the aim that this would support all professionals to maintain their core professional values, including the support to raise concerns when these values were threatened, in other words, to maintain their integrity and enable their professionalism (Francis 2015). The recommendations included the requirement for NHS organisations to appoint someone as their 'Freedom to Speak Up Guardian', that is, someone to whom all care staff could go if they had concerns about care standards.

All NHS organisations now have a Freedom to Speak Up Guardian and most will also have other individuals who are there to support and enable professional values, including organisational leaders and teams who have a lead role in safeguarding. Nurses should be familiar with these people and with the policies and procedures for raising concerns in order to protect themselves and patients. This includes an understanding of responsibilities under the 'Duty of Candour'. The intention of the Duty of Candour legislation (Health and Social Care Act 2008 (Regulated Activities) Regulations 2014: Regulation 20) (HM Government 2014) is to ensure that nurses are open with people who use services when things go wrong with care and treatment. This includes informing people about the adverse incident, providing support and providing truthful information and an apology. Guidance related to the Duty of Candour can be found on the Care Quality Commission (CQC) website (CQC 2022).

Additionally, nurses are supported to maintain their professionalism and values by the presence of good nursing leaders. Many studies and reports have established that the development and support of nurse leaders are key to ensuring the quality of nursing care (Francis 2013). Strong clinical leaders help nurses to define and deliver high quality of care and maintain their professional integrity in busy and complex environments. Clinical nurse leaders will articulate and uphold nursing values, giving nurses support to reaffirm and follow these. It is important to say that to lead in nursing does not need an individual to be in a position of power or seniority. Newly qualified nurses can take leadership roles, as indeed can student nurses. Clinical nurse leadership is defined by the values and beliefs that the leader holds about care, nursing and respect for others, and therefore, any nurse can lead the team in enhancing care and improving quality: a team will be inspired by and follow an individual who reflects sound nursing values regardless of their rank. Student nurses will observe role models in this respect from their very earliest practice experiences, and it is important to observe and learn how effective nurse leaders live their values and role model excellence in nursing practice.

This chapter has so far summarised some key issues for nurses and nursing. It now continues with the important subject of safeguarding adults and children for which everyone has a responsibility in law. Safeguarding activities are underpinned by the requirements of the Human Rights Act (1998).

The Human Rights Act 1998

The Human Rights Act (HM Government 1998) describes the rights and freedoms that all human beings are entitled to in order that they can lead lives characterised by dignity and respect and this Act underpins safeguarding adults work. The actions of all UK public bodies (including the NHS and its staff) are governed by this Act. Human rights principles have close links to safeguarding values and practice because neglect of these principles can lead to a loss of dignity and to care that does not uphold the principles of equality and autonomy (CQC 2017). Importantly, the principles of the Human Rights Act are also embedded within the NHS Constitution (DHSC 2015) and The Code (NMC 2018).

Safeguarding Adults

Living a life that is free from harm and abuse is a fundamental human right and an essential requirement for health and wellbeing (Department of Health 2011).

The core values of nursing and the responsibilities of nurses include the duty to safeguard people from abuse and/or neglect. 'Safeguarding adults' is a term which embraces a continuum of activities, including prevention, delivering safe and effective care, monitoring others in this endeavour and raising concerns when needed. Safeguarding is central to all nursing practice and is seen throughout all nursing activities. All nurses have a duty to safeguarding people from abuse and neglect across their lifespan. Nurses care for people who may be some of the most vulnerable in our society and when people are vulnerable they may be more at risk of abuse and/or neglect. The NMC Code (NMC 2018) highlights how nurses and NAs must take all reasonable steps to protect someone from harm, neglect or abuse.

However, it is not only individuals who are responsible for safeguarding. Sometimes the quality of nursing care falls short of the expected standard because of failings in organisational systems and processes (including failings in management and leadership). This is called 'organisational abuse'. This kind of environment may not be created by individual nurses but it is their responsibility to speak up when they find themselves working in a culture like this.

In addition, nurses may be the people with whom individuals share concerns about abuse and/or neglect, either historic or current, and all nurses have a duty to take appropriate action if they are in receipt of disclosures of this kind. The action to be taken varies according to the problem disclosed and it is important for nurses to share information and consult with colleagues to ensure that their actions are appropriate and proportionate.

There are a number of key documents which encapsulate the responsibilities of nurses and other care workers with regards to safeguarding their patients.

The Care Act 2014

The Care Act (HM Government 2014) put the duty to safeguard adults at risk of neglect and/or abuse into law for the first time in England, Wales and Northern Ireland. Chapter 7 of the Care and Support Statutory Guidance (HM Government 2022) lays out safeguarding duties in law in relation to adults.

The Care and Support Statutory Guidance (HM Government 2022), the guidance which supports the Care Act (HM Government 2014), lays out 10 categories of abuse. Nurses must be familiar with what constitutes abuse within each of these categories in order that they can understand when to take action to safeguard a person and to raise concerns. The categories of abuse within Care and Support Statutory Guidance (HM Government 2022) are

- Physical Abuse
- Domestic Violence
- Sexual Abuse
- Psychological Abuse
- Financial or Material
- Modern Slavery

- Discriminatory Abuse
- Organisational Abuse
- Neglect and Acts of Omission
- Self-neglect

Safeguarding is a complex area of practice and all concerns and disclosures by patients must be taken seriously. It is vital that all nurses and student nurses are familiar with the safeguarding policy for their organisation and that they know how to raise a concern or respond to a disclosure of abuse, as this knowledge will support nurses in adhering to the Code (NMC 2018).

Safeguarding Children (Under 18s)

Working Together to Safeguard Children (HM Government 2018) lays out the statutory duty to protect children and requirements related to safeguarding children when there are concerns about and abuse or neglect. Safeguarding is therein defined as

- Protecting children from maltreatment
- Preventing impairment of children's mental and physical health or development
- Ensuring that children grow up in circumstances consistent with the provision of safe and effective care
- Taking action to enable all children to have the best outcomes

There are four main categories of child abuse and these are physical abuse, emotional abuse, sexual abuse and neglect. Nurses who work with adult patients still have a duty to safeguard children. Our patients may well have children of their own and have family and/or friends who may also have children. In caring for an adult, concerns about a child may be recognised, and when caring for children, concerns about adults at risk of abuse may arise too. In some cases an older child may pose a risk to an adult. It is important that all concerns are discussed with a more senior person and that any concerns are raised in line with local safeguarding policies.

Information sharing is a key part of ensuring good safeguarding practice but it can be complicated in relation to safeguarding adults and children and, if unsure, nurses should take advice on how to respond to any concerns they may have. Incidences and allegations of abuse and neglect can be emotionally challenging and complex issues to contemplate and respond to, and many organisations have in place a person or team who has specialist knowledge in safeguarding who can be contacted for advice when nurses need to discuss any concerns.

Being in a Position of Trust

Nurses can hold a position of power in comparison to patients for many reasons. Firstly they have professional knowledge and access to private information about their patients. Patients may be vulnerable by virtue of their presenting condition, but even relatively healthy patients can be vulnerable in some way during their healthcare episode. This may be because they have altered levels of consciousness, are bed bound, feel unwell and/or are in pain. Nurses may also be responsible in areas such as supporting patients to manage their money and for protecting a patient's property. Nurses therefore occupy a position of trust which requires high levels of honesty and integrity. In terms of safeguarding patients, should this position of trust be breached, it is considered to be very serious. Nurses must always be aware of the position of trust they hold and their duty to uphold the reputation of the profession.

Mental Capacity

Mental capacity is the ability to make our own decisions. There is legislation which applies to everyone aged 16 years and over, and

therefore children are included under this legislation. The Mental Capacity Act (HM Government 2005) is designed to protect people who cannot make their own decisions due to experiences such as living with dementia, a learning disability, a brain injury or a mental illness. However, it is important to note that because someone may have one of these conditions does not mean they cannot make any decisions for themselves. For example, they may be able to make day-to-day decisions such as what to wear and what to eat but find more complex decisions about their money or where to live difficult.

The Mental Capacity Act (HM Government 2005) says that a person is unable to make a decision if they cannot:
- Understand the information relevant to the decision
- Retain that information
- Use or weigh that information as part of the decision-making process

Adult nurses will often encounter people who have reduced or fluctuating capacity, in particular people who have difficulty in making and expressing decisions about their care and treatment preferences because of intermittent problems with mental capacity. This can make the process of knowing what people want and also the process of ensuring consent difficult. The Mental Capacity Act (HM Government 2005) provides statutory principles for the care of people with problems with their mental capacity and these principles protect patients and guide nurses and other care workers when decisions need to be made about care or treatment for people with reduced or fluctuating capacity. Although the Mental Capacity Act (2005) is often thought of as a requirement when safeguarding activities are required to safeguard the individual, it is a freestanding piece of legislation which must be fully embedded into everyday nursing practice as core business in order to support and protect all individuals who may struggle to make decisions because their mental capacity is impaired.

Knowing how to work effectively with people who have problems with mental capacity is something that requires study and practice, but it is paramount that adult nurses understand how to work with the principles laid down in the Mental Capacity Act, as this understanding is essential to being able to provide ethical and effective care that complies with the law.

Delegation

Delegation is the process by which the registered nurse allocates clinical or nonclinical treatment or care to a person who is deemed competent (for example, an NA or a healthcare assistant). The registered nurse remains responsible for the overall management of the patient and is accountable for the decision to delegate (Cipriano 2010). Delegation must always be in the best interest of the patient and cannot be performed in order to save time or money.

The Code (NMC 2018) makes clear that the registered nurse is accountable for any decision made to delegate tasks or other duties to other people, and when delegating, this must be done in an appropriate manner. Tasks and duties should only be delegated when they are within the other person's scope of competence, ensuring that the person fully understands the instructions given. When tasks are delegated the person being delegated to must be adequately supervised and provided with support so that they can deliver safe and compassionate care. The outcome of the task that has been delegated must meet the required standard.

Full training must have been provided to the person to whom the task has been delegated. There must be clear guidelines and protocols in place so that, for example, a support worker is not required to make a standalone clinical judgement. The whole process of delegation must be assessed to identify any risks. If a registered nurse or the person being delegated to is working within their sphere of competence and within the policies of their employer, the employer accepts vicarious liability for those actions. This means that the employer accepts liability for the employee's acts performed in the course of their duty.

The five Rs of delegation are:
1. Right activity
2. Right circumstances
3. Right person
4. Right communication
5. Right supervision and evaluation

If the delegator adheres to these five principles they have done their best to ensure a patient's safety.

Lifelong Learning

Nursing takes place in dynamic and changing environments, and therefore the requirement to continue to learn is part of being a professional nurse and being able to always practise safely and effectively and to deliver high quality care.

Let us never consider ourselves finished nurses…we must be learning all of our lives.

FLORENCE NIGHTINGALE

Lifelong learning has been said to involve working to gain a new perspective on practice by reviewing the environment in which we practise, our level of knowledge in the situation, our level of skill and our interactions with patients and colleagues (Davis et al. 2014).

The NMC clearly state that nurses must maintain their knowledge and skills for safe and effective practice (NMC 2018). Within clinical nursing practice, on a daily basis, there are multiple opportunities for learning if we keep an open mind and a attitude of curiosity to improving our practise for the benefit of our patients. In addition, reading professional journals and courses both online and face to face can support nurses' ongoing learning. Whichever approach to learning the nurses chooses to use, it is important that the information is current and has an evidence base.

Clinical supervision is also part of lifelong learning. Clinical supervision is a process where the clinical supervisor supports the nurse to review their clinical practice including the emotional responses to practice, those factors impacting on practice from the within the institution or company and levels of skills and knowledge. Clinical supervision is a positive process aimed at supporting the nurse to develop their practice to improve patient care. Central to clinical supervision is the process of reflection on practice.

Part of being a lifelong learner is the ability to be able to undertake 'reflective practice'.

Reflection on professional practice is a key skill for nurses and something with which all nurses, NAs and students of nursing should be familiar: it is central to safe and effective nursing practice and supports life-long learning. Reflective practice supports a nurse to consciously look at a situation with an awareness of their own values and beliefs and to learn from the experience with a core endeavour of improving patient care.

It has been described as

…a self-enquiry into experience to find meaning, gain insight and prompt action that will deepen you. Reflection enables you to understand yourself and, on that basis, to take leadership of your professional life. By leadership I mean the action towards realising your values and vision about your practice (Johns 2017, p. 2).

Registered nurses are required to 'revalidate' their registration with the NMC every 3 years, providing evidence of continuing development and reflection on practice and learning. The NMC therefore acknowledges reflection as a key component of safe and effective nursing practice. Reflection supports nurses to understand *why* something has been successful or problematic so that they can know how to either replicate their actions or to change them when encountering a similar situation again. Reflection is also important to enable the nurse to identify and/or address any positive or difficult emotions that the event has prompted.

There are several ways of reflecting on practice, and these include reflective conversations with a peer or mentor, using a reflective diary or being part of a group reflection. Reflecting with others can support the nurse to really critically think about what happened. Students of nursing may also be asked to write reflective essays which will require reflection on an incident or event in detail. It is important that if a nurse reflects on their own they explore both the positive aspects of the event and the areas which could be improved to avoid reflection becoming a negative experience. Even when reflecting on a negative event, the activity should feel positive as it moves the nurse to improve situations in the future. Nurses tend to choose negative occurrences to reflect on but they should also focus on events which were positive as there is learning in every situation.

Regardless of the method of reflection that is chosen, such as alone or in a group, there are formal models of reflection which help to guide the reflective process to ensure enough depth, understanding and learning. These models take the reflector through a series of steps which helps them to explore their experience in depth, allowing them to identify how it has affected them and what they have learned for future practice. There is no prescribed model for or method of reflection in nursing, and nurses will encounter reflection in a number of ways. Sometimes nurses prefer one model of reflection over another for their own work. However, the key thing to note is that nurses will be able to develop their skills and provide better care if they are given opportunities to reflect on their practice.

Focus on Safety

There are many aspects of good nursing practice that will ensure patients' safety, many of which have been discussed earlier. Two recent areas of research and practice initiative are worthy of particular note. The first is the value of 'civility', and how incivility can endanger lives.

Incivility can be defined as behaviours like rudeness, undermining, dismissiveness, aggressiveness and bullying (Cheetham and Turner 2020, Katz et al. 2019, Riskin et al. 2015). Studies have shown that these types of behaviours, even at a very low level, affect colleagues in a way which impacts on patient safety. The behaviours create distractions in clinical environments and lead to problems in clinical areas such as poor communication between team members, lapses in concentration and decreased ability being able to diagnose and to act flexibly and creatively (Cheetham and Turner 2020, Katz et al. 2019, Riskin et al. 2015), with patients' safety and lives being put at risk.

It is not uncommon to experience incivility in highly pressurised clinical areas but nurses, NAs and students of nursing should raise issues with incivility with a manager if they experience it – doing so could saves lives. Information and advice on this topic can be found on the Civility Saves Lives website.

The second initiative of note is NHS England's Patient Safety Response Framework (PSIRF). The PSIRF is a framework for looking into patient safety incidents so that there is better understanding of what things contribute to risks for patients and how we can make sure that we learn from them.

The PSIRF was developed on the back of a report produced by NHS Improvement (2018) which identified problems in the way in which healthcare providers responded to patient safety events, leading to patients and carers having a lack of trust in how these events are being investigated and responded to. The PSIRF is mandatory for any healthcare services which are under contract to the NHS, including ambulance services, hospitals (physical and mental health) and community services.

Conclusion

The core nursing values that promote focus on holistic and person-centred care have remained constant since the birth of the profession, and with this resolute values base nurses are able to consistently provide care that make a difference to patients and their experience of healthcare, and are emerging as leaders in many areas of healthcare.

Nursing is diverse and brings great rewards to each and every nurse who has the privilege of being present with individuals at times of difficulty and success, joy and sorrow in their lives. The imperative is that nurses remain open hearted and compassionate, holding their unique and special contribution to healthcare as a place where every nursing interaction and action improves the patient experience.

This duty lies with us all.

When I think about all the patients and their loved ones I have worked with over the years, I know most of them don't remember me, nor I them. But I do know that I gave a little piece of myself to each of them, and they to me, and those threads make up the tapestry that is my career in nursing (Wilk Cardillo 2009).

References

Burnell L. Compassionate care: a concept analysis. *Home Health Care Manag Pract.* 2009;21(5):319–324.

Care Quality Commission. What we do. 2017. www.cqc.org.uk/what-we-do.

Care Quality Commission. Regulation 20: duty of candour. Information for all providers: NHS bodies, adult social care, primary medical and dental care, and independent healthcare. 2022. https://www.cqc.org.uk/guidance-providers/all-services/regulation-20-duty-candour.

Cipriano PF. Overview and summary: delegation dilemmas: standards and skills for practice. *The Online Journal of Issues in Nursing.* 2010;15(2). https://ojin.nursingworld.org/MainMenuCategories/ANAMarketplace/ANAPeriodicals/OJIN/TableofContents/Vol152010/No-2May2010/Overview-and-Summary-Delegation-.html.

Cheetham LJE, Turner C. Incivility and the clinical learner. *Future Healthc J.* 2020;7(2):109–111.

Civility Saves Lives. https://www.civilitysaveslives.com/. Accessed 19 October 2022.

Cummings J, Bennett V. *Compassion in Practice. Nursing, Midwifery and Care Staff: Our Vision and Strategy.* DH and NHS Commissioning Board; 2012. https://www.england.nhs.uk/wp-content/uploads/2012/12/compassion-in-practice.pdf.

Curtis K. Compassion is an essential component of good nursing care and can be conveyed through the smallest actions. Evidenced based practice. *Evid Based Nurs.* 2015;18(3):95.

Davis L, Taylor H, Reyes H. Lifelong learning in nursing: a Delphi study. *Nurse Education Today.* 2014;34(3):441–445. https://doi.org/10.1016/j.nedt.2013.04.014.

Department of Health. Safeguarding Adults. The role of Health Service Practitioners. 2011. https://assets.publishing.service.gov.uk/media/5a74a158e5274a44083b838d/dh_125233.pdf.

Department of Health and Social Care. The NHS Constitution for England. 2021. https://www.gov.uk/government/publications/the-nhs-constitution-for-england/the-nhs-constitution-for-england.

Flynn M. Serious Case Review (Winterbourne View). South Gloucester Safeguarding Adults Board; 2012. http://www.southglos.gov.uk/news/serious-case-review-winterbourne-view/.

Francis R. Report of the Mid Staffordshire NHS Foundation Trust Public Inquiry. Chaired by Robert Francis QC. London: TSO; 2013. https://assets.publishing.service.gov.uk/government/uploads/system/uploads/attachment_data/file/279124/0947.pdf.

Francis R. Freedom to Speak Up: An Independent Review Into Creating an Open and Honest Reporting Culture. *Report by Sir Robert Francis QC*; 2015. http://webarchive.nationalarchives.gov.uk/20150218150953/https://freedomtospeakup.org.uk/wp-content/uploads/2014/07/F2SU_web.pdf.

Katz D, Blasius K, Isaak R, et al. Exposure to incivility hinders clinical performance in a simulated operative crisis. *BMJ Qua Saf.* 2019;28(9):750–757.

HM Government. Human Rights Act. 1998. https://www.legislation.gov.uk/ukpga/1998/42/contents.

HM Government. The Mental Capacity Act. 2005. https://www.legislation.gov.uk/ukpga/2005/9/contents.

HM Government. Care Act. 2014. https://www.legislation.gov.uk/ukpga/2014/23/contents. Accessed 18 October 2022.

HM Government. *Working together to safeguard children.* Department of Health and Social Care; 2018. https://www.gov.uk/government/publications/working-together-to-safeguard-children–2.

HM Government. Care and Support Statutory Guidance. 2022. https://www.gov.uk/government/publications/care-act-statutory-guidance/care-and-support-statutory-guidance.

Health Foundation. *Person-Centred Care Made Simple: What Everyone Should Know About Person-Centred Care.* London: The Health Foundation; 2014. https://www.health.org.uk/newsletter-feature/a-quick-guide-to-person-centred-care. Accessed 7 December 2023.

Johns C, ed. *Becoming a Reflective Practitioner.* Oxford: Wiley-Blackwell; 2017.

Karlsson M. Ideas of caring in nursing practice. *Nursing Philosophy.* 2020;21(4). https://onlinelibrary.wiley.com/doi/full/10.1111/nup.12325.

MacDonald MT. Reconciling temporalities: a substantive explanation of the origins of difficulty in the nurse patient encounter. *Dissertation Abstracts International.* 2005;66(3):1397B.

Metcalfe J. *A lonely endeavour: clinical nurse leadership and the older unpopular patient in community settings.* Doctorate dissertation. Portsmouth, England: University of Portsmouth; 2014. https://researchportal.port.ac.uk/portal/files/5948836/Whole_thesis_completefinal.pdf.

Moore C, Gino F. Ethically adrift: how others pull our moral compass from true North and how we can fix it. *Research in Organizational Behavior.* 2013;33:53–77. https://www.researchgate.net/publication/318759331/download Cited in Johnston M.J. (2013) Setting nursing's moral compass. *Australian Nursing & Midwifery Journal,* 25 (1): 16.

NHS England (2012). Compassion in Practice. 2012. https://www.england.nhs.uk/wp-content/uploads/2012/12/compassion-in-practice.pdf.

NHS Improvement. The future of NHS patient safety investigation: engagement feedback. 2018. https://webarchive.nationalarchives.gov.uk/ukgwa/20200501110534/https://improvement.nhs.uk/documents/3519/Future_of_NHS_patient_safety_investigations_engagement_feedback_FINAL.pdf.

Nursing and Midwifery Council. The Code: Professional Standards of Practice and Behaviour for Nurses, Midwives and Nursing Associates. 2018. https://www.nmc.org.uk/globalassets/sitedocuments/nmc-publications/nmc-code.pdf.

Ockenden Report. House of Commons. 2022. https://www.ockenden-maternityreview.org.uk/wp-content/uploads/2022/03/final_independent_maternity_review_of_maternity_services_report.pdf.

Riskin A, Erez A, Foulk TA, et al. The impact of rudeness on medical team performance: a randomised trial. *Paediatrics.* 2015;136(3):487–495.

SCIE. Prevention and wellbeing. Person centred care. 2022. https://www.scie.org.uk/prevention/choice/person-centred-care.

Stockwell F. *The Unpopular Patient.* Kent: Croom Helm Ltd; 1984.

Wilk Cardillo D. *A Daybook for Beginning Nurses.* Indiana polis, IN: Nursing Knowledge International; 2009.

SECTION 1

Care of Patients With Common Disorders

2

Nursing Patients With Cardiovascular Disorders

EMMA MENZIES-GOW

CHAPTER OUTLINE

Introduction

Cardiovascular disease (CVD) is a term used to describe all conditions affecting the heart and circulatory system. The two main diseases in this category are coronary heart disease (CHD) and stroke, but CVD also includes congenital heart disease, arrhythmias, heart failure, valvular heart disease, aortic disease, peripheral vascular disease and many other conditions. Approximately 7.6 million people are living in the UK with CVD, with CVD responsible for the deaths of over 168,000 people in 2020 (British Heart Foundation (BHF) 2022). The National Health Service (NHS) Long-Term Plan identifies these conditions as the largest area of care where the NHS can save lives (NHS 2019). While still a major cause of death in the UK, the mortality rate from CVD has fallen dramatically in the past 50 years due to improved survival rates following acute cardiovascular events, despite the population growing and more people living into old age (Cheema et al. 2022). The COVID-19 global pandemic significantly impacted on access to early interventions for patients with acute cardiovascular presentations, which has led to excess deaths, increased disease burden for these patients and an increase in the number living with CVD. It is currently estimated that there are more than 7 million people living with CVD in the UK (BHF 2022).

CVD has an immense impact on society in human terms. In the UK, healthcare costs are estimated at £9 billion per year, with an estimated cost to the UK economy of £19 billion per annum, as a result of premature death or disability affecting working-age people (BHF 2022). Many CVDs, such as heart failure, take the form of progressive debilitating illness, often becoming chronic with intermittent acute episodes. In contrast, a heart attack (known as acute coronary syndrome (ACS) or myocardial infarction (MI)) is often sudden and unexpected, causing acute distress to the individual and their family as they confront a life-threatening crisis.

Cardiovascular nursing is continuously evolving, with nurses developing more advanced skills sets and leading patient care. Nurses will encounter patients with CVD in a variety of care settings as the prevalence of CVD means that it is not simply a condition seen in patients in emergency care. CVD can affect people cared for within mental health, learning disability and community settings as well as in the acute hospital setting. Most recently, it has become apparent that CVD and cardiovascular risk factors are associated with higher mortality in patients with COVID-19 (Bae et al. 2021). With an increasingly ageing population and life-lengthening interventions, the prevalence of heart and circulatory disease is expected to continue to rise (BHF 2022). Cardiovascular nursing is continuously evolving as nurses move on from practising skills of advanced life support and 12-lead electrocardiogram (ECG) interpretation, to leading patient care as nurse specialists.

ANATOMY AND PHYSIOLOGY OF THE HEART

The heart is a hollow, four-chambered muscular organ that generates pressure changes resulting in the propulsion of blood around the vascular system. The right side of the heart pumps blood around the pulmonary circulation where gaseous exchange takes place and then on to the left side of the heart. The left side of the heart operates under much greater pressure to enable it to pump blood around the systemic circulation. The chambers of the heart are illustrated in Fig. 2.1.

The heart wall is composed of different layers of tissue:

Pericardium – a double-layered sac that protects the heart from injury and infection.

Epicardium – the visceral layer of serous pericardium that lies immediately on top of the myocardium.

Myocardium – specialised, involuntary muscle cells (myocytes) that form the main mass of the heart. The atria, which act as filling chambers, have a thin layer of myocardium as they do not have to generate high pressures. In the ventricles, the muscular layer is better developed, particularly on the left side, as a more forceful contraction is required to pump blood through the systemic circulation.

Endocardium – a thin layer of endothelium and connective tissue that lines the inner chambers of the heart and coats the valves, which open and close to ensure forward blood flow.

Cardiac Valves

The cardiac valves are situated on the annulus fibrous, often referred to as the atrioventricular (AV) ring (see Fig. 2.1). Each

Figure 2.1 The internal anatomy of the heart.

valve consists of an annulus, or ring and two or three leaflets, known as cusps, of fibrous and collagenous tissue.

The tricuspid and mitral valves (AV valves) separate the atria from the right and left ventricle respectively, and work in a similar manner. During ventricular diastole, when the chamber is relaxed, the valves open to allow blood to flow from the atria acting as a funnel to promote rapid filling of the ventricles. During ventricular systole (contraction), the valves remain closed as the leaflets are restrained by the chordae tendineae that are attached to the papillary muscles within each ventricle, and thus prevent backflow of blood into the atria during ventricular systole.

There are two 'semilunar' valves. The pulmonary valve separates the right ventricle from the pulmonary artery, and the aortic valve lies between the left ventricle and aorta. Both valves are closed during ventricular diastole, permitting the rise in intraventricular pressure brought about by myocardial contraction. When the pressure in the ventricles becomes greater than that in the aorta and the pulmonary artery, the semilunar valves are forced open and blood is ejected. After ventricular systole, the pressure in the aorta and pulmonary artery is greater than that in the left and right ventricles, resulting in a small amount of retrograde blood flow that closes the valve cusps.

The closure of the valves produces the sounds referred to as heart sounds. Mitral and tricuspid valve closure produces the first heart sound (S1) which precedes that of the aortic and pulmonary valves, known as the second heart sound (S2).

Coronary Circulation

Like all major organs, the heart requires blood flow to maintain cellular activity. The heart is supplied with blood from the left and right coronary arteries which arise from the aorta, just behind the leaflets of the aortic valve, and run over the outer surface of the heart (Fig. 2.2).

The left coronary artery, or left main stem, runs towards the left side of the heart and divides into two major branches: the left anterior descending artery (LAD) and the circumflex artery (Cx). The LAD follows the anterior ventricular sulcus (AV groove)

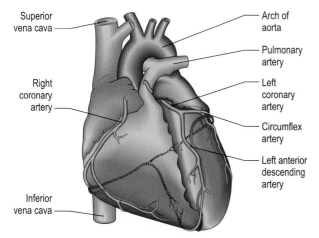

Figure 2.2 The coronary circulation.

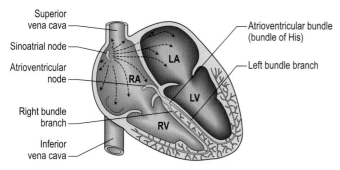

Figure 2.3 The conduction system of the heart. *LA,* Left atrium; *LV,* left ventricle; *RA,* right atrium; *RV,* right ventricle.

and supplies blood to the interventricular septum and the anterior walls of the left ventricle. The Cx supplies blood to the lateral region of the left atrium and left ventricle. The right coronary artery (RCA) runs to the right side of the heart and supplies blood to the right ventricle and inferior portion of the left ventricle. In approximately 80%–85% of cases, the posterior descending artery emerges from the RCA, supplying both the posterior wall of the left ventricle and the AV node.

After passing through the cardiac capillary bed, deoxygenated blood drains into the cardiac veins which merge to form the coronary sinus on the posterior surface of the heart, from where venous blood drains into the right atrium and is carried to the pulmonary circulation (Klabunde 2021).

Cardiac Conduction System

The contraction and relaxation of the muscles of the atria and ventricles need to be coordinated to ensure that the filling and emptying of the chambers are optimally timed and responsive to changing conditions and metabolic demands of the body (Klabunde 2021). The cardiac conduction system coordinates contraction of the chambers using a collection of specialised heart muscle (myocardial) cells. These cells are capable of generating and transmitting electrical activity to initiate and coordinate myocardial cell (myocyte) contraction (Huff 2022).

The cardiac conduction system consists of (Fig. 2.3):
- the sinoatrial (SA) node, located in the posterior wall of the right atrium
- the AV node, located in the annulus fibrous that separates the atria and ventricles

- the His–Purkinje system (bundle of His) emerges from the AV node and splits in the two bundle branches (left and right) from which a network of conduction tissue spreads out across the ventricles (Purkinje fibres).

The SA node is the principal pacemaker of the heart, which sets the heart rate (HR). Electrical activation spreads from the SA node through both atria in approximately 120 ms, resulting in atrial contraction. When the impulse reaches the AV node, there is a delay of approximately 40 ms to allow the ventricles to fill sufficiently with blood from the atria above during diastole. From the AV node, the impulse enters the rapidly conducting tissue of the bundle of His, the right and left bundle branches and Purkinje fibres, causing the entire ventricular mass to become depolarised within 120 ms, resulting in simultaneous right and left ventricular contraction.

The autonomic nervous system alters the rate of impulse generation by the SA node, the speed of impulse conduction and the strength of cardiac contraction. It regulates the heart through both sympathetic and parasympathetic nerve fibres. The sympathetic fibres supply all areas of the atria and ventricles, and the effects on the heart include increased HR, increased conduction speed through the AV node and increased force of contraction. Parasympathetic impulses are conducted to the heart via the vagus nerve and affect primarily the SA and AV nodes. Parasympathetic stimulation produces decreased HR, decreased conduction rate through the AV node and decreased force of atrial contraction (Aaronson et al. 2020).

Sympathetic and parasympathetic control of the heart is coordinated in the medulla oblongata of the brain. The group of neurones in the brain that affects heart activity and the blood vessels is known as the cardiovascular centre. This centre receives information from various sensory receptors. Baroreceptors, located in the atria, the aortic arch and carotid sinuses, alter their rate of impulse generation in response to changes in blood pressure; chemoreceptors, located for example in the carotid artery, respond to changes in the chemical composition of the blood (Klabunde 2021).

Cardiac Action Potential

Electrical activity of myocytes results from the movement of electrically charged particles, known as ions, across the cell membrane, altering the electrical charge within the cell, known as the cardiac action potential. The main ions involved are sodium (Na+), potassium (K+) and calcium (Ca2+), which move across the cell membrane either by the process of diffusion or by active transport, where energy is needed to transport the ions against a concentration gradient. Myocytes at rest (known as polarised) are negatively charged on the inside of the cell. The movement of ions across the cell membrane results in a positive electrical charge within the cell, at which point the cell becomes polarised (known as depolarisation) and results in the contraction of the cell. Further movement of ions across the cell membrane eventually returns the myocyte to its resting state (repolarisation) (Huff 2022).

Both specialised cardiac conduction tissue and myocytes transmit electrical impulses in this way, but the cells within the conduction system do so in a more rapid and coordinated way. They possess three specific properties:
- Automaticity – the ability to generate action potentials, spontaneously and regularly
- Excitability – the ability to respond to electrical stimulation by generating an action potential
- Conductivity – the ability to propagate action potentials to surrounding cells.

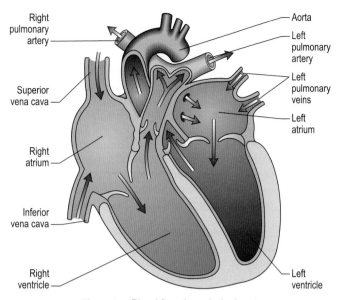

Figure 2.4 Blood flow through the heart.

Cardiac Cycle

The cardiac cycle is the cyclical contraction (systole) and relaxation (diastole) of the two atria and the two ventricles. Each cycle is initiated by the spontaneous generation of an action potential in the SA node. The blood flow through the heart is illustrated in Fig. 2.4 and described in the following paragragh.

Deoxygenated blood returns to the right atrium via the vena cava; oxygenated blood flows from the pulmonary veins into the left atrium. In response to the electrical stimulus originating in the SA node, the atria contract, completing ventricular filling (diastole). As the ventricles begin to contract, ventricular pressure increases and for a short time (isometric phase) all four valves are closed and the volume of blood in the ventricles remains constant. Increasing pressure eventually forces the pulmonary and aortic valves to open and blood is ejected into the pulmonary artery and aorta. When the ventricles stop contracting, the pressure within them falls below that in the major blood vessels, the aortic and pulmonary valves close and the cycle begins again with diastole (Lilly 2021).

The *normal HR* in an adult at rest is approximately 60–100 bpm (beats per minute). With each ventricular contraction, 65%–75% of the blood in the ventricle at the end of diastole is ejected. This is usually approximately 70–80 mL, and is known as the stroke volume (SV).

Cardiac output is the volume of blood ejected from the left ventricle in 1 minute, calculated by multiplying HR by SV (HR × SV) (Aaronson et al. 2020). Normal cardiac output is approximately 4–7 L/min. Although cardiac output is a traditional measure of cardiac function, it differs markedly with body size. Thus a more informative measure is the cardiac index, which is the cardiac output per minute per square metre of body surface area. Usually, it is about 2.5–4.0 L/min/m^2.

The primary factors that determine cardiac output are:
- *Preload* – the amount of tension on the ventricular muscle fibres before they contract, determined primarily by the end-diastolic volume (EDV)
- *Afterload* – the resistance against which the heart must pump. It is determined by blood pressure in the aorta, resistance in the peripheral vessels, the size of the aortic valve opening, left ventricular size, contractility of the heart and the HR.

Within physiological limits, the volume of blood pumped out by a ventricle is the same as that entering the atrium on the same side of the heart; i.e. cardiac output matches venous return. This means that the heart is able to adapt to changing loads of inflowing blood from the systemic and pulmonary circulations. Within certain limits, cardiac muscle fibres contract more forcibly the more they are stretched before the start of contraction; this is referred to as Frank–Starling's law. Once the venous return increases beyond a certain limit, the myocardium begins to fail.

Circulatory System

The systemic circulation is a high-pressure system that supplies all the tissues of the body with blood. It consists of the arteries, arterioles, capillaries, venules and veins. Blood flows through the system because of a downward pressure gradient from the aorta to the superior and inferior venae cavae. Arteries distribute oxygenated blood from the left side of the heart to the tissues, and veins convey deoxygenated blood from the tissues to the right side of the heart. Adequate perfusion resulting in oxygenation and nutrition of body tissues is dependent in part upon patent and responsive blood vessels and adequate blood flow.

Arteries are thick-walled structures that carry blood from the heart to the tissues. The major arteries leading from the heart branch to form smaller ones, which eventually give rise to arterioles. The walls of the arteries are lined with endothelial cells and have three distinct layers:
- The inner layer (tunica intima) provides a smooth surface in contact with the flowing blood.
- The middle layer (tunica media), the thickest, consists of elastic fibres and muscle fibres; the elasticity of the arterial wall enables it to recoil during ventricular relaxation and maintain blood flow.
- The outer layer (tunica adventitia) of connective tissue anchors the vessel to its surrounding structures.

Arterioles contain significantly less elastic tissue than the arteries and have a middle layer of predominantly smooth muscle that controls the vessel's diameter. The arterioles are able to respond to local changes in concentrations of oxygen, carbon dioxide and other waste products and changes in blood pressure. This process is known as autoregulation, which works to maintain adequate blood flow in changing circumstances.

Capillaries consist of a thin single layer of cells with a large total surface area. The velocity of blood is at its slowest in the capillaries to allow efficient transport of nutrients to the cells and the removal of metabolic wastes.

Veins and venules. Capillaries join together to form larger vessels called venules, which in turn join to form veins. The walls of the veins are thinner and much less muscular than the arteries, allowing them to distend more and permitting storage of large volumes of blood under low pressure. Approximately 75% of total blood volume is contained in the veins. Some veins are equipped with valves to prevent the reflux of blood as it is propelled towards the heart. The sympathetic nervous system can stimulate venoconstriction, thereby reducing venous volume and increasing the general circulating blood volume. This adjustment of the total volume of the circulatory system to the amount of blood available to fill it is part of the process of regulating blood pressure.

Blood Pressure Regulation

Blood pressure refers to the hydrostatic pressure exerted by the blood on the blood vessel walls and is a consequence of blood flow and vascular resistance. As most of the resistance to blood flow is due to the peripheral vessels, especially the arterioles, it is often described as the total peripheral resistance, as in the equation:

$$\text{mean arterial pressure} = \text{cardiac output} \times \text{total peripheral resistance}$$

Blood pressure varies in different blood vessels. However, clinically, the term 'blood pressure' refers to systemic *arterial* blood pressure. It is the pressure of blood that makes the exchange of fluid and nutrients between capillaries and tissues possible.

Arterial blood pressure fluctuates throughout the cardiac cycle. The maximum pressure occurs during ventricular systole and is known as the *systolic* pressure (SBP), which ideally should fall in the range of 90–120 mmHg. Systolic pressure is dependent on the SV, the force of contraction and the stiffness of the arterial walls. SBP normally falls a little on standing and this fall may be particularly marked in those with autonomic failure, who are taking vasodilator medication or are in shock. The level to which arterial pressure falls before the next ventricular contraction is the minimum pressure, known as the *diastolic* pressure (DBP) and is normally between 60 and 80 mmHg. Diastolic pressure varies according to the degree of vasoconstriction and is dependent on the level of the systolic pressure, the elasticity of the arteries and the viscosity of the blood. Normally, the diastolic blood pressure rises a little on standing. Alterations in HR will also affect diastolic pressure. A slower HR produces a lower diastolic pressure as there is more time for the blood to flow out of the arteries. The difference between the systolic and diastolic blood pressures is known as the 'pulse pressure', calculated using the following formula:

$$\text{SBP} - \text{DBP} = \text{pulse pressure} \quad [\text{normal values} = 30{-}50 \text{ mmHg}]$$

The average pressure of blood flow through the circulatory system is known as the 'mean arterial pressure'. This can be calculated using the following equation:

$$(2\text{DBP} + \text{SBP}) \div 3 = \text{mean arterial pressure}$$
$$[\text{normal values} = 70{-}100 \text{ mmHg}]$$

Blood pressure should be measured when the patient has been seated for at least 5 minutes, using an appropriately sized cuff. Automated devices may record an inaccurate measurement if the patient has an irregular pulse, in which case a sphygmomanometer should be used (NICE 2022a). Factors such as age, gender and ethnicity can influence blood pressure values. Pressure also varies with exercise, emotional reactions, sleep, digestion and time of day. If high blood pressure is found, a diagnosis of hypertension is made by measuring the blood pressure in both arms followed by ambulatory monitoring (NICE 2022a).

The predominant mechanisms that control arterial pressure within the 'normal' range are the autonomic nervous system and the renin–angiotensin–aldosterone system (RAAS). Baroreceptors in the aortic arch and carotid sinus respond to changes in arterial pressure and relay impulses to the cardiovascular centre in the medulla oblongata. When the arterial pressure is increased, baroreceptor endings are stretched and relay impulses that inhibit the sympathetic outflow to the heart and circulatory system. This results in a decreased HR, arteriolar dilatation and the arterial pressure returning to its former level. If the blood pressure remains chronically high, the baroreceptors are reset at a higher level and respond as though the new level were normal.

When blood pressure falls, blood flow to the kidneys decreases and renin is released from the juxtoglomerular cells. Renin is an enzyme that acts on the blood protein angiotensinogen, which is converted to angiotensin I in the liver and then, by the angiotensin-converting enzyme (ACE), to angiotensin II. Angiotensin II produces an elevation in blood pressure by direct constriction of arterioles. Angiotensin II also directly stimulates the release of the hormone aldosterone from the adrenal cortex which leads to retention of sodium and water in the distal convoluted tubule and collecting duct in the nephrons. This increases extracellular volume, which increases the venous return to the heart, thereby raising SV, cardiac output and arterial blood pressure. The kidneys respond to an increase in arterial pressure by excreting a greater volume of fluid. This decreases the extracellular fluid, resulting in a lower venous return and reduced cardiac output until arterial pressure returns towards normal.

CARDIAC ARRHYTHMIAS

The term 'arrhythmia' is used to imply an abnormality in either electrical impulse formation or electrical impulse conduction within the heart.

Electrocardiography

A patient's heart rhythm can be determined using electrocardiography. Electrocardiography is the graphic recording from the body surface of potential differences resulting from electrical currents generated in the heart (vertical axis) plotted against time (horizontal axis) (Goldberger et al. 2018). This recording may be displayed on special graph paper or on a monitor (oscilloscope) and is known as an ECG. The ECG is a valuable tool in the detection and interpretation of cardiac arrhythmias and the diagnosis of ACSs.

A range of equipment can be used, such as a cardiac monitor, a Holter monitor and a 12-lead ECG. The equipment uses electrodes to detect the heart's electrical current through the patient's skin which is transposed onto a cardiac monitor or ECG paper. The ECG equipment is usually standardised to record electrical activity at a rate of 25 mm/s, with the voltage calibrated to 10 mm/mV. When ECG graph paper is used, this will mean that one small square on the horizontal axis of the graph represents 40 ms; one small square on the vertical axis represents 0.1 mV. These settings are used to measure the waveforms of P, QRS complex and T waves (Fig. 2.5). These waveforms, when repeated regularly and in sequence, make up the normal, regular rhythm of the heart, known as sinus rhythm.

ECG Waveforms

The electrical waveforms produced with each heartbeat in normal sinus rhythm have arbitrarily been labelled P, Q, R, S and T. Each waveform emerges from a flat (isoelectric) line, which occurs when no electrical activity is present.

The electrical impulse originates in the SA node, which is the primary pacemaker of the heart. The impulse is conducted across

Figure 2.5 Electrocardiogram recording of one cardiac cycle.

the atria, causing the atria to contract. This is seen as a P wave on the ECG, a rounded waveform that lasts for less than 120 ms (three small boxes on the horizontal axis of the ECG). When the impulse reaches the AV node, there is a slight delay to allow the ventricles to sufficiently fill before contraction. The PR interval, measured from the beginning of the P wave to the beginning of the first deflection of the QRS complex, represents the total time taken for atrial activation and AV nodal delay. After the brief delay at the AV node, the impulse is passed down into the bundle branches, Purkinje fibres and finally the ventricular myocytes, causing them to depolarise and contract. This is seen as a QRS complex, a larger waveform of less than 120 ms duration. The ventricles go through a comparatively slow process of repolarisation when they go back into their resting state. This is seen on the ECG as the ST segment, a flat isoelectric line after the QRS, followed by a rounded T wave, which may vary in duration. The QT interval is a measurement taken from the beginning of the QRS complex to the end of the T (or U) wave, which reflects the time taken from depolarisation of the ventricles until repolarisation is complete. This interval varies with HR, and therefore, the corrected QT (QTc) interval is most useful measurement for clinical practice. In men, the QTc should be less than 440 ms and in women, 460 ms. Many drugs, including antiarrhythmic drugs, can lengthen the QT interval, which increases the risk of life-threatening arrhythmias, e.g. torsade de pointes and ventricular fibrillation (VF).

Normal Sinus Rhythm

Normal sinus rhythm has a ventricular (QRS) rate (or pulse rate) of between 60 and 100 bpm which is regular (Rowlands and Sargent 2019). Each QRS complex should be preceded by a P wave, and followed by a T wave. The PR interval, a measurement taken from where the P wave begins to where the QRS complex begins, should be between 120 and 200 ms in duration (Fig. 2.6).

Sinus bradycardia is present when the ventricular/pulse rate is less than 60 bpm. This is common among athletes and people who undertake regular, intensive exercise. It also occurs during sleep, when the vagus nerve decreases the firing rate of the SA node. However, sinus bradycardia may also indicate an abnormality, such as electrolyte imbalance, hypoxia, ACS, hypothyroidism and hypothermia, and therefore in the acutely unwell adult may also be associated with haemodynamic instability.

Sinus tachycardia is present when the ventricular/pulse rate exceeds 100 bpm. This is expected during exercise, and stress may also result from a range of conditions, including pain, infection, sepsis, shock, hypoxia, ACS, excess alcohol, caffeine or recreational drug intake, specific inotropic agents, acute heart failure, hyperthyroidism and pregnancy. It may be associated with haemodynamic instability, and therefore, close monitoring of the patient is necessary, along with rapid identification of the cause of the tachycardia.

Causes of Cardiac Arrhythmias

Arrhythmias can occur due to a variety of causes, and therefore, it is necessary to identify the cause in most patients, such as electrolyte imbalance, myocardial ischaemia and ACSs, intake of alcohol,

Figure 2.6 Sinus rhythm. (Reproduced with permission from Aaronson P, Ward J, Connolly M. *The Cardiovascular System at a Glance.* 4th ed. Wiley-Blackwell; 2012.)

caffeine or recreational drugs. Some arrhythmias occur as a result of a congenital conduction defect, such as supraventricular tachycardia (SVT), or because of abnormal shape or structure of the heart, e.g. ventricular tachycardia (VT). Ascertaining the cause requires taking a history from the patient and conducting a variety of investigations (Menzies-Gow and Spiers 2018).

Patient Assessment

Rapid assessment of the patient with a suspected arrhythmia should include pulse, blood pressure, respiratory rate and oxygen saturation levels as these may indicate the onset of haemodynamic instability due to a reduction in cardiac arrest. If the patient is found to be unstable, continuous cardiac monitoring should be commenced with regular assessment of observations as arrhythmias may result in cardiac arrest.

Symptoms reported by patients with arrhythmias vary considerably. Some may be unaware of the occurrence of the arrhythmias, whereas others may develop severe haemodynamic dysfunction, evidenced as marked hypotension and shortness of breath; some may deteriorate into cardiac arrest. Symptoms include:

- palpitations
- dizziness
- faintness
- shortness of breath
- chest pain
- headache
- reduced exercise tolerance
- anxiety.

Holter monitoring, 12-lead ECGs and cardiac monitors are some examples of monitoring equipment that can identify arrhythmias. Systematic assessment of the ECG recording should be undertaken to identify the presence of sinus rhythm, and to recognise the presence of an arrhythmia.

❖ Nursing Management and Health Promotion: Cardiac Arrhythmias

Table 2.1 outlines the steps to assess cardiac rhythm on an ECG recording or cardiac monitor. The features of each rhythm are outlined later, along with the specific evidence-based care.

Nursing assessment of the patient presenting with symptoms associated with arrhythmias should start with a rapid, prioritised

TABLE 2.1	Assessing Cardiac Rhythm
Parameter	**Aspect to Note**
Electrical activity	Is it present? Are the leads and electrodes effectively connected to the patient and ECG? If no electrical activity present, assess patient using ABCDE approach and commence advanced life support measures.
Rhythm	Is it regular/irregular?
Rate	Is it fast/slow/normal?
QRS complex	Is it normal duration (narrow) or prolonged (wide)?
P waves	Are they present/absent?
P:QRS relationship	Is each QRS complex preceded by a P wave?
Intervals: PR and QTc	Is it normal/prolonged?
Identify the rhythm	Is it sinus rhythm or not?

ECG, Electrocardiogram.

assessment using the ABCDE approach and recorded using NEWS2 scoring. It is helpful to ascertain a history of any past experiences of the problem, knowledge of any relevant medications or other treatments and identification of any possible precipitating factors. An ECG should be recorded and continuous cardiac monitoring commenced, with regular observations recorded frequently (5–15 minutes) until the patient is stable, when 1–4-hourly observations can be recorded. Close monitoring is required as the patient's condition may deteriorate at any time, even if they are initially haemodynamically stable. Nursing management involves anticipating and resolving patient problems, monitoring the patient and their response to treatment, providing information and support and assisting the patient with activities of living that are compromised by the symptoms associated with arrhythmias.

Treatments for Patients With Cardiac Arrhythmias

Treatment will vary, dependent upon the type of arrhythmia, how badly it is affecting the patient and whether the cause can be effectively corrected. Treatment often aims to restore sinus rhythm and prevent recurrence of the arrhythmia by identifying and addressing the cause, but first and foremost, the haemodynamic stability of the patient must be restored (Resuscitation Council UK 2021). The approach to treating arrhythmias, discussed later in relation to specific arrhythmias, often depends on how the arrhythmia has affected cardiac function, and addressing the cause, such as electrolyte imbalance or ACS. Antiarrhythmic drugs may be selected to either terminate an arrhythmia with a rapid ventricular rate, known as tachyarrhythmia, or to simply slow the HR in order to restore haemodynamic stability. However, if the patient is severely unstable, direct current cardioversion (DCCV) may be used as it can rapidly restore normal sinus rhythm. In arrhythmias with a slow ventricular response (bradyarrhythmias), drugs such as atropine or isoprenaline can be used to accelerate the rhythm, but if the patient is haemodynamically unstable, then temporary cardiac pacing will rapidly restore a ventricular rate that provides a normal cardiac output and blood pressure.

Antiarrhythmic Drugs

These drugs are used for the pharmacological treatment of arrhythmias. They inhibit depolarisation or prolong repolarisation of the myocardial cells. Their effects include:

- reducing HR in a tachyarrhythmia (examples: beta-blockers, verapamil, digoxin)
- increasing HR in a bradyarrhythmia (examples: atropine, isoprenaline)
- inhibiting the generation of the arrhythmia (examples: amiodarone, flecainide)
- terminating the arrhythmia to enable sinus rhythm to be restored (examples: adenosine, verapamil, amiodarone).

Many antiarrhythmic drugs prolong ventricular repolarisation to inhibit arrhythmias, and in doing so, the QT interval will be lengthened. QT prolongation can induce life-threatening arrhythmias, such as torsade de pointes and VF, and therefore, it is essential to monitor the QTc interval in patients on these drugs, e.g. amiodarone and flecainide, and to avoid combining these with other drugs that also prolong the QT interval, e.g. macrolide antibiotics, methadone and haloperidol.

Stasis of blood within the atria can occur in the absence of atrial contraction, particularly with atrial fibrillation and atrial flutter. This results in the formation of a thrombus, usually formed within the atrial appendages. There is a high risk that the thrombus may embolise; i.e. a small section may break off and be carried through the circulation until it lodges within a blood vessel, and this can result in a stroke. Therefore, NICE (2021a) recommends that patients with atrial fibrillation and atrial flutter are considered for long-term anticoagulation with a non-vitamin K antagonist oral anticoagulant (NOAC) such as rivaroxaban, to reduce the risk of stroke. Due to the increased risk of bleeding associated with anticoagulation, patients should have an individualised stroke risk assessment (CHA_2DS_2-VASc score) and bleeding risk assessment (ORBIT score) before therapy is commenced. Heparin may be administered to the patient in the short term until the anticoagulant has reached therapeutic levels.

Temporary Cardiac Pacing

This is a short-term intervention that provides a means of ensuring a patient has an HR that will generate sufficient cardiac output to maintain a normal blood pressure. It is only used if the patient develops signs and symptoms caused by severe haemodynamic compromise resulting from bradycardia, such as hypotension, dyspnoea or reduced level of consciousness (Glikson et al. 2021). In an emergency, transcutaneous pacing can be quickly set up using a defibrillator with a synchronised pacing function. Defibrillator pads are applied to the patient's chest, through which low-energy shocks are delivered to stimulate the heart to contract at the rate set on the defibrillator, e.g. 70 bpm. As this can be extremely painful for the patient, they should be offered sedation and pain relief at the earliest opportunity.

Transvenous pacing requires a pacing wire to be inserted via the venous circulation into the right ventricle, usually via the subclavian vein. The wire is connected to a pulse generator known as a pacing box that will discharge an electrical impulse down the wire into the right ventricle causing the ventricle to depolarise and contract. This is referred to as 'capture'. The pulse generator will continuously monitor for underlying electrical activity and will not discharge an impulse if an intrinsic beat has occurred. This is known as 'sensing'. It is necessary to establish the minimum amount of electricity required to achieve 'capture' at least once every 24 hours, to ensure that the pulse generator is set to emit sufficient electrical energy (voltage).

Epicardial pacing is the preferred form of temporary pacing for patients immediately following cardiac surgery, such as coronary artery bypass grafts and valve replacement surgery.

Patients should be closely monitored while temporary pacing is in progress. If transvenous or epicardial pacing is used, the insertion site should be closely monitored for signs of infection. Removal of the transvenous or epicardial wires is performed at the patient's bedside under aseptic conditions.

Permanent Pacemakers

These may be offered to patients with bradyarrhythmias that are causing haemodynamic instability, such as complete heart block and a 'slow' atrial fibrillation (Glikson et al. 2021). A pacemaker is a small device, implanted in the patient under local or general anaesthetic in a pocket made underneath pectoral muscle. The device contains a battery, with a life of approximately 10–12 years, and sensors that are able to detect electrical activity in the heart using wires that extend into the right atrium and right ventricle. If electrical activity is not detected, the pacemaker will discharge a small amount of electricity, which will stimulate the atria or ventricular chambers to depolarise and contract. The pacemaker therefore ensures the patient has a consistent HR that will generate a normal cardiac output, which enables the person to live life without experiencing symptoms associated with bradycardia.

Implantable Cardioverter Defibrillators (ICDs)

These have the capabilities of a pacemaker but, in addition, are able to detect and treat ventricular tachyarrhythmias (VT and VF) using defibrillation. The device will detect rapid electrical activity using the ventricular lead, and will firstly discharge a rapid burst of low-energy shocks, known as anti-tachycardia pacing, but if this fails to correct the arrhythmia, the ICD will discharge an electric shock down the ventricular lead to defibrillate the heart to restore normal sinus rhythm.

Patients receiving device therapy for arrhythmias require advice and specialist counselling before giving informed consent for the procedure.

Cardiac Ablation

This is an intervention offering permanent treatment for patients experiencing atrial fibrillation, atrial flutter, SVT or VT. An electrophysiology study (EPS) would first establish the origin of the arrhythmia. EPS involves the introduction of an intravenous (IV) or intra-arterial catheter with multiple electrodes positioned at various intracardiac sites for the purpose of recording or initiating electrical activity from specific areas of the atria or ventricles. Once the site of the arrhythmia within the myocardium has been identified, radiofrequency ablation or cryoablation may be used to produce localised tissue damage to the cells, to inhibit the production of the arrhythmia.

Synchronised Cardioversion

This may be offered to patients with haemodynamic instability caused by a tachyarrhythmia such as SVT or VT, or as an elective procedure for patients with atrial fibrillation or flutter who continue to have symptoms despite antiarrhythmic drug therapies. The purpose of electrical cardioversion is to suppress the activity of the cells causing the arrhythmia to enable the SA node to restore sinus rhythm. Sedation or general anaesthesia is required prior to delivering the shock as the procedure is extremely painful (Resuscitation Council UK 2021). Electrodes are placed on the patient's chest and connected to a defibrillator with the capability of delivering a synchronised shock. Delivery of a shock while the ventricles are repolarising during the T wave on the ECG may induce torsade de pointes or VF (known as the R on T phenomenon). Therefore, a 'synchronised' shock is required to ensure it is delivered on the QRS complex, well away from the vulnerable T wave.

Rhythm Recognition and Associated Patient Care

Atrial Fibrillation (AF)

Atrial fibrillation is an irregular rhythm, with a ventricular rate between 30 and 180 bpm (Fig. 2.7). It is characterised by the absence of P waves and can occur due to a vast range of causes, including heart failure and mitral valve disease and excess drug,

alcohol or caffeine intake and commonly presents with ischaemic changes in old age. Patients will typically have an irregular pulse that may be described as weak and thready.

Rapid excitation of a large number of atrial cells is often seen on the ECG as low-frequency 'fibrillatory' waves. The AV node will filter the impulses arriving from the SA node and will allow up to 180 impulses through to the ventricles each minute, resulting in the irregular tachyarrhythmia known as fast AF. However, damage to the AV node as a result of advanced age or ischaemia may severely limit conduction of atrial impulses into the ventricles, resulting in an irregular bradycardia.

Atrial fibrillation can severely compromise cardiac output, as the loss of the effect of atrial contraction impacts on ventricular filling, reducing SV by up to 25%. Therefore, a substantial fall in blood pressure may occur resulting in severe haemodynamic instability. The danger of the formation of a thrombus within the fibrillating atria is high, and may result in stroke if part of the embolus dislodges and is carried to the cerebral vasculature.

Treatment is aimed at reducing the rapid ventricular rate using antiarrhythmic drugs such as beta-blockers. Normal sinus rhythm may be restored using DCCV, although this is usually reserved for patients who are severely unstable or who have long-standing AF. Anticoagulation in the form of heparin, warfarin or a non-vitamin K antagonist (NOAC) should be considered for all patients with paroxysmal or permanent AF to reduce the risk of stroke (NICE 2021a).

Atrial Flutter

This is usually a regular rhythm with a ventricular rate of 75, 100 or 150 bpm (Fig. 2.8). It is characterised by rapid and regular beats originating within the atria at a rate of 300/min, resulting in a regular, repeated atrial waveform that has a sawtooth appearance known as 'flutter waves'. The AV node cannot conduct each flutter wave down to the ventricles and so exerts a block that is described as a ratio, e.g. 4:1, meaning four flutter waves per QRS complex. A variable block within the AV node will result in an irregular rhythm. Atrial flutter may cause haemodynamic instability and can progress to atrial fibrillation. The approach to treatment is the same as AF (NICE 2021a).

Supraventricular Tachycardia (SVT)

This arrhythmia is a fast, regular rhythm of more than 140 bpm with a normal duration QRS complex of less than 120 ms and no visible P waves (Fig. 2.9). It usually occurs as a result of a congenital abnormality that results in an additional conduction pathway linking the atria and ventricles, usually found within the AV node, or across the annulus fibrosus (AV ring).

Figure 2.8 Atrial flutter. (Reproduced with permission from Aaronson P, Ward J, Connolly M. *The Cardiovascular System at a Glance.* 4th ed. Wiley-Blackwell; 2012.)

Figure 2.7 Atrial fibrillation. (Reproduced with permission from Aaronson P, Ward J, Connolly M. *The Cardiovascular System at a Glance.* 4th ed. Wiley-Blackwell; 2012.)

Figure 2.9 Supraventricular tachycardia. (Reproduced with permission from Aaronson P, Ward J, Connolly M. *The Cardiovascular System at a Glance.* 4th ed. Wiley-Blackwell; 2012.)

SVT is usually triggered by an extra heartbeat, known as an ectopic, arising within the atria or ventricles. Ectopic beats are often caused by stimulants such as caffeine, alcohol, recreational drugs or during emotional stress or exercise. SVT may spontaneously resolve back to sinus rhythm but interventions, such as a vagal manoeuvre, adenosine or DCCV, are often required. Antiarrhythmic drugs may be prescribed regularly to prevent recurrence, or patients may be prescribed medication to be administered when their symptoms occur.

Heart Block

This occurs when there is a delay or interruption of impulse conduction from the atria to the ventricles at the AV node. It manifests as:
- first-degree heart block
- second-degree heart block
- third-degree (complete) heart block (see Fig. 2.10).

First-Degree Heart Block

Appears as sinus rhythm but with a prolonged PR interval in excess of 200 ms. Patients rarely experience symptoms with this and it is often associated with high levels of fitness but may be caused by drug treatments such as beta-blockers or digoxin, acute MI or endocarditis.

Second-Degree Heart Block

This is an irregular bradycardia in which occasional QRS complexes are 'dropped'. The SA node fires regularly, causing atrial depolarisation seen as regular P waves, most of which are conducted through to the ventricles but occasionally the AV node blocks the transmission of the impulse, resulting in an irregular rhythm. It has two forms:
- Mobitz Type I (Wenckebach pattern), in which the patient has a PR interval that increases in length until a QRS complex is 'dropped'

- Mobitz Type II, in which the PR interval is fixed, and often within normal parameters (120–200 ms) but a QRS complex is suddenly 'dropped'.

If a fall in blood pressure or other signs of reduced cardiac output develop, that patient may require temporary or permanent pacing if they do not respond to atropine.

Complete Heart Block

Complete heart block occurs when the AV node is not transferring any impulses from the atria through to the ventricles. The patient's heart rhythm is generated by a pacemaker located in the ventricles, resulting in a QRS rate of 20–40 bpm. Cardiac output may be reduced as the ventricles often contract at a rate of less than 40 bpm, causing the patient to become haemodynamically compromised. Effective treatment may be achieved with atropine or isoprenaline but usually temporary pacing is required to restore cardiac output. The exact cause of the arrhythmia, such as electrolyte imbalance, drug treatments, MI or age-related degeneration, should be identified and, if possible, treated. Many patients will require a permanent cardiac pacemaker if the cause is irreversible.

Ventricular Tachycardia (VT)

This is a broad complex tachycardia with a QRS complex that looks wide and bizarre (Fig. 2.11). The rate is regular but the speed may vary between 100 and 250 bpm, and cardiac arrest may ensue in some patients. It is generally caused by ischaemic myocardium, and therefore may be a sign of acute MI, but may also occur due to electrolyte imbalance, channelopathies such as Brugada syndrome or structural abnormalities such as cardiomyopathy. If the patient maintains a pulse but is haemodynamically unstable, treatment is with immediate synchronised DCCV. The VT/VF algorithm should be followed if the patient has pulseless VT (Fig. 2.13) (Resuscitation Council UK 2021). Antiarrhythmic agents such as amiodarone and lidocaine may be used, alongside correction of electrolyte imbalance. Persistent episodes of VT may be treated with ablation where the ectopic focus or source of the arrhythmia can be removed. Patients may be offered an ICD if the risk of VT or VF remains high.

Ventricular Fibrillation

This occurs when there are no discernible waveforms present and the patient is unresponsive with no pulse (Fig. 2.12). Treatment is by immediate initiation of resuscitation procedures and defibrillation (Fig. 2.13). The cause of VF should be investigated and survivors may be offered an ICD.

Asystole

This occurs when no electrical current is generated from within the heart. Therefore, there is no electrical activity present on the monitor, the patient will be pulseless and should therefore be treated

Figure 2.10 Heart blocks. (A) First-degree (1 degree) atrioventricular (AV) block: features of sinus rhythm but PR interval >0.2 s. (B) Second-degree (2 degrees) AV block (Mobitz Type I, Wenkebach): PR interval lengthens until P wave is unconducted (i.e. no QRS). (C) Second-degree (2 degrees) AV block (Mobitz Type II): PR interval is fixed, occasional P waves are unconducted (i.e. no QRS). (D) Third-degree (3 degrees) AV block (complete heart block): P wave rate is regular, QRS rate is regular but there is no co-ordination between P waves and QRS complexes. (Reproduced with permission from Aaronson P, Ward J, Connolly M. *The Cardiovascular System at a Glance*. 4th ed. Wiley-Blackwell; 2012.)

Figure 2.11 Ventricular tachycardia. (Reproduced with permission from Aaronson P, Ward J, Connolly M. *The Cardiovascular System at a Glance*. 4th ed. Wiley-Blackwell; 2012.)

Figure 2.12 Ventricular fibrillation. (Reproduced with permission from Aaronson P, Ward J, Connolly M. *The Cardiovascular System at a Glance*. 4th ed. Wiley-Blackwell; 2012.)

Figure 2.13 Resuscitation Council UK Advanced Life Support algorithms. *CPR,* Cardiopulmonary resuscitation; *ECG,* electrocardiogram; *PEA,* pulseless electrical activity; *VF,* ventricular fibrillation; *VT,* ventricular tachycardia. (Reproduced with the kind permission of the Resuscitation Council UK, https://lms.resus.org.uk/modules/m25-v2-als-algorithm/11118/resources/chapter_6.pdf.)

following the Resuscitation Council UK's (2021) asystolic/pulseless electrical activity (PEA) cardiac arrest algorithm (Fig. 2.13).

Pulseless Electrical Activity (PEA)

This occurs when electrical conduction of the heart is not resulting in ventricular contraction. Therefore, even though a rhythm may be visible on the monitor, the patient's pulse will be absent and the situation should be treated as a cardiac arrest (Fig. 2.13).

CARDIOVASCULAR DISEASE

Atherosclerosis

Atherosclerosis is a complex disorder responsible for most CHD, peripheral and cerebrovascular disease. It is characterised by the progressive accumulation of cholesterol within the arterial wall. Atherosclerosis is an inflammatory condition, thought to evolve following injury to the endothelial lining of the artery caused by cardiovascular risk factors, such as diabetes or hypertension, resulting in the accumulation of cholesterol and fibrous tissue forming atheromatous plaques within the intimal layer of the artery wall (Lilly 2021). These plaques evolve over decades, with a soft lipid-rich core and a thin fibrous cap that harden and thicken over time, resulting in loss of elasticity, that can increase blood pressure (Fig. 2.14). Vessels may become blocked or stenosed leading to reduced perfusion and ischaemic tissue. High blood pressure may cause the stenosed arterial wall to become permanently dilated and weakened, forming an aneurysm. In the coronary arteries, the endothelial lining of the vessel wall and the atherosclerotic cap surrounding the plaque may become eroded or even rupture,

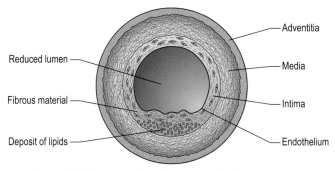

Figure 2.14 Cross-section of an artery with atherosclerosis.

resulting in platelet aggregation and adhesion, vasoconstriction and thrombus formation resulting in an acute ischaemic event known as an ACS (Collet et al. 2021).

❖ Nursing Management and Health Promotion: Cardiovascular Risk Factors

Epidemiological studies have sought to find associations between CVD and the biomedical, behavioural and psychosocial characteristics of a population or individuals. As a result, predictive variables termed 'risk factors' have been defined, which have been shown to be associated with the development of atherosclerosis that results in CVD. Cardiovascular risk factors are known to be cumulative, i.e. the more risk factors in one individual, the greater the risk of developing CVD, although it does not follow that risk factors will result in an acute cardiovascular event. It is also important to remember that a significant number of patients presenting with CVD do not have identifiable risk factors (Table 2.2).

Nonmodifiable risk factors include increasing age, ethnicity and a family history of premature CVD and, to some extent, type 1 and 2 diabetes, which are often considered modifiable with effective glycaemic control. Modifiable risk factors include tobacco smoking, raised serum cholesterol levels/dyslipidaemia (disruption in the amount of lipids in the blood), being overweight/obese, chronic kidney disease (CKD), smoking, physical inactivity, poor nutrition, excessive alcohol consumption, anxiety and depression, social isolation and stress.

TABLE 2.2	Modifiable and Nonmodifiable Risk Factors for Coronary Heart Disease	
Nonmodifiable Risk Factors	**Modifiable Risk Factors**
Age	Smoking and other tobacco use
Gender	High cholesterol
Ethnicity	High blood pressure
History	Elevated BMI Diabetes mellitus Alcohol consumption
Hormonal factors, e.g. hyperthyroidism	Physical inactivity Chronic kidney disease Pollution Social deprivation and isolation Stress, anxiety and depression

BMI, Body mass index.

Strategies for managing CVD are linked to the probability or risk of individuals developing the disease over time. Several cardiovascular risk assessment tools exist to inform the assessment of overall risk and the most effective and cost-effective use of treatment (NICE 2016b). Cardiovascular risk calculation tools include:

- QRISK3 – risk calculator. https://qrisk.org
- Joint British Societies for the Prevention of Cardiovascular Disease (JBS3) – risk calculator. http://www.jbs3risk.com/pages/risk_calculator.htm
- European Systemic Coronary Risk Estimation (SCORE) – used to estimate fatal cardiovascular events over 10 years in low- and high-risk individuals. https://www.escardio.org/Education/Practice-Tools/CVD-prevention-toolbox/SCORE-Risk-Charts

Hypertension

Hypertension is the clinical term used to describe high blood pressure, which in the UK is currently defined as persistently raised blood pressure above 140/90 mmHg (NICE 2022a). Above this level, blood pressure is known to significantly increase the risk of developing complications of CVD, such as stroke, CHD and peripheral vascular disease and therefore, once identified, specific interventions are recommended to reduce this risk.

🫀 Pathophysiology

Following ejection of blood from the left ventricle, blood flows through the arterial circulation, and in response to the increase in volume, the arteries dilate and thereby prevent an increase in SBP. Ideally, the systolic value should be less than 120 mmHg (NICE 2022a). However, atherosclerosis, the most common cause of hypertension, causes the arteries to become stiff and rigid, reducing their ability to dilate when blood flows through them, resulting in an increase in the pressure of flow, measured as an increase in the systolic pressure value, in mmHg. The diastolic blood pressure value should ideally be less than 80 mmHg (NICE 2022a). It represents the pressure within the arterial circulation when the left ventricle is at rest, when it fills with blood in advance of the next contraction. However, the diastolic pressure may increase if the left ventricle becomes stiffened, for example due to previous MI or aortic valve disease.

Therefore, many factors that contribute to the development of hypertension are also cardiovascular risk factors, such as smoking, lack of exercise, obesity, consumption of large amounts of alcohol and a family history of hypertension. Age increases risk, as does ethnicity; African or Caribbean descent is known to increase the risk of developing hypertension. High salt intake is a significant cause of raised blood pressure, and therefore, lifestyle and dietary modification forms the mainstay of early intervention for hypertension.

Specific conditions, such as CKD, diabetes and lupus, are known to cause hypertension, as well as certain medications, such as the oral contraceptive pill.

Patient Assessment

Accurate blood pressure assessment is essential for effective clinical assessment. Blood pressure is usually measured at the brachial artery using an automated device or a manual sphygmomanometer and stethoscope. Ideally, patients should be in a calm, comfortable, temperate environment with their arm stretched out and supported. Tight clothing that might constrict the arm should be removed. The patient should have been resting for at least 5 minutes before the recording (NICE 2022a).

Selection of the correct cuff size for the patient is essential for accuracy. The cuff bladder should cover 80%–100% of the circumference of the upper arm, with the centre of the bladder placed directly over the brachial artery pulse. Automated devices can make assessment considerably easier; however, they may not record blood pressure accurately, particularly if the patient has hypotension or an irregular pulse when a 'manual' blood pressure should be recorded. It is recommended that the patient's pulse is palpated first to allow the correct device to be used.

If elevated blood pressure is found, the assessment should be repeated in the other arm. It is important to ensure you do not alarm the patient in any way. If a blood pressure difference between the arms is found to be more than 20 mmHg, this should be escalated urgently as the patient requires urgent assessment for the possibility of an aortic dissection.

If the patient's blood pressure is found to be higher than 140/90 mmHg, it must be reported to ensure that further investigations are conducted, including repeating the measurements again. The patient will require ambulatory or home blood pressure monitoring to record a series of readings over the course of 24 hours from which an average of daytime recordings is taken for diagnosis.

High blood pressure increases the perfusion pressure of vital organs within the body, such as the heart, kidneys and eyes, and as a result, organ damage may occur. The left ventricular myocardium may thicken and enlarge in response to hypertension, known as hypertrophy. This can increase the risk of the patient developing angina or arrhythmias and therefore should be identified through early assessment with a 12-lead ECG and echocardiogram. Patients should have regular urinalysis and blood tests, including urea, electrolytes and estimated glomerular filtration rate (eGFR), to assess renal function and regular eye examinations to check for retinopathy.

❖ Nursing Management and Health Promotion: Hypertension

Hypertension is known to increase the risk of developing an acute cardiovascular condition, such as ACS or stroke. Therefore, patients found to have it should have a 10-year cardiovascular risk assessment using, for example, the QRISK score.

Lifestyle modification measures are essential to the reduction in blood pressure and nurses are frequently involved in providing patients with personalised advice to support this. Patients should be advised to undertake moderate-intensity aerobic exercise for 30 minutes at least five times per week. Dietary intake should include consumption of at least five portions of fruit and vegetables per day but patients should be advised to reduce their intake of total and saturated fat and alcohol. Importantly, salt intake should be restricted to a maximum of 5–6 g/day and it is helpful to advise patients of where salt may be hidden in foods, such as cheese and ham. Smoking cessation guidance and support should be offered if appropriate, and weight loss reduction if the patient has a body mass index (BMI) greater than 25 kg/m². Further information regarding lifestyle modification to prevent CVD is provided within this chapter under 'Cardiac Rehabilitation'.

Treatments for Patients With Hypertension

In addition to the lifestyle measures identified earlier, pharmacological treatment can effectively reduce elevated blood pressure.

Current NICE guidance (2022a) recommends drug treatments for patients who have stage 1 hypertension and at least one risk factor such as target organ damage, CVD, kidney disease, diabetes or a 10-year cardiovascular risk score ≥20%. Drug therapies should be selected based on the patient and any comorbidities present, such as diabetes or renal dysfunction. At present, NICE (2022a) recommends starting with an ACE inhibitor, such as ramipril, or an angiotensin-receptor blocker, such as losartan, for patients aged under 55 years and for people with diabetes. Patients over 55 years or those of African or Caribbean ethnicity of any age should be offered a calcium channel blocker, such as amlodipine. If the patient's blood pressure does not fall below the recommended target level, the drugs may be combined and a diuretic, such as Bendroflumethiazide, added to their treatment. Expert help may be necessary in drug-resistant hypertension.

Coronary Heart Disease

'Coronary heart disease' (CHD) is the term used when atherosclerosis affects the arterial circulation of the heart, manifesting as symptoms of angina due to myocardial ischaemia, ACS, heart failure, arrhythmias or sudden death. CHD is one of the leading causes of death in the UK, and was the leading cause of death worldwide in 2019 prior to the COVID-19 pandemic. It is responsible for approximately 66,000 deaths in the UK each year, accounting for 1 in 8 deaths in men and 1 in 14 deaths in women (BHF 2022).

The prevalence of CHD is falling due to advances preventative measures and treatments (Cheema et al. 2022). However, it is estimated that approximately 2.3 million people live with CHD in the UK and marked regional variations in mortality remain evident with the lowest rates in the South of England and the highest rates in Scotland (BHF 2022). There is also a clear difference between socioeconomic groups in the prevalence of CHD, with pollution, loneliness and social isolation emerging as risk factors for CHD (Alun and Murphy 2019). The risk of CHD in women is often underestimated, as women tend to develop heart disease later in life than men, as it is thought premenopausal hormones may provide some protection from the disease but mortality remains highest among men. Ethnic background is also a significant factor. In the UK, people of South Asian family origin are at greater risk of CHD than those of European descent, although people of African Caribbean family origin are known to have a lower risk (Tillin et al. 2013).

Ischaemia

Ischaemia is defined as a condition in which there is an imbalance between oxygen supply and demand. Oxygen supply to the tissues of the body varies with blood flow and may be compromised by abnormalities of the vessel wall, the blood flow or the blood itself. Peripheral artery occlusion can occur as a result of an embolus, atherosclerosis, diabetic vascular disease, vasculitis and vasospastic conditions. Myocardial blood supply can be reduced through atherosclerosis, thrombosis and arterial spasm. It is thought that a coronary artery must be narrowed by at least 50% before coronary blood flow fails to meet the demands of the heart during exertion. Severe anaemia and hypoxia can also result in a decreased oxygen supply. For the myocardium, oxygen demand depends mainly upon HR, myocardial contractility and tension in the myocardial wall, with increased oxygen demand occurring in a variety of clinical conditions, including tachycardia, hypertension, valvular disease, left ventricular hypertrophy and hyperthyroidism. Insufficient perfusion of the myocardium results in anaerobic respiration leading to the accumulation of lactic acid, usually triggering discomfort in the chest or shortness of breath. This symptom is commonly referred to as 'angina'. Localised myocardial ischaemia may be intermittent and have reversible effects, but it inevitably causes myocardial dysfunction. If untreated, the affected area of myocardium will die, leading to infarction.

Angina

Angina is a symptom, rather than a disease, describing discomfort, pain or shortness of breath resulting from a transient but reversible episode of myocardial ischaemia. This occurs when the coronary artery blood supply does not meet the demand for oxygen within the myocardium, usually during exertion. In the absence of sufficient oxygen supply, the myocytes create energy using anaerobic respiration, resulting in accumulation of lactic acid that results in the typical angina symptoms. If the symptoms disperse with rest in a patient with stable angina, because the HR slows and myocardial oxygen demand falls, it may be caused by coronary artery disease or other conditions that lead to increased myocardial oxygen demand on exertion, such as tachyarrhythmias and aortic stenosis. If the angina symptoms continue despite rest, the patient should be immediately assessed for an ACS.

Patient Assessment

Angina is diagnosed by the nature of the symptoms, history and examination, the perceived likelihood of coronary artery disease in that individual and the results of various diagnostic tests. Cardiac biomarkers will be negative, as no myocardial necrosis (damage) will occur as a result of the episode. Where a diagnosis of angina is suspected, patients should have rapid access to a cardiology clinic, which frequently may be nurse led (NICE 2016a).

The presentation and history may be misleading but is frequently one of discomfort that is brought on by exertion. The location, character, duration and any relationship of the symptoms to exertion need to be determined, and often, mnemonics, such as SOCRATES (Box 2.1), provide a helpful aide-memoire for a comprehensive assessment (Menzies-Gow and Spiers 2018). Stable angina is typically episodic pain and discomfort occurring centrally in the chest, often described as 'dull', 'aching', 'heaviness' and 'tightness' and is often confused with indigestion. The discomfort may radiate to the arms, lower jaw or neck and can be associated with breathlessness, which may also be the only symptom. It is often induced by exercise or emotion and relieved by rest and/or glyceryl trinitrate (GTN). Myocardial ischaemia may also be 'silent' especially in older adults, and women in particular, or those with diabetes. Symptoms may vary from day to day and there is no link between symptom severity and the extent of underlying disease.

Establishing an overview of the patient's medical history provides subjective information about the presenting symptoms, previous patterns of health and illness and the activities of living. It is important to explore the patient's history to establish the cause of the symptoms; angina symptoms can frequently occur as a result of other conditions, such as aortic stenosis or atrial fibrillation. The characteristics of the pain, as well as any associated symptoms, should be established, and risk factors should be identified, such as a family history of CHD, smoking, hypertension, diabetes and CKD, as well as social and psychological background, which adds to the picture. Physical examination needs to include calculation of BMI and measurement of the waist circumference, an assessment for diabetes and renal disease which can increase the risk of CHD.

Diagnostic Investigations

A 12-lead electrocardiogram should be recorded at rest for patients with symptoms of suspected angina (NICE 2016a). If possible, the ECG should be obtained when there are angina symptoms, when the segment between the end of the QRS complex and the beginning of the T wave may be depressed (ST depression) and the T wave may also be flattened or inverted (Fig. 2.15). A right-sided ECG, and a posterior lead ECG, should also be recorded in patients whose standard 12-lead ECG does not reveal any evidence of ischaemia (NICE 2016a). (For more information on how to record an ECG, see Richley 2016; Menzies-Gow 2018.)

Blood samples should be taken to assess a full blood count, fasting lipid profile, eGFR and a fasting glucose level to give an

---

• BOX 2.1	**Structured Symptom Assessment Using SOCRATES**

S Site
O Onset
C Character
R Radiation
A Associated symptoms
T Timing
E Exacerbating factors
S Severity

0–6 h post-infarction
ST elevation

6–24 h post-infarction
Abnormal Q wave
ST elevation
T-wave inversion

12 h–14 days post-infarction
Abnormal Q wave
ST elevation less than previously
T-wave inversion

Long term – abnormal Q waves usually persist indefinitely but may resolve in inferior infarcts

– ST elevation resolves in inferior infarcts in 2 weeks but persists in 40% of all infarcts and may be associated with aneurysm formation

– T-wave inversion may persist or resolve

Figure 2.15 Electrocardiogram changes in myocardial infarction.

indication of the risk profile for CHD. These tests should be repeated at least annually.

Computed tomography (CT) coronary angiogram is recommended to establish a diagnosis of angina by detecting and quantifying coronary calcification (NICE 2016c). If this is inconclusive, the patient may be offered myocardial perfusion scintigraphy, which is a noninvasive method of obtaining images and assessing myocardial perfusion by IV injection of a radioisotope, usually thallium or technetium, which is taken up by the heart and distributed throughout the myocardium in proportion to regional blood flow. Alternatively, stress-echocardiography may be used, which involves the imaging of altered myocardial contractility during exercise or pharmacological stress or a cardiac MRI.

Coronary angiogram is a procedure carried out under local anaesthetic that involves the injection of contrast medium into the heart and coronary arteries (Information 2.1). The procedure

---

INFORMATION 2.1

Coronary Catheterisation (Angiogram)

Coronary catheterisation can be used to perform an angiogram that visualises the patency of the coronary arteries and identifies atherosclerotic lesions significantly inhibiting coronary blood flow and to determine which intervention would be the most suitable for the individual patient. The patient may be offered angioplasty, where a balloon is used to dilate the artery at the point of the narrowing, and stent deployed to maintain patency. Collectively this procedure is known as PCI, which if used while a patient experiencing an acute STEMI is known as PPCI. CABG may be a more suitable intervention for the patient if the angiogram reveals multiple lesions across two or more arteries. Cardiac catheterisation may also be used to measure pressure within the right and left ventricles and to measure left ventricular ejection fraction.

The patient must give written informed consent for the procedure, which takes place in a purpose built theatre known as a Cardiac Catheterisation Laboratory (Cath Lab). The patient is usually asked to fast prior to the procedure, wear a gown and if femoral access is to be used, the right side of the groin area should be shaved. The patient should be prepared to lie flat on their back on a hard table during the procedure. Under sterile conditions and with local anaesthetic, a needle will be inserted into the patient's radial or femoral artery, followed by a sheath that will remain in situ during the procedure, and the needle removed. A catheter, which is a fine radio-opaque wire, is inserted into the sheath and advanced along the artery to the aorta and the aortic root, where the coronary arteries emerge behind the aortic valve. Dye is injected via the catheter into each of the coronary arteries while live X-rays are recorded to establish vessel patency and identify the location of stenotic lesions that are severely reducing blood flow to the myocardium. Intravascular imaging techniques such as ultrasound (IVUS) or optical coherence tomography (OCT) and assessment of fractional flow reserve (FFR) may be used to guide decision-making for the patient's suitability for PCI or CABG.

Following the procedure, regular observations should be recorded that include assessment of the access site, which may bleed or develop a haematoma, and perfusion of the limb by checking warmth and pulses. Frequently, the sheath will be removed at the end of the procedure and a closure device inserted. However, patients often return from the procedure with the arterial sheath still in situ, which will require careful removal by trained nurses. Sustained pressure to the access site must be applied to prevent bleeding. Manual pressure that is gradually reduced may be effective but usually a device will be necessary to deliver prolonged pressure to the site, such as a TR band used for radial access or a Femostop for femoral access. The patient may require analgesia and bed rest for a few hours before discharge and should be encouraged to drink plenty of fluids to encourage excretion of the dye.

---

provides reliable anatomical information to identify the presence of coronary artery stenosis and inform treatment options. The patient should be fully informed about each procedure, its findings and their implications. If a narrowing in the coronary artery is found, the cardiologist may proceed to open the artery using a special catheter with an inflatable balloon (angioplasty) and may deploy a stent to remain embedded within the coronary artery to keep it open, or patent. If diffuse disease is found across several coronary arteries, the patient may be referred for coronary artery bypass surgery.

❖ Nursing Management and Health Promotion: Stable Angina

The approach to managing patients with stable angina involves alleviating symptoms and prevention of life-threatening cardiac events, such as ACS. Individuals who develop new symptoms of angina should be assessed by a specialist within 2 weeks of referral, and rapid access chest pain clinics (NICE 2016a), which are frequently nurse led, are examples of how such patients can be seen promptly. Practice nurses, nursing associates and healthcare assistants may be the main source of professional information and support for those in the community.

Patients should be offered a clear explanation of what stable angina is; the factors that may possibly provoke an episode, such as exertion, stress and eating a large meal; and how their symptoms will be managed. They should be advised to seek professional help if their symptoms worsen in severity or frequency, or if their angina symptoms occur at rest (Aaronson et al. 2020). Nurses are frequently involved in delivering lifestyle advice and psychological support. Relatives or carers should be involved in the discussions, and all should be offered the chance to ask questions.

Treatments for Patients With Stable Angina

During an episode of angina, the patient should be advised to rest from the activity that provoked it, which may be sufficient to relieve their symptoms. The use of a sublingual glyceryl GTN spray will dilate the coronary arteries, to restore perfusion to the myocardium. However, if symptoms persist for more than 10–15 minutes despite rest and sublingual GTN, the patient should be advised to call for an ambulance, as this may be an ACS.

Secondary prevention, in this context, is the term used to describe an approach to clinical care for patients with stable angina that aims to prevent an acute cardiac event, such as an ACS that may occur as a result of atherosclerosis. A multifactorial approach is used that includes medication, risk factor modification and revascularisation using interventions such as percutaneous coronary intervention (PCI) and coronary artery bypass graft surgery (CABG), discussed later in this chapter.

In addition to a sublingual GTN spray for symptom relief, patients are likely to be prescribed a range of drug treatments to prevent worsening of CVD. Pharmacological therapies may include aspirin, lipid modification therapies such as statins and ACE inhibitors for patients who also have diabetes (NICE 2016c). Blood pressure needs to be controlled, especially in patients with diabetes for whom target levels of blood pressure are set lower. Recurrence of symptoms may be prevented with the use of a long-acting nitrate or with beta-blockers or calcium antagonist, which will slow HR and reduce myocardial oxygen demand (NICE 2016c).

Comprehensive assessment of an individual's cardiovascular risk is an essential aspect of CVD prevention. Particular attention should be paid to elements of the patient's lifestyle that could have contributed to the condition and that could affect prognosis. Patients with angina benefit from a management plan to address modifiable risk factors, in particular smoking, physical activity and dietary habits. Close monitoring and treatment of comorbidities such as hypertension and diabetes that can accelerate atherosclerosis are also necessary (NICE 2016c). Cardiovascular risk factor assessment and strategies for lifestyle and pharmacological modification are discussed in detail later in this chapter.

Acute Coronary Syndromes

The term 'acute coronary syndrome' (ACS) is an umbrella term encapsulating three acute life-threatening conditions: unstable angina, non-ST elevation myocardial infarction (NSTEMI) and ST elevation myocardial infarction (STEMI) (Thygesen et al. 2018). An ACS can be diagnosed from assessment of the patient's symptoms and history alongside a 12-lead ECG. Elevated cardiac biomarkers, such as troponin, and echocardiography may be used to provide supplemental information if the diagnosis is unclear; however, prompt revascularisation is essential to reduce the risk of mortality.

● Pathophysiology

ACSs occur when there is a prolonged interruption to blood flow through a coronary artery, most often caused by the formation of a thrombus in the intracoronary lumen. There are three forms of ACS: STEMI, NSTEMI and unstable angina. STEMI occurs when a coronary atherosclerotic plaque ruptures, resulting in rapid platelet aggregation, vasoconstriction and thrombus formation. Unstable angina and non-STEMI occur when the plaque is slightly damaged through erosion, resulting in gradual platelet aggregation, but usually some blood supply can still pass through the artery to perfuse the myocardium beyond. NSTEMI results in some myocardial damage, resulting in a raised serum troponin level; unstable angina does not cause myocardial damage, and so the cardiac troponin level remains within normal limits.

In STEMI, the myocardial damage most frequently results from total occlusion of a coronary artery by a thrombus, usually at the site of a recently cracked or fissured atheromatous plaque (Lilly 2021). If the lumen of an artery is blocked for about 20 minutes, and blood supply by the small vessels of the surrounding collateral circulation is inadequate, the myocardial tissue will die; this is known as necrosis, or infarction. Surrounding the area of necrotic tissue there is usually a zone of injury (Fig. 2.16). This injured myocardium cannot contract but may be salvaged if an adequate blood supply can be quickly established; this is sometimes known as 'hibernating' myocardium. During the first 6 hours after the onset of symptoms, the affected myocardium becomes oedematous. Electrolytes, such as sodium and potassium ions, leak out from the myocardium, leading to an increased risk of arrhythmias, such as VT or VF, which may cause death within the first hour of symptoms, which may be before help arrives (Menzies-Gow and Spiers 2018). The infarcted area is replaced by fibrous scar tissue over the course of 6–7 weeks. The site of infarction depends on which coronary artery has become occluded. The extent of infarction, and therefore the amount of muscle involved, depends on the artery involved, the previous rate of progression of the disease and the effectiveness of the surrounding collateral circulation.

Patient Assessment

Rapid, prioritised assessment is essential and a systematic ABCDE approach should be used to assess the patient with suspected ACS

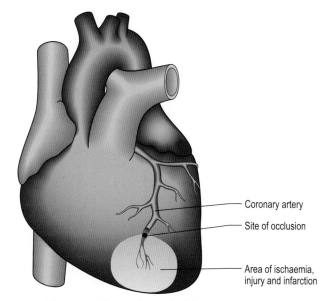

Figure 2.16 Zones of necrosis, injury and ischaemia.

(Creed and Spiers 2020). Some patients may present in cardiac arrest; often this will be a shockable rhythm, such as VT or VF. Atrial fibrillation may also occur with ACS, as well as bradyarrhythmias such as heart blocks. Changes in respiratory rate or reduced urine output can be early signs of deterioration associated with the presence of heart failure, which is a serious complication. The patient's blood pressure may be lower than normal with reduced cardiac output or high due to pain and anxiety; slight pyrexia is a common response to the inflammatory process around atherosclerotic plaque rupture. On examination, patients may appear pale, sweaty and distressed with cool extremities due to the sympathetic neural response.

Continuous cardiac monitoring using 3, 5 or 12 leads should be commenced promptly as the patient is at risk of life-threatening arrhythmias. The patient's haemodynamic status should be closely monitored for signs of deterioration, that could occur at any time. Observations should be repeated every 5–15 minutes and recorded using NEWS2 scoring (Creed and Spiers 2020). Assessment should include AVPU, airway assessment, respiratory rate, peripheral oxygen saturations, pulse and blood pressure measurement, capillary refill, capillary blood glucose (CBG) and examination of the patient's ankles for signs of oedema. A standard 12-lead ECG should be recorded and interpreted by a competent practitioner urgently as this will be used for evidence of ACS (Collet et al. 2021).

Angina associated with ACS often occurs suddenly, while the patient is at rest, or on exercise. It may typically be described as a central, retrosternal crushing pain, that radiates to other regions such as the arms, neck and lower jaw. However, patients may also describe a dull ache, heaviness, burning sensation that they associate with indigestion symptoms or frequently no pain at all, something that is common among women, older adults and people with diabetes. ACS may be 'silent', suggesting no pain was experienced, but often the event is not entirely silent, as patients often experience associated symptoms, such as shortness of breath, fatigue, nausea and vomiting or severe distress. Risk stratification tools, such as the Heart Score, can support clinical decision-making in this situation (Stepinska et al. 2020).

Therefore, it is essential that patients are not asked to describe their 'pain'; open questioning should be used to encourage the patient to describe their 'symptoms' to ensure that nothing is missed (Menzies-Gow and Spiers 2018). The onset, duration, location, nature of symptoms, any relieving or aggravating factors and any attempted methods of pain relief should be ascertained (Box 2.1). It is essential that the patient is asked to rate their pain, for example on a scale of 0–10, so that the effectiveness of pain relief can be assessed (Collet et al. 2021).

The pain is not usually affected by movement or breathing in deeply. It may not be relieved by GTN. Associated symptoms include shortness of breath, nausea, sweating and dizziness. The discomfort and fear around what is causing the symptoms can mean that patients are anxious and distressed. Atypical presentations can make the diagnosis unclear; these may include not experiencing any chest pain, sudden loss of consciousness, confusion, profound weakness or arrhythmia.

Exploring the patient's history is necessary to build a picture of the likelihood of the symptoms being due to an ACS, as chest pain can be caused by a wide range of conditions (Stepinska et al. 2020). A family history of CHD, together with the patient's age, risk factor identification and social and psychological background, adds to the picture. It may be inappropriate to obtain a full history if the patient is in pain or acutely ill or would benefit from prompt revascularisation. An initial assessment can be enough to set early priorities, without a full physical examination or diagnostic tests.

Diagnostic Investigations

The 12-lead ECG should be recorded as a matter of priority and assessed for signs of myocardial ischaemia. When myocardium is damaged, electrolytes leak out of the cells, resulting in changes to the ST segment and T waves. Early signs include T-wave inversion and ST depression; both are associated with NSTEMI and unstable angina. STEMI is diagnosed in the presence of ST elevation on the 12-lead ECG, or new onset of bundle branch block (Ibanez et al. 2017). VT and VF are also indicative of ACS. In the very early stages of ACS, the ECG may be normal, at least initially, and repeat ECGs should be performed if the clinical history and presentation suggest that the problem is cardiac. The ECG changes can pinpoint the area of ventricle affected and help nurses identify and prepare for potential complication such as AV blocks (Olson 2021).

Blood tests are needed to confirm the diagnosis and to identify possible modifiable cardiovascular risk factors. Troponins (T and I) are proteins released into the bloodstream when heart muscle, myocardium, is damaged, often referred to as 'cardiac biomarkers'. A rise in serum troponin above normal parameters will therefore occur in STEMI and NSTEMI; in unstable angina, as there is no myocardial damage, the troponin level will remain normal. A negative troponin in the presence of chest pain enables ACS to be ruled out. High-sensitivity troponins are now recommended for faster identification of ACS (NICE 2016a).

Close monitoring of key electrolytes, such as potassium and magnesium, is essential as the patient is at high risk of arrhythmias that may be life-threatening, such as VT or VF. Correction of electrolyte imbalance can help prevent occurrence. This blood test also enables estimation of glomerular filtration rate (eGFR). Thyroid function tests (TFTs), liver function tests (LFTs) and lipid profiles should also be assessed, as these may enable identification of cardiovascular risk factors that may require addressing later on. The patient's CBG should be monitored hourly during the acute phase of the ACS. Hyperglycaemia may occur in patients who are not known to have diabetes as well as in individuals with known

diabetes. Tight glycaemic control using intensive insulin and glucose therapy is necessary for patients whose CBG >11 mmol/L during the acute phase of the illness. Patients should have an HbA1C blood test before discharge, which should not be fasting unless it is more than 4 days after the ACS event (NICE 2020a).

Transthoracic Echocardiogram

This should be recorded before the patient is discharged to establish the extent of left, and possibly right, ventricular dysfunction (NICE 2020a). This test can enable estimation of ejection fraction, which is the percentage of blood that is ejected from the heart with each stroke compared with the volume at the end of diastole (Aaronson et al. 2020). Risk stratification tools, such as the Global Registry of Acute Cardiovascular Events (GRACE) score, should be used in patients with NSTEMI or unstable angina to estimate the risk to the patient from major adverse cardiovascular events (MACE), such as STEMI or death. This risk assessment can help guide the timing of invasive treatment, in the form of PCI (NICE 2020a). Patients with hyperglycaemia but no diabetes are at increased risk of developing type II diabetes and should therefore be offered lifestyle advice.

❖ Nursing Management and Health Promotion: Acute Coronary Syndromes

Nursing priorities include rapid assessment to inform diagnosis and identification of complications, administering pain relief and ensuring the cardiology team are engaged in assessing the patient's suitability for reperfusion interventions at the earliest opportunity. Preparations should be made for the immediate transfer of the patient to the Cath Lab, which may require interhospital transfer to a Heart Attack Centre for primary PCI (PPCI).

An ABCDE approach and NEWS2 scoring should be used to assess and frequently reassess the patient with an ACS. The patient will require close observations during the acute phase of their illness as they are at high risk of complications, including cardiac arrest. Information and reassurance should be offered throughout the episode of patient care, especially as patients often experience extreme anxiety during the acute phase of ACS, often referred to as 'a sense of impending doom'.

The patient must be positioned in a bed where high-dependency care can be delivered in a calm environment with resuscitation equipment immediately available, such as a coronary care unit. Continuous cardiac monitoring will be required as the patient is at high risk of arrhythmias, such as VT, VF which may cause cardiac arrest, as well as atrial fibrillation and heart blocks (Ibanez et al. 2017). Airway assessment, respiratory rate, peripheral oxygen saturations (SpO_2) levels, pulse and blood pressure should be recorded every 5–15 minutes. A 12-lead ECG should be recorded and repeated, using the same electrodes if possible, at close intervals, particularly when the patient reports symptoms. In addition, right-sided and posterior lead ECGs should also be recorded in patients presenting with an inferior STEMI or in patients with suspected ACS with a normal 12-lead ECG (Rowlands and Sargent 2019). Patients should be encouraged to report any change in their symptoms, which should be explored using a chest pain assessment tool, such as SOCRATES (Box 2.1) and a set of observations including a 12-lead ECG. IV access should be established as early as possible, and blood tests recorded as stated previously. A fluid balance chart should be commenced to observe urine output, which may decrease indicating a reduction in cardiac output, and hourly CBG recorded to observe for hyperglycaemia.

The patient's temperature should be recorded regularly, which may be slightly elevated due to the inflammation underlying the ACS.

Treatments for Patients With Acute Coronary Syndromes

Oxygen therapy may be required if the patient's pulse oximeter reads less than 94% (O'Driscoll et al. 2017), although recent evidence proposes delivering oxygen if the SpO_2 is less than 90% (Ibanez et al. 2017). Pain relief using IV opiates such as morphine may address symptoms associated with ischaemia. IV morphine can be administered in small incremental doses until the pain is completely relieved, assessed using pain scoring. If residual pain continues, an IV infusion of GTN may be prescribed, which can be titrated to the patient's pain, but close monitoring of the patient's blood pressure is essential, as severe hypotension may ensue.

Patients should be offered dual antiplatelet therapy in the form of aspirin and a P2Y12 inhibitor, such as prasugrel, ticagrelor or clopidogrel, at the earliest possible opportunity with antithrombin therapy commenced during or after PPCI (NICE 2020a).

Patients diagnosed with a STEMI should be immediately assessed for eligibility for coronary reperfusion with PPCI, which should be delivered as soon as possible to limit the extent of myocardial damage. It is the intervention of choice when the patient presents within 12 hours of onset of symptoms and can access the service within 120 minutes (Ibanez et al. 2017; NICE 2020a). STEMI is often diagnosed by paramedics, who will divert the ambulance to take the patient directly to a 'Heart Attack Centre', which has 24-hour facilities for PPCI available. PPCI usually involves coronary angiography to locate the obstruction in the coronary artery, removal of the thrombus with aspiration, angioplasty to dilate the narrowed vessel and drug-eluting stent deployment to ensure arterial patency is maintained (Information 2.1). If PPCI cannot be delivered within 2 hours of first medical contact, the patient should be offered IV thrombolysis to dissolve the obstructive thrombus followed up with PCI as soon as possible. Where the patient's symptoms began more than 12 hours previously, urgent angiography may be necessary especially if there is evidence of ischaemia, haemodynamic instability or cardiogenic shock (NICE 2020a).

Patients diagnosed with NSTEMI or unstable angina require the same pharmacological therapies as those with STEMI, but PCI can be delivered within 72 hours unless the patient is clinically unstable (NICE 2020a). Until PCI is delivered, the patient remains at significant risk of developing STEMI or possibly cardiac arrest. Therefore, risk stratification tools, such as GRACE scoring, should be used to identify those at high risk (Collet et al. 2021). Therefore, patients must remain on bed rest until they have been pain-free for 24 hours and monitored continuously for signs of instability, such as hypotension, tachycardia, dyspnoea; refractory chest pain; dynamic changes to the ST–T segment on the 12-lead ECG; and arrhythmias such as AF, VT and VF. If any of these occur, PCI should be expedited, ideally within 2 hours (NICE 2020a), which may mean preparing the patient for a rapid transfer to a Heart Attack Centre.

Secondary prevention therapies should be started as soon as it is safe to do so, dependent upon the haemodynamic status of the patient. This usually includes the administration of a beta-blocker, such as bisoprolol (or calcium channel blocker, such as diltiazem), to reduce myocardial work; an ACE inhibitor, such as ramipril, to prevent cardiac remodelling; and a statin, such as atorvastatin, to reduce circulating low-density lipoprotein (LDL) cholesterol and to strengthen the fibrous caps of atherosclerotic plaques to prevent plaque rupture. In addition, patients are usually advised to continue taking a low dose of aspirin daily for the rest of their life, and PY12 inhibitor such as prasugrel or ticagrelor for a year after stent implantation.

Percutaneous Coronary Intervention (PCI)

This treatment is appropriate for patients with life-limiting symptoms of angina despite optimal medical treatment and for those with atherosclerosis causing narrowing of one or two of the coronary arteries. It is known as PPCI when used urgently for patients in the acute phase of STEMI.

PCI is an umbrella term referring to a procedure that involves firstly using coronary angiography to identify and evaluate the exact location in the coronary artery where the lumen has narrowed due to atherosclerosis, followed by intervention to open the narrowed arteries (Information 2.1). Next, a balloon catheter is advanced to the site of the narrowing, via the radial or femoral artery. Once at the site, the balloon is inflated for a very short time, dilating the narrowed artery to restore adequate perfusion. Finally, an intracoronary stent is deployed and left at the site, acting as scaffolding to maintain the open artery. Drug-eluting stents are used, which discharge a small amount of immunosuppressive medication to prevent the stent from becoming blocked through restenosis.

Postprocedure care involves close monitoring of the patient, who should be advised to remain on bed rest, lying flat if femoral access has been used, for several hours after the procedure; patients will be able to mobilise sooner if radial access has been used. The patient should be placed on a cardiac monitor with regular observations recorded that include regular review of the access site for signs of bleeding, bruising or development of haematoma. The affected limb should be assessed regularly for warmth, colour and pulse (using Doppler if necessary) as evidence of adequate perfusion; if the limb whitens, becomes cold or a pulse cannot be found, immediate escalation of care is essential. Patients sometimes return to the ward with the arterial sheath in situ which should be removed at a specified time using a device that can apply sustained pressure to the site, such as the TR band for radial puncture or Femostop for femoral puncture, as the patient is likely to have received antithrombin therapies during the procedure which may delay clotting and increase the risk of haematoma formation. The patient should be encouraged to report any symptoms they experience after the procedure, and to drink plenty of fluids to facilitate excretion of the dye used during the angiogram (Olson 2021).

Coronary Artery Bypass Graft Surgery (CABG)

This surgery is appropriate for patients who have severe atherosclerosis in three or more coronary arteries, often referred to as triple vessel disease. Coronary artery bypass surgery requires a sternotomy to expose the patient's heart and to enable cardiopulmonary bypass, a procedure necessary to ensure continuous circulation while the heart remains completely still during the procedure. This allows the surgeon to graft native arteries or veins from the aorta to below (distal) the narrowings in the coronary arteries, which effectively bypasses the stenosed portions of the arteries and restores perfusion to the myocardium. Minimally invasive direct coronary artery bypass surgery (MIDCAB) is an alternative approach suitable for single-vessel bypass grafting without cardiopulmonary bypass or sternotomy. A small incision is made in the thoracic wall, through which surgeons use videoscopic guidance to create the bypass grafts on a beating heart.

Shared decision-making for patients with multivessel coronary disease is made by a multidisciplinary 'Heart Team' to establish whether CABG or PCI is the most suitable approach to revascularisation. The team usually includes a cardiologist, cardiac surgeons, an anaesthetist and perfusionists who will agree on the best approach to revascularisation based on the patient's clinical profile and potential risks (Neumann et al. 2018). Preoperative assessment clinics, run by experienced nurses, offer education for patients and their relatives or carers about what to expect before, during and after the procedure.

Initial postoperative care may be delivered in intensive or high-dependency care while the patient remains intubated and sedated for several hours after the procedure. The nurse's role involves close monitoring of the patient for signs of haemodynamic instability that may arise due to dehydration, internal bleeding, arrhythmias, heart failure and renal dysfunction. Patients usually have chest drains and epicardial pacing wires in situ which must be closely monitored, along with fluid balance. The patient will require regular pain relief and clear instructions and support to enable them to move around without placing pressure on their sternum. Patients will require assistance with activities of daily living, care of their sternal or thoracic wounds as well as the sites where the veins or arteries were removed, usually in the legs or arms. Patients should be encouraged to mobilise with assistance early in their postoperative stay. Some may experience some confusion or 'postpump' delirium, which must be identified early on so that effective psychological support can be offered.

Patients will be advised to expect some degree of pain from the sternotomy for several weeks, discomfort on coughing or lifting the hands above the head, and leg swelling. Short-term anxiety and depression may occur if patients feel that recovery is slower than anticipated. Partners and other family members will also need ongoing information and support and the patient should be offered cardiac rehabilitation.

Complications Arising From Acute Coronary Syndromes

There are a considerable number of complications of ACSs ranging from hyperglycaemia to myocardial rupture. Some complications arise due as a result of PCI, such as acute kidney injury due to poor excretion of the radio-opaque dye, haematoma developing at the site of arterial puncture or in-stent stenosis causing occlusion of the coronary artery. The nurse should be able to recognise these and other major complications outlined here, escalating care as required.

Cardiac Arrest

Cardiac arrest, when the heart stops contracting, results in the sudden loss of blood flow to vital organs and death will occur within minutes without urgent intervention (Menzies-Gow and Spiers 2018). This is an emergency, and every nurse is responsible for recognising that cardiac arrest has occurred, knowing the procedure for summoning help within the clinical setting or in the community and commencing effective cardiopulmonary resuscitation (CPR). In ACSs, sudden onset of pulseless VT or VF can occur due to myocardial hypoxia; however, other causes, such as pulmonary embolus, may induce asystole and PEA which also cause cardiac arrest. The Chain of Survival (Fig. 2.17) (Resuscitation Council UK 2021) indicates that early identification of warning signs, activation of emergency services, initiation of basic life support, defibrillation and Advanced Cardiac Life Support are necessary to optimise the chance of successfully resuscitating the patient. Therefore, summoning urgent help is essential; if in hospital, a cardiac arrest call should be made to alert the in-hospital resuscitation team.

The latest guidance on Adult Advanced Cardiac Life Support is issued by the Resuscitation Council (2021). These guidelines are regularly reviewed and updated, and their specific guidance should be adhered to.

Rapid assessment of the collapsed patient with suspected cardiac arrest should include:
- Checking that it is safe before approaching the patient
- Assessing responsiveness by shouting in both ears, 'Can you hear me?'
- Opening the patient's airway and observing for signs of obstruction
- Checking for signs of breathing by looking for a rise and fall in the chest wall, listening for any breath sounds and feeling for any expelled air for a maximum of 10 seconds
- Checking for a carotid pulse
- Connecting the patient to an automated external defibrillator and a cardiac monitor

Advanced Cardiac Life Support

These measures (see Fig. 2.13) include commencing effective CPR: repeated cycles of 30 regular chest compressions (depth of 5–6 cm at a rate of 100–120/min), followed by two effective breaths using a bag-valve mask or more advanced airway support through which high-flow oxygen can be delivered. Defibrillation should be administered as soon as possible if the patient is in VT or VF to enable restoration of sinus rhythm; if VT or VF continues, adrenaline and amiodarone may be given via IV access after three shocks. If the patient is in asystole or PEA, defibrillation is not indicated. CPR should continue while IV access is obtained to enable immediate delivery of adrenaline and repeated every 3–5 minutes.

Figure 2.17 Chain of survival. (Reproduced with the kind permission of the Resuscitation Council UK.)

Causes of cardiac arrest should be considered and addressed, e.g. hypovolaemia, hypoxia, hyper/hypokalaemia, hypothermia, pulmonary thromboembolism, tension pneumothorax, cardiac tamponade and toxins. Thrombolysis may be administered where pulmonary embolus is the cause, and where ACS is suspected, the patient should be urgently transferred for PPCI while in cardiac arrest to enable restoration of myocardial blood flow and, consequently, normal sinus rhythm.

Patients may require a range of supportive interventions on return of spontaneous circulation (ROSC), dependent upon the severity of organ ischaemia resulting from cardiac arrest. Patients may have a reduced level of consciousness or be comatose, require intubation and ventilation to support their airway and breathing, and inotropes or other forms of circulatory support, such as extracorporeal membrane oxygenation (ECMO). While postarrest care should start immediately, it may be necessary to transfer the patient to intensive care or coronary care (Resuscitation Council UK 2021). A 12-lead ECG will reveal ST elevation or new bundle branch block as indicators of MI as the cause, which should prompt urgent patient transfer for PPCI.

Acute Heart Failure and Cardiogenic Shock

Damage to the left ventricle of the heart as a result of an ACS can rapidly, or gradually, lead to reduced myocardial contraction during systole and a fall in cardiac output, resulting in hypotension, tachycardia and pulmonary oedema, indicating acute heart failure (for further information see section on acute heart failure). Cardiogenic shock is a severe form of heart failure that results from sustained hypotension (SBP less than 90 mmHg) and causes a significant reduction in perfusion of the vital organs leading to multiorgan failure (Aaronson et al. 2020). Cardiogenic shock is explored in detail in Chapter 20, Recognising and Managing Shock.

ABCDE assessment of the patient will reveal the early signs associated with shock: reduction in urine output due to reduced perfusion of the kidneys, vasoconstriction leads to cold clammy skin; later tachycardia and hypotension become evident. Hypoxia ensues due to inadequate oxygenation, despite tachypnoea, caused by pulmonary oedema. The patient's pulse will be fast and thready as a compensatory response to the falling cardiac output and the associated rhythm may be sinus tachycardia, atrial fibrillation or VT. Lactic acid is produced in the skeletal muscle beds as the metabolism changes, giving rise to a metabolic acidosis. This process is cyclical, with the heart continually trying to pump harder for an ever-falling SV.

The patient should have continuous cardiac monitoring and haemodynamic assessment, including close monitoring of blood pressure using noninvasive or invasive techniques, e.g. an arterial line, which can also be used for arterial blood gas analysis. IV access must be established early to permit cautious administration of IV diuretics, such as furosemide, to reduce circulating volume. A central line is essential for central venous pressure (CVP) monitoring, as well as administration of inotropic drugs to improve left ventricular contraction, such as dobutamine. A fluid balance chart must be maintained and a urinary catheter will be necessary to monitor output. Blood samples should include natriuretic peptides or the pro-hormone N-terminal pro-B type natriuretic peptide (N-terminal prohormone of brain natriuretic peptide (NT-proBNP)), troponins and eGFR. Continuous positive airway pressure (CPAP) may be beneficial to patients in respiratory distress but without hypotension, while an intra-aortic balloon pump (IABP) may be indicated as haemodynamic support for patients with severe hypotension in cardiogenic shock (Ibanez et al. 2017).

Mechanical devices, such as a left ventricular assist device, or ECMO may be considered in severe cases when the patient does not respond to treatment.

Arrhythmias

Arrhythmias, such as AF, VT, VF and heart blocks, are common during and immediately after an ACS, and therefore, close cardiac monitoring is essential in the first few days after the acute event. Reperfusion of the myocardium during PCI may also induce arrhythmias, such as junctional arrhythmias. If ventricular arrhythmias repeatedly occur after an ACS, the patient may require insertion of a device such as a permanent pacemaker or an ICD device. See the earlier discussion concerning 'Cardiac arrhythmias' for detailed information.

Myocardial Damage

Extensive, permanent damage to the myocardium as a result of an ACS can result in severe mechanical complications, such as creation of a ventricular septal defect, myocardial rupture, papillary muscle rupture and formation of a ventricular aneurysm. These complications are often life-threatening and require urgent surgical correction for any chance of survival (Ibanez et al. 2017). Pericarditis may develop in the first couple of weeks following STEMI, when it is referred to as Dressler's syndrome, but eventually subsides.

Cardiac Rehabilitation

Cardiac rehabilitation is a programme of activities offered to all patients who have experienced an ACS. The programme of activities and classes aims to enable patients to resume activities associated with normal life and to prevent recurrence of an acute cardiac event in a non-judgemental and respectful environment (British Association for Cardiovascular Prevention and Rehabilitation [BACPR] 2023). The programme begins while the patient is in hospital, when a specialist nurse, or other members of the multidisciplinary team, meet with the patient, and ideally a close family member or carer, to offer personalised education, advice and individualised goal setting to help them understand the acute event they have just experienced and to adjust to life immediately after the event. Following discharge home, patients may be contacted by the rehabilitation team for follow-up support and are invited to attend home-based or centre-based rehabilitation classes approximately 3–4 weeks later which provide the opportunity to engage in physical exercise under the supervision of nurses and physiotherapists (Cowie et al. 2019). There is also specialist input from dieticians, occupational therapists as well as physios and nurses offering patient education to support behaviour change and lifestyle modification, as well as psychosocial support.

NICE (2020a) currently recommends that individualised advice and support be given to patients to enable them to change their lifestyles to prevent future cardiac events which may include the following:

Smoking cessation should be encouraged and an explanation of the associated benefits provided. Advice should be offered to patients prior to discharge home, with a referral to specialist services, if appropriate. Patients may be offered nicotine replacement therapy. The NICE guidance on treating tobacco dependence provides specific information on approaches to therapy (NICE 2022b).

Weight management. Each patient should have their BMI calculated to identify those who are overweight or obese. Advice on physical exercise and diet should be offered to help patients achieve and maintain a healthy weight. The NICE guidance on obesity prevention (NICE 2015) provides additional information on specific strategies to support this.

Dietary advice recommending healthy eating that follows a Mediterranean style diet should be offered to the patient and their closest family member/partner. Guidance should be offered to help them replace foods that are high in saturated fat (LDL cholesterol) such as meat and cheese with plant-based alternatives. The Eatwell Guide (Public Health England 2016) provides a useful guide, including intake of two portions of oily fish a week, and at least five fruit and vegetables per day should be advised (Fig. 2.18). Salt intake should be limited to less than 6 g per day, to reduce the risk of developing hypertension.

Alcohol consumption advice should adhere to the current guidance on alcohol: a maximum of 14 units per week, spread evenly across three or more days. Several days each week should be alcohol free, with at least 2 days with no alcohol consumption at all (Department of Health [DH] 2016).

Physical activity reduces the risk of a range of diseases, helps to maintain a healthy weight, can improve self-esteem and can limit the symptoms associated with depression and anxiety (Department of Health and Social Care [DHSC] 2019). However, exercising after having a life-threatening cardiac event may be daunting for the patient, and their carers. Exercise should be gently reintroduced once the patient has returned home. Following cardiac rehabilitation classes, where moderate-intensity aerobic exercise is gently introduced, patients may be advised to gradually increase the amount they exercise daily, aiming to be physically active for 20–30 minutes a day for at least 5 days of the week, although this may be individually tailored to suit the patient's condition. Patients should be reassured that sexual activity poses no greater risk of MI, and therefore can be advised that they can resume sexual activity when they feel ready to do so.

Psychological and social support Patients and their families, particularly partners, are likely to be anxious at the time of the acute event, on discharge home from hospital and during recovery. They need individualised and appropriately timed information about what is happening to them and the likely pattern of recovery to enable them to feel more in control and be able to cope. Planned periods of rest and relaxation, graded exercise, instructions on stress management and individual and group support sessions may help. Anxiety and depression are common after a cardiac event and patients and their carers should be made aware of the signs that might indicate onset.

Figure 2.18 The Eatwell Guide. (From Public Health England in association with the Welsh Government, Food Standards Scotland and the Food Standards Agency in Northern Ireland.)

Valvular Heart Disease

There are two main types of valvular dysfunction: regurgitation and stenosis. These two abnormalities can affect any of the four valves, but this book will simply explore the two valves most commonly affected: aortic and mitral valve.

Aortic Valve Disease

The aortic valve normally has three cusps or leaflets, which open fully during ventricular systole to approximately 3 cm in diameter. Immediately following ventricular systole, the valve will close, with the leaflets meeting tightly together to prevent back flow of blood from the aorta into the left ventricle.

In aortic stenosis, the valve cusps have become sclerosed and calcified, leaving them rigid, affecting their ability to fully open during systole and potentially reducing SV and cardiac output. In response, left ventricular contraction becomes more forceful, resulting in myocardial hypertrophy (thickening) known as left ventricular hypertrophy (LVH), to facilitate the generation of sufficient preload to force blood through the narrowed valve. Patients usually remain asymptomatic until the valve opening has diminished to approximately 1 cm^2, when patients may experience symptoms of dizziness (presyncope) or loss of consciousness (syncope). LVH may induce symptoms such as angina and dyspnoea on exertion as the myocardium does not receive sufficient oxygen to meet the increased demand, which in turn may result in potentially life-threatening arrhythmias arising from the ventricles, such as VT or VF.

Aortic stenosis is diagnosed using the patient's clinical history and an echocardiogram. The 12-lead ECG may reveal signs of left ventricular enlargement. Pharmacological treatment includes beta-blockers to prevent progression, but ultimately most patients require surgical replacement of the valve. Aortic valve replacement usually requires the patient to have a full sternotomy and be placed on cardiopulmonary bypass before suturing in a new prosthetic or homograft valve into position. In patients for whom invasive surgery carries considerable risk, transcutaneous aortic valve implantation may be suitable. This is a percutaneous procedure conducted under X-ray guidance in which a prosthetic valve is positioned directly over the existing aortic valve using a catheter inserted in the femoral artery and advanced to the aortic root.

In aortic regurgitation, the valve cusps fail to close tightly, and as a result, during ventricular diastole, blood will be able to re-enter the left ventricle from the aorta. Often this is due to prolonged hypertension that has resulted in widening of the aorta, which dilates the annulus on which the valve cusps sit. Congenital connective tissue disorders such as Ehlers–Danlos and Marfan syndromes can result in dilatation of the aortic root, leading to severe aortic regurgitation.

Symptoms such as breathlessness emerge due to the fall in cardiac output, and patients sometimes develop arrhythmias such as atrial fibrillation. Diagnosis is made using echocardiography, and early intervention includes treatments to prevent and manage heart failure. Surgical replacement of the aortic valve is currently recommended for patients.

Mitral Valve Disease

The mitral valve has two cusps or leaflets, which can also become regurgitant or stenotic. Many people are born with mitral valve prolapse but remain asymptomatic, never requiring treatment. Infections, such as rheumatic fever and endocarditis, can damage the valve cusps causing regurgitation of blood through the mitral valve during ventricular systole. Symptoms are associated with the ensuing heart failure, including breathlessness, and the patient may develop atrial arrhythmias such as AF. Interventions include the percutaneous 'mitraclip' procedure or surgical replacement of the mitral valve, as described in the section on aortic stenosis.

Mitral stenosis, where the cusps become rigid, preventing full opening of the valve, may also result in symptoms of heart failure and atrial fibrillation. Surgical replacement of the valve is usually necessary, although less invasive valvuloplasty procedures can be used to open and separate the rigid valve cusps to restore blood flow.

Heart Failure

Heart failure is a complex syndrome with clinical signs and symptoms that occur when the heart is unable to provide sufficient cardiac output to meet the body's metabolic requirements. Heart failure is secondary to an underlying condition which is most commonly cardiovascular, such as CHD, arrhythmias, hypertension and inherited conditions such as cardiomyopathy. It can also result from noncardiac causes, including specific forms of chemotherapy, substance use disorder and infection, and is strongly associated with comorbidities such as stroke, diabetes and chronic kidney dysfunction (McDonagh et al. 2021). As a result, the prevalence in the UK is high, with around 200,000 new diagnoses made each year, and as society ages, it is anticipated the prevalence of heart failure will continue to rise (BHF 2022). Around 920,000 people live with heart failure in the UK (BHF 2022), their symptoms of breathlessness, fatigue, ankle oedema, lack of appetite, cognitive dysfunction or depression managed using a range of therapies and lifestyle modifications to optimise cardiac function (British Society for Heart Failure [BSH] 2022).

The trajectory for patients living with heart failure is unpredictable, usually involving periods of stability and good health interjected with episodes of acute heart failure where a deterioration in cardiac function leads to decompensation and hospital admission. The typical course for the patient from diagnosis to death is illustrated in Fig. 2.19 (Goodlin 2009). Most patients with heart failure receive therapies aimed at prolonging life and relief from symptoms. Over weeks, months or even years, cardiac dysfunction will gradually deteriorate and is most often the cause of death. Therefore, early palliative and end-of-life care planning is an essential element of patient care (BSH 2022). Patients may be referred for a detailed suitability assessment for cardiac transplantation if they meet specified criteria, which can be curative but requires long-term immunosuppressive therapy.

Acute heart failure has been identified as the most common reason for hospitalisation in the world (Ferreira et al. 2019), with patients usually presenting with pulmonary oedema due to acute decompensation. The diagnosis of heart failure remains most frequently made in hospital during an episode of acute decompensation despite advances in diagnostics and therapies (NCEPOD 2018). Patients have often been living with signs of heart failure for some time, such as breathlessness on exertion or fatigue, which can be either misdiagnosed or overlooked. Recent campaigns have sought to raise awareness of heart failure with the aim of improving diagnosis in the community, which is associated with significantly improved patient outcomes compared with those first diagnosed during an acute admission (NICOR 2021).

Classification of Heart Failure

Heart failure is clinically defined using the measure of left ventricular ejection fraction. Heart failure with a reduced ejection

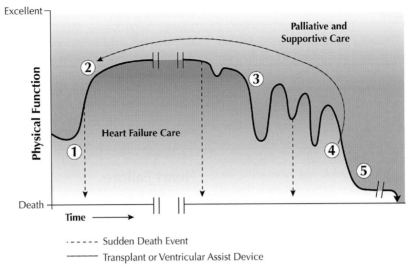

Figure 2.19 Clinical effects of the decompensatory phase of left ventricular failure.

fraction (HFrEF) is diagnosed in patients with structural heart disease or diastolic dysfunction that causes symptoms and signs of left ventricular failure and an ejection fraction less than 40%. Heart failure with a mildly reduced ejection fraction (HFmrEF) is diagnosed where patients have an ejection fraction of 40%–49% and heart failure with a preserved ejection fraction (HFpEF) where the ejection fraction is more than 50%. Both require evidence of structural heart disease and elevated natriuretic peptides to confirm the diagnosis (McDonagh et al. 2021). The New York Heart Association classification provides a useful means of classifying the effects that the symptoms patients are living with have on their exercise tolerance and quality of life at any point in time. Both classifications are used to direct the use of specific drug and device therapies, such as sacubitril/valsartan, eplerenone, dapaglifozcin and cardiac resynchronisation therapy (McDonagh et al. 2021).

In diastolic heart failure, the left ventricular wall is stiffened, impairing diastolic filling of the ventricle that reduces cardiac output. This often results in HFpEF, which may eventually cause systolic dysfunction and HFrEF. Right ventricular systolic dysfunction may occur as a result of left ventricular failure, as described earlier, or due to any condition that increases the pressure within the pulmonary vasculature and right ventricle, such as a pulmonary embolus, pulmonary hypertension or specific forms of adult congenital heart disease.

Pathophysiology

CHD, and ACSs in particular, is the most common cause of heart failure. The reduction or cessation of blood flow as a result of a severely narrowed or obstructed coronary artery leads to myocardial cell injury and necrosis (Lilly 2021). The portion of dead tissue (infarct) is unable to contract, which reduces the SV from the left ventricle. Other conditions, including tachycardias such as atrial fibrillation, shorten diastolic filling time, reducing SV and cardiac output. Neurohormonal mechanisms can maintain blood pressure and cardiac output through haemodynamic compensation. Triggered in response to a fall in systemic blood pressure, which is detected by baroreceptors located in the aortic arch and carotid arteries, compensatory mechanisms will be activated to maintain sufficient cardiac output and therefore systemic perfusion. These include increased HR (as cardiac output = HR × SV), increased force of myocardial contraction,

vasoconstriction and activation of the RAAS to retain water to increase blood volume.

However, these mechanisms will eventually fail, resulting in symptoms associated with reduced cardiac output, such as pulmonary oedema, hypotension, reduced urine output, fatigue and confusion (Fig. 2.20). Blood will accumulate within the left ventricle, left atrium (leading to atrial fibrillation) and the pulmonary circulation, where the increased osmotic pressure forces fluid to move across from the pulmonary capillaries surrounding the alveoli into the alveoli themselves, resulting in symptoms of breathlessness, sputum production and acute anxiety associated with pulmonary oedema. This increases the pressure exerted on the right side of the heart, resulting in accumulation of blood within the right ventricle, right atrium and venous circulation which will eventually begin to fail, too, known as right-sided heart failure. This is evident through assessment of the internal jugular vein, which would be distended and also the examination of the lower limbs and sacrum for signs of oedema. In severe cases, the oedema may extend to the liver and abdomen (Aaronson et al. 2020).

Patient Assessment

Acute heart failure is a medical emergency. It may be an episode of decompensation in patients known to have heart failure or be the first occurrence of pulmonary oedema associated with an acute cardiac event, such as ACS, aortic dissection, sepsis, new-onset AF or a pulmonary embolus. A rapid, initial assessment of the breathless patient should be undertaken using the ABCDE approach and a history taken from the patient in an attempt to identify the underlying cause of the condition (O'Driscoll et al. 2017). An episode of acute heart failure may cause the patient to be very distressed with a range of clinical symptoms, including reduced level of consciousness, shortness of breath with tachypnoea, low peripheral oxygen saturations and a cough, often expectorating white, frothy sputum associated with pulmonary oedema (Lilly 2021). The cardiac monitor can reveal sinus tachycardia or possibly tachyarrhythmias such as atrial flutter or fibrillation and show signs of haemodynamic instability including hypotension, prolonged cardiac resynchronisation therapy (CRT), cool extremities, with evidence of pallor and a cold sweat (diaphoresis). Examination of their ankles, legs, sacrum and abdomen may

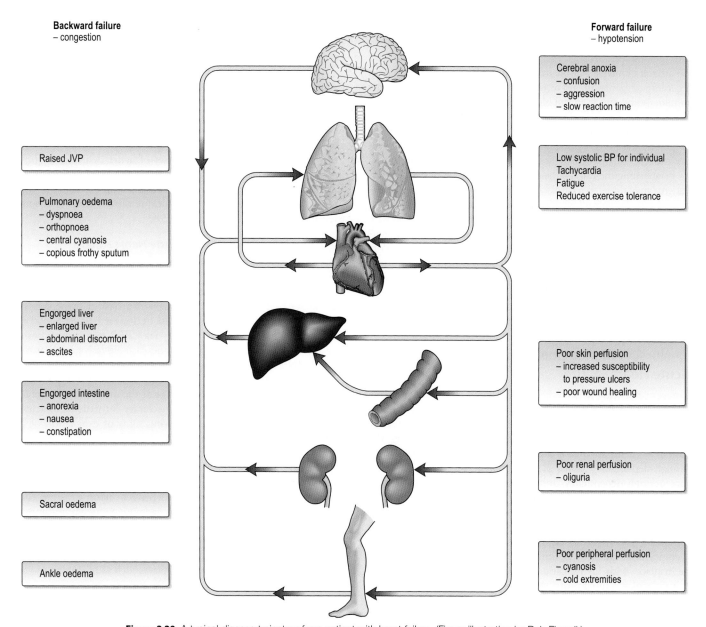

Backward failure
– congestion

Forward failure
– hypotension

Raised JVP

Pulmonary oedema
– dyspnoea
– orthopnoea
– central cyanosis
– copious frothy sputum

Engorged liver
– enlarged liver
– abdominal discomfort
– ascites

Engorged intestine
– anorexia
– nausea
– constipation

Sacral oedema

Ankle oedema

Cerebral anoxia
– confusion
– aggression
– slow reaction time

Low systolic BP for individual
Tachycardia
Fatigue
Reduced exercise tolerance

Poor skin perfusion
– increased susceptibility
  to pressure ulcers
– poor wound healing

Poor renal perfusion
– oliguria

Poor peripheral perfusion
– cyanosis
– cold extremities

Figure 2.20 A typical disease trajectory for a patient with heart failure. (Figure illustration by Rob Flewell.)

reveal oedema. The patient may also show signs of the underlying condition responsible for the episode of acute heart failure, such as sepsis (Menzies-Gow and Spiers 2018).

Chronic heart failure causes the patient to have symptoms associated with reduced cardiac output, which can limit perfusion to the systemic circulation which manifests as a wide range of debilitating symptoms that can significantly impact on the patient's quality life. These can include an often overlooked symptom of fatigue, particularly on exertion, that may gradually diminish the amount of exercise the patient can comfortably undertake, measured as the distance that can be walked without symptoms occurring (known as exercise tolerance). Reduced perfusion to the brain may impair cognition and lead to symptoms of confusion and disorientation; diminished perfusion to the kidneys can cause oliguria and initiate or worsen CKD. Pulmonary oedema will cause dyspnoea, particularly at night (nocturnal dyspnoea), with patients unable to sleep lying flat, requiring several pillows to sleep sitting up to avoid waking with breathlessness (orthopnoea). Auscultation of the chest may reveal pulmonary

crepitations, associated with oedema, which may cause a cough which may be productive of white frothy sputum. With right-sided heart failure, oedema initially builds within the tissue around ankles but may spread towards the sacral area, especially in patients lying in bed. Engorgement of the intestines may cause gastrointestinal symptoms such as bloating, loss of appetite and nausea, and the patient may develop signs of liver dysfunction such as ascites. As oedema will result in weight gain, recording regular weights at the same time of day can help detect early signs of fluid overload. However, heart failure may eventually cause cardiac cachexia (McDonagh et al. 2021).

Diagnostic Investigations

A full systematic assessment of the patient should include history taking and physical examination which may reveal jugular venous distension and signs of lower limb or sacral oedema. Auscultation of the lung fields may reveal signs associated with pulmonary oedema (Aaronson et al. 2020). Measurement of serum natriuretic peptides (BNP or NT-proBNP) is essential for diagnosis and a range of additional tests are recommended to confirm the presence of heart failure, including 12-lead ECG, urinalysis, chest X-ray and blood tests including electrolytes, urea, creatine and eGFR (NICE 2021b). An arterial blood gas sample may also provide valuable information regarding oxygenation and reveal metabolic acidosis. Blood samples should also be sent for a full blood count and to assess thyroid and liver function, with fasting samples taken for lipids and glucose. Where the natriuretic peptides are found to be elevated, echocardiography should be carried out to establish the cause of heart failure and to evaluate the patient's left ventricular ejection fraction.

Establishing the cause of heart failure is essential for patient care. Patients may undergo a cardiac magnetic resonance imaging (MRI) scan or stress echocardiography to assess the structure of the heart, and to identify any myocardial damage that may be reversible with reperfusion, known as 'hibernating myocardium'. Cardiac catheterisation or CT coronary angiogram may be undertaken to explore whether coronary revascularisation may be of benefit (see Information 3.1), or a cardiac biopsy may be necessary to establish a diagnosis of rarer causes of heart failure, such as amyloidosis or cardiomyopathy. Ambulatory 24-hour Holter (ECG) monitoring may be offered to patients with suspected arrhythmias (McDonagh et al. 2021).

❖ Nursing Management and Health Promotion: Acute Heart Failure

Patients presenting in acute heart failure with pulmonary oedema and haemodynamic instability may feel very anxious and frightened, with signs and symptoms of respiratory failure caused by this life-threatening condition, and therefore, supporting the patient with reassurance is an essential element of nursing care. A high-dependency (level 2) environment such as a coronary care or high-dependency unit is recommended to ensure close monitoring and proximity to resuscitation equipment, as acute deterioration of their condition into cardiogenic shock or cardiac arrest could occur at any time (NICE 2021b). The patient should be advised to remain in bed and helped to sit upright in a comfortable position. Continuous cardiac monitoring should be in place, with identification of any arrhythmias such as atrial or ventricular ectopic beats, atrial fibrillation or VT, which must be treated immediately. Often, defibrillator pads are positioned on the patient when the risk of cardiac arrest is considered to be high to enable defibrillation to be rapidly implemented. Regular observations should be recorded using NEWS2 scoring, including AVPU (with GCS if necessary) and airway assessment, respiratory rate, pulse oximetry, pulse and blood pressure, with hourly assessment of temperature and CBG. Maintenance of patent IV access is essential as it will be required for drug administration. A central line can provide invasive monitoring of venous pressure, and if the patient is very unstable or requires inotropic support, an arterial line should be used for continuous arterial blood pressure monitoring and also facilitate regular assessment of arterial blood gases; metabolic acidosis may develop as a result of tissue hypoxia.

Fluid balance and renal function should be closely monitored throughout using fluid balance charts, blood samples to assess urea, creatinine and eGFR, BNP or NT-pro-BNP and daily weights recorded at the same time each day once the patient is mobile. Restricting fluid and dietary salt intake may be necessary to help reduce fluid overload. Discussing with the patient how best to manage the diuresis that will ensue following diuretic therapy is essential; a urinary catheter may be beneficial to help the patient cope, especially where mobility is impaired, which will also facilitate close monitoring of urine output. As with any acutely unwell patient, risk assessments for venous thromboembolism (VTE), pressure ulcers and malnutrition should be conducted at the earliest opportunity.

Older adults with heart failure may be very frail and suffer from a wide range of comorbidities, such as diabetes, CKD or cognitive impairment, which will necessitate individualised nursing care and involvement of the heart failure team. The existence of multiple comorbidities and frailty increases the likelihood of hospital admission, length of stay and risk of mortality. Acute heart failure may cause sudden onset of acute delirium, requiring assessment of cognitive function using the Mini-Mental State Examination. Patients may therefore require considerable nursing care and the involvement of the multidisciplinary team to ensure their individual needs are fully addressed.

Treatments for Patients With Acute Heart Failure

Oxygen therapy should be titrated to achieve a target saturation of 94%–98% (O'Driscoll et al. 2017), and using a reservoir mask, a Venturi face mask or nasal cannulae is recommended for patients with acute heart failure. If the patient is at risk of hypercapnic respiratory failure, the target should be lowered to 88%–92%. Patients may require oxygen delivery via CPAP, noninvasive positive pressure ventilation and in some cases invasive ventilatory support (NiPPV) (McDonagh et al. 2021). CPAP may be beneficial in patients with a satisfactory SBP who are not responding sufficiently well to diuretic therapy, or at the onset of cardiogenic shock. Invasive ventilation may be necessary for patients in acute respiratory failure or who are showing signs of exhaustion or a reduction in level of consciousness.

For patients with acute pulmonary oedema, NICE (2021b) and the European Society of Cardiology (McDonagh et al. 2021) recommend the IV loop diuretic furosemide as first-line therapy, administered as a bolus or infusion dependent upon the dose, the patient's symptoms and the level of haemodynamic compromise. An IV vasodilator, e.g. GTN, may be suitable for patients with myocardial ischaemia if their SBP is above 90 mmHg. Acute pulmonary oedema can cause the patient significant distress, which may be relieved through administration of opiates such as morphine.

If the patient's SBP falls below 90 mmHg, the patient may develop cardiogenic shock, a syndrome caused by low cardiac output causing significant reduction in perfusion to vital organs that can lead to multiorgan failure. IV therapies may be used such as inotropes, e.g. dobutamine, which will increase the force of myocardial contraction to improve cardiac output, and vasopressors such as noradrenaline, which can raise blood pressure and improve organ perfusion. Mechanical circulatory support may also be necessary. Treatment of any reversible cause of heart failure such as ACS or an arrhythmia that accompanies acute heart failure, often atrial fibrillation or flutter, will be necessary. Some patients with severe heart failure that is potentially reversible or for whom transplantation is a treatment option may be offered a left ventricular mechanical assist device to provide circulatory support (NICE 2021b).

Once the patient is haemodynamically stable, they should be offered the pharmacological and nonpharmacological measures outlined later for chronic heart failure to prevent further episodes of acute decompensation and to optimise quality of life.

Drug Therapies and Interventions for Patients Living With Heart Failure

Drug and device therapies for patients with chronic heart failure will not provide a cure but should help reduce symptoms and improve quality of life, slow disease progression, prevent episodes of acute decompensation and potentially fatal arrhythmias. The package of care is generally guided by the patient's left ventricular ejection fraction, measured using an echocardiogram and elevated natriuretic peptides. Until recently, almost all research evidence supported therapies for patients with HFrEF, but now more studies are exploring interventions for patients diagnosed with HFpEF.

NICE (2018) recommends offering patients with reduced ejection fraction (HFrEF) low-dose ACE inhibitors such as ramipril or beta-blockers, such as bisoprolol, as first-line drug therapies. An angiotensin II receptor antagonist (ARB), e.g. valsartan, may be more suitable for patients experiencing side-effects associated with ACE inhibitors, such as a persistent dry cough. Both drugs induce vasodilation and reduce salt retention in the kidneys, thereby increasing diuresis. An alternative option to these agents for specific patients is sacubitril/valsartan, which combines the ARB with sacubitril, an angiotensin receptor neprilysin inhibitor which inhibits the breakdown of natriuretic peptides responsible for diuresis. Diuretics such as bumetanide can help relieve symptoms of fluid retention and congestion associated with pulmonary oedema. These may also be offered to patients with HFpEF as well. Novel drug therapies have emerged that have demonstrated huge benefits in terms of limiting the progression of the disease. Dapagliflozin is one example of the sodium–glucose cotransporter 2 (SGLT2) inhibitor drugs that have been found to reduce the risk of worsening heart failure for patients with HFrEF (McMurray et al. 2019). SGLT2 inhibitors are already widely offered to patients with diabetes because they block reabsorption of glucose in the kidneys, reducing blood sugar. Excretion of water accompanies the increased excretion of glucose which can aid fluid balance, and therefore, several drugs from this class are now recommended for patients with HFrEF with and without diabetes (NICE 2021c). Establishing and addressing the cause of heart failure in each patient are essential aspects of care. Surgical and pharmacological interventions for CHD, hypertension, tachyarrhythmias and valvular heart disease should be considered alongside the therapies for heart failure. Atrial fibrillation or flutter may occur as a result of heart failure and should be treated with amiodarone or digoxin as recommended, and anticoagulation to prevent thromboembolism (NICE 2021a). CRT, using a biventricular pacemaker, may be suitable for some patients to augment and optimise cardiac output, often providing considerable symptomatic relief. ICD devices or CRT with defibrillator capabilities (CRT-D) may be offered for patients considered to be at high risk of cardiac arrest, which may be in the early or late stages of heart failure. Cardiac transplantation may be considered for patients with end-stage heart failure.

Cardiac rehabilitation classes are recommended to provide the opportunity to exercise in a supervised environment, as well as psychological support, dietary advice and information to support lifestyle modification to limit disease progression (NICE 2021b). Exercise training can improve exercise tolerance and reduce symptoms of breathless on exertion, which in turn can improve quality of life. Cardiac rehabilitation has been shown to reduce the frequency of hospitalisations due to heart failure (Bozkurt et al. 2021). Education should offer specific guidance to enable patients to self-care by recognising their symptoms, taking treatments appropriately and adjusting their lifestyle.

❖ Nursing Management and Health Promotion: Chronic Heart Failure

Receiving a diagnosis of heart failure may be distressing for many patients, their relatives and caregivers, with term itself inferring

death may be imminent. Therefore, considerable care must be taken in delivering information and providing support, especially with newly diagnosed patients. Understanding heart failure is relevant for nurses in all clinical settings, as it affects patients in the community, in mental health settings or in acute hospital settings, even if heart failure is not the cause of their admission. For example, a patient with known chronic heart failure admitted with sepsis will have specific care needs to prevent an acute decompensation of heart failure.

Patients diagnosed with heart failure in the UK are referred to specialist nurses or Heart Failure Multidisciplinary Teams for monitoring which can be done in person or remotely using advances in digital technology (NICE 2018). Heart failure nurse specialists based in primary and secondary care provide support for patients living with the condition through outpatient and home visits, delivering advanced clinical care including prescribing (Masters et al. 2019).

Patients are usually prescribed a large number of medications, and therefore, encouraging the patient to learn about their condition and the purpose of the treatments is important to encourage adherence, but patients should also be made aware of the possible side-effects, and who to contact for support, e.g. heart failure specialist nurses, general practitioner (GP) or pharmacist. The patient should be guided towards establishing the optimal timing of administration of each of the drug therapies, which can often be adjusted to suit their lifestyle or activities of daily living. This is especially important for drugs with diuretic effects (BSH 2022).

Patients may be advised to restrict their fluid intake to between 1.5 and 2 L/day to help manage their circulatory volume as their cardiac function declines. It is helpful to enable patients to understand the volume of the cups and glasses they use at home to help them effectively control their intake. However, they should also be advised of the need to increase their intake during hot or humid weather, or following diarrhoea or vomiting and to abstain from or restrict intake of alcohol. Dietary advice should also be provided to guide the patient towards reducing their salt intake to less than 6 g/day (McDonagh et al. 2021), to lose weight or maintain a healthy body weight and to avoid malnutrition. The advice recommended for patients to prevent CVD is also relevant for patients with heart failure including smoking cessation. Vaccinations to prevent influenza and pneumonia should also be offered to patients.

Much of this advice can be delivered during cardiac rehabilitation classes, which combine exercise with education and support. Regular exercise that causes mild breathlessness is encouraged where patients are able, and initiating this in a clinical setting can provide the patient, and their families, with support and encouragement. Patients can be offered advice regarding sexual activity, and options for addressing erectile dysfunction, which may be caused by the use of beta-blockers. Heart failure can cause anxiety and depression, for which the patient may require pharmacological treatments and/or talking therapies. Cardiac support groups may be available to patients in their local area and it is helpful to provide patients with this information, if possible.

Supporting the patient to understand their condition and the importance of adherence to self-monitoring and drug treatments is key to improving patient outcomes including quality of life. Simple techniques, such as daily weights using the same set of scales at the same time each day to identify fluid overload early, or remote monitoring using digital apps, can empower the patient to manage their own condition. With support from heart failure nurse specialists, patients can identify a deterioration in their condition early to enable up-titration of drug therapies that could prevent hospital admission for acute decompensation as well as identifying common complications associated with heart failure such as anaemia or depression (NICE 2018a). Many patients with heart failure experience depression and anxiety as a result of living with their condition, and therefore, early identification and interventions including psychological support are an important aspect of the nurses' role (Sharp and McCowat 2019). Patients waiting for cardiac transplantation will also need support from specialist teams; there is no guarantee a donor organ will become available while they remain well enough to undergo the surgery.

For patients who are not suitable for cardiac transplantation, palliative and end-of-life care will inevitably become necessary. Planning for this should be introduced at an appropriate point early in the anticipated trajectory of their condition and revisited frequently to ensure patients are offered the opportunity to be fully involved in decision-making for their care (Fig. 2.20). This may include withdrawal of specific drug therapies and device deactivation, and establishing their preferred location for their death, e.g. hospice or home. Heart failure nurse specialists are pivotal in this important aspect of patient care, coordinating healthcare professionals based in primary and secondary care including the cardiology team, the patient's GP, palliative care services and hospice (BSH 2021; McDonagh et al. 2021).

Aortic Aneurysms and Acute Aortic Syndromes

The aorta is the largest artery in the body, made from three distinct layers: tunica intima, media and adventitia. It begins at the aortic root at the site of the aortic valve annulus, where it ascends from the left ventricle (ascending aorta), then arches round (aortic arch) to form the descending thoracic aorta, which extends through the chest and into the abdomen. Conditions that can affect the aorta include aneurysms, which can occur anywhere from the aortic root through to the abdominal aorta, and acute aortic syndromes such as dissection and intramural haematoma.

An aneurysm is a localised dilatation of an artery that results in a permanent bulge along the vessel wall. Aortic aneurysms may affect the abdominal or thoracic portions of the aorta. Aneurysms often cause patients little or no symptoms but cause a life-threatening emergency if they rupture. Therefore, once they have been identified, patient care aims to reduce the risk of rupture through medical management or surgical repair.

A dissection occurs when a tear within the lumen of the aorta creates a false channel for blood to flow through within the arterial wall, which may lead to rupture. This is a life-threatening condition that requires urgent treatment to maintain the stability of the patient.

Thoracic Aortic Aneurysms and Rupture

Thoracic aortic aneurysms may affect the ascending, descending thoracic aorta or the aortic arch. Age-related degeneration, hypertension and specific connective tissue disorders, such as Marfan syndrome, can lead to degeneration of elastin fibres within the wall of the ascending aorta, weakening of all three layers of the wall, resulting in widening of the aortic lumen. Atherosclerosis is a common cause of aneurysms affecting the thoracic aorta. A significantly widened aorta is at high risk of dissection or rupture, and therefore once found, close monitoring with timely surgical intervention is required to prevent aortic dissection (Sharples et al. 2022).

Patient Assessment and Investigations

Patients with thoracic aortic aneurysms are often asymptomatic; often the finding is incidental on imaging, such as a chest X-ray, conducted for other reasons. Patients with connective tissue disorders such as Marfan syndrome, who have a mutation in the gene responsible for fibrillin production, are regularly screened for aortic dilatation as the risk of aortic dissection is high. Rapid enlargement of the diameter of the aorta may compress adjacent structures, causing symptoms such as chest pain, stridor, haemoptysis and hoarseness.

If a thoracic aortic aneurysm is suspected, a chest X-ray and echocardiogram can be used for initial diagnosis but a CT is needed to identify and evaluate the extent of the dilated aorta and may identify patients at risk of dissection (Chetter and Alexiou 2022).

The risk of rupture increases significantly once the width of the ascending aorta exceeds 6 cm, or 7 cm for the descending aorta (Erbel et al. 2014). Rupture of the aortic aneurysm may cause a slow trickle of blood loss, or be an abrupt gush and is therefore life-threatening. Most commonly, this causes the patient to develop sudden onset of severe chest pain, that radiates to the upper back. It will cause acute deterioration of the patient, who will rapidly develop signs of shock, including hypotension and tachycardia.

❖ Nursing Management and Health Promotion: Thoracic Aortic Aneurysms

For patients with a ruptured aortic aneurysm, the risk of death is extremely high and therefore this is a medical emergency. Rapid assessment, continuous monitoring and escalation of care are essential to maintaining the safety of the patient, as well as ensuring provision of reassurance and sufficient pain relief to address the distressing symptoms associated with the condition. The only curative treatment is surgical repair, but this must be delivered rapidly, and therefore, the patient and their families must be prepared and supported accordingly.

Patients diagnosed with a thoracic aortic aneurysm will require regular follow-up clinic appointments, that will include repeat imaging to enable the team to observe for any changes in the width of the lumen of the aorta. Dietary and lifestyle modification advice may be offered to the patient to address hypertension and atherosclerosis, and medical therapy may be needed to maintain a normal blood pressure to prevent worsening of the aneurysm.

Treatments for Patients With Thoracic Aortic Aneurysms

Close monitoring of the diameter of the aortic lumen is necessary for patients diagnosed with an aortic aneurysm. Hypertension will worsen the condition, and therefore medical therapy and lifestyle measures may be advised to maintain a normal blood pressure and therefore hopefully prevent worsening of the condition. The decision to use surgical intervention to treat an aortic aneurysm is guided by the diameter of the lumen; the wider the lumen becomes, the greater the chance of rupture. Rupture can be prevented either by surgical replacement of the affected portion of the aorta with a prosthetic graft or by using thoracic endovascular aortic repair (TEVAR) that uses a minimally invasive approach to deploy an intravascular stent (Erbel et al. 2014). The use of TEVAR is expanding and is particularly useful for patients unsuitable for cardiac surgery.

Aortic Dissection

An aortic dissection occurs when a tear in the intimal layer of the aorta creates a false channel within the tunica media, through which blood can flow, further worsening the tear. Aortic dissections are classified anatomically. The Stanford classification uses type A to describe an aortic dissection affecting the aortic root, ascending aorta and aortic arch which may extend down into the descending thoracic aorta. Type B dissection affects the descending thoracic aorta and may extend to affect the abdominal aorta (Erbel et al. 2014). Treatment is typically directed by the location of the tear; urgent surgical repair is recommended for patients with a type A dissection and medical therapy alone to control HR and blood pressure for patients with type B unless the patient has complications such as rupture, ischaemia or recurrent pain (Bossone et al. 2018).

Patient Assessment and Investigations

Sudden onset of severe pain, often described as 'tearing', is the characteristic symptom associated with aortic dissection. The pain may be located in the central chest, often associated with a type A aortic dissection, the most common form, or between the scapulae for a type B dissection. Rapid patient assessment is necessary, and should include a prioritised ABCDE approach as the patient is at high risk of shock and death. If the aortic arch is affected by the dissection, the patient may have a marked difference in blood pressure recordings between their right and left arms. Patients may show signs associated with aortic regurgitation, myocardial ischaemia, heart failure or neurological symptoms. NEWS2 scoring should be used to identify early deterioration of the patient and to guide escalation of care. A record of fluid balance should be maintained, as the patient may require a blood transfusion or IV fluids and the patient will require a urinary catheter. Blood tests should be taken and should include a cross-match prior to surgery. Continuous cardiac and haemodynamic monitoring is essential, and a 12-lead ECG should be recorded to rule out ACS, which is associated with a similar presentation. A chest X-ray may quickly reveal the widened mediastinum but a CT scan, transoesophageal echocardiogram (TOE) or cardiac MRI will be needed to confirm the diagnosis, and to guide treatment (Bossone et al. 2018).

❖ Nursing Management and Health Promotion: Aortic Dissection

Continuous cardiac and haemodynamic monitoring will be essential to maintain the safety of the patient. The patient's SBP will be closely monitored, either invasively with an arterial line or noninvasively. Treatments, such as IV GTN infusion or IV beta-blockers, may be necessary to control HR and maintain SBP between 100 and 120 mmHg to prevent worsening of the dissection. However, if the patient develops signs of shock, medical therapies such as IV fluids and inotropes may be required to treat hypotension. The patient's symptoms should be closely monitored and pain relief offered, and the effectiveness of it recorded using a pain chart. The patient is likely to be extremely anxious, and therefore, providing reassurance, information and advice for both the patient and their family/carers will be essential throughout the episode of care. Preparation for emergency surgical intervention may be necessary.

Treatments for Patients With Aortic Dissection

Urgent surgical repair is indicated for a type A aortic dissection as the condition is associated with a 50% mortality rate within the first 48 hours if untreated (Erbel et al. 2014). Surgical repair with a graft may be suitable for some patients. TEVAR is increasingly used to implant a stent covered with a membrane at the point of the origin of the tear (dissection) to block off the entrance to the false channel. Patients with a type B aortic dissection may be offered conservative management with close monitoring and medical therapy to prevent worsening of the tear. However, if the type B dissection is affecting perfusion of major arteries, emergency surgical repair or TEVAR will be necessary.

Abdominal Aortic Aneurysms and Rupture

Abdominal aortic aneurysms (AAAs) are large, irreversible dilatations of the aorta most commonly occurring below the origin of the renal arteries, known as infrarenal. They are usually identified when the diameter of the aorta is found to be greater than 3 cm (McMahon 2022). The highest incidence of AAAs in the UK is found among White-British men, and as this carries significant risk of rupture, men over the age of 66 years in England can refer themselves for a routine screening programme (NICE 2020b). Risk factors can include advancing age, prior CVD, smoking, dyslipidaemia (high LDL cholesterol and triglycerides), hypertension and high BMI (Hellawell et al. 2021). Weakening of the wall of the aorta can be caused by inflammatory conditions or connective tissue disorders which are associated with degradation of the collagen and elastin within the media and adventitia layers, reducing the strength of the arterial wall (McMahon 2022).

Patient Assessment and Investigations

AAAs are most often detected through routine screening using abdominal ultrasound or are an incidental finding appearing during investigations. Most AAAs do not cause the patient any symptoms at all, although the bulging vessel wall may affect other structures, such as the ureter, duodenum and vena cava, which can result in a range of symptoms. Exploration of key risk factors, such as smoking, hypertension and a family history of AAA, should be carried out. Abdominal examination may reveal a pulsatile mass, which can be visualised on an abdominal ultrasound and CT scans; auscultation of the abdominal aorta may reveal bruits associated with atherosclerotic disease (Hellawell et al. 2021). An MRI is recommended prior to surgical intervention (NICE 2020b).

Rupture of an abdominal aortic aneurysm will cause severe epigastric pain that radiates to the patient's back. AAA rupture will cause catastrophic internal bleeding, resulting in hypotension, tachycardia, low haemoglobin levels and, if urgent surgical repair is not available, the patient is unlikely to survive.

❖ Nursing Management and Health Promotion: Abdominal Aortic Aneurysms

A ruptured AAA is a life-threatening emergency for which only urgent surgical repair is curative. Therefore, patients must be rapidly assessed using the ABCDE approach. Close monitoring in a high-dependency environment is essential as the patient is at high risk of cardiac arrest. Cardiac monitoring should be commenced, and observations recorded every 5–15 minutes including airway assessment (including AVPU), respiratory rate, oxygen saturation levels, pulse and blood pressure. A 12-lead ECG should be taken and the CBG recorded. Establishing IV access is essential, ideally with a central venous catheter, to facilitate pressure monitoring and administration of fluids and blood products. An arterial line will enable close monitoring of mean arterial pressure (target 50–70 mmHg). The surgical team should be informed at the earliest opportunity.

Treatments for Patients With Abdominal Aortic Aneurysms

Patients diagnosed with ruptured aortic aneurysm may require tracheal intubation and ventilatory support. Fluid management to maintain the target mean arterial pressure should be administered with caution, as it may exacerbate bleeding. Endovascular aneurysm repair (EVAR), in which stent-grafts are advanced along the aorta via femoral or iliac artery access, is the recommended treatment for all patients with ruptured AAA, with open-surgical repair advised for patients where this is not a suitable approach (NICE 2020b). However, many patients will not survive long enough for the procedure to be undertaken.

The care of patients with asymptomatic AAA aims to prevent catastrophic rupture. Prevention of worsening dilation can be addressed through careful blood pressure control, smoking cessation and lipid-lowering medications. Regular monitoring of the aneurysm is necessary, as surgical repair with EVAR or Dacron graft implantation using an open surgical approach will be considered if the diameter of the aorta is growing rapidly by more than 1 cm in a year, or exceeds 5.5 cm or the patients becomes symptomatic (NICE 2020b).

PERIPHERAL VASCULAR DISEASE

Peripheral vascular disease includes pathological processes affecting both the arterial and venous circulations. Arterial and venous disease can occur alone or together and it is important to be able to differentiate between the two.

Peripheral Arterial Disease

Pathophysiology

Peripheral arterial disease (PAD) is most commonly caused by atherosclerosis, whereby plaques that have developed within the arterial system partially reduce or obstruct blood flow to the tissue beyond, resulting in ischaemia affecting the lower limbs. Risk factors for developing chronic lower limb ischaemia include smoking, diabetes, high BMI, high cholesterol, hypertension and sedentary lifestyle. Critical limb ischaemia can occur in patients with PAD and is associated with pain at rest, tissue loss or nonhealing wounds with increased risk of amputation in patients with diabetes (Criqui et al. 2021).

Patient Assessment

Signs of PAD include patients who have difficulty walking accompanied by unexplained leg pain or nonhealing wounds on the legs and feet, particularly in patients with diabetes. Intermittent claudication is a clinical term used to describe pain in the leg, most commonly in the calf, that occurs on exertion due to ischaemia. The pain is usually relieved by rest. Some patients with more severe disease develop pain at rest in their foot, often at night time, which may be relieved by standing on a cold floor or hanging the foot off the side of the bed. On examination the leg may appear cold with dry skin. Femoral, popliteal and foot pulses should be palpated, for which Doppler may be required (NICE 2018b). The presence of ulceration or tissue necrosis, known as gangrene, suggests severe disease.

Diagnostic Investigations

The severity of the disease should be assessed using the 'ankle brachial pressure index' (ABPI), which compares the pressure of blood flow within the lower limb with blood pressure within the brachial artery (Criqui et al. 2021).

Diagnostic imaging techniques, such as duplex ultrasound, contrast-enhanced magnetic resonance angiography and CT angiography can be used to directly view the extent of the disease prior to re-vascularisation.

❖ Nursing Management and Health Promotion: Peripheral Arterial Disease

Patients with PAD will require regular assessment of the affected limbs, as described earlier, to closely monitor progression of the condition. Written information that explains the causes of their symptoms, how to effectively manage their pain and to prevent disease progression should be provided. It is essential to remember that the presence of PAD indicates that the patient has atherosclerosis that is highly likely to also affect other organs, and therefore, the patient is at increased risk of acute cardiovascular event, such as MI or stroke. Addressing key modifiable risk factors, such as smoking, and supporting tight glycaemic control in patients with diabetes are essential aspects of care.

Treatments for Patients With Peripheral Arterial Disease

Patients with intermittent claudication should be offered a supervised exercise programme that encourages them to exercise to the point of maximal pain (NICE 2018b). Cardiovascular risk factors should also be addressed, as the patients are at high risk of a cardiovascular event.

Interventions for intermittent claudication include percutaneous transluminal angioplasty, with stent placement, which may be offered to patients for whom the exercise programme has not improved their calf pain. Bypass surgery using vein grafts may be considered for patients with severe symptoms to facilitate perfusion to the distal vessels. Pharmacological therapy may be suitable for patients for whom surgical intervention is not an option. Naftidrofuryl oxalate is recommended by NICE (2018b). It is a vasodilator agent, which can improve blood flow and reduce lactic acid accumulation due to ischaemia to reduce symptoms of pain and may improve the patient's walking distance. Patients with critical limb ischaemia should be referred to a specialist pain management service to address the severe pain associated with the condition. Limb amputation may be necessary for patients with critical limb ischaemia but should only be considered if all revascularisation options have been considered (NICE 2018b).

Acute Lower Limb Ischaemia

Acute lower limb ischaemia is a medical emergency as the patient is at high risk of limb loss and death. It may occur from an embolism lodging within an artery (NB this is different from *venous* thromboembolism) which may have occurred due to an arrhythmia, such as atrial fibrillation, or be dislodged from a thrombus formed on an aneurysm. Acute lower limb ischaemia can also occur as a result of an endovascular procedure in which an artery is cannulated, such as PCI, and therefore, regular observation of the lower limb is an essential part of postprocedure care.

Acute (sudden onset) lower limb ischaemia will cause the patient to have pain in their leg, associated with a white discolouration (pallor), abnormal sensation or paralysis. The leg will feel very cold with mottled or marbled skin. Rapid assessment of the leg and foot is essential and should include examination, pulse assessment (femoral, popliteal and foot), which may be diminished or absent, a duplex ultrasound and a CT angiogram. The patient's pain can be managed with paracetamol or opioids but they may require referral to a specialist pain team. Treatment must be instigated rapidly to limit the damage to the affected limb. Anticoagulation medications will be prescribed alongside treatments that will target the underlying cause of the embolism. Revascularisation may be achieved in a variety of ways, including angioplasty intraarterial thrombolysis, embolectomy or bypass grafting (Natarajan et al. 2020). Reperfusion of the limb may result in 'compartment syndrome', in which oedema accumulates, increasing pressure within the muscles causing pain, numbness and poor perfusion to the limb. Therefore, close monitoring is necessary postprocedure to ensure early recognition. Prompt decompression is necessary to avoid the development of ischaemia and rhabdomyolysis (Schinco and Hassid 2019).

Peripheral Venous Disease

Venous return from the lower limbs relies on muscular contraction and effective action of the valves. Venous insufficiency occurs due to persistent elevation of venous pressure in the lower limbs, caused by a deep vein thrombosis (DVT) or incompetency of the valves, resulting in leg pain, muscle fatigue, heaviness and cramps when standing for long periods. Chronic venous insufficiency may cause dry, scaly skin, dilation of superficial veins, ankle oedema and leg ulcers (Mills and Armstrong 2020).

Varicose Veins

Varicose veins are the painful manifestation of venous insufficiency and are strongly associated with prolonged periods of standing. They appear most commonly in the legs as permanently dilated veins of more than 3-mm diameter, measured on standing, that cause severe itching, dry skin and pain. Compression hosiery may provide symptomatic relief, although NICE currently advises that this should only be offered if surgical interventions, such as endothermal ablation or endovenous laser treatment, are unsuitable (NICE 2013).

Venous Thromboembolism (VTE)

VTE is the term used to describe a thrombus (blood clot) that has formed within a vein that may present as a DVT or pulmonary embolism (PE). When this occurs within the deep veins of the leg or pelvis, it is known as DVT. The thrombus, or a part of the thrombus, may dislodge and be carried in the venous circulation until it lodges within a smaller vessel, most commonly within the pulmonary arterial circulation resulting in a PE, which can be fatal.

❖ Nursing Management and Health Promotion: Prevention of VTE

All patients admitted to hospital should be assessed for their risk of developing VTE and bleeding as soon as possible after admission (NICE 2019) using a tool such as the Department of Health VTE Risk Assessment Tool (Department of Health 2018). This includes all patients with acute medical conditions, trauma, psychiatric conditions, elective or emergency surgery, pregnant women and women who have given birth or had a miscarriage. Reassessment should be part of patient review or if the patient's condition changes.

Encouraging mobilisation and ensuring adequate hydration are key to preventing VTE. However, patients admitted with a medical condition, undergoing major surgery or following trauma are at high risk of developing a VTE, and therefore, consideration for VTE prophylaxis (prevention) with antiembolism stockings and/or anticoagulation therapy must be prioritised on admission (NICE 2019). Drug therapy with low-molecular-weight heparin should be commenced for medical patients within 14 hours of admission (NICE 2019).

Antiembolism stockings provide mechanical prophylaxis but are not be suitable for patients with PAD, peripheral neuropathy, severely oedematous legs or skin damage. They should not be offered to patients admitted with acute stroke, for whom intermittent pneumatic compression may be more suitable, and are usually unnecessary for patients with ACS, as VTE prophylaxis is already addressed by the dual antiplatelet therapy and anticoagulation that is the mainstay of treatment. Accurate measurements should be taken to ensure the correct stocking size is selected for use. Remeasurement and refitting may be necessary for patients with oedema. Patients should be advised on how to use the stockings and, if discharged home with them, advised to wear them day and night, to remove them once daily for a short period for hygiene purposes and to inspect the integrity of the skin, particularly over the heels (NICE 2019).

Deep Vein Thrombosis (DVT)

The development of a DVT is characterised by unilateral calf swelling and pain on palpation, that may track along the path of the vein. Many are at increased risk of DVT due to active cancer, trauma, major surgery, pregnancy or oral contraceptive use, and following prolonged periods of immobilisation (Kakkos et al. 2021). Comparing calf circumference is an essential part of assessment, as frequently the circumference of the affected calf will be more than 3 cm larger than the unaffected calf. The Wells' clinical probability tool is a useful test to establish the likelihood of DVT; the presence of a DVT is likely if two or more specific criteria are found, such as active cancer, calf swelling, prominent superficial veins, pitting oedema, recent bed rest for more than 3 days or a recent anaesthetic. A score of 1 or lower suggests DVT is unlikely.

Current national guidance recommends that if the Wells score is higher than 2, an ultrasound of the proximal leg vein should be carried out within 4 hours, but if this is not possible, a D-dimer test should be conducted and anticoagulant therapy prescribed, with the test conducted within 24 hours (NICE 2019). In those patients with an 'unlikely' Wells score, a D-dimer blood test should be carried out, and if found to be positive, an ultrasound of the leg vein conducted as soon as possible.

Interim anticoagulation therapy, usually with low-molecular-weight heparin, should be administered to patients with suspected DVT. Waiting for results from blood tests and further investigations should not delay administration but it can be stopped once DVT has been excluded. If confirmed, treatment for DVT usually involves anticoagulation for approximately 3 months, usually with a direct oral anticoagulant (DOAC), such as rivaroxaban. Specific comorbidities, such as cancer and CKD, and contraindications such as increased bleeding risk established through risk scoring using HAS-BLED, should be considered before initiating long-term treatment, along with the patient's preference (NICE 2019). Rarely, thrombolysis may be offered to the patient, delivered directly to the thrombus via an IV catheter (Merli et al. 2018). It is usually safe for patients to mobilise after diagnosis, and patients are frequently not admitted to hospital for treatment.

Pulmonary Embolism (PE)

A DVT may embolise, in which a part of the thrombus breaks away and travels within the venous circulation until it lodges in a small vessel, most commonly in the pulmonary arterial vasculature causing a PE, or multiple emboli.

❖ Nursing Management and Health Promotion: Suspected Pulmonary Embolism

Patients with suspected PE may be acutely well, with shortness of breath, localised chest pain, a cough and acute anxiety associated with tachycardia and hypotension. Patients may present in cardiac arrest.

Rapid assessment using the ABCDE approach is essential. Physical examination, history taking, 12-lead ECG and a chest X-ray are required to rule out other conditions, and patients should have a point of care or laboratory D-dimer test. The clinical probability of a PE should be assessed using the two-level PE Wells score, in which the presence of specific criteria scoring a total of 4 or higher indicates high probability. The criteria include suspected presence of a DVT (3 points) and HR greater than 100 bpm (1 point), haemoptysis (1 point), prolonged immobilisation or recent surgery (1.5 points).

A computed tomographic pulmonary angiogram (CTPA) is indicated for patients with a high probability of PE (NICE 2020c). Patients unable to tolerate the contrast dye may be offered a V/Q scan.

The treatment of PE is dictated by the severity of the presentation. Patients who are haemodynamically stable may simply be offered anticoagulation therapy with low-molecular-weight heparin or a DOAC such as rivaroxaban, prescribed for 3 months.

Patients with acute PE require urgent treatment, as they are at high risk of cardiac arrest. High-flow oxygen therapy is indicated if the patient's peripheral oxygen saturations are less than 94% (or less than 88% in those with known hypercapnic respiratory failure) (O'Driscoll et al. 2017). Patients who are haemodynamically stable may simply be offered interim low-molecular-weight heparin followed by a 3-month course of anticoagulation therapy with a DOAC such as rivaroxaban. Where patients are haemodynamically stable, or presenting in shock, evidenced by tachycardia and an SBP of less than 90 mmHg, they will require IV fluids and IV inotropic support. Systemic thrombolysis to break down the clot is currently recommended for patients with severe haemodynamic compromise (NICE 2020c), but this carries a significant risk of major bleeding, such as gastrointestinal bleed or stroke. Some patients may be offered surgical removal of the thrombus (embolectomy) or catheter-directed therapy to break up the thrombus.

❖ Nursing Management and Health Promotion: Anticoagulation Therapy

Anticoagulation pharmacological therapy may be indicated for VTE prophylaxis or treatment for a range of conditions, including VTE, PE and following surgical valve replacement. Anticoagulation is associated with an increased risk of bleeding, and therefore, it may not be recommended for some patients, particularly those following surgery or trauma. DOACs, such as rivaroxaban and apixaban, are non-vitamin K antagonists that are now widely used to treat VTE and PE. They do not necessitate regular blood testing but may not be suitable for some patients. A HAS-BLED risk assessment score should be completed before commencing therapy, along with baseline blood tests including full blood count, urea and electrolytes, LFTs, prothrombin time and activated partial thromboplastin time (APTT) (NICE 2020a). Low-molecular-weight heparin is recommended.

Providing accurate patient information relating to anticoagulation is an essential aspect of care. It should address how to administer the medication, the potential side effects, the effect of food and other medications, what to do if the patient is planning a pregnancy or undertaking sporting activities and when to seek medical help. It is important to advise patients that heparins are an animal product, and DOACs contain lactose and therefore some patients may wish to use a synthetic alternative.

Summary: Key Nursing Issues

- CVD is an umbrella term used to describe a range of conditions affecting the heart and circulatory system, including MI, stroke, arrhythmias, heart failure and peripheral vascular disease. Mortality rates have fallen due to improved treatment for acute cardiovascular conditions, despite the increasingly aging population.
- Atherosclerosis is most often the cause of CHD, hypertension, peripheral vascular disease and cerebrovascular disease. It is characterised by the accumulation of cholesterol within the arterial wall lining, driven by an inflammatory response to damage. Cardiovascular risk factors are specific characteristics known to contribute to the development of atherosclerosis such as diabetes, smoking, ethnic origin and dyslipidaemia.
- CHD remains one of the leading causes of death in the UK. It often manifests as symptoms of myocardial ischaemia on exertion, such as breathlessness or angina, but it can also lead to ACSs, heart failure and arrhythmias.
- 'Acute coronary syndromes' (ACS) is the term used to describe STEMI, non-STEMI and unstable angina, which all require emergency management. Diagnosis is usually made from the patient's clinical history, 12-lead ECG recordings and measurement of cardiac biomarkers, such as troponin.

- In unstable angina, the coronary artery occlusion tends to be episodic and transient but if permanent muscle damage occurs, it will be identified as a non-STEMI. This is recognised as a rise in serum troponin levels. STEMI occurs due to rupture of an atherosclerotic plaque, resulting in total occlusion of a coronary artery and substantial myocardial damage.
- Expediting treatment for patients presenting with ACS is essential. Patients found to have STEMI require urgent PPCI and patients are often taken directly by ambulance to a Heart Attack Centre for this treatment.
- Around 920,000 people live with heart failure in the UK, with approximately 200,000 new cases diagnosed each year (BHF 2022), most often caused by an underlying cardiovascular condition such as ACS or hypertension. Heart failure is strongly associated with CKD, diabetes and stroke. Early detection, in combination with a range of therapies and interventions, can provide symptomatic relief and improve quality of life.
- Cardiogenic shock is a serious form of heart failure, precipitated by extensive left ventricular damage in which the cardiac output is not sufficient to maintain blood pressure and organ perfusion, that can lead to multiorgan failure.

- Monitoring of vital signs and the use of early warning strategies such as NEWS 2 are important in order to identify the deteriorating patient prior to cardiac arrest.
- All patients admitted to hospital should be assessed for their risk of development VTE as soon as possible after admission. Encouraging mobilisation and adequate hydration may reduce risk, but many patients require prophylactic interventions such as antiembolism stockings or anticoagulation therapy.

Reflection and Learning – What Next?

- **Test** your knowledge by visiting the website 🌐 and answering the multiple-choice questions and critical thinking questions.
- **Consolidate** your learning by looking at some of the further reading suggestions, references and specialist websites.
- **Revisit** some of the additional material on the website.
- **Consider** what you have learnt and how this will help your professional development.
- **Reflect** on how you can apply this knowledge to the care of patients.
- **Discuss** your learning with your practice assessor/supervisor, lecturer and colleagues.

References

Aaronson P, Ward J, Connolly M. *The Cardiovascular System at a Glance*. 5th ed. Chichester: Wiley-Blackwell; 2020.

Bae S, Kim SR, Kim M-N, Shim WJ, Park S-M. Impact of cardiovascular disease and risk factors on fatal outcomes in patients with COVID-19 according to age: a systematic review and meta-analysis. *Heart*. 2021;107(5):373–380.

Alun J, Murphy B. Loneliness, social isolation and cardiovascular risk. *Br J Car Nurs*. 2019;14(10):1–8.

Bossone E, LaBounty T, Eagle K. Acute aortic syndromes: diagnosis and management, an update. *Eur Heart J*. 2018;39(9):739–749.

Bozkurt B, Fonarow G, Goldberg L, et al. Cardiac rehabilitation for patients with heart failure: JACC Expert Panel. *J Am Coll Cardiol*. 2021;77(11):1454–1469.

British Association for Cardiovascular Prevention and Rehabilitation (BACPR). *The BACPR Standards and Core Components for Cardiovascular Disease Prevention and Rehabilitation*. 3rd ed.; 2023. https://www.bacpr.org/news/bacpr-standards-and-core-components-2023-edition.

British Heart Foundation (BHF). Heart and circulatory disease statistics 2022. https://www.bhf.org.uk/what-we-do/our-research/heart-statistics/heart-statistics-publications/cardiovascular-disease-statistics-2022.

British Society for Heart Failure (BSH). The BSH Heart Failure Care Pathway. 2022. http://bshpathway.org.uk/rationale_detection.html.

CHA2DS2-VASc score. MD+CALCCHA2DS2-VASc score. MD+CALC. https://www.mdcalc.com/calc/801/cha2ds2-vasc-score-atrial-fibrillation-stroke-risk.

Cheema KM, Dicks E, Pearson J, Samani NJ. Long-term trends in the epidemiology of cardiovascular diseases in the UK: insights from the British Heart Foundation statistical compendium. *Cardiovasc Res*. 2022;118(10):2267–2280.

Chetter I, Alexiou A. BMJ Best Practice: Aortic Dissection. 2022. Available at https://bestpractice.bmj.com/topics/en-gb/3000226.

Collet J-P, Thiele H, Barbato E, et al. ESC guidelines for the management of acute coronary syndromes in patients presenting without persistent ST-segment elevation: the Task Force for the Management of Acute Coronary Syndromes in Patients Presenting Without Persistent ST-Segment Elevation of the European Society of Cardiology. *Eur Heart J*. 2021;42(14):1289–1367. https://academic.oup.com/eurheartj/article/42/14/1289/5898842.

Cowie A, Buckley J, Doherty P, et al. Standards and core components for cardiovascular disease prevention and rehabilitation. *Heart*. 2019;105(7):510–515. https://heart.bmj.com/content/105/7/510.

Creed F, Spiers C. *Care of the Acutely Ill Adult: An Essential Guide for Nurses*. 2nd ed. Oxford: Oxford University Press; 2020.

Criqui M, Matsushita K, Aboyans V, et al. Lower extremity peripheral artery disease: contemporary epidemiology, management gaps and future directions: a scientific statement from the American Heart Association. *Circulation*. 2021;144(9):e171–e191.

Department of Health (DH). *UK Chief Medical Officers' Alcohol Guidelines Review*. Summary of the Proposed New Guidelines; 2016. https://assets.publishing.service.gov.uk/government/uploads/system/uploads/attachment_data/file/489795/summary.pdf.

Department of Health (DH). Venous Thromboembolism (VTE) Risk Assessment Tool. 2018. https://www.nice.org.uk/guidance/ng89/resources/department-of-health-vte-risk-assessment-tool-pdf-4787149213.

Department of Health and Social Care (DHSC). UK Chief Medical Officers' Physical Activity Guidelines. 2019. https://assets.publishing.service.gov.uk/government/uploads/system/uploads/attachment_data/file/832868/uk-chief-medical-officers-physical-activity-guidelines.pdf.

Erbel R, Aboyans V, Boileau C, et al. ESC guidelines on the diagnosis and treatment of aortic diseases. *Eur Heart J*. 2014;35:2873–2926.

European Society of Cardiology. European Systemic Coronary Risk Estimation (SCORE). n.d. https://www.escardio.org/Education/Practice-Tools/CVD-prevention-toolbox/SCORE-Risk-Charts.

Ferreira JP, Kraus S, Mitchell S, et al. World Heart Federation roadmap for heart failure. *Glob Heart*. 2019;14(3):197–214.

Glikson M, Nielson J, Kronberg M, et al. ESC guidelines on cardiac pacing and cardiac resynchronization therapy. *Eur Heart J*. 2021;42(35):3427–3520.

Goldberger AL, Goldberger ZD, Shvilkin A. *Goldberger's Clinical Electrocardiography: A Simplified Approach*. 9th ed. Philadelphia: Elsevier; 2018.

Goodlin SJ. Palliative care in congestive cardiac failure. *JACC Clin Electrophysiol*. 2009;54(5):386–396. https://www.sciencedirect.com/science/article/pii/S0735109709015228?via%3Dihub.

Hellawell H, Mostafa A, Kyriacou H, et al. Abdominal aortic aneurysms part one: epidemiology, presentation and preoperative considerations. *J Perioper Pract*. 2021;31(7-8):274–280.

Huff J. *ECG Workout*. 8th ed. Philadelphia: Wolters Kluwer; 2022.

Ibanez B, James S, Agewall S, et al. ESC guidelines for the management of acute myocardial infarction in patients presenting with ST-segment elevation. *Eur Heart J*. 2017;39(2):119–177.

Joint British Societies for the Prevention of Cardiovascular Disease (JBS3). Risk calculator. n.d. http://www.jbs3risk.com/pages/risk_calculator.htm.

Kakkos S, Gohel M, Baekgaard N, et al. European Society for Vascular Surgery (ESVS) clinical practice guidelines on the management of venous thrombosis. *Eur J Vasc Endovasc Surg*. 2021;61(1):9–82.

Klabunde R. *Cardiac Physiology Concepts*. 3rd ed. Philadelphia: Wolters Kluwer; 2021.

Lilly LS. *Pathophysiology of Heart Disease: an Introduction to Cardiovascular Medicine*. 7th ed. Philadelphia, PA: Wolters Kluwer; 2021.

Masters J, Barton C, Blue L, Welstand J. Increasing the heart failure nursing workforce: recommendations by the British Society for Heart Failure Nurse Forum. *Br J Card Nurs*. 2019;14(11):1–12.

McDonagh T, Metra M, Adamo M, et al. European Society of Cardiology guidelines for the diagnosis and treatment of acute and chronic heart failure. *Eur Heart J*. 2021;42(36):3559–3726.

McMahon G. Abdominal aortic aneurysm. 2022. https://bestpractice.bmj.com/topics/en-gb/145.

McMurray J, Solomon S, Inzucchi S, et al. Dapagliflozin in patients with heart failure and reduced ejection fraction. *N Engl J Med.* 2019;381(21):1995–2008.

Menzies-Gow E. How to record a 12-lead ECG. *Nurs Stand.* 2018;33(2):38–42. https://journals.rcni.com/nursing-standard/evidence-and-practice/how-to-record-a-12lead-electrocardiogram-ns.2018.e11066/print/abs.

Menzies-Gow E, Spiers C. *Rapid Cardiac Care.* Chichester: Wiley-Blackwell; 2018.

Merli G, Galanis T, Earso L, Ouma G. Deep vein thrombosis. *BMJ Best Practice.* 2018. https://bestpractice.bmj.com/topics/en-gb/70.

Mills J, Armstrong D. BMJ best practice: chronic venous insufficiency. 2020. https://bestpractice.bmj.com/topics/en-gb/507.

Natarajan B, Patel P, Mukherjee A. Acute lower limb ischaemia – etiology, pathology and management. *Int J Angiol.* 2020;29(3):168–174.

NCEPOD (National Confidential Enquiry into Patient Outcome and Death). Acute heart failure: failure to function. 2018. https://www.ncepod.org.uk/2018ahf.html.

Neumann F-J, Sousa-Uva M, Ahlsson A. ESC/EACTS guidelines on myocardial revascularization. *Eur Heart J.* 2018;40(2):87–165. https://academic.oup.com/eurheartj/article/40/2/87/5079120?login=false.

NHS (National Health Service). Long term plan. Cardiovascular disease. 2019. https://www.longtermplan.nhs.uk/online-version/chapter-3-further-progress-on-care-quality-and-outcomes/better-care-for-major-health-conditions/cardiovascular-disease/.

NHS (National Health Service). The Eatwell Guide. 2022. https://www.nhs.uk/live-well/eat-well/food-guidelines-and-food-labels/the-eatwell-guide/.

NICE (National Institute for Health and Care Excellence). Varicose veins: diagnosis and management. *Clinical guideline [CG168].* 2013. https://www.nice.org.uk/guidance/cg168.

NICE (National Institute for Health and Care Excellence). Obesity prevention. Clinical guideline [CG43]. 2015. https://www.nice.org.uk/guidance/cg43.

NICE (National Institute for Health and Care Excellence). Recent-onset chest pain of suspected cardiac origin: assessment and diagnosis. *Clinical guideline [CG95].* 2016. https://www.nice.org.uk/guidance/cg95.

NICE (National Institute for Health and Care Excellence). Cardiovascular disease: risk assessment and reduction, including lipid modification. *Clinical guideline [CG181].* 2016. https://www.nice.org.uk/guidance/cg181.

NICE (National Institute for Health and Care Excellence). Stable angina: management. *Clinical guideline [CG126].* 2016. https://www.nice.org.uk/guidance/cg126.

NICE (National Institute for Health and Clinical Excellence). Chronic heart failure in adults: diagnosis and management. *NICE guideline [NG106].* 2018. https://www.nice.org.uk/guidance/ng106.

NICE (National Institute for Health and Care Excellence). Peripheral arterial disease: diagnosis and management. *Clinical guideline [CG147].* 2018. https://www.nice.org.uk/guidance/cg147/chapter/Recommendations#imaging-for-revascularisation.

NICE (National Institute for Health and Care Excellence). Venous thromboembolism in over 16s: reducing the risk of hospital-acquired deep vein thrombosis or pulmonary embolism. *NICE guideline [NG89].* 2019. https://www.nice.org.uk/guidance/ng89/chapter/Recommendations#risk-assessment.

NICE (National Institute for Health and Clinical Excellence). Acute coronary syndromes. *NICE guideline [NG185].* 2020a. https://www.nice.org.uk/guidance/ng185.

NICE (National Institute for Health and Care Excellence). *Abdominal aortic aneurysm: diagnosis and management [NG156].* 2020b. https://www.nice.org.uk/guidance/NG156.

NICE (National Institute for Health and Care Excellence). Venous thromboembolic disease: diagnosis, management and thrombophilia. *Clinical guideline [NG158].* 2020c. https://www.nice.org.uk/guidance/ng158.

NICE (National Institute for Health and Care Excellence). Atrial fibrillation: management. *Clinical guideline [NG196].* 2021. https://www.nice.org.uk/guidance/ng196.

NICE (National Institute for Health and Care Excellence). Acute heart failure: diagnosis and management. *Clinical guideline [CG187].* 2021. https://www.nice.org.uk/guidance/cg187.

NICE (National Institute for Health and Care Excellence). Dapagliflozin for chronic heart failure with reduced ejection fraction. *Technology appraisal [TA679].* 2021. https://www.nice.org.uk/guidance/ta679.

NICE (National Institute for Health and Care Excellence). Hypertension in adults: diagnosis and management. *Clinical guideline [CG127].* 2022. https://www.nice.org.uk/guidance/ng136/chapter/Recommendations#measuring-blood-pressurehttps://www.nice.org.uk/guidance/ng136/chapter/Recommendations#measuring-blood-pressure.

NICE (National Institute for Health and Care Excellence). Tobacco: preventing uptake, promoting quitting and treating dependence. *NICE guideline [NG209].* 2022. https://www.nice.org.uk/guidance/ng209.

NICOR (National Institute for Cardiovascular Outcomes Research). Heart failure (heart failure audit). 2021 https://www.nicor.org.uk/heart-failure-heart-failure-audit/.

O'Driscoll B, Howard L, Earis J, Mak V. British Thoracic Society Guideline for oxygen use in adults in healthcare and emergency settings. *BMJ Open Respir Res.* 2017;4(1):1–20.

Olson K. *Oxford Handbook of Cardiac Nursing.* 3rd ed. Oxford: Oxford University Press; 2021.

ORBIT Score. MD+CALC. Available at https://www.mdcalc.com/calc/10227/orbit-bleeding-risk-score-atrial-fibrillation.

Public Health England. Eatwell Guide. 2016. ttps://assets.publishing.service.gov.uk/government/uploads/system/uploads/attachment_data/file/528193/Eatwell_guide_colour.pdf.

QRISK. QRISK3-2018 risk calculator. 2018. https://qrisk.org/.

Resuscitation Council UK. Adult Advanced Life Support. 2021. https://www.resus.org.uk/library/2021-resuscitation-guidelines .

Richley D. ECG recording in primary care: the challenges getting it right. *Pract Nurs.* 2016;27(2):60–64.

Rowlands A, Sargent A. *The ECG Workbook.* 4th ed. Keswick: M&K Publishing; 2019.

Sampson M. Continuous ECG monitoring in hospital: part 1: indications. *Br J Card Nurs.* 2018;13(2):80–85.

Schinco M, Hassid V. BMJ best practice: compartment syndrome of extremities. 2019. https://bestpractice.bmj.com/topics/en-gb/502.

Stepinska J, Lettino M, Ahrens, et al. Diagnosis and risk stratification of chest pain in the emergency department: focus on acute coronary syndromes. A position paper of the Acute Cardiovascular Care Association. *Eur Heart j.* 2020;9(1):76–89.

Sharples L, Sastry P, Freeman, C. et al. Aneurysm growth, survival and quality life in untreated thoracic aortic aneurysms: the effective treatments for thoracic aneurysms study. *Eur Heart j.* 2022;43(25):2356–69.

Sharp J, McCowat M. Depression in heart failure. *Br J Card Nurs.* 2019;14(6):1–11.

Thygesen K, Alpert JS, Jaffe AS, et al. Fourth universal definition of myocardial infarction. *Eur Heart J.* 2018;40(3):237–269. https://www.escardio.org/Guidelines/Clinical-Practice-Guidelines/Fourth-Universal-Definition-of-Myocardial-Infarction.

Tillin T, Hughes A, Whincup P, et al. Ethnicity and prediction of cardiovascular disease: performance of QRISK2 and Framingham scores in a UK tri-ethnic prospective cohort study (SABRE – Southall and Brent Revisited). *Heart.* 2013;100(1):60–67.

Further Reading

Huff J. *ECG Workout.* 8th ed. London: Lippincott, Williams and Wilkins; 2021.

Kandan S, Johns W. Management of percutaneous coronary intervention complications. *Heart.* 2019;105:75–86.

Lilly L, ed. *Pathophysiology of Heart Disease: an Introduction for Cardiovascular Medicine.* 7th ed. London: Wolters Kluwer; 2021.

Macdonald N, Jones J, Leslie SJ. Acute coronary syndromes – the role of the CCU nurse. Part I: initial management. *Br J Card Nurs*. 2016;11(9):453–458.

Macdonald N, Jones J, Leslie SJ. Acute coronary syndromes – the role of the CCU nurse. Part II: a look at inpatient recovery and discharge. *Br J Card Nurs*. 2016;11(11):544–547.

Olson K. *Oxford Handbook of Cardiac Nursing*. 3rd ed. Oxford: Oxford University Press.

Reed G, Rossi J, Cannon C. Acute myocardial infarction. *Lancet*. 2018;389(10065):197–210.

Useful Websites

Arrhythmia Alliance: http://www.heartrhythmalliance.org/aa/uk

British Association for Cardiovascular Prevention and Rehabilitation: https://www.bacpr.org/

British Heart Foundation: www.bhf.org.uk

British Society for Heart Failure: https://www.bsh.org.uk/

Cardiac Risk in the Young: www.c-r-y.org.uk

European Society of Cardiology: https://www.escardio.org/

Life in the Fast Lane: https://lifeinthefastlane.com/

3

Nursing Patients With Respiratory Disorders

ANTHONY WHEELDON

CHAPTER OUTLINE

Introduction

The primary function of the respiratory system is to extract oxygen from the atmosphere and deliver it to cells. It is, therefore, one of the most important systems in the human body. In health, it functions automatically and usually without our awareness. However, there are several diseases, both acute and chronic, which have a disruptive effect on the respiratory system. The most common causes of respiratory disease are related to smoking, infection, allergens, genetics and poverty. In the UK, one in five people live with a respiratory condition, 10,000 people receive a new respiratory diagnosis every week, and someone dies from respiratory disease every 5 minutes. In the UK, respiratory disease accounts for 6 million bed days each year (British Lung Foundation 2023). The impact on the individual is more difficult to measure, although it has been recognised that disability is a frequent consequence of respiratory impairment and people living in poverty are at the greatest risk of developing long-term respiratory disease (Young et al. 2019).

Respiratory nursing encompasses roles within primary, community and acute care. Nurses are developing new independent and interdependent roles to meet the demands of new approaches to healthcare delivery. Increasingly, they are being employed in community and specialist clinics to screen, advise, immunise and treat patients and to promote disease prevention and health education. At the same time, technological and medical advances are demanding a higher level of clinical nursing skills.

This chapter will review the anatomy and physiology of the respiratory system and address two of the major principles of nursing management of respiratory disorders: disease prevention and health promotion. It will explore the nursing care and assessment skills required when caring for patients with respiratory disorders and the psychological and social impact of chronic respiratory illness upon the individual, their family and friends. It will also identify and evaluate strategies to promote respiratory treatment concordance and explore the function of specialist nurses and the interprofessional team in providing holistic respiratory care. Although the emphasis is on nursing management, the implicit assumption is always that nurses work in close collaboration with other healthcare professionals and, in many instances, will be responsible for coordinating the work of the whole team.

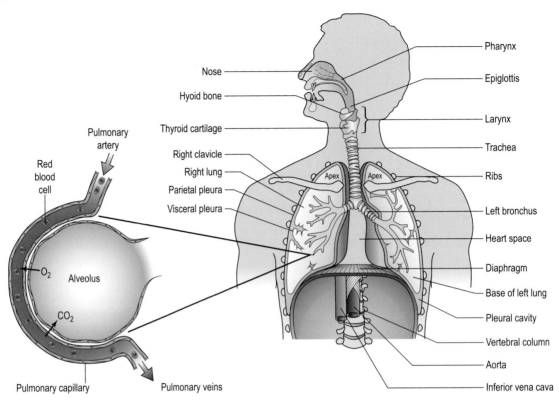

Figure 3.1 Respiratory system. (Reproduced from Esmond G. Respiratory Nursing. Edinburgh: Baillière Tindall; 2001, with permission.)

Anatomy and Physiology: Overview

This section is intended as an overview of the most relevant points relating to normal respiratory function. For a more detailed discussion please consult a textbook such as Peate I, Evans S. *Fundamentals of Anatomy and Physiology: For Nursing and Healthcare Students.* 2020.

The respiratory system comprises the upper and lower airways and the thoracic cage (Fig. 3.1).

The upper airway includes the nose, mouth, nasopharynx, oropharynx, laryngopharynx and larynx and has a protective role. The nasopharynx filters, warms and moistens the air before it enters the lungs, protecting the lung from exposure to microorganisms, toxic gases and particulates larger than 10 μm (microns) in diameter. Any particles that are deposited in the airways are propelled upwards towards the oropharynx by the mucociliary system. The mucus traps the particles and the cilia (microscopic hair-like projections) sweep the mucus upwards so that it can be expectorated. Ciliary movement can be impaired by tobacco smoke, pollution and excessive mucus production. The larynx protects the lower airways by closing during swallowing to prevent food entering the lower airways. It is also responsible for initiating the cough reflex, as it is sensitive to particles that cause irritation.

The lower airways include the trachea, bronchi, lungs, bronchioles, which are conducting air passages, and the alveoli, which are small grape-like sacs that extend from alveolar ducts, responsible for the passage of gases between the lungs and bloodstream. These structures work in combination with the thoracic cage, which includes the ribs, sternum and vertebrae, in promoting the exchange of oxygen and carbon dioxide in the lungs.

Control of Breathing

The rate and depth of breathing, which is mostly involuntary, are controlled by complex interactions between many physiological processes to allow an adequate exchange of oxygen and carbon dioxide.

Respiratory Centre

The medullary respiratory centre, situated in the medulla oblongata in the brain stem, primarily controls breathing through stimulating the contraction of the diaphragm and the external intercostal muscles, which expand and contract the thoracic cavity. During inspiration the diaphragm contracts and flattens, causing the thoracic cavity to lengthen, whilst the external intercostal muscles contract to expand the chest. This creates a negative intrapulmonary pressure. During expiration the diaphragm rises, and the intercostal muscles relax, resulting in a positive intrapulmonary pressure. Air pressure differences allow the movement of air in and out of the lungs. All gases move from an area of greater pressure to one of lesser pressure. During inspiration, air is drawn into the lungs. It flows through the bronchi and then into the bronchioles, alveolar ducts and alveolar sacs until it reaches the alveolar capillary membrane. The lungs can expand and move easily because the visceral pleura that lines the lungs and the parietal pleura that lines the mediastinum and chest wall create a potential space, known as the pleural cavity. It contains a small amount of lubricating fluid that allows easy movement between the pleura when the lungs expand.

Pulmonary Stretch Receptors

Pulmonary stretch receptors are in the smooth muscle of the bronchi and bronchioles and respond to inspiration by sending impulses through the vagus nerve to the medullary respiratory centre when the lungs are filled with air, inhibiting further inflation of the lungs. This is known as the Hering–Breuer reflex and prevents overinflation of the lungs.

Chemoreceptors

Peripheral chemoreceptors located in the aorta at the aortic arch (aortic body) and at the carotid bifurcation (carotid body) send impulses by sensory nerves to the medullary respiratory centre in response to a decrease in oxygen and pH, and an increase in carbon dioxide in the blood. The chemoreceptors in the carotid bodies are the main oxygen sensors and are stimulated to increase the breathing rate when there is a significant decrease in oxygen levels, i.e. below 90% or 8 kPa.

The normal stimulus to breathe is the rising level of carbon dioxide that easily crosses the blood–brain barrier into cerebrospinal fluid where it hydrates to form carbonic acid and then dissociates into bicarbonate and hydrogen ions. The hydrogen ions stimulate the central chemoreceptors in the medulla oblongata to send impulses to the medullary respiratory centre to increase the respiratory rate, thereby eliminating excess carbon dioxide.

Gas Transport

The main function of the respiratory system is the transfer of gases, principally oxygen and carbon dioxide. Gas transfer occurs by diffusion and includes the movement of oxygen from the alveolar capillary membrane to the mitochondria within the cells, and the movement of carbon dioxide from tissue capillaries to the alveolar capillary membrane. There are millions of alveoli, each surrounded by pulmonary capillaries and lined by a single layer of epithelium. This allows maximal gas exchange because the barrier between the gas in the alveoli and the blood in the capillaries is very thin (0.5 µm thick).

Oxygen Transport

During inspiration, air containing 21% oxygen is taken into the lungs and passes down the trachea and bronchi and into the alveoli, where it meets pulmonary circulation. Once the oxygen diffuses across the alveolar capillary membrane, it is carried in arterial blood to the heart and pumped around the body in two ways. Approximately 3% dissolves in the plasma, with the remaining 97% being carried in erythrocytes, bound to haemoglobin. Each haemoglobin molecule can reversibly bind (i.e. can give up again) four molecules of oxygen to form oxyhaemoglobin. The maximum amount of oxygen that can chemically combine with haemoglobin is called the oxygen capacity. The oxygen capacity, plus the oxygen carried as dissolved oxygen, is termed the oxygen content (CaO_2).

Carbon Dioxide Transport

Carbon dioxide, the waste product of metabolism, is transported in the blood in three forms: dissolved carbon dioxide, bicarbonate ions and carbamino compounds (carbaminohaemoglobin). The carbon dioxide diffuses from the blood capillaries across the alveolar capillary membrane to the alveoli to be exhaled. Because of the properties of haemoglobin, the unloading of oxygen and the loading of carbon dioxide are reciprocal events. When the carbon dioxide levels rise the affinity of haemoglobin for oxygen decreases.

Ventilation and Perfusion

Adequate alveolar ventilation and perfusion are required for normal gas exchange. Alveolar ventilation ($\dot{V}$) is the volume of gas that reaches the alveoli per minute and is approximately 4 L/min.

The perfusion (Q) is the amount of blood that flows through the pulmonary capillaries per minute and is approximately 5 L/min. The normal ratio is minus which is 0.8, although this will change in various parts of the lung due to gravitational forces. In healthy individuals, these gravitational differences do not affect adequate gaseous exchange; however, in lung disease, the mismatch is wider and is the most common cause of low oxygen levels in arterial blood (hypoxaemia). With effective ventilation and perfusion, oxygen can diffuse from the alveoli into the blood to achieve a partial pressure (PaO_2) of between 10 and 13 kPa.

Acid–Base Balance

The respiratory system also has an important role in maintaining acid–base balance. The regulation of acid–base balance is expressed as pH, which measures acidity and alkalinity, or hydrogen ion (H^+) concentration in the body. The normal pH of arterial blood is 7.35–7.45. A fall in pH (<7.35) indicates an increase in hydrogen ions, causing an acidosis. In respiratory disease this is due to raised carbon dioxide levels, caused by alveolar hypoventilation. This situation can be corrected through increasing ventilation, but if the respiratory acidosis continues, the action of buffers and the renal system will be activated to maintain homeostasis. Buffers (bicarbonate, proteins and phosphate) combine with the acid to prevent excessive changes in hydrogen ion concentration. The kidneys contribute to the regulation of acid–base balance by increasing or decreasing the bicarbonate concentration. This is the most efficient mechanism; however, it takes several hours or even days for the renal system to change the plasma bicarbonate level.

Pulmonary Function

Lung Volume Capacity and Compliance

The volume of air breathed in and out and the number of breaths per minute vary from one individual to another according to age, size and activity. Normal, quiet breathing gives about 15 complete cycles per minute in the adult. Lung volume can be assessed in the following terms (Fig. 3.2):

- Tidal volume (TV) – this is the amount of air that passes in and out of the lungs during each cycle of quiet breathing (approximately 500 mL in the adult). Exchange of gases takes place only in the alveolar ducts and sacs. The rest of the air passages are known as 'dead space' and contain about 150 mL of air.
- Inspiratory capacity – this is the amount of air that can be inspired with maximum effort. This consists of TV plus the inspiratory reserve volume (IRV).

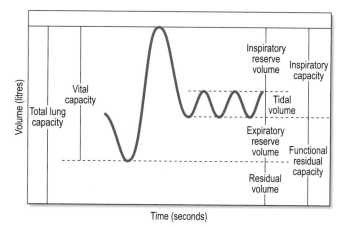

Figure 3.2 Lung volumes and capacity. (Reproduced from Esmond G. Respiratory Nursing. Edinburgh: Baillière Tindall; 2001, with permission.)

- Functional residual capacity (FRC) – this is the amount of air remaining in the air passages and alveoli at the end of quiet respiration; it is composed of expiratory reserve volume (ERV) and residual volume (RV). The RV prevents collapse of the alveoli and makes continuous gaseous exchange possible as the alveolar gas mix remains constant.
- Vital capacity (VC) – this is the TV plus the IRV and ERV.
- Total lung capacity (TLC) – with maximum effort, the adult lungs can hold 4–6 L of air. Most of this can be forcibly expelled, leaving an RV of about 1 L.

Lung Expansion and Recoil

Elastic fibres in lung tissue and the surface tension of the fluid lining the alveoli give the lungs their natural recoil tendency. Ease of expansion and recoil depends on normal compliance and elasticity and on the presence of surfactant in the fluid lining the alveoli. Compliance can be reduced by the stiffening of normally soft alveolar tissue due to pulmonary oedema or to the ageing process. Conversely, compliance can be increased by extreme softening due to loss of lung tissue, as in emphysema.

Principles of Nursing Management in the Prevention and Treatment of Respiratory Disorders

There are two main nursing priorities:
- health promotion and disease prevention.
- developing clinical skills to ensure competent care.

Health Promotion and Disease Prevention

Promoting health and preventing disease are vital to the social and economic well-being of our society, and their importance is reflected in government legislation and the development of large-scale screening and health education programmes (Public Health England 2019). With the cost of healthcare soaring, it makes good sense to prevent disease where possible rather than just treating the consequences.

Tobacco smoke, which contains nicotine, tar, carbon monoxide and 4000 chemicals, is currently the leading cause of respiratory ill-health and premature death. In susceptible individuals smoking may affect the respiratory system and cause:
- Recurrent infections in the airways.
- Damage and loss of efficiency in the lungs.
- Lung cancer.
- Chronic bronchitis and emphysema.

Smoking accelerates the normal decline in lung function due to the ageing process from about 30 mL per year to 45 mL per year (Fig. 3.3). The consequence of this increased loss of lung function is that functional impairment occurs leading to fatigue and breathlessness which impacts on the individual's ability to perform normal activities of living (ALs). Furthermore, smoking in pregnancy leads to an increased risk of spontaneous abortion, premature birth, smaller babies and sudden infant death syndrome. Children who are subject to passive smoking from parental smoking are more likely to experience acute respiratory illness, chronic middle ear infection, asthma, chronic cough and wheezy chest.

Nurses are well placed in their many roles in the hospital and community to have an active and expanding role in primary health prevention through health promotion activities in relation to tobacco control (Mendes 2022).

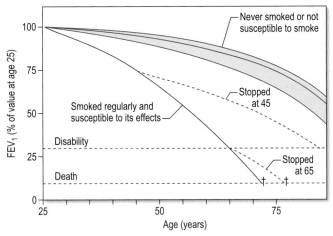

Figure 3.3 The effects of smoking on the decline in lung function. (Reproduced from Fletcher CM, Peto R. The natural history of chronic airflow obstruction. BMJ. 1977;1:1645-1648, with permission.)

Smoking Cessation

In 2021, around 12.7% of the UK population smoked cigarettes, around 55% of whom expressed a wish to quit (Office for National Statistics 2022). Of this 55%, less than half stated they intend to stop in the next 3 months. Stopping smoking requires motivation, effort, commitment and stamina to be successful therefore it must be the right time for the smoker to try. Helping people to stop smoking is a challenge faced by many nurses as it requires facilitating change and supporting patients through the process rather than actively providing care. Behaviour change required for smoking cessation is complex, with nicotine addiction as well as many other factors including social and psychological influences playing their part. Evidence-based smoking cessation guidelines have been developed to assist healthcare professionals to develop smoking cessation strategies that fit in with the overall tobacco control (National Institute for Health and Care Excellence [NICE] 2021).

Nurses are in an ideal position to encourage and enable smokers to quit the habit through applying the 5 As for anybody who smokes:
- Ask about smoking.
- Assess the smoker's motivation to stop smoking.
- Advise all smokers to stop smoking.
- Assist motivated smokers in stopping smoking.
- Arrange follow-up.

This approach is supported by NICE (2021), and it will ensure that patients are referred to smoking cessation services, often run by practice nurses or specially trained smoking cessation advisors. There are two main strategies used in smoking cessation: pharmacological interventions and lifestyle behavioural change.

Pharmacological Interventions. The use of pharmacological agents alongside behavioural interventions increases the likelihood of successful smoking cessation (NICE 2022) and, provided they are used in sufficient quantity and for a long enough period, to reduce the withdrawal symptoms as outlined in Table 3.1.

Currently, there are two pharmacological preparations that can be used for smokers who have been assessed as being ready to quit:
- Nicotine replacement therapy.
- Bupropion.

Pharmacological interventions should be used as part of a programme that includes advice and support from a healthcare professional which will assist with lifestyle behavioural changes.

TABLE 3.1	Withdrawal Symptoms After Smoking Cessation	
Symptoms	Duration	Prevalence
Irritability/aggression (nicotine withdrawal)	−4 weeks	50%
Depression	−4 weeks	60%
Restlessness	−4 weeks	60%
Poor concentration	−2 weeks	60%
Cough (clearing lungs out)	−2 weeks	60%
Increased appetite (food taste better)	+10 weeks	70%
Lightheadedness (more oxygen to brain)	−48 hours	10%
Night-time awakenings	−1 week	25%
Urges to smoke	+2 weeks	70%
Anxiety	−1 week	50%

− = in the first number of hours/weeks; + = after the number of weeks.

TABLE 3.2	Effects of Smoking Cessation
The effects of giving up smoking begin as soon as the cigarette is stubbed out	
Short-Term (7–14 days)	
Nicotine levels in the blood begin to fall	
20 minutes	Stimulation of adrenaline and noradrenaline ceases and blood pressure and heart rate return to normal.
2 hours	Nicotine levels continue to fall in the blood.
8 hours	Carbon monoxide and nicotine levels in the blood are reduced by half. Oxygen levels return to normal.
24 hours	Carbon monoxide levels will be eliminated from the body A CO reading will be at normal levels.
3–4 days	Smooth muscle in the bronchioles begins to relax. Breathing improves. Energy levels increase.
5–14 days	Mucus glands are no longer being overstimulated. Mucus clearance begins.
Medium Term (2–12 weeks)	
Circulation, sense of smell and taste improves.	
3–9 months	Respiratory symptoms improve.
	Nasal congestion, cough and sputum production reduces.
12 months	Risk of small cell lung cancer is halved.

Lung function cannot be reversed after years of damage; however, stopping smoking means that the rate of decline reverts to the age decline of a nonsmoker (30 mL per year) and prevents further damage. The reduction in mucus production helps to reduce exacerbations

Further reading (British National Formulary, NICE smoking cessation guidance) is recommended for familiarisation with medication doses, side-effects and the advantages and disadvantages of each of the products.

Lifestyle Behavioural Change. Smoking is a complex habit, and dealing with the nicotine withdrawal alone may not be sufficient to quit smoking. Emphasis needs to be placed on the psychological and social aspects of the habit as well as the management of the nicotine withdrawal symptoms if smoking cessation is to be achieved (Table 3.2). Techniques to change smoking habits include talking therapies and have been shown to increase the likelihood of smoking cessation for periods of 6 months when compared to quitting with no behavioural support. Counselling is also considered the most effective method, but support via text and offering money for successful cessation have also been shown to be effective (Hartmann-Boyce et al. 2021).

Respiratory Assessment and Investigations

While causative factors, organisms and irritants differ, the clinical manifestations can appear similar, therefore an important aspect to respiratory care is assessment and specialised investigations to enable a differential diagnosis to be made and the severity of symptoms identified.

Nursing Assessment of Respiratory Status

The assessment of respiratory status is important in determining the severity of the respiratory problem to prioritise care. During the acute phase of respiratory illness (i.e. acute asthma 'attack' or acute infective exacerbation of chronic obstructive pulmonary disease (COPD)), the emphasis is placed on physiological assessment to detect life-threatening situations that require immediate treatment. However, the impact of the respiratory problem on ALs, because of breathlessness, and the psychosocial aspects are equally important if the patient and family are to cope with the consequences of chronic respiratory illness. Respiratory assessment requires observation, communication and clinical skills and should include assessment of physiological factors, mental state, causative factors, symptoms, impact on ALs and psychosocial factors.

Respiratory Rate, Rhythm and Depth

Normal breathing should be regular and appear effortless, with a respiratory rate in adults between 12 and 20 breaths per minute. Many patients with underlying respiratory disease will have an elevated respiratory rate (>20 breaths per minute) to facilitate adequate oxygenation and ventilation. Respiratory depression (<12 breaths per minute) may occur due to exhaustion and fatigued respiratory muscles caused by the work of breathing. The use of sedatives and opioid analgesics may also cause respiratory depression. Observation of the rhythm and depth of breathing should be assessed, as this will indicate the quality of each breath. Slow, shallow breathing is a sign of respiratory depression and indicates that there is an insufficient number and quality of breaths to sustain adequate ventilation. Equally, a rapid, irregular breathing pattern which does not allow expansion of the lower lobes of the lungs will also result in ventilatory failure.

Chest Movement

The chest movements should be symmetrical and are best observed by standing in front of the patient rather than to one side. If one side of the chest is not expanding as well as the other, this may indicate a collapsed lung due to pneumothorax (air in the pleural space) or the presence of bronchial obstruction. The patient's use of accessory muscles in the neck and shoulders (the sternocleidomastoid and trapezius muscles) should also be noted as this indicates that the patient is unable to use the diaphragm and external intercostal muscles sufficiently to maintain ventilation.

Oxygen Levels

Observation of skin colour and pulse oximetry (oxygen saturation) will indicate whether the patient is receiving adequate oxygenation. The patient's skin should be observed for blueness of the lips, tongue and oral mucosa, as this indicates the presence of central cyanosis caused by hypoxaemia (low oxygen levels in arterial blood). In patients with dark skin, it may not be possible to see changes in lip colour and therefore the oral mucosa and tongue should always be examined. Hypoxaemia will also be detected through performing pulse oximetry as this will measure oxygen saturation levels. According to the British Thoracic Society (2017a) the normal ranges are:

- 96%–98% for adults <70 years of age.
- 94%–98% for adults >70 years of age.

When examining the skin, the presence of peripheral oedema should be noted as this may indicate the presence of cor pulmonale (right ventricular hypertrophy and failure) due to vasoconstriction of the pulmonary circulation because of local hypoxia in the lungs. Another sign of chronic tissue hypoxia is finger clubbing, which is where the terminal phalanges of the fingers become enlarged, and the base of the nail feels spongy.

Mental State

Respiratory assessment should include assessment of mental state because confusion and disorientation may be a sign of severe hypoxia resulting in a reduced supply of oxygen to the brain. Asking relatives and friends if they have noticed a change in mental state may be helpful when the nurse has not previously known the patient. The patient's level of alertness also needs to be assessed as drowsiness may indicate hypercapnia (raised levels of carbon dioxide in arterial blood).

Causative Factors

Factors that influence the patient's respiratory health status, such as allergens, the environment and smoking, should be identified so that potential health education strategies can be implemented. As smoking is a major cause of respiratory illness, a thorough smoking history should include current and past smoking habits, with the total pack years of smoking being estimated. The number of pack years can be calculated as follows:

$$\text{Pack years} = \text{Rough sum of cigarettes smoked per day} \times \text{Number of years smoked})/20$$

The patient's present and past occupation may indicate exposure to toxic substances, such as asbestos and industrial chemicals. Through identifying exposure as the causative factor of respiratory disease, the patient and their family may be eligible for compensation.

Symptoms

The most common symptom associated with respiratory disease is breathlessness, although wheeze – often described by patients as chest tightness, cough and muscular chest pain – can be equally troublesome. Through assessing symptoms at regular intervals, it is possible to monitor treatment effectiveness. Assessment for the presence of infection is important as it causes much respiratory disease, such as pneumonia and tuberculosis (TB). A raised temperature and pulse rate, a raised white blood cell count, positive blood cultures and a productive cough with yellow or green sputum indicate the presence of infection.

Impact on Activities of Living

Assessing the impact of breathlessness on all the ALs will allow the nurse to plan care effectively, identifying the need for referral to occupational therapy, physiotherapy, dietetics and social services as appropriate. Particular attention to mobility and nutritional status is essential, as breathlessness has been shown to cause immobility, and malnutrition due to increased energy requirements and poor appetite (Keogh and Williams 2021).

Patients with underlying respiratory disease should be observed for increasing breathlessness and oxygen desaturation (lowering of oxygen levels) on exertion, as this may indicate the need for supplementary oxygen to prevent complications of immobility. Assessment of the patient's nutritional status should include body mass index (BMI; see Chapter 22, Nutrition and Health), identification of recent significant weight loss, eating habits and changes in appetite. Patients found to have a BMI less than 20 or those with a recent weight loss greater than 10% should be referred to a dietitian.

Psychosocial Factors

The chronic nature of much respiratory disease can affect the patient's psychological state and relationships with family and friends. Through assessing the patient's perceptions and concerns, coping strategies, such as relaxation techniques to alleviate fear and anxiety or activity pacing to allow greater mobility, can be identified to assist with adaptation to chronic respiratory illness. The introduction of nurse-led clinics, usually run by practice nurses or respiratory nurse specialists, has assisted those suffering from chronic respiratory illness to feel at ease to discuss psychosocial issues. This is usually achieved through the nurse building a therapeutic trusting relationship with the patient over time so that a profile of perceptions and concerns can be developed. Consideration of current social issues and need for referral to social services or community nursing should be continually assessed so that interventions can be identified at the earliest opportunity.

Respiratory Investigations

The symptoms of breathlessness, wheeze, chest tightness and cough can be associated with many different respiratory conditions. Respiratory investigations are used to determine the cause of respiratory symptoms, allowing appropriate treatment to be commenced, to monitor disease progression and to assess treatment effectiveness. The most used respiratory investigations are:

- Lung function tests.
- Pulse oximetry.
- Chest X-ray.
- CT scan of thorax.
- Sputum microscopy, culture and sensitivity.
- Bronchoscopy.

Lung Function Tests

Lung function tests assess the functioning of the lungs and can be used to confirm a diagnosis through measuring flow rates and lung volumes. They include the following, which are collectively called spirometry:

- *Peak expiratory flow (PEF)*, commonly referred to as 'peak flow', is measured in litres per minute and is an objective measure that detects airflow obstruction in the larger airways. If the airways are narrowed, then the rate of expiration is limited, and the PEF will be lower than the predicted normal value for the person's age, height and sex. To ensure the measurement is accurate, the patient must be taught how to perform the test (Fig. 3.4). The patient must be standing or sitting in an upright position and is required to make a seal with his/her lips around the mouthpiece before exhaling forcibly. The test is repeated three times and the highest result recorded.
- *Forced expiratory volume in 1 second (FEV1) and forced vital capacity (FVC).* FEV_1 determines the amount of air that is exhaled in the first second of a forced expiration. FVC is the total amount of air exhaled from maximal inspiration to maximal expiration. A spirometer is the instrument used to measure FEV_1 and FVC and can detect obstructive patterns of breathing which occur in asthma, COPD, cystic fibrosis (CF) and bronchiectasis, and restrictive patterns of breathing due to pulmonary fibrosis, sarcoid, asbestosis, kyphoscoliosis and muscular dystrophies.
- *Reversibility testing.* Respiratory function tests can also be used to determine the extent to which airflow obstruction can be reversed with bronchodilators. The respiratory function test is performed before and 15 minutes after administration of a bronchodilator, and the two results are compared. An increase in FEV_1 or PEF of greater than 15% is representative of a positive response and indicates the presence of asthma. This is not the case in COPD, where the airflow is fixed, and the respiratory function test will either show limited (<15%) or no reversibility following bronchodilators.

Pulse Oximetry

Pulse oximetry is a simple, noninvasive way of measuring peripheral oxygen saturation of arterial blood (SpO_2) to determine whether the values are within the normal range. A probe consisting of a small light-emitting diode (LED) on one side and a light detector on the other is placed on the patient's finger. The technique works because of the light-absorbing characteristics of haemoglobin. In hypoxaemia the 'blueness' of the blood will be measured by the pulse oximeter. Although clearly useful, pulse oximetry has its limitations. It is unable to detect changes in carbon dioxide levels and produces inaccurate readings at saturation levels below 82%, and so may not be reliable in severe respiratory disease. Furthermore, recent studies suggest that pulse oximetry can overestimate oxygen levels in people with darker skin tones (Fawzy et al. 2022). Inaccurate readings may also be due to several other factors, including:
- Peripheral vasoconstriction (insufficient perfusion to detect pulse).
- Anaemia (if vasoconstriction occurs).
- Movement, i.e. shivering or fitting (affects the ability of the light to travel from the LED to the photodetector).
- Nail varnish/false nails (blockage of the light detector).
- Dark skin pigment (blockage of the light detector).
- Intravenous dyes (reduce readings by absorbing light).
- Severe hypoxaemia (not accurate below 82%).
- High levels of carboxyhaemoglobin due to smoking (due to vasoconstriction).
- Exposure to carbon monoxide.

1. Fit disposable mouthpiece to peak flow meter

2. Ensure patient stands up or sits upright and holds peak flow meter horizontally without restricting movement of the marker. Ensure the marker is at the bottom of the scale

3. Ask patient to breathe in deeply, seal lips around mouthpiece and breathe out as quickly as possible

4. Repeat steps 2 and 3 twice more. Choose and record the highest of the three readings

Figure 3.4 Measuring peak expiratory flow rate using a peak flow meter. (Reproduced from Brooker C, Nicol M. Nursing Adults: The Practice of Caring. Edinburgh: Mosby; 2003, with permission.)

Chest X-ray

Chest X-ray is a valuable aid to diagnosis of respiratory disease and will show the lung fields, pleura, rib cage, diaphragm shape and size of the heart. Chest X-ray is usually performed when patients present with persistent cough, chest pain, unexplained breathlessness, haemoptysis (coughing up blood), weight loss and pyrexia.

Computerised Tomography (CT)

CT scanning of the thorax is a radiological investigation that uses X-rays to obtain thin 'slices' that are put together to form images of the lung tissue. CT is mostly used to diagnose lung cancer, bronchiectasis and interstitial lung disease (ILD). It is also used to stage the disease progression, allowing the most appropriate treatment to be determined.

Sputum

Observations of sputum colour, viscosity, odour and amount can establish the effectiveness of antibiotic therapies. Patients who are producing sputum require:

- A sputum pot with a lid, as swallowing the sputum may cause nausea.
- Tissues to wipe excess secretions from the mouth and nose.
- Mouthwash/regular mouth care, as sputum is often foul tasting.
- Encouragement with fluid intake, as dehydration will increase the viscosity of the sputum.

The diagnosis of respiratory infections can be achieved through microbiological analysis of sputum. A specimen of mucopurulent or purulent sputum, not saliva, should be collected in a sterile container, to prevent contamination, prior to the commencement of antibiotic therapy. Sputum should never be left for long periods before being transferred to a laboratory; otherwise, an overgrowth with gram-negative organisms may occur. The patient should be asked to rinse their mouth before the specimen is obtained to prevent contamination of the sputum with food, which renders it unusable by the laboratory. The laboratory will perform microscopy, culture and sensitivity to antibiotics.

Bronchoscopy

Flexible fibreoptic bronchoscopy is an invasive procedure that is commonly used to diagnose:

- lung cancer,
- TB,
- pneumonia and other respiratory infections.

Bronchoscopy and related procedures (lung biopsy, brushing and lavage) are usually performed under sedation and local anaesthetic to the throat. Sedatives, such as midazolam, may cause respiratory depression, hypoventilation and hypotension, and local anaesthetics applied to the throat may lead to laryngospasm and bronchospasm. The patient therefore needs careful monitoring during the procedure and for 6–8 hours afterwards as bronchoscopy can cause bronchospasm, hypoxaemia, fever, pneumonia, pneumothorax and haemorrhage. On discharge, the patient should be given information (usually a postbronchoscopy leaflet) explaining how they should feel during the first 12 hours and detailing what to do if prevailing symptoms worsen or new symptoms develop. It is not usually necessary to admit patients to hospital following bronchoscopy unless significant postbronchoscopic bleeding, pneumothorax and/or respiratory distress occur.

Common Respiratory Disorders

Asthma

Asthma is a common chronic inflammatory condition of the airways, characterised by bronchospasm, severe dyspnoea, wheezing, chest tightness and expiratory exertion. As a result of inflammation, the airways are hyperresponsive and narrow easily in response to a wide range of provoking stimuli.

Pathophysiology

Immunoglobulin E (IgE) is present in small amounts in normal blood but in increased amounts in asthma sufferers. In allergic extrinsic asthma, the disease process involves inhalation of antigens (allergens) which are absorbed by the bronchial mucosa and trigger production of IgE antibodies. These antibodies bind to mast cells and basophils around the bronchial blood vessels. When the allergen is encountered again, the antigen–antibody reaction releases histamines and bradykinin, resulting in bronchial muscle spasm, oedema and excessive secretion of thick mucus. In many cases, the severity of attacks lessens with age and good treatment, unless other factors are involved. There are various theories of the pathogenesis of intrinsic asthma, including the impact of allergens. Whatever the cause, the bronchi and bronchioles are chronically inflamed, oedematous, full of mucus and subject to bronchospasm.

Clinical features are produced in response to the narrowing of the airways and include wheeze; chest tightness; dry, nonproductive cough; and breathlessness. Symptoms of uncontrolled asthma are often worse at night and early morning.

Investigations are used to confirm the diagnosis based on clinical presentation and past medical history, and will include spirometry (FEV_1, FVC, PEF). Furthermore, once a diagnosis has been established, PEF using a peak flow meter will be used to monitor asthma. Skin sensitivity tests and a history of exposure to specific allergens may help in isolating and avoiding triggering factors.

Treatment

The aim of treatment is to control symptoms and prevent asthma 'attacks'; thus, treatment needs to be targeted at prevention and control of inflammation and bronchoconstriction. The British Guidelines on Asthma Management (British Thoracic Society and Scottish Intercollegiate Guidelines Network [SIGN] 2019) recommend a stepwise approach that corresponds to the severity of asthma based on symptoms and peak flow measurements (Fig. 3.5). The main treatment used to control asthma is corticosteroids. For further information on asthma medication, see http://www.brit-thoracic.org.uk/standards-of-care/guidelines/btssign-british-guideline-on-the-management-of-asthma.

Acute Severe Asthma

It is important that both patient and nurse can detect acute severe asthma as delay in recognising deterioration may be fatal. Table 3.3 outlines the symptoms of acute asthma and classifies them into acute severe asthma, life-threatening asthma and near-fatal asthma.

The aim of treatment is to prevent hypoxia and to reduce bronchoconstriction and inflammation of the airway, and therefore the patient will immediately require:

- Supplementary oxygen to maintain an SpO_2 of 94%–98%. Administration of oxygen should not be delayed.
- Nebulised bronchodilators delivered via oxygen at a flow rate of 6 L/min as early as possible.
- Steroid therapy, i.e. prednisolone 40–50 mg orally daily (British Thoracic Society/SIGN 2019).

Patients with an acute exacerbation of their asthma *must* receive oxygen via a face mask or nasal cannula at concentrations large enough to maintain oxygen saturations above 94%. Hypercapnia may occur due to exhaustion and fatigue of respiratory muscles and may lead to respiratory arrest if not reversed. Nebulised β_2 agonists (e.g. salbutamol) and anticholinergics (ipratropium bromide) in high doses will be administered to ensure bronchoconstriction is alleviated as quickly as possible. A single dose of intravenous

STEP 1 Regular preventer	STEP 2 Initial add-on therapy	STEP 3 Additional add-on therapies	STEP 4 High dose therapy	STEP 5 Continuous or frequent use of oral steroids
Low dose inhaled steroid (ICS)	Add inhaled long acting bronchodilator (LABA) to low dose inhaled steroid (ICS) Consider leukotriene receptor antagonist (LTRA) (If allergy/atopy present)	No response to LABA Stop long acting bronchodilator (LABA) & consider increasing dose of inhaled steroid (ICS) If benefit from LABA but inadequate control Stop long acting bronchodilator (LABA) & increase inhaled steroids (ICS) to medium dose If benefit from long acting bronchodilator (LABA) but inadequate control Continue LABA & ICS & consider trial of other therapy (i.e. leukotriene receptor, LAMA, SR theophylline)	Consider trials of: Increasing inhaled steroid (ICS) up to high dose Addition of a fourth drug. • Leukotriene receptor antagonist (LTRA) • SR theophylline • Beta agonist tablet • Long acting muscarinic antagonist (LAMA)	Use daily steroid tablet in the lowest dose providing adequate control Maintain high-dose ICS Consider other treatments to minimise use of steroid tablets

↑Stepping up treatment as necessary (consider moving up if using three doses or more of short acting β2 agonists a week
↓Stepping down when control is good

Figure 3.5 Stepwise asthma management.

TABLE 3.3	Levels of Severity of Acute Asthma

Near-Fatal Asthma

Raised $PaCO_2$ and/or requiring mechanical ventilation with raised inflation pressures

Life-Threatening Asthma

Any one of the following in a patient with severe asthma:

• PEF <33% best or predicted • SpO_2 <92% • PaO_2 <8 kPa • Normal $PaCO_2$ (4.6–6.0 kPa)	• Silent chest • Cyanosis • Feeble respiratory effort • Bradycardia	• Dysrhythmia • Hypotension • Exhaustion • Confusion • Coma

Acute Severe Asthma

Any one of the following:

• PEF 33%–50% best or predicted • Respiratory rate ≥25/min	• Heart rate ≥110/min • Inability to complete sentences in one breath

Moderate Asthma Exacerbation

• Increasing symptoms • PEF >50%–75% best or predicted	• No features of acute severe asthma

Brittle Asthma

• Type 1: wide PEF variability (>40% diurnal variation for >50% of the time over a period >150 days) despite intense therapy
• Type 2: sudden severe attacks on a background of apparently well-controlled asthma

PEF, Peak expiratory flow.

magnesium sulphate is considered in patients with acute severe asthma who have not had a good initial response to inhaled bronchodilator therapy (British Thoracic Society/SIGN 2019).

Asthma Mortality

There are several factors that have been identified as increasing the risk of premature death from asthma (British Thoracic Society/SIGN 2019). They are:

• Inadequate treatment with inhaled or oral steroids – as asthma control will be poor.
• Nonadherence with treatment and monitoring – as signs of deterioration may be ignored.
• Failure to attend appointments and self-discharge – this may indicate denial about the life-threatening consequences of uncontrolled asthma.
• Mental health problems, which include psychiatric illness, current or recent tranquilliser use, deliberate self-harm and alcohol or drug use disorder.
• Learning disabilities – because symptoms are often underreported.
  When assessing a patient, it is important to consider whether the patient with acute asthma has any additional risk factors so that discharge planning can be as effective as possible. For example, early discharge would not be appropriate for the high-risk patient as they are unlikely to complete the course of treatment.

❖ Nursing Management and Health Promotion: Asthma

The role of the nurse in asthma care will depend on the severity of the patient's symptoms. Most people with asthma are cared for by practice nurses in the community who provide preventative asthma care. This is achieved by:

• monitoring symptoms;

(A)

How to use:
- Remove cap and shake inhaler and place into spacer
- Gently breathe out
- Make seal with lips around mouthpiece
- Press the canister once to release dose of drug
- Breathe in and out slowly and gently (tidal breathing) five times.
  This will make a clicking sound as the valve opens and closes

(B)

How to use:
- Unscrew and remove cap
- Hold the device upright
- Twist the grip forwards and backwards. A click should be heard
- Gently breathe out
- Make seal with lips around mouthpiece
- Breathe in steadily and deeply through the mouthpiece
- Remove inhaler from mouth and hold breath for at least 10 seconds

(C)

How to use:
- Shake the inhaler and remove cap
- Gently breathe out
- Hold the inhaler upright and do not occlude air holes
- Make seal with lips around the mouthpiece
- Once inhaler is activated take a deep breath
- Hold breath for at least 10 seconds
- Close the cap

Figure 3.6 Inhaler delivery devices. (Reproduced from Brooker C, Nicol M. Nursing Adults: The Practice of Caring. Edinburgh: Mosby; 2003, with permission.)

- peak flow monitoring (see Fig. 3.4);
- checking inhaler technique (Fig. 3.6);
- providing allergy avoidance advice;
- identification of acute severe asthma requiring emergency treatment; and
- developing a personal asthma action plan (PAAP).

Self-management Plans

Patients with acute severe asthma will require hospital admission as this is life-threatening. Respiratory nurse specialists should be involved with discharge planning as they provide liaison between primary and secondary care to ensure that continuity of care is achieved. They will also continue to monitor patients with severe asthma in nurse-led asthma clinics where they provide education and support in developing PAAPs. Self-management has become an integral part of asthma management (British Thoracic Society/SIGN 2019) and empowers the patient to make changes to their own treatment without consulting a healthcare professional. The nurse has an important patient education role, as acquisition of knowledge and skills is necessary for the patient to have the confidence and ability to take control of their asthma care. For a PAAP to be developed, it is necessary that the patient:
- Understands the disease process.
- Can perform and interpret peak flow measurements.
- Can recognise symptoms.
- Has the confidence to adjust medication.
- Has sufficient insight to know when professional advice is required.

Asthma UK produces preprinted PAAPs that can be individualised for the patient, but this will only be successful when combined with education, support and agreement between the healthcare professional and patient.

 See website Critical thinking question 3.1.

Chronic Obstructive Pulmonary Disease

COPD is defined as a heterogeneous lung condition characterised by chronic respiratory symptoms due to abnormalities of the airways and/or alveoli that cause persistent often progressive airflow obstruction (Global Initiative for Chronic Obstructive Lung Disease 2023). Tobacco smoke is the most important risk factor for the development of COPD, although occupational exposure (e.g. coal mining and welding) and α_1-antitrypsin deficiency can also cause COPD.

Pathophysiology

COPD is a term used to describe several overlapping conditions:
- Chronic bronchitis – chronic inflammation of the membranes of the trachea and bronchi resulting in a productive cough on most days for at least 3 months in at least two consecutive years.
- Emphysema – abnormal, permanent enlargement of the terminal airspaces due to destruction of the alveolar wall.
- Chronic asthma that has become unresponsive to treatment.

Clinical Features

The clinical features will depend upon disease severity but usually include chronic cough, wheeze and breathlessness. In advanced cases the slightest physical activity can cause severe respiratory distress and cyanosis. Abnormal ventilation results in chronic hypoxaemia (low oxygen), hypercapnia (high CO_2) and polycythaemia (raised red blood cell count), which cause cyanosis and facial flushing, because CO_2 is a vasodilator. The patient is weakened by constant respiratory effort and becomes unable to tolerate normal basic AL.

Investigations

Lung function tests (spirometry) are used to confirm the diagnosis based on history, symptoms and clinical examination. Spirometry

(FEV$_1$, FVC, FEV$_1$/FVC), blood gas analysis and chest X-ray will confirm the stage and effects of the disease and influence treatment.

❖ Nursing Management and Health Promotion: COPD

The aim of treatment is to prevent further deterioration in lung function, control unpleasant symptoms, increase physical activity and improve the individual's quality of life. Most of the treatment will take place in the community or outpatient setting. It is during acute exacerbations, usually because of respiratory infection, that patients may require hospital intervention or admission, although some acute exacerbations can be managed through 'hospital at home' schemes.

The management of COPD is dependent on the severity of the disease process and the associated symptoms. Fig. 3.7 outlines the treatments used to manage each stage of COPD, based on the NICE COPD guidelines (NICE 2019a) and GOLD guidelines (Global Initiative for Chronic Obstructive Lung Disease 2023).

As well as medication the other mainstay treatments for severe COPD are:
- Smoking cessation.
- Long-term oxygen therapy.
- Pulmonary rehabilitation.

Long-term Oxygen Therapy

The benefits of long-term oxygen therapy in patients with chronic hypoxaemia (PaO_2 ≤7.3 kPa) due to COPD are well established (Khor et al. 2019). The reason for low concentrations of oxygen being administered to COPD patients is that they develop sensitivity to falling oxygen levels in the blood rather than raised levels of carbon dioxide. If a higher percentage of oxygen is administered, this may reduce the stimulus to breathe and lead to carbon dioxide retention.

Long-term oxygen therapy is delivered by an oxygen concentrator rather than oxygen cylinders. This frees the patient from relying on the delivery of the cylinders, allows the patient to be more mobile around the home and eliminates the need for storage of numerous cylinders. Patients who need to use oxygen outside the home can be provided with portable oxygen cylinders, although not all patients are willing to wear nasal cannulae in public. According to the British Thoracic Society's Home Oxygen Guidance (British Thoracic Society 2017a) the patient newly started on long-term oxygen therapy should have written instructions and outpatient or community follow-up so that the following aspects of care can be addressed:
- Safe use of oxygen (e.g. fire risk and smoking, falls due to tubing).
- Oxygen saturation (SaO_2) monitored to ensure that oxygen therapy is correcting hypoxaemia (SaO_2 >92%).
- Adherence to treatment.
- Monitoring of patient's condition and observation for signs of deterioration.

Respiratory Nurse Specialist

The respiratory nurse specialist is often the most appropriate person to provide the education, support and follow-up required for patients recently commenced on long-term oxygen therapy as they have clinical expertise and a liaison role.

Pulmonary Rehabilitation

Pulmonary rehabilitation is different from rehabilitation offered to patients with other conditions (e.g. cardiac or musculoskeletal rehabilitation); there is no cure, and the patient does not have the potential to return to a predisease state because the lung damage is not reversible. It is all about the patient achieving their own maximum potential within the limits of their disease and being able to live with and cope with a respiratory disability.

The aim of pulmonary rehabilitation is to reduce respiratory symptoms, increase exercise tolerance, improve psychological coping and improve overall quality of life (British Thoracic Society 2014). The common components of pulmonary rehabilitation programmes include:
- *Education* – increasing the patient's knowledge so that they are empowered to make decisions about their health needs, including modification of high-risk behaviours such as smoking.
- *Exercise* – many rehabilitation programmes use interval training which consists of 2–3 minutes of high-intensity training (e.g. bicycle or step-ups) alternating with equal periods of rest. This allows the patient to exercise safely and learn how to control their dyspnoea whilst exercising.
- *Breathing control* – patients are taught breathing techniques using their diaphragm, designed to slow respiratory rate while increasing their TV.
- *Psychosocial interventions* – patients with COPD have a high incidence of depression and anxiety and therefore need to develop coping strategies to deal with the impact of respiratory disability on their lives.
- *Nutritional intervention* – patients with COPD require nutritional advice and support as they are at high risk of malnutrition. Both the practical aspects of preparing meals as well as the physiological barriers, such as breathlessness and reduced appetite due to infection, need to be addressed. Usually, small regular high-calorie meals or snacks are better tolerated than two large main meals per day (see Chapter 22, Nutrition and Health).

For pulmonary rehabilitation to be successful, a multiprofessional approach is essential (British Thoracic Society 2014). The programme is usually undertaken by the respiratory physiotherapists with input from the respiratory nurse specialists and other disciplines, including dietitian and psychologist as appropriate.

Management of Acute Respiratory Exacerbation of COPD

A patient with an acute exacerbation of COPD presents with worsening symptoms of a previously stable condition and two of the following three symptoms:
1. increased breathlessness;
2. increased sputum volume; and
3. purulent sputum.

As the underlying cause of the acute exacerbation is usually infection, the patient is usually commenced on antibiotic therapy. If breathless, patients will also start oral corticosteroids and be given increased doses of bronchodilators, often nebulised (see Information 3.1).

During acute exacerbations, COPD patients are at risk of either type I respiratory failure (low oxygen levels in arterial blood) or type II respiratory failure (low oxygen and high carbon dioxide levels in arterial blood). It is therefore necessary to monitor arterial blood gases (ABGs) and treat with oxygen therapy and, if necessary, noninvasive ventilation (NIV) (see Chapter 28, Nursing the Critically Ill Patient).

Patients may require admission to hospital during an acute exacerbation; however, increasing numbers of patients are being cared

COPD CLASSIFICATION AND TREATMENT

Spirometric classification	**C** **LAMA** *If continued frequent exacerbations:* LABA/ICS or LAMA/LABA	**D** **LABA/ICS or LAMA/LABA** *If continued frequent exacerbations or breathlessness:* LABA/ICS + LAMA	**Exacerbations per year**
	A **SABA or SAMA** *If persistent breathlessness:* LAMA or LABA	**B** **LAMA or LABA** *If persistent breathlessness:* LAMA/LABA	
	Symptom severity		

Patient group	Risk & symptoms	Spirometric classification	Exacerbations per year	CAT score	MRC grade
A	Low risk, less symptoms	GOLD/NICE 1–2	0–1 no hospitalisation	<10	1–2
B	Low risk, more symptoms	GOLD/NICE 1–2	0–1 no hospitalisation	≥10	≥3
C	High risk, less symptoms	GOLD/NICE 3–4	≥2 or ≥1 with hospitalisation	<10	1–2
D	High risk, more symptoms	GOLD/NICE 3–4	≥2 or ≥1 with hospitalisation	≥10	≥3

Spirometric classification of airflow limitation in COPD (FEV1/FVC <0.7)	
Stage & severity	**FEV1 predicted**
GOLD/NICE Mild	≥80%
GOLD/NICE Moderate	50–79%
GOLD/NICE Severe	30–49%
GOLD/NICE Very Severe	<30%

Figure 3.7 COPD classification and treatment. *CAT,* COPD assessment test; *COPD,* chronic obstructive pulmonary disease; *FEV1,* forced expiratory volume in 1 second; *FVC,* forced vital capacity; *GOLD,* Global Initiative for Chronic Obstructive Lung Disease; *ICS,* inhaled corticosteroid; *LABA,* long-acting beta agonist; *LAMA,* long-acting muscarinic antagonists; *MRC,* modified medical research council; *NICE,* National Institute for Health and Care Excellence; *SABA,* short acting beta agonist; *SAMA,* short-acting muscarinic antagonist.

for at home by respiratory nurses providing 'hospital at home' or early supported discharge. Patients assessed as suitable for home treatment will be provided with an oxygen concentrator, nebuliser and home visits from the respiratory nurses who will monitor progress and provide advice and support. Once recovered from their acute exacerbation, the patient will be discharged back into the care of the general practitioner (GP) and community nurses (i.e. respiratory nurse specialist, practice nurse, community matron).

⊕ **See website Critical thinking question 3.2.**

Respiratory Failure

If impending respiratory failure is recognised early, the actual state can be avoided; nurses should be alert for the following clinical signs:
- restlessness and confusion
- increase in respiratory rate with laboured ventilatory effort and use of ancillary respiratory muscles (sternocleidomastoid and abdominal muscles)
- forced and abnormal movement of the diaphragm
- pronounced flaring of the nostrils with each breath
- pale or deeply cyanosed and clammy skin.

INFORMATION 3.1

Nebulisers

A nebuliser is a device that administers medication (i.e., bronchodilators, antibiotics) by converting a liquid into a mist that can be inhaled into the lungs. It is commonly used in treating patients with cystic fibrosis or acute asthma and during exacerbations of COPD. The jet nebuliser is the most widely used device. Compressed gas (oxygen or air) is forced through a narrow opening in the base of the nebuliser unit, creating the negative pressure required to draw up the drug solution from its reservoir. When the liquid collides with the jet of gas, it fragments into droplets that then impact on a baffle. The smallest particles form a therapeutic mist for the patient to inhale, while larger particles return to the reservoir and are recycled until the prescribed dose has been given, usually about 10 minutes. A flow rate of 6–8 L/min produces 50% of the particles at a diameter of less than 5 μm which allows deposition of the drug in the lungs.

Compressed air is the most common source for driving a nebuliser unless a high rate of inspired oxygen (i.e. patients with asthmatic) is indicated and prescribed. To prevent worsening of carbon dioxide retention, patients at risk of carbon dioxide retention (i.e. COPD patients) should use compressed air to drive the nebuliser. The use of nasal cannulae to deliver the prescribed flow rate of oxygen during nebulisation will prevent hypoxaemia.

Where impending respiratory failure is suspected ABGs will be taken to confirm if the patient has respiratory failure and whether it is:

- type I respiratory failure – PaO_2 <8 kPa
- type II respiratory failure – PaO_2 <8 kPa, $PaCO_2$ >6 kPa
- respiratory acidosis – PaO_2 <8 kPa, $PaCO_2$ >6 kPa, pH <7.35.

Untreated, the condition will worsen steadily, and increasingly difficult ventilatory effort will leave the patient exhausted and hypoxic, which will eventually lead to the patient becoming comatose and to death. However, respiratory support techniques can be used for patients with impending respiratory failure. The treatment options are:

Type I respiratory failure.
- Oxygen therapy to maintain SpO_2 greater than 94%.
- Continuous positive airway pressure (CPAP) (see Chapter 28, Nursing the Critically Ill Patient).

Type II respiratory failure.
- Oxygen therapy.
- NIV.
- Endotracheal intermittent positive pressure ventilation (IPPV) (see Chapter 28, Nursing the Critically Ill Patient).

Oxygen Therapy

The aim of oxygen therapy is to increase the fractional inspired oxygen (FiO_2) above 21% (air) to ensure adequate saturation of haemoglobin.

In the presence of type I respiratory failure, oxygen therapy must be prescribed at a level that will correct hypoxaemia, and a patient with severe asthma or pulmonary embolism may require 60%–100% oxygen initially to prevent hypoxia, until specific disease management is initiated.

In the presence of type II respiratory failure, the low levels of oxygen are providing the respiratory drive, i.e. the stimulus to the respiratory centre in the medulla. High percentages of oxygen can reduce the hypoxic respiratory drive causing carbon dioxide retention and a respiratory acidosis. This is because patients with underlying respiratory disease such as COPD develop sensitivity to falling oxygen levels in the blood rather than raised levels of carbon dioxide. If a higher percentage of oxygen is administered, this may reduce their stimulus to breathe and lead to carbon dioxide retention. If the rising levels of carbon dioxide remain untreated, narcosis, disorientation and ultimately death due to respiratory acidosis will occur. These patients require low percentage oxygen (24%–28%) initially. The oxygen can be gradually increased based on repeated ABGs whereby carbon dioxide levels can be monitored. Patients with COPD can receive more than 28% oxygen, provided ABGs indicate that there is no evidence of carbon dioxide retention (hypercapnia).

Oxygen Delivery Devices

A variety of oxygen devices are available. They can be categorised into two types:

- *Variable performance devices* (nasal cannula, Hudson mask and any system that does not incorporate a 'Venturi' mechanism) deliver a percentage of oxygen that varies according to the rate and depth of the patient's respirations.
- *Fixed performance devices* include in the delivery circuit a 'Venturi' coloured adaptor or the use of the Venturi principle incorporated in the humidification delivery device (e.g. Respiflow humidification system). The 'Venturi' supplies oxygen to the patient at a precise flow rate that causes mixing of the oxygen with air drawn

into the system through holes in the adaptor. This system is more accurate and is not dependent on the patient's rate and depth of respirations. During acute respiratory episodes, these are the masks of choice as they provide accurate concentrations of oxygen and prevent patients rebreathing their own carbon dioxide.

Humidification of Oxygen

When oxygen is delivered at low flow rates of <4 L/min and in the absence of respiratory tract infections, the oropharynx or nasopharynx may be able to provide adequate humidification. However, oxygen is very drying, and therefore, humidification should be considered for patients with:

- flow rates above 4 L/min
- respiratory infections
- tracheostomy (see Chapter 16, Nursing Patients With Disorders of the Ear, Nose and Throat)
- nasal discomfort/dryness.

❖ Nursing Management and Health Promotion: Oxygen Therapy

As well as ensuring the patient is receiving the prescribed percentage of oxygen using an appropriate oxygen device, the nurse needs to consider the comfort of the patient. As oxygen can cause mucosal drying, the development of mouth ulcers is not uncommon in patients receiving continuous oxygen therapy. The nurse needs to offer/perform regular mouth care to prevent the development of mouth ulcers as the resulting pain and difficulty with eating and drinking can have a significantly adverse effect on the patient's recovery. The use of humidification helps to counteract the drying effect and is indicated if the patient complains of discomfort or there are signs of mouth ulceration. An oxygen mask creates a barrier when speaking and the noise of the oxygen may interfere with the patient's ability to hear, which means that some patients may have difficulty with communication. Facing the patient, taking time and speaking clearly can improve communication, prevent isolation and facilitate the patient to express concerns and care needs. The nurse also needs to be aware that pressure ulcers can occur under the straps of the oxygen mask and therefore regular inspection behind the ears for redness and ulceration is necessary. If the straps are causing pressure and/or discomfort, padding behind the ears may help. The risks associated with oxygen therapy, particularly fire and falls, can be mitigated through ensuring a risk assessment is undertaken and acted upon (British Thoracic Society 2017b).

Continuous Positive Airway Pressure (CPAP)

Oxygenation can be enhanced by using CPAP which increases lung volume and keeps the alveoli open at the end of each breath to allow more time for gaseous exchange. A full-face mask is strapped in position and needs to be tight fitting, as any leaks will reduce the effectiveness of the positive pressure. The aim of treatment is to increase functional lung capacity and compliance, decrease the work of breathing, improve ventilation and perfusion, increase oxygen saturations, mobilise secretions and reexpand collapsed alveoli. CPAP relies on the patient's own respiratory effort and therefore is indicated for treatment of type I respiratory failure when there is:

- A restrictive pattern of breathing (e.g. fractured ribs, pain).
- Atelectasis (collapse of lung tissue affecting part or all of one lung) often secondary to pneumonia.

- Increased work of breathing due to the respiratory effort required to maintain adequate oxygen levels.
- Difficulty with clearing secretions, particularly when the cough reflex is reduced due to fatigue.

CPAP needs to be used with caution and by experienced practitioners as it is contraindicated in patients with pneumothorax, bullae (air cysts inside the lung), lung abscess, haemoptysis and hypotension. Most patients receiving CPAP will be cared for in a critical care environment, such as the high-dependency unit (HDU) or intensive care unit (ICU) (see Chapter 28, Nursing the Critically Ill Patient).

Noninvasive Ventilation (NIV)

NIV is a form of ventilation using a well-fitting nasal or full-face mask and unlike CPAP does not rely on the ability of the patient to breathe spontaneously as the machine has an inspiratory and expiratory phase. It is used to treat patients in type II respiratory failure and has the advantages of being noninvasive, able to provide adequate oxygen levels with carbon dioxide clearance and able to decrease work of breathing and improve quality of sleep. For it to be successful the patient must be able to adhere to treatment, have normal swallowing reflexes and haemodynamic stability and the ability to clear bronchial secretions. Nurses caring for patients receiving NIV need to be skilled so that they can troubleshoot problems such as mask problems, dry nose, air leaks, eye irritation and gastric distension. Patients will require psychological support to deal with the effects of altered body image due to needing to wear a facial mask.

Infections of the Respiratory System

Infections of the upper respiratory tract are addressed in Chapter 16, Nursing Patients With Disorders of the Ear, Nose and Throat. This chapter will focus on pneumonia and TB.

Pneumonia

Pneumonia is an infection of the lung caused by bacteria, viruses or fungi. There is parenchymal/alveolar inflammation, and the alveoli fill with fluid which leads to consolidation and exudation.

Pathophysiology

Pneumonia may be acquired in the community or in hospital, when it is known as a nosocomial infection (hospital acquired) as it has been acquired from other patients, the environment or healthcare workers. The type of pneumonia is determined by the causative organism, e.g. pneumococcal pneumonia, *Streptococcus pneumoniae* and *Pneumocystis* pneumonia (PCP).

Pneumonia can occur in previously healthy people although there is a higher incidence amongst the elderly and those with comorbidities. Complications of pneumonia include meningitis, empyema (pus in the pleural space), lung abscess and septicaemia. Death occurs most often in the elderly and those with debilitating chronic conditions, especially when pneumonia is secondary to recent influenza.

Clinical Features

Clinical presentation will vary in severity depending on the overall condition of the patient but includes varying degrees of pyrexia, cough with copious purulent sputum, breathlessness and tachypnoea (rapid respiratory rate).

Investigations

Investigations will include chest X-ray, sputum microscopy, culture and sensitivity, blood cultures, white cell count (WBC), C-reactive protein (CRP), pleural fluid microscopy, culture and sensitivity, pneumococcal antigen tests and serological tests.

Treatment

The aim of treatment is to identify the cause of the pneumonia, deliver appropriate treatment and rule out other causes of disease. Pneumonia will require treatment with antibiotics that are effective against the causative organism. In accordance with the NICE guidelines on antimicrobial prescribing in community-acquired pneumonia, the choice and route of administration will depend on the severity, presentation and previous antibiotic use (NICE 2019b).

Nursing Management and Health Promotion: Pneumonia

The needs of the patient with pneumonia will be determined by the causative factors and symptoms experienced by the patient, but most patients will require the following care:

- Monitoring temperature, pulse, respirations, blood pressure (BP), peak flow rate and oxygen saturation and reporting changes.
- Positioning the patient in an upright position supported by pillows or leaning against a bed table will help to alleviate dyspnoea by allowing effective lung expansion.
- Administration of oxygen to manage hypoxaemia (low oxygen levels). The dryness of oxygen will restrict the expectoration of sputum, so it is advisable to use humidified oxygen therapy and offer frequent drinks or mouth washes.
- Assistance with sputum clearance and encouraging the patient to expectorate the sputum. Chest physiotherapy will also be initiated to assist with airway clearance and usually consists of postural drainage, percussion and breathing control.
- The patient with pyrexia requires sufficient fluid intake to replace fluid lost in sweat; this will assist with excretion of toxins from the body. An antipyretic, such as paracetamol, may be used to control body temperature and make the patient more comfortable.
- Additional analgesia may be required, as paracetamol alone may be insufficient to manage pleuritic chest pain, which is caused by inflammation of the pleura.
- Nutritional support, as pyrexia and pain may have an adverse effect on nutrition.
- Psychological support, as having pneumonia can be a very frightening experience. Listening to fears and anxieties can be very supportive. During severe breathless episodes, the patient may be reassured by the presence of the nurse or family member.

Prevention of Pneumonia

A pneumococcal vaccine is available and is recommended for high-risk groups such as the elderly and those with underlying respiratory disease (Public Health England 2020). The polyvalent vaccine is usually a single 'one-off' injection. Vaccination against influenza ('flu' vaccine) is also recommended and needs to be administered annually. In addition, causative risk factors such as poverty, poor housing, malnutrition, environment exposure to pollutants, smoking (both active and passive) and excessive alcohol consumption need to be addressed if mortality rates are to be reduced (Reflection 3.1).

Tuberculosis

TB is a notifiable disease, which in accordance with the Public Health Act (Department of Health 1984) requires individuals diagnosed with TB to be notified to the Consultant in Community Diseases Control (CCDC) or Director of Public Health who is responsible for TB surveillance and control of spread of TB within the local community.

Pathophysiology

TB is a chronic infectious disease caused by the tubercle bacillus, *Mycobacterium tuberculosis*. It mainly affects the lungs as it is transmitted by inhalation of infected droplets of sputum coughed up by someone with active TB. However, other parts of the body (extrapulmonary) can be affected, through the bacterium entering the bloodstream via the lymphatic system. The most common forms of extrapulmonary disease are lymphadenopathy, pleural effusion, pericardial TB, miliary TB and TB meningitis.

Most people infected with *M. tuberculosis* never develop active disease as the body's immune system makes the bacterium dormant. Soon after the primary infection enters the lung, the inflammatory response occurs, and a calcified lesion is left. The primary infection remains dormant and is known as latent TB but may be reactivated (postprimary infection) to become active TB if the immune system is weakened.

The risk factors for developing active TB are associated with exposure to infectious TB and immune system weakening; this includes immunodeficiency (i.e. human immunodeficiency virus (HIV)), close contact with someone newly diagnosed with infectious TB, homelessness, particularly with a history of alcohol misuse and malnutrition, the elderly and those with chronic respiratory disease.

Clinical Features of TB are those associated with infection: chronic cough, pyrexia, weight loss, night sweats, general malaise and haemoptysis (blood in the sputum).

Investigations will include a chest X-ray, a tuberculin skin test (Mantoux) or interferon gamma release assay (IGRA) to detect past or present TB infection and sputum microbiological analysis; acid–fast bacillus (AFB) in sputum indicates that the patient has active (smear-positive) TB. A smear-negative result cannot exclude the presence of TB until the sputum culture, which takes approximately 8 weeks, also proves negative.

Treatment

The NICE produced guidelines on the treatment and management of TB in the UK (NICE 2019c). Currently, first-line treatment for TB consists of a 6-month treatment regimen of rifampicin, isoniazid, pyrazinamide and ethambutol for 2 months and then rifampicin and isoniazid for a further 4 months. The fourth drug, ethambutol, can be omitted when patients have a low risk of developing resistance to isoniazid.

Multidrug-Resistant TB

Pulmonary TB is a treatable condition, but multidrug-resistant TB (MDR-TB) can develop for the following reasons:
- Inadequate initial therapy (single drug therapy or low dose).
- Failure to complete the course of antibiotics because of poor adherence to treatment.
- Patients become asymptomatic after 2–4 weeks of treatment and so believe they no longer need the medication.
- Lack of knowledge and understanding of TB and its treatment.
- Inability to access healthcare, which is prevalent amongst the homeless and minority ethnic groups if there are language problems.

❖ Nursing Management and Health Promotion: Tuberculosis

Treatment of TB usually takes place at home; only those with severe illness, secondary complications (e.g. pleural effusion or adverse drug reactions) or social problems are admitted to hospital. The nursing priorities are:
- *Prevention* – based upon public health education and on screening and vaccination to protect those at risk. Specialist TB nurses, working closely with health visitors, public health nurses, school nurses, GPs, microbiologists and CCDCs, are key in the prevention and control of TB.
- *Infection control* – when a patient with suspected TB is admitted to hospital, they should be nursed in a single room so that isolation precautions for airborne infections can be implemented. If the patient needs to leave their room, they should wear a face mask. Once the patient has commenced TB treatment and has three consecutive smear-negative sputum results, they can be nursed in an open ward. Patients with, or suspected to have, MDR-TB should be cared for in a negative-pressure room and, because of the serious consequences of contracting MDR-TB, staff caring for the patient should wear dust mist-fume masks as these provide greater protection (see Chapter 18, Infection Prevention and Control).
- *Contact tracing* – people who have been in close contact with the person diagnosed with TB (index or source case) will be contacted and screened for TB. Contact screening is usually done by the TB nurse specialist who will screen close contacts (people living in the same house and very close associates such as boyfriend/girlfriend) of the index or source case.
- *Treatment supervision* – adherence to therapy is essential if TB is to be controlled and MDR-TB is to be prevented. Causes of nonadherence may include lack of knowledge, social problems, health beliefs, cultural beliefs and chaotic lifestyle. By working in partnership with the patient, strategies to improve adherence can be individualised.

- Directly observed therapy (DOT) is where the patient is observed taking their therapy by a healthcare professional (NICE 2019c). This strategy is labour-intensive and often difficult to achieve; in the UK it is only implemented if the patient is assessed to be at high risk of nonadherence. Homeless people are a group at high risk of nonadherence as they have difficulty accessing healthcare and obtaining medication. Incentives such as provision of meals and taxis have been used in association with DOT to encourage homeless people to attend appointments.

Cystic Fibrosis

CF is the most common life-threatening genetic disorder in the UK. It affects approximately 1 in 2500 live births because 1 in 25 of the White ethnic group in the UK are carriers of the *CF* gene. As it is a recessive genetic disorder, when both parents are carriers of the abnormal gene there is a one in four chance of each pregnancy producing a child with CF.

Pathophysiology

CF involves a basic dysfunction of the exocrine glands ducts due to altered sodium and chloride channel function at the epithelial cell surface. This results in the production of abnormally concentrated secretions that tend to block exocrine ducts. CF is a multisystem disorder that primarily affects the respiratory and digestive system, although there are often associated problems of liver disease, CF-related diabetes (CFRD), arthropathy and male infertility. The main cause of morbidity and mortality in CF is bacterial lung infections (Keogh and Bilton 2018). A background of chronic lung sepsis, usually due to *Staphylococcus aureus*, *Haemophilus influenzae* or *Pseudomonas aeruginosa*, is punctuated at increasingly frequent intervals by acute infective exacerbations. In response to persistent inflammation, pulmonary fibrosis and bronchiectasis (collection of necrotic material and bronchial secretions in dilated bronchi) progress, culminating in respiratory failure and death.

Investigations

The diagnosis of CF is based on history and clinical examination and will be confirmed by a sweat test and genotyping. Once the diagnosis is made, the severity will be determined by performing spirometry, chest X-ray, sputum cultures and pancreatic function tests.

Treatment

Treatment is aimed at delaying progression of the disease by maintaining lung function through preventing and controlling lung infections (NICE 2017). This involves:
- Physiotherapy to assist mucus clearance from the lungs.
- Administration of a combination of oral, nebulised and intravenous antibiotics to control infection.
- Nebulised bronchodilators (e.g. salbutamol).
- Anti-inflammatory medication (i.e. oral or inhaled steroids).
- Nutritional support consisting of pancreatic enzyme supplementation, fat-soluble vitamin supplementation and 20%–50% increased calorie intake.
- Monitoring disease progression (FEV_1, FVC, SpO_2 and weight).
- Aggressive treatment of acute exacerbation to prevent loss of lung function.

❖ Nursing Management and Health Promotion: Cystic Fibrosis

CF puts many demands on the individual and their family. The treatment regimen can be demanding, symptoms unpleasant and coping with emotions associated with a life-threatening chronic illness often stressful. The CF nurse has an important role in supporting the patient and family and is often the person they contact for support. The CF nurse also has a coordinating role within the multidisciplinary team and often acts as the patient's advocate.

Bronchiectasis

Bronchiectasis is a chronic dilation of the bronchi caused by inflammation. Collections of necrotic material and bronchial secretions in the dilated bronchi result in inflammation that causes secondary bacterial infection and fibrosis in the lung. This will result in recurrent and persistent lower respiratory tract infections causing production of large amounts of purulent sputum, bronchoconstriction, cough and haemoptysis. The main causes of bronchiectasis are:
- childhood infections (i.e. bronchiolitis),
- immunodeficiency syndromes (i.e. hypogammaglobulinaemia),
- allergic bronchopulmonary aspergillosis (ABPA),
- pneumonia,
- CF,
- TB and
- α_1-antitrypsin deficiency.

Treatment

The principles of treatment are the same as CF.

Lung Cancer

Lung cancer can be of primary origin or can occur as secondary metastatic spread from other primary sources.

Pathophysiology

Lung cancer is classified according to basic cell type, i.e. squamous cell adenocarcinoma (the most common), undifferentiated carcinoma and large and small cell carcinoma. The tumour may present as a cauliflower-shaped mass which slowly infiltrates the lung parenchyma. Because this form of cancer is difficult to detect in the early stages, it has a high potential for metastatic spread before being discovered.

Clinical features include a persistent cough of several months' duration which may be accompanied by haemoptysis (bloodstained sputum), chest pain, hoarseness and breathlessness. There may also be weight loss, anaemia, pleural effusion and bone pain. The patient will look generally unwell.

Investigations

Diagnosis is confirmed by clinical examination, chest X-ray, CT scan, positron emission tomography (PET) scan and sputum cytology. A bronchoscopy may be performed to enable a small piece of lung tissue (biopsy) to be taken via the bronchoscope and sent for pathology.

Treatment

A full explanation of the diagnosis and prognosis will be given to the patient and family so that an informed decision can be made regarding treatment. Approximately 15% of primary lung tumours can be treated successfully by surgical removal. This will involve either lobectomy (removal of the affected lobe) or pneumonectomy (removal of the whole lung) followed by cytotoxic chemotherapy. Where there is invasive and metastatic spread, the treatment is usually conservative, involving chemotherapy, radiotherapy, intervention to alleviate symptoms and pain control (see Chapter 31, Nursing the Patient With Cancer).

Pneumothorax

A pneumothorax occurs when the integrity of either layer of the pleura is breached, allowing air to enter the pleural cavity leading to lung collapse. There are two types of pneumothorax:
- Spontaneous pneumothorax – occurs because of the rupture of small blebs, cysts or bullae (air cysts inside the lung).
- Traumatic pneumothorax – caused by blunt chest trauma or a penetrating injury (e.g. stab wound or fractured rib, central line insertion). Trauma, particularly with penetrating injuries, can also cause blood to enter the pleural cavity and this is known as a haemothorax.

Tension Pneumothorax

Both spontaneous and traumatic pneumothorax can develop into a tension pneumothorax. This is a life-threatening event because air enters the pleural space on inspiration but cannot leave on expiration. The increased pressure causes the mediastinum to shift, moving the heart towards the opposite side.

Signs and Symptoms

The first sign of pneumothorax is the sudden onset of dyspnoea with unilateral chest pain that may radiate to the shoulder or arm and becomes worse on inspiration. On physical examination, there is hyperresonance and decreased breath sounds on the affected side and chest movement is asymmetrical. Severe dyspnoea, cyanosis, hypotension and tachycardia signify a tension pneumothorax, requiring immediate treatment.

A chest X-ray will confirm the presence and the amount of air in the pleural cavity and will be performed before initiation of treatment unless there is a tension pneumothorax, in which case the treatment is required immediately. The chest X-ray, along with the signs and symptoms, will determine the management of the pneumothorax.

INFORMATION 3.2

Nursing Management of an Underwater-Sealed Chest Drain

The underwater-sealed drainage system acts as a one-way valve, allowing air to bubble out through the water during expiration, but because the end of the tube is under water, air is prevented from being drawn back into the pleural cavity during inspiration. If at any point the seal is broken, air can enter the pleural cavity causing the lung to collapse again. The nurse has an important role in caring for patients with a chest drain as many of the potential complications can be prevented if principles of chest drain management are understood and implemented. The nurse needs to ensure that:
- The water level in the chest drain bottle covers the end of the tube.
- Connections are secure and not leaking.
- The chest drain bottle is kept below the chest level to prevent fluid entering the pleural cavity.
- The chest drain remains patent by checking that the water in the tube is 'swinging' and 'bubbling' as the patient breathes.
- Tubing is not routinely clamped (unless the connection becomes disconnected) because this prevents air escaping and may lead to lung collapse.
- Infection is prevented by adhering to asepsis and checking that the drain site dressing is kept clean and dry.
- When removing the chest drain, air is prevented from re-entering the pleural cavity by getting the patient to take a deep breath and hold it while the drain is pulled out and the 'purse-string' suture tied to seal the wound.

Treatment

The size of a pneumothorax, along with the symptoms, will guide treatment. According to the British Thoracic Society pleural disease guidelines (British Thoracic Society 2010), a pneumothorax is described as small (<2 cm) or large (>2 cm). Treatment options for pneumothorax include:
- Observation for a small, closed pneumothorax without significant breathlessness.
- Simple needle aspiration for a small (<2 cm) pneumothorax not associated with breathlessness.
- Intercostal chest-drain for a large (>2 cm) pneumothorax, or small (<2 cm) when associated with breathlessness (Information 3.2).
- Pleurodesis or pleurectomy when the lung has failed to re-expand after insertion of intercostal chest drainage or after two or more recurrences.

Summary: Key Nursing Issues

- Lung disease affects around 12 million people in the UK and results in tens of thousands of deaths annually, with a higher incidence of respiratory disease in the lower socioeconomic groups.
- The overwhelming cause of respiratory disease is tobacco smoking.
- Breathlessness is the main cause of disability associated with respiratory disease and impacts on the individual's ability to perform activities of daily living.
- Due to the chronic nature of much respiratory disease, self-management skills need to be taught so that individuals are empowered to manage their condition and make decisions about their health.
- Nurses have an important role in improving the quality of life of people with respiratory disease through holistic care.
- Respiratory nurse specialist roles provide continuity of care and a focal point for patients to seek advice and support.

Reflection and Learning – What Next?

- **Test** your knowledge by visiting the website 🌐 and answering the multiple-choice questions and critical thinking questions.
- **Consolidate** your learning by looking at some of the further reading suggestions, references and specialist websites.
- **Revisit** some of the additional material on the website.

- **Consider** what you have learnt and how this will help your professional development.
- **Reflect** on how you can apply this knowledge to the care of your patients.
- **Discuss** your learning with your mentor/supervisor, lecturer and colleagues.

References

British Lung Foundation. *Lung diseases in the UK*; 2023. https://statistics.blf.org.uk/.

British Thoracic Society. BTS pleural disease guideline. 2010. https://www.brit-thoracic.org.uk/quality-improvement/guidelines/pleural-disease/

British Thoracic Society. BTS guideline on pulmonary rehabilitation in adults. *British Thoracic Society Reports*. 2014;6(2). https://www.brit-thoracic.org.uk/quality-improvement/quality-standards/pulmonary-rehabilitation/.

British Thoracic Society. BTS guideline for oxygen use in adults and emergency settings. *Thorax*. 2017a;72(1). https://www.brit-thoracic.org.uk/quality-improvement/guidelines/emergency-oxygen/.

British Thoracic Society. British Thoracic Society quality standards for home oxygen use in adults. *BMJ Open Respiratory Research*. 2017b. https://www.brit-thoracic.org.uk/quality-improvement/quality-standards/home-oxygen/.

British Thoracic Society and Scottish Intercollegiate Guidelines Network. British Guideline on the management of asthma. 2019. https://www.brit-thoracic.org.uk/quality-improvement/guidelines/asthma/.

Brooker C, Nicol M. *Nursing Adults: the Practice of Caring*. Edinburgh: Mosby; 2003.

Department of Health. *Public Health (Control of Disease) Act*. London: The Stationery Office; 1984. http://www.legislation.gov.uk/ukpga/1984/22/pdfs/ukpga_19840022_en.pdf.

Esmond G. *Respiratory Nursing*. Edinburgh: Baillière Tindall; 2001.

Fawzy A, Wu TD, Wang K, et al. Racial and ethnic discrepancy in pulse-oximetry and delayed identification of treatment eligibility among patients with COVID-19. *JAMA Internal Medicine*. 2022;182(7):730–738.

Fletcher CM, Peto R. The natural history of chronic airflow obstruction. *BMJ*. 1977;1:1645–1648.

Global Initiative for Chronic Obstructive Lung Disease. *Management, and Prevention of Chronic Obstructive Pulmonary Disease (2023 Report)*; 2023. https://goldcopd.org/2023-gold-report-2/.

Hartmann-Boyce J, Livingstone-Banks J, Ordonez-Mena JM, et al. Behavioural interventions for smoking cessation: an overview and network meta-analysis. *Cochrane Database Syst Rev*. 2021;1:CD013229. doi:10.1002/14651858.CD013229.pub2.

Keogh RH, Bilton D. Up-to-date and projected estimates of survival for people with cystic fibrosis using baseline characteristics: a longitudinal study using UK registry data. *J Cyst Fibros*. 2018;17(2):218–227.

Keogh E, Williams EM. Managing malnutrition in COPD: a review. *Respiratory Medicine*. 2021;176:106248. doi:10.1016/j.med.2020.106248.

Khor YH, Renzoni EA, Visca D, McDonald CF, Goh NSL. Oxygen therapy in COPD and interstitial lung disease: navigating the knowns and unknowns. *ERJ Open Research*. 2019;5(3):00118–02019. doi:10.1183/23120541.00118-2019.

Mendes A. Nurses' role in smoking cessation interventions. *Br J Community Nurs*. 2022;27(11):525–526. doi:10.12968/bjcn.2022.27.11.525.

NICE (National Institute for Health and Care Excellence). Cystic fibrosis: diagnosis and management. NICE guideline [NG78]. 2017. https://www.nice.org.uk/guidance/ng78.

NICE (National Institute for Health and Clinical Excellence). Chronic obstructive pulmonary disease in over 16s: diagnosis and management. Clinical guideline [CG115]. 2019a. https://www.nice.org.uk/guidance/ng115.

NICE (National Institute for Health and Care Excellence). Pneumonia (community-acquired: antimicrobial prescribing [NG138]. 2019b. https://www.nice.org.uk/guidance/ng138.

NICE (National Institute for Health and Care Excellence). Tuberculosis. NICE guideline [NG33]. 2019c. https://www.nice.org.uk/guidance/ng33.

NICE (National Institution for Health and Clinical Excellence). Tobacco: preventing uptake, promoting quitting and treating dependence. NICE Guideline [NG209]. 2021. https://www.nice.org.uk/guidance/ng209/resources/tobacco-preventing-uptake-promoting-quitting-and-treating-dependence-pdf-66143723132869.

NICE (National Institution for Health and Clinical Excellence). Tobacco: treating dependence. Quality Standard [QS207]. 2022. https://www.nice.org.uk/guidance/qs207/resources/tobacco-treating-dependence-pdf-75547419465157.

Office for National Statistics (ONS). Adult Smoking Habits in the UK: 2021. 2022. file:///C:/Users/midqarw/Downloads/Adult%20smoking%20habits%20in%20the%20UK%202021.pdf.

Public Health England. PHE strategy 2020 to 2025. 2019. https://assets.publishing.service.gov.uk/government/uploads/system/uploads/attachment_data/file/831562/PHE_Strategy_2020-25.pdf.

Public Health England. Immunisation against infectious diseases. Pneumococcal: The Green Book. 2020. https://www.gov.uk/government/publications/pneumococcal-the-green-book-chapter-25.

Young SL, Jee YO, Kyung HM, Sung L, Kyung HH, Jae JS. The association between living below the relative poverty line and prevalence of chronic obstructive pulmonary disease. *J Thorac Dis*. 2019;11(2):427–437.

Useful Websites

Asthma UK, www.asthma.org.uk
British Lung Foundation, www.lunguk.org
British National Formulary, www.bnf.org
British Thoracic Society, www.brit-thoracic.org.uk
Global Initiative for Chronic Obstructive Lung Disease, www.goldcopd.org
NICE (National Institute for Health and Care Excellence), www.nice.org.uk
Thorax (Journal of the British Thoracic Society), www.thorajnl.com
World Health Organisation, www.who.int/health

4

Nursing Patients With Gastrointestinal, Liver and Biliary Disorders

SALLY PANNIFEX, JOHANNES MELLINGHOFF

CHAPTER OUTLINE

Introduction

Gastrointestinal (GI) disorders are the number one complaint requiring medical attention in various settings; knowledge of the anatomy and physiology of the GI system is essential for nursing practice. There is an increased need for knowledgeable, competent and confident nurses to assess, diagnose, plan, implement and evaluate the sometimes complex and challenging nursing care that patients require.

The GI system comprises several organs with a range of interrelated functions and disorders and as such can produce diverse and often distressing symptoms, for example, pain, dysphagia, anorexia, weight loss, dyspepsia, nausea and vomiting, constipation and diarrhoea, causing considerable embarrassment and restricting a person's activities.

GI system disorders may present as acute, life-threatening emergencies or chronic long-term illnesses, requiring long-term management and sometimes admission to hospital for more intensive treatment and/or surgical intervention. Whilst the specific needs of patients vary, the general principles of preoperative and postoperative care are standard and require skilled nursing care. Nurses are ideally placed to offer explanations of investigations, treatments, diagnosis and prognosis, and to follow up any information given by other health and social care providers. When offering nursing care to patients with GI disorders a process of continuous assessment, planning, intervention and evaluation should be carried out. This should be a dynamic process, allowing priorities to be changed as the patient's condition and circumstances change.

This chapter provides an overview of the important anatomy and physiology of the GI tract and related structures, outlining the fundamental functions of the system and how the organs and tissues contribute to effective functioning. Readers are encouraged to read Waugh and Grant (2023) for a more in-depth discussion of the anatomy and physiology of the GI system. The disorders of the GI system, liver and biliary tract most commonly encountered by nurses in hospital or community settings are described and the essential nursing care required by patients is described.

Anatomy and Physiology of the Gastrointestinal Tract

The GI tract begins at the mouth and ends at the anal canal and includes the oesophagus, stomach, duodenum and small and large intestines. The ancillary organs of digestion – the liver, pancreas and gallbladder – are connected to, but not part of, the digestive tract. The digestive tract is responsible for the ingestion of food and fluids at the mouth, breaking the food into pieces of a manageable size, moving the food along the canal, before digestion and absorption of the nutritional content of the food occurs, and finally expelling residues and waste products by defaecation. This section will briefly describe the structure and function of the different components of the digestive tract.

The Mouth

The mouth has three functions in the process of digestion: mastication (the mechanical chewing of food), salivation (moistening of the food) and deglutition (swallowing of the food).

The tongue, composed mainly of skeletal muscle covered with mucous membrane, manoeuvres and shapes food within the mouth for swallowing; it is also a sensory organ, allowing the taste, texture and temperature of food and fluids to be perceived. The upper surface is covered with filiform papillae (or taste buds) and sensory nerve endings (Drake et al. 2015).

Saliva, composed of 99.5% water and 0.5% solutes, is released from three pairs of glands: the parotid, the submandibular and the sublingual glands located around the lower jaw. The submandibular glands secrete about 70% of saliva in the absence of a food stimulus to keep the mucous membranes moist and lubricate the tongue and lips during speech. The sight, smell or presence of food in the mouth stimulates the parotid glands also to secrete saliva. In digestion, saliva helps to lubricate food prior to swallowing and initiating the digestion of starch.

Swallowing

There are three stages of swallowing (deglutition). After food has been sufficiently chewed, it is formed into a bolus between the palate and the tongue. The tongue rolls the bolus, pushing it into the pharynx. This is a voluntary reaction, known as the buccal stage of swallowing. The bolus passes over the glottis at the entrance of the larynx and trachea. When swallowing occurs, a small flap of cartilage, the epiglottis, covers the glottis. This stage of swallowing is the pharyngeal stage and is involuntary. Once the bolus has passed safely over the epiglottis it enters the oesophagus; this is known as the oesophageal stage of swallowing (Waugh and Grant 2023).

The Oesophagus

The oesophagus is a muscular tube connecting the pharynx to the stomach. It has three layers of tissue: an inner mucosal layer with an underlying submucosal layer, a middle muscular layer and an outer connective tissue layer. The mucosal layer secretes mucus for the lubrication of food as it passes down the oesophagus. The submucosal layer provides a nerve and blood supply. The muscles of the middle layer are arranged circularly and longitudinally. The composition of this layer changes throughout the length of the oesophagus in such a way that there is more striated, or voluntary, muscle at the pharyngeal end. Towards the stomach end, the muscle becomes predominantly and then entirely smooth, or involuntary.

The propulsion of food towards the stomach occurs by peristalsis, a series of relaxations and contractions of the muscles forcing the bolus along the oesophagus. Peristalsis is brought about by waves of contraction of the circular muscle, narrowing the lumen and thereby compressing the bolus of food. This action is preceded by a contraction of the longitudinal muscles, widening the lumen in order to receive the bolus of food. Peristalsis is entirely under involuntary control. Relaxation of the lower oesophageal sphincter permits food to enter the stomach (Drake et al. 2015).

The Stomach

The stomach is a J-shaped enlargement of the GI tract connecting the oesophagus to the duodenum, made up of four parts:

- Cardia
- Fundus
- Body
- Pylorus (including the pyloric antrum and pyloric canal)

Between the pylorus and the duodenum is the pyloric sphincter. The stomach wall is composed of four layers, similar to the remainder of the GI tract: mucosa, submucosa, muscularis and serosa. The basic structure of the stomach is illustrated in Fig. 4.1.

Digestion continues in the stomach when the bolus of food enters via the lower oesophageal sphincter. On the inner surface of the stomach, the mucosal layer of tissue is supplied with blood vessels and lymph glands by the underlying submucosal layer. Between the mucosal layer and the outermost peritoneal layer lies a muscular layer composed of three layers: an inner layer of oblique fibres, a middle layer of circular fibres and an outer layer of longitudinal fibres. These layers of muscle allow increasingly stronger waves of contraction in three directions, mixing the food in the stomach and allowing maximal contact with gastric juice. Innervation of the stomach is from a branch of cranial nerve X (vagus) providing parasympathetic nerve endings stimulating the secretory cells of the stomach. The internal surface area of the stomach is increased by the arrangement of rugae in the lining (Waugh and Grant 2023).

Gastric Juice

Cells in the mucosa of the stomach produce mucus, hydrochloric acid and pepsinogen, referred to as 'gastric juice' which when combined with food in the stomach, is known as 'chyme'. Hydrochloric acid helps maintain the acidity of the stomach at a pH of about 2. At this level of acidity, pepsinogen, an inactive precursor, is converted to pepsin, a protein-digesting enzyme that works best at this pH level. The stomach is primarily responsible for initiating protein digestion, although some carbohydrate digestion may continue by the action of any salivary amylase that has not yet become inactivated by the acidity of the stomach.

Release of gastric juice by the stomach mucosa is stimulated by the sight, smell and thought of food, known as the cephalic phase of digestion. The gastric phase of digestion commences when food reaches the stomach and continues until chyme enters the duodenum where the intestinal phase of gastric digestion begins. The length of time taken to empty the stomach is variable and depends on the composition of the meal eaten. The average time for emptying of the stomach after a meal is around 4 hours. Emptying takes place through the pylorus. The pyloric region holds about 30 mL of chyme; with each wave of contraction in the stomach, approximately 3 mL of chyme is released into the duodenum. The process is regulated by the pyloric sphincter (Waugh and Grant 2023).

Digestion

Digestion in the stomach is controlled by several factors. The presence of food in the stomach stretches the stomach wall, activating stretch receptors and stimulating the release of gastric juice. Gastrin (a hormone) is released by the stomach walls, stimulating the release of gastric juice. The presence of some specific food substances such as protein and caffeine further stimulates gastrin release. Contractions in the stomach are increased by stretching of the stomach wall and by the presence of protein. Low pH will inhibit gastrin release. The cephalic and gastric phases of digestion can also be inhibited by emotional factors. The stomach is not involved in the main process of absorption, although some water, alcohol and some medications such as aspirin are absorbed in the gastric phase.

The intestinal phase of digestion commences when chyme enters the duodenum. Entry of food into the duodenum leads to the inhibition of gastric secretion by the enterogastric reflex, mediated via the medulla. Enterogastrone relates to any hormone secreted by the mucosa of the duodenum inhibiting the forward movement of chyme. The enterogastric reflex is one of the three extrinsic reflexes of the GI tract. When it is stimulated, the release of the hormone 'gastrin' from the G-cells in the antrum of the stomach is inhibited, thereby further inhibiting gastric motility and secretion of gastric acid. In addition, the presence of food in the duodenum stimulates the release of three hormones, specifically secretin, cholecystokinin and gastric inhibitory peptide, all of which inhibit gastric juice secretion and reduce gastric motility (Fig. 4.2).

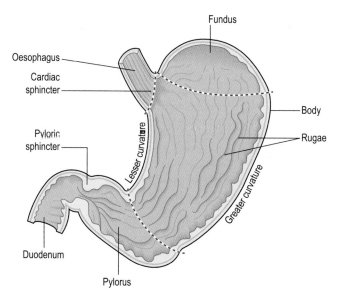

Figure 4.1 Longitudinal section of the stomach. (Reproduced with permission from Waugh A, Grant A. Ross and Wilson: anatomy and physiology. In: *Health and Illness*. 13th ed. Edinburgh: Churchill Livingstone Elsevier; 2018.)

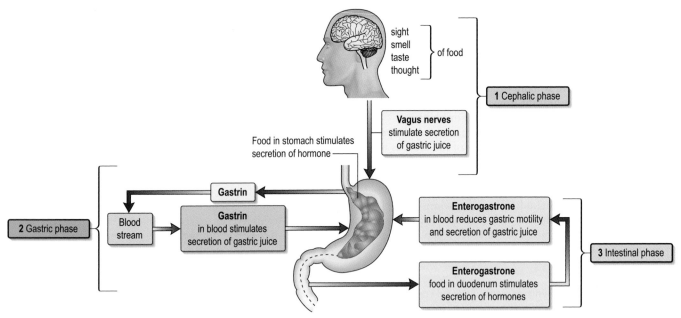

Figure 4.2 The phases of secretion of gastric juices.

The Small Intestine

The small intestine extends from the pyloric sphincter to the ileocaecal valve. It is responsible for the completion of digestion, with the absorption of nutrients and the reabsorption of most of the water that enters the digestive tract. The duodenum is the first section of the small intestine; it is approximately 25 cm in length. Secretions from the gallbladder and the pancreas are mixed with chyme and enter the duodenum through the ampulla of Vater, the joining of the common bile duct and the pancreatic duct. Gallbladder emptying is regulated by the sphincter of Oddi (Waugh and Grant 2023).

The Duodenum

The duodenum has a mucosal layer, a submucosal layer, a muscular layer and a peritoneal layer (Drake et al. 2015). Unlike the remainder of the small intestine, the duodenum is relatively immobile. Its regulatory role is fulfilled when the stimulus of chyme entering the duodenum triggers the enterogastric reflex as well as stimulating the release of gastrin, secretin, cholecystokinin and gastric inhibitory peptide. Secretin stimulates the cells of the liver to secrete bile, and cholecystokinin stimulates the release of digestive enzymes by the small intestine.

Chyme is very acidic, due to its high concentration of hydrochloric acid; when entering the duodenum, it becomes neutralised by the effect of alkaline bicarbonate released by the pancreas. Bile emulsifies fats in the chyme, breaking up fat globules into smaller particles. The enzymes of the pancreatic juice then begin to digest respective food substances in the duodenum. This action continues as chyme is passed down the small intestine (Waugh and Grant 2023).

The Jejunum and Ileum

The first two-fifths of the small intestine after the duodenum is the jejunum, and the remaining three-fifths, the ileum. Two types of movement, known as segmentation and peristalsis, mix and move food along the small intestine. Secretory cells of the mucosa of the small intestine release a slightly alkaline juice containing mainly water and mucus. The remaining enzymes of digestion in the GI tract are located on the microvilli, microscopic finger-like projections of the cell membrane. The enzymes of the small intestine complete the digestion of all components of the diet, including protein, fat, carbohydrate and nucleic acids (Burch and Collins 2021).

Absorption of Nutrients

Absorption occurs along the full length of the small intestine, with 90% of all the products of digestion absorbed here. Products of digestion are amino acids and peptides from protein, fatty acids and monoglycerides from fats, hexose sugars from carbohydrates and pentose sugars and nitrogen-containing bases from nucleic acids. Around 7.5 L of water are secreted into the small intestine daily and 1.5 L ingested. As only about 1 L enters the large intestine, the major portion of the water is reabsorbed in the small intestine. Absorption occurs by two main processes: diffusion and active transport. Absorption takes place at the villi. Each villus contains an arteriole and a venule connected by a capillary network, and a central lacteal, a projection of the lymphatic system (Fig. 4.3). Short-chain fatty acids, amino acids and carbohydrates are absorbed directly into the bloodstream. Triglycerides form structures called chylomicrons, which are also absorbed into the lacteals and then enter the bloodstream where the thoracic lymphatic duct empties into the left subclavian vein. Monosaccharides, amino acids, fatty acids and glycerol are actively transported into the villi. Disaccharides, dipeptides and tripeptides are also actively transported into the enterocytes and digestion is completed before transfer into the capillaries of the villi (Waugh and Grant 2023).

The Large Intestine

With most nutrients removed, the indigestible residue of food from the small intestine passes through the ileocaecal valve, entering the large intestine. The mesentery, a double layer of peritoneum, attaches both the small and large intestines to the rear wall of the abdomen, providing both with their blood supply.

The large intestine is divided into four portions:
1. Ascending colon
2. Transverse colon
3. Descending colon
4. Sigmoid colon

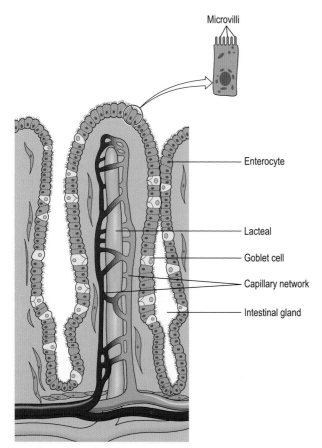

Figure 4.3 A highly magnified view of one complete villus in the intestine. (Reproduced with permission from Waugh A, Grant A. Ross and Wilson: anatomy and physiology. In: *Health and Illness*. 13th ed. Edinburgh: Churchill Livingstone Elsevier; 2018.)

The curves joining the ascending with the transverse colon and the transverse with the descending colon are referred to as the hepatic and splenic flexures, respectively. Two features can be identified near the ileocaecal valve: the caecum, a pouch below the ileocaecal valve, and the appendix, a finger-like projection of the caecum. The descending colon leads to the sigmoid colon, terminating in the rectum. Three muscular bands called the taeniae coli run the length of the large intestine. They maintain a slight longitudinal tension in the large intestine, giving the colon its characteristic segmented appearance. The rectum stores food residue as faeces before expulsion via the anus. The anal canal opens externally at the anus, controls evacuation and has an internal anal sphincter of smooth muscle and an external anal sphincter of skeletal muscle (Drake et al. 2015).

The large intestine, like the small intestine, has mucosal, submucosal, muscular and peritoneal layers; it differs in appearance from the small intestine in that there are no villi. The large intestine is designed primarily to absorb water and lubricate food residue as it is passed through the ileocaecal valve to the rectum. Any nutrients entering the large intestine are broken down by commensal bacteria, causing the gases methane, hydrogen, carbon dioxide and sulphur dioxide to be produced. Food may take up to 24 hours to pass through the large intestine.

Defaecation

When faeces reach the rectum, a reflex is initiated, and stretch receptors in the wall of the rectum send signals to the brain informing it of the presence of faeces. Defaecation can be suppressed until the time and place are appropriate. When appropriate to defaecate, the internal anal sphincter relaxes automatically, and the external anal sphincter, under voluntary control, is relaxed. Intraabdominal pressure is increased as the individual breathes in and holds the breath against a closed glottis (Valsalva's manoeuvre); faeces are expelled from the rectum via the anal canal (Waugh and Grant 2023).

DISORDERS OF THE GASTROINTESTINAL TRACT

Disorders of the Mouth

The mouth and tongue are often examined during clinical examination, as local abnormalities or indications of disease elsewhere can often be detected. For example, a dry, furred tongue can indicate the presence of a digestive problem or dehydration.

Patients with GI and liver disease require meticulous attention to oral hygiene as the mouth can be affected directly, such as in Crohn's disease (CD), and indirectly, such as in vitamin and iron deficiency in malabsorption and GI haemorrhage. Patients receiving steroid and immunosuppressive therapy are prone to infections of the mouth and oesophagus.

The principles of mouth care and the treatment of a range of disorders affecting the mouth and related structures are described in detail in Nicol et al. (2012).

Disorders of the Oesophagus

As the oesophagus has a relatively narrow lumen, any obstruction quickly impacts the passage of food. The two most common symptoms experienced by patients with disease of the oesophagus are dysphagia (difficulty in swallowing) and pain. Dysphagia may present in varying degrees, ranging from slight and intermittent difficulty in swallowing solid food to total occlusion of the oesophagus, preventing the patient even from swallowing saliva. Oesophageal pain can be extremely severe, and it should not be underestimated. There are three main presentations:

- A burning pain ('heartburn') felt high in the epigastrium and behind the sternum. Often due to the reflux of gastric contents, sometimes radiating to the neck and to one or both arms.
- A deep, boring, gripping pain across the front of the chest, may radiate to the back, neck or arms. Often due to spasm of the oesophageal muscle, similar in nature to the pain of angina pectoris (see Chapter 2).
- Pain behind the sternum on swallowing, especially hot liquids. Usually due to oesophagitis.

Gastro-Oesophageal Reflux Disease

Gastro-oesophageal reflux disease (GORD) is a common condition where the reflux of the contents of the stomach causes troublesome symptoms that may have a significant impact on the physical, social and emotional life quality of those living with it (Information 4.1). The prevalence of GORD is increasing globally.

Pathophysiology and Risk Factors

Normally, the action of swallowing stimulates the relaxation of the lower oesophageal sphincter (LOS), permitting food to pass into the stomach. In GORD, however, there is prolonged or inappropriate relaxation of the LOS, resulting in reflux of gastric contents into the oesophagus. British Medical Journal (BMJ) Best Practice (2022) suggests that those with mild to moderate GORD do not necessarily have more transient LOS relaxations but structural changes at the gastro-oesophageal junction reduce the resistance to reflux during these events. As structural changes become more marked the risk of reflux increases and the reflux volume rises, extending further up the oesophagus. The regurgitation of the highly acidic (pH of 1–4) contents is abrasive to the oesophageal lining resulting in the characteristic symptoms of GORD. Patients suffering from GORD for prolonged periods are at increased risk of developing further complications including Barrett's oesophagus (Information 4.2), a pre-malignant condition which can lead to oesophageal cancer.

Hiatus Hernia

In those with severe GORD symptoms, a hiatus hernia, a condition whereby a portion of the stomach protrudes upwards into the chest through an opening in the diaphragm, is often present (BMJ Best Practice 2022). In this condition, a large amount of gastric contents pass unhindered into the hiatal sac with ensuing severe symptoms. Hiatus hernias occur most frequently from middle age onwards. They are four times more common in women than in men and often found in association with obesity. However, they can also result from a congenital abnormality presenting in early infancy. Hiatus hernias are described as 'sliding' or 'rolling' (para-oesophageal), the former being the more common. In sliding hernias, the oesophageal sphincter mechanism is defective, causing reflux of acid-peptic stomach contents and, as their name suggests, the herniated stomach tends to slide back and forth into and out of the chest. In the less common 'rolling' or para-oesophageal hernia, the gastro-oesophageal junction remains where it belongs but part of the stomach is squeezed up beside the oesophagus. These hernias remain in the chest at all times.

Although the primary cause of GORD is the compromised functioning of the LOS, genetic, environmental, behavioural and comorbid risk factors may also be associated with the development of the condition (Dent et al. 2005). Whilst lifestyle factors such as smoking, alcohol consumption and drugs impairing sphincter pressure (anticholinergics, theophylline, nitrates, calcium channel blockers, progestogens, nicotine replacement therapy) do not cause GORD, they may worsen the symptoms. Obesity has also been associated with GORD, particularly where there is a tendency to consume larger meals and rich, energy-dense foods, increasing the risk of reflux. Dent et al. (2005) found no clear association between certain foods and GORD; however some patients report that fatty foods, citrus fruits, coffee, chocolate etc. can trigger an episode and therefore they avoid them (BMJ Best Practice 2022). Reflux is very common in pregnancy due to progesterone relaxing the gastro-oesophageal sphincter smooth muscle as well as the increased pressure on the stomach as the fetus grows.

Diagnosis

Traditionally, the diagnosis of GORD is based on a combination of clinical evaluation, medical history and diagnostic tests. What is considered important is that treatment and management options are based on patients' reports of symptoms and the impact on their lives.

Pharmacological and lifestyle management is the first line of treatment and routine endoscopic investigation is not considered necessary for those who do not present with 'alarm' symptoms. However, urgent referral for endoscopic investigation is recommended (Information 4.3) in cases where alarm features are present. These include GI bleeding, iron deficiency anaemia, unexplained and unintentional weight loss, progressive dysphagia, persistent vomiting, palpable epigastric mass, a family history of GI cancer, previous documented peptic ulcer or suspicious imaging results (NICE 2019).

Treatment Options

Lifestyle modifications alone are not usually considered effective for the relief of GORD symptoms; they are generally recommended as an adjunct to pharmacological therapy, the backbone of nonsurgical intervention. However, certain factors such as smoking, alcohol consumption and obesity can contribute to frequency and severity of symptoms; so modifications are usually recommended. Dietary adjustments, for example avoiding alcohol and foods that may trigger symptoms, are strategies that patients adopt. Avoiding large meals and eating several hours before going to bed are suggested. For those who are overweight or obese, weight loss can be effective in improving symptoms, elevating the head of the bed is also helpful for some (BMJ Best Practice 2022). Smoking cessation is advised (see Reflection 4.1).

In those with a hiatus hernia and whose symptoms are considered mild, additional advice and education include taking small meals more frequently, wearing loose clothing and avoiding bending over from the waist. Sleeping well supported by pillows is also helpful.

Pharmacological Interventions

Pharmacological intervention forms the mainstay of treatment. The aim of treatment is to manage the symptoms of GORD and reduce the risk of recurrence and complications associated with the disease.

Proton Pump Inhibitors (PPIs). Those with reflux symptoms are given initial treatment with proton pump inhibitors (PPIs). PPIs (e.g. omeprazole, lansoprazole, esomeprazole) are effective acid suppressants and heal reflux oesophagitis in many patients. There is a high rate of symptom recurrence in GORD when PPIs are discontinued and when this occurs long-term and maintenance therapy is required (NICE 2019).

PPIs are considered to be safe and effective and are not associated with the development of abnormal cells or neoplasms (Thomson et al. 2010). However, recent evidence suggests that long term use of PPIs may be associated with the development of abnormal lesions (Lv et. al 2023). More lage scale trials are required to assess this increased risk.

In a minority of patients where PPI therapy is ineffective, altering the medication and dosage under supervision must be undertaken to achieve a level of symptom control.

Histamine H_2-Receptor Antagonists (H_2RAs). Although histamine H_2-receptor antagonists (H_2RAs) such as famotidine and nizatidine also suppress acid, they are considered less effective than PPIs in healing oesophagitis and maintaining remission from mucosal symptoms and injury (BMJ Best Practice 2022). However, they are sometimes used before bed if GORD symptoms are problematic at night.

Gastroprotective Agents. Alginates and antacids (e.g. Gaviscon and Maalox Plus) are widely used because of their over-the-counter availability; they provide instant and temporary relief from symptoms. However, their value in symptom relief is questioned as they have no effect on the healing of erosive oesophagitis. (Leiman et al. 2017)

Surgical Interventions

Most people with GORD respond to pharmacological therapy and lifestyle adjustments or modifications. However, for some, they are ineffective and surgery is an option offering a permanent resolution for symptoms. Surgery is also recommended for those who have volume reflux, respiratory symptoms (e.g. cough/asthma) and Barrett's CLO.

Anti-reflux surgery aims to recreate the LOS, and surgery is commonly performed laparoscopically, enabling a more rapid recovery and reduced hospital stay. It is also associated with reduced pain as there is no abdominal or chest incision and an improved respiratory function postoperatively. Essentially, laparoscopic anti-reflux surgery (LARS) mobilises the lower end of the oesophagus, reduces the oesophageal hiatus using sutures and wraps the fundus of the stomach partially or completely around it (fundoplication).

❖ Nursing Management and Health Promotion: GORD

The majority of patients presenting with GORD are managed in primary and secondary care settings. In many instances the patient may be managed solely by their GP. However, community or practice nurses have the opportunity to provide information and education ensuring the patient understands the role of medication management. Taking time to assess the patient's understanding ensures medication is taken appropriately and can enhance patient adherence to any regimen. Health promotion may involve educating the patient regarding lifestyle modifications including dietary choices and management and smoking cessation.

🔹 Preoperative Management

Preparation for LARS surgery will be as for elective abdominal surgery on the GI tract as described in Chapter 25, Nursing the Patient Undergoing Surgery. In addition, the patient must be given information about the surgery and the risks associated with it. The short- and long-term effects of the surgery and the changes in diet required should be explained in sufficient detail so the patient has a clear understanding of the implications and is making an informed choice to undergo the procedure.

🔹 Postoperative Management

Those undergoing LARS surgery normally stay in hospital for approximately 24–48 hours postsurgery depending on the type of surgery. Nursing management in the postoperative period centres on early detection of and minimising the risk of complications (Information 4.4).

Monitoring of vital signs (temperature, pulse, respirations, blood pressure (BP), oxygen saturation and assessment and management of postoperative pain and nausea and vomiting are key in reducing the potential for complications. Vital sign monitoring should be undertaken half-hourly in the immediate postoperative period; this is gradually reduced to 4-hourly if the patient's vital signs remain within normal parameters.

Pain assessment and documentation should be carried out using a pain assessment tool such as the visual analogue scale (see Chapter 20). Analgesia, for example diclofenac, is commonly used to control pain and is usually administered intravenously. If needed, opiates may be given; should the patient have patient-controlled analgesia (PCA), this will not remove the need for evaluation of the effectiveness of pain relief. This should be undertaken at the same time as vital sign monitoring. Sedation level must also be monitored. The patient should also be offered antiemetics intravenously, minimising the risk of nausea and vomiting. Local policy is adhered to regarding the fasting period. Intravenous (IV) fluids are administered to maintain hydration. The introduction of oral fluids and liquid diet is done in accordance with local policy.

Dietary Advice

If the patient's vital signs are within normal limits, signs of dysphagia are absent and postoperative pain is well controlled, the patient is discharged and written information about lifestyle and dietary modifications is provided. Early dysphagia following LARS is common; patients may be advised to adhere to a liquid diet initially. As symptoms resolve and patients no longer experience food 'sticking', they progress towards a normal diet. In a small number of cases, symptoms persist and may require oesophageal dilatation or surgical revision of the fundoplication.

Patients are advised to eat small, frequent meals in the first few weeks following surgery to counter early feelings of fullness; this usually diminishes over time. Patients who have this type of surgery often lose the ability to belch and may have a tendency to increased bloating and flatulence. They should be advised to chew food thoroughly and avoid excessive swallowing while chewing. Eating large meals should be discouraged and 'fizzy' drinks are not recommended. Where possible, nausea, vomiting and coughing should be prevented, as these increase abdominal pressure and may result in herniation of the stomach into the chest. Antiemetics are used to reduce this. Additionally, patients should avoid heavy lifting, straining and excessive exercise in the early postoperative period.

Carcinoma of the Oesophagus

In 2016–2018, there were around 9300 new oesophageal cancer cases in the UK. Oesophageal cancer is the 14th most common cancer in the UK, accounting for 2% of all new cancer cases (2016–2018). The lower third of the oesophagus is the most common specific location for oesophageal cancers in the UK. Thirty-one per cent of oesophageal cancer cases in the UK are in females, and 69% are in males. In England, there are approximately 1200 cases of oesophageal cancer that are each linked with deprivation. Between 2013 and 2017, in England, it was estimated that rates for oesophageal cancer were lower in the Asian and Black ethnic groups, compared with the White ethnic group (Cancer Research UK 2021).

This form of cancer is extremely unpleasant and distressing, with surgery on its own or in conjunction with chemotherapy offering the only possibility of cure. The prognosis remains poor, and around 12% survive oesophageal cancer for 10 or more years (2013–2017). This has been associated with the late presentation of symptoms in this condition (Cancer Research UK 2021).

● Pathophysiology and Risk Factors

The two main types of oesophageal cancer are squamous cell cancer and adenocarcinoma. The way in which oesophageal squamous cell cancers are staged is different from how oesophageal adenocarcinomas are staged. Treatment may also be different for the two types.

Adenocarcinomas are the most common type of oesophageal cancer in the UK. They are more common in men than women and are linked to being overweight and having a long history of acid reflux. Oesophageal adenocarcinomas mainly affect the lower part of the oesophagus. Squamous cell cancer develops from squamous cells that make up the inner lining of the oesophagus. This is the second most common type of oesophageal cancer in the UK and tends to develop in the upper and middle part of the oesophagus.

The primary tumour can spread locally, up or down the oesophagus, and through its wall to the trachea, bronchi, pleura, aorta and lymph vessels. Distant metastases may occur in the liver and lungs.

Several predisposing factors for oesophageal cancer have been identified (Cancer Research UK 2023a):
- Lifestyle factors such as smoking, alcohol consumption, a diet high in fat and obesity.
- Oesophageal adenocarcinoma risk is more than 11 times higher in people with Barrett's oesophagus versus the general population.
- Around 3%–13% of people with Barrett's oesophagus in the UK will develop oesophageal adenocarcinoma in their lifetime.

Clinical Features

The most prominent presenting feature is dysphagia. In the initial stages, this only occurs occasionally and the individual will probably not seek medical help. However, as the tumour increases in size, it occludes the lumen of the oesophagus. Dyspepsia after eating may also occur. Although pain on swallowing or reflux is less common, their occurrence tends to indicate a spread of the cancer. Poor oral intake due to dysphagia and cancer cachexia causes weight loss. Many patients develop a cough due to pressure on the bronchus, and a chest infection due to aspiration of oesophageal contents. Haematemesis (vomiting of blood which may appear bright red or dark and blackish) and melaena (abnormally dark tarry faeces containing blood) occasionally occur due to bleeding from an ulcerated tumour. The patient will rapidly become emaciated due to difficulty in eating and drinking, and skilled nursing care is essential for comforting and supporting the patient in coping with these and other effects of the illness.

Diagnosis

Where oesophageal carcinoma is suspected, an urgent referral for GI endoscopy is recommended (NICE 2021).

NICE (2023) guidance provides information on the assessment and management of oesophago-gastric cancer, addressing the staging and management of oesophago-gastric cancer.

This approach provides information regarding the location and size of the primary tumour, whether or not it is operable and whether or not metastatic disease exists. If the tumour is deemed to be operable, endoscopic ultrasound (EUS) assesses and stages the tumour. Bronchoscopy may be performed if the tumour is in the upper zone, identifying whether the bronchus has been invaded and will have a bearing on treatment and care.

Treatment Options

Despite the generally poor prognosis, there are a number of treatment options for those with oesophageal cancer. These include surgery and chemotherapy, surgery alone, endoscopic resection, chemotherapy, chemoradiotherapy and palliative care. These options depend primarily on the location, histology and spread of the tumour, as well as patient characteristics and the existence of comorbidities. Each patient is carefully assessed as to the extent of the disease before a treatment plan is chosen and commenced. Surgery remains the standard treatment where the tumour is localised or operable. However, chemotherapy is now commonly administered preoperatively as it has been demonstrated not only to improve outcome in respect of survival but also helps in reducing the tumour size, improving tumour-related symptoms and improving nutritional status and weight gain. Chemoradiotherapy is administered if the tumour is radiosensitive, i.e. a squamous cell carcinoma. This treatment is usually used for tumours of the upper third of the oesophagus, but is also sometimes used for the relief of pain. For those with inoperable carcinoma of the oesophagus, the focus of palliative treatment is on symptom relief. Malignant dysphagia may be relieved by oesophageal dilatation, endoluminal stenting, endoscopic or open insertion of a stent, or tumour ablation with laser, heat, diathermy or injection of cytotoxic substances (Hanna et al. 2012).

❖ Nursing Management and Health Promotion: Oesophageal Carcinoma

Nursing management will depend on whether treatment is surgical or nonsurgical.

● Surgical: Preoperative Management

In addition to the standard preoperative preparation for all patients who are undergoing GI surgery (see Chapter 25), there are particular considerations that must be attended to in the patient who is to have an oesophagectomy. There are several types of oesophagectomy (Information 4.5), and the choice is determined by the location and size of the tumour as well as the level of fitness to tolerate what is a physically demanding surgery. Oesophagectomy is procedurally difficult; it involves the cardiovascular system and carries with it a significant morbidity. Therefore thorough physiological assessment and preparation must be undertaken in order to minimise the impact for the patient.

In patients who are experiencing nutritional deficits due to dysphagia, nutritional assessment using a tool such as the Malnutrition Universal Screening Tool (MUST) (British Association for Parenteral and Enteral Nutrition (BAPEN) 2018) is fundamental, and it is essential that any deficiencies are addressed preoperatively. This can be undertaken by encouraging the patient to sip nutritional supplements or, where deemed necessary, through the use of fine-bore nasogastric tube feeding.

Psychological and emotional preparation is extremely important for these patients and their families. Patients should be educated as to what to expect in the immediate postoperative period but should also be counselled as to the impact on lifestyle and quality of life in the medium and long term.

● Surgical: Postoperative Management

In addition to standard postoperative care (see Chapter 25), there are specific management considerations for patients following oesophagectomy. Given the significant risk of a number of complications, patients are often nursed in intensive care for approximately 2 days after surgery. Intensive cardiopulmonary monitoring is undertaken as the risk of respiratory complications is high. Physiotherapy, humidified oxygen for several days and nursing the patient in a semiupright position are some additional strategies that are used to reduce the incidence of respiratory complications. Given the nature and complexity of the surgery, pain intensity is high following oesophagectomy. Failure to adequately control pain can contribute to poor inspiration and ventilation, which increases the likelihood of respiratory problems. Thus, epidural analgesia (see Chapter 20) is one method of pain control (Royal College of Surgeons 2014). Careful assessment and monitoring of the patient's wound(s) and wound drains must also be undertaken.

Nutrition

Oral fluids and diet are withheld for the first 5–7 days following surgery. The patient will have a nasogastric tube on free drainage to ensure the stomach remains decompressed in order to facilitate healing. In order to combat further nutritional depletion, enteral feeding is commenced using a feeding tube such as a jejunostomy that can be inserted at the time of surgery. Feeding continues until the patient is able to take sufficient oral intake. Fluids are given intravenously whilst the patient is nil by mouth. Careful monitoring and accurate recording of fluids and enteral feeding are required throughout. Postoperative feeding via the jejunal route is routine in some centres and this may improve nutritional status, although evidence to show improved clinical outcomes compared with standard care is currently lacking. It is recommended that nutritional support be provided for all patients who are malnourished or at risk of malnutrition and have an inadequate oral intake, defined as having eaten little or nothing for more than 5 days and/or likely to eat little or nothing for the next 5 days or longer. Preferably this should be given via the GI tract if it is functioning and adequate access can be obtained National Institute for Health and Care Excellence (2006/2017). A barium swallow is performed to determine there is no leaking of the anastomosis. Once a leak has been discounted the patient may commence on progressive fluids, only gradually progressing on to a soft and finally normal diet.

Psychological Support

In addition, in the initial postoperative period, the nurse will be required to provide considerable assistance to the patient with meeting their activities of living. The patient can expect to remain in hospital for up to 2 weeks. However, convalescence and recovery are slow and it can take the patient several months to adjust to the negative physical, psychological and social effects of the surgery. In 2006, Verschuur et al. (2006) found that physical issues were perceived by patients as most problematic and were cited as early satiety (fullness), eating problems, fatigue,

---

INFORMATION 4.5

Types of oesophagectomy

- Two-phase subtotal oesophagectomy via a right thoracotomy (Ivor-Lewis)
- Three-phase subtotal oesophagectomy (McKeown)
- Left-sided subtotal oesophagectomy
- Transhiatal oesophagectomy

For further information see van Baalen (2009).

constipation/diarrhoea, pain and weight loss. Because of physical problems, patients can find it difficult to return to normal social activity. Fear of a return of the cancer or the development of metastases tends to cause patients to have low moods associated with an unpredictable future. Patients can also feel frustrated at being dependent on others or being unable to resume normal activities.

It is essential therefore that continued support either through specialist nurse follow-up and/or community nurse should form part of the overall care of patients following oesophagectomy. Education and advice regarding strategies for management of physical problems should continue in the follow-up period. Moreover patients should be given the opportunity to discuss the psychological and social implications of the surgery. Given the ultimately poor prognosis, it is important that patients and their families feel supported throughout.

Nonsurgical Management

Many patients with this form of cancer will be very distressed and emaciated, their life dominated by the symptoms of the disease and by the thought that there is no cure. However, by adopting a caring and sensitive approach, the nurse can do much to alleviate the patient's physical and emotional suffering.

Nutrition and Weight Loss

Some patients experience significant weight loss, for example several kilograms over a period of months. Weight should be recorded weekly and noted in relation to pre-illness weight. An accurate account of daily dietary intake should be recorded with the dietitian's help. Consistency of food is important and the patient should avoid large pieces of meat, 'stringy' foods such as oranges and 'stodgy' foods such as scones and pastries, as these food choices may lead to blocking of the oesophageal lumen. The patient should be encouraged to take fluids with meals and to chew foods thoroughly, for example, twice as long as normal. In order to ensure adequate nutrition it may be necessary to provide a liquidised diet. Nutritional assessment and specialist dietetic support should be provided to people with oesophago-gastric cancer prior to, during and post radical treatments. Further guidance concerning nutritional support for adults is provided by NICE (2017).

As the disease advances, the patient will be able to swallow liquids only and should be supplied with a variety of nutritionally supplemented liquids. Supplementary drinks are now available in a variety of sweet and savoury flavours. Eventually, total dysphagia will occur. It cannot be overemphasised how distressing this is for the patient and family. See Chapter 22, Nutrition and Health, for more information on nutritional care.

Oesophageal Stent

In the case of a bolus obstruction, it may be necessary to perform an endoscopy to relieve the obstruction. The insertion of a stent is often used to relieve dysphagic symptoms. The oesophagus is dilated at endoscopy and the tube inserted. Following this procedure, the patient will lose the action of the gastro-oesophageal sphincter and will therefore suffer from reflux. The head of the bed should be elevated at all times. The patient will be prescribed an H_2 blocking agent, e.g. cimetidine, to help prevent reflux oesophagitis. This should be given in syrup form. Encouragement should be given to eat a semi-solid diet and to chew food well. The patient should take carbonated drinks, e.g. soda or tonic water, with every meal as this helps keep the stent clear.

Immediately after the insertion of a stent, the patient may suffer quite severe discomfort and analgesics may be necessary. A chest X-ray will be performed and the patient should not be allowed any food or fluid until this has been done in case perforation of the oesophagus has occurred.

Pain

In the earlier stages of oesophageal cancer, if pain is present, mild analgesics such as paracetamol given in dispersible form may be all that is necessary. As disease advances, opiates may be required. Initially, the patient may be able to swallow a morphine suspension, but if total occlusion of the oesophagus occurs, morphine by injection may be needed. The most effective and convenient way of administering this is by the subcutaneous route using a syringe driver. This delivers a constant level of opioid and allows for a 'booster' dose to be given as necessary, to avoid the distress of breakthrough pain. If circumstances allow, the patient will be able to be at home with a community nurse support to change the syringe. If necessary, an antiemetic can also be added to the syringe driver.

Time must be set aside to allow these patients to express their thoughts, fears and anger, which may be directed towards either the distressing nature of their symptoms or the poor prognosis of the disease, or perhaps both. In the final stages of the disease, every effort should be made to allow the patient to die in the environment of their own choosing. If the patient's choice is to remain at home, a Macmillan or Marie Curie nurse can provide the support and care required.

Disorders of the Stomach and Duodenum

Disorders of the stomach and duodenum are the most common organic disorders of the GI tract. They are considered together here because disorders of one organ commonly affect the other.

Peptic Ulcer

It is difficult to establish the exact prevalence of peptic ulcer disease, as the definitions used vary between studies, and endoscopy is needed to make a formal diagnosis (NICE 2019).

A peptic ulcer occurs in those parts of the digestive tract that are exposed to gastric secretions, namely the stomach and duodenum. Previously, peptic ulcer disease was thought to be a chronic relapsing condition that required long-term acid suppression therapy and often major surgical intervention. There was also an associated mortality due to major GI haemorrhage and development of gastric cancer. The identification of the *Helicobacter pylori* bacterium by Marshall and Warren in 1984, and its association with peptic ulcer disease, radically altered the management of this condition, especially with the shift in focus in the National Health Service (NHS) from secondary to primary care.

Pathophysiology and Risk Factors

Peptic ulcer formation requires both the presence of gastric acid and damage to the mucosal defence barrier. *H. pylori* is known to be a major factor in causing this damage; the pathogen has been isolated in 50% of the world population and is present in over 95% of all patients with duodenal ulcers and 80%–90% of those with gastric ulcers (Banning 2012). Gastric irritant medications such as aspirin and nonsteroidal anti-inflammatory drugs (NSAIDs) are also known to cause mucosal damage. Cigarette smoking is considered to be a causative influence in the development of peptic ulcers and there is growing evidence that smoking prevents the healing of gastric and duodenal ulcers (Prabhu and Shivani 2014). The exact mechanisms by which this occurs are not clear, but it is known that long-term smoking increases gastric secretion and interferes with the actions of H_2RAs.

The gastric mucosa is protected, in part, by being buffered by food but erratic dietary habits may contribute to ulcer formation. There is conflicting evidence as to whether emotional factors such as stress and anxiety are also causative factors.

In *H. pylori* infection, the bacteria burrow beneath the mucosal layer and release a toxin that results in a local inflammatory and systemic immune response. Consequently there is inhibition of the release of somatostatin, a gastric hormone that inhibits gastric acid formation, and oversecretion results. *H. pylori* survives in this acid climate by enzymatically creating an alkaline microenvironment.

Chronic peptic ulcers penetrate through the mucosa to the muscle layers and may damage blood vessels, causing bleeding. In the duodenum, they are found immediately beyond the pylorus and in 10%–15% of cases are multiple. The resulting fibrosis can lead to pyloric stenosis, which in turn can lead to gastric outlet obstruction. Gastric ulcers are found on the lesser curvature of the stomach in most cases.

Clinical Features

The person with a chronic peptic ulcer will describe a pattern of episodic pain and dyspepsia. Pain is a classic symptom and is described as a burning or boring pain in the epigastrium; often patients point directly to where the pain is felt. The pain is sometimes more diffuse or radiates through to the back. Patients sometimes experience 'water brash', which is saliva filling the mouth.

While studies show that the relationship to food and mealtimes is variable, the person with a duodenal ulcer is more likely to feel pain and 'hunger feelings' about 2–3 hours after a meal, whereas with a gastric ulcer pain is felt about 30–60 minutes after a meal and is not relieved by more food. Sometimes patients explain that they have induced vomiting in an attempt to relieve the pain. Persistent noninduced vomiting of large amounts indicates an obstruction to the pylorus: pyloric stenosis. Other common features are belching and regurgitation which causes heartburn.

Diagnosis

An accurate diagnosis of peptic ulceration is made by endoscopy and/or barium meal. A full blood count (FBC) is taken for haemoglobin (Hb) estimation. Diagnosis of *H. pylori* infection is commonly made using the noninvasive ^{13}C-urea breath test. *H. pylori* produces urease as a source of protection from the harmful effects of gastric hydrochloric acid. The breath test detects isotopic carbon dioxide after ingestion of radiocarbon-labelled urea. The *H. pylori* enzyme splits the carbon from the urea. It is then carried as carbon dioxide via the blood to the lungs, where it can be detected in exhaled breath. This test is specific and has 80%–90% sensitivity as no other bacterium is known to produce the urease enzyme. Moreover the test can be undertaken in a GP's surgery and reduces patient discomfort and distress associated with an endoscopy.

Alternatively, the diagnosis of *H. pylori* infection can be made by blood or serum tests for antibodies, and at endoscopy by taking a biopsy from the stomach lining and subjecting it to the rapid urease test, which detects the enzyme that *H. pylori* produces.

Treatment Options

Treatment is dependent on the cause and severity of the ulcer. Removal of the causative factor followed by healing of the ulcer is the main aim of treatment, e.g. eradication therapy in *H. pylori* or discontinuation of NSAIDs or aspirin, followed by acid-suppressing medication.

Advice should be given about avoiding known aggravating factors such as smoking and erratic dietary patterns. Patient adherence to medication regimens is crucial to the success of *H. pylori* eradication and ulcer healing. Therefore patient education is essential (Reflection 4.2).

Pharmacological therapy may include:
- A PPI, e.g. omeprazole, esomeprazole to inhibit the release of hydrochloric acid from the parietal cells.
- H_2RAs, e.g. nizatidine, famotidine. These assist in ulcer healing by preventing histamine from stimulating the gastric parietal cells to secrete hydrochloric acid.
- Antacids for the relief of dyspepsia. Many preparations are based on magnesium and may result in a degree of diarrhoea.
- Misoprostol two to four times a day. Misoprostol inhibits gastric acid secretion by acting directly on the parietal cells. It is also used to prevent the gastric damage that can occur from long-term use of NSAIDs.
- Where the existence of *H. pylori* is confirmed, eradication therapy (combined/triple therapy) is the first-line treatment. It is given for a period of 7 days and consists of:
  - a PPI (e.g. lansoprazole/omeprazole) twice daily in conjunction with two antibiotics, commonly:
  - clarithromycin three times a day and/or
  - amoxicillin three times daily and/or
  - metronidazole three times daily.

In patients with penicillin allergy, it is common practice to use clarithromycin instead of amoxicillin. Substitution is also necessary where bacterial resistance is suspected. This regimen is effective in eradicating *H. pylori* in 75%–90% of cases and can be assessed by a resolution of the symptoms and confirmed with a repeat ^{13}C-urea breath test. If the test is still positive a further course of eradication therapy should be given but with different antibiotics.

In some cases of *H. pylori*, antisecretory treatment (PPIs or H_2RAs) is continued for 4–8 weeks to ensure ulcer healing. Long-term acid-lowering therapy such as NSAID therapy may be required if there are complicating factors.

Surgical intervention may be necessary for patients with peptic ulcer and the indications are as follows:
- failure to respond to medical therapy
- recurrence
- development of complications such as perforation, haemorrhage and pyloric stenosis.

REFLECTION 4.2

Identifying priorities of care for the patient with a duodenal ulcer

Mr R, who lives alone, has been diagnosed as having a duodenal ulcer. He is 54 years old. He has lost a lot of weight over the last few months as a result of vomiting and does not eat much now. He is very thin and is also very anxious. He admits that he smokes 30–40 cigarettes a day and has difficulty sleeping.

Activity
- Reflect on what the priorities of care may be for Mr R.

The aim of surgical intervention is to reduce acid and pepsin secretion. This is achieved by interrupting the vagus nerve or by resection of the gastric acid-producing section of the stomach.

❖ Nursing Management and Health Promotion: Peptic Ulcer

Surgery for peptic ulceration is rarely necessary and is used only for complications. Although the incidence of perforation is decreasing, duodenal ulcers perforate more often than gastric ulcers and usually into the peritoneal sac causing peritonitis. Surgery is performed to close the perforation and drain the abdomen. In recurrent uncontrolled haemorrhage, the bleeding vessel is ligated.

◉ Preoperative Management

The patient who is to undergo an elective procedure may be admitted 1 day prior to surgery or, if otherwise healthy, may be requested to attend a pre-admission clinic. This allows time for medical examination to be made regarding the individual's fitness for the operation and a general anaesthetic. A blood sample is required for grouping and cross-matching in case blood transfusion is required. Other tests are undertaken as per local policy and procedure.

A full nursing assessment is made and a care plan formulated to meet the specific needs identified and to fulfil standard preoperative nursing requirements (see Chapter 25). Explanations are given of the timescale for the preparation that will take place. If the patient is a smoker, the importance of smoking cessation is emphasised and support to do so is offered.

Preparation of the GI tract will be based on local preference. On the morning of the operation, the patient is prepared for theatre. Prior to surgery, regular vital signs recordings are made in order to detect any deterioration in the patient's condition. Analgesics are given for pain relief, and clear, concise explanations are given to the patient and the relatives regarding treatment.

◉ Postoperative Management

On the patient's return to the ward, the nurse will monitor and/or observe the following:
- Airway, respiratory rate, skin colour, BP, pulse, temperature, oxygen saturation level and bleeding/drainage from the wound and the wound drain if present. Careful monitoring of these is important during the first 24–48 hours, decreasing in frequency as haemodynamic stability is regained.
- Nasogastric aspirate. The nasogastric tube is usually left on free drainage between aspirations to allow air to escape. The aspirate should be observed for colour and amount. Normally, the volume of aspirate reduces and reduced bowel sounds (borborygmi) are heard within 24–48 hours. Should large amounts of aspirate continue, this would indicate that absorption from the stomach is not occurring; it may also indicate the onset of paralytic ileus (see Chapter 25). Care should be taken that the nasogastric tube is positioned comfortably and well supported. Nasal care is given as required. The nurse should be cautious when assessing a patient to determine if bowel sounds have returned (however assessing for bowel sounds has been questioned by some authors).
- IV infusion and cannula site. The IV infusion must be maintained as prescribed, to preserve fluid and electrolyte balance and to prevent dehydration while oral fluids are not being taken.
- Urinary output. Renal function is a good indicator of tissue perfusion.

- National Early Warning Score 2 (NEWS2) (Royal College of Physicians (RCP) 2018) is implemented in order to monitor and detect any deterioration in the patient's condition.

Nutrition and Hydration

Fluids are usually withheld for at least 24 hours, after which period, sips of water or ice chips may be given according to local policy and procedure. Fluids may then be given at increasing frequency and gradually increasing until free amounts of fluid are well tolerated. Light, easily digested food is gradually introduced and the patient is encouraged to eat, but is asked to avoid drinking fluids for at least 30 minutes after meals (see 'dumping syndrome', below). Oral hygiene is also important and the patient's mouth should be kept clean and moist using mouthwashes or by brushing the teeth if the patient can tolerate this.

Mobilisation

Following surgery, patients should be encouraged to sit up, get out of bed and take a few steps as soon as possible. They should also be encouraged to breathe deeply and cough regularly to clear the lungs of anaesthetic gases and excess mucus. These measures will help to prevent chest infection. Regular gentle leg activity, even when in bed, can also help to prevent the development of deep vein thrombosis. Adequate analgesia and holding the wound firmly when moving or coughing will encourage the patient to cooperate actively with postoperative therapy.

Dumping Syndrome (Rapid Gastric Emptying)

Dumping syndrome is a postoperative complication of gastric surgery that may occur following eating. It can be separated into early and late forms according to how soon it occurs after eating a meal. Dumping syndrome occurs when the undigested contents of the stomach are transported or 'dumped' too quickly into the small intestine. The sudden emptying of hyperosmolar solutions into the small bowel results in rapid distension of the jejunal loop anastomosed to the stomach and a withdrawal of water from the circulating blood volume into the jejunum to dilute the high concentration of electrolytes and sugars. Symptoms of early dumping include nausea, vomiting, bloating, cramping, diarrhoea, dizziness and fatigue. They tend to occur within 10–15 minutes of eating and usually settle within 30–60 minutes. Symptoms of late epigastric fullness and dumping include weakness, excessive sweating and dizziness (Cudd 2018).

In order to delay stomach emptying and minimise the occurrence of dumping symptoms, patients should be educated to eat with their head at a 15–45 degree elevation. They should eat small meals more frequently and where possible these should be of a dry consistency. Fluids should be consumed up to 1 hour before or after eating but should not be taken with meals. Concentrated sources of carbohydrate such as high-energy snacks and drinks should be avoided, but fat can be consumed as tolerated. After meals, patients should lie down for 20–30 minutes or until symptoms subside. If symptoms persist, changes in dietary intake and further surgery may eventually be indicated.

Discharge Planning

Patients who have undergone surgery for peptic ulceration are assessed for safe discharge usually within a week of the operation. However, those with concurrent disease may need a longer period in hospital. Therefore, it is important for the nurse to be fully aware of the patient's social circumstances so that from the time of admission adequate preparation for discharge can be made and potential problems anticipated. Early communication with the patient's family or friends is essential in planning for discharge.

An outpatient follow-up appointment may be arranged to ensure that a satisfactory recovery has been achieved, to discuss any ongoing management and to monitor the patient's rehabilitation. The GP is always given details of the patient's surgery and discharge and of any special aftercare that may be required. If continuing care of the wound is required, this should be arranged with the community nursing team or practice nurse prior to discharge.

Complications of Peptic Ulceration

The three major complications of peptic ulcer are:
- haemorrhage
- perforation
- pyloric stenosis.

Carcinoma of the Stomach

Gastric cancer (stomach cancer, cancer that starts anywhere inside the stomach or the stomach wall) is often asymptomatic until the disease is advanced (de Wit et al. 2017).

Stomach cancer is more common in men than women, with more than 50% occurring in people aged 75 or over. Most stomach cancers are linked to lifestyle or environmental factors and this includes diet. Stomach cancer is linked with the bacterium *H. pylori* which lives in the stomach; however, not everyone with *H. pylori* will develop stomach cancer.

In the year 2016–17, there were around 6500 new stomach cancer cases in the UK; it is the 17th most common cancer. Incidence rates (2016–18) are highest in people aged 85 to 89 years. Around 1300 cases of stomach cancer each year in England are linked with deprivation; incidence rates are lower in the Asian ethnic group, higher in the Black ethnic group and similar in people of mixed or multiple ethnicity, compared with the White ethnic group, in England (Cancer Research UK 2023b).

The most common specific location for stomach cancers in the UK is the cardia.

Tobacco smoking is classified by the International Agency for Research on Cancer (IARC 2017) as a cause of stomach cancer, with 15% of stomach cancer cases in the UK being caused by smoking (Brown et al. 2018).

Stomach cancer risk is 2–10 times higher in people with a family history of the disease (Yaghoobi et al. 2010).

Pathophysiology and Risk Factors

Gastric carcinomas are almost always adenocarcinomas derived from the mucus-secreting cells of the gastric glands; 60% occur at the pylorus or in the antrum, 20%–30% in the body of the stomach and 5%–20% in the cardia. The tumour spreads along the gastric wall to the duodenum and oesophagus and through the wall to the peritoneum. Adjacent organs become infiltrated. Metastatic spread may occur locally to neighbouring organs within the peritoneal cavity, or via the lymphatic or blood vessels to the liver, lungs and bones.

Clinical Features

In the initial stages, symptoms do not differ significantly from indigestion or a feeling of having an 'upset stomach'. Individuals report feeling full or distended after eating. Common symptoms include anorexia, loss of weight and epigastric pain. These are often tolerated despite the distress they cause, with the result that there may be considerable delay before the patient seeks medical help. Nausea and vomiting may also occur whilst weakness, anaemia, retrosternal back pain and darkened stool or melaena have also been reported. By the time the person seeks medical help, the disease may be well advanced and may have spread to adjacent organs. Tumours that are located in the cardia or fundus of the stomach can cause dysphagia, among other symptoms. If a tumour obstructs the pylorus, the individual will experience dramatic weight loss and dehydration and is likely to vomit small amounts of undigested food on a regular basis.

Diagnosis

Around a third of stomach cancer cases in England are diagnosed after presenting as an emergency. Overall, around 60% of those with gastric cancer will not be eligible for curative treatment due to late presentation or comorbidities (Lordick et al. 2022).

Diagnosis can be made by medical history, clinical examination and a barium meal, usually confirmed by computed tomography (CT) scanning. Fibreoptic gastroscopy allows direct inspection and a biopsy to be taken.

Treatment Options

The prognosis for those with gastric cancer remains poor. Surgery still offers the best hope of a cure and even in more advanced stages is undertaken to relieve symptoms. A partial or total gastrectomy, which is either palliative or so-called 'curative', depending on the extent of the tumour, may be undertaken. The treatment option available will depend on:
- Where the cancer is.
- How far it has grown or spread (the stage).
- The type of cancer.
- How abnormal the cells look under a microscope (the grade).
- The patient's general health and level of fitness.

The multidisciplinary team (MDT), a team of nurses, doctors and other professionals, discuss the best treatment and care for the patient and with the patient (and if appropriate the family).

The results of a large clinical trial on operable tumours (the MAGIC trial) examined the benefits of chemotherapy before and after surgery (Choi and Kim 2015). It was found that chemotherapy before surgery reduced the size of the tumour, making it easier to resect. Similarly, in patients with what are initially considered to be inoperable tumours, resection can be made possible with chemotherapy. In patients with advanced disease, palliative chemotherapy may be used to shrink or slow down progression of the tumour or relieve symptoms. Radiotherapy may also shrink a tumour and is used to relieve pain or stop bleeding.

Although multiple phase trials have been performed globally, no standard of care exists for the treatment of gastric cancer. Choi and Kim (2015) suggest that ongoing prospective randomised trials may help better refine clinical factors to best determine the timing of chemotherapy and radiation in relation to surgery for gastric cancer.

Nursing Management and Health Promotion: Carcinoma of the Stomach

Preoperative Management

For details of perioperative nursing priorities in abdominal surgery see Chapter 25, Nursing the Patient Undergoing Surgery.

Similar to those undergoing surgery for oesophageal cancer, there are particular considerations that must be attended to in the patient who is to have a partial or complete gastrectomy. In addition to the thorough physiological assessment needed prior to surgery, these patients may require nutritional support preoperatively. Nutritional assessment using a tool such as MUST (BAPEN 2018) is essential in order to identify actual and potential deficiencies such as weight loss, nausea and vomiting, dietary changes or impediments to sufficient calorific intake. Changes to elimination pattern should also be assessed. Where the patient is found to be debilitated or undernourished, parenteral nutrition should be considered.

Psychological and emotional preparation is a fundamental aspect of care as these patients are undergoing major surgery whilst already living with a traumatising diagnosis. Primarily, some effort should be directed at allaying the patient's fears and anxieties regarding the impending surgery. Time should be taken to answer questions and the patient and their family should be encouraged to verbalise fears and concerns. Patients and their families will require explanations and a discussion of what to expect in the immediate postoperative period.

🔴 Postoperative Management

Partial or total gastrectomy is major surgery and intensive monitoring of vital signs and the recording of NEWS2 are required in the immediate postoperative period. Pain management and evaluation of the effectiveness of analgesia are fundamental. Where the patient has a PCA pump, it should not be assumed that it is effective. Pain relief should be sufficient to enable the patient to mobilise, perform deep breathing and coughing and undertake leg exercises (see Chapter 20).

The patient will have a nasogastric tube and strict monitoring of the type and amount of drainage is required. Some bloody drainage for the first 12 hours is expected, but excessive bleeding should be reported. Drainage is less following a total gastrectomy as there is no longer a reservoir. Ensure the tube is secured to prevent dislocation as this would result in increased pain and distension.

Parenteral nutrition may already be in place or commenced following surgery to meet the patient's calorific needs, to replace fluids lost through drainage and vomiting and to support the patient metabolically until oral intake is adequate. Patients who have had abdominal surgery will experience paralytic ileus following handling of the bowel (see Chapter 25). Care provision must be based on best available evidence and in alignment with local policy and procedure. Therefore, oral intake will not be resumed until borborygmi returns and the patient will require supplementary IV fluids. After the return of bowel sounds and removal of the nasogastric tube, fluids may be commenced. Food in small portions should be gradually introduced and added until the patient is able to eat six small meals a day and drink 120 mL of fluid between meals; this must all be tailored to meet the needs of the individual patient.

Following gastrectomy, patients may have a urinary catheter in situ in order to accurately measure kidney function and output. Depending on the type of gastrectomy performed, patients may have a thoracic and/or abdominal incision. The dressing should be observed for signs of bleeding and output from wound drains strictly monitored and recorded.

Patients should be assisted with mobilising as soon as possible postoperatively. Whilst in bed, the patient should be positioned in a low Fowler's position (head elevation 15–45 degrees) to promote comfort and aid gastric emptying.

Complications of gastric surgery include dysphagia, gastric retention, bile reflux, dumping syndrome and vitamin and mineral deficiencies. Gastric retention causes abdominal distension, nausea and vomiting and it may be necessary to reinstate nil by mouth status and nasogastric drainage. Regurgitation may occur if the patient eats too much or too quickly. At times, oedema along the suture line may prevent fluids and food from moving into the intestinal tract. It is important that pressure remains low in the remaining portion of the stomach or the pouch to avoid disrupting the sutures.

Discharge Planning

Detailed information about diet, pain management and monitoring for the onset of complications should be given in verbal and written form when preparing the patient and their family for discharge. Teaching the patient about dietary self-management is essential. The nurse should ensure that the patient understands the strategies for prevention and management of dumping syndrome (see earlier). In addition, patients should be encouraged to eat a diet that is high in protein with reduced sugar and salt. They should also be encouraged to monitor their weight. Anaemia is common in those who have had a total gastrectomy as there is a reduction in gastric acid production and a deficiency of intrinsic factor. These patients will require vitamin B_{12} injections at 3-monthly intervals.

Patients and their families should be informed of the signs and symptoms of complications such as bleeding, obstruction and perforation and should have impressed upon them the importance of seeking medical help where symptoms worsen or do not resolve.

Long-Term Care After Palliative Surgery

After the patient has been discharged home, it is very likely that the symptoms of the cancer will gradually increase. Skilful and sensitive nursing care will be required to help the patient to remain as comfortable and as free from anxiety as possible.

Pain from the tumour, metastases and ascites can be relieved initially by oral morphine sulphate (MST), progressing, as the need arises, to the judicious use of opioid analgesics, usually diamorphine, given subcutaneously via a syringe driver. Such delivery gives a consistent level of analgesia and is often the key factor in enabling the patient to be pain-free and to remain at home.

Dietary intake may prove a problem. Persistent nausea and vomiting may develop and be difficult to control. Regular and pre-emptive antiemetic medication can be most beneficial. Meals should be small and ideally served at times when the effect of antiemetics is at its optimal level. Nutritious drinks (containing vitamins, minerals, protein and high in calories) can help to supplement nutrition without extra effort on the part of the patient.

Diarrhoea and constipation can both occur. A common side-effect of opiate analgesics is constipation, for which an oral laxative should be prescribed. Orally or rectally administered medications can help to control these symptoms, as can dietary advice.

Mouth infections such as candidiasis are very common and occur in all malignant disease. Nystatin lozenges or suspensions may be given after meals and oral hygiene and dental/denture care must be meticulously maintained.

For some patients there may be the added distress of ascites, which is an accumulation of serous fluid within the peritoneal cavity that can cause pressure on other abdominal organs and the respiratory system. Abdominal paracentesis (see Information 4.6),

INFORMATION 4.6

Abdominal paracentesis

In intractable ascites, i.e. when sodium restrictions and diuretic therapy have little effect, it is possible to drain the fluid from the peritoneal cavity by means of a catheter inserted through the abdominal wall. This procedure is known as abdominal paracentesis. Such patients are already hypoproteinaemic and the sudden loss of fluid and protein by paracentesis is likely to lead to a shift of both from the rest of the body into the abdominal cavity, sometimes with consequent hypovolaemia, shock and even death. The protein is therefore replaced at the time of paracentesis by an infusion of salt-poor albumin.

The patient's blood pressure should be monitored closely and the fluid drained no more quickly than at a rate of approximately 2 L/h. Strict aseptic technique should be used when inserting the catheter to avoid introducing infection that can lead to bacterial peritonitis. This procedure requires cooperation from the patient to lie relatively still in bed while the catheter is in situ over several hours. Help will be required from the nursing staff to maintain comfort over this period. Any leakage on removal of the catheter can be collected in a drainable bag until the puncture site heals (usually within 48 hours).

Nursing management of a patient during paracentesis

Monitor and record vital signs for baseline data prior to the procedure. Vital signs should be recorded every 15 minutes during the procedure, thereafter 15–30 minutes for the first hour, and hourly for the following 2 hours until the patient is cardiovascularly stable. The paracentesis catheter may be in place for 4–6 hours. Monitor neurological signs for signs of increased confusion, i.e. hepatic encephalopathy. Monitor for signs of infection. Record intake and output including ascitic drainage, replacement albumin if required and urine output. Notify the physician/medical team if any signs of deterioration occur. The INR, prothrombin time and platelet counts should be checked and corrected prior to large-volume paracentesis (LVP) (Steen-Pedersen et al., 2015). Patients may require LVP every 2–4 weeks, and the procedure can be undertaken in the outpatient setting.

whereby the ascitic fluid can be drained off, may be preferred to relieve the symptoms. Diuretics may also be used.

Patients with incurable gastric cancer are likely to experience psychological distress. The support of the community nursing team and where possible the Macmillan or Marie Curie nursing services can prove indispensable in giving the patient the confidence to remain at home rather than in hospital. Visits by such a nurse, as well as ensuring that the practical aspects of care are achieved, give the patient and the family the opportunity to talk about fears and worries. The visiting nurse is in an ideal position to monitor the well-being of all parties and to recognise when plans of care should be reviewed. Chapter 31, Nursing the Patient With Cancer, and Chapter 32, Nursing Patients Who Need Palliative Care, explore many ways in which a sensitive continuity of care can be achieved, whether in hospital, at home or in a hospice.

Disorders of the Small and Large Intestines

Unlike disorders of the upper GI tract, in which the major problem is that of ingestion of nutrients, disorders of the small and large intestines result in problems of absorption of nutrients or the transit and elimination of bowel contents. People suffering from such problems complain of varying degrees of abdominal pain and discomfort, diarrhoea and/or constipation. Often the symptoms are insidious and/or embarrassing, such that they are ignored or tolerated and not mentioned even to close relatives.

Malabsorption Syndromes

Malabsorption is a consequence of impaired digestion or absorption of nutrients from the intestinal lumen.

● Pathophysiology and Risk Factors

Malabsorption is caused by a number of conditions. These include:
- Lack of digestive enzyme activity, as in chronic pancreatitis (CP) and hypolactasia.
- Lack of bile salts, as in common bile duct obstruction and liver disease.
- Loss or damage to the absorptive area, as in coeliac disease, extensive bowel resection or CD.
- Failure of adequate removal from the interstitial fluid of absorbed nutrients, as in obstruction of lymphatic drainage.

Clinical Features

Whatever the cause, the presenting signs and symptoms of malabsorption are essentially the same. Patients may complain of frothy, greasy and bulky stools that are difficult to flush away (steatorrhoea), diarrhoea, weight loss and abdominal distension.

Vitamin and mineral deficiencies due to malabsorption may result in anaemia, lack of iron, folate and vitamin B_{12}, bleeding disorders and purpura due to lack of vitamin K, and peripheral neuropathy due to lack of vitamins A and B. Protein deficiency can result in oedema and the musculoskeletal system may also be affected by osteopenia due to lack of calcium, vitamin D and phosphate and tetany due to lack of calcium.

Diagnosis

When a careful history and clinical examination suggest malabsorption, the following diagnostic tests will be carried out to determine the cause:
- faecal fat estimation,
- glucose and lactose tolerance tests,
- haematological studies,
- radiological and barium studies and
- endoscopic examination and biopsy.

Treatment Options

The form of treatment offered will clearly depend upon the cause of the malabsorption. In coeliac disease, where there is sensitivity to gluten, or in lactose intolerance, the advice seems simple: avoid foods containing the offending element. However, for the individual, such advice is not always easy to follow and the condition can potentially cause disruption and stress in everyday life, undermining the sense of well-being. Where malabsorption is part of, or has resulted from, some other disorder, nutritional supplementation may be required on a temporary or permanent basis.

❖ Nursing Management and Health Promotion: Malabsorption Syndromes

The assessment and planning of care will necessarily focus on the problems of nutritional impairment, diarrhoea and any associated feeling of embarrassment, anger or despair. For some, pain will be a distinctive feature, in which case providing analgesics must be a priority.

A full nutritional assessment should be made with the assistance of the dietitian. While assessing elimination function, efforts should be made to minimise the physical misery and embarrassment caused by diarrhoea. Attention to hygiene and the provision of soothing creams for any excoriation can make all the difference.

Ensuring rest and relaxation can help general malaise. This is not always easy, as the investigations may be many and frequent. Supporting the patient through such tests and ensuring full understanding will help in maintaining a positive attitude.

Counselling and teaching will be a priority once the diagnosis and management have been determined. This is especially important as discharge approaches and the patient begins to take responsibility for dietary modification. The community nurse, GP and self-help groups can give support in the community, but probably the best support can be gained from those closest to the patient. The involvement of family and significant friends in any teaching and health promotion programme should be encouraged.

Irritable Bowel Syndrome

Irritable bowel syndrome (IBS) is the name for a group of unexplained symptoms related to disturbance of the large bowel. IBS is a chronic, relapsing and often lifelong condition; the prevalence of IBS in the general population is estimated to be 5%–20%, but as many people with symptoms do not seek medical advice, this may be an underestimate (NICE 2017).

The condition commonly affects those in the 20–39 year age group, with twice as many women being affected than men. Recent trends also suggest there is a notable prevalence among older adults (NICE 2017).

Clinical Features

Individuals with IBS characteristically complain of abdominal pain or distension (bloating) and nausea often worse after eating. There may be an increase in flatulence and frequency of bowel motion including incontinence. People with IBS can present with a wide range of symptoms but there is a tendency to be either 'diarrhoea dominant' or 'constipation dominant' or alternating (NICE 2017). Some people also experience backache and lethargy and find the symptoms distressing and/or embarrassing so are often reluctant to discuss them with others.

Diagnosis

According to the NICE guidelines for IBS (NICE 2017), any person presenting with abdominal pain or bloating or a change in bowel habit for a period of longer than 6 months should be assessed for IBS. However, organic bowel disease must be excluded when making the diagnosis. Unintentional or unexplained weight loss, rectal bleeding, a family history of bowel or ovarian cancer, anaemia, abdominal or rectal masses, markers for inflammatory bowel disease (IBD) and an altered bowel habit that includes more frequent and/or looser stools in a person over the age of 60 years require referral for further investigation.

In making the diagnosis, it is important that the level of distress and frequency of symptoms are assessed, particularly in relation to altered bowel habit or stool passage. NICE (2017) recommends the use of the Bristol Stool Form Scale (Information 4.7) to assist the individual with stool descriptors. Diagnosis of IBS is made on the basis of the clinical features presented earlier. Investigations in those who meet the criteria for IBS include an FBC, erythrocyte sedimentation rate (ESR), C-reactive protein (may be raised if there is active inflammation and infection) and antibody testing for coeliac disease.

Treatment Options

Once the diagnosis of IBS is confirmed, time is spent discussing the symptoms and findings and reassuring the patient that there is

---

> ### INFORMATION 4.7
>
> **Bristol stool form chart (Lewis and Heaton 1997)**
>
> Type 1 Separate hard lumps, like nuts (hard to pass)
> Type 2 Sausage-shaped, but lumpy
> Type 3 Like a sausage but with cracks on its surface
> Type 4 Like a sausage or snake, smooth and soft
> Type 5 Soft blobs with clear cut edges (passed easily)
> Type 6 Fluffy pieces with ragged edges, a mushy stool
> Type 7 Watery, no solid pieces. Entirely liquid

no underlying pathology. The focus of treatment for IBS is aimed at control of the predominant symptoms. This is primarily directed towards dietary and lifestyle changes but at times supplemented by pharmacological therapy and psychological interventions.

Pharmacological therapy is based on the nature and severity of the symptoms being experienced. Antispasmodics are used sometimes in conjunction with dietary and lifestyle management. For those with constipation, laxatives should be considered but lactulose is contraindicated in IBS because of the increased risk of abdominal symptoms (e.g. abdominal cramping and diarrhoea) (NICE 2017). Loperamide is the drug of choice for those with diarrhoea. Where pain management is unsuccessful with antispasmodics, laxatives and loperamide, tricyclic antidepressants may be considered. Peppermint oil or buscopan may also provide some relief.

Psychological interventions such as cognitive behavioural therapy (CBT), hypnotherapy and/or psychological therapy should be considered if the person does not respond to pharmacological treatments after 12 months.

❖ Nursing Management and Health Promotion: Irritable Bowel Syndrome

Once a diagnosis of IBS has been made, the majority of those with the condition are managed within the community setting. For the most part, the focus of care should be on education to promote and enhance self-management. The focus of education is related to diet, lifestyle, physical activity and medication to manage their symptoms.

Nutritional assessment should be undertaken and the person should be advised to keep a food diary and to eat regularly avoiding long gaps between meals. At least 1.5 L of water and noncaffeinated drinks should be consumed daily, and coffee, tea, alcohol and carbonated drinks should be avoided. Eating fresh home-cooked meals instead of highly processed foods, limiting high-fibre foods and confining fruit to three portions a day may also help. The use of oral aloe vera should also be avoided by those who have IBS because of its laxative effects and the potential for abdominal cramps and diarrhoea (NICE 2017). Where necessary, the person should be referred to a dietitian.

The person's level of physical activity should also be assessed and advice given where there is an identified need to increase activity levels. In addition, the person should be encouraged to identify leisure time and take time to relax.

Patients who are receiving pharmacological therapy require education to develop an understanding that medication doses should be adjusted in order to achieve a soft well-formed stool.

The nurse should discuss a range of coping strategies with the person but should be realistic as alternative therapies are not readily available on the NHS and can be very expensive. However, alternative therapies such as hypnotherapy have been shown to have significant and long-term value in symptom control in IBS; acupuncture and reflexology are not recommended due to a lack of evidence to support their efficacy (NICE 2017). For further information on the management of IBS, refer to the NICE clinical guideline (NICE 2017).

Inflammatory Bowel Disease: Crohn's Disease and Ulcerative Colitis

Inflammatory bowel disease is the term used to describe two chronic and debilitating conditions: CD and ulcerative colitis (UC). Although they are often described together, each has its own unique pathology, characteristics and treatments (Information 4.8), so they will be discussed separately. Both disorders are relatively common in developed countries and usually affect people in young adulthood. The incidence of both conditions has risen in Western populations over the last century. As yet no definitive cause has been found but it is currently believed that a combination of genetic susceptibility and environmental factors such as bacteria, drugs, smoking and perhaps diet is implicated (Mowat et al. 2010). IBD is characterised by unintentional weight loss and increased frequency of stool, with more than six times per day considered to be severe. Stool samples should be investigated promptly for infective causes as well as faecal elastase and faecal calprotectin to aid diagnosis. The psychological impacts of IBD can be an excessive lack of energy due to malabsorption, and the need to access toilets urgently can disrupt individuals' ability to work and enjoy activities of daily living. Encouraging them to join support groups such as Crohn's and Colitis UK is recommended for access to peer support.

🔵 Pathophysiology and Risk Factors

UC is an autoimmune disease where the immune system triggered by an infection fails to switch off once the infection clears, causing inflammatory changes to occur in the mucosa and submucosa. These changes are diffuse, with widespread superficial ulceration. The rectum is almost always involved (proctitis), but there is potential for the entire colon to be affected. If the disease fails to respond to medical treatment, then colonoscopy may be considered as a curative option. An increased incidence of primary sclerosing cholangitis (PSC) with inflammation and damage to the bile ducts can be seen in this group. UC is diagnosed by sigmoidoscopy and biopsy. This is a short 15-minute procedure under light sedation following laxatives to clear the colon and can usually be undertaken as a day case. The extent of the disease is generally divided into four categories (Information 4.9). The inflammatory process primarily affects the mucosa and is continuous. Initially, there is reddening and oedema of the mucosa with bleeding points. This is followed by ulceration. In acute disease, especially of the transverse colon, there may be gross dilatation (toxic dilatation) causing the bowel wall to become thin and rupture which is life-threatening. The occurrence of severe abdominal pain accompanied by high fever and tachycardia requires urgent medical attention and treatment with antibiotics and IV fluids. Steroids and/or lifesaving colectomy may also be indicated. Patients should be offered information and empowered to know when to seek help; nurse-led advice lines are often in place to ensure prompt pathways to urgent treatment in event of UC flares.

UC can respond to 5-aminosalicylic acid (ASA) and some immunosuppressants, but there is an associated risk of osteoporosis,

INFORMATION 4.8
Distinguishing features of inflammatory bowel disease

Ulcerative colitis	Crohn's disease
Colon only	Any part of the gut (from the mouth to the anus)
Rectum is involved	Rectum is usually spared
Usually starts in the rectum	Not continuous with alternating normal areas in between diseased areas
Deep layers of the gut not involved – mucosa and submucosa only	Full thickness – affects all layers
Bleeding is evident	Up to 1/3 have no bleeding
No perianal disease	Perianal disease
No granuloma	Granuloma

INFORMATION 4.9
Ulcerative colitis: extent of the disease (Norton et al. 2008)

- Distal disease – affecting the rectum (proctitis) or the rectum and sigmoid colon (proctosigmoiditis)
- Left-sided disease – affecting up to the splenic flexure (left-sided) colitis and distal colitis (affects 33% of UC patients in the UK)
- Pancolitis – affecting the whole colon (19% of patients in the UK)
- Proctitis – affects the rectum only (48% of patients in UK)

so dual-energy X-ray absorptiometry (DEXA) scans and vitamin D and calcium supplements are needed. It can affect growth and delay puberty. It can be linked to PSC with inflammation and damage to the bile ducts and itching is also common.

The risk of developing bowel cancer in this group increases over time so regular colonoscopy every 5 years depending on severity is recommended, and taking aminosalicylates such as balsalazide, mesalazine, olsalazine and sulfasalazine. CD presents with recurring diarrhoea and abdominal cramping which gets worse after eating. The causes of CD are widely debated; no factor has consistently met the criteria necessary to be recognised as the sole or major cause of the condition (National Clinical Guideline Centre 2019).

Those with CD often have extreme fatigue and weight loss, with nausea vomiting and maybe fever. Arthritis, uveitis and painful mouth ulcers can also occur. With CD, the inflammatory changes affect isolated segments of all layers of the intestinal tract. The damaged mucosa develops granulomas, which give the bowel a cobblestoned appearance. Fibrosis and narrowing of the tract can occur and the transmural damage can lead to fistula formation whereby abnormal passageways develop between loops of the bowel.

Clinical Features

Bloody diarrhoea with frequency, urgency and abdominal cramping is characteristic of UC. Pain may be relieved by defaecation. Pus and mucus may be present in the stool. Attacks vary in severity from being troublesome to life-threatening (Information 4.10).

The symptoms of CD depend on the site of inflammation and, as with UC, the severity of the attacks varies. In small bowel disease the patient may present with nausea and vomiting, bloating/abdominal distension, canker sores (a type of oral ulcer that presents inside the mouth or upper throat and is caused by a break in the mucous membrane) and duodenal ulcers. Patients may also experience abdominal pain, and an abdominal mass is sometimes palpable, particularly in the right iliac fossa. In large bowel disease, patients can experience severe diarrhoea, rectal bleeding or passing mucus rectally. In perianal CD, patients can experience varying bowel habits from diarrhoea to constipation and severe rectal pain. They may also develop recurrent fistulae, abscesses and skin tags (Burch and Collins 2021) (see Information 4.10).

Both conditions may be associated with extra-intestinal symptoms that include arthritis, skin lesions and eye inflammation. Whilst both conditions have minimal mortality rates, they can have a substantial negative affect on the person's social and psychological well-being.

Sometimes the disease is in quite an advanced state before help is sought. In such situations, the symptoms may reflect the more serious complications of rectal abscesses, fissures, fistulae or even obstruction and perforation, which will constitute an abdominal emergency.

Diagnosis

History and examination suggesting IBD prompt hospital admission for diagnostic tests. There are no specific blood tests for IBD, but haematological studies may support a diagnosis. These can reveal a raised white cell count (WBC), a raised ESR and C-reactive protein, a raised platelet count and lowered Hb, B_{12} and zinc. There is often hypoproteinaemia.

Specialist assessment permits consideration of a possible diagnosis of IBD by using a number of investigations. These include clinical evaluation and a combination of biochemical, endoscopic, radiological and histological investigations so as to confirm a diagnosis (NICE 2015).

Other investigations will include:

- Examination of the diarrhoea for blood, fat and infective agents.
- Radiological and barium examination to reveal characteristic features of IBD.
- Endoscopic examination – proctoscopy, sigmoidoscopy and colonoscopy; great care must be taken with such examinations, which are in fact contraindicated in fulminating disease due to the risk of perforation of the bowel.
- Ultrasound and CT scanning to determine the presence of abscess formation.

Treatment Options

As there is no real cure for IBD, with the exception of total colectomy in UC, the aim of treatment is to bring about remission of active disease and maintain this for as long as possible. This may involve the initial correction of fluid and electrolyte imbalance (see Chapter 21), malnutrition and anaemia, and relief of abdominal pain as well as pharmacological interventions (Information 4.11). Please refer to the Evolve website and www.bsg.org.uk for additional information on pharmacological management in UC and CD.

Close observation will be required for signs of obstruction or perforation.

In fulminating disease, enteral nutrition may not be possible and parenteral nutrition will be required (see Chapter 22). If enteral nutrition is possible, an elemental diet free of residue may be necessary for a short while before a low-residue diet can be reintroduced. As the inflammation settles, dietary restrictions can be reduced. During any quiescent phase, a 'normal' healthy diet is recommended. Such a diet should have sufficient kilocalories to restore and maintain weight, as well as being high in protein and carbohydrate and low in fat. Supplements of vitamins, iron, folic acid, zinc and potassium may be required.

🔴 Surgical Management

Surgery is required in 20%–30% of patients with UC and up to 50% with CD, but it is always preferred that any surgery be postponed for as long as possible. As a result, living with this condition can mean living with the constant anxiety that symptoms will

---

INFORMATION 4.10

Clinical features of ulcerative colitis and Crohn's disease

Ulcerative colitis	Crohn's disease
Characterised by relapses and remissions	Characterised by episodes of remission and relapse, which are unpredictable
Lifelong condition that is treatable	Symptoms are dependent on the site, severity and pathological process of the disease
Bloody diarrhoea	Diarrhoea and/or bleeding (altered bowel habits)
Frequency, urgency, abdominal cramps (usually pre-defecation)	Cramping abdominal pain
Passing mucus rectally	Anorexia and weight loss
May be pus in the stools	Pyrexia (fever)
Loss of appetite (anorexia)	Anal and perianal lesions
Blood loss can vary from mild to causing shock	Slowed growth in children
Malaise (lethargy)	Malaise (lethargy), anorexia
Tenesmus	Subacute GI obstruction
Malodorous flatus	Susceptible to extra-intestinal manifestations

---

INFORMATION 4.11

Non-surgical treatment in inflammatory bowel disease

Ulcerative colitis	Crohn's disease
Pharmacological treatments (corticosteroids, aminosalicylates, thiopurines, infliximab)	Pharmacological treatments (corticosteroids, aminosalicylates, thiopurines, methotrexate, infliximab) – antibiotics, e.g. metronidazole
Fluid replacement/blood transfusion	Nutritional assessment and nutritional replacements/ supplements
Local disease – topical therapy of salicylates and steroid enemas	Elemental diet
20%–30% of patients require surgery	50% of patients will require surgery in the first 10 years

become severe and complications arise. Surgery becomes unavoidable when:

- Acute episodes become more frequent or fail to respond to medical treatment and there is a deterioration, leading to generalised debility, malnutrition, fluid and electrolyte disturbance and anaemia.
- Obstruction is acute and/or fails to resolve by conservative means.
- Perforation occurs.
- Toxic megacolon occurs – the colon hypertrophies, dilates and could rupture.
- Fistulae develop – these may be internal or enterocutaneous.
- Abscesses fail to respond to intensive treatment.
- Malignant changes are considered to be a risk.

The choice of operation will depend on the extent and severity of the disease. It is generally accepted that the emergency operation of choice is colectomy (removal of the colon) with terminal ileostomy (opening into the ileum) and preservation of the rectum. Preserving the rectum means that it may be possible to have the ileostomy reversed in the future.

Ileal–anal pouch surgery (formation of a pouch/reservoir from the ileum that is joined to the anus) has changed greatly the treatment of UC and it has become standard care for those with the condition (see also NICE 2017; Lamb et al. 2019). Patients are advocates of this type of surgery as it removes the necessity of having a stoma.

In CD, the patient may undergo more than one operation over many years, as surgery may initially be limited to resection of the affected segments of the bowel. However, because the disease affects the total GI tract, alternatives to stoma formation are less easily achieved.

❖ Nursing Management and Health Promotion: Inflammatory Bowel Disease

The nursing care of patients with IBD is essentially symptomatic and must be individualised. Assessment and nursing management will focus on nutritional status, pain and discomfort, bowel function, patient knowledge and ability to cope with the condition, body image and self-esteem, and work and social implications. Education and inclusion of the patient in their care are essential throughout their hospitalisation, both in terms of enabling them to cope with the stress of undergoing a range of often exhausting investigations for which fasting and bowel preparation is required and in preparing them to live with the condition (Reflection 4.3).

Nursing monitoring should focus on early detection of deterioration in the patient's condition, particularly any elevation in temperature or pulse rate or signs of impending shock. During fulminating episodes, the patient may be acutely ill. Abdominal pain can be severe and diarrhoea unremitting, and the presence of fissures, fistulae and rectal abscesses may make the symptoms worse. The patient will be prone to infection, and the nurse should be alert for signs of pyrexia and tachycardia that may indicate the presence of infection. Alteration in vital signs in conjunction with increasing abdominal tenderness could also indicate the advent of colonic dilatation, toxic megacolon or perforation.

Accurate intake and output recording is essential as these patients are prone to dehydration from fluid and electrolytes lost through diarrhoea. Muscle weakness, cramps, tachycardia and pyrexia can indicate electrolyte imbalance. Dehydration and electrolyte imbalance must be corrected, usually through the IV route.

> ## REFLECTION 4.3
>
> ### The person living with Crohn's disease
>
> Margaret is a 23-year-old hotel receptionist who was diagnosed with Crohn's disease when she was 17 years old. Margaret has been in and out of hospital regularly due to her condition. Margaret attended an outpatient appointment and was admitted to the GI ward after her appointment. When Margaret met her admitting nurse she burst into tears, explaining how she had developed an embarrassing and 'horrible' faecal discharge from her vagina and uncontrollable diarrhoea. On admission, Margaret was pyrexial with a temperature of 38.4°C, pale, clammy and very distressed. The nurse offered her a single room as she was obviously distressed by her diarrhoea.
>
> Her consultant suggested a fistula was the cause of Margaret's problem and advised that the best plan of action would be to surgically repair it. Margaret was also informed that there was a possibility she would require a defunctioning stoma or proctectomy. Margaret was unable to sleep and spent most of the night talking to the night nurses about her condition and her options. She also told the nursing staff that she had ended her relationship with her boyfriend of 2 years because of her present condition.
>
> - Refer to website Critical thinking question 4.2 in relation to this case.
>
> 🌐 See website for Critical thinking question 4.2

Patients should also be observed for signs of prolonged bleeding such as lethargy, tiredness, breathlessness and pale mucosa.

Patients with IBD experience loose frequent stools, sometimes with the presence of blood and mucus, up to 20 times per day. These episodes are often accompanied by abdominal pain and cramps that are made worse by food and fluids. These patients are not only incapacitated by these episodes, they also are often embarrassed and self-conscious about odours. Ideally, they should have easy access to a toilet or commode, and privacy should be ensured. Advice on good perianal care is essential as the area is prone to excoriation and patients should be encouraged to maintain a high standard of personal hygiene. A barrier cream may be helpful. Patients may request a continence pad as a precautionary measure. A stool chart should be maintained to record the number and character of bowel movements (see Information 4.7), including the presence or absence of blood/mucus. Although antidiarrhoeal medication should not be given in the acute phase, antispasmodics are sometimes helpful.

Nutritional assessment and management are fundamental for patients with IBD. They are often malnourished or afraid to eat for fear of exacerbating already debilitating symptoms. A nutritional assessment tool such as MUST (BAPEN 2018) should be maintained. There is no definitive advice regarding what foods to eat, but patients should be encouraged to eat small, regular meals and supplements may be beneficial. Small snacks between meals will help to increase calorie intake. The provision of regular oral hygiene and antiseptic mouthwashes is essential to prevent candidiasis. For some, particularly those with CD, supportive therapy in the form of nasogastric, enteral or parenteral feeding may be required to correct malnutrition.

In order to offer education and support that is individualised, it is important that the nurse gets to know the patient's lifestyle, likes and dislikes, and to identify any sources of stress in their daily life. Fatigue will be a constant feature and the patient should be encouraged and facilitated to rest. A tactful approach when disturbing an exhausted patient in order to carry out essential care is helpful in gaining cooperation, despite the patient appearing unappreciative of the nursing care being carried out.

The patient will have to accept the reality of a condition that is with them for life. Time must be spent on a regular basis helping them to adjust and to plan positively for the future. The National Association for Colitis and Crohn's Disease (NACC) can offer a great deal of support to both patients and their families. Psychological and social adjustment is central to successful self-management in the person with IBD. The impact on self-esteem and body image of the condition can be devastating. Not only does the patient have to cope with the indignity of having faecal urgency and the risk of soiling themselves, they can also experience negative changes in their physical experience as a result of malnutrition, prolonged steroid use or surgery (e.g. formation of a stoma). There are also actual and potential work and social implications. People may refuse certain employment or their ability to sustain their job might be affected by the cyclical nature of remissions and acute phases of the condition. Social implications include the potential for isolation due to a lack of willingness to engage in social activities or intimate relationships.

Perioperative Management

The principles of perioperative care are discussed in Chapter 25. In IBD, there are additional concerns of which the nurse must be aware. Many patients are physically debilitated and, should they present as an abdominal emergency, it may not be possible to improve this state prior to surgery. The psychological preparation for surgery that may involve stoma formation is essential, even if time is limited. Patients and their families are likely to already have conceptions or misconceptions about life with a stoma and may be distressed. If optimal time is available, preparation, in which the stoma nurse specialist plays a key role, centres on assessment of the person's ability to live with the stoma postoperatively. This preparation encompasses both physiological and psychological factors that include assessment of the person's emotional wellbeing, their knowledge levels regarding surgery, the impact of the surgery on sexual functioning and activity, their physical abilities (e.g. existence of comorbidities, eyesight and manual dexterity), cultural considerations and the positioning of the stoma. Further information on the role of the stoma nurse specialist can be found on the Evolve website.

For more information about the pre- and postoperative care of a patient with a stoma and for the psychological, sexual and cultural issues that must be considered when caring for such a patient, see White (2019).

Stoma Care

Postoperatively, the nurse must maintain close observation of the stoma to ensure that it is viable and has a good blood supply. The stoma should be pink; if it darkens in colour this indicates that the blood supply is threatened. Initially the stoma will be oedematous, but this should reduce over a few days. A clear drainage stoma bag should be used to allow good observation of the stoma. Daily assessment should include:

- Observation of the mucocutaneous junction (where the mucosa of the bowel joins the skin) for signs of separation.
- Assessment of the condition of the peristomal skin for redness, inflammation and broken areas.
- Monitoring the surrounding area for any indication that the stoma is receding into an indentation or crease on the abdomen.

If an ileostomy has been formed, digestive enzymes will be present and fluid faeces will become copious; care must be taken that the skin is protected by the correct application of the stoma bags. The stoma is formed so that it is approximately 3.5 cm long, thus protecting the surrounding skin. However, care is still necessary to protect the skin and position the appliance. No pressure should be put on the stoma during care.

The patient should be reassured that the output from the stoma will reduce and become more 'paste-like' in consistency as the small intestine recovers and adjusts. The stoma nurse specialist can demonstrate the various appliances available so that the patient has a supply of those most suitable prior to discharge. Initial care of the stoma is given by the nursing staff, with the patient gradually taking over under supervision and then performing care independently before going home.

It is fundamental that the patient has knowledge and understanding of the potential adjustments to lifestyle that may need to be made in respect to food, medications, maintenance of general health, work life and hobbies. Moreover there may be implications for sexual functioning depending on the type of surgery that has been undertaken as well as the parallel issues of the impact on body image and self-esteem (White 2019).

Dietary advice should be given by the dietitian and the stoma nurse specialist before discharge, and the patient and family should be advised of the likely protracted recovery and adjustment time that will be required before a return to good health and a full lifestyle can be achieved. Continuity of care is key to supporting and enabling the patient and their family and is provided in the community by the primary healthcare team and the stoma nurse specialist.

Diverticular Disease

Diverticular disease presents as small hernias or outpouchings of the mucosa through the muscular wall of the bowel. These occur predominantly in the sigmoid and descending colon. The presence of uncomplicated diverticula with minimal or no symptoms is known as diverticulosis. The precise prevalence of diverticulosis is unknown, as most people are asymptomatic. It is estimated that around 80%–85% of people with diverticula remain asymptomatic, approximately 10%–15% develop symptomatic diverticular disease, and the remainder develop diverticulitis (Sartelli et al., 2020).

However, three-quarters of these people remain asymptomatic throughout their lives. In the presence of symptoms the condition is referred to as diverticular disease. When inflammation occurs, it is known as diverticulitis and, if persistent, is considered a chronic inflammatory disease.

Pathophysiology and Risk Factors

Although the pathogenesis of diverticular disease is not fully understood, there is an inverse relationship between its incidence and fibre content in the diet. Those with diverticular disease often have diets low in fresh fruit and vegetables, brown bread and potatoes and high in meat and milk products. Chronic constipation and the excessive use of purgatives may also cause diverticular disease by raising intraluminal pressure.

It is thought that a low volume of colonic content leads to a reduction in the diameter of the colon. Increased luminal pressure during segmentation causes herniation of the mucosa through the muscle wall. Faeces may collect in the hernia(e), causing inflammation, perforation and abscess formation, the formation of fistulae into the small intestine, bladder or vagina and peritonitis. Repeated attacks can eventually lead to obstruction.

Clinical Features

Clinical features include the presence of intermittent grumbling, spasmodic pain in the left iliac fossa or suprapubic region and a mass that is palpable on abdominal or rectal examination. Constipation, intermittent constipation or intermittent diarrhoea is common. The majority of patients with diverticular disease are asymptomatic.

Diagnosis

Diagnosis is made by barium enema. Flexible sigmoidoscopy (visualisation of the rectum and sigmoid colon) is undertaken to exclude cancer. Colonoscopy (visualisation of the colonic mucosa) is indicated when there is rectal bleeding or where a carcinoma is suspected. Most individuals are treated in the community by their GP.

Treatment Options

The main treatment is dietary. The individual should be encouraged to increase fibre intake, including unprocessed bran, wholemeal bread, fruit and vegetables, and should drink plenty of water. Antispasmodics such as propantheline bromide can be used. It must be emphasised that stimulant laxatives should not be used, as they increase the pressure in the muscular wall of the colon and can cause more herniation of the mucosa.

In severe exacerbations, admission to hospital may be necessary if there is marked abdominal pain and pyrexia. Treatment will include broad-spectrum antibiotics, IV infusion and nasogastric aspiration until the inflammation subsides. Although many people who live with diverticular disease feel able to cope and have no difficulty adhering to dietary advice, complications do occur in some people and surgical intervention will be required. Depending on the nature and severity of the problem, resection and temporary or permanent stoma formation may be necessary.

Surgical procedures for diverticular disease might include:
- Colectomy (removal of the entire colon).
- Hartmann's procedure (formation of an end colostomy through surgical resection of the descending or sigmoid colon with closure of the rectal stump and formation of a colostomy).
- Transverse loop colostomy (formation of a colostomy in the right upper quadrant – may be a temporary measure).

Appendicitis

The vermiform appendix is a blind-ended, worm-like tube that projects into the caecum in the right iliac fossa. It has a large amount of lymphoid tissue in its walls and is covered by the peritoneum. The appendix is described as vestigial in that it constitutes the remnant of a structure whose function is no longer required. In adulthood it is about the size of an adult's little finger (5–6 cm) (Fig. 4.4).

Inflammation of the appendix is the most common cause of abdominal sepsis in developed countries. The concern is always that the inflamed appendix might rupture, causing peritonitis. Appendicitis is a life-threatening condition and constitutes a surgical emergency.

Pathophysiology and Risk Factors

Although in many people the appendix has virtually disappeared by their middle years, appendicitis can occur at any age. It is rare in infancy and less common in later life. Acute appendicitis is the most common abdominal surgical emergency in the world;

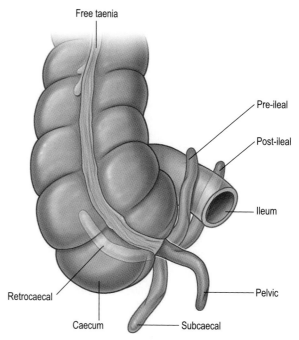

Figure 4.4 Position of the appendix. (Reproduced with permission from Drake RL, Vogl W, Mitchell AWM. *Gray's Anatomy for Students*. 3rd ed. Philadelphia: Elsevier; 2015.)

in the UK, there are around 50,000 acute appendicectomies performed annually (Baird et al. 2017). Its prevalence is thought to be closely related to refined Western diets where faecolith (hard faecal matter) residues may be retained in and obstruct the lumen of the blind-ended appendix. The incidence of appendicitis does appear to have fallen significantly over the past 10 years, perhaps reflecting the promotion of a healthier diet that is high in fibre. Less commonly, viral infections, contaminated food and intestinal (tape) worms can precipitate appendicitis.

When the lumen of the appendix becomes obstructed, bacteria proliferate and cause an acute inflammatory response. The local end-arteries become thrombosed and gangrene sets in. This in turn leads to perforation and localised peritonitis. If left untreated, this becomes generalised peritonitis (Information 4.12).

Clinical Features

For many, appendicitis occurs suddenly, but for others symptoms of colic and fever may 'grumble' on for some time before an acute episode occurs. In such cases, the obstruction has perhaps been partial and the inflammation transitory. These recurrent episodes can result in formation of adhesions, which can cause further problems.

Because of the mobile position of the appendix (see Fig. 4.4), clinical presentation can vary. Typically, however, the patient experiences central abdominal pain localising to the right iliac fossa in the first few hours. There may be rebound tenderness and guarding of the abdomen. The patient may experience nausea and vomiting and have a mild pyrexia, furred tongue and/or unpleasant-smelling breath.

Diagnosis

Following a careful history and examination, only essential investigations will be carried out to confirm diagnosis. If this is in doubt, an ultrasound scan may be undertaken.

INFORMATION 4.12

Peritonitis (inflammation of the peritoneum)

Acute peritonitis

Acute peritonitis is commonly caused by irritating substances, often bacterial in nature, entering the abdominal cavity due to:

- perforation of an organ by either trauma or disease, e.g. a penetrating injury, a perforated appendix, duodenal ulcer, or ruptured fallopian tube as a result of an ectopic pregnancy
- gangrene of an organ such as might occur in a strangulated hernia
- septicaemia, which may have originated in another part of the body.

The peritoneum becomes inflamed, inciting a dramatic increase in the production of serous fluid. This rapidly becomes infected and purulent in the presence of bacteria (typically *Escherichia coli* and *Bacteroides*). Toxins are absorbed from the inflamed and oedematous peritoneum and large amounts of fluid are lost into the peritoneal cavity, leading to paralytic ileus, abdominal distension, hypovolaemia, fluid and electrolyte imbalance and loss of protein.

Immediate and intense pain is felt at the site, followed by vomiting, pyrexia, extreme weakness and shock. Diagnosis is essentially clinical, supported by X-ray examination to detect the presence of free air, fluid levels, abdominal masses and perforations.

Treatment is by a combination of surgery, intravenous antibiotic therapy and specific intervention for the underlying cause. The peritoneal cavity may need to be opened to remove the toxic material and allow drainage of the peritoneal cavity. Supportive therapy includes intravenous fluids to maintain fluid and electrolyte balance, nasogastric aspiration to relieve distension, oxygen therapy and analgesics. If the patient continues to remain pyrexial, tachycardic and in pain, an abdominal abscess should be suspected as a complication.

Chronic peritonitis

This is far less common than acute peritonitis but may occur in association with tuberculosis or as a complication of some long-standing irritant such as peritoneal dialysis or a foreign body. Symptoms are less severe and include low-grade fever, vague pain and malaise. Treatment will depend on the cause.

REFLECTION 4.4

Identifying the nursing care of a patient with appendicitis

Read the case history of an adolescent with appendicitis on the website and answer the Critical thinking question.

🌐 **See website Critical thinking question 4.3**

Treatment Options

Surgical appendicectomy, either through an open incision or laparoscopically, is the treatment of choice. The appendix is removed and the remaining stump is sutured. The cavity will be irrigated and a drainage tube inserted if any infected material is evident.

❖ Nursing Management and Health Promotion: Appendicitis

◉ *Preoperative Management*

As appendicitis so often presents as an emergency, the patient may have to be prepared quickly for surgery. Nonetheless, safe physical preparation must be attended to with appropriate psychological and emotional support being offered. The preoperative nursing assessment should focus on establishing baseline data and identifying factors that may increase the potential for postoperative complications. Vital signs should be monitored to assess if there is infection (peritonitis) or signs of septic shock. Pain assessment is important in determining whether the patient's condition is deteriorating and should be undertaken using a pain assessment tool. Enemas or aperients must not be given as induced peristalsis can cause a perforation of the bowel. Heat should not be applied

directly over the area of the pain as it may cause the appendix to rupture and peritonitis to develop. In the past, withholding analgesia has been standard practice in those suspected of having appendicitis.

◉ *Postoperative Management*

In the majority of cases, postoperative recovery will be uneventful and rapid. In addition to the standard postoperative care of all patients following surgery (see Chapter 25), patients who have had an appendicectomy should be placed in a semi-sitting position to reduce tension on the incision, thus helping to reduce pain. Pain assessment and management should be undertaken and opiates such as morphine administered if the patient does not have PCA. Vital signs should be monitored for signs of complications. Diet and fluids can be commenced when bowel sounds are present.

Discharge is usually early if the surgery was uncomplicated. The patient should be advised on meeting their hygiene needs and caring for the wound and/or laparoscopic puncture sites. Where necessary, arrangements should be made for sutures to be removed. The nurse should ensure the patient understands the need for a gradual return to normal activity within 2–4 weeks but that heavy lifting must be avoided in that period.

Complications

Should perforation and peritonitis occur (see Information 4.12), the patient may become seriously ill. Intestinal peristalsis will be halted and the risks of dehydration, electrolyte imbalance and septic shock are very real. Treatment will involve the removal of the appendix and toxic material, drainage of any abscess and the administration of systemic antibiotics. Oxygen therapy may be necessary and vascular volume will be restored and maintained intravenously. Opiate analgesics will be given to ensure that pain is not allowed to exacerbate an already serious situation. With effective and prompt intervention, the mortality rate of such complications is low (Reflection 4.4).

Abdominal Hernias

A hernia is the protrusion of an organ through the structures that normally contain it. Abdominal hernias occur where there is an acquired or congenital weakness in the muscle wall of the abdomen, allowing an outpouching of peritoneum to form a sac. Acquired weakness can occur in any condition that may result in chronically raised intra-abdominal pressure, e.g. chronic cough, constipation or heavy lifting, or where abdominal muscle weakness has developed, e.g. obesity, old age, illness or pregnancy.

An untreated hernia may progress to contain peritoneal contents, typically the small or large bowel. The major concern is that, due to twisting and/or constriction at the neck of the sac, the blood supply may become impaired at that site. Unless this is immediately resolved, all of the symptoms of intestinal obstruction will occur (Information 4.13).

INFORMATION 4.13

Intestinal obstruction

Intestinal obstruction occurs when the normal transit of intestinal contents is impeded due to mechanical obstruction, vascular occlusion or impaired innervation. Obstruction may be partial or complete.

Causes
Mechanical obstruction
- Intraluminal causes
- Neoplasms
- Strictures
- Foreign bodies
- Faeces
- Intussusception: a telescoping of one part of the bowel into another part

Extramural causes
- Adhesions
- Strangulated hernia
- Volvulus: twisting of the bowel
- Neoplasms outwith the intestinal tract
  When the obstruction occurs, the affected intestine becomes distended with GI secretions (as much as 8 litres is formed each day). As the fluid accumulates, the pressure rises and the bowel responds by attempting to propel the contents forward. This serves only to increase secretions; eventually, the increase in pressure increases capillary permeability and fluid is forced out into the peritoneal cavity. The distension may cause respiratory embarrassment. Severe abdominal colic is experienced. If the obstruction is in the small bowel, vomiting occurs. Obstruction in the large bowel results in distension with air and faeces, and the eventual increase in pressure results in necrosis and the threat of perforation. The outcome of unresolved obstruction will be electrolyte imbalance, hypovolaemia and possibly peritonitis.

Vascular occlusion
Obstruction may occur if there is vascular occlusion of the major mesenteric blood supply by a thrombus or embolus. It is the resulting ischaemia that leads to obstruction. Although there is pain, there is no distension. As the condition deteriorates, the pain may actually decrease. If undiagnosed, gangrene and bacteraemia develop as toxins from the lumen invade the peritoneum and are absorbed into the bloodstream. If surgical intervention is not prompt, death may result. It should also be noted that any mechanical obstruction (e.g. strangulation) that impairs blood supply carries with it a significant mortality risk.

Impaired innervation: paralytic ileus
Paralytic ileus will occur when trauma, inflammation or pain in the thoracolumbar region interferes with the normal innervation of the bowel. It can therefore be a complication of such conditions as back and chest injury, renal pathology and peritonitis. Temporary (paralytic) ileus that follows the necessary handling of the bowel in certain abdominal surgical procedures usually resolves in 12–48 hours (see Chapter 24 , Nursing the patient undergoing surgery). Paralytic ileus will result in marked distension, causing discomfort and respiratory embarrassment.

Treatment
Treatment will involve the correction of fluid and electrolyte imbalance, the relief of the distension and pain, and surgical intervention to address the cause.

Pathophysiology and Risk Factors

The most commonly occurring types of abdominal hernia may be described as follows:

Inguinal Hernia. May be indirect or direct, the former being the more common. In indirect inguinal hernia, congenital abdominal weakness causes the hernial sac to protrude through the inguinal ring and follow the round ligament or spermatic cord. A direct inguinal hernia protrudes directly through the posterior ring. Inguinal hernias are far more common in men than in women.

Femoral Hernia. Femoral hernia is considered to be acquired, resulting from herniation through the femoral canal. This canal is wider in women, making such herniation more commonly a female complaint. Femoral hernias also have a greater risk of complications.

Umbilical Hernia. Many infants are born with an umbilical hernia. This normally disappears in the first year of life without surgical repair. Acquired umbilical hernias can develop in overweight individuals or in those with abdominal ascites.

Incisional Hernia. Following abdominal surgery, the incision site is a point of potential weakness. This becomes a problem if the patient experiences postoperative problems such as impaired healing, especially if drainage of the wound has been required, abdominal distension or generalised debility.

Reducible and Irreducible Hernias. In the early stages a hernia may often be reducible, i.e. with manual palpation or a change to standing posture, the sac will return to the abdominal cavity. However, as the hernia becomes larger and adhesions form, reduction becomes impossible and the hernia is described as irreducible or incarcerated. If the blood flow is then impaired and obstruction occurs, the hernia is described as strangulated.

Colorectal Cancer

Cancers that occur in the large bowel, rectum and anus are collectively referred to as colorectal cancers. In the UK each year, there are around 42,900 new bowel cancer cases; this cancer is the fourth most common cancer in the UK, accounting for 11% of all new cancer cases (2016–2018). In the UK, bowel cancer accounts for 10% of all new female cancer cases, and 12% of all new male cancer cases. Incidence rates for bowel cancer in the UK (2016–2018) are highest in those aged 85 to 89 years. The most common specific location for bowel cancers in the UK is the rectum. In England (2013–2017), incidence rates for bowel cancer are lower in the Asian and Black ethnic groups, and in people of mixed or multiple ethnicity, compared with the White ethnic group (Cancer Research UK 2023c).

Pathophysiology and Risk Factors

Colorectal cancer is more common in relatives of those who have had the disease than those who have not. Genetic syndromes such as familial adenomatous polyposis (FAP) and hereditary nonpolyposis colorectal cancer (HNPCC) cause colorectal cancer. People who have FAP tend to develop hundreds of polyps, and by the age of 40 years, most will have cancer unless the colon is surgically removed. IBD is also associated with an increased risk, particularly where the condition has been present for more than 10 years. Colorectal cancer is increasingly associated with lifestyle and environmental factors, particularly in developed countries. Those that have been identified include a high consumption of processed meat, low consumption of vegetables, very low intake of fibre, alcohol consumption, obesity and smoking (Burch and Collins 2021).

More than 90% of cases of colorectal cancer are adenocarcinomas, where the tumours arise from the epithelial cells of glandular tissue. As they grow, they progressively obstruct the bowel by extending into the lumen or spreading circumferentially to form a ring-like stricture. Metastatic spread is by direct infiltration of local tissues and organs via the lymphatic and portal circulation, or by implantation during surgery.

Clinical Features

The symptoms are subtle, gradual and easily ignored or explained away and, unfortunately, patients tend not to present until the disease is at an advanced stage. Symptoms will vary somewhat according to the site of the tumour. Those with right-sided tumours may experience anaemia, weight loss, ill-defined abdominal pain, alteration in bowel habit and perhaps a felt abdominal mass. Those who have left-sided tumours can have abdominal cramping and an alternating bowel habit, i.e. constipation alternating with diarrhoea with or without the presence of mucus or blood. In people with rectal tumours, bright red blood in the stool, tenesmus (feeling of the need to evacuate) and a change in bowel habit may occur. Pain is not a common feature in the early stages and, perhaps due to this, medical advice is often not sought until either the patient is anaemic and debilitated or the symptoms associated with obstruction are marked. More rarely, patients may present with a fistula, bowel obstruction, haemorrhage or even perforation of the bowel.

Diagnosis

Many patients will present with a palpable mass that can be detected on abdominal or rectal examination. Specific investigations to confirm diagnosis will include barium studies, sigmoidoscopy, colonoscopy colon capsule endoscopy and biopsies. CT colonoscopy, CT scan, PET scan, chest X-ray and ultrasound scan will be necessary to seek out metastases, particularly in the lung and liver. For the latter, liver function tests (LFTs) will also be carried out.

Staging

The staging of the carcinoma is based on histological examination of a resected specimen. For colorectal cancer, Dukes' staging is the most widely used and, at its simplest, it describes four stages (Information 4.14).

Treatment

Surgical removal of the tumour is the only effective management and is curative in 50% of patients diagnosed with colon cancer (Burch and Collins 2021). The type and extent of surgery will depend on the site of the tumour (Information 4.15), but during resection, a segment of the bowel is removed and includes margins above and below the location of the tumour, the vascular supply to the area and the part of the mesentery including lymphatics and lymph nodes. It may be possible for resection and end-to-end anastomosis to be performed, but often stoma formation is necessary on a temporary or permanent basis.

Radiotherapy and chemotherapy are also used either alone or in conjunction with surgery (either before or after) to control recurrence or reduce the size of the tumour before/after surgery, as a means of controlling symptoms and improving quality of life in patients whose condition is advanced.

❖ Nursing Management and Health Promotion: Colorectal Cancer

Psychological Support

The realisation that seemingly minor ailments are actually symptoms of cancer is most stressful for any individual. The patient is

---

INFORMATION 4.14

Dukes' classification of bowel cancer

Stage A The cancer is only affecting the innermost lining of the colon or rectum or slightly growing into the muscle layer.
Stage B The cancer has grown through the muscle layer of the colon or rectum.
Stage C The cancer has spread to at least one lymph node in the area.
Stage D The cancer has spread to somewhere else in the body, like the liver or lung. Some doctors prefer to call this cancer Stage 4, or advanced bowel cancer.

INFORMATION 4.15

Surgery for colorectal cancer

Type/location of colorectal cancer/tumours	Type of surgery
Right colon (caecum, ascending, proximal transverse colon)	Right hemicolectomy
Transverse colon	Transverse hemicolectomy
Left colon	Left hemicolectomy
Sigmoid colon	Sigmoid hemicolectomy
High rectum or low sigmoid colon	Anterior resection – a colonic pouch is created to enable the patient to have a normal bowel function or a temporary colostomy or ileostomy to allow the anastomosis to heal and to prevent complications
Lower rectum	Abdominoperineal resection – results in the formation of a permanent colostomy. In some cases it is possible to preserve the sphincter muscles and reconstruct the rectum in tumours situated above 5 cm from the anal verge

---

usually shocked, bewildered and frightened and will rely on family members or carers for emotional support. From the moment a patient is referred, as an outpatient or inpatient, a sensitive and tactful approach is of paramount importance. Psychological care needs to include the family and significant others in order to develop a trusting relationship. The beneficial effect of spending time to allow fears to be expressed and explanations and support to be given cannot be overstated.

⦿ Perioperative Management

The principles of perioperative nursing care are discussed in Chapter 25. If surgery is to include stoma formation, this will present a further source of stress. A cooperative team approach by the various healthcare professionals involved will greatly assist the patient's physical and psychological recovery and adjustment to what may prove to be major and perhaps only palliative surgery. See the website for the specific input of the stoma nurse specialist.

Discharge Planning

For those patients for whom cure is not a possibility, planning for discharge and home care should aim to maximise their independence and quality of life for as long as possible. This requires the coordination and integration of hospital and community services, and a respect for the wishes of both the patient and the family.

Health Promotion

Great efforts are being made to detect colorectal cancer early, when its prognosis is so much more favourable. Bowel cancer survival has more than doubled in the last 50 years in the UK; 51.9% of males and 53.8% of females are predicted to survive their disease for 10 years or more, as shown by age-standardised net survival for patients diagnosed with bowel cancer during 2013–2017 in England (Office for National Statistics 2019).

Factors being addressed include fostering awareness of early warning signs and information for those especially at risk. Preventive measures also include providing advice concerning diet and health screening. In the UK, the NHS Bowel Cancer Screening Programme has been rolled out, with men and women between the ages of 60 and 74 being invited for screening every 2 years.

Anorectal Disorders

Anorectal conditions such as haemorrhoids, abscesses, fissures, fistulae and sinuses are relatively common and always distressing, but are often tolerated for many months or even years before professional help and advice are sought.

Haemorrhoids

Haemorrhoids, commonly called 'piles', are generally varices of the superior haemorrhoidal veins occurring as a result of congestion of the venous plexus.

Pathophysiology and Risk Factors

It would seem that a lack of dietary fibre is the most important predisposing factor. The resulting chronic constipation and straining during bowel movements raises intra-abdominal pressure, leading to venous plexus engorgement (Information 4.16). The bulging mucosa is dragged down and, as the condition worsens, the haemorrhoids prolapse into the anal canal. Other conditions that can lead to or aggravate the congestion are pregnancy (where the development of haemorrhoids is often neglected), tumours and cardiac failure.

Haemorrhoids may be internal or external. Internal haemorrhoids are classified according to the degree to which they prolapse into the anal canal. External haemorrhoids occur outside the anal canal and are less common.

Clinical Features

Commonly the patient complains of 'fresh' blood in bowel movements, which at first may be thought to be due simply to the passing of constipated motions. The experience of prolapse, at first transient, becomes increasingly frequent and is associated with pain, the discharge of mucus and pruritus (intense itching). Often such symptoms have been managed by over-the-counter remedies such as creams to reduce the itching and pain. Education of the patient in order to achieve the passing of soft bulky stools with minimal effort often yields more relief in the long

term than conventional treatments. The addition of supplementary dietary fibre and ensuring an adequate fluid intake are often seen as more acceptable (Burch and Collins 2021). However, many people find the adjustment of diet too much of a change in lifestyle. Should the haemorrhoidal vessels thrombose, pain is always severe and it may only be at this stage that the patient seeks help.

Diagnosis

Diagnosis is confirmed by:
- History and examination to exclude other pathologies, particularly a carcinoma.
- Rectal examination, proctoscopy and/or sigmoidoscopy.

Treatment Options

If the haemorrhoids are identified in their early stages, management requires no more than attention to the patient's diet and perhaps a bulk laxative. If the constipation is corrected, the problem will usually resolve but the patient must understand this and feel confident in diet alteration. The practice nurse can play an important part in patient education and in arranging a follow-up appointment to monitor the patient's well-being.

Surgical Management

The following surgical treatments may be used to resolve haemorrhoids that do not respond to conservative management:
- *Injection* – for haemorrhoids in the early stages, injection of the haemorrhoidal veins with an irritant solution provokes fibrosis and atrophy with minimal discomfort.
- *Band ligation* – bands are applied to the mucosa-covered haemorrhoidal pedicle, constricting the vessels, which eventually shrink.
- *Infrared coagulation* – infrared radiation is applied in pulses to the haemorrhoid by means of a fibreoptic probe, causing coagulation and shrinkage.
- *Haemorrhoidectomy.* The previous interventions are the most commonly used and can be carried out on an outpatient basis. If, however, the haemorrhoids are not amenable to such therapies, haemorrhoidectomy to ligate and excise the haemorrhoids may be required. If thrombosis has occurred, this procedure will be required immediately.

Nursing Management and Health Promotion: Haemorrhoids

Whether it is the cause or the effect, it is most important that difficulty with defaecation is effectively corrected. Measures to achieve this include:
- increasing dietary fibre
- maintaining a high fluid intake (2–3 L/day)
- prescribing a stool softener to facilitate water and fat absorption into the faeces
- ensuring sufficient exercise and activity.

In addition, nursing priorities must include measures to alleviate pain and itching, to ensure good personal hygiene, to provide appropriate privacy in a hospital setting and to prevent infection.

Preoperative Management

If surgery is required, the aim of nursing care in the preoperative period is to control the acute symptoms and to ensure that the patient feels comfortable and free from any distress when

---

INFORMATION 4.16

Constipation

Constipation may be defined as difficult and infrequent defecation. The following factors can contribute to its development.

Diet

A diet that is low in fibre and bulk predisposes to small faecal bulk. A low fluid intake also contributes to small bulk. Small bulk predisposes the GI tract to reduced peristaltic action and slow passage of contents along the colon. Epidemiological studies indicate that low-fibre diets contribute to many of the GI diseases found in the Western world, such as diverticulosis, appendicitis and haemorrhoids.

Exercise

Lack of exercise contributes to reduced peristalsis, due to reduced muscle tone of the bowel and abdominal muscles. Individuals who take less exercise include the older person and those who are ill or have a physical disability. Hospital patients are, in general, restricted in their mobility, given their environment and their medical condition, and investigations and treatment often predispose patients to constipation.

Elimination habits

Neglecting to empty the rectum when the stimulation caused by faeces therein (the 'call to stool') is ignored results in constipation. If this occurs repeatedly, faecal impaction can result. Watery diarrhoea, caused by the breakdown of faecal material proximal to the hard impacted mass, can bypass the mass. Impacted faeces can press on the urethra and cause retention of urine.

Socioeconomic factors

Nutritional and dietary intake is determined by eating patterns formed in childhood and influenced by familial and social norms and income levels. A low income can result in the exclusion from the diet of fresh fruit and vegetables, which can be relatively expensive. Low-income families and older people living alone may have to make difficult choices in spending their limited resources on food, heating and clothing. Lack of transport or reduced mobility can also limit shopping expeditions and therefore the choice of foods. The older person living alone may be less likely to cook nutritious meals for a number of reasons, e.g. lack of motivation, poor appetite and limited mobility.

Medication

Many medications have side-effects that cause constipation; these include ganglion-blocking drugs, psychotropic drugs, muscle relaxants, and morphine and its derivatives.

Dentition

Poor dentition makes chewing difficult, especially where there has been dental clearance and dentures do not fit well or comfortably. This can result in the avoidance of fresh fruit and vegetables, and an emphasis on soft, easily chewed foods that do not add fibre to the diet.

Motility of colon

Eating results in increased colonic motor activity that may be perceived by the individual as an urge to defecate, but lack of mobility or regular exercise decreases gut motility and may contribute to constipation.

The bowel may become obstructed by a growth, a hernia or by adhesions following surgery. In addition, spasticity can occur in inflammatory conditions such as appendicitis or diverticulitis.

Rectal conditions

Local conditions such as haemorrhoids or anal fissure, which cause pain on defecation, can result in avoidance of defecation with eventual constipation.

Prevention and treatment

Dietary advice is important in the prevention of constipation. Wholemeal bread, fresh fruit and vegetables, and cereals such as porridge oats and All Bran are important. Unprocessed bran can also be added to soups or stews. The individual should be advised to drink plenty of fluid throughout the day. Older people who have urinary incontinence tend to take inadequate fluid in an attempt to avoid being incontinent of urine.

The importance of emptying the bowel regularly and of not ignoring the call to stool should be emphasised. The individual should be encouraged to take as much physical exercise as possible.

The initial treatment of constipation can include the use of laxatives. Bulkforming preparations such as Fybogel and stimulant laxatives such as bisacodyl by mouth or by rectum may be used initially. Where there is a faecal mass, rectally administered faecal softeners such as arachis oil may be necessary.

Any condition, such as haemorrhoids, anal fissure or diverticulosis, which is predisposing the individual to constipation, should be treated.

---

defaecating. One of the major postoperative fears in any form of anorectal surgery is the pain that might be experienced upon the first bowel movement. Time is well spent explaining postoperative care and how any pain and discomfort will be relieved or minimised. Patients are very often comforted merely by the fact that the nurse understands their fears and has the knowledge and skill to help them to manage the problem.

🔊 Postoperative Management

Care priorities in the postoperative period include:
- relief of pain and promotion of comfort,
- prevention of postoperative haemorrhage,
- prevention of postoperative urinary retention,
- prevention of infection,
- promotion of optimal faecal elimination and
- patient education prior to discharge regarding lifestyle and diet.

DISORDERS OF THE HEPATOBILIARY SYSTEM: AN INTRODUCTION

Anatomy and Physiology of the Liver

The liver, weighing approximately 1.5 kg, is the largest single gland in the body and is located mainly in the upper right quadrant of the abdomen just below the diaphragm. The liver is a compact lobular organ with large right and left lobes and two smaller caudate and quadrate lobes (Fig. 4.5). Blood is supplied to the liver by the hepatic artery and the hepatic portal vein which carry blood containing the products of digestion from the small intestine directly to the liver. The hepatic portal system also collects blood from the lower oesophagus, the stomach, the spleen and the large intestine.

Each lobe of the liver is subdivided into functional units called lobules. In these lobules, branches of the hepatic artery, the hepatic portal vein and a bile duct run concurrently in a structure known as

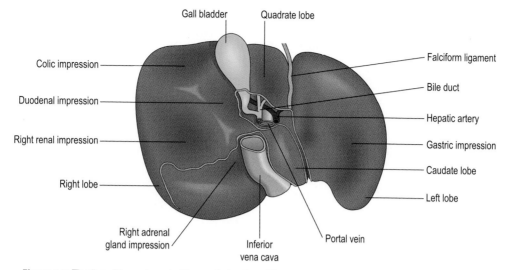

Figure 4.5 The liver. (Reproduced with permission from Waugh A, Grant A. Ross and Wilson: anatomy and physiology. In: *Health and Illness*. 13th ed. Edinburgh: Churchill Livingstone Elsevier; 2018.)

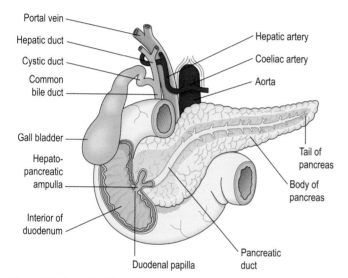

Figure 4.6 The gallbladder and related structures. (Reproduced with permission from Waugh A, Grant A. Ross and Wilson: anatomy and physiology. In: *Health and Illness*. 13th ed. Edinburgh: Churchill Livingstone Elsevier; 2018.)

the portal triad. All of the blood entering the liver mixes in spaces called sinusoids and then drains into a central vein. The multiple functions of the liver are carried out mainly by two types of cells: the parenchymal cells or hepatocytes, which release substances into bile canaliculi, into blood and lymph channels, and the Kupffer cells, which form a part of the lining of blood sinusoids and are phagocytic.

Functions of the Liver

Due to its size and unique structure the liver has both endocrine and exocrine functions. The exocrine functions include the production of bile consisting of water, inorganic electrolytes and bile salts. Bile assists in the neutralisation of acid chyme in the duodenum. The endocrine functions of the liver include the detoxification of drugs and other noxious substances, carbohydrate metabolism, protein and fat metabolism, synthesis of plasma proteins and most blood clotting factors from amino acids, the breakdown of erythrocytes and defence against microbes, the inactivation of hormones including insulin, glucagons, cortisol, aldosterone, the

thyroid and sex hormones (Waugh and Grant 2023), production of heat and the storage of glycogen, fat-soluble vitamins (A, D, E and K), iron, copper and vitamin B12.

Anatomy and Physiology of the Gallbladder

Lying beneath the liver, the gallbladder is a pear-shaped sac approximately 10 cm long attached to the posterior surface of the liver. It has a middle muscular layer comprising of smooth muscle under vagal and hormonal control. Vagal stimulation causes the gallbladder to contract. The mucosal surface area of the gallbladder is increased by the presence of rugae, promoting the reabsorption of water and a 10-fold concentration of the bile that enters from the cystic duct. As the muscular walls of the gallbladder contract, bile is expelled, the sphincter of Oddi (also known as the hepatopancreatic sphincter) relaxes and bile is ejected via the bile duct into the duodenum (Fig. 4.6). The functions of the gallbladder include storing bile and releasing the stored bile. Bile is composed principally of bilirubin, derived from the breakdown of haemoglobin from erythrocytes, and bile salts, formed from excess steroid hormones. The release of bile is stimulated by cholecystokinin and secretin.

The liver has a remarkable ability to repair itself, depending on the extent and duration of the damage it sustains (Fig. 4.7). A brief mild insult, such as viral infection, toxins, hereditary conditions, or autoimmune processes causes inflammation known as hepatitis, which may resolve completely. If an insult is sudden and significant, it can cause acute liver injury (ALI). If that injury is severe, it can quickly progress to acute liver failure (ALF), which is very rare but catastrophic without specialist treatment. Still, the majority of liver disease we see in the clinical setting has developed over months or years leading to chronic liver disease and sometimes permanent scarring known as cirrhosis. In compensated cirrhosis, the liver is still able to function adequately, and blood results may be normal, with the patient unaware there is a problem. If the insult continues, they may develop decompensated cirrhosis with distressing symptoms that lead them to seek medical attention.

Liver disease is rising globally (Sepanlou et al. 2020), while the leading causes of liver-related morbidity and mortality are almost entirely preventable. They include unhealthy diet and/or alcohol excess along with viral hepatitis. The burden of disease is much higher in those from a low socioeconomic background acknowledging

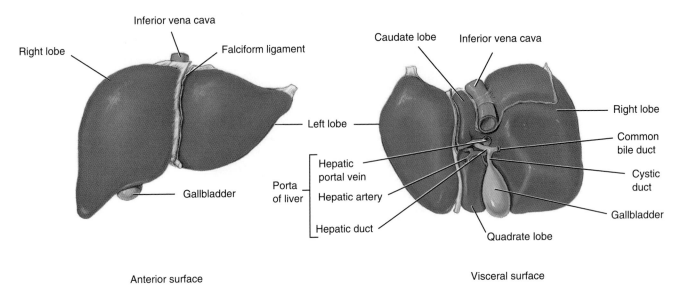

Figure 4.7 Features of the liver.

health inequalities (Williams et al. 2018). Health promotion aims to screen those at risk of developing liver disease to prevent or reverse it. Treatment of those presenting with liver disease is aimed at identifying and addressing the underlying cause, managing symptoms and preventing complications (Tsochatzis et al. 2014).

Poorer survival outcomes seen in patients with liver disease treated outside specialist centres have led to the development of evidence-based guidelines and quality standards to make specialist knowledge widely and freely available to benchmark best practices. The UK has established an accreditation program to promote best practice with the aim of Improving Quality in Liver Services (IQILS). It requires centers to measure their performance against evidence-based standards of care, drawn from the British Association for the Study of the Liver (BASL) and European Association for the Study of the Liver (EASL) guidelines. Specifically, for the context of this chapter, the BASL Decompensated Cirrhosis care bundle is a concise yet comprehensive guide for the optimal treatment for this patient group and forms the basis of care and nursing considerations, which will be outlined in this chapter (McPherson et al. 2014).

It can help to simplify management approaches if we consider liver disease within the following distinct groups based on the speed of insult and severity, rather than the underlying cause. This is because management approaches are broadly similar within these groups which are as followed:

- Hepatitis
- ALI, ALF, subacute liver failure
- Chronic: fibrosis
- Cirrhosis: including compensated (stable) versus decompensated (liver failure)
- Acute on chronic liver failure (ACLF)
- Primary liver cancer

Aetiology

We can consider the underlying causes and ensure treatment is targeted to address them. These include:

Drug toxicity: Drug-induced liver injury (DILI), paracetamol overdose, alcohol excess, magic mushrooms, 3,4-methylenedioxymethamphetamine (MDMA)

Viral hepatitis: A, B, C, D + E

Autoimmune: Autoimmune hepatitis (AIH), primary biliary cholangitis (PBC), PSC, alcoholic hepatitis (AH)

Metabolic: Metabolic Associated Fatty Liver Disease (MAFLD) formerly known as Nonalcoholic Fatty Liver Disease (NAFLD), nonalcoholic steatotic hepatitis (NASH), Wilson's disease, haemochromatosis, alpha-1-antitrypsin deficiency

Pregnancy related: fatty liver of pregnancy (FLOP), cholestasis of pregnancy, haemolysis elevated liver enzymes and low platelets (HELLP) syndrome

Ischaemia: Hypotension, hypoperfusion, major trauma

Prothrombotic: Hepatic artery thrombosis (HAT), hepatic vein thrombosis (Budd–Chiari syndrome), portal vein thrombosis

Presentation

Patients with liver disease tend to present with tiredness and flu-like symptoms including nausea, malaise or reduced appetite. They may have right upper quadrant and/or abdominal pain and sometimes fever.

Stigmata of liver disease include subtle signs suggestive of liver cirrhosis that the patient may not be aware of, such as Palmer erythema and Kayser–Fleischer rings. Spider naïve and caput medusa are more obvious and common in patients with decompensated liver cirrhosis who usually present with abdominal distension, jaundice and significant muscle wasting (Møller and Bendtsen 2018).

Many patients are found to have liver disease during routine investigations and may be surprised and alarmed by their diagnosis.

Assessment

This begins with taking a comprehensive history from the patient or relative, exploring the presenting symptoms including bowel habits, weight or dietary changes and any previous medical history. Diabetes, hypertension and obesity (body mass index (BMI) >30) are significant risk factors for metabolic syndrome and NAFLD (Radu et al. 2023). In addition, prescribed medications, herbal remedies, alcohol and illicit drug use should also be explored (Mansour and McPherson 2018).

Recent travel history and evidence of tattoos or piercings may reveal the source of viral hepatitis. Blood transfusions prior to 1991, surgery or organ transplantation prior to 1992 should be noted because of the risk of acquiring a blood-borne virus. Unprotected sex and previous intravenous drug use (IVDU) are also risk factors, and a family history of liver disease is important to note. As liver disease affects most other body systems, an ABCDE approach to clinical assessment is recommended for the clinical examination process (Mansour and McPherson 2018).

Nursing Assessment

Conducting routine observations using the NEWS2 or similar, in addition to local policies/guidelines, helps guide the nurse through the assessment process.

Airway: If the patient is drowsy, is difficult to rouse, has a weak cough or is actively vomiting or bleeding from the mouth, their airway may be compromised. Patients with liver disease are at risk of hepatic encephalopathy (HE), which can lead to airway compromise. In addition, patients with severe alcohol withdrawal symptoms may develop seizures requiring immediate airway management. A Glasgow Coma Scale (GCS) score of lower than 8 requires airway adjuncts due to risk of airway obstruction. Compromised patients should be nursed with their head elevated at least to 30 degrees and should avoid lying flat. Consider the recovery position if they are not able to reposition independently.

Breathing: In addition to the respiratory rate, oxygen saturation and auscultation, notice the patient's breathing pattern and use of accessory muscles. Patients unable to speak in full sentences and with breathlessness require close monitoring. Furthermore, patients with liver disease have weak muscles and large distended abdomen due to ascites which can increase the work of breathing and can lead to exhaustion. Encourage them to sit upright to reduce the impact of gravity on their breathing and allow for greater lung expansion. If breathing improves when lying flat, this suggests hepatopulmonary syndrome, a pulmonary vascular complication of liver disease (Raevens et al. 2022).

Circulation: Patients with cirrhosis are typically hyperdynamic indicated by a low BP and elevated heart rate with low systemic vascular resistance due to changes to the circulation related to impaired liver function and portal hypertension (Møller and Bendtsen 2018). If the patient is taking beta-blockers, this may mask tachycardia in the context of hypovolaemia as a consequence of GI bleeding (Mansour and McPherson 2018).

Although patients often have outward signs of fluid retention, such as peripheral oedema, they may be intravascularly volume depleted. As a result, strict and timely fluid balance monitoring is essential. If the urine output falls below 0.5 mL/kg/per hour or sustained hypotension develops, a urinary catheter should be considered to monitor urine output hourly, and their renal function monitored closely. Assessment of dynamic indicators such as capillary refill time (CRT), visual inspection of skin colour, Hb and lactate are critical to identify patient deterioration. Immune dysfunction is common in liver disease, therefore screening for and preventing infection are important. Responding to high or very low temperatures should be a priority and include a septic screen and medical review.

Disability: Patients with liver disease are at risk of HE. They may present with specific signs such as asterixis, also referred to as liver flap, which is the inability to maintain sustained posture with subsequent brief, shock-like, involuntary movements (Ellul et al. 2017). Disability assessment should include blood glucose levels, nutritional assessment and problems with activities of living.

Exposure: The acutely ill patient with liver disease may not be able to acknowledge what is wrong with them. Therefore, exposure whilst maintaining dignity and privacy can help reveal the complete clinical picture. Findings such as the passing of black stool or blood clots suggest bleeding via the GI tract and are a medical emergency (Ralston et al. 2018). Old dressings should be removed and swabbed for possible sources of infection. Other findings may include cellulitis, skin breaks and/or evidence of bruising or rashes.

Jaundice and Pruritus

Pruritus or itching is related to jaundice, occurring mainly in patients with cholestatic liver disease such as PBC and if severe can be an indication for a liver transplant. The underlying cause is complex and multifactorial; it relates to the build-up of bile salts, histamines and endogenous opioids.

Symptoms tend to be worse in the evening and overnight and exacerbated by stress and hormones that regulate the menstrual cycle and tend not to be relieved by scratching; primarily affecting the limbs and palms of hands and soles of feet. The degree of pruritus experienced is individualised and does not relate to the severity of jaundice. In severe cases, it causes disrupted sleep, anxiety and depression, the person being generally unwell.

Although ursodeoxycholic acid (URSO) has a role in treating cholestatic liver disease, it does not improve symptoms of pruritus, nor do antihistamines. Aqueous creams with 1% menthol help to soothe and moisturise the skin and provide a cooling effect that may be sufficient if symptoms are mild.

First-line treatment is with cholestyramine; this should be taken in the morning at least 4 hours on either side of other medications and has an unpleasant taste, therefore is best taken with fruit juice. Other options include rifampicin, naltrexone or sertraline, which should be tried in a stepwise fashion but also have potential side effects and require special license (Hegade et al. 2015).

Blood Tests

Liver function tests (LFTs) include bilirubin and albumin but also enzymes reflecting liver injury known as aminotransferases. These include aspartate amino transferase (AST), alkaline phosphatase (ALP) and alanine transaminase (ALT) which become elevated in ALI or other liver failure but may be unremarkable in someone with compensated cirrhosis (Ralston et al. 2018).

Albumin makes up a large proportion of the proteins present in plasma. It has a long half-life so may initially be normal in someone with ALF. Low albumin reflects poor nutrition and/or impaired liver function and is a feature of decompensated liver disease. Low albumin contributes to the formation of peripheral oedema and ascites, common with chronic liver disease because of reduced oncotic pressure within the vascular system, making it more likely for fluid to leak into the interstitial tissues (Ralston et al. 2018).

International normalisation ratio (INR) is a useful marker of synthetic liver function, often abnormal in liver disease. It has a short half-life, becoming deranged within days of the initial insult. INR is a key marker used to calculate prognostic scores in liver disease and determine whether a patient with ALF will fulfil the listing criteria for urgent liver transplantation. Consequently, the INR should not be corrected routinely in this context (Wendon et al. 2017). Despite significant INR derangement being a feature of liver failure, routine correction of INR with fresh frozen plasma (FFP) is not recommended and may be harmful (Northup et al. 2021).

Gamma Glutamyl Transferase (GGT) and **FBC** are useful along with **alpha feta protein** (AFP) which if elevated can suggest liver cancer. **Urea and electrolytes** (U&Es), **coagulation screen** and **bone profile** are relevant to guide overall management (Mansour and McPherson 2018).

Bilirubin: When the normal pathway for excretion of bilirubin is disrupted, it accumulates in the blood, causing jaundice, the characteristic yellowing of the skin and sclera seen when bilirubin levels exceed 35–50 μmol/L. Bilirubin is a normal by-product of red cell breakdown and is conjugated by the hepatocytes to make it water soluble enabling excretion via the gut. A split bilirubin is useful to establish the amount of unconjugated and conjugated bilirubin which helps to determine the underlying cause of jaundice (Tortora et al. 2017). Hepatocellular jaundice is characterised by elevated conjugated bilirubin, and due to the failure of the hepatocytes to transport bilirubin into the bile, it builds up in the blood (Ralston et al. 2018). Obstructive jaundice caused by gallstones or external compression of the biliary tree by tumours can cause bilirubin to become elevated. In cases of jaundice where INR is also elevated, administering 10 mg of vitamin K daily for 3 days helps to establish the underlying cause of the jaundice. If INR does not respond to IV vitamin K administration, this confirms hepatocyte failure as the cause for jaundice.

Patterns Commonly Seen in Liver Disease Blood Tests
Obstructive jaundice/cholestatic liver disease: Bilirubin, ALP and GGT are commonly elevated.

Alcohol-related liver disease (ARLD): elevated GGT, ferritin, mean corpuscular volume (MCV) (even if the synthetic function is still normal), AST:ALT ratio of >2.

Compensated cirrhosis: All blood tests may be normal, and cirrhosis may not be detected.

In cases in which liver disease is suspected, a **noninvasive liver screen (NILS)** examines all possible causes of liver disease establishing underlying causes and guiding appropriate treatment.

Additional Screening for Liver Disease
Liver Ultrasound With Doppler. Patients presenting with signs of liver disease should have an urgent liver ultrasound with Doppler to ensure that the flow in all liver vessels is not obstructed. It should be conducted on an empty stomach to allow for views of the gall bladder. Simple gallstones may be noted in the gallbladder, but duct dilatation is a concern warranting further investigation. A normal liver has a smooth outline, and an irregular nodular outline is consistent with cirrhosis. Evidence of free fluid (ascites) is an abnormal finding. Cysts are not uncommon and usually stable, but focal lesions require urgent investigation and treatment (Ralston et al. 2018).

Fibroscan. This is a quick, noninvasive scan to determine a liver stiffness measurement (LSM). This helps stage the degree of fibrosis/cirrhosis and measures the amount of fat in the liver by way of a controlled attenuation parameter (CAP) score. The result of the scan directs what follow-up is required. Patients with NAFLD and an LSM of less than 8 kPa can usually be discharged from liver clinics with dietary and lifestyle advice. A sustained reduction of 7%–10% of body weight is sufficient to mobilise excess fat in the liver and reverse fibrosis (Brunner et al. 2019). Higher readings may require a liver biopsy to exclude other causes (Angeli et al. 2018). An LSM of above 20 kPa is consistent with portal hypertension and cirrhosis.

Liver Biopsy
Liver biopsies are conducted in a specialist liver centre at the request of a hepatologist (Harrison et al. 2016). Most percutaneous liver biopsies are conducted as a day case in the outpatient setting, but those who are medically unwell with Alcoholic Hepatitis (AH) should have a transjugular biopsy (TJB) to reduce the risk of complications.

Other Investigations
Further imaging of the biliary system may be required to guide the treatment for obstructive jaundice. Options include magnetic resonance cholangiopancreatography (MRCP), EUS, endoscopic retrograde cholangiopancreatography (ERCP) and percutaneous transhepatic cholangiography (PTC). If possible, gallstones are removed during ERCP and biliary stents are inserted to open up blockages and allow bile to flow again (Ralston et al. 2018). Nursing care following such procedures includes providing pain relief and monitoring for signs of bleeding or infection. Documenting the volume and characteristics of fluid drained and ensuring that drains are not dislodged are part of the overall care.

❖ Nursing Considerations for Pre- and Postinvasive Liver Investigations

Invasive interventions such as those mentioned previously require preparation and informed consent. Preprocedural assessment is recommended to establish baseline blood results and to review medications, particularly those that may increase the risk of bleeding. Local guidelines vary, but the consensus is that warfarin should be stopped 5 days prior to invasive procedures and bridged with low-molecular-weight heparin if necessary. Aspirin should be held 2–3 days prior to the procedure and based on the lead clinician's advice with an individualised approach based on risk (Neuberger et al. 2020, Veitch et al. 2021).

Some procedures may require the patient to fast for at least 6 hours prior to the procedure. Check with the medical team whether specific oral medications should be withheld or prescribed intravenously instead.

Emerging evidence suggests that attempts to normalise the INR by giving FFP to cirrhotic patients prior to invasive procedures is of no benefit and may cause harm (Baruah and Bajpai 2018, Rassi et al. 2020). Even though coagulation test results are often deranged, homeostasis is usually rebalanced, while patients present prothrombotic. Liver patients should generally receive deep vein prophylaxis (DVT) prophylaxis, which should be stopped prior to planned invasive procedures or if active bleeding occurs. Providing vitamin K 10 mg if the INR is abnormal is reasonable but FFP should not be given routinely (Angeli et al. 2018, Northup et al. 2021).

Invasive procedures are likely to cause a degree of pain and other unforeseen complications. Consequently the specific nursing care of patients following invasive procedures should include assessing vital signs, looking out for bleeding and infection and ensuring adequate analgesic support. If drains were inserted, care should be taken to monitor the insertion sites and document the volume and characteristics of drainage fluid. The nurse shall ensure that drains are labelled and secured to avoid accidental dislodgment.

Hepatitis

The term 'hepatitis' denotes inflammation of the liver, irrespective of the cause. Globally, blood-borne viruses such as hepatitis B and C or hepatitis A and E virus spread via the faecal/oral route and are the most common cause of hepatitis (Torre et al. 2021). In high-income countries with improved hygiene and well-resourced health services, hepatitis is more likely to be triggered by alcohol excess (Huang et al. 2023).

Viral Hepatitis
Viral hepatitis management has improved greatly in recent years with a well-tolerated cure for hepatitis C available, and there are hopes to eradicate it by 2030 (World Health Organization 2016). Well-resourced health systems, such as the UK, are on track to achieve this by 2025 (England 2022). There is no vaccination for hepatitis C. Successful eradication of the disease following treatment requires education and resources to prevent re-infection. Whilst there is a vaccination to prevent Hepatitis B transmission, there is no cure and it is highly infectious. Management focuses on prevention, screening and close monitoring by a hepatologist for those found to have the virus. Treatment with combination therapy to suppress the virus from replication is highly effective in preventing disease progression. Vertical transmission from a hepatitis B-positive mother to a child

has a 70%–90% risk of infection and the newborn should be vaccinated at birth to prevent chronic infection (Veronese et al. 2021).

Regular review of patients with chronic hepatitis in hepatology outpatient clinics allows for early detection of viral replication and immune-driven inflammation, which can cause fibrosis. This enables timely treatment with medications such as entecavir or tenofovir, which prevent viral replication and further damage. Compliance with this medication is essential to prevent viral replication from reoccurring (Ralston et al. 2018). Viral hepatitis clinics should offer hepatoma surveillance by way of blood tests and ultrasound scans because there is an increased risk of cancer developing in patients with viral hepatitis and/or cirrhosis compared to the general population (Angeli et al. 2018, NICE 2013).

Autoimmune Hepatitis

AIH is rare, and its primary cause is unknown (Muratori et al. 2023). It is thought to be immune mediated whereby the body's immune system attacks liver cells. The prognosis is dependent on the severity of the inflammatory activity. Patients with severe multilobular necrosis, detected by a liver biopsy, generally develop cirrhosis within 5 years. With early referral to a hepatology centre, progression can be prevented with immune-suppressant treatment and lifelong monitoring. The disease may present suddenly in people who are otherwise fit and well and support from groups such as the British Liver Trust can help patients adapt to their new diagnosis.

Alcoholic Hepatitis

AH is increasingly common in the UK and is likely to be encountered in the hospital setting (Office for National Statistics 2022). As such, it is a subset of ARLD. It occurs in patients who have been binge drinking and/or drinking to excess for prolonged periods even if they have stopped drinking alcohol a few weeks prior to presentation to a healthcare professional. They may also be at risk of alcohol dependence which should be screened for upon presentation and managed concurrently (Angeli et al. 2018).

Patients with AH tend to present with jaundice (bilirubin above 50 µmol/L), fever (with or without infection), lethargy and abdominal pain. In severe cases, coagulation may be deranged, indicated by a low platelet count and with elevated INR (>1.5). They often have a poor appetite, nausea and vomiting or present with nose bleeds (epistaxis) or GI bleeding. Clinical history and NILS should be taken including liver ultrasound with Dopplers to detect any underlying liver disease and a liver biopsy may also be indicated. A TJB is considered the safest route if a biopsy is indicated to confirm diagnosis as the risk of bleeding is less than by the percutaneous route (Angeli et al. 2018). If patients are clinically unstable or require organ support, a further insult of undertaking a liver biopsy may be too risky and a delay may be necessary. Features of inflammation including neutrophil and hepatocyte ballooning can be seen in biopsy samples, confirming the diagnosis. The degree of fatty change, fibrosis or early cirrhosis may also be identified (Buchanan and Sinclair 2021).

Survival from AH is poor and ultimately depends on sustained abstinence from alcohol and optimal nutrition (Buchanan and Sinclair 2021, Philips et al. 2019). The only treatment proven to improve short-term outcomes in some patients is a month's course of oral prednisone 40 mg (Thursz et al. 2015). The Maddrey Discriminant Function (MDF) score is calculated, and those with a score >32 may benefit from steroids (Maddrey et al. 1978). Once an infection is ruled out, a week-long trial of steroids is commenced usually whilst the patient remains in the hospital. The Lille score is then calculated after 7 days of treatment and captures an improving

trend in bilirubin and INR (Louvet et al. 2007). 'Steroid responders' have a Lille score between 0.16 and 0.56 and may benefit from completing the steroid course (Foncea et al. 2021). Steroids should otherwise be discontinued as the risks outweigh any benefits.

Nursing Considerations

- Give steroids in the morning with breakfast.
- Do not administer on an empty stomach because it can disrupt stomach mucosa.
- Monitor blood sugar levels which may become elevated. Appetite may also increase, which is usually positive.
- Monitor closely for signs of infection, i.e. increase in oxygen requirements, new onset of confusion, abdominal pain, fever, tachycardia, hypotension and elevated CRP.
- Strict infection control including hand hygiene and aseptic nontouch techniques (ANTTs) with IV access must be always maintained.
- Adverse effects might present as aggression or confusion.

With good nutrition and complete abstinence, the steroid responder's prognosis is good. Bilirubin levels and deranged coagulation screens tend to normalise, and patients may make a full recovery. Nonresponders have a poor prognosis and are unlikely to recover with only 25% survival after 6 months (Thursz et al. 2015). It is important to be open with the patient and family about the prognosis to allow for advanced care planning (ACP) (Deng et al. 2022). The clinical condition can deteriorate rapidly, so timely discussions surrounding ceilings of care and involvement of the palliative care team are appropriate to help with symptom control and psychological impact which can be devastating.

Alcohol-Related Liver Disease

The importance of complete and sustained abstinence from alcohol should be made clear to the patient with ARLD when it is first diagnosed. The degree of underlying liver damage will influence the liver's capacity to repair assuming abstinence is sustained. In many cases, good nutrition combined with abstinence enables significant recovery so that a liver transplant will not be required. Because proven abstinence is usually a prerequisite for consideration of a liver transplant, overcoming alcohol dependence should be a priority to ensure that all treatment options remain open.

Alcohol Use Disorder

In the UK, nearly a quarter of the population drinks to harmful levels, well above the recommended safe limit (Office for National Statistics 2018). Physical dependence on alcohol develops in people who drink to excess on a daily basis for a prolonged period. A healthy liver can metabolise alcohol at a rate of 10 g per hour. In the UK, 1 unit of alcohol equates to 8 g, with the chief medical officer recommending that safe alcohol consumption should be within 14 units/week and include alcohol-free days to prevent alcohol-related harm (Ralston et al. 2018). Alcohol excess overwhelms the usual metabolic pathways, this causes inflammation and may progress to a fatty change in the liver parenchyma, which may further progress to fibrosis and permanent scarring if the alcohol excess continues (Buchanan and Sinclair 2021). If alcohol intake suddenly stops then life-threatening alcohol withdrawal can develop, which is a medical emergency.

Alcohol dependence can be psychological and/or physical; reasons for this vary, including boredom, social isolation or anxiety and depression (Clay et al. 2023). It is important that those who fall ill due to their alcohol consumption are treated with compassion, empathy and understanding and are empowered to believe that with the right support, recovery is possible. Nurses must avoid judgment and perpetuating stigma, which can be a barrier to patients from accessing treatment (Nursing & Midwifery Council 2018), and the term 'alcoholic' should be avoided. Patients sometimes minimise their alcohol use or compare it to others who drink more than they do. Nurses can help service users recognise harm due to their level of alcohol usage.

Once an individual patient has completed detoxification and has withdrawal symptoms controlled, motivational interviewing techniques have been shown to be effective to promote behaviour change (Foxcroft et al. 2016). Facilitating referral to free confidential community services that can support individuals to achieve abstinence as well as peer support groups such as Alcoholics Anonymous can make all the difference in sustaining behaviour change (see NICE 2011 Clinical Guideline).

Recommendations (NICE 2011)

All patients should be screened for risk of harmful alcohol use on admission using a validated tool such as the Alcohol Use Disorder Identification Test: AUDIT C (Dawson et al. 2005) (Fig. 4.8). Patients should be given brief advice regarding the risk of harm attached to their alcohol usage and signposted to community resources for support if appropriate. AUDIT C scores above 12 suggest harmful drinking levels and risk of alcohol withdrawal.

Patients who are at risk of alcohol withdrawal and require admission due to medical problems should be closely monitored for objective signs of alcohol withdrawal using a validated score such as the CIWA-Ar (Mirijello et al. 2015, Sullivan et al. 1989) (see Table 4.1). Those with elevated scores should be treated with a benzodiazepine such as chlordiazepoxide to control withdrawal symptoms. In addition, they should also receive high-dose vitamins Pabrinex intravenously for 5–7 days to manage the risk of Wernicke's encephalopathy. This is often referred to as a 'detox'. Detox can be managed using a fixed-dose regimen or symptomatically depending on local policy. Poorly managed alcohol withdrawal symptoms can lead to delirium tremens (DTs) which is a medical emergency. DTs can quickly progress to seizures which may be life-threatening and very distressing. Prompt recognition and treatment of those at risk of DTs are therefore recommended.

Cirrhosis

Cirrhosis is the term used to denote when the liver has become scarred due to sustained damage over time. On ultrasound scanning, the liver will have a nodular irregular outline and specific

Score	0	1	2	3	4
How often do you have a drink containing alcohol?	Never	Monthly or less	2-4 times per month	2-3 times per week	4+ times per week
How many units of alcohol do you drink on a typical day when you are drinking?	1-2	3-4	5-6	7-9	10+
How often have you had 6 or more units if female, or 8 or more if male, on a single occasion in last year?	Never	Less than monthly	Monthly	Weekly	Daily or almost daily

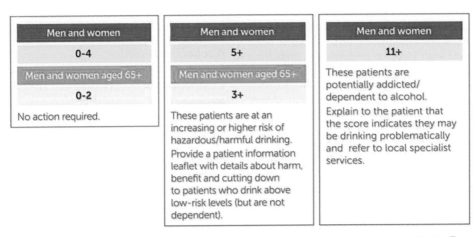

Men and women	Men and women	Men and women
0-4	5+	11+
Men and women aged 65+	Men and women aged 65+	These patients are potentially addicted/ dependent to alcohol.
0-2	3+	Explain to the patient that the score indicates they may be drinking problematically and refer to local specialist services.
No action required.	These patients are at an increasing or higher risk of hazardous/harmful drinking. Provide a patient information leaflet with details about harm, benefit and cutting down to patients who drink above low-risk levels (but are not dependent).	

Figure 4.8 Audit-C alcohol scoring system and key. (1. AUDIT: the Alcohol Use Disorders Identification Test: guidelines for use in primary health care [Internet]. "http://www.who.int. Available from: https://www.who.int/publications/i/item/WHO-MSD-MSB-01.6a. 2. Bush K, Kivlahan DR, McDonell MB, Fihn SD, Bradley KA. The AUDIT alcohol consumption questions (AUDIT-C): an effective brief screening test for problem drinking. Ambulatory Care Quality Improvement Project (ACQUIP). Alcohol Use Disorders Identification Test. *Arch Intern Med*. 1998 Sep 14;158(16):1789–1795. doi: 10.1001/archinte.158.16.1789. PMID: 9738608 3. Alcohol use disorders identification test for consumption (AUDIT C) (publishing.service.gov.uk) Alcohol use screening tests – GOV.UK http://www.gov.uk) https://www.gov.uk/government/publications/alcohol-use-screening-tests.)

TABLE 4.1 Clinical Institute Withdrawal Assessment for Alcohol–Revised (CIWA-Ar) Scale

Symptoms	Range of Scores
Nausea or vomiting	0 (no nausea, no vomiting)–7 (constant nausea and/or vomiting)
Tremor	0 (no tremor)–7 (severe tremors, even with arms not extended)
Paroxysmal sweats	0 (no sweat visible)–7 (drenching sweats)
Anxiety	0 (no anxiety, at ease)– 7 (acute panic states)
Agitation	0 (normal activity)– 7 (constantly trashes about)
Tactile disturbances	0 (none)–7 (continuous hallucinations)
Auditory disturbances	0 (not present)–7 (continuous hallucinations)
Visual disturbances	0 (not present)–7 (continuous hallucinations)
Headache	0 (not present)–7 (extremely severe)
Orientation/clouding of sensorium	0 (orientated, can do serial additions)–4 (disorientated for place and/or person)

Modified from: Sullivan JT, Sykora K, Schneiderman J, Naranjo CA, Sellers EM. Assessment of alcohol withdrawal: the revised Clinical Institute Withdrawal Assessment for Alcohol Scale (CIWA-Ar). *Br J Addict.* 1989;84:1353–1357.

features of portal hypertension may be seen (Liu and Chen 2022) (Fig. 4.9).

Patients with compensated cirrhosis can have normal liver blood tests and enough functioning hepatocytes to meet day-to-day requirements. They have no symptoms and are unaware that they have underlying liver disease. If this fine balance is disrupted by an insult such as trauma, infection, surgery (particularly to the abdomen) or being overwhelmed by ongoing alcohol excess, signs of decompensated cirrhosis emerge. Patients with cirrhosis are also at risk of ACLF, which can be catastrophic if multiorgan failure develops. In such cases, chances of survival depend on early detection and treatment of precipitating causes (Hernaez et al. 2017).

Fibrosis 4 (FIB 4) and enhanced liver fibrosis (ELF) testing are used in the community to help identify those at risk and refer them to a liver specialist. Outpatient investigations for those patients should include a noninvasive fibro scan and blood tests (Ralston et al. 2018).

The **Child–Pugh score** (Child and Turcotte 1964; Pugh et al. 1973) (Table 4.2) is widely used to classify cirrhosis into three main groups based on objective scores for liver function and clinical severity. Those within group A have compensated cirrhosis with preserved liver function and no symptoms of liver failure with good long-term survival outcomes. Those in group B are beginning to develop outward signs of liver failure but if the cause

TABLE 4.2 Staging of Liver Disease: Child–Pugh Score

Measure		1 Point	2 Points	3 Points
Total bilirubin, µmol/L (mg/dL)		<34 (<2)	34–50 (2–3)	>50 (>3)
Serum albumin, g/dL		>3.5	2.8–3.5	<2.8
OR	Prothrombin time, prolongation (s)	< 4.0	4.0–6.0	>6.0
	INR	<1.7	1.7–2.3	> 2.3
Ascites		None	Mild (or suppressed with medication)	Moderate to severe (or refractory)
Hepatic encephalopathy		None	Grade I–II	Grade III–IV

INR, International normalised ratio.
Points 5–6 = Class A (1-year survival 100%; 2-year survival 85%); Points 7-9 = Class B (1-year survival 80%; 2-year survival 60%); Points 10-15 = Class C (1-year survival 45%; 2-year survival 35%)

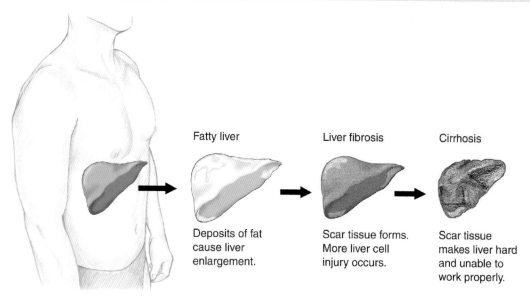

Figure 4.9 Schematic of development of cirrhosis.

of the deterioration is diagnosed and addressed, they may recompensate. Those in group C have developed decompensated liver failure with features like jaundice, ascites, varices, GI bleeds and HE and their survival options are bleak. The United Kingdom Model for End-Stage Liver Disease (UKLED) is another scoring system which is used to assess prognosis and guide clinicians on when to refer for liver transplantation assessment (Barber 2011).

In PSC and PBC, some use a modified Child–Pugh score where the bilirubin references are changed to reflect the fact that these diseases feature high conjugated bilirubin levels. The upper limit for 1 point is 68 μmol/L (4 mg/dL) and the upper limit for 2 points is 170 μmol/L (10 mg/dL).[1]

Chronic liver disease is classified into Child–Pugh class A to C, employing the added score from earlier.[2]

Portal Hypertension

Portal hypertension refers to the increased resistance to blood flow through the liver caused most commonly by excess scar tissue present in cirrhosis (Oliver et al. 2023). It can also occur in the absence of cirrhosis if there is an obstruction to blood flow due to thrombosis or compression by a tumour. Normally, the liver is a low-pressure system with normal fibroscan LSMs being less than 7 kPa. An LSM of above 20 kPa is consistent with portal hypertension (De Franchis et al. 2022) which is responsible for the main feature in patients with decompensated liver cirrhosis. Low platelets and an enlarged spleen are also commonly associated with portal hypertension.

The arterial vasodilation theory (Schrier et al. 1988) suggests an explanation for how portal hypertension leads to splanchnic vasodilation and the triggering of the renin–angiotensin–aldosterone system (RAAS). Please refer to Waugh and Grant (2023) for further information on the RASS system. This results in renal vasoconstriction and sodium/water retention to compensate for splanchnic vasodilation. Whilst this mechanism is helpful during hypovolaemia, as commonly seen in shock or bleeding, with portal hypertension, it impairs renal perfusion and exacerbates sodium and fluid retention.

Medications used to manage the symptoms of portal hypertension or fluid retention seen in cirrhosis target the underlying principles of this theory. Terlipressin and carvedilol target splanchnic vasodilation causing vasoconstriction which reduces portal pressure and splanchnic blood flow (Qi et al. 2022, Sakiani et al. 2022). Human albumin solution (HAS) 20% and 4.5% are volume expanders that help to restore renal perfusion. Spironolactone acts on the distal tubules in the kidneys to reduce sodium and water retention and promote diuresis.

Portal hypertension reflects significant cumulative liver damage. Its impact on collateral circulation is largely responsible for the development of most symptoms of decompensated cirrhosis as previously mentioned. The BASL guidance on the decompensated cirrhosis care bundle recommends a standardised evidence-based approach to caring for this group of patients.

Ascites

Ascites refers to the build-up of fluid in the peritoneal cavity causing the abdomen to become distended and is the most common symptom of decompensated cirrhosis. Mortality in this group is 50% within 2 years (Angeli et al. 2018). It is caused by a combination of low albumin and high portal vein pressures causing fluid to accumulate in the abdomen. Eighty-five per cent of the time it is due to cirrhosis, but tuberculosis (TB), pancreatitis and malignancy need to be excluded. A serum ascites albumin gradient (SAAG) of above 11 g/L is consistent with cirrhosis as the underlying cause (Mansour and McPherson 2018).

Small-volume ascites can be detected by liver ultrasound, and the patient may only become aware of abdominal swelling once moderate ascites has developed. In the case of ARLD, patients may not present until they have tense ascites, with significant physical discomfort and reduced exercise tolerance or dyspnoea due to the lungs being compressed by the build-up of fluid under the diaphragm. Pleural effusions may also develop and a chest X-ray is required if the patient's breathing or oxygenation is compromised.

A diagnostic tap of ascitic fluid is recommended to screen for spontaneous bacterial peritonitis (SBP) which may present as abdominal pain, fever or vomiting, but most patients are asymptomatic (Mansour and McPherson 2018). If suspected, then urgent treatment with broad-spectrum antibiotics prior to draining the fluid is advised to reduce the risk of damage to the kidneys. With improved detection and treatment of SBP, mortality has reduced from 90% to 20% (Angeli et al. 2018). Refer to the BASL decompensated cirrhosis care bundle for best practices and management guidance (McPherson et al. 2014).

It is preferable to manage ascites using diuretics such as spironolactone and/or furosemide if peripheral oedema is also present. These medications require close monitoring of sodium levels and renal function, and should be avoided if the sodium concentration is less than 130 mEq/L and/or if there is renal impairment.

❖ Nursing Management of Ascites and Peripheral Oedema

- Strict fluid balance monitoring (insert urinary catheter if patients are incontinent or unable to collect urine to be measured).
- Monitor serum creatinine and electrolytes regularly. Stop diuretics if low sodium or renal impairment (Fabrellas et al. 2020).
- Sodium restriction to avoid fluid retention (limit of 4.6–6.9 g sodium/day).
- Daily weighing (fluid loss target: 0.5 kg/day with ascites or up to 1 kg/day if peripheral oedema is also present).
- Administer diuretics (dose titrated based on renal function, sodium levels and BP). Spironolactone takes several days to work; therefore, avoid dose increase until 72 hours.
- Enforce fluid restriction if sodium is low (<130 mEq/L), 1–1.5 L.
- Encourage patients to sit upright, recline on pillows and avoid lying flat.
- Abdominal binders can help support the abdomen particularly if the patient has a hernia (Fabrellas et al. 2020).
- Provide analgesia such as paracetamol three times per day, avoid NSAIDs.

Peripheral Oedema
- Monitor for breaks in skin integrity that pose a risk of infection.
- Keep dry skin moisturised, avoid tight clothing.
- Support patients with body image disturbance. Provide reassurance that compliance with abstinence and adequate nutrition should help symptoms resolve.
- Provide written supportive information.

Large-Volume Paracentesis

Once any infection has been addressed by antibiotics, large-volume paracentesis (LVP) (Fig. 4.10) can be undertaken in patients

---

[1]https://en.wikipedia.org/wiki/Child%E2%80%93Pugh_score#cite_note-2

[2]https://en.wikipedia.org/wiki/Child%E2%80%93Pugh_score#cite_note-Cholongitas-1

Figure 4.10 Abdominal paracentesis.

with tense ascites to drain the ascitic fluid and decompress the abdomen (Harvey et al. 2023). It must be explained to the patient that the fluid is likely to reaccumulate and therefore not to rely on the procedure regularly as a quick fix. LVP is an invasive procedure with risks of bleeding and infection. Ultrasound guidance is used to identify the exact location of fluid and whether it is amenable to drainage. Sometimes, the fluid can be loculated in pockets and consequently not amenable to drainage. A local anaesthetic should be used prior to insertion of the drain and general analgesia may also be considered.

❖ Nursing Management of Large-Volume Paracentesis

- Weigh the patient before the procedure, take blood samples for laboratory investigations, insert the cannula and drain.
- Monitor vital signs, ensure adequate analgesia.
- Consider the possibility of bleeding from drain insertion.
- Ensure HAS 20% is available: 100 mL is given for every 2 L drained.
- Maintain strict fluid balance and record total volume drained.
- If drainage of the ascitic fluid slows or stops, check the catheter is not twisted or blocked. Repositioning the patient can help. Consider medical support.
- Due to the increased risk of infection, the drain should not be left in situ for more than 6 hours.
- The patient's weight should be recorded after the procedure so that their dry and wet weight is known and documented.
- In the case of a pleural drain, it should be clamped after 500 mL is drained to avoid rebound pulmonary oedema.

With good nutrition, abstinence from alcohol and scope for the introduction of diuretics, it is possible that ascites can resolve over time.

Refractory Ascites

Patients who do not tolerate diuretics and require repeated LVP as a consequence of their chronic liver disease should be considered for transplantation and referred to a specialist centre for assessment (Millson et al. 2020). Patients who require regular LVP monthly or weekly are usually seen as a day case, avoiding the need for hospital admission. The value of a nurse-led service for rapport and continuity of care brings many benefits. Refractory ascites has a significant impact on quality of life; it may be appropriate to

consider ACP and referral to palliative care for symptom control (Deng et al. 2022). This is particularly relevant in patients who are not eligible for a liver transplant. In some instances, the insertion of a permanent drain is preferable, allowing the patient to avoid returning to the hospital, with district nurses visiting to drain up to 1 L, two or three times per week (Macken et al. 2022). A continuous drain carries the risk of increased infection and this should be given due consideration.

Upper Gastrointestinal Bleeding

Commonly, patients with liver disease present with melena and/or haematemesis, and this requires urgent assessment and treatment (NICE 2012); this can occur in patients unaware that they have liver disease. Consequently, the underlying disease process should be established, and patients should receive appropriate education and support for their ongoing care. Upper GI bleeding ranges from coffee-ground/blood-streaked vomit to massive haematemesis; this is a medical emergency and may be fatal if not dealt with promptly (Elsayed et al. 2016). The patient and their family are likely to be highly anxious, therefore a calm but urgent approach is likely to provide them with much needed reassurance. Patients are at risk of rapid deterioration and cardiac arrest due to hypovolaemia, and prioritising care whilst taking an ABCDE assessment approach is recommended. Appropriate personal protective equipment (PPE) must be readily available.

Treatment Recommendations

- At least two large-bore cannulas for IV access should be inserted. Blood should be taken for laboratory investigations, including FBC, coagulation screen, blood group and crossmatch. An arterial blood gas (ABG) which includes lactate and Hb helps to establish the clinical severity.
- High-flow Yankauer suction should be readily available to assist with the maintenance of the upper airway patency. The patient should be positioned in an upright position if the BP is maintained to reduce the risk of aspiration of gastric content. If the BP is compromised, the recovery position with the head slightly elevated may be more appropriate.
- Delivery of oxygen therapy by nasal cannula instead of a facemask is easier if intermittent oral suctioning is required.
- Anticipating airway protection by intubation may be required to investigate and control severe bleeding. The endoscopy and anaesthetic team are alerted promptly to prepare for this intervention.

- In case of high blood loss, INR >1.5, this should be corrected by administering FFP, and fibrinogen <1 g/L should be corrected with cryoprecipitate transfusion.
- In case the INR in the clotting screen is >1.5, 10 mg of IV vitamin K should be administered immediately. The platelet count should be maintained above 50 and deranged calcium levels corrected to support the coagulation.
- Active monitoring of vital signs is aided by the insertion of an arterial line. If only noninvasive BP monitoring is available, it should be repeated according to the patient's clinical severity. This will guide the scale of crystalloid volume replacement required to achieve and maintain an adequate BP maintaining overall organ perfusion.
- Targeting a mean arterial blood pressure (MAP) of 65 mmHg and an Hb level of 7–9 g/dL should be sufficient to perfuse organs until bleeding is controlled. Restrictive transfusion strategies are recommended avoiding increasing portal hypertension and further blood loss (Mansour and McPherson 2018).
- Alert the transfusion department as soon as possible especially if volumes of blood loss are excessive. However, a more restrictive blood transfusion policy below normal Hb levels has been found to improve patient outcomes (Orpen-Palmer and Stanley 2022).
- Inserting a urinary catheter and monitoring urine output hourly along with an accurate fluid balance are important. Less than 0.5 mL/kg of urine per hour may herald acute kidney injury (AKI) (Joannidis et al. 2017).
- Guidelines recommend the transfer of patients to specialist centres that can perform emergency endoscopy within 12 hours once vital signs have been stabilised (NICE 2012).
- If vital signs are not compromised and there is no transfusion requirement, out-of-hours emergency endoscopy is not necessary. The Glasgow–Blatchford Bleeding score is the validated tool widely used to help establish this objectively (Blatchford et al. 2000).
- Patients requiring emergency endoscopy are likely to require an intensive care unit (ICU) or recovery bed following the procedure.

The purpose of endoscopy is to visualise the GI tract, to identify the cause of bleeding and target the appropriate treatment. Oesephago gastro duodenoscopy (OGD) i the term used for this procedure, referring to the three regions of the supper GI tract. Varices are the cause of 70% of significant upper GI bleeds in patients who have portal hypertension and should be treated as such until proven otherwise (Angeli et al. 2018). Varices are vessels which become twisted and engorged with blood in patients with portal hypertension. Resembling bunches of grapes, they may rupture and cause extensive haemorrhage and are commonly found in the oesophagus or stomach and graded depending on their size (Abby Philips and Sahney 2016). Bleeding varices are treated by the application of bands to ligate the bleeding vessel known as banding. Gastric varices found in the stomach tend to be injected with glue rather than banded (NICE 2012).

Nursing Responsibilities

- IV terlipressin 2 mg four times daily is recommended for 72 hours causing splanchnic constriction and reducing the chances of further bleeding (NICE 2012).
- An electrocardiogram (ECG) should be performed before administering in patients over 65 years of age with known cardiac dysfunction, as terlipressin can cause cardiac ischaemia.
- Broad-spectrum antibiotics are given three times a day, administered for 72 hours to reduce the risk of infection and help prevent further bleeding.

- The amount and colour of bowel motions must be recorded, old blood and black stool (malena) are to be expected initially. Hb monitoring is an indicator of patient progression.
- Further evidence of active bleeding requires urgent medical review. If Hb continues to drop and the patient requires a blood transfusion, further investigations will be indicated. The endoscopy may also reveal other abnormalities.

Sengstaken Blakemore Tube

In some cases, catastrophic bleeding prevents the endoscopist from seeing anything but blood, so a Sengstaken Blakemore tube is inserted via the mouth as a temporary measure to stop bleeding (Zuckerman et al. 2022). If not placed properly, complications can be life-threatening; its position is confirmed by X-ray. The correct application of this device allows pressure to be applied internally by inflation of the gastric balloon with air. Gentle traction to sustain this pressure is achieved by securing the external portion of the tube to the patient's cheek using tape; care is taken to prevent pressure injuries from developing.

Nursing Considerations

- The oesophageal balloon should only be inflated as a last resort due to the risk of ischaemia and perforation.
- The gastric balloon should be deflated every 4 hours and the gastric port aspirated to quantify any ongoing blood loss.
- The patient should remain sedated and intubated in a critical care setting while the device is in situ for 24–48 hours maximum.
- Once the patient's condition is stable and clotting optimised, the OGD is repeated to identify and resolve the underlying cause of bleeding.
- An event such as variceal bleeding can precipitate other complications in a patient with cirrhosis who is at risk of developing Hepatic Encephalopathy (HE). Close monitoring of cognitive function using tools such as the GCS is pivotal to avoid oversedation while protecting the airway from aspiration.
- Patients who have been treated successfully initially require a repeat OGD within 2–4 weeks, ensuring the varices have healed.
- Maintenance treatment includes nonselective beta-blockers, which may be contraindicated in patients with asthma.
- The dose should be up-titrated with a target heart rate of above 55 bpm if tolerated and the patient is not showing signs of dizziness or hypotension.

Nurses must ensure that patients understand the importance of lifelong compliance with the prescribed medication and offered written information to support their understanding of the condition. The British Liver Trust provides online and written material which may help to reinforce verbal explanation. Progressively, the standards of care delivered have evolved reducing the risk of frightening and life-threatening variceal bleeds occurring and patients known to have portal hypertension are offered screening in the outpatient setting.

Transjugular Intrahepatic Porto-Systemic Shunt

In some patients with significant varices and/or refractory ascites a transjugular intrahepatic porto-systemic shunt (TIPSS) can be inserted under radiological guidance (Büttner et al. 2022). An electroencephalogram (EEG) and cardiac echo form part of the work-up prior to the procedure. TIPSS is an effective treatment for refractory ascites and varices avoiding the need for liver transplant. There is an increased risk of HE developing following TIPSS because less blood flows through the liver, reducing its detoxifying function (Schindler et al. 2020). TIPSS is contraindicated in patients known to have HE; for this reason, it is a side effect that may develop following the procedure. If HE does develop, the shunt may need to be reduced or the procedure reversed altogether.

Hepatic Encephalopathy

In liver disease, HE presents an altered level of consciousness reflecting that the damaged liver's ability to clear toxins is inadequate. This may be due to an exess of toxins building up and/or reduced capacity in a failing liver to deal with the ususal demand. Whilst usually reversible it can be life-threatening so should be considered as a medical emergency. How it is managed depends on whether it presents in ALF or CLD.

In the context of decompensated liver disease, HE is usually reversible but can be life-threatening and therefore must be treated as a medical emergency. It can be subclinical in its mildest form, presenting with subtle signs such as vagueness or reversed sleep cycle seen commonly in Grade 1 HE (Table 4.3) (Vilstrup et al. 2014). However, the presence of asterixis, also referred to as liver flap, indicates serious HE, reflecting the fact that the liver is struggling to detoxify neurotoxins which build up and disrupt motor function. If not treated, it can progress to a deep coma where airway protection is compromised.

Treatment focuses on avoiding triggers and the build-up of toxins. Patients with cirrhosis and their carers need to be aware of the risk of developing HE and understand how it might present. It is important for the nurse to discuss this and provide written information to reinforce key points so patients are empowered to seek help if it develops. It should be suspected in all liver patients who become drowsy or confused. If they fail to respond to treatment, other causes of deterioration such as a cerebral event need to be excluded using brain imaging. Whilst measuring arterial ammonia is useful in ALF because it correlates with the degree of HE, this does not apply in cirrhosis and is of no benefit (Mansour and McPherson 2018).

Prevention
- Avoid triggers.
- Avoid constipation and medications such as loperamide and codeine/opiates that delay gut motility.

TABLE 4.3	Grades of Hepatic Encephalopathy, West Haven Criteria
Covert	Grade 1	Trivial lack of awareness Euphoria or anxiety Shortened attention span Impairment of addition or subtraction Altered sleep rhythm
Overt	Grade 2	Lethargy or apathy Disorientation for time Obvious personality change Inappropriate behavior Dyspraxia Asterixis
	Grade 3	Somnolence to semistupor, responsive to stimuli, time and place disorientation, asterixis, hyperactive DTRs
	Grade 4	Coma

DTR, Deep tendon reflex.
From Vilstrup H, Amodio P, Bajaj J, et al. Hepatic encephalopathy in chronic liver disease: 2014 Practice Guideline by the American Association for the Study of Liver Diseases and the European Association for the Study of the Liver. *Hepatology.* 2014;60:715–735.

- Aim for two to three soft stools per day using lactulose if needed.
- Avoid sedatives such as benzodiazepines and alcohol.

Triggers
- Constipation
- Dehydration
- Infection
- Alcohol excess
- Variceal and gastric bleeding

Treatment. The mainstay of treatment focuses on limiting the development and absorption of neurotoxins such as ammonia via the gut. Regular bowel motions clear the gut and prevent toxins from accumulating and overwhelming the liver. Lactulose, a nonabsorbable disaccharide and is the aperient of choice because it changes the pH of the gut to suppress the activity of the bacteria responsible for producing toxins.

Consider prophylactic treatment with rifaximin, a nonabsorbable antibiotic if a patient has more than two episodes. It acts by suppressing the growth of bacteria responsible for producing endotoxins.

Nursing Considerations

- Vigilance with identifying and treating the underlying cause continues until the patient returns to baseline.
- Ensure bowels open at least 2-3 times a day. Document the response to aperients and consider NG/PR if patient if swallowing is unsafe.
- Consider a nasogastric tube for medication and feeding.
- Nurse with the head elevated to minimise the risk of microaspiration.
- Cognitive responsiveness and an effective cough should be monitored closely using the GCS score and Clinical Hepatic Encephalopathy Staging Scale (CHESS) score (Ortiz et al. 2007).
- Assessment of the patient's risk of falls due to confusion must be completed.
- Ensure close supervision and provide a call bell to hand at the bedside.
- Having a familiar face such as a relative or friend present in hospital may be reassuring.
- Family members are likely to be distressed; therefore, reassurance and education are important.
- Maintain patient dignity and ensure personal care needs are met.
- Assess for risk of developing pressure injuries.
- A urinary catheter may be indicated if the urine output is a concern but insertion of any type of invasive devices is an inherent infection risk and therefore needs to be justified.
- Refractory HE indicates end-stage liver disease and healthcare teams may consider palliative care.

Nutrition in Liver Disease

Ensuring good nutrition, eating little and often, is advised to mitigate protein-energy malnutrition (PEM), which is seen in at least 50% of chronic liver disease patients. Typically, patients have very low albumin levels and profound sarcopenia; encourage the patient to eat snacks in between meals and to take high-calorie snacks before going to bed to avoid muscle breakdown occurring during periods of fasting. Improving nutritional status is a simple and effective way of improving outcomes in chronic liver disease and is a key part of the work-up for patients who are awaiting liver transplantation as frailty is a poor prognostic sign (Bischoff et al. 2020).

The input of a specialist liver dietician is recommended because conventional tools such as the MUST (Weekes et al. 2004) fail to account for excess fluid retention and the impact of poor appetite and early satiety seen in patients with liver disease. Patients with decompensated cirrhosis are in a catabolic state and should eat little and often (six meals daily) with a high-protein, high-caloric diet rich in vitamins and minerals. Those admitted to hospital with alcohol dependence and/or at risk of refeeding syndrome should also receive IV Pabrinex. They should have a food chart if the ability to meet nutritional requirements is in doubt and may require additional nutritional supplements as well as a snack before bed (Bischoff et al. 2020). Usually, once ascitic fluid has been drained, and appetite improves, antiemetics and antinausea medication can be helpful.

Nursing considerations for malnourished liver disease patients include:

- Is there a need a food chart?
- Are IV fluids or nasogastric feeding required?
- Is the person at risk of aspiration?
- Is the person at risk of falling if attempting to mobilise?
- Is the person able to meet hygiene needs?
- Are the person's bowels open regularly? Do they have constipation or diarrhoea?
- Is the person at risk of developing pressure injury?
- Is the person supported by friends and family? Do they seem socially isolated or show signs of self-neglect?

Acute on Chronic Liver Failure

ACLF is a unique category of liver disease with mortality outcomes worse for patients treated outside specialist centres (Jalan et al. 2012). It is an acute deterioration in patients with cirrhosis and is usually triggered by insults such as infection or a variceal bleed. Sometimes, no trigger is identified. It is characterised by systemic inflammation disrupting the microcirculation and mitochondrial function resulting in failure of the immune system. This can quickly progress to organ failure if not detected and treated.

Nursing Considerations

Prompt recognition of the deteriorating cirrhotic patient to treat reversible causes includes:

- Close monitoring using NEWS2 score. Ensure BP is maintained and adequate oxygenation provided.
- Fluid overload leading to respiratory failure is a risk in hypotensive patients receiving fluid boluses.
- Strict fluid balance and hourly urine measurements by way of a urethral catheter are necessary.
- The patient and family are likely to be distressed and anxious, reassurance and timely updates are important.
- Early identification and treatment of the underlying reversible cause can prevent a catastrophic cascade of immune modulation failure leading to multiple organ failure and death which may have been preventable.
- Patients identified as having ACLF benefit from prompt admission to critical care, including fluid optimisation and organ support if they fail to respond within 6 hours of ward-based interventions
- Septic screens and treatment with broad-spectrum antibiotics or antifungals can help to prevent progression to multiple organ failure which heralds poor outcomes.
- ACLF is a dynamic disease requiring prognostication with the CLIF-C ACLF score (Jalan et al. 2014). Failure of improvement after 48 hours of optimal treatment and organ support suggests futility and a consideration of care towards comfort and palliation.

Hepato-Renal Syndrome (HRS)

HRS is a functional renal impairment in patients with liver disease who have no underlying renal pathology (Simonetto et al. 2020). It is diagnosed by excluding other possible causes of renal dysfunction. The impact of the splanchnic vasodilation and the RAAS theory explains the likely pathophysiology. Targeted treatment is needed.

All nephrotoxic medications and diuretics should be withheld until the renal function recovers.

Type 1 HRS occurs when renal function deteriorates rapidly despite stopping diuretics and has a 50% mortality within 1 month. Treatment with terlipressin with colloids such as HAS can prevent further renal dysfunction.

Type 2 HRS develops gradually with creatinine greater than 133 μmol/L and is commonly seen in diuretics-resistant ascites.

Acute Liver Injury/Acute Liver Failure

ALI occurs following an acute insult in a normal liver and is characterised by a deranged INR and significantly elevated liver enzymes reflecting the magnitude of the liver damage (Stravitz and Lee 2019). These patients need close monitoring of blood results and level of consciousness because if HE develops, this heralds the onset of liver failure. If HE develops too, ALF is diagnosed requiring urgent referral to a specialist transplant centre for expert management and timely life-saving care (Aziz et al. 2021). ALF is relatively rare but commonly caused by a paracetamol overdose. Treatment with IV N-acetyl cysteine (NAC) within 8 hours of ingestion of the toxic dose can prevent liver damage developing.

ALF is catastrophic, with systematic deterioration occurring rapidly within days of the insult. HE can progress within hours; a mildly confused or sleepy patient can suddenly become incoherent and agitated. Close monitoring and hourly documentation of the GCS are required, and elective neuroprotective sedation and mechanical ventilation should be anticipated or instigated if HE progresses beyond grade 2. The build-up of toxins such as ammonia causes massive changes in the permeability of the blood–brain barrier leading to cerebral oedema and raised intracranial pressure (ICP). Neuroprotective sedation and intubation to manage the risk of a catastrophic cerebral event are required and should continue until the clinical condition improves significantly.

Fulminant standards of care for this group occur in intensive care.

Patients may develop cardiovascular collapse akin to systemic inflammatory response syndrome (SIRS). In such cases, high-dose inotropic drugs are required to support the individual's BP aiming to preserve end-organ perfusion. If not contraindicated and the patient fulfils the transplantation criteria, they will be urgently listed for a lifesaving orthotopic liver transplant (OLT) replacing the failing liver (Burra et al. 2016). As the INR is a key component of transplantation listing criteria, it is important not to correct it routinely with FFP. Active bleeding is not usually a problem, despite significant coagulation screen derangements. Even after the transplantation, complications such as infection and bleeding can occur along with organ rejection. The psychological impact on patients and families with this critical illness is significant and support should be offered via the clinical services within the specialist centre. Patients at risk of developing ALF require prompt discussion with specialist liver centres who provide initial treatment advice and arrange for transfer (Bernal and Wendon 2013).

Liver Cancer

Liver cancer continues to be a significant challenge with a rising incidence globally (Llovet et al. 2021). Assuming there is no spread, then hepatectomy to cut out lesions is the curative approach in patients with no underlying liver disease. The risk of developing liver cancer is greatest in patients with viral hepatitis and cirrhosis. In higher socioeconomic countries, routine screening in cirrhosis clinics to measure alpha-fetoprotein (AFP) levels and by undertaking a liver ultrasound to determine focal lesions may indicate liver cancer at an early stage.

Patients with cirrhosis are not suitable for hepatectomy because of the risk of inducing liver failure, due to lack of functioning hepatocytes. Treatment options vary depending on the size of the lesions and include radiofrequency ablation (RFA) and transarterial chemoembolisation (TACE) which target tumour cells directly and cut off their blood supply. Liver transplantation may be an option if the lesion is larger with no evidence of metastasis. Timely detection offers the best treatment option.

Orthotopic Liver Transplant

A small proportion of patients requiring liver transplantation are urgently listed for transplantation. Most liver transplants are elective, and with significant improvements in the last decade, 1-year survival is greater than 90% (Ralston et al. 2018). Indications for transplant include liver cirrhosis and some specific variants of hepatocellular carcinoma; 10% of patients listed still die on the waiting list. In the UK, the Model of End-Stage Liver Disease (UKELD) score determines those most likely to have a survival benefit of greater than 50% for 5 years, with a score of 49 or higher being the threshold. Contraindications include sepsis, metastatic disease and inability to overcome substance misuse.

Complications include bleeding, primary graft nonfunction, infection and rejection. Lifelong immunosuppressant medication is usually required (Ralston et al. 2018).

Cholelithiasis

Cholelithiasis or the presence of gallstones is very common. Around 10%–20% of adults are thought to have gallstone disease (EASL 2016). Of these, approximately 80% have asymptomatic gallbladder stones (stones found only in the gallbladder, causing no symptoms). Often, they are found by investigations for other conditions; adults with asymptomatic gallbladder stones may never develop symptoms or complications (NICE 2014).

Pathophysiology and Risk Factors

Gallstones are formed from the constituents of bile salts. Stones vary in size and shape and may be solitary or multiple. Their colour can vary from yellow to dark brown or black pigmentation. There are three main types:
- pure cholesterol stones (a 'solitaire' that fills the gallbladder): 10%
- pigmented stones ('jack stones', black and shiny): 2%–3%
- mixed stones (mainly cholesterol, often with some calcium): 80%. Eleven new subtypes of mixed stone were introduced in 2013 (Qiao et al. 2013).

Shabanzadeh (2018) notes that the incidence of gallstones rises noticeably in people aged over 40 years and is 4–10 times more likely in older people, peaking at 70–79 years.

Other factors related to the development of gallstones include the use of oral contraceptives, diabetes mellitus and genetic history. Of patients found to have gallstones during screening, there is a 2% chance per year of these patients developing symptoms. It is believed that only 10%–30% of gallstones become symptomatic. More often they cause biliary colic or an acute or chronic cholecystitis.

Biliary colic is caused by a transient obstruction of the gallbladder from an impacted stone or stones leading to severe spasms of the gallbladder and/or biliary ducts. Cholecystitis can less commonly be caused by trauma and, even more rarely, by tumours.

Clinical Features

The patient complains of a sudden onset of severe gripping pain in the right hypochondrium that often radiates to the back. The pain, referred to as 'biliary colic', may vary in intensity and can last for several hours. The pain will ease when the stone either passes into the common bile duct or falls back into the gallbladder. Nausea and vomiting are also common.

Diagnosis

Tests that may be used to establish a diagnosis include:
- Blood tests – LFTs, serum amylase and WBC
- Abdominal ultrasound
- CT scanning
- ERCP
- MRCP
- EUS

Ultrasound is now the main investigative procedure for patients with suspected gallstones. It is noninvasive and causes minimal discomfort to the patient. Ultrasound can identify stones in the gallbladder, thickening of the gallbladder wall and both intra- and extrahepatic duct dilatation (Ansaloni et al. 2016).

❖ Nursing Management and Health Promotion: Cholelithiasis

Pain management is the main nursing priority. Using a pain scale, assess the patient's pain score and administer a prescribed intramuscular opioid/narcotic analgesia and an antiemetic. The effect of the analgesia should be evaluated. Following investigations, the patient may require a cholecystectomy.

If the patient refuses surgery or if it is contraindicated (e.g. first trimester of pregnancy), lifestyle changes and dietary modifications are advised. In particular, the reduction of risk factors such as obesity and diabetes are important to manage disease progression and symptoms. While the overall evidence of specific dietary advice is of moderate and low certainty the following advice may help to reduce the formation of gallstones and manage symptoms (Ansaloni et al. 2016, Wang et al. 2022):
- Consume small meals that are low in fat.
- Increase fibre intake such as fruits and vegetables high in vitamin C content as it helps to convert cholesterol to bile acid.
- Reduce the intake of coffee and tea.
- Avoid red meats, raw fish and foods with high nitrate.
- Consuming high-starch foods such as potatoes, bread and rice is recommended.

Acute Cholecystitis

Cholecystitis is inflammation of the gallbladder.

Pathophysiology and Risk Factors

The usual cause of acute cholecystitis is impacted gallstones in the cystic duct or Hartmann's pouch causing severe biliary colic.

Clinical Features

The patient presents with an acute illness that is severe in nature and may be in hypovolaemic shock due to vomiting and pain. The pain is typically described as severe, in the right hypochondrium and frequently radiating to the right scapula. On examination, an abdominal mass may be felt and Murphy's sign, a catching of the breath at the height of inspiration when the gallbladder is palpated, is usually positive. There may also be tenderness and guarding of the whole abdomen and sometimes the patient may not be able to tolerate a physical examination. Sweating and pallor may also be present. Patients often present with a pyrexia and tachycardia due to infection. Jaundice can occur, especially if there is an obstruction of the common bile duct. Frequently, patients describe a history of pale stools and dark urine. Also, they may complain of fat intolerance and describe pain after eating a fatty meal.

Treatment Options

Cholecystectomy is indicated in patients with biliary colic or acute cholecystitis and may be carried out as an urgent case. Surgeons are more likely to operate on patients sooner, as an 'early' cholecystectomy means the patient is not at risk of further attacks of acute cholecystitis while awaiting elective surgery (Bagepally et al. 2021).

Open cholecystectomy was performed commonly in the past, but today laparoscopic (keyhole) procedures are preferred due to a reduced hospital stay. However, it is extremely important that the patient also understands and gives consent for an open laparotomy procedure as laparoscopic removal may not be possible. Operating on an acutely inflamed gallbladder carries a risk of conversion to open surgery due to challenges identifying the biliary tree, common bile duct, cystic duct and cystic artery. Furthermore, patients who have pre-existing medical conditions may not be suitable for laparoscopic surgery.

Removal of gallstones can also be performed by ERCP and sphincterotomy and less commonly by extracorporeal shock wave lithotripsy (ESWL) to break up the stones. Most patients will be prepared for laparoscopic surgery as gallstones almost never spontaneously disappear, except when they are formed under special circumstances, such as pregnancy or sudden weight loss.

The advantages of laparoscopic cholecystectomy include:

- reduced stay in hospital
- early mobilisation with lower risk of complications
- minor nature of surgical wounds
- reduced need for opioid analgesics
- quick return to normal life.

Still, there is inconclusive evidence for the superiority of the laparoscopic approach in certain patient populations such as the obese and the elderly and decisions on surgery need to take individual patient factors and wishes into account (Antoniou et al. 2014, Tiong and Oh 2015).

❖ Nursing Management and Health Promotion: Acute Cholecystitis

⬤ Preoperative Management

If the patient requires surgery, preoperative preparation must be undertaken (see Chapter 25). Preoperatively, pain must be assessed and managed as a priority. Opioid/narcotics such as pethidine and NSAID medications such as diclofenac have been found to be effective for pain management. An antiemetic also should be prescribed and administered. Vomiting can be severe and distressing; hence, a nasogastric tube may be passed and aspirated hourly to promote patient comfort.

Hourly monitoring and recording of the patient's vital signs should be undertaken. The patient should be nil orally and IV fluids should be commenced to maintain hydration. Fluid and electrolyte balance should be monitored carefully. The patient

should also be prescribed and administered an IV broad-spectrum antibiotic prior to surgery.

Nurses should provide assistance with personal hygiene to keep the patient comfortable, particularly as excessive perspiration commonly occurs with acute cholecystitis. Oral hygiene is also a nursing priority as the patient is nil by mouth, may be vomiting and may have a nasogastric tube in situ.

The patient may be restless and uncomfortable due to the severity of the pain and possibly due to fear. It is important to reassure the patient and relieve anxiety by explaining that the condition can be treated and the pain relieved. If the patient is expected to have a laparoscopic cholecystectomy, the nurse should explain that the patient may experience shoulder and neck pain for 2–3 days postoperatively. This is due to phrenic nerve irritation from the carbon dioxide gas used to inflate the peritoneum in laparoscopic surgery. This pain can be eased by moving position, physiotherapy and applying hot packs. Some patients find the symptoms improve by taking peppermint water.

If the patient is due to have an open cholecystectomy, the nurse should explain the importance of deep breathing exercises postoperatively to avoid the development of pneumonia. Preparation of the patient for the immediate postoperative period also includes explanations regarding IV fluids, management of the nasogastric tube and the T-tube and the possibility of having an indwelling urinary catheter. The patient should be informed and educated about the postoperative pain management plan and the use of PCA (see Chapter 20).

⬤ Postoperative Management

Immediate postoperative nursing care for patients following a laparoscopic cholecystectomy is similar to the initial care provided for all other patients following other abdominal surgery requiring general anaesthesia (see Chapter 25). Typically, patients are discharged 8 hours postoperatively and most can resume normal activities, such as returning to work, after 2 weeks.

Following open laparotomy surgery, analgesia is vital so that the patient can perform deep breathing and coughing exercises. Opioid PCA is regularly used to manage postoperative pain. The patient should also be assisted to an upright sitting position and encouraged to perform deep breathing exercises to prevent pulmonary complications.

IV fluids are prescribed and administered until the patient is able to tolerate oral fluids (30–60 mL/h). When bowel sounds return, usually after 24 hours, and if tolerated, free fluids may be given. Diet can then be introduced gradually and increased to normal over the next 3 days. All care provided must be evidence based and related to a patient's individual needs.

Early removal of the indwelling catheter, usually the morning following the surgery, is recommended to reduce the likelihood of the patient developing a urinary tract infection.

Sometimes, the patient returns to the ward with a T-tube inserted to maintain patency and prevent stricture of the biliary duct. The 'T' part of the T-tube is in the common bile duct and the long leg of the tube is brought out through a stab wound in the abdominal wall and connected to a drainage bag. In the first 24 hours the T-tube usually drains approximately 300–500 mL of bile. The drainage will reduce over the consecutive days, to approximately less than 200 mL. The nurse should check for bile leakage from around the tube and wound site. Furthermore, it is vital that the T-tube is not removed accidentally. A T-tube cholangiogram is carried out 8–10 days postoperatively to check the patency of the bile duct and the flow of bile into the duodenum prior to the removal of the T-tube. If the ducts are stone free, the tube will be removed as per local policy and procedure.

Following removal of the tube, the nurse should observe the amount of bile leakage and apply a sterile dressing to the wound. Observation of the patient for any signs of biliary peritonitis should be made for 24 hours. Wound sutures, if present, are removed when the wound is healed, generally 5–7 days postoperatively, unless an absorbable subcutaneous suture is used. If wound sites are dry the wound can be left exposed.

Postoperative Complications

Occasionally, postoperative complications can occur, and it is very important that nurses are aware of the symptoms that indicate their onset. Bile duct injury is one such complication that is more common after laparoscopic surgery. Symptoms include persistent pain accompanied by pyrexia of 38°C or above, abdominal distension and jaundice. The patient may need ERCP to locate the injury and may need to return to the operating theatre for surgical repair. Paralytic ileus can also occur postoperatively as a consequence of the primary procedure or secondary to opioid drug treatment (see Chapter 25). If a paralytic ileus does occur, the patient should be kept fasting, a nasogastric tube passed and the stomach kept empty. IV antibiotics are usually given for 5 days and then discontinued. The nurse must inform the surgical team if any of the above symptoms occur.

Depending on the patient's fitness and age, discharge home normally occurs within 6–10 days. Discharge plans will need to be discussed with relatives or carers. The patient must be instructed to avoid lifting heavy objects and to avoid driving for 4–6 weeks to prevent wound herniation. Explain to the patient that faeces pass quicker through the bowel following a cholecystectomy and bile binders such as colestyramine may be required for chronic diarrhoea. Normal diet is encouraged. In an uncomplicated recovery, the patient should be fit to return to work in 4–6 weeks. A detailed discharge summary will be sent to the GP. A follow-up appointment will be given for 4 weeks after discharge. See Reflection 4.5 to reflect on the nursing care of a patient following a laparoscopic cholecystectomy.

REFLECTION 4.5

Care of a patient following a laparoscopic cholecystectomy

Anne Black is a 52-year-old woman admitted to the GI ward complaining of severe gripping pain radiating to her right shoulder. She is very nauseated and was vomiting on admission. However, the vomiting has subsided following an intramuscular injection of prochlorperazine 12.5 mg. She was also given 75 mg of pethidine intramuscularly for pain relief 30 minutes before her arrival to the ward. She informs the nursing staff that the pain is slightly improved but still distressing. Her vital signs are recorded on arrival (BP 140/80 mm/Hg, pulse rate 86 beats per minute, respiration rate 24 breaths per minute, oxygen saturations 98% on air, temperature 37.6°C). On examination, her sclera are slightly jaundiced, she is guarding her abdomen and has a positive Murphy's sign. The nursing staff prepare the patient for a laparoscopic cholecystectomy.

Activities

- Describe the potential advantages and disadvantages of laparoscopic surgery over an open laparotomy.
- Describe the postoperative nursing care Mrs Black should receive following laparoscopic surgery.
- What discharge advice should the nursing staff give to Mrs Black?

Cancer of the Gallbladder

Pathophysiology and Risk Factors

This is a rare cancer and is predominantly related to gallstones. It is more common in females than in males. Within Europe, rates have stabilised over recent years, while in India and South America, they are increasing (Kanthan et al. 2015).

Clinical Features. Signs and symptoms are consistent with those for gallstones, and a history of persistent obstructive jaundice may be present. A mass may be palpable.

Treatment Options. Surgery is the only cure, but in most cases, it is not a chosen treatment. The development of the cancer is mostly silent and can take between 5 and 10 years, and as a consequence, it is usually found at a late stage (Kanthan et al. 2015). Overall survival rates are poor and dependent on the site of cancer formation. Ninety-eight per cent of gallbladder tumours are adenocarcinomas (Hundal and Shaffer 2014). As with other tumours, the involvement of lymph nodes and the presence of metastases will determine the patient's prognosis.

Cancer of the Bile Duct (Cholangiocarcinoma)

Pathophysiology and Risk Factors

The cause of bile duct cancer is unknown although there are strong associations with IBD and PSC. It is more common in older people, and men are affected more than women. It is a very rare cancer but its incidence appears to be increasing (Banales et al. 2020). Tumours can arise from the intra- or extrahepatic biliary tree. Direct spread and metastases are present in at least 50% of the patients who go for surgery.

Treatment Options. As cancer of the bile ducts carries a very poor prognosis, treatment is usually in the form of palliative therapy. For some patients, palliation can be achieved by the insertion of a stent, either by ERCP or by percutaneous transhepatic techniques, e.g. PTC. In a few cases, where the tumour is at the lower end of the common bile duct, a radical resection in the form of a Whipple's procedure may be possible (Fig. 4.11). This is major surgery and should be considered only if the tumour is localised and the patient is fit for surgery.

Tumours of the upper biliary tract are resectable in only 25% of cases (Banales et al. 2020). Following resection of the tumour, a Roux loop of jejunum is anastomosed to the biliary tract or, in some cases, the left hepatic duct. A hepaticojejunostomy then restores the continuity of the small intestine. It can also be performed to bypass the tumour and achieve palliation. Radiotherapy and chemotherapy have not been shown to improve survival.

Figure 4.11 Whipple's procedure

❖ Nursing Management and Health Promotion: Cholangiocarcinoma

The patient with a diagnosis of cholangiocarcinoma will require specialised nursing care. Only a few of these patients will be considered for major resection, following which they are cared for in a high-dependency ward for approximately 48 hours. In some cases, the patient is prepared for major resection but at the time of surgery, it is discovered that only a bypass of the tumour may be carried out safely. These patients are usually devastated by this turn of events and require a great deal of support. Following palliation, jaundice will subside and the patient's appetite will improve. For a few months patients may feel so well that they become unrealistic about the prognosis. Few patients survive more than a year following palliation. Following resection, the outlook is better. Good family support is necessary and it is important to take an honest approach by giving explanations to the patient and family as they request them. It will be necessary to spend time with the patient and the relatives to answer their questions and offer support. Close communication with the GP is pivotal so that community care can be provided when necessary.

THE PANCREAS

The pancreas has both exocrine and endocrine functions and lies below and behind the stomach, in the epigastric and left hypochondriac region of the abdominal cavity (see Fig. 4.6). The function of the exocrine gland is to produce and release pancreatic juice containing enzymes that digest protein, carbohydrate, fat, nucleic acids and bicarbonate. The exocrine secretory functions of the pancreas are under vagal and hormonal control. The initial stimulus for the release of pancreatic juice is food entering the duodenum and stimulating the release of cholecystokinin and secretin. Cholecystokinin is responsible for stimulating the release of the pancreatic enzyme portion of pancreatic juice and secretin is responsible for the release of bicarbonate. The pancreatic duct, which delivers pancreatic juice to the duodenum, and the common bile duct join at the ampulla of Vater. Release of bile and pancreatic juice into the duodenum is controlled by the sphincter of Oddi. This sphincter, a ring of smooth muscle, is relaxed by cholecystokinin.

The endocrine function of the pancreas is concerned with the secretion of the hormones insulin and glucagon directly into the bloodstream in response to fluctuating blood glucose levels. The islets of Langerhans contain the endocrine hormone-producing cells. Insulin and glucagon are synthesised and secreted by the beta cells and alpha cells, respectively. For further information on the endocrine role of the pancreas, see Chapters 5 & 6, Nursing Patients With Disorders of the Lymphatic and Immune System.

DISORDERS OF THE PANCREAS

Pancreatitis

Broadly speaking, inflammation of the pancreas is classified as either acute or chronic, with the essential difference being that the gland returns to normal after an acute attack. In chronic pancreatitis (CP), the inflammatory process is continuous leading to irreversible damage to the gland and impairment of function. The incidence of CP within the UK BioBank cohort of 4200 patients was 163 per 100,000, while the rate for acute pancreatitis (AP) was 48 per 100,000 (Spagnolo et al. 2022).

Acute Pancreatitis

AP is most commonly caused by gallstones or alcohol misuse, which together account for around 75% of cases (NICE 2018b). Other risk factors for AP are related to:

- postendoscopic procedures
- surgery close to the pancreas such as biliary tract procedures, gastric surgery and splenectomy
- metabolic conditions such as hypertriglyceridaemia and hypercalcaemia
- infections such as mumps
- some drugs
- microlithiasis (small gallstones and biliary sludge)
- anatomical or functional disorders
- autoimmune conditions and pancreatic cancer.
  Ten per cent of cases are idiopathic.

🫀 *Pathophysiology and Risk Factors*

The exact process by which pancreatic necrosis occurs is unclear, but it is a complication of AP and affects approximately 20% of hospitalised patients with a mortality rate of about 25% (Rashid et al. 2019). However, it is thought that premature activation of the enzyme trypsin is the initial step in the process. It is normally activated in the small intestine and causes early activation of other enzymes in the pancreas, resulting in autodigestion of pancreatic tissue. This autodigestion leads to varying degrees of oedema, haemorrhage and necrosis, and abscess and cyst formation in and around the pancreas. Spasm of the sphincter of Oddi with reflux of duodenal contents into the pancreatic duct is thought to be an important factor in this enzyme activation. Gallstones block the papilla of Vater, which in turn blocks the main secretory duct from the pancreas and the common bile duct. The pancreatic enzymes are then backed up. Passage of stones down the common bile duct may also promote reflux of infected bile along the pancreatic duct when these ducts form a common channel to the papilla of Vater. Although not clear, it is thought that ethanol (alcohol) either has a generalised impact on cell physiology or a specific effect on pancreatic enzymes (Gukovsky et al. 2012).

Activated enzymes such as trypsinogen and chymotrypsinogen, phospholipase, elastase and catalase are responsible for increased capillary permeability. This permits large volumes of fluid to escape into the peritoneal and retroperitoneal cavity, causing damage to the surrounding tissue. This severe loss of circulating fluid leads to hypovolaemic shock and predisposes the individual to acute renal failure, which may result from local intravascular coagulation in the renal vascular bed. Development of pulmonary oedema with left-sided pleural effusion may result from release of toxins (Goodchild et al. 2019). The release of lipase causes fat necrosis in the omentum and areas adjacent to the pancreas. Calcium salts become sequestered in areas of fatty necrosis, which may result in the development of hypocalcaemia. In 10%–20% of cases, SIRS occurs, which predisposes to multiorgan failure and/or pancreatic necrosis.

Clinical Features

The clinical presentation of AP varies and may be influenced by factors such as age, the presence of comorbidities and the severity of the attack. However, abdominal pain located in the left upper quadrant epigastrium and often radiating to the back is the most common clinical feature (Goodchild et al. 2019). The pain can be unbearably severe, reaching maximal intensity in approximately 30 minutes, and is resistant to attempts at relieving it. The pain is often accompanied by nausea and vomiting, and eating fatty foods or consuming alcohol can exacerbate it. The patient may be very distressed and anxious due to the pain and may be sweating visibly.

AP is often associated with severe shock. There may be signs of dehydration with rapid pulse and respiration rates, hypotension and pyrexia. Marked abdominal tenderness is usually present in the upper abdomen, which may appear distended. Bruising around the umbilicus (Cullen's sign) and in the loin region (Grey Turner's sign) is a rare late manifestation of AP due to petechial bleeding into the retroperitoneal space.

Diagnosis

Investigations will include blood analysis, urinalysis, ultrasound and a CT scan. Radiographic studies are not indicative of AP but may give clues such as the formation of atelectasis and pleural effusions in a chest X-ray. In AP, there may be an elevated plasma concentration of pancreatic enzymes. However, serum amylase and lipase may not reach the diagnostic threshold as their diagnostic performance decreases in the hours and days after the onset of AP and other tests such as C-reactive protein and WBC are indicative of inflammation and progression.

Plain X-ray films of the abdomen can reveal distended loops of small bowel with paralytic ileus but can be a poor prognostic tool given the difficulty with visualising the pancreas. Ultrasound can reveal dilated pancreatic ducts, ascites and gallstones in patients with biliary-induced disease. U&E levels are important indicators of the state of hydration and are necessary for the correct management of the patient. Hyperglycaemia and glycosuria are often present but are transient. ABGs may reveal severe hypoxia. CT scanning is required where a deterioration in clinical status, signs of sepsis or persistent organ failure is evident (Goodchild et al. 2019).

It is important that patients with a severe attack are identified early as they need admission to a high-dependency unit or ICU. For this reason, a number of scoring systems have been developed to predict the severity of attack, e.g. Modified Glasgow Scoring System, Ranson's criteria, APACHE II and Atlanta Classification.

Treatment Options

The overall goal in the management of AP is to provide supportive therapy, treat complications (Information 4.17) as they occur and limit the severity of the inflammatory response. AP is usually managed conservatively, and in mild attacks treatment is generally symptomatic. The principles of management are as follows:

Pain Relief. This is usually provided in the form of opiates/narcotics. IV administration using PCA is one of the options if the patient can manage it, but a background infusion may be required to maintain adequate pain control. Although epidural analgesia has been effective in some patients, it should be used with caution, particularly in patients with altered coagulation (see Chapter 20).

Correction of Shock. If haemorrhagic pancreatitis is diagnosed, shock is treated by IV administration of large volumes of crystalloids, plasma or blood in order to maintain circulatory blood volume and adequate urine output. Oxygen therapy is essential to correct the associated hypoxia. PO_2 saturation levels should be monitored. Hypoxaemia may develop insidiously such that respiratory failure can develop. ABGs are closely monitored in case ventilatory support is required (see Chapter 28).

Suppression of Pancreatic Function. In cases of the presence of paralytic ileus, the patient is kept nil by mouth to decrease stimulation of pancreatic enzymes and a nasogastric tube is passed to drain

---

INFORMATION 4.17

Major complications of acute pancreatitis

Pancreatic pseudocyst

Pancreatic pseudocysts may develop following acute and chronic pancreatitis and are described as such because they are lined with granulation tissue whilst true cysts are lined with epithelium. A pseudocyst is a sac containing pancreatic juice, debris and blood that may be confined initially to the pancreatic parenchyma. They may regress spontaneously, persist with or without symptoms or result in complications. They can rupture with the result that liquefied necrotic tissue becomes evident and can involve adjacent structures where they can cause pain, nausea, vomiting, haemorrhage following erosion of blood vessels, infection and biliary obstruction (Smith and Fawcett 2006). Further complications include pancreatic fistulae or pancreatic ascites. Ultrasound scan can be used in diagnosis and monitoring. Surgery may be necessary if the cyst is symptomatic, since there is a danger that it may rupture or precipitate haemorrhage. Large cysts can resolve with percutaneous aspiration or drainage but those that communicate with the main pancreatic duct require surgical intervention (Smith and Fawcett 2006).

Pancreatic abscess

A pancreatic abscess is an intra-abdominal collection of pus, usually near or around the pancreas. They arise as a consequence of acute pancreatitis, usually a few weeks after the attack has started. This is a serious complication of acute pancreatitis. The patient is usually very ill, with pyrexia, a raised white blood cell count and tachycardia. Early diagnosis by CT scanning and the use of aggressive surgical intervention have improved survival rates. Surgery consists of extensive drainage and debridement of infected tissues. Multiple large drains are used to drain the abscess cavity. Peritoneal lavage with normal saline 0.9% warmed to body temperature can be used to irrigate the cavity. Adequate nutrition following surgery is vital. Most surgeons establish a feeding jejunostomy and gastrostomy tube during surgery.

Pancreatic necrosis

This complication is a major cause of death in acute pancreatitis with a mortality rate of between 15% and 50% depending on the severity and course of the disease. Early differentiation between non-infected (sterile) or infected pancreatic necrosis is essential in order to determine the most appropriate treatment. This can be done using CT or fine-needle aspiration (Werner et al. 2005). The mortality associated with non-infected necrosis is low and it can be treated conservatively. In infected necrosis, the patient often fails to improve with conservative management. A persistent pyrexia, raised white blood cell count, tachycardia, hypotension and poor respiratory function are ominous signs. There is some controversy over the use of radiological drainage or surgical debridement for pancreatic necrosis. However, at laparotomy, necrotic tissue is removed, peritoneal lavage is carried out and the pancreatic bed adequately drained. A feeding jejunostomy and gastrostomy tube may be inserted.

In some cases, the surgeon may opt to leave the wound open to allow for packing of the wound and to minimise the need for repeated laparotomies to deal with recurrent intra-abdominal sepsis.

Duodenal ileus

Due to persistent pancreatic inflammation, duodenal ileus may persist. Nutritional status will need to be maintained either by parenteral means or by jejunostomy feeding. A gastroenterostomy may need to be performed.

Haemorrhage

Severe bleeding may occur from gastric or duodenal ulceration. Prophylactic intravenous cimetidine is given to patients with acute pancreatitis. On rare occasions, haemorrhage may occur into a pseudocyst or by erosion of a blood vessel by the inflammatory process.

gastric secretions and prevent them from entering the duodenum, thus reducing stimulation. Intraabdominal pressure monitoring may be indicated in those patients suffering from severe abdominal distention. In addition, while these patients are at risk of catabolism, nutritional support is one of the cornerstones of therapy. The guidelines by the European Society for Clinical Nutrition and Metabolism (ESPEN) suggest early oral nutrition with a low-fat, soft oral diet if tolerated and enteral feeding via nasogastric or nasojejunal tube within 24–72 hours if the former is not possible. Parenteral nutrition is indicated for patients who do not tolerate oral/enteral nutrition or have contraindications. It may also be used as supplementary nutritional support if the oral/enteral routes are not sufficient to provide adequate nutritional requirements (Arvanitakis et al. 2020).

Controlling Infection. Bacterial infection of necrotic pancreatic tissue is a major cause of morbidity and mortality. However, the use of antibiotics as prophylaxis is controversial and the guidelines indicate that they should not be used beyond 7–14 days without evidence of bacterial growth on culture (NICE 2020). When there is evidence of infection, a broad-spectrum antibiotic is prescribed.

Monitoring Blood Glucose Levels. This is required because secondary diabetes mellitus can sometimes develop, requiring insulin therapy.

Monitoring Cardiac Status. This will be required if electrolyte derangement is such as to cause potentially lethal dysrhythmias.

For the majority of patients, this supportive treatment will settle the acute attack and surgical treatment will not be necessary. If there is any doubt about the diagnosis, a laparotomy will exclude other causes of peritonitis such as perforated peptic ulcer and mesenteric ischaemia.

Surgical Intervention

At an early stage in management, gallstones as a cause of the acute attack are excluded by ultrasound scanning. Cholecystectomy during the course of the patient's admission is now advocated to avoid recurrent problems following discharge. Patients with gallstone pancreatitis can usually be identified by their slow clinical progress and by the use of various clinical and biochemical prognostic factors.

Early ERCP may demonstrate the presence of stones in the common bile duct, which can be extracted by a small balloon catheter or basket following sphincterotomy. The complication of peripancreatic necrosis or abscess can be detected by radiological imaging. Most patients will require necrosectomy, i.e. the removal of necrotic tissues, and drainage at laparotomy or laparoscopic surgery. It may be wise to put in place a gastrostomy and jejunostomy tube at this time, as recovery is slow and the patient may require prolonged nutritional support (see Chapter 22).

❖ Nursing Management and Health Promotion: Acute Pancreatitis

Care of patients with AP will vary according to the severity of the attack. Whilst those with a severe attack of AP will be nursed in a high-dependency unit or intensive care, most will be nursed on the ward. It should be borne in mind that the severity of the attack is not always easily judged by an initial assessment. Therefore, it is imperative that nurses caring for these patients are vigilant in their monitoring to detect any deterioration in the patient's condition. The priorities of nursing care include the following.

Management of Fear and Anxiety. The sudden onset of pain and the sheer severity of the pain are very frightening for these patients. Added to this, few people will have heard of pancreatitis and the patient is likely to have no knowledge of the condition. Attempts to reduce anxiety and fear through continuity of care, information giving and good pain management are important. It is important to explain the rationale of all procedures and investigations to alleviate anxiety. Showing patient diagrams can be very helpful. Communication with the family is vital and nurses and medical staff should give a full explanation of what has occurred to the patient and relatives where applicable.

Respiratory Monitoring. Patients who are in pain are more likely to have reduced respiratory depth evidenced by shallow breathing. In addition, patients with AP may suffer respiratory distress due to inadequate gaseous exchange and shock. Strict respiratory monitoring should be undertaken, including rate and depth of breathing, oxygen saturation and colour of skin, nail bed and peripheries. If tolerated, the patient should be positioned with the head up in bed so as to promote ventilation, but this may not always be tolerated due to abdominal distension. Chest physiotherapy should be undertaken and deep breathing and coughing of secretions encouraged, although this may be very difficult for the patient if the pain is intense. Humidified oxygen therapy may be administered. Good oral hygiene should be maintained and mouth care given where necessary.

Cardiovascular Monitoring. Cardiovascular monitoring should include BP, pulse, temperature, skin temperature, CRT and colour recording. Patients with AP are also at risk of developing thrombi and for this reason, antiembolism stockings should be worn and/or low-molecular-weight heparin administered.

Pain Management. The pain from AP increases metabolic activity, which in turn increases the release of pancreatic enzymes. Therefore, good pain management and the promotion of patient comfort are essential. Pain should be assessed and evaluated using a recognised pain assessment tool such as a visual analogue scale (VAS). IV administration of opiates/narcotics such as morphine or fentanyl using a PCA system is one of the options. As respiratory depression is the main side-effect of opiate analgesia, respiratory, cardiovascular and sedation level monitoring are important. Similarly, monitoring of abdominal discomfort is indicated due to the risk of the development of a paralytic ileus due to the primary pathology but also as a consequence of opioid administration. Regardless of whether or not the patient is being administered oxygen, oxygen saturation rates must be recorded.

Monitoring Fluid Status and Elimination. IV access is established early in those with AP, and in severe cases a central line is inserted. The choice of IV fluids will depend on the patient's haemodynamic status. The nurse must ensure that strict monitoring of fluid input and output is undertaken. A urinary catheter may be inserted to assist with accurate output measurement. Urinalysis should be performed daily. Patency of the IV infusion is essential and monitoring for redness, inflammation and signs of extravasation must be undertaken. Bowel movements and the presence of flatus should be observed.

Blood Glucose Monitoring. In AP, persistent hyperglycaemia can be an indication of a poor prognosis; it is therefore essential that close monitoring of blood glucose takes place. Capillary testing should be undertaken, making sure that testing sites are rotated to prevent fingers becoming sore. If blood glucose levels become unstable, insulin therapy using a sliding scale (variable regimen) may be required.

Maintaining Nutrition. As alluded to, nutritional support is one of the cornerstones of support for this patient group and is dependent on the severity and progression of the disease. Usually, a nasogastric tube to drain gastric secretions is inserted in the acute stage when abdominal distention is present. Drainage must be recorded accurately and frequent oral care must be undertaken to promote patient comfort. In addition, it is important that the nasogastric tube is properly secured to reduce 'drag' and nasal care should be performed to avoid device-related pressure injuries. In the presence of nausea and vomiting, antiemetics should be administered. Where nutritional support is required, an appropriate route should be used as per ESPEN guidelines. Care and observation of the tube insertion site are important and include observation for signs of inflammation, excoriation and leakage. As the patient's general condition improves, oral nutrition must be introduced with gradual progression to a light diet.

Maintaining Skin Integrity and Hygiene Needs. As many of these patients are acutely ill, they will require assistance and support in maintaining personal hygiene. Skin should be kept clean and dry, especially if the patient is pyrexial or sweating excessively. Particular attention should be paid to the skin and hygiene needs of those who may develop jaundice due to obstruction of the common bile duct. This can be accompanied by discomfort and itching of the skin (pruritus, refer to hepatic section). Cool sponging and the application of a soothing lotion/aqueous cream may help to alleviate symptoms. In addition, during the acute phase when the patient is most incapacitated, it is important that an assessment of susceptibility to pressure ulcer development is undertaken and documented. During periods of intense pain, patients may be reluctant to move and the nurse should ensure that regular repositioning is undertaken. Early mobilisation should be encouraged.

Discharge planning following AP will be determined by the patient's individual situation and the perceived cause of the attack. For patients who have gallstones, treatment must be planned to prevent recurrence. This may involve an open or laparoscopic cholecystectomy with an operative cholangiogram or, for patients who are not fit for surgery, an ERCP and sphincterotomy. The timing of this treatment will depend on the severity of the attack of AP. In the interim, these patients should be referred to a dietitian for advice on a low-fat diet.

Where alcohol is implicated in the onset of AP, the advice is that the person should abstain permanently or risk a life-threatening recurrence (refer to section on hepatitis and alcohol dependence). In a person with alcohol dependency, this can be extremely challenging and without appropriate support and counselling, they are not likely to succeed. Therefore it is imperative that nurses broach the subject in a non-judgemental manner ensuring that the patient has sufficient information and time to consider referral for counselling. Many hospitals now employ alcohol liaison nurse specialists who provide support and advice on abstinence. Continued support in the community should also be explored.

Advice regarding return to work is important. The patient often feels tired and in many cases, it is advisable not to return to work for perhaps 4–6 weeks. The patient may be very worried about work, family and financial situation, and a visit from the social worker may be of value. The patient will be reviewed in the outpatient clinic initially at 3–4 weeks or as per local policy.

Chronic Pancreatitis

CP develops as a consequence of recurrent inflammatory episodes resulting in the replacement of the pancreatic parenchyma by fibrous connective tissue (Herreros-Villanueva et al. 2013, Löhr et al. 2017, NICE 2018b). Recurrent AP is the main underlying cause which can result in various complications such as pancreatic insufficiency,

steatorrhea, diabetes and pancreatic calcification ultimately leading to fibrosis. Although alcohol and its byproducts are not the direct cause of this disease, they can make the pancreas more vulnerable to harm from other seemingly harmless agents. In addition, it has been proposed that genetic predisposition is an important factor in its development. Therefore, alcohol could be described as a cofactor in susceptible people. Other risk factors include metabolic issues (hypercalcaemia, hyperlipidaemia, chronic renal failure, cystic fibrosis and hyperparathyroidism); genetic and hereditary predisposition; idiopathic (no known cause); nutritional or tropical pancreatitis; and obstructive (post-traumatic ductal strictures, pseudocysts, tumours, pancreatic divisum).

Pathophysiology and Risk Factors

CP leads to permanent damage of the gland, with the replacement of the cells by fibrotic tissue and calcification. The ducts become narrowed and the flow of pancreatic juice is obstructed and functional cells slowly stop secreting pancreatic juice. The obstructed ducts can give rise to recurrent attacks of pancreatitis. Irreversible structural damage may have taken place long before the person with CP develops clinical signs and symptoms of exocrine and endocrine dysfunction. In advanced disease, peripancreatic fibrosis can occur that involves the portal and splenic veins. As a result, portal hypertension and occlusion of the lymph nodes develop. Endocrine dysfunction and the development of diabetes mellitus occur later in the process of pancreatic cell destruction. Furthermore, those who are diagnosed with CP can develop pancreatic pseudocysts (see Information 4.17) and are at increased risk of developing pancreatic cancer.

Clinical Features

Although its presentation varies from person to person, pain, either persistent or episodic, is the symptom with which the patient usually presents and has been described as the most distressing. It is classically located in the epigastrium, radiates to the back and can be relieved by sitting forward. The pain is associated with oral intake, and nausea and vomiting may also be present. A history of alcohol use disorder may be given.

The gradual destruction of the pancreas leads to impairment of endocrine and exocrine function, although clinical signs such as malabsorption and steatorrhea may only appear after significant destruction has taken place. In steatorrhea, the stool is pale, offensive and difficult to flush away and is due to a high undigested fat content. Steatorrhea accompanied by weight loss provides evidence of advanced structural damage of the pancreas. It is often a distressing feature for the patient.

Endocrine insufficiency affects approximately 5–10 people per 100,000 population in Europe and manifests itself by the development of diabetes mellitus and patients are at severe risk to develop hypoglycaemia (Löhr et al. 2017). Its management in CP is similar to that of other diabetic patients except that it usually requires treatment with insulin. Transient jaundice may be present due to inflammation of the head of the pancreas, which obstructs the common bile duct.

Diagnosis

Due to the complexity of the disease, diagnosing CP in the early stages is difficult, particularly when trying to differentiate between acute relapsing and CP. Moreover, in the early stages of the illness, there may not be any clinical signs of pancreatic destruction. As a result, investigations may not detect CP unless the condition is at an advanced stage. If the attack that prompts the patient to seek medical help is severe, then blood analysis for serum amylase and lipase may show elevations as seen in AP. However, they are not reliable markers for the presence of CP. A plain abdominal X-ray may show speckled calcification of the pancreas whilst ultrasound scan may show an enlarged, swollen gland. CT gives good detail showing an increased density of the parenchyma, atrophy of the gland, calcification, pseudocysts and irregularities of the main pancreatic duct and its side branches but only in the advanced stages of the disease. Direct tests of pancreatic and duodenal juice via ERCP are no more regarded as a definitive diagnosis and therefore not recommended (Löhr et al. 2017). However, ERCP may be performed to outline the pancreatic duct if surgery is contemplated. Faecal fat estimation, although used less often now, may reveal malabsorption. Fasting blood sugars are assessed and a glucose tolerance test may be necessary.

Treatment Options

Management of CP is mainly symptomatic. The patient should be advised to stop drinking alcohol and may need professional counselling to this end. Replacement of pancreatic enzymes with a commercial preparation may help to alleviate the steatorrhoea and reduce pain. Good control of diabetes will be necessary.

Pain control can be difficult and management advice from a pain control specialist is invaluable. In a small number of patients in whom severe pain persists, surgery will be indicated. It may be necessary to resect the head of the gland (Whipple's procedure; see Fig. 4.11) or the body and tail (distal pancreatectomy). Adequate drainage of the duct (pancreatojejunostomy) may be undertaken where ERCP shows the pancreatic duct to be dilated. A total pancreatectomy is rarely undertaken due to the resulting permanent diabetes mellitus and exocrine insufficiency.

❖ Nursing Management and Health Promotion: Chronic Pancreatitis

Nursing management of an acute attack in CP is similar to that for AP.

Pain. Pain is often constant in nature, radiating through to the back. It is often described as being like a sharp knife twisting in the gut and presents a major challenge to pain control. Pain assessment, using a recognised pain assessment tool, should be undertaken. The analgesic ladder is also an effective tool for determining the level at which the pain is controlled. NSAIDs such as diclofenac sodium (Voltarol) in suppository form can be of value. It is often necessary to use opioid analgesics to alleviate pain and a pain specialist or pain management team can be invaluable in advising about management of what is often intractable pain (see Chapter 20). Assisting the patient into a comfortable position may help. The patient may find that bending forward while leaning on a bed table helps. The use of a heat pad to the back may give some relief.

Alcohol Dependency. Alcohol dependence is commonly implicated in the onset of CP. Total abstinence may help reduce the severity of the pain but it does not always resolve it. If the patient has a known dependency, sudden withdrawal may precipitate DTs. Mild sedation is frequently used to prevent this. Expert help by e.g. alcohol liaison services and continued personal support may assist the patient to overcome an alcohol problem.

Nutrition. The patient diagnosed with CP is at risk of being nutritionally compromised and many will experience significant weight loss as, at times, they are reluctant to eat for fear of exacerbating the pain. In addition, as the function of the pancreas deteriorates, they can experience dyspepsia, malabsorption and steatorrhoea. Therefore nutritional assessment must be undertaken. Once the acute attack is resolved, a dietitian consultation will provide the appropriate information and education about pancreatic enzyme replacement therapy and maintaining a well-balanced diet low in fat and high in carbohydrates. Pancreatic enzyme supplements can be prescribed and taken prior to meals to aid absorption of nutrients. This should also help alleviate the steatorrhoea. Concurrent administration of H_2RA or protein pump inhibitors (PPIs) may improve the efficacy of these supplements. Close monitoring of blood glucose should be undertaken and in the event of the development of diabetes mellitus, the input of a diabetic nurse specialist will provide invaluable assistance.

Health Promotion. Information and education about the implications of living with CP are fundamental in order to facilitate lifestyle adjustments, particularly in respect of maintaining nutritional status and abstaining from alcohol. Smoking cessation is also advocated since smoking is thought to be implicated in increasing the risk of developing pancreatic cancer. For those who do not have an alcohol dependency or where the cause is not known, there is a sense of helplessness associated with not knowing why they have developed this condition. Depending on the severity of the symptoms, CP can have a significant impact on the quality of life of those living with it. Symptoms can be debilitating leading to attendant psychosocial problems, loss of work, reliance on narcotics to manage the pain and significant periods of time spent in hospital. Integrated support across acute and community-based services is essential in enabling these patients to maximise self-management of this lifelong condition. Caring for these patients can present a professional and personal challenge to members of the MDT, who may feel inclined to blame the patient for the illness.

Cancer of the Pancreas

The cause of pancreatic cancer is unknown, but cigarette smoking, pre-existence of diabetes mellitus, chronic or hereditary pancreatitis, stomach ulcer, IBD, previous cancers, family history, diet and being overweight and physically inactive have all demonstrated an increased risk.

In the UK, each year there are around 10,500 new pancreatic cancer cases; this is the 10th most common cancer in the UK, accounting for 3% of all new cancer cases. In females in the UK, pancreatic cancer is the 9th most common cancer, and in males, the 12th most common cancer. The incidence rates for pancreatic cancer in the UK (between 2016 and 2018) are highest in those aged 85 to 89 years. The most common anatomical location for pancreatic cancers is the head of the pancreas. Approximately 540 cases of pancreatic cancer each year in England are linked with deprivation and pancreatic cancer incidence rates are lower in the Asian ethnic group and in people of mixed or multiple ethnicities, but higher in the Black ethnic group, compared with the White ethnic group (England, 2013–2017) (Cancer Research UK 2023).

◆ Pathophysiology and Risk Factors

Tumours of the pancreas can arise from exocrine or endocrine tissue and can be malignant or benign, although the latter is very rare. More than 80% of exocrine pancreatic cancers are adenocarcinomas; the majority of these are ductal adenocarcinomas. They start in the cells lining the ducts of the pancreas (Cancer Research UK 2023). Endocrine tumours also exist and arise from the islets of Langerhans. Tumours of the head of the pancreas account for more than two-thirds of pancreatic cancers. Lesions frequently obstruct the pancreatic duct, causing CP. The carcinoma can also obstruct the bile duct, giving rise to obstructive jaundice. Cancer of the pancreas carries a very poor prognosis because the disease has often spread to nearby organs by the time a diagnosis is made. Surgical resection has not been shown to improve the rate of survival. However, cancer of the duodenum, lower bile duct and periampullary regions often presents earlier with obstructive jaundice, and surgical resection offers a much better prognosis.

Clinical Features

Clinical features will vary according to the location, size in relation to nearby structures and the specific anatomical location of the tumour. Many of the early symptoms are nonspecific and tend to go unrecognised with the result that diagnosis occurs at an advanced stage. However, obstructive jaundice is often the symptom with which the patient first presents to the GP. The urine may be dark in colour, the stool pale and fatty, and the skin and sclera have a yellowish tinge. Severe itch (pruritus, refer to earlier in this chapter) can be a very distressing symptom. Severe weight loss (approximately 2–3 kg per month) and anorexia are associated with vague epigastric pain, often radiating to the back. Initially, pain is intermittent, but gradually it becomes constant and severe.

Diagnosis

Blood is taken for LFTs and to check for the presence of a coagulation defect. The most frequently used biomarker for pancreatic cancer is carbohydrate antigen 19-9 (CA 19-9), however, diagnosis cannot be established solely on its level because other conditions may also cause a rise. Still, it can help with predicting prognosis, assessing treatment response in advanced disease or determining the risk of recurrence following surgery (Lee et al. 2020).

Dual-phase CT scanning is a more sensitive and noninvasive diagnostic tool that has a degree of specificity in detecting a pancreatic mass, local invasion by tumour or metastases. An ultrasound scan will detect a dilated biliary tree and exclude the presence of gallstones. Pancreatic tissue may be obtained for cytology by using CT scan or ultrasound-guided fine-needle aspiration. ERCP can be used to define the site of obstruction and obtain biopsies (NICE 2018a).

Treatment Options

Relief of obstructive jaundice and pain control are all that can be offered to the majority of patients with pancreatic cancer. ERCP with stenting of the biliary tree can relieve obstructive jaundice and may reduce the necessity for surgical intervention. Chemotherapy is used but appears to have little long-term clinical benefit or effect on survival. Where the tumour is not resectable, radiotherapy has been shown to reduce local progression and has an effect on survival time and metastatic spread. Surgery is usually palliative but jaundice may be relieved by cholecystojejunostomy or choledochojejunostomy. The proportion of patients with pancreatic cancer receiving radiotherapy is strongly influenced by the staging outcome at diagnosis. Other important factors include whether the patient is generally well enough to tolerate the treatment, the patient's age and their own treatment preference.

In a minority of cases (8%) where the tumour is deemed to be resectable for curable causes, a Whipple's procedure (pancreatoduodenectomy) (see Fig. 4.11) may be considered. However, this surgery is highly complex with variable results and a high rate of perioperative mortality, although this is improving particularly in hepatobiliary specialist centres. However, the 5-year survival rate is around 30% (NICE 2018a).

❖ Nursing Management and Health Promotion: Cancer of the Pancreas

Investigative procedures are extensive, and surgery in the majority of cases offers palliation only. The nurse has a very important role in helping both the patient and the family to cope as the prognosis is one of the worst and the condition dramatically affects the patient's quality of life.

Anxiety. Patients with pancreatic cancer are usually very anxious. They may have no previous history of illness and often deny the diagnosis. They may have difficulty coming to terms with the diagnosis and are often angry and withdrawn, especially with close family members. Relatives often feel shut out and helpless. The nurse can help by offering support and advice to the patient and family members, who should be given opportunities to discuss the illness and its implications.

If surgery is to be undertaken, extensive discussion with the patient and relatives is necessary. Some patients are prepared for a Whipple's procedure but at surgery, it is found that the disease is more extensive than expected and a bypass is all that can be safely attempted. This is devastating for the patient and family, who will have built up hopes for recovery.

Pain. Pain is often persistent, particularly when the disease is at an advanced stage. Oral opioids may be given and titrated to the patient's specific needs. Progression to subcutaneous diamorphine may be necessary as the disease advances and an oral laxative will also be given to prevent the side-effect of constipation. As the disease advances, pain may become more difficult to control. A coeliac plexus nerve block may also be of benefit (NICE 2018a).

Close monitoring of the effectiveness of pain control is essential to ensure that the best possible quality of life can be maintained for the patient (see Chapter 20). If the patient is discharged home, liaison with the primary healthcare team is essential to ensure that full continuity of care is achieved. Referral to a hospice should be made to ensure that the patient and their family receive the best possible care as the condition deteriorates (see Chapter 32).

Jaundice. Jaundice is usually persistent and accompanied by severe itching (pruritus). The itching (pruritus, see earlier in the chapter) is usually all over the body and the patient may scratch until the skin bleeds. Patients may be so distressed by itch that they feel they are being driven mad. Every effort should be made to relieve itching, which is believed to be caused by a deposition of bile salts in the skin. Antihistamines are used but they can cause sedation. A twice-daily bath with added sodium bicarbonate may be effective but good data on its efficacy are currently not available. Night sedation is important, as itching is often worse at night.

Following ERCP and stenting, the jaundice and itch will subside over 7–10 days. The patient will feel much better as soon as the itch disappears and jaundice fades. Patients should be actively encouraged to drink extra fluids. This helps jaundice to abate by flushing bilirubin and bile salts out of the blood and tissues.

Anorexia and Weight Loss. Poor appetite and subsequent weight loss are further distressing aspects of the disease. Meals should be small and attractively presented. Liaison with the dietitian is necessary. High-protein drinks between meals may be tolerated well. If weight loss is severe, special care should be taken to prevent the development of pressure ulcers. Malaise associated with anorexia and weight loss will increase the patient's dependency and nurses and other carers will need to offer more and more assistance with many aspects of daily life. A food supplement called pancreatin may be prescribed to compensate for the reduced or absent exocrine secretion. The use of fish oil as a nutritional supplement should be avoided (NICE 2018a).

THE SPLEEN

The spleen (Fig. 4.12) is the largest lymph organ in the body and lies in the upper left quadrant of the abdomen, between the

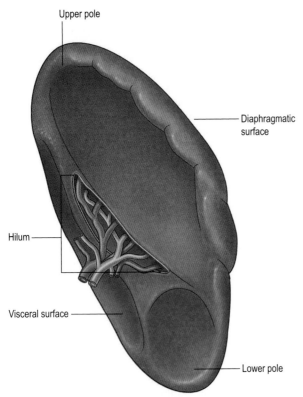

Figure 4.12 Surface and hilum of the spleen. (Reproduced with permission from Drake RL, Vogl W, Mitchell AWM. *Gray's Anatomy for Students*. 3rd ed. Philadelphia: Elsevier; 2015.)

fundus of the stomach and the diaphragm. It is richly supplied with blood via the splenic artery. Blood flow through the spleen is slowed down by the fact that blood must pass through sinuses in which the monophage/macrophage system scavenges old erythrocytes and pathogenic particles and passes the breakdown products on to the liver via the hepatic portal system. The main functions of the spleen include phagocytosis, storage of blood, immune activation in the presence of antigens and erythropoiesis.

DISORDERS OF THE SPLEEN

Splenic Trauma

The spleen is highly vascular and is one of the organs most frequently damaged by abdominal trauma. Fractures of the lower ribs following trauma are often implicated in splenic injury; road traffic collision is one example. These are not always identifiable from an abdominal ultrasound. Furthermore, the spleen is particularly susceptible to injury when it is pathologically enlarged.

Pathophysiology and Risk Factors

Injury to the spleen can result in rupture, evulsion from its pedicle or tearing beneath the capsule, with possible formation of a subcapsular haematoma. Delayed rupture of the spleen occurs in about 5% of patients and is thought to be caused by haematoma bursting through the capsule wall. This usually occurs within 2 weeks of injury, but in a few cases can be delayed for months or even years.

Clinical Features

Rupture and evulsion of the spleen cause immediate intraperitoneal bleeding. As blood spreads throughout the peritoneal cavity, signs

of haemorrhage and hypovolaemic shock (see Chapter 19) may develop. Patients generally present as an acute abdominal emergency. The patient experiences abdominal pain with particular tenderness in the left upper quadrant and percussion dullness of the left flank (Ballance's sign). Referred pain is often felt in the left shoulder tip (Kerh's sign). Bruising to the abdomen is not always evident.

Not all patients with splenic injury present in such a dramatic way. Sometimes, patients may require a splenectomy following lymphatic malignancy, sickle cell disease or malignancy causing infarction of the spleen or due to splenic injury during or as a consequence of surgery.

Treatment Options

If a diagnosis is difficult to establish and splenic injury is suspected, vigilant and careful observation of the patient is vital. Splenic injury due to trauma is frequent but the majority of these (80%–90%) are managed conservatively (Wiik Larsen et al. 2023). Still, injury to the spleen due to blunt trauma may constitute an indication for either splenectomy or embolisation of the splenic artery (Yiannoullou et al. 2017). In addition, if at all possible, conservation by suturing capsular tears or by performing a partial splenectomy is the preferred option, as there is a risk of systemic infection following splenectomy.

❖ Nursing Management and Health Promotion: Splenic Trauma

Following splenic injury, the patient's pain should be monitored, noting the site, type and duration. Whether the pain is increasing or decreasing may be relevant. There is no evidence to support withholding pain relief until a diagnosis is confirmed, hence opioid analgesia should be prescribed and administered. The patient will be nil per mouth during this acute period and so oral hygiene needs will be a nursing priority.

The patient's vital signs should be monitored. Any changes in the patient's condition should be reported immediately as, following rupture, temporary improvement in the patient's condition may precede sudden deterioration.

IV access should be established and IV fluids, blood and blood products should be administered as required. Oxygen therapy may be commenced to raise the circulating oxygen levels, and a urinary catheter is inserted to assess renal function. BP, pulse, respirations and oxygen saturation should be closely monitored and any changes reported immediately. A nasogastric tube may be passed to empty the stomach contents and prevent aspiration.

The nurse should provide reassurance as the patient may be distressed and anxious preoperatively. Relatives should be kept informed and comfort and support should be given during this stressful and worrying time.

Preoperative Management

In preparation for splenectomy, a full assessment of the patient's blood count and coagulation status must be made. In the presence of any bleeding tendency, a transfusion of blood or platelets may be administered. However, in the acute phase of trauma, permissive hypotension is the preferred method, as extensive fluid replacement in the polytrauma patient has shown worse outcomes (Tran et al. 2018). In patients with thrombocytopenia, platelets should be made available for use to cover the intra- and postoperative phase. *Haemophilus influenzae* type B vaccine is also given prophylactically. Preparation for surgery is as for abdominal surgery requiring general anaesthesia (see Chapter 25).

Postoperative Management

Postoperative care is as described for abdominal surgery requiring general anaesthesia (see Chapter 25). The patient will usually be nursed in a high-dependency area until stable enough to return to a general ward.

Nursing observations include monitoring the patient's vital signs and pain levels. The use and effectiveness of the PCA and prescribed antiemetics should be monitored. Ensure the patient's comfort throughout.

The wound should be monitored for signs of inflammation. If wound drains are present, output should be monitored and they should be removed when drainage is minimal. Fluid intake and output should be carefully recorded, and oral fluids should be encouraged when the patient is able to tolerate them.

In the postoperative period, an antipneumococcal vaccine is given to prevent or minimise the risk of developing a chest infection. These patients are more susceptible to chest infection because of the role of the spleen in immune activation. Furthermore, because the spleen is located close to the left lung, there is an increased risk of collapse of the left lower lobe following splenectomy. Therefore, chest physiotherapy is essential. The nurse must also encourage the patient to perform deep breathing exercises and aid expectoration between physiotherapy sessions. Low-dose heparin should be prescribed due to a transient increase in platelet and leucocyte levels. The nurse should perform passive leg exercises whilst the patient is on bed rest and encourage movement and early ambulation. Anti-embolism stockings should be worn to prevent the development of postoperative deep venous thrombosis.

Pancreatitis caused by the handling and bruising of the tail of the pancreas during surgery is a complication of splenic surgery. The serum amylase and lipase should be monitored for 2–4 days postoperatively. Nurses should observe for the signs and symptoms of the development of pancreatitis, i.e. nausea and vomiting, severe abdominal pain and abdominal distension. The nurse must be alert to any increase or change in the nature of the patient's pain.

Due to the loss of lymphoid tissue, there is an increased risk of infection following splenectomy. As most infections occur within 3 years of surgery, prophylactic penicillin for this period or even longer may be prescribed. Antibiotic cover must be based on individual assessment of each patient, and lifelong prophylaxis may be needed for those who are severely immunosuppressed and those who have had a splenectomy for haematological malignancy.

Persistent haemorrhage occurs in less than 1% of patients following a splenectomy and usually occurs in those who have had surgery for the treatment of thrombocytopenia. It is important that the patient is educated about the complications that can occur following a splenectomy and any lifestyle changes that they may need to consider.

Summary: Key Nursing Issues

- The predominant function of the GI and hepatobiliary system is to digest food in order to generate energy for the body.
- Because the GI and hepatobiliary system comprises a large number of organs with a range of interrelated functions, disorders can produce diverse and often distressing symptoms, such as pain, dysphagia, anorexia, weight loss, dyspepsia, nausea and vomiting, constipation and diarrhoea, causing considerable embarrassment and activity restrictions in patients' lives.
- Both surgical and conservative management of patients with GI and hepatobiliary conditions constitute interventions that can result in a reduction in the patient's life quality.
- Deaths from diseases of the GI system are increasing. Malignancies of the GI and hepatobiliary system are among the most common and, given their relationship with nutrition, digestion and excretion, can cause significant suffering for patients and their families.
- In order to provide effective care, nurses must have a good knowledge and understanding of the anatomy and physiology of the GI and hepatobiliary system.
- Nurses have a key role in health promotion such as screening, advising about lifestyle changes, providing educational support, promoting and enabling self-care and monitoring the patient's physical, psychological and social functioning.
- Pain assessment and management are essential nursing skills as pain is severe for many patients presenting with disorders of the GI and hepatobiliary systems.
- A non-judgemental approach is vital when supporting patients suffering from disorders that are linked to obesity, alcohol and recreational drug use and cigarette smoking.
- Nurses specialising in GI nursing need a wide variety of skills and knowledge in order to assess, diagnose, plan, implement and evaluate the sometimes complex and challenging nursing care required by patients with GI, hepatobiliary, pancreatic and splenic disorders.
- Nurses specialising in GI nursing are now performing diagnostic and therapeutic interventions. These advances are in line with evolving technology and the increased demand for rapid access to healthcare services and it is likely that the role will continue to evolve and grow to meet the needs of a modern health service.
- All care provided has to be evidence based with the patient at the centre of all that is done.

Reflection and Learning – What Next?

- **Test** your knowledge by visiting the website 🌐 and answering the multiple-choice questions and critical thinking questions.
- **Consolidate** your learning by looking at some of the further reading suggestions, references and specialist websites.
- **Revisit** some of the additional material on the website.
- **Consider** what you have learnt and how this will help your professional development.
- **Reflect** on how you can apply this knowledge to the care of your patients.
- **Discuss** your learning with your assessor/supervisor, lecturer and colleagues.

References

Abby Philips C, Sahney A. Oesophageal and gastric varices: historical aspects, classification and grading: everything in one place. *Gastroenterol Rep (Oxf)*. 2016;4:186–195.

Angeli P, Bernardi M, Villanueva C, et al. EASL Clinical Practice Guidelines for the management of patients with decompensated cirrhosis. *J Hepatol*. 2018;69:406–460.

Ansaloni L, Pisano M, Coccolini F, et al. 2016 WSES guidelines on acute calculus cholecystitis. *World J Emerg Surg*. 2016;11:25.

Antoniou SA, Antoniou GA, Koch OO, Pointner R, Granderath FA. Meta-analysis of laparoscopic vs open cholecystectomy in elderly patients. *World J Gastroenterol*. 2014;20:17626–17634.

Arvanitakis M, Ockenga J, Bezmarevic M, et al. ESPEN guideline on clinical nutrition in acute and chronic pancreatitis. *Clin Nutr*. 2020;39:612–631.

Aziz R, Price J, Agarwal B. Management of acute liver failure in intensive care. *BJA Education*. 2021;21:110–116.

Bagepally BS, Haridoss M, Sasidharan A, Jagadeesh KV, Oswal NK. Systematic review and meta-analysis of gallstone disease treatment outcomes in early cholecystectomy versus conservative management/delayed cholecystectomy. *BMJ Open Gastroenterol*. 2021;8:e000675.

Baird DL, Simillis C, Kontovounisios C, et al. Acute appendicitis. *BMJ*. 2017;357:1–6.

Banales JM, Marin JJG, Lamarca A, et al. Cholangiocarcinoma 2020: the next horizon in mechanisms and management. *Nat Rev Gastroenterol Hepatol*. 2020;17:557–588.

Banning M. Helicobacter pylori: microbiology, transmission and health significance. *Gastrointest Nurs*. 2012;10(1):45–49.

Barber K, Madden S, Allen J, Collett D, Neuberger J, Gimson A. United Kingdom Liver Transplant Selection and Allocation Working Party. Elective liver transplant list mortality: development of a United Kingdom end-stage liver disease score. *Transplantation*. 2011;92(4):469–476. doi:10.1097/TP.0b013e318225db4d.

Baruah S, Bajpai M. Effect of FFP transfusion on international normalized ratio in liver disease patients. *Indian J Hematol Blood Transfus*. 2018;34:719–722.

Bernal W, Wendon J. Acute liver failure. *N Engl J Med*. 2013;369:2525–2534.

Bischoff SC, Bernal W, Dasarathy S, et al. ESPEN practical guideline: Clinical nutrition in liver disease. *Clin Nutr*. 2020;39:3533–3562.

Blatchford O, Murray WR, Blatchford M. A risk score to predict need for treatment for upper gastrointestinal haemorrhage. *Lancet North Am Ed*. 2000;356:1318–1321.

British Association for Parenteral and Enteral Nutrition (BAPEN). MUST calculator. 2018. Available at: https://www.bapen.org.uk/screening-and-must/must-calculator.

British Medical Journal Best Practice. *Gastro-oesophageal reflux disease*. BMJ Publishing Group; 2022. https://bestpractice.bmj.com/topics/en-gb/82.

Brown KF, Rumgay H, Dunlop C, et al. The fraction of cancer attributable to known risk factors in England, Wales, Scotland, Northern Ireland and the UK overall in 2015. *Br J Cancer*. 2018;118(8):1130–1141.

Brunner KT, Henneberg CJ, Wilechansky RM, Long MT. Nonalcoholic fatty liver disease and obesity treatment. *Curr Obes Rep*. 2019;8:220–228.

Buchanan R, Sinclair JMA. Alcohol use disorder and the liver. *Addiction*. 2021;116:1270–1278.

Burch J, Collins B. *Oxford Handbook of Gastrointestinal Nursing*. 2nd ed. Oxford: Oxford University Press; 2021.

Burra P, Burroughs A, Graziadei I, et al. EASL Clinical Practice Guidelines: Liver transplantation. *J Hepatol*. 2016;64:433–485.

Büttner L, Aigner A, Pick L, et al. 25 years of experience with transjugular intrahepatic portosystemic shunt (TIPS): changes in patient selection and procedural aspects. *Insights Imaging*. 2022;13:73.

Cancer Research UK. Types. https://www.cancerresearchuk.org/about-cancer/oesophageal-cancer/stages-types-and-grades/types; 2019.

Cancer Research UK. Oesophageal cancer incidence statistics. https://www.cancerresearchuk.org/health-professional/cancer-statistics/statistics-by-cancer-type/oesophageal-cancer/incidence#heading-Zero; 2021.

Cancer Research UK, https://www.cancerresearchuk.org/health-professional/cancer-statistics/statistics-by-cancer-type/pancreatic-cancer, Accessed 28 November 2023.

Cancer Research UK. Oesophageal cancer risk. https://www.cancerresearchuk.org/health-professional/cancer-statistics/statistics-by-cancer-type/oesophageal-cancer/risk-factors; 2023a

Cancer Research UK. Stomach cancer statistics. https://www.cancerresearchuk.org/health-professional/cancer-statistics/statistics-by-cancer-type/stomach-cancer?_gl=1*trj3ot*_ga*MTk2NDIwMTk5Ni4xNjc2ODA3OTQ4*_ga_58736Z2GNN*MTY3Njg1ODMyNC40LjEuMTY3Njg1ODkwNi4zOS4wLjA.&_ga=2.132113231.1700408575.1676807948-1964201996.1676807948; 2023b

Cancer Research UK. Bowel cancer statistics. https://www.cancerresearchuk.org/health-professional/cancer-statistics/statistics-by-cancer-type/bowel-cancer/incidence; 2023c

Cancer Research UK. Pancreatic cancer statistics https://www.cancerresearchuk.org/health-professional/cancer-statistics/statistics-by-cancer-type/pancreatic-cancer; 2023d

Cancer Research UK. Types of pancreatic cancer https://www.cancerresearchuk.org/about-cancer/pancreatic-cancer/stages-types-grades/types; 2023e

Cancer Research UK. Pancreatic cancer incidence [online]. Available at: https://www.cancerresearchuk.org/health-professional/cancer-statistics/statistics-by-cancer-type/pancreatic-cancer#heading-Zero; 2023f. Accessed 24 April 2023.

Child CG, Turcotte JG. Surgery and portal hypertension. *Major Probl Clin Surg*. 1964;1:1–85.

Choi AH, Kim J, Chao J. Perioperative chemotherapy for resectable gastric cancer: MAGIC and beyond. *World J Gastroenterol*. 2015;21(24):7343–7348.

Clay JM, Fontana BD, Proserpio C, et al. Drinking during social isolation: investigating associations between stress, inhibitory control, boredom, drinking motives, and alcohol use. *Addiction Research & Theory*. 2023;31:16–28.

Cudd S. The person with a gastrointestinal disorder. In: Peate I, Wild K, eds. *Nursing Practice, Knowledge and Care*. 2nd ed. Oxford: Wiley; 2018:635–661.

Dawson DA, Grant BF, Stinson FS, Zhou Y. Effectiveness of the Derived Alcohol Use Disorders Identification Test (AUDIT-C) in screening for alcohol use disorders and risk drinking in the US general population. *Alcohol Clin Exp Res*. 2005;29:844–854.

de Wit SC, Stromberg HK, Vareeland -Dallred C. *Medical Surgical Nursing: Concepts and Practice*. 3rd ed. St Louis: Elsevier; 2017.

De Franchis R, Bosch J, Garcia-Tsao G, et al. Baveno VII – renewing consensus in portal hypertension. *J Hepatol*. 2022;76:959–974.

Deng LX, Tana MM, Lai JC. Thinking ahead: advance care planning for patients with cirrhosis. *Clin Liver Dis*. 2022;19:7–11.

Dent J, El-Scrag HB, Wallander MA, Johansson S. Epidemiology of gastro-oesophageal reflux disease: a systematic review. *Gut*. 2005;54:710–717.

Drake RL, Vogl W, Mitchell AWM. *Gray's Anatomy for Students*. 3rd ed. Philadelphia: Elsevier; 2015.

EASL. European Association for the Study of the Liver (EASL) Clinical Practice Guidelines on the prevention, diagnosis and treatment of gallstones. *J Hepatol*. 2016;65:146–181.

Ellul MA, Cross TJ, Larner AJ. Asterixis. *Pract Neurol*. 2017;17:60–62.

Elsayed IAS, Battu PK, Irving S. Management of acute upper GI bleeding. *BJA Educ*. 2016;17:117–123.

Fabrellas N, Carol M, Palacio E, et al. Nursing care of patients with cirrhosis: the LiverHope Nursing Project. *Hepatology*. 2020;71:1106–1116.

Foncea CG, Sporea I, Lupuşoru R, et al. Day-4 Lille score is a good prognostic factor and early predictor in assessing therapy response in patients with liver cirrhosis and severe alcoholic hepatitis. *J Clin Med*. 2021;10.

Foxcroft DR, Coombes L, Wood S, et al. Motivational interviewing for the prevention of alcohol misuse in young adults. *Cochrane Database Syst Rev*. 2016.

Goodchild G, Chouhan M, Johnson GJ. Practical guide to the management of acute pancreatitis. *Frontline Gastroenterol*. 2019;10:292–299.

Gukovsky I, Pandol SJ, Mareninova OA, Shalbueva N, Jia W, Gukovskaya AS. Impaired autophagy and organellar dysfunction in pancreatitis. *J Gastroenterol Hepatol.* 2012;27(Suppl 2):27–32.

Hanna WC, Sudarshan M, Roberge D. What is the optimal management of dysphagia in metastatic eosphageal cancer? *Curr Oncol.* 2012;19(9):e60–e66.

Harrison P, Hogan BJ, Floros L, Davies E. Assessment and management of cirrhosis in people older than 16 years: summary of NICE guidance. *BMJ.* 2016;354:i2850.

Harvey JJ, Prentice R, George J. Diagnostic and therapeutic abdominal paracentesis. *Med J Aust.* 2023;218:18–21.

Hegade VS, Kendrick SF, Jones DE. Drug treatment of pruritus in liver diseases. *Clin Med (Lond).* 2015;15:351–357.

Hernaez R, Solà E, Moreau R, Ginès P. Acute-on-chronic liver failure: an update. *Gut.* 2017;66:541–553.

Herreros-Villanueva M, Hijona E, Bañales JM, Cosme A, Bujanda L. Alcohol consumption on pancreatic diseases. *World J Gastroenterol.* 2013;19:638–647.

Huang DQ, Mathurin P, Cortez-Pinto H, Loomba R. Global epidemiology of alcohol-associated cirrhosis and HCC: trends, projections and risk factors. *Nat Rev Gastroenterol Hepatol.* 2023;20:37–49.

Hundal R, Shaffer EA. Gallbladder cancer: epidemiology and outcome. *Clin Epidemiol.* 2014;6:99–109.

International Agency for Research on Cancer. List of classifications by cancer sites with sufficient or limited evidence in humans. *IARC Monogr.* 2017. Volumes 1–132a. https://monographs.iarc.who.int/wp-content/uploads/2019/07/Classifications_by_cancer_site.pdf.

Jalan R, Gines P, Olson JC, et al. Acute-on chronic liver failure. *J Hepatol.* 2012;57:1336–1348.

Jalan R, Saliba F, Pavesi M, et al. Development and validation of a prognostic score to predict mortality in patients with acute-on-chronic liver failure. *J Hepatol.* 2014;61:1038–1047.

Joannidis M, Druml W, Forni LG, et al. Prevention of acute kidney injury and protection of renal function in the intensive care unit: update 2017. *Intensive Care Med.* 2017;43:730–749.

Kanthan R, Senger J-L, Ahmed S, Kanthan SC. Gallbladder cancer in the 21st century. *J Oncol.* 2015:967472. doi: 10.1155/2015/967472

Katz PO, Gerson LB, Vela MF. Guidelines for the diagnosis and management of gastroesophageal reflux disease. *Am J Gastroenterol.* 2013;108(3):308–328.

Lamb CA, Kennedy NA, Raine T, et al. British Society of Gastroenterology consensus guidelines on the management of inflammatory bowel disease in adults. *Gut.* 2019;68:s1–s106. https://gut.bmj.com/content/gutjnl/68/Suppl_3/s1.full.pdf.

Lee T, Teng TZJ, Shelat VG. Carbohydrate antigen 19-9 – tumor marker: past, present, and future. *World J Gastrointest Surg.* 2020;12:468–490.

Leiman DA, Riff BP, Morgan S, Metz DC, Falk GW, French B, Umscheid CA, Lewis JD. Alginate therapy is effective treatment for GERD symptoms: a systematic review and meta-analysis. *Dis Esophagus.* 2017;30(5):1–9. doi:10.1093/dote/dow020.

Lewis SJ, Heaton KW. Stool form scale as a useful guide to intestinal transit time. *Scand J Gastroenterol.* 1997;32(9):920–924.

Liu YB, Chen MK. Epidemiology of liver cirrhosis and associated complications: current knowledge and future directions. *World J Gastroenterol.* 2022;28:5910–5930.

Llovet JM, Kelley RK, Villanueva A, et al. Hepatocellular carcinoma. *Nat Rev Dis Primers.* 2021;7:6.

Löhr JM, Dominguez-Munoz E, Rosendahl J, et al. United European Gastroenterology evidence-based guidelines for the diagnosis and therapy of chronic pancreatitis (HaPanEU). *United European Gastroenterol J.* 2017;5:153–199.

Lordick F, Carneiro F, Cascinu S, et al. Gastric cancer: ESMO Clinical Practice Guideline for diagnosis, treatment and follow-up. *Ann Oncol.* 2022;Vol 33(Issue 10):1005–1020. doi:10.1016/j.annonc.2022.07.004.

Louvet A, Naveau S, Abdelnour M, et al. The Lille model: a new tool for therapeutic strategy in patients with severe alcoholic hepatitis treated with steroids. *Hepatology.* 2007;45:1348–1354.

Lv F, Wang J, Mao L, Zhou X, Zhang T, Zhou S. Whether long-term use of proton pump inhibitor increases the risk of precancerous lesions in the stomach: A systematic review and meta-analysis of randomized controlled trials. *Medicine (Baltimore).* 2023;102(38):e35062. doi:10.1097/MD.0000000000035062.

Macken L, Corrigan M, Prentice W, et al. Palliative long-term abdominal drains for the management of refractory ascites due to cirrhosis: a consensus document. *Frontline Gastroenterol.* 2022;13:e116–e125.

Maddrey WC, Boitnott JK, Bedine MS, Weber Jr FL, Mezey E, White Jr RI. Corticosteroid therapy of alcoholic hepatitis. *Gastroenterology.* 1978;75:193–199.

Mansour D, McPherson S. Management of decompensated cirrhosis. *Clin Med.* 2018;18:s60–s65.

McPherson S, Dyson J, Austin A, Hudson M British Society of Gastroenterology BSG-BASL decompensated cirrhosis care bundle – first 24 hours. 2014. https://www.bsg.org.uk/clinical-resource/bsg-basl-decompensated-cirrhosis-care-bundle-first-24-hours/

Millson C, Considine A, Cramp ME, et al. Adult liver transplantation: a UK clinical guideline – part 1: pre-operation. *Frontline Gastroenterol.* 2020;11:375–384.

Mirijello A, D'Angelo C, Ferrulli A, et al. Identification and management of alcohol withdrawal syndrome. *Drugs.* 2015;75:353–365.

Mowat C, Cole A, Windsor A, et al. Guidelines for the management of inflammatory bowel disease in adults. *Gut.* 2010;60:571–607.

Møller S, Bendtsen F. The pathophysiology of arterial vasodilatation and hyperdynamic circulation in cirrhosis. *Liver Int.* 2018;38:570–580.

Muratori L, Lohse AW, Lenzi M. Diagnosis and management of autoimmune hepatitis. *BMJ.* 2023;380:e070201.

National Clinical Guideline Centre (2019). Crohn's disease management in adults, children and young people. NCGC Template. https://www.nice.org.uk/guidance/ng129.

National Institute for Health and Care Excellence. Nutrition support for adults: oral nutrition support, enteral tube feeding and parenteral nutrition. *Clin Guideline.* 2006/2017;32. Available at: https://www.nice.org.uk/guidance/cg32/resources/nutrition-support-for-adults-oral-nutrition-support-enteral-tube-feeding-and-parenteral-nutrition-pdf-975383198917 (Accessed: 28 November 2023).

Neuberger J, Patel J, Caldwell H, et al. Guidelines on the use of liver biopsy in clinical practice from the British Society of Gastroenterology, the Royal College of Radiologists and the Royal College of Pathology. *Gut.* 2020;69:1382–1403.

NHS England. *News NHS set to eliminate Hepatitis C ahead of rest of the world.* 2022/2023. Available at: https://www.england.nhs.uk/2022/12/nhs-set-to-eliminate-hepatitis-c-ahead-of-rest-of-the-world/ (Accessed: 28 November 2023).

NICE. *Alcohol-Use Disorders: Diagnosis, Assessment and Management of Harmful Drinking (High-Risk Drinking) and Alcohol Dependence.* United Kingdom; 2011.

NICE. *Acute Upper Gastrointestinal Bleeding in Over 16s: Management.* United Kingdom; 2012.

NICE. *Hepatitis B (Chronic): Diagnosis and Management.* UK: National Institute for Health & Care Excellence; 2013.

NICE. *Gallstone Disease: Diagnosis and Management.* UK: National Institute for Health & Care Excellence; 2014.

NICE. Gallstone disease. 2015. https://www.nice.org.uk/guidance/cg188.

NICE. Nutrition support for adults: oral nutrition support, enteral tube feeding and parenteral nutrition. https://www.nice.org.uk/guidance/cg32/resources/nutrition-support-for-adults-oral-nutrition-support-enteral-tube-feeding-and-parenteral-nutrition-pdf-975383198917; 2017.

NICE. *Pancreatic Cancer in Adults: Diagnosis and Management.* National Institute of Health and Care Excellence; 2018.

NICE. *Pancreatitis: National Guideline (NG 104).* National Institute for Health and Care Excellence; 2018.

NICE. *Overview. Gastro-Oesophageal Reflux Disease and Dyspepsia in Adults: Investigation and Management.* National Institute for Health and Care Excellence; 2019. https://www.nice.org.uk/guidance/cg184.

NICE. Pancreatitis. https://www.nice.org.uk/guidance/ng104/resources/pancreatitis-pdf-66141537952453; 2020.

NICE. *Suspected Cancer: Recognition and Referral.* National Institute for Health and Care Excellence; 2021. https://www.nice.org.uk/guidance/ng12.

NICE. *Oesophago-Gastric Cancer: Assessment and Management in Adults*; 2023. https://www.nice.org.uk/guidance/ng83.

Nicol JM, Bavin C, Cronin P, et al. *Essential Nursing Skills.* 4th ed. Edinburgh: Mosby; 2012.

Northup PG, Garcia-Pagan JC, Garcia-Tsao G, et al. Vascular liver disorders, portal vein thrombosis, and procedural bleeding in patients with liver disease: 2020 practice guidance by the American Association for the Study of Liver Diseases. *Hepatology.* 2021;73:366–413.

Norton C, Williams J, Taylor C et al, eds. *Oxford Handbook of Gastrointestinal Nursing.* Oxford: Oxford University Press; 2008.

Nursing & Midwifery Council. The code: professional standards of practice and behaviour for nurses, midwifes and nursing associates. In: Council, N. M. (ed.); 2018. https://www.nmc.org.uk/standards/code/.

Office for National Statistics. Adult drinking habits in Great Britain: 2017. In: Statistics, O. F. N. (ed.). UK: Office for National Statistics; 2018. https://www.ons.gov.uk/peoplepopulationandcommunity/healthandsocialcare/drugusealcoholandsmoking/bulletins/opinionsandlifestylesurveyadultdrinkinghabitsingreatbritain/2017.

Office for National Statistics. Cancer survival in England – adults diagnosed. 2019. https://www.ons.gov.uk/peoplepopulationandcommunity/healthandsocialcare/conditionsanddiseases/bulletins/cancersurvivalinengland/nationalestimatesforpatientsfollowedupto2017.

Office for National Statistics. *Alcohol-Specific Deaths in the Uk: Registered in 2021.* United Kingdom: Office for National Statistics; 2022.

Oliver TI, Sharma B, John S. *Portal Hypertension. StatPearls.* Treasure Island, FL: StatPearls Publishing; 2023.

Orpen-Palmer J, Stanley AJ. Update on the management of upper gastrointestinal bleeding. *BMJ Med.* 2022;1:e000202.

Ortiz M, Córdoba J, Doval E, et al. Development of a Clinical Hepatic Encephalopathy Staging Scale. *Aliment Pharmacol Ther.* 2007;26:859–867.

Philips CA, Augustine P, Yerol PK, Rajesh S, Mahadevan P. Severe alcoholic hepatitis: current perspectives. *Hepat Med.* 2019;11:97–108.

Pugh RN, Murray-Lyon IM, Dawson JL, Pietroni MC, Williams R. Transection of the oesophagus for bleeding oesophageal varices. *Br J Surg.* 1973;60:646–649.

Prabhu V, Shivani A. An overview of history, pathogenesis and treatment of perforated peptic ulcer disease with evaluation of prognostic scoring in adults. *Ann Med Health Sci Res.* 2014;4(1):22–29.

Qi X, Bai Z, Zhu Q, et al. Practice guidance for the use of terlipressin for liver cirrhosis-related complications. *Therap Adv Gastroenterol.* 2022;15:17562848221098253.

Qiao T, Ma RH, Luo XB, Yang LQ, Luo ZL, Zheng PM. The systematic classification of gallbladder stones. *PLoS One.* 2013;8:e74887.

Radu F, Potcovaru C-G, Salmen T, Filip PV, Pop C, Fierbințeanu-Braticievici C. The link between NAFLD and metabolic syndrome. *Diagnostics.* 2023;13:614.

Raevens S, Boret M, Fallon MB. Hepatopulmonary syndrome. *JHEP Rep.* 2022;4:100527.

Ralston SH, Penman ID, Strachan MWJ, Hobson R. *Davidson's Principles and Practice of Medicine.* Philadelphia, United Kingdom: Elsevier; 2018.

Rashid MU, Hussain I, Jehanzeb S, et al. Pancreatic necrosis: complications and changing trend of treatment. *World J Gastrointest Surg.* 2019;11:198–217.

Rassi AB, D'Amico EA, Tripodi A, et al. Fresh frozen plasma transfusion in patients with cirrhosis and coagulopathy: effect on conventional coagulation tests and thrombomodulin-modified thrombin generation. *J Hepatol.* 2020;72:85–94.

Royal College of Physicians (RCP). National Early Warning Score (NEWS) 2. 2018. Available at: https://www.rcplondon.ac.uk/projects/outputs/national-early-warning-score-news-2.

Sakiani S, Heller T, Koh C. Current and investigational drugs in early clinical development for portal hypertension. *Front Med (Lausanne).* 2022;9:974182.

Sartelli M, Weber DG, Kluger Y, et al. 2020 update of the WSES guidelines for the management of acute colonic diverticulitis in the emergency setting. *World J Emerg Surg.* 2020;15(1):32. doi: 10.1186/s13017-020-00313-4.

Schindler P, Heinzow H, Trebicka J, Wildgruber M. Shunt-induced hepatic encephalopathy in tips: current approaches and clinical challenges. *J Clin Med.* 2020;9.

Schrier RW, Arroyo V, Bernardi M, Epstein M, Henriksen JH, Rodés J. Peripheral arterial vasodilation hypothesis: a proposal for the initiation of renal sodium and water retention in cirrhosis. *Hepatology.* 1988;8:1151–1157.

Sepanlou SG, Safiri S, Bisignano C, et al. The global, regional, and national burden of cirrhosis by cause in 195 countries and territories, 1990–2017: a systematic analysis for the Global Burden of Disease Study 2017. *Lancet Gastroenterol Hepatol.* 2020;5:245–266.

Shabanzadeh DM. Incidence of gallstone disease and complications. *Curr Opin Gastroenterol.* 2018;34:81–89. doi:10.1097/MOG.0000000000000418.

Sharma K, Akre S, Chakole S, Wanjari MB. Hepatic encephalopathy and treatment modalities: a review article. *Cureus.* 2022;14:e28016.

Simonetto DA, Gines P, Kamath PS. Hepatorenal syndrome: pathophysiology, diagnosis, and management. *BMJ.* 2020:m2687.

Smith G, Fawcett T. Chronic pancreatitis: pathophysiology and patient care. *Gastrointest Nurs.* 2006;4(7):20–26.

Spagnolo DM, Greer PJ, Ohlsen CS, et al. Acute and chronic pancreatitis disease prevalence, classification, and comorbidities: a cohort study of the UK BioBank. *Clin Transl Gastroenterol.* 2022;13:e00455.

Steen Pedersen J, Bendtsen F, Møller S. Management of cirrhotic ascites. *Ther Adv Chronic Dis.* 2015;6(3):124–137.

Stravitz RT, Lee WM. Acute liver failure. *Lancet North Am Ed.* 2019;394:869–881.

Sullivan JT, Sykora K, Schneiderman J, Naranjo CA, Sellers EM. Assessment of Alcohol Withdrawal: the revised clinical institute withdrawal assessment for alcohol scale (CIWA-Ar). *Br J Addict.* 1989;84:1353–1357.

Thomson AB, Sauve MD, Kassam N, et al. Safety of the long-term use of proton pump inhibitors. *World J Gastroentrol.* 2010;2116(19):2323–2330.

Thursz MR, Richardson P, Allison M. Prednisolone or pentoxifylline for alcoholic hepatitis. *N Engl J Med.* 2015;372:1619–1628.

Tiong L, Oh J. Safety and efficacy of a laparoscopic cholecystectomy in the morbid and super obese patients. *HPB (Oxford).* 2015;17:600–604.

Torre P, Aglitti A, Masarone M, Persico M. Viral hepatitis: Milestones, unresolved issues, and future goals. *World J Gastroenterol.* 2021;27:4603–4638.

Tortora GJ, Derrickson B, Tortora GJ. *Tortora's Principles of Anatomy & Physiology.* Hoboken, NJ: Wiley; 2017.

Tran A, Yates J, Lau A, Lampron J, Matar M. Permissive hypotension versus conventional resuscitation strategies in adult trauma patients with hemorrhagic shock: a systematic review and meta-analysis of randomized controlled trials. *J Trauma Acute Care Surg.* 2018;84:802–808.

Tschatzis EA, Bosch J, Burroughs AK. Liver cirrhosis. *Lancet.* 2014;383:1749–1761.

Veitch AM, Radaelli F, Alikhan R, et al. Endoscopy in patients on antiplatelet or anticoagulant therapy: British Society of Gastroenterology (BSG) and European Society of Gastrointestinal Endoscopy (ESGE) guideline update. *Gut.* 2021;70:1611–1628.

Verschuur EM, Steyerberg EW, Kuipers EJ, Tilanus HW, Siersema PD. Follow-up after surgical treatment for cancer of the gastrointestinal tract. *Dig Liver Dis.* 2006;38(7):479–484. doi:10.1016/j.dld.2006.03.008.

Veronese P, Dodi I, Esposito S, Indolfi G. Prevention of vertical transmission of hepatitis B virus infection. *World J Gastroenterol.* 2021;27:4182–4193.

Vilstrup H, Amodio P, Bajaj J, et al. Hepatic encephalopathy in chronic liver disease: 2014 Practice Guideline by the American Association for the Study of Liver Diseases and the European Association for the Study of the Liver. *Hepatology.* 2014;60:715–735.

Wang Y, Lu J, Wen N, et al. The role of diet and nutrition related indicators in biliary diseases: an umbrella review of systematic review and meta-analysis. *Nutr Metabolism.* 2022;19:51.

Waugh A, Grant A. *Ross & Wilson anatomy and physiology in health and illness*. 14th Edition London: Elsevier; 2023.

Weekes CE, Elia M, Emery PW. The development, validation and reliability of a nutrition screening tool based on the recommendations of the British Association for Parenteral and Enteral Nutrition (BAPEN). *Clin Nutr.* 2004;23:1104–1112.

Wendon J, Cordoba J, Dhawan A, et al. EASL Clinical Practical Guidelines on the management of acute (fulminant) liver failure. *J Hepatol.* 2017;66:1047–1081.

Werner J, Feuerbach S, Uhl W, Buchler M. Management of acute pancreatitis: from surgery to interventional intensive care. *Gut.* 2005;54(3):426–436.

White P. Stoma care clinical nursing standards. www.securicaremedical.co.uk/media/2019-Stoma-Care-Clinical-Nursing-Standards.pdf; 2019.

Wiik Larsen J, Thorsen K, Søreide K. Splenic injury from blunt trauma. *Br J Surg.* 2023;110(9):1035–1038. doi:10.1093/bjs/znad060.

Williams R, Alexander G, Armstrong I, et al. Disease burden and costs from excess alcohol consumption, obesity, and viral hepatitis: fourth report of the Lancet Standing Commission on Liver Disease in the UK. *Lancet (North American Edition).* 2018;391:1097–1107.

World Health Organization. *Global Health Sector Strategy on Viral Hepatitis 2016–2021. Towards Ending Viral Hepatitis.* Geneva: World Health Organization; 2016.

Yaghoobi M, Bijarchi R, Narod SA. Family history and the risk of gastric cancer. *Br J Cancer.* 2010;102:237–242.

Yiannoullou P, Hall C, Newton K, et al. A review of the management of blunt splenic trauma in England and Wales: have regional trauma networks influenced management strategies and outcomes? *Ann R Coll Surg Engl.* 2017;99:63–69.

Zuckerman MJ, Elhanafi S, Mendoza Ladd A. Endoscopic treatment of esophageal varices. *Clin Liver Dis.* 2022;26:21–37.

Useful Websites

American Association for the Study of Liver Disease (AASLD), https://www.aasld.org/practice-guidelines

British Liver Trust, https://britishlivertrust.org.uk/

British Association for the Study of the Liver, https://www.basl.org.uk/

British Society of Gastroenterology, https://www.bsg.org.uk/

European Association for the Study of the Liver (EASL), https://easl.eu/publication-category/clinical-practice-guidelines/

Improving Quality in Liver Services, https://www.iqils.org/

British Liver Nurses Association, https://www.basl.org.uk/index.cfm/content/page/cid/4

The Lancet Liver Commission, https://www.thelancet.com/campaigns/liver

NECEPOD Measuring the Units: a review of patients who died with alcohol-related liver disease, https://www.ncepod.org.uk/2013arld.html; 2013.

BASL/BSG, Decompensated Cirrhosis Care Bundle: First 24 hours, https://www.google.com/url?sa=t&rct=j&q=&esrc=s&source=web&cd=&cad=rja&uact=8&ved=2ahUKEwj_gt22q6T-AhXcRkEAHRufDroQFnoECCIQAQ&url=https%3A%2F%2Fwww.bsg.org.uk%2Fwp-content%2Fuploads%2F2019%2F12%2FBSG-BASL-Decompensated-Cirrhosis-Care-Bundle-First-24-Hours.pdf&usg=AOvVaw3-q5loozFfvONt41qf10R9

BSG Guidelines on the management of abnormal liver blood tests, https://www.bsg.org.uk/clinical-resource/guidelines-on-the-management-of-abnormal-liver-blood-tests/

Alcohol Change UK, https://alcoholchange.org.uk/

British Association of Parenteral and Enteral Nutrition (BAPEN), https://www.bapen.org.uk/

NICE Liver Guidance, https://www.nice.org.uk/guidance/conditions-and-diseases/liver-conditions

5

Nursing Patients With Endocrine Disorders

CARL CLARE

CHAPTER OUTLINE

Introduction

Endocrinology is the study of hormones – chemical messengers secreted by endocrine glands and neurones. Hormones, usually travelling in the bloodstream, help to maintain homeostasis by acting on and coordinating activity within target organs or tissues.

It is a specialty that encompasses many complex chronic diseases. Apart from diabetes mellitus (see Chapter 6) and thyroid disorders, endocrine problems are relatively uncommon. Many endocrine disorders are hidden disorders and may be difficult to diagnose without medical tests. As a result, patients may be referred by their general practitioner or local hospital to specialist centres for investigations and/or treatment by an endocrinologist. For the patient, this has the advantage of offering highly specialised care. It also means that relatively few nurses have the opportunity to care for people with these disorders. However, given the wide-ranging effects of endocrine dysfunction, it is important that all nurses have a general understanding of endocrinology. Endocrine diseases can affect every system of the body, sometimes causing permanent disfigurement and a change in body image and quality of life (QoL) and even, occasionally, posing a threat to life. These disorders can seriously affect the patient's psychological outlook, either as a direct result of the illness or by virtue of the individual's reaction to it.

Basal hormone tests are not always diagnostic and patients may have to undergo a range of tests before a diagnosis is reached. As a general principle, if a hormone deficiency is suspected, stimulation tests will be performed; if an excess of a hormone is suspected, suppression tests will be requested. As the tests and investigations required to establish a diagnosis can be complicated, clear explanations are essential so that the patient understands the need for them and the procedures that must be followed. This will help to reduce anxiety and increase the patient's confidence in the healthcare team. The psychological support that the nurse can offer this group of patients is vitally important. Many patients benefit from referral to a support group (see Useful Websites) and the contact this brings with other patients who have the same condition. Often, these patients are young and may be otherwise in good health, and therefore the impact of endocrine disease on their body image and/or self-esteem should not be underestimated. For example, patients experiencing sexual dysfunction may feel embarrassed to talk to and seek support from family members and friends – in such cases, support from the healthcare professional is crucial.

Anatomy and Physiology

The nature of the endocrine system, being one of control, means that it has far-reaching effects throughout the body on various target organs. This section provides a brief outline of hormonal action and outlines the anatomy and physiology of individual endocrine glands and structures (see Further Reading, e.g. Waugh and Grant 2022). The gonads, ovaries and testes are described in Chapter 8 (Nursing Patients With Disorders of the Female Reproductive System), Chapter 9 (Nursing Patients With Disorders of the Male Reproductive System), and Chapter 10 (Nursing Patients With Urinary Disorders).

Hormones

The endocrine system is one of the two major control systems of the body, the other being the nervous system. The nervous system

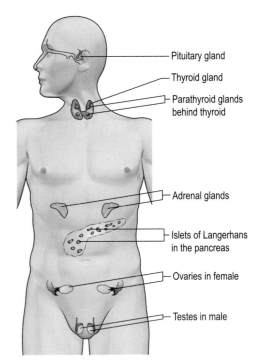

Figure 5.1 The endocrine glands/structures and their location in the body.

- Pituitary gland
- Thyroid gland
- Parathyroid glands behind thyroid
- Adrenal glands
- Islets of Langerhans in the pancreas
- Ovaries in female
- Testes in male

mediates endocrine activity. The endocrine system produces hormones from ductless glands which have no physical connection with each other. These hormones are secreted into the bloodstream for transport to their respective target organs and tissues located throughout the body. The key endocrine glands are the pituitary, the thyroid, the parathyroids, the adrenals, pancreas and gonads (Fig. 5.1). Hormones are either lipid based (e.g. the steroid hormones and the thyroid hormones) or peptides (e.g. adrenaline (epinephrine), insulin and glucagon).

Action

Hormones affect only those cells or organs upon which they have an excitatory or inhibitory action. This system allows individuals to respond to changes in their environment and is important in controlling growth and development, sexual maturation and homeostasis.

Many hormones are bound to proteins within the circulation. Only unbound or free hormones are biologically active, and that binding serves as a buffer against very rapid changes in plasma levels of a hormone. This principle is important in the interpretation of many tests of endocrine function.

Control

Most hormone systems are controlled by a negative feedback system which ensures that hormone levels, whilst fluctuating, remain within a preset range (see Appendix – normal values). Fig. 5.2 illustrates how negative feedback operates in the hypothalamic–pituitary–thyroid axis.

Pattern of Secretion

Hormone secretion is either continuous or intermittent. An example of continuous secretion is thyroxine (T_4) by the thyroid gland, in which hormone levels over a day, month or year show very little variation. Intermittent secretion is seen in three forms: circadian, menstrual and pulsatile.

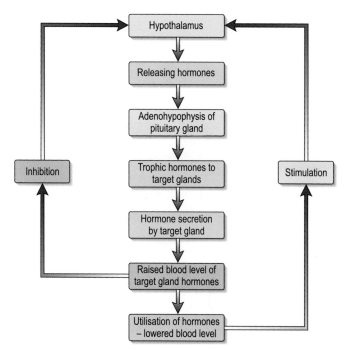

Figure 5.2 Negative feedback regulation of the secretion of anterior pituitary hormones.

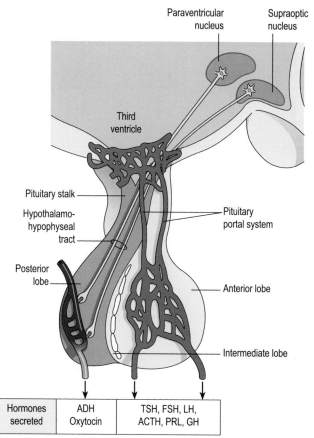

Figure 5.3 The pituitary gland and its relationship with the hypothalamus. *ACTH,* Adrenocorticotrophic hormone; *ADH,* antidiuretic hormone; *FSH,* follicle-stimulating hormone; *GH,* growth hormone; *LH,* luteinising hormone; *PRL,* prolactin; *TSH,* thyroid-stimulating hormone. (Reproduced from Waugh and Grant 2006 with permission.)

Other factors that affect hormone secretion include disease, trauma, surgery, other medications, stress or emotional upset. As in any complex regulatory system, it is likely that disequilibrium in endocrine function will have important consequences. Disorders of the endocrine system may be categorised most simply as those involving overproduction (hypersecretion) and those involving underproduction (hyposecretion).

Pituitary

The pituitary gland lies immediately below the hypothalamus (part of the floor of the third ventricle of the brain) in the pituitary fossa. It is connected to the hypothalamus by the pituitary stalk and comprises two lobes which function independently of each other (Fig. 5.3). During fetal life, the glandular anterior lobe develops from the oropharynx to become the adenohypophysis. The neural posterior lobe is a down-growth from the forebrain, which becomes the neurohypophysis. The posterior pituitary receives nerve fibres from hypothalamic nuclei via the hypothalamohypophyseal tract in the pituitary stalk.

The hypothalamus contains specialised cells or nuclei (paraventricular and supraoptic) which synthesise the hormones antidiuretic hormone (ADH) (also known as arginine vasopressin (AVP) or vasopressin) and oxytocin. The hypothalamus also produces releasing/inhibiting hormones that regulate the secretion of anterior pituitary hormones (Fig. 5.4). The hypothalamus also controls many centres for functions such as appetite, thirst, temperature regulation, sexual activity and sleep/wake cycles.

The pituitary stalk carries blood to both lobes of the pituitary in a portal system by which the hypothalamic releasing/inhibitory hormones are carried to the anterior pituitary. The trophic hormones produced in the anterior pituitary stimulate the other endocrine glands. ADH and oxytocin are stored in the posterior pituitary until released. Table 5.1 outlines the hormones secreted by the pituitary gland.

The optic chiasm sits just above the pituitary fossa. Therefore an expanding lesion from the pituitary or the hypothalamus may result in a defect in the visual fields because of pressure on the optic nerve or optic chiasm.

Thyroid

The thyroid is a gland in the neck sited anteriorly to the larynx and attached to the thyroid cartilages and the trachea. It comprises two lobes connected by an isthmus (Fig. 5.5). Structures in close proximity include the oesophagus, the parathyroid glands, the recurrent laryngeal nerves and the carotid arteries.

The thyroid receives a rich blood supply from the superior thyroid arteries (branch of external carotid arteries) and from the inferior thyroid arteries (branch of subclavian arteries). Each lobe is filled with follicles, which produce and store the two thyroid hormones thyroxine (T_4) and tri-iodothyroxine (T_3). Between the follicles are parafollicular cells (C cells) which secrete the hormone calcitonin; this, together with parathyroid hormone (PTH) from the parathyroid glands, regulates calcium and phosphate homeostasis.

The hormones, thyroxine (T_4) and some circulating tri-iodothyronine (T_3), are synthesised and secreted by the thyroid gland. Thyroid hormone production is dependent on the availability of iodine in the diet (see Chapter 22, Nutrition and Health). More T_4 than T_3 is produced, but T_4 is converted in some tissues to

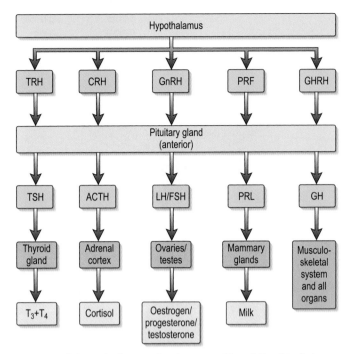

Figure 5.4 Schematic diagram showing some of the relationships between the hypothalamus, the anterior pituitary gland and their target organs. *ACTH*, Adrenocorticotrophic hormone; *CRH*, corticotrophin-releasing hormone; *GH*, growth hormone; *GHRH*, growth hormone releasing hormone; *GnRH*, gonadotrophin-releasing hormone; *LH (ICSH)/FSH*, luteinising hormone/follicle-stimulating hormone; *PRF*, prolactin-releasing factor; *PRL*, prolactin; *TRH*, thyrotrophin-releasing hormone; *TSH*, thyroid-stimulating hormone.

Figure 5.5 The thyroid gland and associated structures.

the more biologically active T_3. Over 99% of all thyroid hormone is bound to plasma thyroid-binding proteins. Only the free hormone is available for use by the tissues. If the levels of T_4 and T_3 in the blood fall, the hypothalamus releases thyrotrophin-releasing hormone (TRH). As the levels of TRH rise, the pituitary gland secretes thyroid-stimulating hormone (TSH) which stimulates the thyroid gland to produce more T_4 and T_3. The principal effect of thyroid hormones is to influence the metabolism of cells and,

TABLE 5.1	Hormones of the Pituitary Gland and Their Action
Hormone	**Action**
Anterior Lobe	
Growth hormone (GH) (*syn.* somatotrophin)	Pulsatile release. Does not have a single target gland but acts on a variety of tissues, e.g. bone, viscera and soft tissues. It is particularly important in children to stimulate growth. Action in adults recently thought to involve maintenance of cardiovascular activity, fat deposition and muscle development
Prolactin (PRL)	Main action is to stimulate lactation in females; also stimulates the corpus luteum of the ovary to secrete progesterone
Adrenocorticotrophic hormone (ACTH)	Secreted under circadian rhythm. Stimulates the adrenal cortex to secrete corticosteroids
Luteinising hormone (LH), known as interstitial cell-stimulating hormone (ICSH) in men (gonadotrophins)	In women, LH promotes ovulation; stimulates formation of the corpus luteum. In men, ICSH stimulates the production of the androgen hormone testosterone
Follicle-stimulating hormone (FSH) (a gonadotrophin)	FSH stimulates the production of sex hormones and contributes to regulation of the menstrual cycle in women. In women, stimulates the production of ovarian follicles and secretion of oestrogen; in men, stimulates spermatogenesis
Thyroid-stimulating hormone (TSH)	Stimulates the thyroid to release the hormone thyroxine
Posterior Lobe	
Antidiuretic hormone (ADH) (also known as arginine vasopressin (AVP) or vasopressin)	Controls water homeostasis in the body by regulating water reabsorption from the distal convoluted tubules of the kidney
Oxytocin	Induces uterine contraction during labour (unusually controlled by a positive feedback mechanism) and ejection of milk from breasts postpartum

therefore, the metabolic rate. Low levels of hormone are associated with a low temperature, i.e. patients will complain of feeling cold, slow heart rate, weight gain, poor concentration and low mood, whereas patients with high concentrations of thyroid hormones experience a rapid heart rate, heat intolerance, anxiety and weight loss despite increased appetite.

Parathyroids

The parathyroid glands are usually situated on the posterior lobes of the thyroid gland. They are usually four in number however, 6% of people have more than four glands. The blood supply is from the inferior and superior thyroid arteries.

The glands secrete PTH, which is the most important hormone involved in calcium and phosphate homeostasis. PTH maintains plasma calcium levels within normal limits (2.12–2.62 mmol/L). It acts predominantly on the renal tubules to increase reabsorption of calcium but also increases gut absorption of calcium and mobilises it from bone. Plasma calcium will therefore rise and in turn suppress PTH secretion; conversely, a fall in plasma calcium will stimulate the secretion of PTH.

Vitamin D and calcitonin are also involved in calcium metabolism (Information 5.1).

Adrenals

The adrenal glands are situated one on the upper part of each kidney (Fig. 5.6A). They are highly vascular and derive their blood supply from the renal arteries, the inferior phrenic arteries and directly from the aorta; they are drained by the suprarenal veins.

The adrenal glands have a composite origin. The cortex, the outer part, has the same embryonic site of origin as the gonads. The medulla, the inner part, is derived from neural crest cells which have migrated from the developing neural tube and have become enclosed within the cortex. The latter can arguably be considered part of the nervous system. The secretions, and therefore the actions, of the two separate parts of the glands are quite different and will be discussed separately.

Adrenal Cortex

The adrenal cortex has three layers (Fig. 5.6B) that produce different hormones, collectively termed corticosteroids:
- mineralocorticoids (in the zona glomerulosa, the outer layer),

---

INFORMATION 5.1

Vitamin D and Calcitonin in Calcium Metabolism

Vitamin D is found in two forms: cholecalciferol (also called calciol or vitamin D_3), which is formed predominantly in the skin by the action of sunlight, and ergocalciferol (vitamin D_2), which is found in some foods and as a synthetic form added to foods. It is the skin-synthesised form which is of greater importance and is perhaps best considered as a hormone.

Vitamin D_3 is biologically inactive; only when it is metabolised by the liver (to form mildly active 25-hydroxycholecalciferol) and the kidney (to form very active 1,25-dihydroxycholecalciferol, also called calcitriol) does it have any action on calcium metabolism. The active metabolite increases calcium absorption from the gut and is essential for bone formation.

If 1,25-dihydroxycholecalciferol is present in excess, it causes increased resorption of calcium from bone, leading to hypercalcaemia. The kidney is sensitive to rising levels and ceases production of the active form, producing an inactive form until the levels drop.

Bone is constantly being re-formed by deposition and reabsorption of calcium. Calcitonin reduces the reabsorption of calcium from bone. Local stress, such as weight bearing, is important in this process. Prolonged inactivity or immobility can result in calcium being lost from bone, while exercise increases bone formation and remodelling.

- glucocorticoids (in the zona fasciculata, the middle layer),
- adrenal sex hormones (androgens) and some glucocorticoids (in the zona reticularis, the inner layer).

Glucocorticoids

Glucocorticoids such as cortisol, the principal glucocorticoid, have varied and wide-ranging actions, many of which are not fully understood. They are essential to life, and in their absence, blood sugar, blood pressure and blood volume fall, sodium excretion increases and muscle contractility decreases. If present in excessive amounts, an opposite set of changes occurs: blood volume expands, blood pressure rises, potassium falls, glycogen storage is increased, blood sugar levels rise, connective tissue is reduced in quality and strength, and immunity is impaired. Wound healing and the inflammatory process are also inhibited.

Mineralocorticoids

The most important of the mineralocorticoids is aldosterone, which is the most potent regulator of sodium and potassium and is important in maintaining acid–base balance. Aldosterone acts on

Figure 5.6 (A) The adrenal glands and associated structures. (B) Layers through the adrenal gland.

the distal convoluted tubules of the kidney and stimulates the cells to reabsorb and thus conserve sodium (see Chapter 10, Nursing Patients With Urinary Disorders, and Chapter 21, Maintaining Fluid, Electrolyte and Acid–Base Balance).

Adrenal Androgens

The adrenal cortex, in addition to the gonads, produces male sex hormones. The effects are appropriate in the male, but in the female, excessive production may have a virilising effect.

Adrenal Medulla

The catecholamines adrenaline (epinephrine), noradrenaline (norepinephrine) and dopamine are secreted by the adrenal medulla. Eighty per cent of adrenomedullary secretion is adrenaline, most noradrenaline and dopamine being secreted by neurones and functions as neurotransmitters.

In normal secretion, adrenaline probably has some effect on mean blood pressure; although it increases systolic pressure, it decreases diastolic pressure. When secreted under the control of the sympathetic nervous system (see Chapter 11, Nursing Patients With Disorders of the Nervous System), it causes tachycardia, decreased gut motility and the closure of sphincters in the gut, pupil dilatation, bronchodilatation and piloerection.

Noradrenaline raises both systolic and diastolic blood pressure.

The difference between the effects of adrenaline and noradrenaline is partly explained by the presence of different receptors (α- and β-adrenoreceptors) on the surface of effector cells. Noradrenaline is most active at α-adrenoreceptors and adrenaline at β-adrenoreceptors.

The main effect of the catecholamines is on the cardiovascular system and the central nervous system, and on carbohydrate and lipid metabolism. Together, adrenaline and noradrenaline prepare the body for the 'fight or flight' response.

DISORDERS OF THE PITUITARY AND HYPOTHALAMUS

Disorders of the endocrine system result in either oversecretion or undersecretion of a hormone. Therefore in principle, treatment should be straightforward, either replacing the missing hormone or removing, or suppressing the source of, the oversecretion, although in reality this is sadly not always the case. Advances have made the treatment of the wide range of endocrine disorders more successful, and the outlook for those affected is becoming ever more hopeful. However, patients with pituitary disease still have a greater mortality due to cardiovascular, cerebrovascular and respiratory causes than the general population and women have a worse outcome than men.

Hypersecretion of a hormone usually arises from a so-called 'functioning' pituitary adenoma. As this adenoma grows, it is likely to disrupt the normal function of other areas of the pituitary, and as a result progressive hypopituitarism occurs. This failure of the pituitary hormones occurs in a characteristic sequence (Penman et al. 2022) – first growth hormone (GH) is lost, followed by the gonadotrophins luteinising hormone (LH) and follicle-stimulating hormone (FSH), adrenocorticotrophic hormone (ACTH) and then TSH. Prolactin (PRL) deficiency is rare except as seen postpartum in Sheehan's syndrome.

Hypersecretion of Anterior Pituitary Hormones

Cushing's disease caused by an excess of glucocorticoid hormones stimulated by an ACTH-producing adenoma of the pituitary is discussed in a later section.

Hypersecretion of Growth Hormone: Acromegaly

Acromegaly is a rare condition caused by prolonged, excessive secretion of GH from a benign adenoma (tumour) of the pituitary gland. It affects both sexes equally. It is associated with significant comorbidities and an increased mortality. The median age at diagnosis is 45 years (Melmed et al. 2022).

🔵 *Pathophysiology*
Clinical Features

The onset of acromegaly is insidious, leading to a delay in diagnosis of several years from the initial onset of symptoms. As a result many patients present with complications of the disease and many other patients are diagnosed while being investigated for an unrelated issue (Boguszewski et al. 2019). Signs and symptoms include:

- excessive sweating (in more than 80% of patients)
- headaches (in 55% of patients)
- visual field defects
- enlargement of the hands and feet
- tiredness and lethargy
- joint pain and osteoarthritis
- coarse facial features, frontal bossing, enlarged nose, protruding jaw and increased interdental separation
- thick oily skin
- deep voice
- macroglossia (tongue enlargement)
- soft tissue swelling
- goitre and other organ enlargement
- features of hyperprolactinaemia (increased PRL in the blood)
- decreased QoL.
  Complications include:
- arterial hypertension (40% of patients)
- insulin resistance, impaired glucose tolerance and diabetes mellitus
- obstructive sleep apnoea
- increased risk of colonic polyps and colorectal cancer
- arrhythmias
- congestive heart failure
- cerebral aneurysms.

Common Presenting Signs/Symptoms

The patient may notice an increase in shoe size or that they have had to have a ring enlarged. Along with their family and friends, they may notice a change in their facial appearance. Women often feel very self-conscious about this, and also about their deepening voice, as they may be mistaken for men on the telephone. The major events that prompt a consultation with their general practitioner (GP) are usually headache and sweating. Visual symptoms may be identified by their optician or their dentist may notice changes to dentition (including separation and jaw malocclusion). Patients may therefore be referred to an endocrinologist by a number of routes.

Medical Management

Investigations

Diagnosis can be confirmed following clinical examination and pituitary function testing. On clinical examination, some or all of the symptoms listed earlier may be present. Magnetic resonance imaging (MRI) usually shows the pituitary adenoma and whether there is enlargement of the pituitary fossa. Most patients have a macroadenoma (more than 1 cm in diameter) and these patients should also have their visual fields checked if the adenoma is close to the optic chiasm.

If acromegaly is suspected, a blood sample should be obtained and insulin-like growth factor 1 (IGF-1) measured. A random GH level is rarely diagnostic due to the pulsatile nature of GH secretion. If the IGF-1 level is 'normal', when compared to age- and sex-matched reference ranges, the diagnosis of acromegaly can be excluded in most patients (Fleseriu et al. 2021). Otherwise, the patient should proceed to have an oral glucose tolerance test (OGTT). The OGTT has been the gold standard for the diagnosis of acromegaly for many years. False-positives may occur if the patient has diabetes mellitus, renal or liver disease or anorexia nervosa. In acromegaly, measurement of GH levels during the OGTT are consistently elevated and fail to suppress to less than 2 mU/L in response to a 75 g oral glucose load. Normally, the level of GH would be undetectable. Acromegaly is therefore diagnosed on the basis of an elevated IGF-1 and failure to suppress GH during the OGTT. Further pituitary function tests may be performed to assess whether the remainder of the pituitary gland has been compromised. PRL is co-secreted in 30% of adenomas.

Treatment

In untreated acromegaly, the mortality is nearly twice that of the normal population; early treatment is therefore essential. The aim is to relieve and, if possible, resolve symptoms associated with elevated GH and IGF-1 levels and the local effects caused by the mass itself, and to prevent comorbidity by lowering mean GH and IGF-1 levels to accepted 'safe' levels with minimal disruption to the patient's lifestyle. Treatment usually takes the form of surgery and/or medical therapy with radiotherapy reserved for patients for whom surgery is not an option or who have persistent disease despite surgery or who have not responded to medical therapy or for whom medical therapy is not available.

Surgery. is currently regarded as the first-line therapy for acromegaly and aims to remove the adenoma. When performed by an experienced pituitary surgeon, it remains the treatment of choice. Hypophysectomy via the trans-sphenoidal route, which has a low morbidity and mortality, is the surgical procedure most commonly used. It results in a rapid fall in GH levels, often with no loss of any other pituitary hormones. Surgery is both rapid and inexpensive when compared to medical therapies. Complete resection of an adenoma is dependent on the involvement of local structures such as the carotid artery and cavernous sinus (Hayhurst et al. 2020).

Medical therapy. has changed radically in recent years. It is now possible to control GH and IGF-1 levels in more than half of patients with a somatostatin analogue, a synthetic compound which acts on the somatostatin (GH-release inhibiting hormone) receptors of the adenoma and suppresses the secretion of GH, e.g. lanreotide (Somatulin Autogel) or octreotide (Sandostatin LAR). These analogues are given by deep intramuscular (IM) injection by a nurse every 28 days and are the most widely used form of medical therapy. A short-acting preparation of octreotide

is also available, which is administered subcutaneously three times daily. Initial side-effects include stomach cramps and diarrhoea but these usually settle. If the patient is resistant to this class of medication, pegvisomant (Somavert), a GH receptor antagonist, i.e. it binds to GH receptors, blocking the impact of excessive circulating GH which in turn causes IGF-1 levels to fall, can be used. It is given by a once daily subcutaneous (SC) injection. However, it is very expensive and is currently used only for patients with active disease who have failed to respond to other medical therapies.

Radiotherapy. Conventional external beam radiotherapy (25 fractions over 5 weeks delivered daily Monday to Friday) results in a delayed fall in GH and IGF-1 levels over the following decade which is paralleled by the development of hypopituitarism. After 5 years, 63% of patients have a normal IGF-1 (Hayhurst et al. 2020). Although used less often nowadays, it is safe, and radiation-induced visual damage is extremely rare. Patients may feel tired during the period of treatment and may experience some temporary hair loss at the site of entry of the beams. It is a useful treatment for patients in whom surgery is contraindicated or if GH/IGF-1 levels are not too high and/or there is a large adenoma or residual adenoma postoperatively, or where medical therapy fails to control GH/IGF-1 levels. Another form of radiotherapy is stereotactic radiotherapy, which may be single fraction radiosurgery or linear accelerator-based stereotactic radiotherapy (multiple fraction). The expense is greater than conventional radiotherapy but is a 'one-off' cost. Long-term data are required, but early results suggest that GH and IGF-1 levels fall more rapidly after radiosurgery than with conventional radiotherapy and there is less damage to surrounding tissues, which may reduce the incidence of radiotherapy-induced hypopituitarism (Mathieu et al. 2021). These two forms of radiotherapy can be given following conventional radiotherapy but cannot be used if the adenoma is close to the optic chiasm.

Nursing Management and Health Promotion: Acromegaly

Change in body image is an important feature of this disorder. The patient may have considerable difficulty in coming to terms with their changed appearance and may be anxious about the investigations they must undergo and the treatment that may be required. Their QoL may be affected.

It is important to create as relaxed an environment as possible and to reduce anxiety by spending time with the patient and their family, explaining the reasons for their changed appearance, the effect of therapy and the expected treatment outcome. They will be reassured to hear that biochemical cure may result in a return to a more normal appearance, although the degree will depend on the stage of the disease at the beginning of treatment. Some symptoms, such as sweating, may be cured almost immediately, while others, e.g. soft tissue swelling, may take longer to resolve. Bony changes are usually not reversible.

There are now specific validated QoL assessment tools for acromegaly. The Acromegaly Quality of Life tool (ACROQoL) is useful in assessing the impact of the disease on a patient's QoL (Coopmans et al. 2022).

Some patients benefit from meeting other patients who have been treated successfully and, if the patient wishes, nursing staff should try to arrange this either directly or through a local patient support group (see Useful Websites, e.g. The Pituitary Foundation).

Prolactin Hypersecretion

Hyperprolactinaemia is a common abnormality (Penman et al. 2022). However, a wide variety of medications and diseases can cause high PRL levels. Before carrying out extensive investigations for pituitary disease, it is important to exclude causes such as hypothyroidism and to take a detailed medication history. Medications that block the dopamine receptor and so elevate PRL levels include tranquillisers, e.g. chlorpromazine; antiemetics, e.g. metoclopramide; and some antidepressants, e.g. amitriptyline and fluoxetine. The other key differential diagnosis is a hypothalamic or suprasellar space-occupying lesion which interferes with dopamine production. Dopamine is the natural PRL inhibitory factor, and therefore, in its absence, hyperprolactinaemia ensues; due to the mechanism, this is known as disconnection hyperprolactinaemia.

◉ Pathophysiology

Hyperprolactinaemia causes galactorrhoea (abnormal/inappropriate flow of milk) and amenorrhoea in women; raised PRL level suppresses gonadotrophin-releasing hormone (GnRH) secretion within the hypothalamus, leading to gonadotrophin deficiency (LH and FSH) and then oestrogen deficiency, resulting in infertility. In men, galactorrhoea is much less frequent, but elevated PRL lowers ICSH and FSH levels, which in turn lowers testosterone levels, resulting in a reduced libido, erectile dysfunction and infertility. Prolactinomas are almost always benign.

Common presenting signs/symptoms in premenopausal women include menstrual disturbances, e.g. amenorrhoea, oligomenorrhoea (infrequent menstruation) and infertility. Galactorrhoea occurs in about 80% of these women (Chanson and Maiter 2022). The majority of prolactinomas in women are small (referred to as microprolactinomas) at the time of diagnosis, so headaches and neurological deficits are rare. Men, on the other hand, may present with headache, visual loss, cranial nerve defects and/or hypopituitarism due to the mass effect of the tumour which tends to be larger at the time of diagnosis (referred to as a macroprolactinoma). In both men and women, elevated levels of PRL over a long period can lead to low bone density which increases when PRL levels are normalised but does not return to normal.

◉ Medical Management

Investigations

When other causes have been excluded, PRL levels should be measured in the unstressed patient. Because venepuncture is stressful, an intravenous (IV) cannula is sited in the patient's arm and the patient allowed to rest for 30 minutes prior to the blood sample being taken. The patient should not smoke or drink tea or coffee in this period. If the PRL levels are raised, an MRI scan is performed. If this shows a large pituitary tumour, tests of other pituitary functions should be done to detect any other pituitary hormone deficits. Visual field tests may also be needed to assess if the tumour mass is causing pressure on the optic chiasm. Pituitary MRI will usually show even a small tumour of only a few millimetres in size.

Treatment

The aim for microprolactinomas is to lower the excessive PRL levels, thereby restoring gonadal function. In macroprolactinomas, the aim is tumour reduction, preventing tumour expansion and restoring gonadal function. Reduction of tumour size and lowering of hormone levels may be achieved by medication alone.

Consequently, this is the treatment of choice and trans-sphenoidal surgery is usually performed only in patients who are resistant to or cannot tolerate dopamine agonists.

Prolactinomas respond well to dopamine agonists, e.g. bromocriptine, cabergoline or quinagolide, resulting in reduced PRL levels (which return to normal in over 90% of cases) and significant reduction in tumour size (in over 75% of cases). This in turn results in the restoration of gonadal function and cessation of galactorrhoea, usually within a few weeks of starting treatment. In most women, menstrual cycles resume and fertility is restored. Patients must therefore be given appropriate contraceptive advice. Dopamine agonists are usually stopped once a woman has become pregnant but this can result in tumour regrowth in some patients who may require surgical debulking of the tumour, restarting the dopamine agonist or delivery if the pregnancy is far enough advanced.

Irradiation of the pituitary gland results in a reduction in PRL secretion, but this takes many years to achieve. Dopamine agonists are therefore continued while waiting for the effects of radiotherapy to occur, but the need for this treatment should be reassessed regularly.

❖ Nursing Management and Health Promotion: Prolactin Hypersecretion

Specific nursing care is aimed at ensuring that the medication regimen is followed correctly in order to avoid side-effects. Dopamine agonists, especially bromocriptine, often cause nausea, vomiting, constipation and postural hypotension mediated by dopamine release. Consequently, there should be a slow increase in dosage, the first doses being given whilst eating and on retiring to prevent the common symptoms of postural hypotension and gastric irritation. The dosage can then be gradually increased. Cabergoline, a longer-acting dopamine agonist, need only be taken once or twice a week. It is more potent than bromocriptine and has a lower profile of side-effects (see Further Reading, e.g. Chanson and Maiter 2022).

Hyposecretion of Anterior Pituitary Hormones

Hypopituitarism

Hypopituitarism is a partial or total deficiency of anterior pituitary hormone secretion. It may be associated with pathology that destroys the pituitary itself or with disturbance of hypothalamic control of the pituitary. Total failure of all hormone production is termed panhypopituitarism.

Hypopituitarism is most commonly caused by a pituitary tumour. These are frequently benign. Pituitary cancer is very rare. Benign microadenomas having no clinical effects are surprisingly common and are found in up to 23% of people at postmortem. Other common causes include head injury and (para-)sellar radiotherapy or surgery.

◉ Pathophysiology

Tumours can vary greatly in size and may extend outside the pituitary fossa to compress surrounding structures. They are generally classified as functioning or nonfunctioning, depending on whether they produce a hormone, e.g. GH.

Common Presenting Signs/Symptoms

Effects caused by local compression may arise (see Chapter 11, Nursing Patients With Disorders of the Nervous System), but people usually present with signs of pituitary hormone deficiency. Presentation may vary and depends on which hormones are deficient (Table 5.2).

Medical Management

Investigations

Diagnostic investigations include visual field testing and biochemical investigation to determine the severity and degree of pituitary failure and to distinguish between isolated hormone failure and complete anterior pituitary failure. MRI is also performed.

Treatment

The choice of treatment will depend on the diagnosis of the cause of the pituitary failure and will aim to relieve the clinical effects and symptoms experienced by the patient. Treatment may involve surgery, radiotherapy to reduce the tumour and medication to replace the deficient hormones (see the following section).

TABLE 5.2 Signs and Symptoms of Anterior Pituitary Hormone Hyposecretion

Hormone Deficiency	Signs and Symptoms
GH	*Children* Growth delay, short stature *Adults* Lethargy Muscle weakness Increased fat mass
Gonadotrophins (LH/ICSH, FSH)	*Men* Reduced libido, erectile dysfunction Reduced need to shave Loss of axillary/pubic hair Later gynaecomastia (breast development) Infertility *Women* Oligomenorrhoea, amenorrhoea Infertility 'Hot flushes' Dyspareunia Breast atrophy Loss of axillary/pubic hair
ACTH	Weakness, tiredness Hypotension Dizziness on standing Hyponatraemia Pallor Hypoglycaemia
TSH	*Children* Growth delay *Adults* Apathy Constipation Intolerance to cold Dry skin Weight gain

ACTH, Adrenocorticotrophic hormone; *FSH*, follicle-stimulating hormone; *GH*, growth hormone; *ICSH*, interstitial cell-stimulating hormone; *LH*, luteinising hormone; *TSH*, thyroid-stimulating hormone.

❖ Nursing Management and Health Promotion: Hypopituitarism

Effective nursing intervention depends upon the establishment of an effective therapeutic relationship in a friendly environment. As the effects of hypopituitarism can be widespread, causing diverse physical and psychological changes which can be difficult to comprehend, it is important to ensure that all of the patient's questions are answered in a way that is understood. Open and frank discussion about changes in body image and sexuality is essential to the individual concerned. Clear, ongoing explanations of the extensive and possibly uncomfortable investigations will help to relieve the patient's anxiety. The presence of a nurse known to the patient during these investigations can be reassuring.

Neurosurgery or radiotherapy is a frightening prospect for most people. Preoperative preparation must include an explanation of procedures, the nature of immediate postoperative care and the expected long-term outcome. Reminding the patient that many of their symptoms will be relieved by surgery, radiotherapy and/or hormone replacement therapy will be of considerable psychological benefit.

Supporting the Patient Taking Ongoing Replacement Therapy

Replacement of deficient hormones should alleviate many symptoms, allowing the patient to lead a near-normal life. It is essential that the individual feels free to contact the appropriate doctor or specialist nurse at any time to discuss their condition or any related anxieties. As pituitary disease is a lifelong condition that will require ongoing monitoring, hospital attendance will continue on at least an annual basis for many years, giving the doctor or nurse the opportunity to build therapeutic relationships with their patients. Encouraging concordance by educating the patient as to the importance of correctly taking their replacement medication is vital (Reflection 5.1).

Anterior Pituitary Hormone Replacement

Cortisol. Hydrocortisone in tablet form is given for ACTH deficiency. It directly replaces the missing hormone and is rapidly absorbed with a short half-life (less than 2 hours). It is usually taken on waking, at midday and in the early evening. Alternative preparations include cortisone acetate, which is metabolised to cortisol, and synthetic preparations, e.g. prednisolone and dexamethasone. It is important to monitor cortisol levels regularly, as overreplacement can be associated with hypertension, hyperglycaemia and hyperinsulinaemia, as well as reduced bone mineral density (BMD). The omission of even one dose may have serious consequences. Patients should be advised to carry a blue 'steroid' card and to wear a MedicAlert bracelet at all times, indicating they are cortisol deficient. Patients should also be given an emergency hydrocortisone pack to keep at home containing a vial of hydrocortisone for IM injection which they have been shown how to use. The nurse should demonstrate how to use this and ensure that the patient has practised and is competent.

See Evolve website Critical thinking question 5.1

Thyroxine. Levothyroxine (thyroxine sodium) is given in tablet form, usually one dose in the morning. In older people or in patients with known heart disease, doses should be reduced to meet individual needs. Levothyroxine replacement should not be started until ACTH deficiency has been excluded or treated as otherwise there is a risk of worsening the cortisol deficiency. As levothyroxine has a very long half-life, the occasional missed dose is not critical.

Hormone Replacement Therapy for Hypopituitarism

Lucy has developed hypopituitarism following surgery for a benign tumour of her pituitary gland. You and your assessor/supervisor are seeing Lucy in the outpatient clinic when she asks about her diagnosis and the different drugs she must now take to replace the hormones she is deficient in. She is concerned about the cost of her prescriptions.

Activities

- Access the resources below and find out:
  - information about the pituitary gland and its hormones
  - about the medications used to replace the anterior pituitary hormones
- Discuss with your supervisor/assessor how you might use the website material to help Lucy understand her condition and its management.
- Reflect on how the need to take medication to replace several hormones may affect Lucy's quality of life.
- What information can you give her that will help to reduce her anxieties about prescription costs?

Resources

The Pituitary Foundation. The Pituitary Gland: Its conditions and hormones explained. https://www.pituitary.org.uk/media/548325/Pituitary-Gland_Sept-17.pdf.

You and Your Hormones: An Educational Resource From the Society for Endocrinology. http://www.yourhormones.info/glands/pituitary-gland/.

You and Your Hormones: An Educational Resource From the Society for Endocrinology. http://www.yourhormones.info/endocrine-conditions/hypopituitarism/.

NHS Business Services Authority. Medical Exemption Certificates. https://www.nhsbsa.nhs.uk/exemption-certificates/medical-exemption-certificates.

Thyroxine levels can be monitored by the practice nurse or GP, who should perform thyroid function tests regularly. Excessive doses of levothyroxine over a long period should be avoided as there is an increased risk of osteoporotic fractures and atrial fibrillation.

Growth Hormone. Studies have shown that replacement GH therapy in patients with adult-onset GH deficiency has profound effects on patients' QoL, vascular morbidity and cardiovascular mortality (Aguiar-Oliveira and Bartke 2019). GH replacement is associated with favourable changes in body composition, bone density, lipid metabolism, physical performance and cardiovascular function. The National Institute for Health and Clinical Excellence (NICE) in 2003 produced guidance for the prescription of GH in England and Wales, which was subsequently ratified for use in Scotland. Eligibility for GH replacement is dependent on patients fulfilling several criteria, which include biochemical evidence of GH deficiency, and demonstrating a reduced QoL, judged by their responses to a disease-specific questionnaire, the Adult Growth Hormone Deficiency Assessment–Quality of Life (AGHDA-QoL). Continuation of therapy is dependent on demonstrating that symptomatic benefit, based on improvement in questionnaire score, has been achieved (NICE 2003). GH is replaced by a daily SC injection which patients are taught to self-administer using a special pen device. Needle-free delivery devices are available. The normal starting dose is 0.3–0.5 mg daily titrated over a 3-month period. During this time, IGF-1 levels are checked every 6 weeks with the aim of keeping the levels within the age-matched reference range. The dosing schedule is adjusted to maximise benefits and minimise side-effects, which can include transient oedema, arthralgia and headaches. Older patients, women and those with a higher body mass index (BMI) can be more prone to side-effects. Patients on GH replacement should be reassessed annually for blood lipids and glucose, body composition (waist circumference, lean body mass and BMD), exercise endurance and well-being using the AGHDA-QoL questionnaire. (See Further Reading, e.g. Melmed 2019.)

Gonadotrophins. Testosterone replacement therapy has been available for many years. Replacement can result in an improvement in sexual function, an increase in BMD and improvements in body composition, e.g. increased lean body mass/decreased fat mass in hypogonadal men. In addition, positive changes are seen in erythropoiesis and lipid profiles. Testosterone replacement is usually commenced when the diagnosis of hypogonadism is established and serum testosterone levels fall below a normal age-matched reference range.

Many testosterone preparations with differing routes of administration are available. The most commonly prescribed are IM injections or transdermal patches or gels though SC pellets inserted under the skin, and oral tablets are also available. IM injections may be given every 3–4 weeks (50–250 mg) or every 3 months (1000 mg) depending on the preparation chosen while pellets (600–800 mg) are replaced every 4–6 months. Depending on their lifestyle and taking in to account other factors, patients can self-medicate using patches (5–10 mg) or gels (50–100 mg) which they apply daily or tablets (40–120 mg) which have to be taken twice a day. Testosterone levels are monitored either immediately prior to an injection/implant or 8 hours after the application of a patch/gel.

IM injections have, for many years, been the most widely used and accepted form of testosterone replacement in the UK, but these can be uncomfortable, are disruptive as the patient must make an appointment to see their practice nurse or GP regularly and can cause fluctuations in mood, energy levels and sexual function due to the changing levels of testosterone, which are high immediately postinjection but then fall off over the next 2–3 weeks. Transdermal patches (scrotal or nonscrotal) and transdermal gels mimic the normal physiological and diurnal variations of testosterone resulting in more stable levels of testosterone (Haymana and Sonmez 2022). Both the patch and the gel are self-applied, making them a popular choice, but both frequently cause skin irritation often causing discontinuation. Other options include testosterone implants. Pellet insertion requires minor surgery every 3–6 months and may be complicated by local infection, extrusion and scarring. Oral replacement requires frequent dosing (two to four times per day) and often does not achieve normal levels of testosterone due to variable absorption.

Ultimately, the choice of testosterone replacement therapy should be made in consultation with the patient once they have the information required to make an informed decision. Younger patients are more likely to choose a long-acting preparation whereas men over the age of 50 should be advised to opt for a short-acting one. This is to ensure that if the preparation has to be stopped due to a contraindication to testosterone replacement therapy, e.g. prostate cancer, levels of serum testosterone will immediately fall.

Whatever the replacement therapy chosen, testosterone levels should always be closely monitored to ensure they remain within physiological parameters. While suboptimal dosing can negatively affect a patient's QoL and sexual function, supra-physiological dosing can promote secondary polycythaemia and progression of prostate cancer (see Chapter 10, Nursing Patients With Urinary Disorders). Prostate-specific antigen (PSA) should be measured in men over 50 before any replacement is commenced and must be checked annually because testosterone can stimulate prostate cancer. In older men, haemoglobin (Hb) levels should also be monitored because testosterone can cause polycythaemia. Patients on testosterone replacement should therefore always have their haemoglobin and PSA levels monitored regularly as well as an annual rectal examination of their prostate gland.

Disorder of Posterior Pituitary/Hypothalamus: Abnormal Antidiuretic Hormone (ADH) Secretion

Diabetes Insipidus

Diabetes insipidus (DI) is defined as the passing of large amounts (over 3 L/24 h) of dilute urine (osmolality less than 300 mOsmol/kg) and exists in two main forms:
- cranial DI – reduced hypothalamic secretion of ADH
- nephrogenic DI – resistance of the renal tubules to ADH.

Causes of both types may be familial or acquired and include pituitary tumours, meningitis, encephalitis, tuberculosis (TB), sarcoidosis, head injury, neurosurgery, Sheehan's syndrome, sickle cell disease, chronic renal disease, hyper/hypocalcaemia, hyperglycaemia and some medications (lithium). Primary polydipsia may be psychological.

Pathophysiology
Clinical Features
Deficiency of ADH leads to polyuria, nocturia and a compensatory polydipsia. Urine output may reach 10–15 L or more per day, leading to severe dehydration if the individual's fluid intake is restricted in any way.

Medical Management
Investigations
Diagnosis is often made by single paired urine and plasma osmolality, obviating the need for the more stressful and prolonged water deprivation test. Plasma osmolality will show high concentration and urine will be dilute. However, sometimes the results are equivocal and a water deprivation test is required to make the diagnosis.

Treatment
Desmopressin (DDAVP), a synthetic vasopressin (see following section), is administered.

Nursing Management and Health Promotion: Diabetes Insipidus

During diagnosis and any further investigations, the nurse's interventions will include accurate recording of fluid balance with the full cooperation and participation of the patient. It is essential for the patient to have easy access to toilet facilities. Samples of urine will be required for osmolality assessment.

The nurse will also be involved in medication administration and education of the patient with regard to self-administration of their DDAVP, continued measurement of fluid balance and regular weight recording. Most patients rapidly become aware if

their DDAVP is no longer effective and will contact their specialist nurse, GP or the doctor.

Posterior pituitary hormone replacement desmopressin (DDAVP) is available orally, sublingually, intranasally and parenterally and should be started as a low dose and gradually increased until urine output is controlled. Doses can vary enormously between individual patients. Blood sodium levels should be checked after starting or altering treatment to detect hyponatraemia.

DISORDERS OF THE THYROID

Simple Goitre
A goitre is an enlargement of the thyroid gland. It can occur without over- or underactivity of the gland. The term 'simple goitre' is a paradox as its cause is poorly understood. In young adults the gland is soft and diffuse, enlarged two to three times its normal size. Thyroid hormones and TSH levels are normal and there is no evidence of autoimmunity. If the stimulus to goitre formation remains, whatever it is, the gland becomes further enlarged and nodular over the ensuing 20 years or so (euthyroid (normal thyroid function) multinodular goitre) and people 60 years of age or beyond may develop hyperthyroidism (toxic multinodular goitre).

Hypersecretion of Thyroid Hormones

Hyperthyroidism, or overactive thyroid (previously known as thyrotoxicosis), is characterised by high levels of circulating thyroid hormones. The most common cause of hyperthyroidism is intrinsic thyroid disease; pituitary-driven hyperthyroidism is extremely rare. Hyperthyroidism mainly affects women aged between 30 and 50 years, but can occur at any age in either gender.

Graves' Disease
Graves' disease is the most common form of hyperthyroidism. It is an autoimmune disorder in which anti-TSH receptor autoantibodies behave like TSH, stimulating thyroid hormone production and in some cases thyroid enlargement or goitre. Graves' disease tends to run in families and may be associated with eye features (Reflection 5.2). The ophthalmopathy of Graves' disease, which affects the majority of patients to some extent, is also autoimmune in aetiology. There are changes in the retro-orbital space, with water accumulation and enlargement of the extraocular muscles and increased fat. The increased pressure behind the eye pushes the eye forward (exophthalmos) and the swollen muscles work inefficiently, causing double vision (diplopia). Vision may be threatened. Swelling of the eyelids is due to prolapse of retrobulbar fat and poor lymphatic and venous drainage. Lid retraction and lid lag are features. In mild cases artificial tear drops can help combat the symptoms of dry and gritty eyes. Attaching prisms to glasses can help with double vision. In more severe cases, corticosteroids or radiotherapy are used to reduce swelling. Patients may also undergo surgery to reduce the pressure behind the eyes, or to remove excess tissue.

Toxic Multinodular Goitre
As mentioned earlier, this is often the outcome of the simple diffuse goitre in the young adult. It is the second most common cause of hyperthyroidism after Graves' disease. Older people with hyperthyroidism may present with cardiovascular effects, e.g. atrial fibrillation and predominating.

Toxic Adenoma (Solitary Nodule)

Toxic adenoma causes about 5% of hyperthyroidism. In these patients, the thyroid nodule acts autonomously and produces excess levels of thyroid hormone, leading to suppression of the normal thyroid gland.

Other Causes of Hyperthyroidism

These include:

- Thyroiditis (infection or inflammation of the thyroid gland). Occurring after a viral infection, postpartum (usually in the first 6 months after childbirth) or may be autoimmune.
- Overtreatment of hypothyroidism with levothyroxine.

Pathophysiology

In hyperthyroidism, high levels of circulating thyroid hormones stimulate cell metabolism, resulting in a high metabolic rate. TSH secretion is suppressed. There is tachycardia and, in older patients, atrial fibrillation and cardiac failure. Patients complain of general fatigue, although for short spells, they may become more active, and find that they are restless.

Common Presenting Symptoms

There is increased irritability, with mood swings or aggressive behaviour and inability to relax and sleep, heat intolerance with hot moist skin and excessive sweating, palpitations and tachycardia, and sometimes a feeling of shakiness and a fine tremor of the hands. By far the most common symptom, however, is weight loss, despite an increased appetite. Patients often complain of excessive watering and grittiness of the eyes. There may also be diarrhoea, thirst, oligomenorrhoea/amenorrhoea and pruritus. Enlargement of the gland may have been noticed.

Medical and Nursing Management

Investigations

Clinical examination will confirm tachycardia and atrial fibrillation, goitre and eye signs. Diagnosis is usually confirmed by elevated serum T_4 and suppressed TSH.

Treatment

Treatment approaches for hyperthyroidism are:

Medication. Medication is usually the first line of treatment. Carbimazole or propylthiouracil is used in one of two ways. The first, known as 'block and replace', occurs when drugs are used to completely inhibit the synthesis of thyroid hormones. Levothyroxine is then added to this regimen as a 'replacement' dose to achieve a euthyroid state. Treatment usually continues for 6 months. Fewer blood tests are required, thyroid function tests are more stable and there is less likelihood of the thyroid gland becoming overactive again once the drugs are stopped or reduced.

The second regimen, known as 'dose titration', occurs when the patient is commenced on drugs until a euthyroid state is achieved. The dose is titrated so that the amount of hormone being produced by the overactive thyroid gland is reduced to normal. Thyroid function tests (serum T_4 and TSH) are performed every 4–8 weeks and the drug dose is adjusted to ensure that the patient remains euthyroid and to avoid over- or undermedication. Treatment usually continues for some 18 months, with regular outpatient visits. Side-effects (see later) are less common because of the lower drug doses and concordance increased as patients only have to remember to take one drug.

Anti-thyroid drugs (ATDs) are usually well tolerated. Occasionally, patients may complain of gastrointestinal symptoms or an altered sense of taste or smell. The most common adverse reaction is an urticarial rash which occurs in about 2% of patients. Other side-effects include fever and arthralgias, usually within the first few months of starting therapy, and are more common in patients treated with higher doses. Patients are asked to report unexplained fever or sore throat as the major side-effect of ATDs, although rare, is agranulocytosis, which occurs in approximately 1 in 300–500 patients (see Chapter 13, Nursing Patients With Blood Disorders). Should fever or sore throat occur, patients are forewarned to stop taking their medication immediately and to seek medical advice.

Symptomatic control of tachycardia is obtained by administration of beta-blockers, such as propranolol, given until thyroid hormone levels are normal.

Surgical Interventions. Indications for surgery include:

- suspicious or malignant thyroid nodule
- pregnant women not adequately controlled on drugs or who develop serious allergic reactions
- patients who refuse radio-iodine
- poor patient concordance
- patients who are not well controlled by antithyroid drugs
- patients with severe Graves' ophthalmopathy or relapsed Graves' disease.

Partial thyroidectomy is performed only after ATDs have produced a euthyroid state. In some centres, the patient is given potassium iodide for 1–2 weeks before surgery, which will inhibit thyroid hormone release, reduce the size and vascularity of the gland and reduce the risk of peri- and postoperative haemorrhage. Approximately 80% of patients are cured by surgery, with the best surgical centres achieving less than 4% recurrence. Partial thyroidectomy is also a useful treatment for patients with large/unsightly goitres.

Specific complications of surgery include:

- compromise of airway
- postoperative haemorrhage
- recurrent laryngeal nerve palsy
- thyroid crisis
- tetany due to damage/removal of parathyroid glands
- hypothyroidism (affecting 10%–20% of patients within 10 years).

A critical thinking question on the Evolve website provides an opportunity for you to consider the early postoperative complications following partial thyroidectomy.

See Evolve website Critical thinking question 5.2

Radioactive Iodine Therapy. Iodine-131 (^{131}I) destroys functioning cells or inhibits cell replication. It is usually administered orally as a single capsule taken with water or as a drink on an outpatient basis. Patients are advised to avoid eating for 3–4 hours after administration to allow adequate absorption of the iodine; they are also advised to drink at least 2 L of fluid over the next 24 hours and to pass urine frequently in order to excrete free circulating radioactive iodine as rapidly as possible. Transient side-effects include nausea, anterior neck pain and increased thyroid hormone levels which can exacerbate heart failure.

Patients present a radiation hazard for approximately 1 week following this treatment and should have no close contact (less than 1 metre) with children under the age of 11 during this time. This type of therapy is used to treat multinodular goitres and relapsed Graves' disease or when surgery is not appropriate, but is not usually offered to women of child-bearing age or patients with Graves' ophthalmopathy as it can exacerbate symptoms, especially in patients who smoke.

Cancer of the Thyroid Gland

Thyroid cancer is the most common endocrine cancer but is still rare, comprising less than 1% of all cancers diagnosed in the UK between 2016 and 2018 (Cancer Research UK 2023). Each year, around 3500 people are diagnosed, with women more affected than men (Macmillan Cancer Support 2023).

The main types of thyroid cancer are:
* papillary (most common type, accounts for 80%–85% of all thyroid cancers, is slow growing and is found mostly in young people especially women)
* follicular (much less common; 5%–10%, found more in middle-aged people)
* Hurthle cell (rare, about 4%, affects women more than men, most commonly found in middle age)
* medullary cell (rare, 3%–10%, may run in families, approximately 25% caused by an inherited gene)
* anaplastic (rare, 1%–3% usually diagnosed in older people and is more common in women, tends to grow more quickly than other types of thyroid cancer)
* lymphoma (usually non Hodgkin lymphoma).

Papillary and follicular thyroid cancers are differentiated cancers (i.e. the cancer cells retain histological features typical of normal thyroid cells), whereas anaplastic thyroid cancer is referred to as undifferentiated because the cancer cells do not resemble normal thyroid cells.

Pathophysiology

Papillary or follicular cancers usually present with a lump which can cause hoarseness or difficulty in swallowing. At night, patients can notice difficulty in breathing. Metastatic spread from follicular cancer commonly involves the brain, liver, lungs and bones.

Common Presenting Symptoms
Often the patient will have noticed a painless small nodule or swelling in the neck. Patients may be euthyroid or may have symptoms of either hyper- or hypothyroidism.

Medical Management
Investigations

T_3, T_4 and TSH levels are measured and an ultrasound scan of the neck is undertaken. Fine-needle biopsy or aspiration is necessary to distinguish cancer from benign pathologies, to give a firm diagnosis and to differentiate between the types of thyroid cancer. Radioactive isotope scanning, using technetium or iodine, is a painless procedure which involves injecting the radioactive isotopes intravenously and then, after 20-minute rest, scanning the thyroid gland with a gamma camera. As cancer cells do not absorb the radioactive liquid as well as normal thyroid cells, any cancer cells will generally appear as 'cold areas' or 'cold nodules' on scanning. However, only 10% of such cold nodules are malignant. Many turn out to be cysts, and surgery may be avoided if aspiration cytology is normal.

Patients with papillary and follicular cancers will be commenced on levothyroxine which decreases the rate of growth of the cancer.

Staging
Staging is the process by which a cancer is described in terms of tumour size (T), spread to lymph nodes (N) and metastatic spread (M) (see Chapter 31, Nursing Patients With Cancer).

The basic TNM stages for differentiated thyroid cancer are:
* tumour size – T1, T2, T3, T4a and T4b
* nodal spread – either N0 (no spread), or nodal spread N1a, N1b
* metastatic spread – either M0 (no spread), or metastatic spread M1.

Postoperatively, the cancer can also be described is terms of whether there is any residual disease (R) – R0 (no residual primary tumour), R1 and R2 (micro or macro residual tumour still present).

Some types of thyroid cancer are staged using number stages. The number of stages used, I–IV, depends upon the cancer type and whether the patient is under or over 45 years of age. Staging information is useful for the clinician in order to select the most appropriate treatment for the patient and assess prognosis (Araque et al. 2020).

Treatment
Surgery, radioactive iodine (^{131}I) or radiotherapy may be given alone or in combination. The treatment chosen will depend on several factors, including the patient's age and general health and the type and stage of the tumour. The treatment of choice is near-total thyroidectomy. This is usually followed by a large dose of ^{131}I to ablate any thyroid remnant. Any tissue showing radio-iodine uptake subsequently must be assumed to be recurrent disease, and further ^{131}I may be taken up therapeutically by the tumour tissue. Follow-up is important and will usually be carried out at 6-monthly intervals initially. At follow-up the tumour marker, serum thyroglobulin (Tg), is measured. It should not be detectable in a patient who has had a total thyroidectomy, ^{131}I ablation of remnant and is taking levothyroxine in a dose sufficient to suppress serum TSH. If detectable, further surgery or ^{131}I therapy may be required.

Nursing Management and Health Promotion: The Patient Receiving ^{131}I Therapy

Before ^{131}I ablative therapy, the patient will have discontinued thyroid hormones for 4–6 weeks to allow TSH to rise, which ensures better uptake of ^{131}I. In those in whom a period of hypothyroidism is best avoided, e.g. an older patient with coronary heart disease, high TSH levels in the blood can be achieved by giving thyrotropin alfa (recombinant human rhTSH). Thyrotropin alfa is given as two IM injections 24 hours apart, prior to commencement of ^{131}I, and negates the need to discontinue thyroid hormone replacement.

The patient and family should be given clear explanations regarding the effect of ^{131}I, the reasons for the patient being nursed alone with restricted access for staff and visitors, and procedures to be followed in the handling of body fluids. It should be explained to the patient that they cannot be discharged until their radiation level is safe (around 3 days). Side-effects from treatment can include a sore throat and neck, a dry mouth, nausea and changes to the patient's sense of taste (usually temporary).

Measures should be taken to prevent constipation, as this inhibits the subsequent excretion of radioactive material. A high fluid intake should be encouraged to promote a good urinary output. Commodes and bedpans should be designated for the patient's exclusive use. All body fluids will be highly radioactive following ^{131}I administration and the patient should be encouraged to shower regularly to remove contaminated perspiration.

The patient should be nursed in a single room, often referred to as an 'isolation chamber', containing a minimum of equipment. Dosimeters should be worn at all times by staff members to indicate radiation exposure. Duties should be coordinated so that each staff member spends a minimum amount of time with the patient.

As with all endocrine disease, prompt treatment should result in complete alleviation of all signs and symptoms; the patient should be reassured of this whilst undergoing treatment. Follow-up after treatment is essential. Nursing staff should encourage the patient to attend outpatient or GP clinics as advised. The patient should be reassured that, particularly with localised disease from a papillary or follicular cancer, the probability of 'cure' is extremely high. (See Further Reading, e.g. Smith et al. 2018.)

Hyposecretion of Thyroid Hormones

Underactivity of the thyroid gland may be primary (70%), resulting from disease of the thyroid, or secondary, due to pituitary failure.

Aetiology and Epidemiology

Primary hypothyroidism resulting from autoimmune disease is the commonest cause of thyroid underactivity. It may be associated with other autoimmune disease. It is six times more common in women than in men and the mean age of diagnosis for women is 57 years.

Hypothyroidism (also known as myxoedema) may also be iatrogenic, i.e. caused by previous treatment for hyperthyroidism by surgery or radioactive iodine.

Iodine deficiency, a major public health issue across the world, is another cause of hypothyroidism and is due to insufficient dietary iodine (see Further Reading, e.g. Berger et al. 2022). This leads to reduced thyroid hormone production. Goitre is a common feature of this condition. The most devastating effects of iodine deficiency are increased perinatal mortality and impaired mental development. Iodine deficiency is the biggest cause of preventable brain damage in childhood. Endemic hypothyroidism is occasionally seen in areas where iodine levels in the water supply are low, usually inland areas far from the sea or in mountainous regions. It is still seen in some areas of the world, such as parts of central Africa, central Asia and central and eastern Europe as well as in the Andes and the Himalayas (Zimmerman and Andersson 2021).

Some medications may also induce hypothyroidism, for example lithium carbonate (used in bipolar disorders) and amiodarone (an antiarrhythmic agent) (Penman et al. 2022).

Congenital hypothyroidism occurs in approximately 1 in 2500–3000 live births, resulting in approximately 200 new cases per year, and usually results from congenital absence of the thyroid gland;

it can also be caused by certain enzyme defects. If congenital hypothyroidism is not detected and treated early, the infant/child will not develop fully either mentally or physically and this can lead to reduced intellectual ability and impaired work capacity. Routine neonatal screening is performed in most developed countries at 5–7 days and is a good example of how endocrinology has significantly contributed to improving the public health of the nation.

🔴 Pathophysiology

In primary hypothyroidism, insufficient T_4 is produced by the thyroid gland. Serum T_4 is low and levels of TSH are high. The onset is slow and insidious. Because the affected individual is often an older person, it may be accepted as a normal part of ageing and it may be some time before a medical opinion is sought. The patient may report sensitivity to cold, weight gain, a general slowing down of body functions, lethargy, depression and an inability to 'think quickly'. The face will be puffy in appearance and hair sparse, coarse and brittle. In severe hypothyroidism, the patient may be admitted in a coma and perhaps be thought to be suffering from hypothermia. This represents a medical emergency in which intensive treatment and care are essential. Diagnosis of hypothyroidism is confirmed by low plasma levels of T_4 and raised TSH levels.

🔴 Medical Management

Treatment

Hypothyroidism is treated with replacement doses of levothyroxine commencing with a low dose of 50 µg (25 µg if the patient is over 50 or there is a history of heart disease/angina) and increasing by increments every 3–4 weeks until serum TSH is normal. Levothyroxine has a stable 24-hour profile and is easy to monitor. A typical adult dose would be 100–150 µg daily. There is an increased requirement during pregnancy. Care should be taken not to over-replace thyroxine as this can result in an increased risk of osteoporosis and/or atrial fibrillation.

Levothyroxine is only partly absorbed after ingestion, and foodstuffs (especially those rich in calcium or iron), other minerals, drugs (e.g. antacids) and tablet composition can all influence its absorption. Tablets should therefore be taken as a single daily dose in the morning on an empty stomach. Conditions such as coeliac disease and nephrotic syndrome will also affect the dose required. Symptomatic relief should become apparent 2–4 weeks after starting replacement therapy with improvements to puffy eyes and a reduction in weight often noticed in this time. However, it will take some 6–8 weeks for a steady state of thyroid hormones to be achieved.

❖ Nursing Management and Health Promotion: Hypothyroidism

The nurse should advise the patient and their family that there will only be a gradual improvement in symptoms until the steady state is reached. Until then, it is important to remind the patient and their family that symptoms of lethargy and mental slowness are part of the disease process. Improvement to hair and skin texture can take 3–6 months. In an attempt to reduce constipation, patients should be advised to eat a high-fibre diet. It is usual to treat patients in the community with a 6-monthly or annual hospital review, often at a specific nurse-led thyroid clinic. Community nursing teams should follow up medical treatment and explanations and ensure that patients understand the reasons for T_4 replacement therapy and the importance of attending for regular check-ups and blood tests to ensure that a euthyroid state is achieved and maintained. The patient should be advised that they will need to take T_4 replacement therapy for life.

Patients requiring lifelong replacement therapy are entitled to free prescriptions in England where charges for prescriptions are still made. This includes not only their T_4 but any other medication they are prescribed. Exemption certificates are obtained in England by completing form FP92A which can be obtained from GPs or pharmacists. Other endocrine conditions such as Addison's disease, hypoparathyroidism, DI and other forms of hypopituitarism also entitle patients to free prescriptions.

Patients often forget to take long-term medications routinely and poor concordance with thyroid replacement is not uncommon. Patients can feel despondent if the T_4 does not make them feel as they did before the onset of their disease and consequently not adhere to their treatment. As the half-life of T_4 is 6–7 days patients may not notice any changes if they miss the odd tablet and consequently bad habits can develop.

Condition-specific questionnaires have been designed and validated for use with patients with hypothyroidism: the Underactive Thyroid-Dependent Quality of Life Questionnaire (ThyDQoL) and the Underactive Thyroid Treatment Satisfaction Questionnaire (ThyTSQ) (Uslar et al. 2022). The ThyDQoL has 18 domains covering QoL measures such as energy levels, physical capabilities, motivation, physical appearance and weight together with other aspects of life affected by hypothyroidism (Uslar et al. 2022). It is an individualised measure of the perceived impact of hypothyroidism on the patient's QoL and is a useful tool to use when assessing a new patient or evaluating the benefits of treatment.

DISORDERS OF THE PARATHYROIDS

This section outlines hypersecretion and hyposecretion of PTH.

Hypersecretion of the Parathyroids

Hypercalcaemia

In most instances, raised plasma calcium levels are caused by primary hyperparathyroidism or are secondary to malignancy. Other causes include myeloma, vitamin D poisoning, TB and thiazide diuretics. Mild hypercalcaemia, which is often asymptomatic, occurs in about 1 in 1000 of the population (Gleeson et al. 2020).

Pathophysiology

Hypercalcaemia impairs renal function by reducing the glomerular filtration rate and by causing nephrogenic DI leading to an inability to conserve water. The resulting dehydration augments sodium reabsorption, leading to enhanced calcium reabsorption and impairing the kidney's ability to excrete the unwanted calcium.

Even mild symptoms can lead to an early diagnosis, due to advanced chemical analysis techniques; this means that it is now extremely rare to see the severe renal and skeletal problems associated with hypercalcaemia that occurred in the past.

Common Presenting Symptoms

Patients may present with symptoms of malignancy or of hypercalcaemia including:

- vague malaise (very easily missed)
- weakness
- depression
- drowsiness, coma
- nausea, vomiting
- anorexia
- constipation
- nocturia
- polydipsia, polyuria
- psychosis.

 Medical Management

Investigations

Diagnosis is based on medical history, clinical examination and tests to ascertain the cause, although initial treatment is often started before all tests are completed.

Treatment

Hypercalcaemia caused by malignancy is usually seen only in patients with advanced cancer when bony metastases have occurred and signifies a poor prognosis. If possible, it should be treated, as this may improve the patient's QoL. Adequate hydration is of great importance and, in itself, is often enough to relieve the symptoms of the hypercalcaemia. Patients should be rehydrated with up to 3 L of 0.9% sodium chloride/day. However, it is now established that bisphosphonates, e.g. disodium pamidronate, are highly effective in lowering malignant hypercalcaemia. These are administered by an IV infusion, but oral preparations, e.g. sodium clodronate or ibandronic acid, can be used in the long term to prevent a recurrence of hypercalcaemia. Other treatments include oral phosphate and corticosteroid therapy.

Primary Hyperparathyroidism

This condition is caused by the overproduction of PTH, such as by a parathyroid adenoma. It affects more women than men and its incidence increases with age.

Medical Management

Treatment

Surgery is indicated for the management of hypercalcaemia due to excessive PTH secretion, as no long-term medication is available. However, asymptomatic hypercalcaemia requires no surgical intervention and can be treated conservatively with simple monitoring of calcium levels on an intermittent basis by the practice nurse, GP or the hospital outpatient department.

Following parathyroidectomy, hypocalcaemia of either a transient or permanent nature may ensue. This should be treated promptly to prevent tetany. If severe hypocalcaemia occurs, IV calcium gluconate (10 mL of 10%) should be given immediately. Vitamin D and oral calcium supplements will be required. Calcium levels should be monitored closely until they have stabilised.

Nursing Management and Health Promotion: Primary Hyperparathyroidism

The investigations for diagnosis of hypercalcaemia may require hospital admission, particularly if the hypercalcaemia is severe and/or is thought to be secondary to malignancy. The patient will probably have been unwell for some time and will be feeling very tired and weak on admission.

Careful explanations of the investigations and treatment are required. These will include a 24-hour urine collection for calcium. As it is particularly important for the accuracy of this test that the urine collection is completed properly, it is essential that this is explained clearly and is fully understood by the patient. If surgery

---

INFORMATION 5.2

Chvostek's and Trousseau's Signs: Tests for Latent Tetany due to Hypocalcaemia

Chvostek's sign

The nurse can test for this sign by tapping the person's facial nerve about 2 cm anterior to the ear lobe. If hypocalcaemia (or hypomagnesaemia) is present, unilateral twitching of facial muscles, especially around the mouth, may be observed.

Trousseau's sign

This is tested by inflating a sphygmomanometer cuff on the upper arm to a pressure above systolic pressure for 2–3 minutes. The constrictive effect of the inflated blood pressure cuff exacerbates the hypocalcaemia in the limb distal to the cuff. Spasm of the forearm muscles (contraction or twitching) will be observed in the limb concerned. This is considered to be the more sensitive test.

---

is undertaken, the perioperative care is the same as for thyroidectomy (see Medical and Nursing Management, Treatment) In addition, regular assessment for latent tetany due to hypocalcaemia is undertaken – Chvostek's and Trousseau's signs (Information 5.2).

Secondary and Tertiary Hyperparathyroidism

Secondary hyperparathyroidism occurs due to disease processes that cause hypocalcaemia, e.g. in vitamin D deficiency or in renal disease. The parathyroid glands strive to keep the calcium levels up, while calcium remains normal or is low. Rarely, this can lead to autonomous secretion of PTH, leading to permanent hypercalcaemia, termed tertiary hyperparathyroidism. This is often seen in patients with renal failure.

Hyposecretion of the Parathyroids

Hypocalcaemia

The most common cause of hypocalcaemia is artefactual due to low albumin levels, i.e. the calcium is normal when the low albumin is corrected for by the laboratory. Other relatively common causes include hypomagnesaemia, renal failure and vitamin D deficiency (see Information 5.1). Autoimmune hypoparathyroidism is rare, but iatrogenic hypoparathyroidism following neck surgery is more common, usually presenting within 24–48 hours of surgery.

Treatment

If hypocalcaemia is mild and the patient asymptomatic, oral calcium replacement should be given. Severe or symptomatic hypocalcaemia should be treated with IV calcium gluconate and vitamin D added if the patient requires IV calcium for more than 2 days.

Rickets and Osteomalacia

These are diseases of calcium and phosphorus metabolism resulting from a deficiency in vitamin D intake and synthesis. As these conditions are usually seen and treated by endocrinologists, as opposed to other physicians, they are considered here.

Vitamin D deficiency during growth produces abnormalities in the growing skeleton known as rickets. In childhood, rickets produces soft, painful bones. The weight-bearing bones bend and may give rise to gross deformities. In the adult, where bone growth is completed, osteomalacia is the result; symptoms are generally diffuse bone pain and myopathy.

Rickets is not now commonly seen in the UK, due to better nutrition and, possibly, to a reduction in industrial pollution which allows more sunlight through. It is, however, sometimes seen in the communities who tend to cover up and avoid exposing themselves to sunlight, particularly those individuals with an increased vitamin D requirement, e.g. babies, children and pregnant women.

Treatment is by vitamin D replacement, and prevention is the aim, particularly targeted to known vulnerable groups.

DISORDERS OF THE ADRENALS

This section outlines hypersecretion of the adrenal medulla and cortex, cortical hyposecretion and congenital adrenal hyperplasia (CAH).

Hypersecretion of the Adrenals

Adrenal Medulla – Phaeochromocytoma

Phaeochromocytoma is a very rare condition which causes about 1 in 1000 cases of secondary hypertension (Gleeson et al. 2020). A tumour of the adrenal medulla produces excessive adrenaline and noradrenaline. The tumour is small, with about 10% being multiple tumours and 10% being malignant.

🔹 *Pathophysiology*
Clinical Features

The tumour produces the clinical effects of excessive catecholamine secretion which include hypertension and palpitations.

Common Presenting Symptoms

Patients may present with anxiety, tachycardia, palpitations and panic attacks. Headaches, sweating and pallor may also occur. There may be a history of high blood pressure, which may be labile. Patients may present as an emergency with a hypertensive crisis or may be asymptomatic.

🔹 *Medical Management*
Investigations

A careful history and clinical examination may lead the healthcare practitioner to suspect a phaeochromocytoma. Investigations include 24-hour urine collections for urinary free noradrenaline (norepinephrine, NE) and adrenaline (epinephrine, E) and dopamine or their two major metabolites, metanephrine and vanillylmandelic acid (VMA). Normal levels of NE/E and catecholamine secretion usually exclude a diagnosis of phaeochromocytoma. Abdominal X-rays and a computed tomography (CT) scan may show a tumour of the medulla.

Treatment

This includes surgical removal of the tumour and administration of α- and β-adrenoreceptor blocking medications, e.g. phenoxybenzamine and propranolol.

❖ Nursing Management and Health Promotion: Phaeochromocytoma

The first priority of care is to limit anxiety as much as possible and to nurse the patient in a quiet, nonstressful environment. Clear, concise explanations of the reasons for the symptoms will help to relieve the anxiety.

Blood pressure and pulse should be recorded 4-hourly and any sweating or flushing noted. Antihypertensive medication must be maintained as the risk of postoperative hypotensive collapse is reduced by adequate preparation with adrenoreceptor blocking medication.

A care plan should be devised such that the patient can be as independent as possible in self-care tasks. Preoperative preparation is as for general abdominal surgery (see Chapter 25, Nursing the Patient Undergoing Surgery). Specific postoperative care includes ½-hourly recording of blood pressure to observe for immediate postoperative hypotensive collapse brought on by the reduced blood volume characteristic of chronic vasoconstriction. Specialist medication such as sodium nitroprusside, a potent vasoconstrictor, should be available to control blood pressure in a hypotensive crisis.

Adrenal Cortex – Cushing's Syndrome/Disease

Cushing's syndrome/disease is caused by the excessive and inappropriate circulation of glucocorticoids. It most commonly occurs when synthetic corticosteroids are prescribed.

Spontaneous causes of Cushing's syndrome are extremely rare. The major causes, excluding iatrogenic causes, are (Gleeson et al. 2020):

- pituitary-dependent disease (Cushing's disease)
- ectopic ACTH production
- adrenal adenoma or cancer
- alcohol induced.

⬤ Pathophysiology

Clinical Features

Increased plasma cortisol levels have wide-ranging clinical effects on most systems of the body, i.e. altered fat and carbohydrate metabolism, diabetes mellitus, central obesity, muscle wasting, sodium retention leading to hypertension, oedema, immunosuppression and osteoporosis. Comprehensive coverage of the signs and symptoms is provided in Table 5.3.

Common Presenting Symptoms

Because of the wide-ranging clinical effects of Cushing's syndrome/disease, the patient can present with varying symptoms. Frequently, the patient will complain of infections that will not resolve, weight gain, bruising and discolouration of the skin.

⬤ Medical and Surgical Management

Investigations

Diagnosis is confirmed by radiological (e.g. CT or MRI scan of head and pituitary fossa) and biochemical (e.g. dexamethasone suppression test) investigations.

The differential diagnosis between pituitary disease, ectopic ACTH production and primary adrenal hypersecretion is important as the treatment and management will vary considerably.

Treatment

Metyrapone is commonly used to lower cortisol levels. An alternative approach is to remove completely endogenous cortisol by adrenalectomy and to supplement levels with an oral corticosteroid.

Trans-sphenoidal surgery is used to remove an ACTH-producing pituitary tumour. Ketoconazole (antifungal medication) may be used, as it inhibits the cortisol synthesis pathway. Surgical removal of a benign adrenal adenoma offers a good chance of cure, but adrenal cancer carries a poor prognosis. The medication

TABLE 5.3	Signs and Symptoms of Cushing's Syndrome/Disease
Symptoms or Sign	**Aetiology**
Muscle wasting, which can be demonstrated by the patient being unable to stand from a squatting position	Catabolic effect of the corticosteroids
Osteoporosis, which can be so severe as to result in spontaneous fracture of vertebrae or ribs	Protein loss from the skeletal matrix
Skin thinning and purple striae, plethora, easy bruising and purpura	Atrophy of the elastic lamina allows disruption of the dermic co capillaries can be seen below the surface. Weakening of the capillaries leads to easy bruising (often without trauma)
Oedema	Weakening of the capillaries
Poor wound healing, immunosuppression	The lymphocytes are destroyed, lowering the ability to fight infection. Signs of infection, e.g. swelling and redness, are masked
Obesity and 'buffalo hump' (pad of fat across shoulders)	Altered metabolism of fat. Fat is laid down over the trunk. Lipid levels may be raised
Hypertension	Sodium-retaining properties of glucocorticoids
Diabetes mellitus	Alteration in the normal metabolism of carbohydrate and the increased conversion of protein to carbohydrate
Depression, euphoria and frank psychosis	Unknown
Change in libido, erectile dysfunction, oligomenorrhoea and infertility	Due to the general hormone imbalance that is occurring
Excess hair growth, hair loss (particularly of the male pattern type in women)	This is seen in Cushing's disease/syndrome but is not solely due to cortisol overproduction

mitotane is licensed for the symptomatic treatment of adrenal cortical cancer.

Following adrenalectomy, patients will require lifelong hydrocortisone and mineralocorticoid replacement therapy. They must always wear a MedicAlert bracelet and carry a 'steroid' card, and be informed of the dangers of hypocortisolaemia, a life-threatening condition.

Ectopic ACTH Syndrome

This condition most often occurs in patients with an oat cell cancer of the lung. The cancer cells themselves produce ACTH and give rise to Cushing's syndrome. Care is as for cancer, taking into account the additional complications of Cushing's syndrome. A subgroup of patients with ectopic ACTH production from less malignant carcinoid tumours present with more classical Cushing's syndrome and may survive for many years with appropriate treatment.

❖ Nursing Management and Health Promotion: Cushing's Syndrome

The main aim of nursing care is to relieve the symptoms of the disease. On admission, a full nursing history is taken and the patient's needs thoroughly assessed to provide a basis for a care plan (Nursing Care Plan 5.1).

A major consideration will be the psychological impact of the illness, e.g. related to a change in body image. Providing clear ongoing explanations of the hormonal changes that the patient is experiencing, the investigations and the subsequent treatment that they will undergo helps provide optimal psychological support.

5.1 **Nursing Care Plan** *Care of a Patient With Cushing's Syndrome*

Nursing Considerations	Action	Rationale	Expected Outcome
1. Pain from fractured vertebrae or ribs as a result of osteoporosis	• Provide immediate pain relief. Administer as prescribed, noting the efficacy. • Handle and position the patient carefully.	Pain and discomfort will increase anxiety. Pain relief will reduce this. Fractured ribs will cause shallow breathing which increases the risk of chest infection. Gentle handling will reduce distress and prevent further fractures.	The patient should be pain-free and comfortable and anxiety reduced.
2. Infection as a result of immunosuppression	• Make 4-hourly recordings of temperature, pulse, respiration and blood pressure. Report any variation from the normal range immediately.	Death from overwhelming infection can occur. Signs of infection will be masked, so infection may be advanced before signs are seen.	Any infection will be identified early and correct treatment commenced.
3. Damage to skin as a result of skin thinning and oedema or poor wound healing	• If the patient is immobile, care of pressure areas will be required to prevent tissue damage. Legs will need to be elevated to relieve the oedema and any wounds will require aseptic technique when dressed.	Tissue will be rapidly broken down and slow to heal, so preventive measures are essential. Susceptibility to infection requires precautions to prevent introduction of infection.	Further tissue damage will be prevented and any present source of infection removed as rapidly as possible.
4. Hypertension	• Record blood pressure 4-hourly after 10 minutes lying flat and 1 minute standing. Report levels beyond the normal range or postural deficit.	Increasing blood pressure may lead to stroke or heart failure and if persistently high will need to be treated with drugs. Postural deficit will indicate a problem with sodium excretion or retention.	Blood pressure levels will remain within acceptable limits.
5. Diabetes mellitus as a result of abnormal carbohydrate metabolism	• Record pre- and postprandial blood sugar levels and possibly perform daily urinalysis.	Persistently high blood sugars will lead to the complications of diabetes mellitus and may need to be treated with insulin.	Blood sugar levels will remain within the normal range.
6. Psychosis and mental health problems	• Ascertain the patient's mental status early on. A psychiatric opinion should be obtained. Mood swings and bizarre behaviour should be reported. The patient may be so disturbed as to require 24-hour mental health nurse observation.	The patient's psychological state may change rapidly and close observation for this is necessary. Some patients can express suicidal ideation.	The patient will not be a danger to themselves or others and patient safety is maintained at all times.

Ongoing follow-up after discharge from hospital is essential. Initially, 3-monthly tests will be carried out, gradually reducing to an annual check. If adrenalectomy or pituitary surgery has been performed, precautions will need to be taken regarding hydrocortisone replacement; this must be explained in detail. An information leaflet can be useful as a reference for the patient when at home. This should tell the patient when to increase the therapy, e.g. during illness, and when to seek medical advice.

Hyposecretion of the Adrenals

Addison's Disease

Addison's disease is a rare condition in which there is total destruction of the adrenal cortex and failure of cortisol secretion. It may occur at any age, although the most common age of onset is between 30 and 50 years and it is more common in females. Autoimmune adrenalitis is the most common cause in the developed world and is responsible for 80%–90% of cases. Adrenal destruction by medication (e.g. mitotane), TB, HIV or cancer is a rare cause.

● *Pathophysiology*
Clinical Features
High levels of ACTH result in pigmentation of the skin and mucosae. The production of all three types of cortical hormones is reduced. Plasma levels of proteins and sodium are low and that of potassium is high, with serum urea being elevated due to volume depletion.

Common Presenting Symptoms
The onset of the disease is usually insidious, often starting with a feeling of general malaise and weakness. Nonspecific symptoms can make it difficult to distinguish from depression. Skin discolouration may have been noticed, especially in the palmar creases and on the inside of the lips and cheeks. Postural hypotension, salt cravings, hyperpigmentation, unexplained weight loss, headaches, nausea/vomiting, abdominal pain and persistent fatigue are all grounds for suspicion, and the primary care team is vital in the prompt detection of Addison's and subsequent treatment of emergencies.

Approximately 6% of patients every year will require hospital treatment, usually because of a severe episode of vomiting and diarrhoea. Some patients will first present as medical emergencies with an Addisonian crisis (see later). Untreated, this can be fatal.

● *Medical Management*
Investigations
Diagnosis is by clinical examination and blood tests to confirm high levels of ACTH and low levels of cortisol. In the short Synacthen test (SST), tetracosactide (synthetic ACTH) is given IV or IM, and blood samples for plasma cortisol taken at 0, 30 and 60 minutes after its administration will show a failure of the adrenal glands to respond to the stimulus of the parenteral ACTH. Once this has been demonstrated, the cause of the adrenal failure needs to be identified. The most common cause, i.e. autoimmune, can be diagnosed from an assay to detect the presence of 21-hydroxylase antibodies. If there are no antibodies present, other causes are investigated. Tests will include an MRI of the adrenal glands and screening for TB, HIV and cancer.

Treatment
Treatment is by long-term replacement doses of glucocorticoid and mineralocorticoid. This should lead to an improvement in the patient's well-being. Glucocorticoid replacement is with hydrocortisone (in two or three divided doses throughout the day; on waking, at lunchtime and before 1800 h) and levels of hydrocortisone should be checked regularly to ensure the dose is correct by performing a hydrocortisone day curve. Mineralocorticoid replacement with fludrocortisone (taken as a single morning dose) should be checked by regular blood pressure readings, which should show no postural hypotension, and by measurement of plasma renin.

Early administration by the patient or a family member of IM hydrocortisone will often stabilise an acute episode of vomiting and diarrhoea. Patients should be provided with emergency hydrocortisone packs and educated in their use (see later).

Addisonian Crisis
This is a life-threatening event. It occurs in such situations as injury, infections, anaesthesia and surgical procedures where, unlike in the healthy individual, the stress response does not occur. The absence of the cortisol surge to a major stressor results in severe shock. Addisonian crisis requires immediate intervention. Symptoms may include:
- sudden penetrating pain in the abdomen, legs or lower back
- fever
- severe vomiting and diarrhoea leading to dehydration
- hypotension
- hypoglycaemia
- altered consciousness.

Treatment aims to restore steroid, sodium and glucose levels to within normal range by IV administration of 100 mg hydrocortisone, and IV infusion of 0.9% sodium chloride given quickly with dextrose if glucose levels are low. Hydrocortisone is then given IV or IM 6-hourly until the patient is stable, following which steroid replacement can be given orally and mineralocorticoids introduced.

❖ Nursing Management and Health Promotion: Addison's Disease

Careful observation of temperature, pulse, and standing and lying blood pressure should be made. A raised temperature will indicate signs of infection which the patient may not be able to fight effectively. Any postural drop in blood pressure should be reported immediately.

The corticosteroid replacement therapy should be administered with the patient's full involvement so that they have a full knowledge of dosage and timing and techniques for self-administration before discharge. The patient should be given a 'steroid' card and advised to carry this and to wear a MedicAlert bracelet on their wrist or ankle at all times (Reflection 5.3). They should be provided with a thorough education of the 'sick day rules' that they must follow in case of an intercurrent illness or other stressful life events.

An emergency hydrocortisone pack should be kept at home in case of serious illness or trauma. Ideally, it should be self-administered by the patient, or the practice nurse, GP or community nurse called to administer it. It may be sensible also to teach a member of the family how to do this. Patients should also be encouraged to 'get red flagged' with their local ambulance service (where this service is available) to ensure that they are electronically flagged as being steroid dependent and at risk of an adrenal crisis. This ensures that in the event of such an emergency, the response vehicle comes equipped with IV hydrocortisone. If in doubt, it is better to administer hydrocortisone than to withhold it (Joint Royal Colleges Ambulance Liaison and Association of Ambulance Chief Executives 2022).

See Evolve website Critical thinking question 5.1

It is vital that the patient and family have a thorough understanding of their condition and the symptoms associated with complications. This will help to restore confidence and enable the patient to return to a full and active life.

Congenital Adrenal Hyperplasia (CAH)

This is a group of inherited disorders caused by a deficiency of one of the five enzymes involved in cortisol synthesis. It is one of the most common autosomal recessive disorders, with a prevalence in the USA and Europe of approximately 1 in 15,000–16,000 (Claahsen-van der Grinten et al. 2022).

Pathophysiology

To understand CAH, it is necessary to understand the biosynthesis of steroids (Fig. 5.7). The most common deficiency (accounting for 95% of cases; Claahsen-van der Grinten et al. 2022) occurs if the enzyme 21-hydroxylase (CYP21) is absent because of a gene defect; cortisol will not be produced in sufficient quantity. By means of the negative feedback system, ACTH production will be increased to stimulate cortisol production. This in turn leads to hypertrophy of the adrenal cortex and elevated levels of 17-hydroxyprogesterone, androstenedione and testosterone – the hormones occurring before the enzyme block. This will result ultimately in virilisation.

CAH disorders can be divided into three main groups:
- severe or classic – with or without salt wasting (SW)
- moderate/less severe – simple virilising (SV)
- mild – nonclassic (NC).

Common Presenting Signs and Symptoms

Classical CAH presents at birth or in early infancy with sexual ambiguity and SW due to mineralocorticoid deficiency. Life-threatening vomiting and dehydration, resulting in hyponatraemia and hyperkalaemia, and collapse can occur in the neonatal period. In the female infant, the high level of androgens present causes clitoral hypertrophy and fusion of the labial folds, resulting

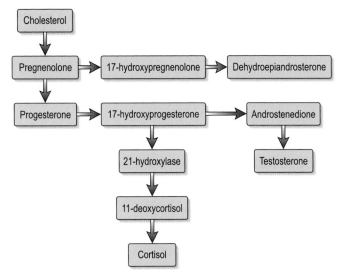

Figure 5.7 Simplified schematisation of cortisol synthesis.

in ambiguous genitalia. Internal genitalia may develop normally. The syndrome may not be recognised in the male infant, who will have normal genitalia. If a diagnosis is not made at birth, a genotypical female (XX) may be labelled male. Gender assignment should therefore wait until adequate anatomical and biochemical information is available.

Moderate or SV CAH is typically recognised by signs of virilisation in prepubertal children. Effects can include premature development of pubic hair (precocious puberty), advanced bone age, accelerated growth velocity and diminished final height in both sexes as a result of premature fusion of the bony epiphyses.

Mild or NC CAH, because prenatal virilisation does not occur, presents in late childhood or early adulthood (Claahsen-van der Grinten et al. 2022). Symptoms of androgen excess include hirsutism, severe acne, temporal baldness and infertility in adolescents and adult women. Menarche may be normal or delayed and secondary amenorrhoea is common. Polycystic ovarian syndrome (PCOS) may also be present. In young men, early beard growth, acne and a growth spurt may prompt the diagnosis. Men may also present with oligozoospermia or diminished fertility despite appearing asymptomatic and are only diagnosed when efforts to conceive fail.

Medical Management

Investigations

These include blood tests to confirm high levels of ACTH and 17-hydroxyprogesterone. In the infant a thorough physical examination together with an abdominal ultrasound should be performed to ascertain the presence of internal female reproductive organs.

Treatment

Replacement of the glucocorticoid is usually given in the form of prednisolone to suppress the ACTH production and thereby reduce the overstimulation of the adrenals. Other requirements frequently include mineralocorticoids, e.g. fludrocortisone. Reconstructive surgery for females is usually initiated between the ages of 3 and 6 months and, while specific to each child's individual anatomy, may involve clitoroplasty, labioscrotal reduction and vaginal exteriorisation.

❖ Nursing Management and Health Promotion: Congenital Adrenal Hyperplasia

Information should be given regarding corticosteroid replacement therapy. Nursing care should concentrate on the psychological support that will be required by both the parents and the child, and for individuals diagnosed during adulthood.

The psychosocial and psychosexual implications of CAH are considerable and formal counselling and psychotherapy should be made available. In female patients, hirsutism and acne can be especially distressing. Antiandrogens, e.g. cyproterone acetate, are now the treatment of choice. Other important issues for women which need discussion include menstruation, sexuality, fertility and the possible need for plastic surgery, as some effects of virilisation are not reversible by medication (Engberg et al. 2020). This is particularly important as the patient approaches adulthood, as sexual intercourse may be rendered difficult, painful or impossible. Prevention of subfertility should be implemented as a treatment goal from the start of puberty. Effective transition of care for the patient from the paediatric to adult endocrinologist is of utmost importance.

THE GONADS – DISORDERS OF SEXUAL DIFFERENTIATION

In normal development, gonadal and phenotypic sex follows an orderly process of development determined by chromosomal sex at the moment of conception.

During the early stages of fetal life, the gonad has the potential to develop female or male characteristics. In the presence of another X chromosome (i.e. 46, XX) or the absence of another chromosome (i.e. 45, XO), development will follow the female pattern. The presence of two X chromosomes is, however, necessary for normal ovarian function.

By the second month of fetal development, the genital organs are undifferentiated duct systems, termed the müllerian (paramesonephric) and wolffian (mesonephric) ducts. In the normal female, as development progresses, the wolffian system regresses and the müllerian system develops to form the uterine tubes, the uterus and the upper vagina. The external genitalia undergo little change.

In the male, the Müllerian system regresses and the wolffian system develops to form the testes, vas deferens, prostate and seminiferous tubules. The genital tubercle present in both systems forms the clitoris in the female and the penis in the male.

There is evidence to suggest that the normal development of a male fetus is hormone-dependent. It appears that testosterone inhibits the regression of the wolffian duct and stimulates its development into the male sexual structures. In contrast to this, the ovary is unaffected by hormones in utero.

Abnormalities of sexual differentiation may present with abnormal genitalia at birth, growth disturbance in childhood or abnormal secondary sexual development.

Abnormalities of Gonadal Development

True hermaphroditism, i.e. the presence of both male and female sexual characteristics in the same individual, is extremely rare. It occurs when both the Müllerian and Wolffian systems continue to develop. Diagnosis requires a high index of suspicion for subtle abnormalities of the genitalia. Ovotestes may exist or an ovary on one side and a testis on the other.

Chromosomal Abnormalities

There are several chromosomal abnormalities that affect sexual differentiation. This section outlines four such disorders.

Klinefelter's Syndrome. A condition in which phenotypical males have one or more extra X chromosomes and one Y chromosome. Eighty per cent of patients display the classic karyotype (47, XXY) but additional X or Y chromosomes may be present. The greater the number of additional chromosomes present, the greater the severity of the condition. It is the most prevalent sex chromosome disorder in men with an incidence of 1 in 600 male newborns (Vukina and Sangster 2020). Symptoms and presentation depend on when the diagnosis is made as this can be antenatal, during childhood or adolescence, or late into adulthood.

Adult patients present with low testosterone and elevated LH and FSH, often during investigations for infertility or following an unexpected fracture. Men with Klinefelter's syndrome are typically tall with long legs compared to upper body length, due to delayed epiphyseal closure of their long bones, exhibit excessive fat, especially around the trunk, and are infertile. They may exhibit a varying degree of interstitial (Leydig) cell failure resulting in testosterone deficiency (Ridder et al. 2023). Almost 40% of patients show some degree of intellectual disability. Adolescence can be a particularly stressful time as boys have to come to terms with hormone replacement therapy, possible breast development and infertility. Counselling should be offered and information provided about support groups.

Turner's Syndrome. A condition in which the individual is phenotypically female but has the genotype XO, i.e. complete or partial absence of one X chromosome. It is the most commonly occurring chromosomal abnormality in females, with an incidence of approximately 50 in 100,000 (Fuchs et al. 2019). Affected individuals have short stature with a 'web neck' and low-set ears and may have widely spaced nipples and peripheral oedema. The ovaries are atrophic and serum LH and FSH levels are elevated. These individuals are prone to a variety of serious cardiac problems including coarctation of the aorta and aortic dissection. Women with Turner's syndrome are thought to have a reduced life expectancy, mainly due to these serious cardiac problems, but they may also have multiple comorbidities, which can include hypothyroidism, deafness, osteoporosis, oestrogen deficiency and infertility (Gravholt et al. 2023).

Kallman's Syndrome. In this condition, there is a normal karyotype but a genetic defect in the pathway leading to gonadotrophin secretion; thus, there is a deficiency of gonadotrophins and therefore sex steroid secretion is reduced. This condition is sometimes termed congenital hypogonadotrophic hypogonadism. Typically, the individual has anosmia (absence of the sense of smell). Normal gonadal function can be restored with replacement of LH and FSH, meaning that fertility is possible. Otherwise, treatment is either oestrogen or testosterone replacement.

Testicular Feminisation. This is a syndrome of androgen resistance or complete androgen insensitivity (CAI syndrome) caused by mutations in the androgen receptor gene. While the karyotype is male (46, XY), the phenotype is female. Testes are present, but because of tissue resistance to circulating androgens but not oestrogen at puberty, breast tissue develops although pubic hair does not. Regression of the müllerian system occurs due to tissue insensitivity but the wolffian system does not develop and a blind-ended vagina results. The gonads may become malignant and are usually removed at the onset of adult life.

❖ Nursing Management and Health Promotion: Disorders of Sexual Differentiation

Whilst disorders of the gonads are rarely life-threatening or require admission to hospital, the psychological and social implications for the individual and their family cannot be overemphasised.

The role of the nurse in the investigation and treatment of these conditions is to offer psychological support to the individual, and, if they agree, their family, in an environment that is both relaxed and supportive.

Counselling on an informal and formal basis is essential during investigations, when complete privacy must be ensured. Feelings of inadequacy regarding sexuality and low self-esteem are common. An approach that demonstrates empathy with the individual helps to create a positive image during the initial examinations and investigations and during subsequent treatment.

POLYCYSTIC OVARIAN SYNDROME (PCOS)

PCOS is the most common endocrine condition in women of reproductive age and is associated with a wide range of signs and symptoms and an increased risk of cardiovascular disease and type 2 diabetes. Signs and symptoms include excessive hair growth (hirsutism), male pattern balding, acne, obesity, menstrual irregularities and reduced fertility. Women with this condition may be more anxious about it as a cosmetic issue rather than a gynaecological one depending on whether or not they have/want to have a family. In the UK and Europe, a diagnosis of PCOS is usually made based on the Rotterdam diagnostic criteria (Vural et al. 2023). This requires women to have any two of the following three symptoms: oligomenorrhea and/or anovulation, hirsutism and/or acne and polycystic ovaries diagnosed by an ultrasound scan. Other endocrine disorders should have been excluded. Despite, or because of, these diagnostic criteria, it is thought that many women with PCOS remain undiagnosed.

Once diagnosed, treatment should be individualised based on the woman's presenting symptoms and agreed treatment goals. Lifestyle modification is considered first-line treatment for patients who are overweight as this can reduce insulin resistance and improve ovulation. Medication, e.g. metformin, can be prescribed for insulin resistance and clomiphene to induce ovulation. If a patient does not want to become pregnant, oral contraceptives are prescribed to treat menstrual irregularities and can help to treat acne and/or hirsutism. Hirsutism may also be treated using spironolactone, an antiandrogenic, or flutamide, a nonsteroidal antiandrogen. Other treatments include eflornithine (Vaniqa cream), electrolysis or laser treatment, although not all of these are available on the National Health Service (NHS).

Summary: Key Nursing Issues

- The endocrine system is one of the major control systems of the body, the other being the nervous system.
- As endocrine diseases are not common, patients may have had a long 'journey' before receiving a diagnosis and may have seen many different health professionals before they come to you.
- Altered body image is an important feature of endocrine disease and some patients may have considerable difficulty in coming to terms with their changed appearance. Providing opportunities to talk about such matters is an important part of the nurse's role.
- A patient's QoL can be severely affected by endocrine disease. Many disease-specific questionnaires are available to assess the impact of disease on patients and to monitor response to treatment. Together with a careful assessment of patients, these can provide valuable information for the nurse when planning care.
- Many patients benefit from joining a local support group specific to their condition and the contact with others with similar histories.
- The majority of patients, once diagnosed, will require long-term follow-up. Establishing an ongoing nurse–patient relationship built on trust is therefore crucial.

- Nurses have an important role in ensuring that patients are aware of the importance of correctly taking their hormone replacement therapy and other prescribed medications. Ensuring patient concordance with treatment is a key nursing role to ensure optimal benefit to the patient and reduce the possibility of side-effects or emergencies. This is especially true for patients on hydrocortisone replacement who must be made aware of the 'sick day' rules and be trained in the emergency self-administration of IM hydrocortisone. All patients should also be encouraged to become members of MedicAlert.
- Nursing initiatives within endocrinology include nurse-led clinics, telephone help-lines and the auditing of services to ensure best practice.
- All nurses working in endocrinology should ensure they keep up-to-date with advances in their field by regularly attending local, national or international conferences. They should strive to disseminate their local knowledge and expertise by presenting at these meetings and by publishing their research, audit or patient cases.
- Good links and effective communication between primary and secondary care teams are important to ensure that patients feel well supported by both their practice nurse/GP and their specialist endocrine team, thus ensuring that care is streamlined.

Reflection and Learning – What Next?

- **Test** your knowledge by visiting the Evolve website ⊕ and answering the multiple-choice questions and critical thinking questions.
- **Consolidate** your learning by looking at some of the further reading suggestions, references and specialist websites.
- **Revisit** some of the additional material on the Evolve website.

- **Consider** what you have learnt and how this will help your professional development.
- **Reflect** on how you can apply this knowledge to the care of your patients.
- **Discuss** your learning with your assessor/supervisor, lecturer and colleagues.

References

Aguiar-Oliveira MH, Bartke A. Growth hormone deficiency: health and longevity. *Endocr Rev.* 2019;40(2):575–601.

Araque KA, Gubbi S, Klubo-Gwiezdzinska J. Updates on the management of thyroid cancer. *Horm Metab Res.* 2020;52(08):562–577.

Boguszewski CL, de Castro Musolino NR, Kasuki L. Management of pituitary incidentaloma. *Best Pract Res Clin Endocrinol Metab.* 2019;33(2):101268.

Cancer Research UK. Thyroid cancer incidence statistics; 2016–2018. 2023. https://www.cancerresearchuk.org/health-professional/cancer-statistics/statistics-by-cancer-type/thyroid-cancer/incidence.

Chanson P, Maiter D. Prolactinoma. In: Melmed S, ed. *The Pituitary*. 5th ed. Academic Press; 2022:495–543.

Claahsen-van der Grinten HL, Speiser PW, Ahmed SF, et al. Congenital adrenal hyperplasia—current insights in pathophysiology, diagnostics, and management. *Endocr Rev.* 2022;43(1):91–159.

Coopmans EC, Andela CD, Claessen KM, Biermasz NR. Evaluating the impact of acromegaly on quality of life. *Endocrinol Metab Clin.* 2022;51(4):709–725.

Engberg H, Möller A, Hagenfeldt K, Nordenskjöld A, Frisén L. Identity, sexuality, and parenthood in women with congenital adrenal hyperplasia. *J Pediatr Adolesc Gynecol.* 2020;33(5):470–476.

Fleseriu M, Biller BM, Freda PU, et al. A pituitary society update to acromegaly management guidelines. *Pituitary.* 2021;24:1–3.

Fuchs MM, Attenhofer Jost C, Babovic-Vuksanovic D, Connolly HM, Egbe A, Longbe A. Longegaly management guidelines. Pituiome: a 68-year follow-up. *J Am Heart Assoc.* 2019;8(11):e011501.

Gleeson H, Reddy N, Levy M. Endocrinology. In: Feather A, Randall D, Waterhouse M, eds. *Kumar and Clark's Clinical Medicine;* Edinburgh: Elsevier; 2020:583–650.

Gravholt CH, Viuff M, Just J, et al. The changing face of Turner syndrome. *Endocr Rev.* 2023;44(1):33–69.

Hayhurst C, Taylor PN, Lansdown AJ, Palaniappan N, Rees DA, Davies JS. Current perspectives on recurrent pituitary adenoma: the role and timing of surgery vs adjuvant treatment. *Clin Endocrinol (Oxf).* 2020;92(2):89–97.

Haymana C, Sonmez A. Testosterone replacement therapy. In: Sarikaya S, Russo G, Ralph D, eds. *Andrology and Sexual Medicine: 419-431.* Springer International Publishing; 2022.

Joint Royal Colleges Ambulance Liaison Committee (JRCALC) and Association of Ambulance Chief Executives. *JRCALC Clinical Guidelines.* Class Publishing; 2022.

Macmillan Cancer Support. Thyroid cancer. 2023. https://www.macmillan.org.uk/information-and-support/thyroid-cancer.

Mathieu D, Kotecha R, Sahgal A, et al. Stereotactic radiosurgery for secretory pituitary adenomas: systematic review and International Stereotactic Radiosurgery Society practice recommendations. *J Neurosurg.* 2021;136(3):801–812.

Melmed S, Kaiser UB, Lopes MB, et al. Clinical biology of the pituitary adenoma. *Endocr Rev.* 2022;43(6):1003–1037.

NICE (National Institute for Health and Clinical Excellence). *Growth hormone deficiency (adults) – human growth hormone.* Technology Appraisal [TA64]; 2003. https://www.nice.org.uk/guidance/ta64/resources/human-growth-hormone-somatropin-in-adults-with-growth-hormone-deficiency-pdf-2294698052293.

Penman I, Ralston SH, Strachan M, Hobson R. *Davidson's Principles and Practice of Medicine.* 24th ed. Edinburgh: Elsevier; 2022.

Ridder LO, Berglund A, Stochholm K, Chang S, Gravholt CH. Morbidity, mortality, and socioeconomics in Klinefelter syndrome and 47, XYY syndrome: a comparative review. *Endocr Connect.* 2023;12(5):e230024.

Uslar V, Becker C, Weyhe D, Tabriz N. Thyroid disease-specific quality of life questionnaires – a systematic review. *Endoc Diabet Metab.* 2022;5(5):e357.

Vukina J, Sangster P. Klinefelter's syndrome. *Urology News.* 2020;13:18.

Vural F, Vural B, Kardaş E. Ertürk Coşkun AD, Yildirim İ. The diagnostic performance of antimullerian hormone for polycystic ovarian syndrome and polycystic ovarian morphology. *Arch Gynecol Obstet.* 2023;307(4):1083–1090.

Zimmermann MB, Andersson M. Global endocrinology: global perspectives in endocrinology: coverage of iodized salt programs and iodine status in 2020. *Eur J Endocrinol.* 2021;185(1):R13–R21.

Further Reading

Azziz R. Diagnostic criteria for polycystic ovary syndrome: a reappraisal. *Fertil Steril.* 2005;83(5):1343–1346.

Baines A. Adrenal insufficiency: improving paramedic practice. *J Paramedic Pract.* 2015;7(4):192–200.

Berger MM, Shenkin A, Schweinlin A, et al. ESPEN micronutrient guideline. *Clin Nutr.* 2022;41(6):1357–1424.

Braverman LE, Utiger RD, eds. *Werner and Ingbar's the Thyroid: A Fundamental and Clinical Text.* 9th ed. Philadelphia: Lippincott Williams and Wilkins; 2004.

Carson MN. Assessment and management of patients with hypothyroidism. *Nurs Stand.* 2009;23(18):48–56.

Casanueva FF, Molitch ME, Schlechte JA, et al. Guidelines of the Pituitary Society for the diagnosis and management of prolactinomas. *Clin Endocrinol (Oxf).* 2006;65:265–273.

Grove E. Thyroid problems. *InnovAiT.* 2018;11(4):206–211.

Melmed S. Pathogenesis and diagnosis of growth hormone deficiency in adults. *N Engl J Med.* 2019;380(26):2551–2562.

Mills J, Dalleywater W. Thyroid cancer. *InnovAiT..* 2018;11(4):212–217.

Perros P, Kendall-Taylor P. Medical treatment for thyroid-associated ophthalmopathy. *Thyroid.* 2002;12:241–244.

Rees A, Levy M, Landsdown A. *Clinical Endocrinology and Diabetes at a Glance.* Oxford: Wiley Blackwell; 2017.

Smith S, Eatough V, Smith J, et al. 'I know I'm not invincible': an interpretive phenomenological analysis of thyroid cancer in young people. *Br J Health Psychol.* 2018;23:352–370.

Waugh A, Grant A. *Ross and Wilson: Anatomy and Physiology in Health and Illness.* 14th ed. Edinburgh: Elsevier; 2022.

Useful Websites

Addison's Disease Self Help Group (ADSHG), www.addisons.org.uk,.

Association for Multiple Endocrine Neoplasia Disorders (AMEND), www.amend.org.uk

British Thyroid Foundation (BTF), www.btf-thyroid.org

Climb: Congenital Adrenal Hyperplasia (CAH) Support Group, www.livingwithcah.com

Klinefelter's Syndrome Association UK(eXtra), www.ksa-uk.net

The Pituitary Foundation, www.pituitary.org.uk

Thyroid Eye Disease Charitable Trust (TEDct), http://tedct.org.uk

Verity (sharing the truth about PCOS), www.verity-pcos.org.uk

6

Nursing Patients With Diabetes Mellitus

CARL CLARE

CHAPTER OUTLINE

Introduction

Diabetes mellitus is defined as a metabolic disorder of multiple aetiology. It is characterised by chronic hyperglycaemia (increased blood glucose) with disturbances of carbohydrate (CHO), protein and fat metabolism which results from defects in insulin secretion, insulin action or both (World Health Organisation [WHO] 2016). Diabetes UK (2019) estimates that there are around 3.9 million people diagnosed with the condition in the UK and there are more than half a million individuals who are unaware that they have diabetes. Diabetes is associated with several long-term complications that include sight impairment, renal failure, neuropathy and cardiovascular diseases. The care of people with diabetes represents a large proportion of health resources (Reflection 6.1).

The terms insulin-dependent and non-insulin-dependent diabetes have been replaced by the WHO classification (WHO 2016), which recognises the main types of diabetes as follows:

- type 1 diabetes (formerly insulin-dependent diabetes or juvenile diabetes)
- type 2 diabetes (formerly noninsulin-dependent diabetes)
- gestational diabetes
- impaired glucose regulation (IGR) (or impaired glucose tolerance (IGT))
- other specific types.

The chapter briefly outlines the anatomy and physiology of the pancreas and the hormonal regulation of blood glucose levels. The types, pathophysiology, clinical presentation, medical management and the acute metabolic and chronic complications of diabetes are covered. Key issues of nursing management and health promotion of diabetes and its complications are discussed in some depth.

Anatomy and Physiology

The Pancreas

The pancreas has both endocrine and exocrine functions. The endocrine function of the pancreas is concerned with the secretion of several hormones. The hormone-secreting islets of Langerhans are found scattered throughout the pancreas. There are four types of cell contained within the islets. Alpha (α) cells secrete glucagon and beta (β) cells secrete insulin; each has a key role in regulating blood glucose. Other islet cells include those that secrete pancreatic polypeptides and delta (δ) cells that secrete somatostatin (also known as growth hormone release-inhibiting hormone (GHRIH)) which contributes to the regulation of a variety of hormones throughout the body, including insulin and glucagon.

Exocrine tissue is responsible for the secretion of digestive enzymes that leave the pancreas in ducts to enter the duodenum (see Chapter 4 Nursing Patients with Gastrointestinal, Liver and Biliary Disorders).

Blood Glucose Regulation

Within a 24-hour period, the healthy human will alternate between the fed state and the fasting state several times. Two hours following a meal, blood glucose will tend to rise as absorption of nutrients takes place, which is the postprandial or fed state. Once glucose has been taken up into the cells, blood glucose levels will tend to fall and will not rise again until the next meal is taken, which is the preprandial or fasting state. In health, these fluctuations are slight, as insulin is secreted at a low (basal) level throughout the whole day, only rising to an increased stimulated level at mealtimes. Insulin and glucagon are principally (but not exclusively) responsible for blood glucose regulation.

Insulin

Insulin, an anabolic hormone, is secreted in response to a rising blood glucose level. Insulin has effects on the metabolism of CHO, fat and protein. Its physiological effects in different tissues include the following.

Carbohydrate

- increased glucose uptake by the cells
- increased glycolysis (breakdown of glucose)
- increased glycogenesis (conversion of glucose to glycogen for storage in the liver and skeletal muscle)
- decreased glycogenolysis (breakdown of glycogen back into glucose)
- decreased gluconeogenesis (formation of glucose from non-CHO sources, e.g. amino acids, lactate, glycerol).

Fat

- increased lipogenesis (formation of triglycerides from glucose and amino acids before storage in adipose tissue)
- decreased lipolysis (breakdown of stored fat for energy)
- increased synthesis of low-density lipoproteins (LDLs) and cholesterol.
- protein
- increased protein synthesis
- decreased protein breakdown.

All of these effects have the effect of preventing an abnormal rise in blood glucose during the postprandial period. Insulin secretion is highest in the fed state and lowest in the fasting state (Fig. 6.1).

Glucagon

Glucagon, a catabolic hormone, is secreted in response to a falling blood glucose level and its physiological effects include:

- increased glycogenolysis and the release of glucose from the liver
- increased fat and protein breakdown in order to provide an alternative source of glucose via lipolysis and gluconeogenesis
- influence on the production of ketone bodies (ketogenesis); in total or near-total insulin lack, these weak acids are produced as a result of the chemical processes involved in fat breakdown.

The actions of glucagon and the other counter-regulatory hormones are all geared towards preventing an abnormal fall in blood glucose (hypoglycaemia). Glucagon secretion is highest in the fasting state and lowest in the fed state (see Fig. 6.1).

Other Influences on Blood Glucose Regulation

Anterior Pituitary Gland. The pituitary hormones influencing glucose regulation include:

- Growth hormone (somatotrophin) – this hormone tends to raise blood glucose. It is diabetogenic in action and anti-insulin in effect. It influences blood glucose in two main ways – by increasing glycogenolysis and by inhibiting muscle glycogen storage.
- Adrenocorticotrophic hormone (ACTH) – this hormone stimulates the adrenal cortex to release the glucocorticoid hormone

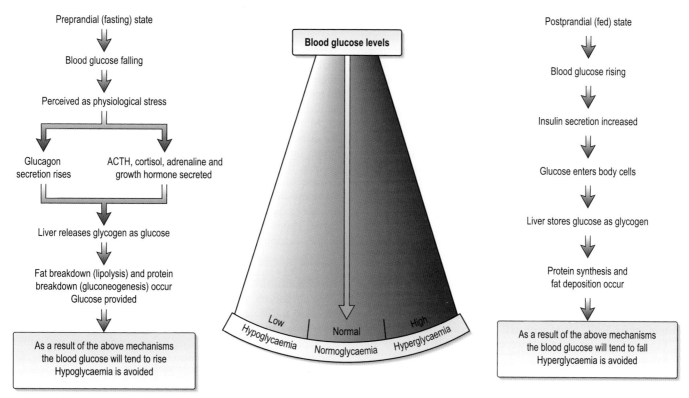

Figure 6.1 The regulation of blood glucose in health.

cortisol (see later). A negative feedback mechanism operates in response to the circulating levels of cortisol in the blood.

Adrenal Cortex. Secretes a group of glucocorticoid hormones, the most significant of which is cortisol. Cortisol is a catabolic hormone. Secretion is increased during prolonged periods of physical or psychological stress, when its effect is to raise the blood glucose level in order to meet the additional metabolic demands of the stressed state. Cortisol increases glycogenolysis, lipolysis and the breakdown of protein to provide amino acids for gluconeogenesis, providing an alternative source of glucose to meet cell energy needs.

Adrenal Medulla. Secretes the catecholamines adrenaline (epinephrine) and noradrenaline (norepinephrine). These 'fight or flight' hormones are catabolic in their action. In response to stress, they place the body and brain in a state of high alert, causing blood glucose to rise as glycogen stores are released and fat/protein breakdown occurs. This increases the amount of available glucose and helps to prepare the body to meet increased energy demands.

Liver and Skeletal Muscle. About 60% of absorbed nutrients are stored as reserves in order to meet energy demands during fasting. Under the influence of insulin, the liver and, to a lesser extent, skeletal muscle can store glucose in the form of glycogen. The liver is also involved in protein and fat synthesis for subsequent storage.

During fasting or in response to stress, glucagon (and other stress hormones) will increase glycogenolysis in the liver and skeletal muscle to release glucose (see Fig. 6.1).

TYPE 1 DIABETES

The pathogenesis of type 1 diabetes is complex and has been the subject of extensive research. It is currently thought that a genetic predisposition to the disease, possibly combined with environmental triggers, activates an autoimmune attack on the pancreatic islet β cells. Insulin secretion is virtually absent.

● *Pathophysiology*

Islet cell destruction probably begins very early in life and is known to start several years before onset of diabetes (Holt and Kumar 2015). Individuals may present with initial symptoms when the demand for insulin has been increased, e.g. in response to a physical or psychological stress such as illness, trauma, surgery or pregnancy. Additional metabolic demands posed by the stressed state can no longer be met by the failing pancreas and symptoms of diabetes become evident for the first time.

Once insulin therapy is commenced, the remaining β-cell mass can temporarily provide sufficient insulin to meet the body's demands. In this case the exogenous insulin can be reduced, and, on occasion, stopped. This remission or 'honeymoon period' is short lived. As the β-cell mass reduces further, symptoms of hyperglycaemia will reappear, necessitating lifelong treatment with insulin.

Clinical Presentation

In general terms, the lack of insulin means that body cells are unable to use glucose for metabolism. The signs, symptoms and clinical features of type 1 diabetes can best be explained in terms of the specific effects of insulin lack, as follows:

- Hyperglycaemia – glucose is unable to enter cells and accumulates in the blood, causing an abnormally high blood glucose level.

- Glycosuria (glucose in the urine) – increased amounts of glucose are filtered in the glomeruli. The capacity of the kidneys to reabsorb glucose is exceeded and glucose appears in the urine.
- Polyuria (excretion of excessive volumes of urine) – this occurs because glucose is highly osmotic, and as glucose is lost in the urine, large volumes of water are lost with it.
- Polydipsia (excessive thirst) – as fluid loss continues, signs and symptoms of fluid imbalance occur (see Chapter 21) and copious drinking is noted in response to severe thirst.
- Cell glucose requirements are unmet. The counterregulatory response is increased secretion of glucagon and other stress hormones in an attempt to increase glucose availability. Under the influence of these hormones there is:
  - glycogenolysis
  - gluconeogenesis.
- Increasing blood glucose – the efforts to meet the cellular demands for glucose have the combined effect of raising the blood glucose even higher.
- Polyphagia (increased appetite) – caused by cell requirements for glucose being unmet (see earlier).
- Weight loss – occurs due to the depletion of body fat and protein stores. This, along with cell deprivation of glucose and fluid and electrolyte imbalance, causes muscle weakness and exhaustion.
- Ketonaemia (ketone bodies in the blood) and ketonuria (ketone bodies in the urine) – without insulin, there is fat breakdown which results in the formation of ketone bodies – β-hydroxybutyric acid, acetoacetic acid and acetone (a process known as ketogenesis). The ketone bodies accumulate in the blood and are excreted in the urine.
- Characteristic sweet 'pear drop' odour on the breath – caused by the excretion of acetone by the lungs.
- Metabolic acidosis (see Chapter 21, Maintaining Fluid, Electrolyte and Acid–Base Balance) – ketone bodies are weak acids and release hydrogen ions [H^+] causing disruption to blood pH (normally maintained within a narrow range). The processes leading to acidosis cause the accumulation of excess acid in the blood (acidaemia), resulting in an abnormally low blood pH.
- Kussmaul's respiration (hyperventilation: rapid deep respiration) – acidaemia leads to increased respiratory buffering in an attempt to correct acidaemia by removing more acidic carbon dioxide through increased rate and depth of respiration.
- Diabetic ketoacidosis (DKA) – a life-threatening situation, which without urgent treatment will progress to coma and ultimately to death.
- Uncontrolled lipolysis in the absence of insulin, gluconeogenesis, ketogenesis and glycogenolysis combine to raise the blood glucose level still further, increase osmotic diuresis, and exacerbate fluid imbalance and metabolic acidosis. As a result of these profound biochemical disturbances, the patient may experience nausea and vomiting and unexplained colicky abdominal pain.

Onset and Progress of Type 1 Diabetes

Although the onset of type 1 diabetes may appear abrupt, the patient may have had signs, such as glycosuria, in the absence of overt symptoms over many months. Once symptoms appear, the condition will usually have a rapid progression. However, there will be variations in severity, some patients being much more acutely ill than others at the time of diagnosis.

Although most patients are referred to hospital, admission is not automatic. The majority of newly diagnosed patients with type 1 diabetes will be managed as outpatients. All adults with diabetes will receive high-quality care and support throughout their lifetime, to optimise the control of their blood glucose, blood pressure and other risk factors for developing complications of diabetes (Department of Health [DH] 2001, 2008).

More recently, care of people with type 1 diabetes has focused on diabetes centres and patients require admission to hospital less often, unless particularly unwell. The central objective of care is to help the patient acquire the knowledge and skills needed to resume an independent lifestyle. The patient will usually be asked to attend the diabetes outpatient clinic at specified intervals or, if unable to do so, may be visited at home by the diabetes specialist nurse. This is essential for the ongoing care, treatment supervision and evaluation of progress of these patients.

TYPE 2 DIABETES

Type 2 diabetes seems likely to have a multifactorial aetiology (Forouhi and Wareham, 2022). Although these factors are not fully understood, they differ from those thought to cause type 1 diabetes.

Type 2 diabetes has a strong genetic component, in families and between racial groups. Glucose metabolism becomes less efficient from the third or fourth decade of life onwards and this deterioration accelerates in people over 60 years of age. Whilst this alteration in glucose tolerance may not in itself be pathological, when compounded by other factors, it can contribute to the onset of symptoms of diabetes.

Tissue sensitivity to insulin may decline in type 2 diabetes. The result is that hyperglycaemia can occur even when the circulating levels of insulin are normal or raised. Several reasons have been suggested for the development of insulin resistance: these include resistance in peripheral tissues in obesity, the effects of ageing and the presence of anti-insulin antibodies in the blood.

Whatever the cause, the result is inefficient use of available insulin.

Specific Factors in the Development of Type 2 Diabetes

β-Cell Deficiency. There is a markedly reduced first phase insulin secretion (immediate insulin release lasting approximately 10 minutes) in response to glucose and, in established diabetes, an attenuated second phase (longer phase that reaches its peak release at around 2–3 hours). Insulin pulsatility is also abnormal, thereby reducing tissue insulin sensitivity (Bilous et al. 2021).

Obesity. Obesity is known to induce insulin resistance in body cells. However, only a minority of obese people develop type 2 diabetes and only around 60% of people with the disorder are obese. Glucose tolerance decreases as weight increases and can be reversed as weight loss occurs. Fat distribution appears to be significant in that there is a relationship between central obesity and diabetes. Previous research by authors such as Wei et al. (1997) indicated that waist circumference is the best central obesity-related predictor of type 2 diabetes, suggesting that distribution of body fat, especially abdominal localisation, is a more important determinant than total body fat. However, as more studies are undertaken the picture has become less clear, and amongst other factors, the total visceral fat mass and sex may also be important (Delaney and Santosa, 2022). Current recommendations are tending towards the prevention of type 2 diabetes by adopting a healthy diet and increasing physical activity (Ahmad et al. 2022).

Racial and Environmental Factors. There are wide geographical variations in the incidence of type 2 diabetes. The International Diabetes Federation (IDF) estimates that in Europe in 2021, 7% of adults aged 20–79 had diabetes (IDF 2022). A study by Massó-González et al. (2009) found that in the UK, the incidence of type 2 diabetes increased during the period 1996 to 2005, while the incidence of type 1 diabetes remained comparatively steady during the same period. They also reported that more patients diagnosed with type 2 diabetes between 1996 and 2005 were obese (an increase from 46% to 56%). In certain societies, incidences of up to 40% have been reported, e.g. among the Pima Indians of North America and the Nauru Islanders of the Pacific, where obesity is also very common. These remarkably high prevalences are probably due to the exposure of genetically isolated, diabetes-predisposed populations to influences such as a 'Western' diet and reduced physical activity. The prevalence for diabetes for all age groups worldwide is predicted to rise to 10.2% in 2030 (Saeedi et al. 2019).

Ethnicity and Type 2 Diabetes in the UK

Type 2 diabetes is noted to be 3 to 5 times higher in non-White European communities as compared to the White European population (Goff 2019) with the onset of diabetes being 10–12 years earlier in both the South Asian and Afro-Caribbean population as compared to the white European population. The proposed factors that drive this increase in risk are still unproven, but several mechanisms are reckoned to be involved:

- There is a known difference in the incidence of diabetes between people of South Asian descent who live in urban areas as opposed to rural areas. This difference is even greater (up to 12 times greater incidence) in the urban-based European Afro-Caribbean population versus the indigenous Black African population. This suggests a role of urban living in the development of diabetes in the non-White European population with socioeconomic deprivation being suggested as a potential causative factor.
- Differences in fat deposition patterns in both those of Afro-Caribbean descent (Reed et al. 2022) and South Asian descent (Kapoor et al. 2019).
- Cultural and economic barriers to accessing healthcare, including a lack of cultural sensitivity amongst healthcare professionals (Goff 2019).

Thus given the increased population risk of type 2 diabetes (and its onset at an earlier age), there is a need for preventive healthcare, health education and risk monitoring that recognises cultural differences and shows cultural sensitivity in both the form of delivery and the point of delivery (for instance faith/church-based programmes).

Pathophysiology

Traditionally, type 2 diabetes was known to present in those over the age of 40 and most commonly in people over 60 however, recent trends have shown an increase in the onset of type 2 diabetes in children and adolescents, with the first child being diagnosed with type 2 diabetes in 2000 (Whicher et al. 2020). The signs, symptoms and clinical features of type 2 diabetes, although still marked, are less severe than those of type 1 diabetes and are due to the more gradual onset and the effects of hyperglycaemia arising from a relative deficiency of insulin. There is still some insulin being secreted; as a result, ketogenesis is inhibited and, as the hyperglycaemia is less severe, dehydration is also much less common.

Clinical Presentation

The effects of a relative lack of insulin include:

- Hyperglycaemia-related symptoms – nocturia, polyuria and polydipsia may develop gradually. Obese patients may initially be gratified to note that weight loss is occurring.
- Genital or oral fungal infections – candidal infections are common and result in the distressing symptoms of pruritus vulvae in the female and balanitis in the male. The glucose-rich urine around the genitalia appears to provide the microorganism with favourable conditions in which to multiply.
- Staphylococcal skin infections – these commonly result in boils and abscesses, and may provide the initial stimulus for the patient to visit their GP.
- Nonspecific symptoms – such as tiredness and lethargy – are also frequently reported. The cause is uncertain, but altered fluid and electrolyte balance may be responsible. Visual disturbance may occasionally be reported, as hyperglycaemia may cause lens opacity and accommodation may be affected by alterations of the lens fluid.

Onset and Progress of the Disease

At the time the patient first seeks medical attention, evidence of vascular and neurological complications such as proteinuria, sexual dysfunction, retinopathy and peripheral neuropathy may already have developed. Such patients have probably had asymptomatic diabetes with persistent hyperglycaemia for several years prior to diagnosis. A diagnosis will usually be made on the evidence of glycosuria and a fasting or random venous plasma blood glucose concentration of ≥ 7.0 mmol/L and ≥ 11.1 mmol/L, respectively.

Ketonuria is not a feature of type 2 diabetes, as ketogenesis is inhibited by the presence of even small amounts of insulin.

Asymptomatic glycosuria may be discovered as an incidental finding, e.g. during a routine medical examination. Such a finding would normally prompt capillary and then venous blood glucose analysis. In the absence of symptoms, these results should be confirmed by repeat testing on a different day.

The WHO (2006) has set glucose values for diagnosing diabetes (Table 6.1), and these values have remained the standard to the present day.

Impaired Glucose Tolerance and Impaired Fasting Glycaemia

Impaired glucose tolerance (IGT) and impaired fasting (hyper)glycaemia (IFG) are recognised as stages in the natural history of diabetes rather than as a class of diabetes (WHO 2006). It is not clear why some people may have blood glucose results at or just above the upper limit of normal and therefore inconclusive results in the absence of symptoms may not necessarily be judged abnormal. It is known that some people with IGT or IFG will go on to develop diabetes mellitus and that they may have a greater risk of developing atherosclerosis.

Onset and Progress of the Disease

Although it is clearly desirable that people should be spared the negative consequences of being inappropriately labelled as 'having diabetes', they should nonetheless have access to regular medical screening. Health promotion should be carried out, usually by the practice nurse or the GP, or the patient may also be asked to attend a diabetes clinic for an annual review.

TABLE 6.1	Diagnostic Glucose Concentrations		
Diagnosis	Venous Whole Blood (mmol/L)	Capillary Whole Blood (mmol/L)	Venous Plasma Blood (mmol/L)
Diabetes mellitus			
Fasting	≥6.1	≥6.1	≥7.0
2-hour postprandial	≥10.0	≥11.1	≥11.1
Impaired glucose tolerance (IGT)			
Fasting	<6.1	<6.1	<7.0
2-hour postprandial	≥6.7	≥7.8	<11.1
Impaired fasting glycaemia (IFG)			
Fasting	≥5.6 and <6.1	≥5.6 and <6.1	≥6.1 and <7.0
2-hour postprandial	<6.7	<7.8	<7.8

In the absence of symptoms, abnormality in both 2-hour postprandial and fasting blood glucose is required to establish the diagnosis of diabetes mellitus. The 2-hour postprandial test should be performed following the oral glucose tolerance test using 75 g glucose load (WHO 2006).

IGT has implications for women who are planning to conceive. Current evidence suggests that it is important to correct hyperglycaemia and ensure tight control of blood glucose prior to conception to reduce the risk of fetal abnormality (Gabbay-Benziv et al. 2015). Preconception advice should be made available and the woman's blood glucose brought within normal limits before conception and closely monitored throughout pregnancy. This care may be provided at a combined diabetes obstetric clinic.

Diabetes Mellitus Secondary to Other Conditions

Pancreatitis and cancer of the pancreas may greatly reduce the number of functioning β cells and result in impaired insulin secretion. Chronic liver disease will have considerable consequences for the metabolism of nutrients. Glycogenesis and glycogenolysis may both be impaired and consequently hyper- and hypoglycaemia frequently feature in chronic disorders of the liver. Chronic renal failure can cause IGT and insulin resistance, although the underlying mechanism by which this occurs remains unclear.

Some drugs, notably corticosteroids, have a diabetogenic effect. The thiazide group of diuretics has been known to worsen established diabetes and in some older patients may actually hasten the onset of the disease. Excess secretion or administration of glucocorticoids, aldosterone, catecholamines or growth hormone will have a diabetogenic effect and can result in hyperglycaemia. Diabetes may therefore be a feature of Cushing's syndrome/disease, phaeochromocytoma, primary aldosteronism and acromegaly (see Chapter 5).

There are other rare genetic disorders which give rise to secondary diabetes (Bilous et al. 2021). Friedreich's ataxia, an inherited disorder of balance and movement, is one example. Another is Wolfram syndrome with autosomal recessive inheritance. This disease is generally referred to as DIDMOAD (diabetes insipidus, diabetes mellitus, optic atrophy and deafness).

MANAGEMENT STRATEGIES IN DIABETES MELLITUS

Diabetes care in the UK and Europe has been strongly influenced by the St Vincent declaration (Khunti et al. 2023). Countries concerned pledged to deploy resources for its resolutions and to intensify research into prevention and cure of diabetes and its complications.

Diabetes management requires a multidisciplinary approach. For patients who are not acutely ill at the time of diagnosis, management may be provided entirely within the community or outpatient setting. However, many patients are more acutely ill at the time of diagnosis and require hospital care to allow close monitoring of the effects of early treatment.

The diabetes care team share common goals, each contributing expertise in accordance with the patient's individual needs. The patient is the most important member of the diabetes care team, and full participation by the patient is necessary to achieve the following aims:
- attaining and maintaining normoglycaemia (blood glucose within the normal range)
- monitoring response to therapy
- preventing and detecting the acute metabolic complications of diabetes
- preventing and detecting the chronic complications of diabetes
- facilitating self-care through education
- promoting social and psychological adjustment.

Attaining and Maintaining Normoglycaemia

There are three main therapeutic approaches:
- dietary therapy – nutritional advice
- noninsulin therapy
- insulin therapy.

Nutritional Advice for People With Diabetes

Appropriate dietary advice is essential in the effective management of diabetes. The aim is to give people with diabetes information to enable them to make informed choices about the type and quantity of food they eat. It is important that all newly diagnosed patients should be offered a consultation with a registered dietitian at the time of diagnosis. Dietitians are skilled in translating nutritional guidelines into practice. Dietary recommendations are the same as those given to the general population (see Chapter 22, Nutrition and Health) (Reflection 6.2).

Carbohydrate

All food that contains CHO will cause blood glucose levels to rise. The extent of the glycaemic response (the rise in blood glucose after eating) caused by food varies. This is affected by the amount of food consumed, the source of the CHO such as glucose or starch, the cooking method and other components of the meal.

The glycaemic index (GI) may explain some of the differences caused by different CHOs on blood glucose levels. It allows the glycaemic effect of foods to be ranked against a standard such as glucose. It is suggested that foods with a high GI cause a rapid rise in blood glucose levels, whereas lower GI foods are reckoned to cause a more gradual glycaemic response and if taken as part of a meal can lower the glycaemic effect of the whole meal (Sainsbury et al. 2018). However, further studies have failed to show a

REFLECTION 6.2

Eating Well

Eating a healthy balanced diet as recommended for the general population is also important in the management of both type 1 and type 2 diabetes and the prevention of complications.

Activities

- Access the following resources and consider the nutritional advice offered to people with type 1 and type 2 diabetes.
- Reflect on the benefits of such a diet, for example better blood glucose control, and discuss with your supervisor/assessor how you might use the resources when educating people newly diagnosed with diabetes.

Resources

Diabetes UK. I have type 1 diabetes – what can I eat? 2023. https://www.diabetes.org.uk/diabetes-the-basics/food-and-diabetes/i-have-type-1-diabetes.

Diabetes UK. I have type 2 diabetes – what can I eat? 2023. https://www.diabetes.org.uk/diabetes-the-basics/food-and-diabetes/i-have-type-2-diabetes.

TABLE 6.2	Sources of Fat
Type of Fat	**Food Source**
Saturated fat	Fatty meat, meat pies, sausages Butter, lard, suet, ghee, coconut oil, palm oil Cocoa butter – chocolate Cheese Cream Pastries, cakes, biscuits made with saturated fats Savoury snack foods
Monounsaturated fat	Olive oil Rapeseed oil Peanut oil (groundnut oil) Some soft margarines
Polyunsaturated fat	Sunflower oil and seeds Flaxseed oil and seeds Corn oil Soybean oil Some soft margarines Oily fish Poultry Eggs from hens fed a special diet

significant clinical effect of GI in glycaemic management and so the value of GI in diabetes control remains unproven (Evert et al. 2019) and the use of the GI should not obscure the need for a healthy, balanced, diet.

Sucrose (a disaccharide – ordinary table sugar) is no longer considered to be any more harmful to blood glucose levels than other CHOs. However, it is an empty calorie source, harmful for teeth and should be taken sparingly as part of a meal.

Fructose (a monosaccharide) is present in some fruit and vegetables and in honey. Fruit consumption should be encouraged as fructose has a low glycaemic effect. People with diabetes should be encouraged to eat five servings of fruit and vegetables per day. However, excessive fruit intake can significantly increase blood glucose levels, and therefore a sensible intake level should be encouraged. These foods are a good source of soluble fibre, which is also found in oats, pulses, nuts and grains.

Carbohydrate restriction is not recommended but some measure of control may be discussed, particularly in those with type 1 diabetes. Historically, dietitians advised people to measure their intake in 10 g exchanges to rigidly control their intake. This became less common in the 1980s when advice focused more on healthy eating guidelines. Quantifying CHO is now being used more frequently in view of the Dose Adjustment For Normal Eating (DAFNE) project findings (DAFNE Study Group 2002). The DAFNE education programme teaches people to adjust their insulin injections to fit their lifestyle, instead of adjusting their lifestyle to a particular insulin regimen, thus improving glycaemic control and quality of life in people with type 1 diabetes. However, the emphasis is markedly different, with the educated patient adjusting the amount of insulin given for the amount of CHO consumed, irrespective of the source of CHO.

Fat

Fat intake should not be overlooked when providing dietary advice to people with diabetes. A reduction in intake is generally necessary for weight control. People with diabetes should generally be encouraged to eat less fat and, where possible, to choose fats from monounsaturated sources, e.g. olive oil (Table 6.2).

Weight Management

Obesity increases insulin resistance and therefore correction of obesity can increase the sensitivity of cells to insulin. Weight reduction alone may bring the blood glucose down within normal limits. Weight management is particularly important in people with type 2 diabetes, where obesity is a well-recognised problem. Losing weight is notoriously difficult and social attitudes can lead to overweight people feeling stigmatised. As a result, guilt or low self-esteem may affect the patient's response to dietary advice. Drugs for the treatment for obesity have been developed (orlistat, sibutramine) and must be used according to national guidelines (see Useful Websites, e.g. British National Formulary, National Institute for Health and Clinical Excellence (NICE)).

Weight is not a sensitive indicator of glycaemic control. However, the negative significance of rapid weight loss accompanied by thirst, glycosuria and ketonuria should be recognised. Similarly, it can be a positive sign if the patient's weight is stable and within an acceptable range. Body mass index (BMI) calculation can provide a picture of the patient's weight in relation to their height and thereby an indication of whether they are overweight or obese (see Chapter 22, Nutrition and Health). A patient is considered to be overweight if their BMI is >25 kg/m^2 and obese if it is >30 kg/m^2 (see for information about monitoring central obesity). It is important that nurses involved in monitoring the patient's weight in the home, clinic or hospital adopt a sensitive approach. For hospital inpatients, weekly weighing should be adequate. Routine weighing at each outpatient clinic appointment is advisable. Frequency of self-weighing by a patient at home will be at the patient's discretion and in relation to the advice offered and the goals which have been set. On the whole, weighing more frequently than once a week is neither psychologically desirable nor valuable as a monitoring tool.

Advice on increasing physical activity should also be included.

Alcohol

It is not necessary to avoid alcohol completely with diabetes. As with the adult population in general, a maximum of 14 units of alcohol per week for women and men should not be exceeded. Further advice from the Chief Medical Officer (2016) suggests that alcohol intake should be spread over the week. Those treated with insulin should avoid hypoglycaemia when consuming alcohol by ensuring adequate CHO intake.

Noninsulin Therapies

Noninsulin therapies are only effective if cells are capable of secreting some insulin. These forms of therapies are used exclusively for patients with type 2 diabetes.

In the absence of persistent symptoms, dietary treatment should continue for at least 3 months before drug therapy is commenced. Oral hypoglycaemic therapy would then be reserved for those with type 2 diabetes who have persistent hyperglycaemia despite a period of dietary adjustment (NICE 2022, SIGN 2017) (Table 6.3).

Sulphonylureas

Drugs such as gliclazide stimulate β cells of the pancreas to secrete more insulin in response to blood glucose levels, increase insulin sensitivity and reduce liver metabolism of insulin.

Side-Effects. The most common side-effect is hypoglycaemia. This can be minimised by starting on the lowest dose possible and gradually increasing the amount over a period of weeks. It is essential that both the patient and carers are aware of the risks of hypoglycaemia. Sulphonylureas should be taken 20–30 minutes before food. The relationship between exercise, medication and diet will form an important part of the patient education programme.

Weight gain, gastrointestinal disturbance and skin rash can occur. Facial flushing following alcohol ingestion can occur with chlorpropamide. The effect of sulphonylureas is potentiated by other protein-bound medication, e.g. warfarin. This interaction increases the amount of available sulphonylurea and may therefore cause hypoglycaemia.

Biguanides

The drug metformin reduces glucose absorption in the gut, reduces peripheral insulin resistance and inhibits liver gluconeogenesis. Guidelines recommend first-line use of metformin following findings of a survival benefit in this group (SIGN 2017).

Side-Effects. Gastrointestinal upset is the most common. Medication-induced hypoglycaemia is very uncommon with biguanide therapy, as is vitamin B_{12} malabsorption. Lactic acidosis is a rare occurrence but should be noted and metformin is contraindicated in patients with renal, liver and severe cardiovascular disease or serious systemic illness.

Dipeptidyl Peptidase 4 Inhibitors (DPP-4 Inhibitors)

These are a relatively new form of oral agents, e.g. sitagliptin. They improve glycaemic control by increasing the levels of active incretin peptide hormones, e.g. glucagon-like peptide 1 (GLP-1), in the intestine. They can be used in combination with other oral hypoglycaemic agents.

Side-Effects. These include gastrointestinal disturbances, peripheral oedema and upper respiratory tract infection. They may cause hypoglycaemia if used with a sulphonylurea.

TABLE 6.3	Noninsulin Agents
Drug Groups and Examples	**Points to Note**
Sulphonylureas	
Gliclazide Glipizide Glimepiride Gliquidone Tolbutamide Chlorpropamide Glibenclamide	Stimulation of β cells to produce insulin and increase insulin sensitivity Avoid use in older people – risk of hypoglycaemia
Biguanides	
Metformin	Inhibition of liver gluconeogenesis. Increases peripheral uptake of insulin Treatment of choice for overweight patients with type 2 diabetes Contraindicated in renal, liver and cardiac disease
Dipeptidyl Peptidase 4 Inhibitors (DPP-4 Inhibitors)	
Sitagliptin Vildagliptin Vildagliptin/metformin	Do not need to be taken with food. Given twice daily
Glucagon-Like Peptide-1 (GLP-1) Mimetics	
(similar glucoregulatory actions to those of the incretin GLP-1)	
Exenatide	Must be injected SC twice daily up to 1 hour before 2 meals in the day, at least 8 hours apart, i.e. breakfast and evening meal. Can cause hypoglycaemia when used with sulphonylureas. Contraindicated in severe gastrointestinal disease
Prandial Glucose Regulators	
Nateglinide Repaglinide	β-cell stimulation. Shorter acting than sulphonylureas – fewer 'hypos'. Take only at meals
Thiazolidinediones	
Pioglitazone	Combats insulin resistance. Increases insulin sensitivity. Increases peripheral uptake of glucose. Reduces liver production. Contraindicated in heart failure and poor liver function. Used in conjunction with other agents
Alpha-Glucosidase Inhibitor	
Acarbose	Delays carbohydrate absorption. Poorly tolerated due to gastrointestinal side-effects

Glucagon-Like Peptide-1 (GLP-1) Mimetics

GLP-1 mimetics, e.g. exenatide, increase the secretion of insulin from the pancreas on a glucose-dependent basis. These drugs are injected subcutaneously.

Side-Effects. Gastrointestinal disturbances are most common in the first few days of starting treatment and usually subside. If used with sulphonylureas, there may be a risk of hypoglycaemia. Other side-effects include decreased appetite, headache and increased sweating. Observe injection sites for any local reaction.

Prandial Glucose Regulators

These drugs, e.g. repaglinide, are designed to stimulate extra insulin release to coincide with meal digestion. They should be taken up to 15 minutes before each meal and are rapidly absorbed. As they are also quickly eliminated from the body, the insulin effect is short lived, thus reducing the risk of hypoglycaemia.

Side-Effects. Side effects are uncommon but can include gastrointestinal upset, nausea and skin rash.

Thiazolidinediones

The thiazolidinediones (glitazones), e.g. pioglitazone, tackle insulin resistance and act by increasing insulin sensitivity within the peripheral tissue, increasing peripheral glucose uptake and reducing liver glucose production. They are used in conjunction with other oral agents.

Side-Effects. These can include weight gain, headache and fluid retention. Use of thiazolidinediones is therefore not advised in patients with cardiac failure or poor liver function.

Alpha-Glucosidase Inhibitor

The drug acarbose can be used alone or in combination with other oral agents. Acarbose acts by delaying the breakdown of starch and sucrose into monosaccharides which can be absorbed in the small intestine. The effect is to reduce the postprandial peak in blood glucose. Acarbose is poorly tolerated due to prominent side-effects and is now less commonly used.

Side-Effects. The most common side-effects are flatulence and diarrhoea.

Insulin Therapy

In type 1 diabetes, insulin therapy is essential to maintain life, and will be required throughout life. Insulin cannot be given orally as its amino acid structure would be inactivated by digestive enzymes. Parenteral administration is absolutely necessary and usually takes the form of subcutaneous (SC) injection.

In type 2 diabetes, glycaemic control deteriorates as the condition progresses and over 30% of patients will eventually require insulin therapy (Gentile et al. 2018). Others may require insulin therapy during periods of stress or illness but this does not change the classification of diabetes.

The objectives of insulin therapy are to:
- maintain blood glucose within normal limits
- relieve hyperglycaemia-associated symptoms
- correct metabolic/biochemical disturbances
- prevent diabetes-associated complications.

In the past, all insulin preparations were derived from beef (bovine) and pork (porcine) sources. Recombinant DNA technology and other advanced techniques have resulted in the production of biosynthetic human insulin and purified or highly purified porcine and bovine insulin.

Types and Duration of Action

There are many insulin preparations on the market. These may be categorised as rapid-acting analogue, short-acting, intermediate-acting, long-acting (including long-acting analogue) and biphasic (Fig. 6.2).
- **Rapid-acting analogue insulin (insulin lispro, insulin aspart, insulin glulisine)**. These are clear, colourless solutions. They have a rapid onset of action and therefore should be injected 0–15 minutes before meals. They are also licensed to be given up to 15 minutes after a meal.
- **Short-acting insulin (soluble insulin)**. These are clear solutions. The onset of action is delayed for 30 minutes when injected SC; their maximal effect occurs in 3–4 hours but can last up to 8–10 hours.

Figure 6.2 Duration of action for short-, intermediate- and long-acting insulins and rapid- and long-acting analogue insulins.

- **Intermediate-acting insulin (isophane insulin)**. These are cloudy in appearance. Their onset of effect is delayed for 1–2 hours. The intermediate-acting insulins achieve maximum effect in 4–6 hours and have a duration of action of 12–20 hours.
- **Long-acting analogue insulin (insulin glargine, insulin detemir)**. This is slowly absorbed, providing a continuous level of insulin over a 24-hour period. It is a true basal insulin with a peakless action profile, which therefore reduces the risk of hypoglycaemia. It may also be used in conjunction with oral hypoglycaemic agents in the treatment of people with type 2 diabetes.
- **Biphasic insulin**. These ready-mixed insulins include a combination of short-acting or rapid-acting analogue and intermediate-acting insulin in set ratios. Examples include Humulin M3 and NovoMix 30 (insulin aspart and insulin aspart protamine).

Administering Insulin

The overall aim in administering insulin therapy is to achieve the best possible control of blood glucose throughout the 24-hour period. The treatment should mimic the physiological response to normal variations in blood glucose. Patients can self-administer insulin using an insulin injecting device in the form of a syringe or pen device with a pen needle attached (Reflection 6.3). There are also insulin pumps available to those who meet NICE guidance criteria for pump therapy. Self-administration of insulin can

Thighs   Abdomen   Arms   Buttocks

Figure 6.3 Suitable injection sites for insulin.

be quick and discreet, enabling adaptability for the day-to-day changes in the patient's activity levels, eating pattern and lifestyle.

Timing and Frequency of Injections

Long-acting analogues must be administered once daily, every 24 hours. This can be at any time of the day to fit in with the patient's life. For many patients, twice-daily injections remain the preferred regimen. These are administered with breakfast and with evening meal. Older patients, who have perhaps been required to progress to insulin from diet and/or oral therapy, may be more willing to accept once-daily injections.

To mimic normal blood glucose fluctuations, a single injection of insulin with a 24-hour period of action could be given once daily in combination with rapid-acting insulin with a short (4–5 hour) duration of action, with each meal. This multiple injection system has considerable advantages, giving flexibility of mealtimes and meal size. This system is most effective if blood glucose levels are regularly monitored and patients are taught to adjust diet, exercise and insulin accordingly. It does, however, not suit everyone.

Injection Sites

Insulin is given by SC injection. Common sites for injection are the upper thighs and the abdominal wall. The outer aspect of the upper arms and buttocks can also be used, but this may prove difficult especially for those with limited range of movement. Overuse of one site can lead to lipohypertrophy, loss of sensitivity and impaired or erratic absorption of insulin. For this reason, injection site rotation is advised (Fig. 6.3).

Injection Technique

Cleansing the skin with alcohol prior to injection is unnecessary. The site must be visibly clean. Insulin syringes and pen needles currently in use in the UK have a variety of needle lengths and gauges, and it is important to select the appropriate needle for the body weight of the patient to ensure a SC injection. A mound of skin should be gently pinched up to avoid intramuscular injection. The skin should not be pinched if a 4 mm, 5 mm or 6 mm needle

is used. The syringe or pen device should be held as illustrated in the appropriate device leaflets and the needle inserted straight into the SC tissue at a 90-degree angle. The insulin should be injected steadily and the needle held in position for a further count of at least 6 seconds before withdrawing smoothly. (See Useful Websites, e.g. BD Medical – Living with Diabetes.)

Monitoring Response to Therapy

The methods used for monitoring glycaemic control include:
- glycated (glycosylated) haemoglobin (HbA_{1c})
- self blood glucose monitoring (SBGM)
- continuous glucose monitoring system (CGMS)
- blood ketone monitoring
- urinalysis
- body weight monitoring.

Glycated (Glycosylated) Haemoglobin Estimation (HbA_{1c})

Glucose in solution is bound to the proteins of haemoglobin. The rate at which proteins bind to glucose is directly related to the current glucose concentration in the blood. It gives an indication of control over a period of time, normally 2–3 months, and not merely a one-off recording as in plasma glucose estimation. Anything that interferes with normal haemoglobin levels, such as haemorrhage or anaemia, could potentially distort glycated haemoglobin results. Similarly, conditions that influence serum albumin levels, such as renal or hepatic disease, may result in problems in interpreting glycated albumin results.

HbA_{1c} should be below 7.5% in patients with type 1 diabetes. In type 2 diabetes, individual targets should be set between 6.5% and 7.5%. Other risk factors such as vascular complications and hypoglycaemia risk should be taken into consideration. This result should be discussed with the patient, who should be actively encouraged to manage their diabetes effectively (NICE 2022).

Changes to HbA_{1c} Measurements

HbA_{1c} testing has been standardised and is reported in mmol/mol (correct scientific value) in line with the International Federation of Clinical Chemists (IFCC) reference method. This change will occur worldwide. For example, an HbA_{1c} of 7% will now be reported as 53 mmol/mol. Most laboratories will give results in both mmol/mol and percentages. (See Useful Websites, e.g. IDF.)

Self Blood Glucose Monitoring (SBGM)

SBGM is the most widely used method of testing glucose levels. It provides a simple and, if performed correctly, reliable method of monitoring glycaemic control. Results may be downloaded from a blood glucose meter or written into the patient's monitoring diary. Training by the diabetes specialist nurse or other trained healthcare professional must be given to the patient. Importantly patients should agree their individual target levels with the diabetes team; Diabetes UK (2023) offers some targets as a guide. Diabetes UK (2023) currently recommends that people with diabetes should keep blood glucose levels as near normal as possible (in the range of a person without diabetes, although individual targets may be set by clinicians. (See Useful Websites, e.g. Diabetes UK.)

Near-patient blood glucose testing in hospital requires a standardised system throughout, with a quality assurance programme in place involving internal and external quality control. Results are recorded on a chart and should be regularly monitored.

(See Useful Websites for information on blood glucose meter systems.)

Advantages

Blood glucose monitoring offers increased patient involvement in diabetes management and helps to improve day-to-day glycaemic control. It is used by patients to adjust their insulin levels, assess if blood glucose level is acceptable for driving or exercise and monitor the effect of certain amounts and types of food eaten. It can also give warning of impending metabolic crisis and guide subsequent intervention.

Blood glucose meters are inexpensive and often provided by NHS diabetes clinics. Each model has different functions to suit the individual patient's capabilities. Some have integrated test strips with capillary-fill dosing, most have a large memory store for downloading results. Quality control solution is supplied with some meters to check the accuracy of the meter. For visually impaired individuals, there are talking meters. Intensive training is required from a diabetes specialist nurse in the use of these devices.

Disadvantages

Blood glucose monitoring requires a fair degree of manual dexterity, visual acuity, cognitive ability and motivation (Reflection 6.4). There may be cost implications for test strip prescriptions in some countries.

Frequency

For patients with type 1 diabetes, preprandial and prebedtime tests, with the occasional postprandial test, can provide important

---

REFLECTION 6.4

Monitoring Blood Glucose: Physical Problems

Think about some physical problems (such as arthritis affecting the hands, a tremor caused by Parkinson's disease or a stroke affecting the dominant hand) leading to poor manual dexterity that make it difficult for a patient who needs/wants to monitor blood glucose as part of managing their diabetes.

Activities

- Use the Useful Websites to investigate whether there are blood glucose meters that meet the needs of people with poor manual dexterity. Discuss your findings with a specialist nurse or another member of the diabetes care team.

---

feedback and aid learning for all seriously motivated people with diabetes and can be an essential tool in achieving tight diabetic control (Holt and Kumar 2015).

Continuous Glucose Monitoring System (CGMS)

Some patients with excessively fluctuating blood glucose levels may require continuous glucose monitoring. This uses a sensor inserted under the skin in the abdomen, measuring interstitial glucose every 10 seconds. This gives a 6-day profile of blood glucose. Results can be interpreted by the diabetes team and discussed with the patient, suggesting ways to improve glucose levels.

Blood Ketone Monitoring

The ketone body β-hydroxybutyrate can be measured with a blood ketone meter. It can be detected quickly and simply by using a blood ketone meter and test strips (the same principles as the blood glucose meter). Patients with newly diagnosed or established type 1 diabetes can be taught to test for blood ketones at home, in times of stress and illness in particular, along with 'sick day rules'. This is useful as insulin treatment can be altered to eliminate ketones with the assistance of the diabetes team. If ketone levels are too high, this can lead to DKA, requiring hospital admission.

Urinalysis

Urine can be tested to detect the presence of glucose and ketones. However, with the increasing use of blood glucose meters for glycaemic control, the use of urine testing is declining. Testing the urine for glucose is not completely accurate as it does not reflect the current blood glucose level. If there is any reason to suspect that the patient is suffering from, or is at risk of, episodes of hypoglycaemia, then instruction in blood glucose monitoring should be considered. Urine ketone testing can aid in initial diagnosis of type 1 diabetes, or to monitor ketone production in illness or stress.

A potential renal complication (diabetic nephropathy) associated with diabetes can be detected by the presence of very small amounts of albumin in the urine (microalbuminuria). Commercial dipstick strips are available that detect the low level of albumin that would not be revealed by a standard dipstick.

Chemically impregnated dipsticks are the usual means of screening for various conditions on admission to hospital. The manufacturer's instructions for use and storage of urine testing materials must be followed precisely. Results of urinalysis should be accurately recorded in the appropriate chart.

Body Weight Monitoring

See earlier section Nutritional Advice for People With Diabetes.

Preventing and Detecting Acute Metabolic Complications of Diabetes

The acute metabolic complications arising from diabetes are:
- DKA
- hyperosmolar hyperglycaemic state (HHS)
- hypoglycaemia.

Diabetic Ketoacidosis

DKA is characterised by uncontrolled hyperglycaemia and uncontrolled lipolysis caused by an insulin deficiency, accompanied by dehydration and acidosis. Individuals with longstanding diabetes can usually recognise the signs and symptoms of impending ketoacidosis and will seek medical help at a much earlier stage in its development. Those newly diagnosed with type 1 diabetes are taught how to recognise and respond to indications of hyperglycaemia and ketoacidosis.

Epidemiology

In the UK, DKA is the most common cause of death for people with diabetes below the age of 20 years. There is very little recent research showing the incidence of DKA; recent estimates suggest that the rate of DKA is rising (Dhatariya 2019). With the onset of the COVID-19 pandemic, it was noted that patients with diabetes who were admitted to hospital with COVID-19 were shown to have a higher rate of DKA than those with no infection (Goldman et al. 2020). Any patient presenting with DKA will be at risk of cerebral oedema, and must be managed in a high dependency environment.

Aetiology

Newly presenting diabetes may lead to DKA where there may have been a delay in diagnosis. In patients with established diabetes, DKA can be precipitated by infection, myocardial infarction (MI), stroke or physical or emotional trauma, as these increase stress hormone secretion. Stress hormones raise the blood glucose and increase insulin requirements. DKA is caused by an inadequate dosage of insulin being taken during intercurrent illness or other major stress, or by insulin being omitted altogether. Inadequate concordance with treatment regimens can be a particular contributing factor, often associated with repeated hospital admissions.

● Pathophysiology and Presentation

The symptoms of DKA are a consequence of the combined effect of insulin lack and increased secretion of catabolic, counter-regulatory stress hormones. As a result, two major biochemical disturbances occur simultaneously:

• Increased lipolysis results in the formation of ketone bodies which are weak acids and cause metabolic acidosis
• Accelerated gluconeogenesis and glycogenolysis cause hyperglycaemia, which in turn results in osmotic diuresis, dehydration and electrolyte imbalance with a loss of sodium (hyponatraemia) and potassium (hypokalaemia).

Note that hyperkalaemia may be evident in the very early stages due to severe metabolic acidosis, but once rehydration is under way, hypokalaemia is usual and may be severe.

Information 6.1 provides further information about the development, presentation and effects of DKA.

● Medical Management

Reversing Hyperglycaemia. Short-acting, soluble insulin is administered to lower blood glucose. Initially, 50 units of short-acting insulin in 50 mL of sodium chloride 0.9% (1 unit/mL) are administered intravenously via syringe driver infusion at 6 units/h. The insulin dose will later be varied in accordance with the blood glucose level; the aim should be a gradual reduction in blood glucose over a period of 12 hours.

Capillary blood glucose should be checked hourly and venous blood glucose and plasma potassium are measured at appropriate intervals by the laboratory.

INFORMATION 6.1

The Development of Diabetic Ketoacidosis

The key precipitating factors for DKA are inadequate supply of insulin and increased demand for insulin, often in combination. These are often triggered by:

• newly presenting type 1 diabetes
• infection, especially respiratory, urinary or abscesses
• trauma or surgery
• severe illness, e.g. myocardial infarction or stroke
• failure to take sufficient insulin – this may be accidental or deliberate. Patients can discover that ketosis will cause rapid weight loss.

As a result of reduced insulin and increased stress hormone levels, cells will be unable to utilise glucose, glycogen will be converted to glucose, gluconeogenesis provides glucose from non-CHO sources (such as protein) and lipolysis occurs, releasing ketone bodies. The combined effects of these events are:

• hyperglycaemia and hyperketonaemia
• osmotic diuresis
• fluid and electrolyte imbalance (see Chapter 21)
• catabolism/wasting
• acid–base imbalance – acidaemia caused by the process of metabolic acidosis (see Chapter 21).

As a result the patient will present with the following signs and symptoms:

Signs and Symptoms

• Polyuria progressing to oliguria
• Polydipsia
• Lethargy/weakness
• Nausea/vomiting
• Abdominal colic
• Muscle cramps
• Blurred vision
• Hyperglycaemia
• Glycosuria
• Ketonuria
• Ketone breath (sweet 'pear drop' fruity odour)
• Weight loss
• Electrolyte imbalance – hypokalaemia, hyponatraemia
• Hypotension and tachycardia
• Acidaemia (a high level of acid (hydrogen ions) in the blood)
• Rapid, deep (Kussmaul's) respirations
• Evidence of intercurrent infection/illness
• Skin flushed and warm
• Hypothermia may develop
• Confusion and drowsiness progressing to coma.

Complications

• Cerebral oedema
• Adult/acute respiratory distress syndrome (ARDS)
• Thromboembolism.

Rehydration. Rapid restoration of circulating fluid volume is necessary, followed by gradual correction of the interstitial and intracellular deficit. Sodium chloride (NaCl) 0.9% is given by intravenous (IV) infusion with potassium chloride (KCl) included if hypokalaemia is present or anticipated (see later). When blood glucose falls to approximately 10 mmol/L, the sodium chloride is replaced by IV glucose 5%, but the insulin infusion continues (British National Formulary 2023).

Replacing Potassium. Derangements in plasma potassium can vary. Hyperkalaemia may be evident in the very early stages due to severe metabolic acidosis, but once rehydration is under way, hypokalaemia is usual and may be severe. IV potassium chloride is prescribed in accordance with the blood biochemistry. This must be administered by a regulated infusion delivery system.

Monitoring. The patient will be closely monitored for the following:

Cardiac monitoring should be commenced and a 12-lead electrocardiogram (ECG) is performed to detect cardiac arrhythmias associated with an imbalance of serum potassium.

Monitoring acidaemia (caused by metabolic acidosis). Arterial blood gases (ABGs) are checked initially, but venous bicarbonate levels are adequate for monitoring 1- to 2-hourly thereafter.

Monitoring fluid and electrolyte imbalance. Blood urea, electrolytes and osmolality.

Response to fluid and potassium replacement. Blood pressure and pulse are measured hourly as a guide to blood volume. Although becoming much less common, central venous pressure (CVP) or pulmonary artery occlusion pressure (PAOP) (also known as pulmonary capillary wedge pressure [PCWP]) may be initiated and measured in the older patient or those with renal or heart failure.

Monitoring ketosis and renal function. Urine is tested for glucose, ketones and protein.

Oxygen therapy. Oxygen will be prescribed and administered in accordance with blood gas results and local policy.

Nasogastric aspiration may be necessary to protect the airway if the patient is vomiting, drowsy or unconscious.

Investigating underlying infection. A chest X-ray is performed. Blood cultures, full blood count, urine and sputum specimens are sent to microbiology.

Observation of vital signs. Temperature, pulse, blood pressure, pulse oximetry, colour and respiration are recorded hourly. Fluid intake and output is measured and recorded.

Additional Therapy. Additional therapy which may be required in the management of DKA includes:

Alkaline – sodium bicarbonate. This is rarely used as it may exacerbate tissue hypoxia and hypokalaemia. As overcorrection may result in alkalosis, sodium bicarbonate is usually reserved for the treatment of very severe acidosis, and then only if the patient does not respond to adequate treatment with fluids and insulin.

Broad-spectrum antibiotics. These may be given only if infection is suspected.

Anticoagulants. Low-molecular-weight heparin may be administered according to local guidelines.

Urinary catheterisation. It may be necessary to facilitate the hourly measurement of urinary output as severe dehydration carries a risk of acute renal failure. However, catheterisation should be avoided if possible because of the risk of urinary tract infection (UTI) (see Chapter 10. Nursing Patients With Urinary Disorders).

❖ Nursing Management and Health Promotion: Diabetic Ketoacidosis

The biochemical disruption of DKA is profound and life threatening. Each patient admitted with DKA will have unique problems and needs. The newly admitted patient with DKA is vulnerable in a variety of ways. Once the patient's condition is stable, every effort should be made to establish the cause of DKA and, where appropriate, the patient should be referred to the diabetes specialist nurse to discuss any changes to medication and issues of self-management in an effort

INFORMATION 6.2

Katie's Story and Part 1 of Her Nursing Care Plan

Katie is a lively 18-year-old and the eldest of three children. She lives with her family but is soon to leave home to start university some 30 miles away.

Katie and her two brothers have recently had gastroenteritis. The boys are now fully fit but Katie is far from well. She has been passing an excessive amount of urine and is constantly thirsty. She has lost weight and has recently been complaining of feeling tired all the time.

This morning she is very drowsy. Her skin feels hot and dry and she looks flushed. She has vomited several times and has complained of abdominal pain and cramps in her limbs. Her breath has a peculiar sweet smell and her mouth is very dry. She has also been complaining of blurred vision.

Her parents are alarmed and have called the GP to request an urgent visit. Alerted by the 'acetone breath', her symptoms and the history of recent illness, the GP checks Katie's capillary blood glucose and finds it to be greater than the upper limit on his blood glucose meter (33.3 mmol/L). She is too drowsy to produce a urine specimen to check for ketones but the GP is in little doubt about the diagnosis. An ambulance is summoned and Katie and her parents are taken to hospital. The ward is alerted to expect an unconscious patient with DKA.

On admission, Katie is acutely ill and has complex care requirements. A nurse who has the appropriate levels of knowledge and skill is assigned to care for her. She has prepared for Katie's admission and will subsequently assess her nursing needs and plan and evaluate her care.

to prevent recurrence. For many patients, however, the experience of DKA is what first makes them aware that they have diabetes.

Priorities for nursing care will be strongly influenced by the prescribed medical therapy and the need for complex monitoring (see earlier in the chapter) and many hospitals have adopted DKA protocols to ensure fluids and insulin are initiated for these patients within a certain timeframe, and ongoing management is monitored.

Whilst the nurse must draw upon technical skills in such a situation, it is vitally important to maintain a holistic approach to care. The nurse should be sensitive to the vulnerability of the patient and try to accommodate individual needs when planning and implementing care.

Katie's story and Part 1 of her Nursing Care Plan for the first 24 hours after admission is provided as an example of how a patient may present with severe DKA and how nursing priorities may be met following admission and until consciousness is regained (Information 6.2). Although Katie was unconscious on admission, the vast majority of patients presenting with DKA will not be unconscious.

Part 2 of Katie's Nursing Care Plan is presented as a critical thinking question on the companion Evolve website and provides an opportunity for you to complete the remaining nursing considerations and related care.

🌐 **See Evolve website Critical thinking question 6.1**

Further information relevant to the subsequent care of a patient with DKA is provided with that required by a patient with HHS (see Nursing Management and Health Promotion: Subsequent Care in DKA and HHS).

Hyperosmolar Hyperglycaemic State (HHS)

HHS refers to the serious metabolic disruption characterised by marked hyperglycaemia (>33 mmol/L) in the absence of DKA in addition to high serum osmolality. It was previously known as hyperosmolar nonketotic coma (HONK). However, it is

Part 1 of Nursing Care Plan for Katie During the first 24 hours After Admission

Nursing Considerations	Action	Rationale	Evaluation
Impaired consciousness	Position and support Katie in a semiprone or lateral position Keep artificial airway in position until voluntarily expelled Perform oropharyngeal suction if secretions are audible Provide nasogastric (NG) aspiration Continuously monitor colour, pulse oximetry and respiration Administer oxygen as prescribed, ensuring that fire safety rules are observed Monitor neurological status hourly. Record/report findings	To prevent asphyxia and prevent aspiration of secretion/vomitus Due to unconscious state and recent vomiting To correct hypoxia and prevent oxygen combustion To detect change in conscious level	Skin colour and respirations are normal Risk factors eliminated Blood gases improving Katie is progressively more responsive
Hyperglycaemia and ketonaemia	Administer prescribed short-acting insulin IV by infusion pump Monitor capillary blood glucose hourly: record/report findings	To correct hyperglycaemia and ketonaemia To evaluate response to insulin therapy and prevent hypoglycaemia	Trends indicate blood glucose returning towards the normal range
Fluid deficit/ replacement	Administer IV fluids as prescribed. Observe venepuncture site for redness, swelling or extravasation. Record all fluids in fluid balance chart Monitor CVP, BP, breathing, temperature: observe neck veins, skin colour and urine volume Catheterisation usually prescribed if unconsciousness persists and if the patient is oliguric Test urine hourly for ketones: record results	To correct hypovolaemia To monitor the effects of fluid replacement To monitor renal function and detect renal insufficiency (urine <30 mL/h)	No discomfort or swelling of venepuncture site Vital signs are returning to normal ranges Urine volume >30 mL/h Ketonuria diminishing
Electrolyte imbalance/ replacement	Observe the effects of potassium replacement; provide continuous cardiac monitoring Report tall peaked T wave on ECG (indicates hyperkalaemia) Report flattened or inverted T wave (indicates hypokalaemia) REPORT ECG CHANGES PROMPTLY	Overzealous potassium replacement can cause ventricular fibrillation, and cardiac arrest Persistent hypokalaemia due to inadequate potassium replacement can result in heart block, which may lead to cardiac arrest	Potassium should be 3.3–4.7 mmol/L Cardiac monitor should display normal tracing
Probable current infection/potential risk of infection	Collect throat swab, catheter specimen of urine and, when consciousness returns, a specimen of sputum. Monitor Temperature, Pulse, and Respiration (TPR). Take venous blood specimen for culture and full blood count Administer prescribed antibiotics and note/report side-effects Reduce risks of infection by high standards of nursing care (e.g. personal, hand and catheter hygiene)	To detect/monitor current infection To safely administer therapy To prevent healthcare-associated infection	Specimen analysis Blood culture results and TPR normal Patient infection-free

recognised that a minor degree of ketosis and acidosis could also occur, hence the revision of the term hyperglycaemic hyperosmolar nonketotic state or coma.

Pathophysiology

HHS is a consequence of relative deficiency of insulin in conjunction with the rise in counterregulatory stress hormones (cortisol, adrenaline, glucagon and growth hormone) with the resultant increase in liver glucose output and decreased peripheral glucose uptake. Rise in blood glucose levels leads to glycosuria, osmotic diuresis and dehydration with ensuing hyperosmolarity and hypernatraemia. The underlying reason for the lack of ketosis in HHS remains unclear. HHS typically presents in individuals with type 2 diabetes, and therefore patients tend to be older than those with DKA. Unlike DKA, osmotic symptoms could have evolved over several days or weeks. Mental obtundation (blunting, reduced alertness and pain sensation) or altered consciousness is more frequent due

to hyperosmolarity. Focal neurological signs or seizures may be a clinical feature in some patients. Physical examination reveals signs of dehydration, tachycardia and hypotension.

The commonest precipitating factor of HHS is infection. Other precipitating factors include MI, stroke and nonconcordance with treatment, pancreatitis or medications, particularly corticosteroid therapy. Mortality rate remains high (5%–20%), reflecting in many cases the underlying causes and the advanced age at presentation.

Medical Management

Insulin Therapy and Blood Glucose Monitoring. Insulin infusion of 50 units of soluble insulin in 50 mL of sodium chloride 0.9% should be commenced. High doses of insulin are rarely needed. An insulin rate of 0.3 U/h is reasonable, although the rate may have to be reduced further if the fall of blood glucose is too rapid. Capillary blood glucose monitoring should be performed hourly to monitor response to insulin and also to avoid hypoglycaemia. However, capillary blood glucose measurement may not be accurate in severe hyperglycaemia and dehydration. Therefore venous samples should be sent to the laboratory during the initial phase of treatment.

Rehydration. The fluid deficit is considerable with estimated fluid deficit of 8–12 L. Fluid replacement in HHS should be slower and must be approached with a degree of caution taking into consideration coexisting conditions and the age of the patient.

The most appropriate initial fluid is 0.9% sodium chloride. Colloid should be considered in hypotensive patients with systolic blood pressure <100 mmHg. If plasma sodium is higher than 155 mmol/L after initial fluid replacement, 0.45% sodium chloride should be considered. Once blood glucose is less than <15 mmol/L, 5% dextrose should be initiated; 0.9% saline should be continued at a slower rate to complete rehydration.

Replacing Potassium. Potassium replacement should commence once hyperkalaemia is excluded or reversed with rehydration and insulin therapy. Hyperosmolarity causes a shift of potassium from within the cells to the extracellular space.

Cardiac Monitoring. Should be commenced and a 12-lead ECG is performed to detect cardiac arrhythmias associated with serum potassium lack or excess.

Oxygen Therapy. This will be administered in accordance with blood gas results and local policy.

Monitoring Level of Consciousness. This is vitally important as there is a risk of a stroke (cerebral thrombosis) and cerebral oedema. Cerebral oedema can develop with rapid fall in osmolality, particularly with the use of 0.45% sodium chloride.

Additional Therapy. Additional therapy which may be required in the management of HHS includes:

Anticoagulants. Low-molecular-weight heparin will be administered per local protocol.

Urinary catheterisation. It may be necessary to facilitate the hourly measurement of urinary output as severe dehydration carries a risk of acute renal failure. However, catheterisation should be avoided if possible because of the risk of UTI (see Chapter 10 Nursing Patients With Urinary Disorders).

Nasogastric tube to protect the airway if the patient is unconscious or drowsy and vomiting.

Treatment of the coexisting morbidity or the underlying precipitating factors.

❖ Nursing Management and Health Promotion: Subsequent Care in DKA and HHS

When the patient is alert and able to respond, the focus of care will change. The nurse will work with the patient, the dietitian and the medical staff to stabilise blood glucose and to monitor the effects of therapy. The subsequent care of the patient with a hyperglycaemic crisis, whether due to DKA or HHS, will be similar in many respects. Appropriate nursing interventions will be required to ensure the patient's safety and comfort, such as meeting hygiene needs. The patient is likely to be vulnerable due to an impaired level of consciousness, dehydration, electrolyte imbalance, the hazards of immobility and diabetes-associated risk factors. The level of consciousness in HHS is important as there is a risk of cerebral thrombosis due to combined effects of immobility, dehydration and diabetes-associated atherosclerosis. A patient with DKA may not necessarily be unconscious. The nurse should promptly report any evidence of deterioration in the patient's level of consciousness or any neurological function (see Chapter 11, Nursing Patients With Disorders of the Nervous System).

Restoration of Self-Care. The diabetes specialist nurse, ward nurses, dietitian and medical staff will initiate the process of preparing the patient to assume responsibility for self-care, along with the contribution made by the community nurses and GP once the patient returns home.

Patient Education. The newly diagnosed patient will require information about how a balance between activity, food and medication can be achieved with the help of frequent blood glucose monitoring. This is especially important for patients with type 1 diabetes.

Once the crisis has passed, perhaps the most important aspect of care is to prevent further episodes of DKA or HHS. This involves identifying the events which led up to the crisis and discussing with the patient where action might have been taken to avert the crisis or obtain help at an earlier stage. Glycated haemoglobin estimation can provide useful information about glycaemic control over the preceding weeks, as can the patient's record of blood glucose or urinalysis results.

Providing Psychological Support. The experience of a hyperglycaemic crisis can cause great distress, not only to the patient but also to family and friends. Adopting a warm empathic approach and accepting the fears of the patient are important if trust and rapport are to be established. The nurse should first ascertain the level of the person's existing knowledge and provide essential information using brief, clear explanations, checking that these are understood. Access to medical staff and information about the ward should be provided.

It is all too easy to be wise after the event and it is unhelpful for the patient to feel that they were to blame for any episode of DKA or HHS. The main aims should be to help the patient understand their diabetes and have confidence in its management; therefore time should be spent reassessing their knowledge and addressing any issues which may help to prevent further episodes of illness. If severe underlying emotional distress or disturbance has precipitated the metabolic crisis, then the patient's difficulties may need to be sensitively explored. In accordance with the patient's wishes, appropriate counselling facilities may be provided. The newly diagnosed patient will require emotional support in meeting the immediate practical demands imposed by the condition. Information about the services and publications provided by Diabetes UK can be very useful.

Hypoglycaemia

Hypoglycaemia is a common complication of insulin treatment and occurs when blood glucose falls below 4 mmol/L. Of people with insulin-treated diabetes, 25%–30% suffer one or more severe hypoglycaemic episodes every year (Bilous et al. 2021).

There are several causes of hypoglycaemia. The three main causes are:

- excess insulin
- insufficient food
- increased exercise/activity.

Information 6.3 outlines the classification, causes and risk factors for hypoglycaemia.

🔴 Pathophysiology and Presentation

Symptoms are idiosyncratic, developing over a very short period of time (5–15 minutes).

Endocrine/Autonomic Response. Glucagon and counterregulatory hormones are secreted in response to falling blood glucose and act to restore blood glucose to normal. Activation of the

Hypoglycaemia: Classification, Causes and Risk Factors

Classification

- *Asymptomatic* – biochemical hypoglycaemia without symptoms
- *Mild* – easily recognised and corrected by the patient
- *Moderate* – patient conscious but requiring help from others
- *Severe (leading to loss of consciousness)* – cerebral function severely affected by glucose lack

Causes

- Excess insulin
- Wrong type of insulin
- Inappropriate combination of insulin
- Excess dosage of oral sulphonylureas
- Delayed or missed meal
- More than usual amount of exercise
- Alcohol ingestion, especially when hungry
- Stress, such as hypothermia

Risk Factors

- Impaired awareness of hypoglycaemia
- Strict glycaemic control
- Excess alcohol consumption
- Drug misuse

autonomic nervous system in response to the stress of hypoglycaemia provokes autonomic symptoms of hypoglycaemia (Heller and Chow 2014). These hormones potentiate the effects of the sympathetic nervous system to cause the following symptoms:

- pounding heart and palpitations
- sweating
- trembling
- sensation of hunger
- sensation of anxiety.

Central Nervous System Response. As brain cells are unable to metabolise alternatives to glucose for energy, a fall below the normal blood glucose will cause neuroglycopenic symptoms, including:

- lack of concentration
- dizziness
- unsteady gait
- slurred speech
- tingling around the lips.

Other nonspecific symptoms, including headache and nausea, can occur. In addition, observers may notice abnormalities such as:

- pallor
- irrational behaviour
- muscle twitching/seizures
- extreme drowsiness or coma.

Some of these symptoms and signs could, with disastrous consequences, be mistakenly attributed to excess intake of alcohol.

Loss of Sensitivity to Symptoms. Recently diagnosed patients may rely on autonomic symptoms such as sweating, tremor and pounding heart to alert them to a fall in blood glucose. However, after some years, patients may become less sensitive to these symptoms and come to rely on neuroglycopenic features to alert them to impending hypoglycaemia.

In longstanding insulin-treated diabetes, perception of the onset of symptoms of hypoglycaemia may become blunted, due

to autonomic neuropathy or the effect of intensified insulin treatment (Bilous et al. 2021). The patient may remain asymptomatic even when the blood glucose falls below 2 mmol/L, although at this level some signs may be obvious to others. This is known as impaired awareness of hypoglycaemia. Symptoms can also be masked by the following:

- *Alcohol* – if the patient is known to have consumed alcohol or smells of alcohol, this can lead to mistaking hypoglycaemia for intoxication, particularly as many symptoms and clinical features are similar.
- *Ageing* – in older people hypoglycaemia may cause neurological disturbances and the presenting symptoms can be mistaken for failing mental function or transient ischaemic attacks (cerebrovascular disease).
- *Time of day* – hypoglycaemia during sleep can be asymptomatic. It is often not detected although features such as night sweats, restlessness, nightmares, snoring and headaches on waking may give the patient an indication of its occurrence. Rebound hyperglycaemia can occur and is attributed to an increase in the release of counterregulatory hormones during the night to correct the hypoglycaemia. This is known as the Somogyi phenomenon.
- *Sulphonylurea-induced hypoglycaemia* – chlorpropamide and glibenclamide, even at normal therapeutic doses, have been implicated in severe, prolonged hypoglycaemic coma. This risk is increased in older people, particularly when they may be unwell and not eating, and in those with poor renal function. Subsequent prolonged hypoglycaemia may be fatal.

Medical Management

Treatment of hypoglycaemia is simple and the effects are usually dramatic and gratifying. Nevertheless, the risks posed by hypoglycaemia and the importance of early detection and intervention must be stressed.

Hypoglycaemia can be treated with oral CHO, SC or IM glucagon, or IV glucose depending on the stage and severity.

The conscious patient should be given rapidly absorbed glucose as a glucose drink or as sweets, followed by a more gradually absorbed form of CHO, e.g. glucose tablets or a glass of fruit juice, followed by biscuits or a sandwich. Hypoglycaemia can recur if food is not consumed after initial treatment with glucose.

The Confused or Drowsy Patient. If the patient cannot eat or drink safely, glucagon by IM injection can be given. This will have the effect of raising the blood glucose. Where possible, relatives should be taught how to administer glucagon.

The Unconscious Patient. Medical help should always be sought for the unconscious patient, although if hypoglycaemia is known to be the problem, glucagon IM should be given while the paramedic or doctor is awaited and the patient should be placed in the recovery position until consciousness returns. Nothing should be given orally whilst the patient is unconscious.

If glucagon is unavailable, or fails to bring a response within 10–15 minutes, IV dextrose in a dose of 30–50 mL of glucose 50% is required, which will usually raise the blood glucose sufficiently for consciousness to be regained. Caution should be exercised in the use of 50% glucose solution as it is very hyperosmolar and will damage peripheral veins; therefore a central vein must always be used. When coma persists, hospital admission will be necessary.

The Hospitalised Patient With Hypoglycaemia. Unconscious hypoglycaemia in the hospitalised patient may be treated by IV dextrose as first-line treatment. Venous blood must be taken for laboratory estimation of blood glucose. Continuous IV infusion of dextrose 10%–20% will be commenced and the patient's response monitored by regular measurement of blood glucose. Approximately 1%–2% of patients with hypoglycaemic coma fail to respond promptly to parenteral therapy. For these patients, other causes of coma such as alcohol or drug overdose, hypothermia or cerebral haemorrhage should be excluded. Cerebral oedema can accompany prolonged hypoglycaemia; an IV infusion of mannitol (a hyperosmotic fluid that acts as an osmotic diuretic) may be required and oxygen therapy administered.

❖ Nursing Management and Health Promotion: Hypoglycaemia

In hypoglycaemic coma the period of unconsciousness and extreme vulnerability tends to be short. The nurse must:

- ensure the airway is clear
- monitor conscious level
- administer prescribed therapy
- monitor capillary blood glucose
- explore the possible cause of the hypoglycaemic coma
- provide information and encouragement for the patient to help improve diabetes management.

The acute metabolic complications of diabetes vary in cause, severity and outcome. All indicate a lack of stability of diabetes management requiring further assessment and investigation. Modification of treatment or lifestyle with the assistance of the diabetes team should be offered.

Preventing and Detecting the Chronic Complications of Diabetes

The Diabetes Control and Complications Trial (DCCT) conducted in the early 1990s (Diabetes Control and Complications Research Group 1993) is considered to be one of the most important pieces of diabetes research in diabetes care. It demonstrated that tight control of blood glucose prevented or delayed the onset of complications in type 1 diabetes, particularly retinopathy, neuropathy and nephropathy. However, the risk of severe hypoglycaemic attacks increased three-fold.

The reduction of long-term complications in patients with type 2 diabetes is through tight control of blood glucose and maintenance of blood pressure within normal limits. Furthermore, the long-term complications of diabetes such as heart disease and stroke and the loss of sight and kidney damage could also be reduced.

Chronic complications of diabetes mellitus have important implications for the planning of nursing care. Whatever the setting, the nurse should carefully assess the individual's nursing needs, giving special consideration to risks associated with impaired circulation and sensation, increased risk of infection and delayed healing. Recognition of these risk factors will enable care to accommodate the patient's particular vulnerabilities and will help to ensure that suitable educational support is provided.

This section outlines the following chronic complications associated with diabetes:

- atherosclerosis (see Chapter 2)
- cardiovascular disease (see Chapter 2)
- cerebrovascular disease (see Chapter 11)
- diabetic retinopathy (see Chapter 15)
- diabetic nephropathy (see Chapter 10)

Atherosclerosis

Although atherosclerosis is not peculiar to diabetes, it is known that MI, stroke and peripheral vascular disease leading to gangrene are relatively frequent complications and are major causes of death in people with diabetes. Atherosclerosis develops at a much younger age in people with diabetes. This is most noticeable in females.

Both types of diabetes carry increased risk, but those with type 2 diabetes show the strongest tendency to develop atherosclerosis. This is potentially due to age-related factors and the effects of longstanding asymptomatic hyperglycaemia prior to diagnosis. In type 1 diabetes, microvascular disease such as retinopathy usually precedes evidence of atherosclerosis.

Aetiology
A significant proportion of adults with type 2 diabetes have raised blood pressure and/or abnormal cholesterol levels (Song et al. 2016). Risk factors for coronary artery disease are:

- increased concentrations of LDL cholesterol
- decreased concentrations of high-density lipoprotein (HDL) cholesterol
- hypertension
- hyperglycaemia
- smoking.

People with diabetes should focus on managing these risk factors.

Onset and Progress of the Disease
The development and vascular distribution of atherosclerosis in diabetes are similar to that found in the population without diabetes, except the more severe peripheral arterial involvement which may affect the lower limbs of some people with diabetes.

Cardiovascular Disease

Compared with the general population, diabetes in men is associated with a two- to three-fold risk of developing coronary heart disease. In premenopausal women, this is increased to four to five times the risk if the woman has diabetes.

Myocardial Infarction
Atherosclerosis of the coronary arteries causes narrowing which can impair oxygen delivery to the myocardium, resulting in angina pectoris or MI. Due to the effects of autonomic neuropathy, the patient with diabetes may develop a cardiac arrhythmia and may have a 'silent' (painless) MI. Indeed, MI is considered to be more often fatal in people with diabetes compared with MI in those without diabetes, although it seems to be more related to hyperglycaemia on admission than diabetes (Hayıroğlu et al. 2019).

Cerebrovascular Disease

The incidence of stroke in patients with diabetes is also high, and mortality following stroke is increased compared to the population without diabetes. Hypertension is probably the most important of those factors which contribute to the development of atherosclerosis.

Retinopathy

Diabetic retinopathy is one of the leading causes of blindness, with an estimated 37 million cases worldwide (Ting et al. 2016). By 20 years after the onset of diabetes, almost all patients with type 1 diabetes and over 60% of patients with type 2 diabetes will have some degree of retinopathy.

Retinopathy results from changes in the basement membrane of small blood vessels of the retina (retinal microangiopathy) and can take two forms:

- background (nonproliferative) retinopathy including maculopathy
- proliferative retinopathy.

Background Retinopathy and Maculopathy

Background retinopathy rarely causes a major threat to vision unless the macula is affected. In the early stages of retinopathy, the capillaries of the retina become more permeable. This can cause fluid exudation (hard exudate) into the retina.

🌐 **See Evolve website Fig. 6.1**

Retinal veins swell at localised spots, giving the appearance of 'beading'. Microaneurysms can develop; these can rupture, causing small bleeds. Arteriolar occlusions cause retinal infarcts or 'cotton wool spots' on the retina. More spots occur in rapidly developing retinopathy or where there is coexisting hypertension. Evidence of venous bleeding and 'cotton wool' spots suggests progression to preproliferative retinopathy. Maculopathy can cause severe loss of central vision and is most common in type 2 diabetes. In this condition, oedema, haemorrhages and exudates are concentrated on the macular area of the retina.

Proliferative Retinopathy

Microvascular disease of the retina can result in areas of hypoxia. As a compensatory development, new, abnormal blood vessels (neovascularisation) grow forward from the retina to invade the vitreous body.

🌐 **See Evolve website Fig. 6.1**

These new vessels are fragile and poorly supported; consequently, haemorrhages into the vitreous body are common. Progressive traction on the retina can result in retinal detachment. Proliferative retinopathy and retinal detachment will seriously threaten vision.

🔵 Medical Management

The main priorities in the treatment of diabetic retinopathy are to reduce the risk of haemorrhage and to limit new vessel growth into the vitreous body. Photocoagulation by means of laser technology can be used to treat proliferative and pre-proliferative retinopathy.

Screening. Retinal photography should be carried out annually. Many health authorities are using mobile units to carry out retinal screening in the community. Annual ophthalmoscopic examination for those with no identified retinopathy and 6-monthly for those with background retinopathy are strongly advised. This will enable swift and appropriate treatment to help prevent blindness. Where glycaemic control is poor, or where hypertension or renal involvement is more frequent, eye examinations may be recommended. Referral to an ophthalmologist should be made for maculopathy, proliferative and pre-proliferative retinopathy, a reduction in visual acuity, retinal detachment or rubeosis iridis (development of new, abnormal blood vessels on the front of the iris).

🌐 **See Evolve website Fig. 6.3**

Prevention. The patient should be aware of the established link between poor blood glucose control and retinopathy and of the importance of promptly reporting changes in vision. The risks of retinopathy increase if the patient is hypertensive.

Other Eye Disorders

Although retinopathy poses an important threat to vision in diabetes, approximately 50% of visual loss in people affected by type 2 diabetes will be due to other causes that include cataract, age-related macular degeneration, glaucoma, optic neuropathy and occlusion of retinal blood vessels (Holt and Kumar 2015) (see Chapter 15, Nursing Patients With Disorders of the Eye and Sight Impairment).

Unfortunately, many patients with diabetes do ultimately suffer partial or total blindness. Maintaining independence in relation to diabetes management and general self-care will present quite a challenge, but patients may be referred to local visual impairment services and the Royal National Institute of Blind People (RNIB). Various devices are now available which can enable the blind or partially sighted patient to administer insulin and monitor blood glucose. The nurse and the visually impaired patient with diabetes should work together to seek out ways of reducing the patient's dependence on others.

Diabetic Nephropathy

Approximately 30% of patients with type 1 diabetes develop diabetic nephropathy after a disease duration of 20 years (Ting et al. 2016) and up to 40% of patients with type 2 diabetes will eventually develop diabetic nephropathy, the incidence of which is related to the duration of their diabetes (Thomas et al. 2015).

🔵 Aetiology and Pathophysiology

The kidneys of people with diabetes are vulnerable with respect to the following:

- Microvascular changes – damage to the capillaries in the glomeruli can occur. The basement membrane initially thickens and, in the later stages, nodules of glycoprotein are deposited in the glomerular capsule. As a result, the filtering capacity of the glomeruli is reduced.
- Macrovascular changes – atheromatous changes in renal vessels can lead to poor renal perfusion which will ultimately impair renal function.
- Hypertension – a common feature in diabetes, hypertension can contribute to kidney damage and, conversely, can also result from kidney damage.
- UTI can occur for several reasons that include:
  - diabetes-associated predisposition to infection
  - damaged renal tissue vulnerable to infection
  - the need for catheterisation during metabolic crisis
  - atonic bladder associated with autonomic neuropathy, causing urinary stasis and ascending UTI.

🔵 Medical Management

All patients with diabetes should be screened for early renal damage.

Screening involves the measurement of urinary albumin concentration and serum creatinine at regular intervals, usually annually, and this should be measured using an early morning urine sample. Urinary albumin:creatinine ratio should be measured by a laboratory method or a 'near-patient' test specific for albumin at low concentration. Any abnormal result should be confirmed by a further sample (SIGN 2017).

Microalbuminuria is defined as a rise in urinary albumin loss of between 30 mg/day and 300 mg/day. This is the earliest sign of diabetic nephropathy and predicts increased total mortality, cardiovascular mortality and morbidity and end-stage renal failure (SIGN 2017).

All patients with proteinuria should have their blood pressure measured at every clinic or surgery visit. It has been demonstrated that reducing blood pressure from 154/87 mmHg to 144/82 mmHg in type 2 diabetes led to a risk reduction of 8% in developing microalbuminuria over 6 years. Therefore tight blood pressure control (<140/80 mmHg) in patients with type 2 diabetes should be maintained (SIGN 2017). Long-term follow-up studies have shown that a reduction in mean HbA_{1c} (glycated haemoglobin) was associated with a reduction in the occurrence of microalbuminuria and proteinuria (Agrawal et al. 2018).

Established diabetic renal disease is treated in the same way as renal disease in the population without diabetes (see Chapter 10, Nursing Patients With Urinary Disorders).

Treatment choices for the patient in end-stage renal failure include haemodialysis, continuous ambulatory peritoneal dialysis (CAPD) or renal transplant using live or cadaver donors.

Renal transplantation using a live donor offers the best treatment for suitable patients. Careful selection of patients is important, given that other major diabetes-related complications usually coexist with the renal disease. Virtually all patients with end-stage renal failure have retinopathy, and 20%–30% are blind. Retinopathy alone would not militate against active treatment by dialysis or renal transplantation but the presence of widespread cancer, advanced dementia or severe cerebrovascular disease may do so.

Due to the danger of lactic acidosis, the oral hypoglycaemic drug metformin (a biguanide) should not be used for patients with renal impairment. Chlorpropamide (a sulphonylurea) should also be avoided as it is mainly excreted by the kidneys and in renal failure can accumulate in the blood, causing serious hypoglycaemia. For some patients in renal failure, whose diabetes was previously controlled by oral medication, insulin therapy may be indicated.

❖ Nursing Management and Health Promotion: Diabetic Nephropathy

Diabetes control should be closely monitored by regular blood glucose measurement. Measurement and recording of fluid intake and output and body weight may be required to monitor renal function. Dietary and fluid restrictions may be necessary. Patients and their families should be made aware of the vital importance of these measures.

Prevention of Renal Failure

By identifying early renal impairment by screening for microalbuminuria, making efforts to improve diabetes control and detecting and treating hypertension, it is possible to prevent or delay the progression of renal disease (Agrawal et al. 2018).

Nursing and medical staff should exercise extreme caution in the introduction and subsequent care of urinary catheters in order to prevent infection. Prompt treatment of any established UTI will normally be required to minimise damage (Li et al. 2019).

Diabetic Neuropathy

Although the cause of diabetic neuropathy is uncertain, it is a common complication of diabetes with up to 30% (Ziegler et al.

2021). The incidence of diabetic neuropathy is known to rise in line with duration of diabetes and increasing age.

● Pathophysiology

Structural damage to the neurones affecting the Schwann cells causes segmental areas of demyelination to appear, thus impairing conduction of the nerve impulses. There is no widely accepted classification of diabetic neuropathy, but a number of clinical syndromes are recognisable.

Peripheral Neuropathy. This is a distal symmetrical neuropathy, principally affecting the lower extremities and playing a major part in the aetiology of diabetic foot problems. It affects either sensory or motor nerves and the patient's symptoms will reflect this.

Polyneuropathy. This is widespread neuropathic changes affecting many nerves. Again, the lower extremities are often affected (peripheral polyneuropathy).

Mononeuropathies. Single nerves or their roots are affected. The condition is often of rapid onset and reversible, suggesting an acute vascular origin rather than chronic metabolic disturbance (Bilous et al. 2021). Examples of mononeuropathy include ptosis (drooping eyelid) and diplopia (double vision) which can occur as a result of damage to the oculomotor nerves (cranial nerve III).

Autonomic Neuropathies. Damage to autonomic nerves causes numerous abnormalities in many areas of the body. Common manifestations are abnormal sweating, postural hypotension, diarrhoea and erectile dysfunction. Less common are gastroparesis (delayed gastric emptying due to poor motility) and bladder dysfunction (Bilous et al. 2021).

● Medical Management

Prevention of diabetic neuropathy is important and major benchmark studies such as the DCCT have shown that strict glycaemic control can decrease the risk of complications, including neuropathy. Other sensible measures such as avoiding smoking and tight control of blood pressure, blood cholesterol and triglycerides are advised (see Chapter 2, Nursing Patients With Cardiovascular Disorders).

Diabetic neuropathy affects many systems of the body. Management, which is essentially symptomatic, may involve the multidisciplinary efforts of the diabetes care team. A variety of treatment approaches may be adopted, including medication, surgery and physiotherapy.

❖ Nursing Management and Health Promotion: Diabetic Neuropathy

Meeting the particular comfort needs of the patient will be a central focus for nursing care. Reducing the risk of accidental tissue damage arising from severe sensory impairment will also be a priority.

Neuropathies can seriously interfere with lifestyle and emotional well-being. An example of this is erectile dysfunction, which affects up to 35% of all men with diabetes. Erectile dysfunction can be devastating for both the patient and his partner. Many men with diabetes and erectile dysfunction would like help for this problem but are reluctant to seek advice. Once the diagnosis has been made, there are several treatment options available, including professional sexual counselling, vacuum devices, penile injections and oral agents such as sildenafil (see Chapter 9). The choice of treatment will depend on local circumstances, personal

TABLE 6.4	Clinical Signs of the Diabetic Foot	
Sign	Neuropathic Foot	Ischaemic Foot
Temperature	Warm	Cool
Peripheral pulses	Present	Absent
Pain	Loss of sensation	Intermittent claudication and rest pain
Skin	Dry cracking skin	Blanches on elevation
Deformity	Present	Absent
Position of ulcer	Plantar surface, toes or high pressure areas	Margins of foot and toes

experience and, most importantly, the patient's own preference (Hazir et al. 2022).

The Diabetic Foot

People with diabetes are at particular risk of foot problems, either neuropathic or caused by ischaemia. People with diabetes must be screened, at least annually, for foot disease. Based on UK population surveys, diabetic foot problems are a common complication of diabetes, with prevalences of 23%–42% for neuropathy, 9%–23% for vascular disease (ischaemic foot) and 5%–7% for foot ulceration (SIGN 2017) (Table 6.4). Education of the patient is vital to prevent problems (Information 6.4).

Screening – foot examination by trained professionals should consist of foot inspection for appearance and footwear, and assessment of sensation using a 10 g monofilament. Palpation of foot pulses and use of Doppler ultrasound should be undertaken if possible.

Painful peripheral neuropathy can be a major problem for many people, particularly at night. It can be treated with some success by tricyclic antidepressants such as amitriptyline. Gabapentin has also been shown to be effective, with fewer side-effects. Topical capsaicin should also be considered for localised neuropathic pain.

Deformity of the foot can lead to ulceration, particularly in the absence of protective pain sensation and with the contribution of unsuitable footwear. Early detection can initiate properly fitting shoes before ulceration occurs.

Charcot foot/Charcot joint is a neuroarthropathic syndrome with osteoporosis, fracture, acute inflammation and disorganisation of foot architecture (SIGN 2017). Signs and symptoms include a hot, red and swollen foot with, or often without, pain. Immobilisation of the limb, usually by casting of the foot, and reduction of stress by decreasing the amount of weight-bearing on the affected limb through use of crutches are the current mainstays of treatment. However, other treatment options are being considered, including drug intervention.

Management of Ulcers

Neuropathic ulcers are most frequently caused from callus build-up and potentially thermal injury, e.g. stepping into hot water, and chemical injury, such as from use of corn plasters. The injury is usually not perceived by the patient, due to loss of pain sensation. The treatment aim is to redistribute plantar pressures by

some form of cast or cradled insole. However, in the neuroischaemic foot, the aim is to protect the vulnerable margins of the foot such as by the use of a wide-fitting shoe.

The ulcer will require initial debridement and management of exudate with an appropriate wound dressing product (see Chapter 23, Tissue Viability and Managing Chronic Wounds). Biological debridement using larval therapy can be very effective. The larvae (maggots) of the sterile blowfly (*Lucilia serricata*) are applied to the wound where the enzymes they produce remove slough and necrotic tissue thereby providing more favourable conditions for healing (see Chapter 23).

Infection. The use of broad-spectrum antibiotics is vital to help improve healing. A wound swab for culture should be taken before antibiotics are commenced. Progression to cellulitis and osteomyelitis will require hospital admission for administration of IV antibiotics, immobilisation and appropriate wound management. Stress hormones are released in response to severe infection, causing hyperglycaemia. The resulting increase in insulin demand will present an increased challenge to the pancreas, increasing the risk of metabolic crisis. IV fluids and insulin may be required.

Necrosis. The ischaemic foot results from atherosclerotic changes in the distal arteries of the legs. Revascularisation of the infected neuroischaemic foot should be explored. Angioplasty is indicated in the treatment of single or multiple stenosis or short segment occlusions of blood vessels. If angioplasty is not possible because of long arterial occlusions, bypass should be considered. Patients with a neuropathic foot in which there is necrosis will probably require surgical debridement. However, severely affected patients may eventually require digital amputation or, in even more serious cases, a below-knee amputation (see Chapter 12, Nursing Patients With Musculoskeletal Disorders).

Nurses involved in the care of people with diabetes should undertake regular monitoring of the patient's feet and commence appropriate and timely treatment whenever necessary.

Facilitating Self-Care Through Education

In both hospital and community settings, overall coordination of patient learning is undertaken by the diabetes specialist nurse working closely with the specialist dietitian and the patient's physician. Care of patients, with type 2 diabetes in particular, will be undertaken by community and hospital nurses who are not specialists in diabetes care. All such nurses may be required to undertake a teaching role and must therefore ensure that their own knowledge base is adequate.

Assessment

By establishing a rapport with the patient and family, the nurse will be equipped to assess the patient's needs in relation to:
- current level of knowledge about diabetes
- understanding of the reasons for prescribed treatment
- knowledge and skills required for self-care
- emotional response to the diagnosis
- social support from family and friends
- barriers to learning, e.g. sensory loss, mobility and manipulation problems, language difficulties, reading and writing difficulties and intellectual impairment.

🌐 **See Evolve website Critical thinking question 6.2**

Planning a Teaching Programme

Staff members must show consistency in the information they provide. Any member of the diabetes care team may be involved in coaching the patient and family in diabetes management. It is likely that the majority of this will rest with the nursing staff, including the diabetes specialist nurse who will work in partnership with the patient and family. The most important team member is of course the patient.

Sessions should be short and information presented in small, easily assimilated and integrated sections with teaching points categorised into lists. Ordering presentation so that the most important point is always raised first can help the patient to prioritise information. Being direct and specific will aid retention, as will using simple words and brief sentences.

Clarifying points and ensuring comprehension before moving to a new topic are very important. Interactive participation is encouraged, although not everyone will feel comfortable with this approach.

Adopting a friendly manner and taking time to talk about non-medical matters can relax the patient and set the scene for a more productive session. It is important to consider the age group for which teaching materials have been designed in order to avoid giving inappropriate information.

An impressive array of informative and attractive booklets is available, many of which are sponsored by manufacturers and written by diabetes healthcare professionals. These provide back-up for teaching and discussion and aide memoires for patients. Conversation maps, patient-orientated websites and DVDs can be sourced for patients to view individually or in groups. DAFNE in type 1 diabetes and Diabetes Education and Self-Management for Ongoing and Newly Diagnosed (DESMOND) in type 2 diabetes are structured education packages used throughout the UK (Reflection 6.5).

The Programme
The teaching programme should be tailored to suit the patient's individual needs but is likely to include some of the following topics:
- What is diabetes? Type 1 and type 2
- Treatment of diabetes
  - oral hypoglycaemics
  - insulin therapy
- Why insulin and how does it work?
- Types of insulin
- Storage and administration of insulin
- Diet–insulin–exercise balance – insulin dose adjustment (Information 6.5)
- Monitoring blood glucose
- Recognising and treating hypo- and hyperglycaemia
- What to do during illness
- Testing for ketones
- Avoiding complications
- Health screening
- Lifestyle factors – sport, alcohol, smoking, illicit drugs, driving, travel, pregnancy and sexual health.

Exercise and People With Diabetes

Exercise and increasing activity can provide many health benefits for the person with diabetes, such as improving insulin sensitivity, weight management and reduction, heart and circulatory protection, strengthening of joints and bones and many other benefits. Exercise will reduce blood glucose levels, and a clear understanding of the role of exercise in blood glucose control is essential for every patient with diabetes. The nurse must find a way of explaining this role that is appropriate to the learning needs of individual patients. The analogy of 'fuel intake' (food) and 'energy output' (activity/exercise) is often useful for the purposes of illustration.

What Happens During Exercise?

When energy output is low, the demand for fuel in the form of glucose is also low. However, during bursts of physical activity the demand for glucose will rise and it is then drawn from the glycogen reserves in the liver and muscles. The rate at which glucose is taken up by the cells is influenced by medication (insulin or tablets). If available supplies of glucose are depleted and are not replaced, the patient's blood glucose will fall and may continue to fall for several hours after prolonged or intense exercise, thus increasing the risk of hypoglycaemia.

Avoiding Exercise-Induced Hypoglycaemia

Insulin-treated patients should be advised to monitor blood glucose before and after exercise and when to take extra carbohydrate to avoid hypoglycaemia. A quickly absorbable form of glucose such as glucose tablets or a glucose drink may be used to augment diet and help prevent an abrupt fall in blood glucose. Another strategy to avoid exercise-induced hypoglycaemia is for the insulin dose to be reduced prior to planned and prolonged strenuous activity. Insulin dose adjustment in relation to exercise is an important aspect of the patient's education programme when commencing insulin therapy. Blood glucose should then be monitored to gauge the effects of any reduction. Patients controlled with oral hypoglycaemic therapy may, less frequently, also experience exercise-induced hypoglycaemia and consequently may need to adjust their carbohydrate intake to meet the additional energy demands imposed by the exercise.

Patients with type 1 diabetes should also be made aware that hyperglycaemia (blood glucose >14.0 mmol/L) with ketonuria is an absolute contraindication to exercise as this can indicate that there is a lack of circulating insulin and that the patient is metabolically unstable. Exercise in this situation could cause higher blood glucose levels.

Promoting Psychological and Social Adjustment

A diagnosis of diabetes has an emotional impact on those affected. The shock of a diagnosis of diabetes has been likened to the experience of bereavement (DeCosta et al. 2020). People newly diagnosed with diabetes may experience the following responses:
- shock and disbelief of diagnosis
- anxiety about different aspects of managing the condition
- confusion about all the information given at diagnosis
- fear about the future and possible development of complications
- anger that it has happened and a feeling of 'why me?'
- sadness at the loss of the person before diagnosis
- stress at not being able to cope.

Psychosocial Factors Influencing Self-management of Diabetes

Diabetes self-management is seen as mostly the patient's responsibility. This is an enormous demand on the person with diabetes and their family. One of the purposes of diabetes education is to impart knowledge and skills that enable the person with diabetes to make informed decisions about how they are going to lead their life with diabetes. However, there are other determinants of behaviour which can influence behavioural choices. These include health beliefs, the person's locus of control (Nuccitelli et al. 2018), self-efficacy, behavioural intentions, quality of life and emotional well-being and depression (SIGN 2017). (See Further Reading, e.g. Wills 2022.)

Behaviour Changes

The empowerment model (Gómez-Velasco et al. 2019) is the model of choice which acknowledges the patient's expertise, their personal responsibilities in self-management and their right to informed choice (see Further Reading, e.g. Wills 2022).

Lifestyle Implications

The charity Diabetes UK works to raise funds for diabetes research and to increase the awareness of diabetes and its implications. Vitally, it also provides information and advice for people with diabetes and professionals involved in their care. It is a national organisation with local branches throughout the UK. Different sections cater for particular groups, e.g. teenagers and those with visual impairment. Diabetes UK offers help and advice on a wide variety of topics such as monitoring and treatment approaches, insurance, holidays and travelling abroad.

Employment

In view of the risk of hypoglycaemia, people with diabetes who are treated with insulin are excluded from some areas of employment, e.g. those which involve certain categories of vocational driving (see next section), airline piloting and air traffic control, deep sea diving, working on offshore oil rigs, working down coal mines, at heights or near dangerous moving machinery. Diabetes would also exclude an applicant from joining the UK armed forces, whereas police forces will review applications on a case-by-case basis. However, in many cases, if diabetes develops while in the job, it is sometimes possible to continue employment. (See Useful Websites, e.g. Diabetes UK.)

Driving and Motor Vehicle Insurance

The UK Driver Vehicle Licensing Authority (DVLA) must, by law, be informed when a driver is diagnosed as having diabetes and is receiving treatment with insulin; the requirement to inform the DVLA when treated with oral therapies is dependent on the specific treatment. A medical practitioner may be required to advise on the stability of the driver's diabetes control prior to relicensing. The DVLA must be informed if any problems or diabetic complications develop which may affect safety.

Different regulations apply to different groups of vehicles; for example the medical standard is more stringent for a group 2 licence covering Large Goods Vehicle (LGV) and/or a Passenger Carrying Vehicle (PCV). People will have their group 2 licence removed when they commence insulin therapy. There are also restrictions on lighter goods and smaller passenger vehicle licences. Hypoglycaemia is the main danger when driving. People with diabetes should receive education about how to avoid and effectively manage hypoglycaemia when driving.

Patients whose diabetes is treated with medication must inform their insurer. Failure to notify the insurer can result in withdrawal of insurance cover, invalidate any claim and lead to the offence of driving without third party insurance.

The regulations concerning driving and mandatory third-party insurance for people with diabetes are complex and readers are directed to the helpful information produced by Diabetes UK (see Useful Websites, e.g. Diabetes UK Diabetes Information Driving and Diabetes).

Travel

Altered mealtimes, travelling across different time zones and dietary and climatic changes may all have an effect on diabetes management. It is essential for the person with diabetes to monitor their diabetes closely whilst travelling. They must seek specific advice from their GP or the diabetes team regarding insulin adjustment. All medication and monitoring equipment should be carried in hand luggage to allow for ready access and to reduce risk of loss. Also, the extremely low temperature of the cargo hold can adversely affect the action of insulin. A doctor's letter detailing the need to carry injecting equipment and blood glucose monitoring equipment in their hand luggage is required for air travel. (See Useful Websites, e.g. Fit for Travel.)

Eating Out

Flexible insulin regimens, insulin pen devices and SBGM have simplified eating out for people with diabetes. People having insulin therapy are advised as to appropriate insulin adjustment to allow more freedom of choice when eating out.

Smoking

Having diabetes increases the risk of developing vascular and neuropathic disorders. Smoking compounds these risks. The diabetes team should encourage smoking cessation and should discuss the availability of resources to provide support whilst the patient is trying to stop smoking. However, it must be accepted that the patient may decide to continue to smoke against advice.

Identification

Patients should be strongly advised to carry a card or wear a MediCAlert pendant or bracelet to identify themselves and give details of the type of diabetes they have and its management.

Future Developments

Research in diabetes care is at an exciting stage. Combined kidney and pancreas transplants are now undertaken in a number of centres in the UK for those with renal failure as a complication of type 1 diabetes. Successful transplantation allows the patient to be free of the restrictions of renal dialysis as well as daily injections of insulin.

Pancreatic islet cell transplantation offers people with type 1 diabetes hope for a cure. This is the subject of intensive research trials. Islet cells are isolated from the donor pancreas and injected into the liver of the recipient. The cells develop a blood supply and begin to produce insulin, a process called the Edmonton protocol. New combinations of immunosuppressive agents prevent the body rejecting the transplanted islet cells, eliminating the need for corticosteroid therapy which could damage the newly transplanted cells. A major drawback to the increasing availability of this advance is that the equivalent of two donated pancreases is required to provide sufficient islet cells for transplantation.

Over the years, feasibility studies into the effectiveness of non-enteral routes of delivering insulin have been attempted. These have included ocular, buccal, rectal, vaginal, oral, nasal and uterine delivery systems. A body of evidence suggested that inhaled insulin was an effective, well-tolerated, noninvasive alternative to SC soluble insulin for patients with type 1 and type 2 diabetes (Home and Mehta 2021). Inhaled insulin became available on prescription to patients in the UK in 2006, but was discontinued in 2007 due to economic reasons.

Research is ongoing into the closed loop system or 'artificial pancreas'. It consists of a continuous glucose meter and an insulin pump, allowing communication between the devices. It is hoped to develop a system that will automatically check blood glucose and administer an appropriate dose of insulin, thus allowing more freedom and greater diabetes control for the user (Zhou and Isaacs, 2022).

The ultimate hope is that diabetes will at some future date be preventable. Researchers continue to seek definitive answers to the questions surrounding aetiological factors, with a view to finding ways of manipulating these factors to prevent the disease developing.

Trends in Diabetes Care Provision

Over recent years, there have been significant changes in the structure and function of the primary care team and a shift of focus with more healthcare provided in community settings. Emphasis has been on developing further the role of the diabetes specialist nurse who 'can transform the standard of diabetic care, achieving liaison between hospital, GP and patients at home and offering a wide range of clinical and educational expertise' (Watkins et al. 2003).

The growth in the number of practice nurses has made it possible for many GP practices to run their own clinics for people with diabetes. In some areas, dietitians and podiatrists are available in the health centres where clinics are run.

Community nurses and health visitors may find themselves taking high-quality diabetes care directly into the patient's home. Effective hospital–community liaison will become especially important to ensure continuity for the patient in 'shared care'.

Whatever the care setting, it is important that the patient has access to facilities for estimation of glycated haemoglobin and microalbuminuria and for screening for retinopathy and foot-threatening neuropathic or vascular disease. It appears likely that integrated hospital and community care will offer the best use of resources for diabetes screening. However, dealing with a severe metabolic crisis such as DKA will remain the province of the hospital.

Continuing education for all members of the diabetes care team must be a priority. National standards and guidelines and frameworks are necessary to create best practice through a firm research base and to support provision of the highest possible quality of care for people with diabetes. Diabetes specialist nurses and community diabetes facilitators make a significant contribution in the education of their colleagues. Providing education and support which will enable the patient to move away from the despondency and fear which frequently accompany diagnosis, towards independence and autonomy, is surely both the science and the art of nursing care in diabetes.

Summary: Key Nursing Issues

- Diabetes is often referred to as an 'epidemic'. Diabetes UK (2019) estimates that there are around 3.9 million people diagnosed with the condition in the UK and there are more than half a million individuals who are unaware that they have diabetes.
- Diabetes is a metabolic disease which results from defects in insulin secretion, insulin action or both (WHO 2016). The two main types are type 1 and type 2.
- All nurses, wherever they practise, will encounter people with diabetes.
- Nurses have a vital health promotion role in the prevention and early detection of type 2 diabetes.
- Diabetes specialist nurses are key in the education of people diagnosed with diabetes so they can understand and manage their condition.

- Lifestyle and healthy eating are the cornerstones of effective glycaemic control. Patient-centred care is paramount.
- Acute life-threatening complications, e.g. hyperglycaemia leading to DKA, can occur.
- Diabetes is associated with several long-term complications that include sight impairment, renal failure, neuropathy and cardiovascular diseases.
- People with diabetes require tailored care to reduce complications.
- Diabetes management is constantly evolving, as new evidence emerges. Research continues into the possibility of manipulating aetiological factors to prevent diabetes developing.

Reflection and Learning – What Next?

- **Test** your knowledge by visiting the Evolve website 🌐 and answering the multiple-choice questions and critical thinking questions.
- **Consolidate** your learning by looking at some of the further reading suggestions, references and specialist websites.
- **Revisit** some of the additional material on the Evolve website.
- **Consider** what you have learnt and how this will help your professional development.

- **Reflect** on how you can apply this knowledge to the care of your patients.
- **Discuss** your learning with your supervisor/assessor, lecturer and colleagues.

References

Agrawal L, Azad N, Bahn GD, Ge L, et al. Long-term follow-up of intensive glycaemic control on renal outcomes in the Veterans Affairs Diabetes Trial (VADT). *Diabetologia.* 2018;61(2):295–299.

Ahmad E, Lim S, Lamptey R, Webb DR, Davies MJ. Type 2 diabetes. *Lancet North Am Ed.* 2022;400(10365):1803–1820.

Bilous R, Donnelly R, Idris I. *Handbook of Diabetes.* 5th ed. Oxford: Wiley-Blackwell; 2021.

Chief Medical Officer. UK Chief Medical Officer's Alcohol Guideline Review: Summary of the Proposed New Guidelines. 2016. https://assets.publishing.service.gov.uk/government/uploads/system/uploads/attachment_data/file/489795/summary.pdf

DAFNE Study Group. Training in flexible, intensive insulin management to enable dietary freedom in people with type 1 diabetes: Dose Adjustment For Normal Eating (DAFNE) randomised controlled trial. *BMJ.* 2002;325:746–749.

DeCosta P, Grabowski D, Skinner TC. The psychosocial experience and needs of children newly diagnosed with type 1 diabetes from their own perspective: a systematic and narrative review. *Diabet Med.* 2020;37(10):1640–1652.

Delaney KZ, Santosa S. Sex differences in regional adipose tissue depots pose different threats for the development of type 2 diabetes in males and females. *Obes Rev.* 2022;23(3):e13393.

Department of Health. National Service Framework for Diabetes: Standards. 2001. https://assets.publishing.service.gov.uk/government/uploads/system/uploads/attachment_data/file/198836/National_Service_Framework_for_Diabetes.pdf.

Department of Health. Five years on: delivering the Diabetes National Service Framework. 2008. http://webarchive.nationalarchives.gov.uk/20130123201230/http://www.dh.gov.uk/en/Publicationsandstatistics/Publications/PublicationsPolicyAndGuidance/DH_112509.

Dhatariya KK. Defining and characterising diabetic ketoacidosis in adults. *Diabetes Res Clin Pract.* 2019;155:107797.

Diabetes Control and Complications Research Group. The effect of diabetes on the development and progression of long term complications in insulin dependent diabetes. *N Engl J Med.* 1993;329:977–986.

Diabetes UK. Diabetes prevalence 2019. 2019. https://www.diabetes.org.uk/professionals/position-statements-reports/statistics/diabetes-prevalence-2019.

Diabetes UK. Diabetes and checking your blood sugars. 2023. https://www.diabetes.org.uk/guide-to-diabetes/managing-your-diabetes/testing.

Evert AB, Dennison M, Gardner CD, et al. Nutrition therapy for adults with diabetes or prediabetes: a consensus report. *Diabetes Care.* 2019;42(5):731–754.

Forouhi NG, Wareham NJ. Epidemiology of diabetes. *Med (Baltimore).* 2022;50(10):638–643.

Gabbay-Benziv R, Reece EA, Wang F, Yang P. Birth defects in pregestational diabetes: Defect range, glycemic threshold and pathogenesis. *World J Diabetes.* 2015;6(3):481–488.

Gentile S, Strollo F, Viazzi F, et al. Five-year predictors of insulin initiation in people with type 2 diabetes under real-life conditions. *J Diabetes Res.* 2018;Sep 19:2018. https://doi.org/10.1155/2018/7153087.

Goff LM. Ethnicity and type 2 diabetes in the UK. *Diabet Med.* 2019;36(8):927–938.

Goldman N, Fink D, Cai J, Lee YN, Davies Z. High prevalence of COVID-19-associated diabetic ketoacidosis in UK secondary care. *Diabetes Res Clin Pract.* 2020;166:108291.

Gómez-Velasco DV, Almeda-Valdes P, Martagón AJ, Galán-Ramírez GA, Aguilar-Salinas CA. Empowerment of patients with type 2 diabetes: current perspectives. *Diabetes Metab Syndr Obes: Targets and Therapy.* 2019:1311–1321.

Hayıroğlu Mİ, Keskin M, Uzun AO, et al. Predictors of in-hospital mortality in patients with ST-segment elevation myocardial infarction complicated with cardiogenic shock. *Heart Lung Circ.* 2019;28(2):237–244.

Hazir B, Haberal HB, Asci A, Muneer A, Gudeloglu A. Erectile dysfunction management: a critical appraisal of clinical practice guidelines with the AGREE II instrument. *Int J Impot Res.* 2022;34(5):471–476.

Heller S, Chow E. Hypoglycaemia in diabetes. *Med (Baltimore)*. 2014;42(12):727–731.

Holt T, Kumar S. *ABC of Diabetes*. 7th ed. Oxford: BMJ Books Wiley-Blackwell; 2015.

Home PD, Mehta R. Insulin therapy development beyond 100 years. The Lancet Diabetes & Endocrinology. 2021; 9(10):695–707.

International Diabetes Federation (IDF). 2022. IDF Diabetes Atlas. https://diabetesatlas.org/

Kapoor N, Furler J, Paul TV, Thomas N, Oldenburg B. Normal weight obesity: an underrecognized problem in individuals of South Asian descent. *Clin Ther*. 2019;41(8):1638–1642.

Khunti K, Mathieu C, Torbeyns B, et al. Diabetes registries and high-quality diabetes care. *Lancet Diabetes Endocrinol*. 2023;11(2):70–72.

Li F, Song M, Xu L, Deng B, Zhu S, Li X. Risk factors for catheter-associated urinary tract infection among hospitalized patients: a systematic review and meta-analysis of observational studies. *J Adv Nurs*. 2019;75(3):517–527.

Massó-González EL, Johansson S, Wallander M, García-Rodríguez LA. Trends in the prevalence and incidence of Diabetes in the UK –1996 to 2005. *Epidemiol Community Health*. 2009;63(4):332–336.

NICE (National Institute for Health and Care Excellence). *Type 2 diabetes in adults: management*. NICE guideline [NG28]; 2022. https://www.nice.org.uk/guidance/ng28.

Nuccitelli C, Valentini A, Caletti MT, et al. Sense of coherence, self-esteem, and health locus of control in subjects with type 1 diabetes mellitus with/without satisfactory metabolic control. *J Endocrinol Invest*. 2018;41(3):307–314.

Reed RM, Nevitt SJ, Kemp GJ, Cuthbertson DJ, Whyte MB, Goff LM. Ectopic fat deposition in populations of black African ancestry: a systematic review and meta-analysis. *Acta Diabetol*. 2022;1:1–7.

Saeedi P, Petersohn I, Salpea P, et al. Global and regional diabetes prevalence estimates for 2019 and projections for 2030 and 2045: results from the International Diabetes Federation Diabetes Atlas. *Diabetes Res Clin Pract*. 2019;157:107843.

Sainsbury E, Kizirian NV, Partridge SR, et al. Effect of dietary carbohydrate restriction on glycemic control in adults with diabetes: a systematic review and meta-analysis. *Diabetes Res Clin Pract*. 2018;139:239–252.

Scottish Intercollegiate Guidelines Network (SIGN). Management of diabetes: a national clinical guideline. No. 116; 2017. https://www.sign.ac.uk/assets/sign116.pdf.

Song Y, Liu X, Zhu X, et al. Increasing trend of diabetes combined with hypertension or hypercholesterolemia: NHANES data analysis 1999–2012. *Sci Rep*. 2016;6(1):36093.

Thomas MC, Brownlee M, Susztak K, et al. Diabetic kidney disease. *Nat Rev Dis Primers*. 2015;1:15018.

Ting DSW, Cheung GCM, Wong TY. Diabetic retinopathy: global prevalence, major risk factors, screening practices and public health challenges: a review. *Clin Experiment Ophthalmol*. 2016;44(4):260–277.

Watkins PJ, Amiel SA, Howell SL. *Diabetes and Its Management*. 6th ed. Oxford: Blackwell; 2003.

Wei M, Gaskill SP, Haffner SM, Stern MP. Waist circumference as the best predictor of non-insulin dependent diabetes mellitus (NIDDM) compared to body mass index, waist/hip ratio and other anthropometric measurements in Mexican Americans: a 7 year prospective study. *Obes Res*. 1997;5(1):16–23.

Whicher CA, O'Neill S, Holt RG. Diabetes in the UK: 2019. *Diabet Med*. 2020;37(2):242–247.

World Health Organisation (WHO). Global report on diabetes. 2016. Available from: http://apps.who.int/iris/bitstream/handle/10665/204871/9789241565257_eng.pdf;jsessionid=D45D4403D8B0E34D73EF5AF1A320314E?sequence=1.

World Health Organization. Definition and diagnosis of diabetes mellitus and intermediate hyperglycaemia: report of a WHO/IDF consultation. 2006. Available from http://apps.who.int/iris/bitstream/handle/10665/43588/9241594934_eng.pdf?sequence=1.

Zhou K, Isaacs D. Closed-loop artificial pancreas therapy for type 1 diabetes. *Curr Cardiol Rep*. 2022;24(9):1159–1167.

Ziegler D, Papanas N, Schnell O, ET AL. Current concepts in the management of diabetic polyneuropathy. *J Diabetes Investig*. 2021;12(4):464–475.

Further Reading

Barnard KD, Lloyd CE. *Psychology and Diabetes Care: A Practical Guide*. London: Springer; 2012.

British National Formulary. 2023. https://bnf.nice.org.uk/

Department of Health. Five years on: delivering the Diabetes National Service Framework. 2008. http://webarchive.nationalarchives.gov.uk/20130123201230/http://www.dh.gov.uk/en/Publicationsandstatistics/Publications/PublicationsPolicyAndGuidance/DH_112509.

Diabetes UK. Pregnancy Care for Women With Diabetes 2015; 2015. https://www.diabetes.org.uk/resources-s3/2017-09/NPID15_Easy_Report_V10.pdf?

Dunning T, Sinclair A. *Care of People With Diabetes: A Manual of Nursing Practice*. 5th ed. Oxford: Wiley-Blackwell; 2020.

Edmonds ME, Foster AVM. *Managing the Diabetic Foot*. 3rd ed. Oxford: Wiley-Blackwell; 2014.

Fisher M. *Heart Disease and Diabetes*. 2nd ed. Oxford: OUP; 2012.

Frier BM, Heller S, McCrimmon R. *Hypoglycaemia in Clinical Diabetes*. 3rd ed. Oxford: Wiley-Blackwell; 2014.

National Institute for Health and Care Excellence (NICE). *Diabetic foot problems: prevention and management*. NICE guideline [NG19]; 2019. https://www.nice.org.uk/guidance/ng19.

Scanlon P, Sallam A, van Wijngaarden P. *A Practical Manual of Diabetic Retinopathy Management*. Oxford: Wiley-Blackwell; 2017.

Tortora GJ. Principles of Anatomy and Physiology. *Global Edition*. 15th ed. New York: John Wiley & Sons; 2017.

Wills J. *Foundations for Health Promotion (Public Health and Health Promotion)*. Elsevier; 2022.

Useful Websites

Abbott Diabetes Care (Abbott Laboratories), https://www.diabetes.co.uk/diabetes_industries/Abbott-Diabetes-Care.html

British National Formulary, https://bnf.nice.org.uk/BD Living with Diabetes, https://livingwithdiabetes.bd.com/.

Diabetes Education and Self-Management for Ongoing and Newly Diagnosed (DESMOND), https://www.desmond.nhs.uk/

Diabetes UK, www.diabetes.org.uk

Driving With Diabetes, www.diabetes.org.uk/guide-to-diabetes/life-with-diabetes/driving

Dose Adjustment For Normal Eating (DAFNE), https://dafne.nhs.uk/

Fit for Travel, https://www.fitfortravel.nhs.uk/advice/general-travel-health-advice/diabetes

Gov.UK, https://www.gov.uk/browse/driving/disability-health-condition

International Diabetes Federation, www.idf.org

National Institute for Health and Care Excellence (NICE), www.nice.org.uk

Royal National Institute of Blind People (RNIB), www.rnib.org.uk

Scottish Intercollegiate Guidelines Network (SIGN), www.sign.ac.uk

World Health Organisation (WHO) Diabetes, https://www.who.int/health-topics/diabetes#tab=tab_1

7

Nursing Patients With Disorders of the Lymphatic and Immune Systems

BARRY HILL

CHAPTER OUTLINE

Introduction

The immune system, acting as the body's safeguard, counteracts a multitude of threats, encompassing external pathogens such as bacteria and viruses, and internal dangers like cancer. Comprising a complex network of tissues and cells, it efficiently contains or eradicates these potential threats. Nevertheless, the immune system's powerful mechanisms can sometimes go awry, resulting in autoimmune diseases where it erroneously attacks the body. Additionally, the lymphatic system, an intricate assembly of vessels, cells and organs, diligently conducts fluid from the tissues to the circulatory system. Given this function, it is optimally positioned to survey the tissues for signs of infection or damage and relay this critical information to the immune system. Although these two systems are discussed separately later, it is paramount to note their intimate connection.

This chapter aims to discuss the immune and lymphatic systems, explain their collaborative role in body defence and briefly address potential illnesses that may occur if the immune system malfunctions.

The Immune System and the Concept of Self vs Non-Self

At its core, the immune system's primary function is the defence of the body. Constituting specialised cells, tissues and a plethora of chemical messengers and signals, it works in unison to amplify and coordinate immune responses. The origin of immune system cells is traced back to the bone marrow, where the process of haematopoiesis occurs. However, certain immune cell types mature in tissues outside the bone marrow. Collectively, the immune system cells that circulate in the bloodstream are known as leucocytes.

A valuable framework to understand the immune system is through the lens of the self and non-self-paradigm. In this construct, the immune system's role is to distinguish between self (elements intrinsic to you) and non-self (elements foreign to you). Anything perceived as non-self is deemed a health threat, prompting the immune system to contain or eliminate it.

This is discernible in the case of bacterial infections; invading bacteria, classified as non-self, should be contained or eradicated before causing harm to the body. Nevertheless, there are circumstances where the self/non-self paradigm falls short, such as during ingestion. Ingesting food introduces non-self elements into the body (self), yet the immune system does not react adversely. This phenomenon, known as oral tolerance, is utilised in certain treatments for food allergies. However, leveraging oral tolerance entails the risk of severe allergic reactions (anaphylaxis) and should always be administered under medical supervision.

Pregnancy is another scenario where the self/non-self paradigm falters. Although the fetus is fundamentally non-self, it is typically not targeted by the immune system. To accommodate the fetus and placenta, the maternal immune system undergoes various adaptations leading to tolerance. In certain instances, these mechanisms can malfunction, resulting in spontaneous abortion or pre-eclampsia.

The concept of self/non-self also holds clinical significance in organ transplants. Often, the host's immune system perceives the transplanted organ as non-self and attempts to reject it. In bone marrow transplants (commonly used in leukaemia treatment), the immune system operates against the host. Since all immune cells originate from bone marrow, the recipient effectively inherits the donor's immune system. Upon finding itself in a new body, the donor's immune system, recognising the body as non-self, triggers various symptoms indicating an attack on the body.

❖ Nursing Management and Health Promotion: Reduced Immune System – General Principles

Due to the integral nature of the immune system, its thorough and effective functioning is crucial in averting illnesses. It is generally acknowledged that any individual suffering from any ailment is likely to have some level of immunocompromise. As such, healthcare providers, particularly nurses, must recognise that patients could be more susceptible to infections and an elevated likelihood of both external (e.g. skin) and internal (e.g. mucous membrane) barrier disruptions. Both young and elderly patients possess an augmented risk of infection. Several organisms, such as Candida and bacteria, can give rise to opportunistic infections in ill individuals. Given the escalating concern of antibiotic resistance, these infections can be profoundly severe. Thus, measures to mitigate such risks should be judiciously employed. Mastery and application of fundamental infection and aseptic techniques become paramount. Key actions, such as meticulous handwashing and diligent sterilisation of equipment shared between patients (e.g. trolleys), are indispensable.

In the following sections, we shall delve into the anatomy and physiology of the immune system and explore nursing care for a variety of immune system-related concerns.

The Innate Immune System

Broadly speaking, there are two branches of the immune system – the innate immune system and the adaptive immune system. The innate branch includes all the defences we are born with. These include the skin and mucosal (epithelial) barriers – structures we would not normally consider part of the immune system. However, a moment's thought should convince you that without your skin and the mucosal barriers, it would be easy for any external pathogen or toxin to enter your body and do damage. There are also specialised cells that are part of the innate immune system. These include the macrophages and monocytes, the neutrophils, natural killer cells, eosinophils and basophils. Macrophages and neutrophils are specialised to ingest invading pathogens by a process called phagocytosis and are collectively called phagocytes. The phagocytes and other cells of the innate immune system play roles in both frontline defence and in communicating information about threats to other parts of the immune system. The cells of the innate immune system either circulate in the bloodstream, are resident in tissues or are resident in lymphatic tissue (e.g. lymph nodes, the spleen – see later). Finally, there are various proteins and signalling molecules that are components of the innate immune system as well. These proteins and signalling molecules serve various purposes from marking potential pathogens (so they are more easily recognised and destroyed) to communicating information about the state of tissue damage and the activation of the immune system. The innate system often deals with threats before we even know they are present because it works very quickly. The characteristic sign of an innate immune response is inflammation.

Inflammation

Inflammation is often described in terms of four cardinal signs. These are redness, swelling, heat and pain. Sometimes loss of function (due to the other signs) is also included. How do these arise? Tissue damage, like a wound – a breach in innate skin defences – may result in bacteria entering the body. The skin cells around the wound release various damage signals (these include molecules like histamine and prostaglandins). The purpose of these chemicals is to signal to the innate immune system that there has been a breach in the 'outer defences'. These signals summon the cells of the innate immune system, especially the phagocytes, to the site of damage to deal with damaged tissue and any invading pathogens. Since the innate immune cells circulate in the bloodstream, we want to get a lot of blood into the area. Therefore the damage signals also cause nearby blood vessels to dilate, bringing in more blood leading to local redness and an increase in local temperature (heat). The dilated blood vessels alter their lining to make themselves stickier. Innate immune cells which would normally rush through these vessels with blood flow begin to stick to the vessel walls near the site of injury. These cells need to get out of the bloodstream and into the site of injury. Consequently, the vessels also become leakier – they increase the gaps in their walls. This allows the innate immune cells to squeeze out but it also allows a lot of fluid out into the area which leads to swelling. This fluid contains antimicrobial compounds (e.g. complement) and will also serve to wash the area. The tissue damage signals also trigger pain receptors, and this leads to the sensation of pain at the site of injury. Drugs like aspirin and ibuprofen work by preventing the manufacture of these tissue damage signals; this is why they have analgesic and other anti-inflammatory effects. The inflammatory response happens extremely quickly and is usually apparent a few seconds after the wound or other stimulus occurs.

Importance of External Barriers

The natural barriers between our body and the external environment are the most basic defence mechanisms we have. These barriers prevent the establishment of infection. The skin and mucus membranes make up the first line of defence against potential pathogens. The surface layer of the skin is composed of dead cells which are continually lost. Any potential pathogen that can cause tissue damage that lands on the skin is thus swept off. In addition, skin secretions and sweat serve to wash off contaminating organisms and contain several antibacterial and antifungal substances. Saliva in the mouth contains various substances that contribute to innate immunity. In particular the enzyme lysozyme can destroy some bacterial cell walls. Pathogens we ingest with food are subject to the harsh acidic environment of the stomach. Other mucosal membranes lining the genitourinary tract, the respiratory tract and the gastrointestinal (GI) tract also secrete mucus that contains antibacterial and antifungal substances and also serves to wash off contaminating organisms. The airways are equipped with cilia, tiny hair-like structures that sweep particles including bacterial and fungal spores out of our lungs to keep the potential infection burden low. Damage to these external defences usually results in an innate immune process called inflammation. A full list of these barriers can be found in Information 7.1.

Wound Infections

Organisms including humans protect and repair themselves. Wound healing involves a complex interaction of many types of cells with functions that include both wound healing and infection prevention. Therefore it is important to be able to identify the difference between normal, healthy mechanisms of wound healing and early signs of infection. In a normal, healthy wound, as the wound heals, neutrophils, macrophages and lymphocytes congregate at the site of the wound, to prevent infection and clean the wound of any invading bacteria. These are essential mechanisms and help wound healing. Therefore an important point in wound care is to let the body heal as much as possible on its own. It is often unnecessary to intervene in wound healing, beyond keeping a wound clean to minimise the risk of uncontrolled infection. Aseptic wound care is essential to minimise infection. However, overwhelming infection can prevent a wound from healing. A nonhealing wound occurs when the immune system fails to keep wounds clean and bacteria cause ongoing tissue damage. This can occur as the result of illness, disease (such as diabetes) and malnutrition. As such, wound management should include a degree of clinical judgement considering what the wound looks like, other conditions present and whether the wound looks as though it is healing or not.

The Adaptive Immune System

Whilst the innate response can control many common infections through inflammation, other activity pathogens are always evolving new ways to invade the body or elude the innate immune system. The adaptive immune response is concerned with making very specific immune responses. Therefore the adaptive immune system can engage with almost any pathogen or other threat. The cells of the adaptive immune system are the T and B lymphocytes. The T lymphocytes get their name from the fact that they mature in the thymus gland. In the thymus, T cells are selected for their ability to function and their inability to recognise self. This is an important step since T cells that recognise self will cause an immune reaction against the body and thus illness. There are several subsets of T cells (see Information 7.2). The most important are the helper T cells or Th cells. These cells are responsible for increasing or amplifying the innate immune response against pathogens like bacteria. The second most important class of T cells are the cytotoxic or Tc cells. These are responsible for directed defence against pathogens inside cells, including viruses and some bacteria that can hide inside cells (such as the bacteria responsible for tuberculosis). Th cells, upon activation, release signalling molecules (termed cytokines) that turn up the killing power of cells of the innate immune system. The Tc cells directly engage virally infected cells and many compounds that eliminate the virally infected cell.

INFORMATION 7.1

Host Defences: First-Line Mechanisms

Skin and Mucosae
- Intact skin/mucosae
- Sloughing and constant renewal of skin and other epithelial surfaces
- Low pH of the skin – the 'acid mantle'
- Low water content
- Antibacterial lysozyme and immunoglobulin A (IgA) in sweat
- Normal flora.

Eyes and Ears
- Eye lashes and blink reflex
- Blinking moving tears across the eyeball
- Antibacterial lysozyme and IgA in tears
- Ear secretions trapping foreign particles and containing IgA.

Gastrointestinal Tract
- Saliva containing antibacterial lysozyme
- Hydrochloric acid in gastric juice
- Gastric mucus protecting the gastric lining from acid damage
- Mucosa-associated lymphoid tissue (MALT)
- Peristalsis
- Vomiting reflex when 'bad' food is ingested
- Normal flora.

Female Genital Tract
- Normal flora of the vagina producing an acid environment (pH 4.5) during the reproductive years
- Stratified squamous epithelial lining protecting the vagina from trauma
- Regular shedding of the outer layer of the endometrium (stratum functionalis) during menstruation.

Urinary Tract
- Regular and complete voiding of urine
- Position of the kidneys and length of ureters
- Length of the male urethra
- pH of urine
- MALT.

Respiratory Tract
- Nasal secretions containing antibacterial lysozyme
- Nasal hairs
- Shape of the upper respiratory tract
- Normal flora of nasopharynx
- Sneeze and cough reflexes
- MALT
- Mechanisms that protect the larynx during swallowing
- Mucus production and ciliated epithelium – microbes and other foreign particles are trapped in mucus. The mucociliary escalator/transport moves the mucus upwards and out of the lungs.

Body Secretions
- Secretions such as breast milk, tears and those produced by the ear, urinary, genital, respiratory and GI tracts contain immunoglobulins.

B cells are the other arm of the adaptive immune response. Like the phagocytes of the innate immune system, B cells circulate in the bloodstream, and they are capable of phagocytosing pathogens. B cells are responsible for releasing antibodies. Antibodies are protein molecules that are exquisitely targeted against pathogens. Briefly, antibodies bind to pathogens, making it easy for the innate immune cells to grab and destroy the bacteria. The high specificity of antibodies allows the immune system to respond in a very targeted way. The adaptive system also has an important role in self/non-self recognition, and when this goes wrong, autoimmune disease can result. The adaptive immune system can mount a very strong response once it is properly activated but it can take up to 10 days for this activation to occur the first time. However, the next time you encounter the same pathogen, the adaptive system reacts very quickly. As discussed later in the chapter, T cells are usually resident in lymphatic tissues whilst B cells circulate throughout the body. An essential part of the immune response is communication between the innate and adaptive systems in the lymph nodes, spleen and other organs of the body.

Allergies and Anaphylaxis

Sometimes, the immune system reacts inappropriately to non-threatening non-self substances such as dust or pollen. This leads to a condition called allergy or hypersensitivity. Hypersensitivities are probably the most common diseases caused by a faulty immune system. Allergens are substances that cause allergic reactions. Most allergens are harmless substances the immune system mistakes for threats. Common allergens include some foods (e.g. nuts, fish), pollens, house dust, latex (e.g. rubber gloves), nickel (used in some jewellery) and drugs (e.g. antibiotics). Some household and medical devices contain latex rubber (Information 7.3). See Reflection 7.1 for more about latex allergy. When a person encounters an allergen, the immune system mistakenly sees the allergen as a threat and creates a large quantity of antibodies of a particular class (usually immunoglobulin E) in defence. This antibody binds to the allergen triggering the activation of tissue resident cells called mast cells and basophils. In turn, the mast cells and basophils release substances such as histamine leading to an inflammatory response. The manifestation of allergy can vary in severity from barely worth bothering about to utterly life-threatening. Anaphylaxis is a severe and life-threatening hypersensitivity reaction resulting in systemic shock. Asthma is an example of an allergic reaction. An asthma attack happens when the response to an allergen causes the tissue resident mast cells and eosinophils to release the signals they contain. In the airways, this results in increased mucous secretion and bronchoconstriction which compromises breathing. Anaphylaxis usually results from systemic exposure to an antigen.

The same signals released by mast cells and eosinophils can also lead to a collapse in the peripheral circulation, shock and organ failure. Anaphylaxis is a medical emergency. Insect stings are a common trigger for anaphylaxis. Food is also an important trigger, particularly in children, whilst drugs are often a trigger in older people. The care of anaphylaxis centres initially around the airway, breathing, circulation (ABC) paradigm.

❖ Nursing Management and Health Promotion: Allergy

Common Presenting Signs and Symptoms

Allergy is usually suspected based on a history of reaction to a particular substance. Often, the patient or parent of the patient will notice the association between trigger and symptoms. Allergy can manifest as atopic eczema (e.g. to biological agents in washing powders), GI symptoms (e.g. to fish or nut ingestion) or asthma (e.g. hay fever). Other systems may also be involved. The symptoms of an allergic reaction usually develop rapidly after exposure, but they can also develop gradually over a few hours. The symptoms include:

- allergic rhinitis – sneezing and an itchy or runny nose
- conjunctivitis – itchy, red, watering eyes
- asthma – chest tightness, coughing, wheezing and shortness of breath
- hives – an itchy raised red rash, often raised
- swollen lips, tongue, eyes or face
- GI upset with stomach pain, nausea, vomiting and/or diarrhoea.

These symptoms may vary depending on the cause of the allergy. Hives, swollen lips and GI upset are common in food allergies for example whilst asthma is more likely with hay fever or other allergy to airborne particles.

Diagnosis

Food allergies are often diagnosed by skinprick testing. Skinprick testing involves putting a drop of liquid that contains a substance they may be allergic to onto the forearm or back of the patient. Several drops of different substances may be placed at once. The skin under the drop is then gently pricked. If there is an allergy to the substance, an itchy, red bump will appear within a few minutes. The correspondence between the bumps and the substance in the drops indicates the cause of the allergy. Skin prick testing is painless and safe. However, there is always a chance of severe anaphylactic reaction (see later) and so this procedure should be carried out under medical supervision. Patients who are going to undergo skinprick testing should be reminded not to take medication before the test as this can interfere with the results. Food allergy may also be examined by asking the patient to eliminate certain foods (or food groups) from the diet and assessing whether symptoms ease. Finally, challenge testing may also be used. In this procedure the patient is given small, but increasing, doses of the suspected allergen (e.g. peanuts) to see how they react. This procedure carries a higher risk of anaphylaxis (see later) and should only be carried out under medical supervision and with full resuscitation equipment available. Allergies that manifest as eczema are often tested for patch testing. The principle is the same as skinprick testing earlier but instead of pricking the skin the suspected allergens are added to special metal discs, which are then taped to the skin for up to 48 hours. After this time the skin under the disc is examined for a reaction.

Treatment

Food allergies are usually managed by simply educating the patient about the nature of the allergen and asking them to ensure they do not consume the trigger food. Patients and their carers should be encouraged to read food labels and ask staff who prepare food if they are unsure about food content. Hay fever and allergies to pets/animals are best treated by avoiding the trigger as much as possible. For animals, this can be easy but depending on the season this can be much harder for hay fever, and medication (see later) may be required. Some people are allergic to mites that live in carpets, duvets, etc. The advice to these patients should be to keep the house as dust free as possible.

Allergies like hay fever or house dust mite allergy can be treated with antihistamines. These drugs block the ability of the chemical signal histamine to trigger the immune responses that lead to allergy. Patients should be encouraged to use antihistamines before expected exposure or as early as possible after symptoms appear. In some cases, antihistamine treatment may be combined with decongestant treatment to reduce the discomfort of a blocked nose. Steroids are able to block the immune reactions triggered in allergy. They may be used more regularly than antihistamines and are often used for longer-term management of the condition. Steroid drugs are available as creams or lotions for eczema, inhalers for asthma or nasal sprays for the symptoms of a blocked nose or sinus inflammation.

Associated Emergency Situations

The same signals released by mast cells and eosinophils that cause allergy can also lead to a collapse in the peripheral circulation, shock and organ failure. Anaphylaxis is a medical emergency. Insect stings are a common trigger for anaphylaxis. Food is also an important trigger, particularly in children, whilst drugs are often a trigger in older people. The care of anaphylaxis centres initially around the ABC paradigm if medical support is available. Treatment is based on the administration of adrenaline (epinephrine) to support cardiovascular and respiratory function, chlorphenamine (an antihistamine) to counter the harmful effects of the histamine, hydrocortisone, oxygen and intravenous (IV) fluids. The Resuscitation Council UK (RCUK) publishes guidelines in the form of an anaphylaxis algorithm (RCUK 2021). However, patients may find themselves without medical support when anaphylaxis begins. Patient education is very important here – patients should be educated as to how anaphylaxis can manifest. The RCUK lists a 'sense of impending doom' or anxiety and panic as potential signs of anaphylaxis. If there has been suspected exposure and the patient starts to feel unwell or describe symptoms like those earlier, they should immediately contact the emergency services (or get someone else to do this). Many patients are given adrenalin autoinjectors to carry with them. In the event of an anaphylactic or suspected anaphylactic reaction, they (or their carers) should inject themselves in the thigh with adrenalin. In the UK, the NHS gives advice for patients/carers (see Box 7.1).

Again, both patient and carer education is important to make sure they understand how dangerous anaphylaxis can be and how to use the adrenalin syringe. See Reflection 7.2.

Ongoing Care and Support

In the event of flare-ups of the condition, there may be a requirement for hospitalisation, especially for asthma. Typically though, most allergy patients are monitored in the community if required.

• BOX 7.1   Advice Given to Patients/Carers Regarding Anaphylaxis

1. **Use an adrenaline autoinjector if the person has one** – but make sure you know how to use it correctly first.
2. **Call 999 for an ambulance immediately (even if they start to feel better)** – mention that you think the person has anaphylaxis.
3. **Remove any trigger if possible** – for example, carefully remove any wasp or bee sting stuck in the skin.
4. **Lie the person down flat** – unless they are unconscious, pregnant or having breathing difficulties.
5. **Give another injection after 5–15 minutes** if the symptoms do not improve and a second autoinjector is available.

From NHS 2022. Treatment of anaphylaxis. NHS UK. https://www.nhs.uk/conditions/anaphylaxis/treatment/.

'A Wasp Sting Might Have Killed Me'

'I was out for a run and something flew into my mouth. I spat it out and then realised that it was a wasp as it had stung me on the tongue. The pain was really bad, and my tongue was swelling. No mobile phone and miles from anywhere – I was alone on the fen and there was no one in sight. How did I feel? Panicky and terrified – what should I do, how could this happen, was I going to die? The pain was increasing and spreading to my throat and teeth. I tried to remain calm and quickly ran back home with a mounting sense of panic.'

Activities

- Reflect on the person's feelings of fear and panic and consider how you might feel in similar circumstances.
- Discuss with your assessor/supervisor or colleagues how the nurse can help to reduce fear and anxiety in such a situation.

Asthma and eczema patients may be regularly reviewed in specialist clinics by a practice nurse.

Vaccinations, Measles and Adaptive Immunity

One key feature of the adaptive immune system is that it has 'memory'. The first time you make an adaptive response (e.g. antibody) to an invading pathogen, it takes around 7–10 days to generate the response. Once the response is made though, it is very powerful. The Th, Tc and B cells responsible for this adaptive response persist in the body as memory cells, often over your whole lifetime. On a second exposure to the same pathogen or other threat these cells are activated, and the adaptive response is incredibly rapid – so much so you usually do not even know you were infected. We can use this property of the adaptive immune response to our advantage to control diseases through vaccination. Vaccination is deliberate infection with a nonfunctional version of the pathogen. Your immune system encounters this nonpathogenic non-self material and mounts a slow primary immune response. This results in the generation of memory Th, Tc and B cells. On subsequent exposure to the real pathogen, the body mounts a rapid and strong secondary response resulting in elimination of the infection. One example is the vaccination for influenza. Basically, antigenic (i.e. antibody-stimulating) components from a harmful flu virus are generated in a nonharmful flu virus. This vaccine (i.e. the nonharmful flu virus) looks like the pathogenic version of the flu virus from the immune system point of view. A primary immune response occurs, and this leads to immunological memory for the pathogenic flu virus. If you are actually infected with the pathogenic virus, then a rapid secondary immune response occurs, and the virus is destroyed without any symptoms of disease occurring. The same can be done with bacterial infections.

The Green Book

In the UK, the Green Book contains the most up-to-date information on vaccines (see Further Reading list). This publication contains all information on administration of vaccines including who can administer and advise on the unlikely occurrence of an adverse event. The Green Book also contains up-to-date information on all vaccines administered in the UK, including dosages. Practitioners administering vaccines should be familiar with this publication.

Human Papilloma Virus

The human papillomavirus (HPV) vaccine is the newest addition to the list of available vaccines. As such, there have been several changes in guidelines for administration since it became available. The HPV is commonly sexually transmitted and is a risk factor for cervical cancer as well as genital warts. Usually the viral infection is cleared up without the person being aware they have even had it. Currently, it is thought that at least 40% of women become infected with at least one HPV virus strain within the first 2 years of sexual activity. Two strains of HPV are thought to be responsible for at least 75% of all cervical cancers in Europe. Unless the HPV virus leads to visible symptoms such as genital warts, the presence of the virus is invisible. The mean duration of an HPV infection is thought to be 8 months. Repeatedly contracting HPV is thought to increase the risk of cervical cancer. Although condoms will not prevent contraction of all HPV viruses, it is likely to reduce the chance of infection and prevent transmission of some strains, so people should be encouraged to wear condoms or use other barrier contraceptives.

The UK government currently recommends the use of Gardasil for vaccination against HPV. Ideally, females should be vaccinated before they become sexually active. In the UK the national vaccination programme is recommended for females aged 11 to 14 years, although females can be vaccinated within the national vaccination programme until the age of 18. The HPV vaccination course is not supported within the national programme for those aged 9 and 10 and those over the age of 18. The English government in 2018 announced that adolescent boys will be offered the HPV vaccine to protect them from cancer. The vaccination course consists of two injections of 0.5 mL of Gardasil HPV vaccine, the second injection being 6–24 months after the first. For females aged 15 years and older, three injections are recommended within a 4-month period, the second dose coming 1 month after the first, and the final dose coming 3 months after the second.

Reflection 7.3 provides you with opportunities to explore issues around immunisation.

The Lymphatic System

The major function of the lymphatic system is to drain body fluids from tissues to the circulation. Blood pressure pushing against the walls of vessels in tissues causes fluid to squeeze out into the interstitial spaces between individual cells in the tissues. An estimated 20 L of plasma per day is pushed into the interstitial spaces in this manner. If this were to continue, swelling and tissue damage would occur. A large fraction of this interstitial fluid is reabsorbed by the blood vessels. The function of the lymphatic system is to drain the remaining excess fluid back into the bloodstream via a series of vessels. The interstitial fluid enters small lymphatic vessels and is then referred to as lymph. The lymph drains back into the circulation from large lymphatic vessels in the chest. As the lymph travels from the peripheral tissues back to the central circulation, it passes through structures called lymph nodes that serve as communication points for the immune system. Therefore as lymph travels to the central circulation, it is examined by the immune system for signs of infection or tissue damage. Blockage of the lymphatic system by cancers or infection leads to an accumulation of lymph and interstitial fluid with resultant tissue swelling. This is termed lymphoedema (see later).

Immunisation

During a public health placement, you are invited to accompany your supervisor (a health visitor) to an 'immunisation question and answer' session at the local health centre.

Activities

- Think about the questions that might be asked by people expecting their first baby, those with older children and teenagers, those with immunocompromised disease, people aged 65 years or over and people caring for relatives with chronic diseases. What type of fears might be expressed?
- Using the resources listed below find answers to the following:
  - What vaccines are given and when does the immunisation schedule start?
  - Why are some vaccines given as a course over several weeks?
  - Why are booster doses needed?
  - What minor and major side-effects can occur?
  - When is vaccination contraindicated?
  - Which vaccines are offered to healthy people aged 65 years or over?
- Find out which vaccines are under consideration for addition to the list of those routinely offered.

Resources

Barr B. The impact of NHS resource allocation policy on health inequalities in England 2001–11: longitudinal ecological study. *BMJ*. 2017;348:g3231.

Blanco-Melo D, et al. Imbalanced host response to SARS-CoV-2 drives development of COVID-19. *Cell*. 2020;181(5):1036-1045.e9.

British National Formulary (BNF). 2023. https://www.bnf.org/products/bnf-online/ (the section on active immunity is particularly informative).

British Society for Immunology. Publications. 2023. https://www.immunology.org/.

Department of Health. Immunisation against infectious disease – 'The Green Book'. 2020. https://www.gov.uk/government/collections/immunisation-against-infectious-disease-the-green-book.

Department of Health. Immunisation. 2023. https://www.gov.uk/government/collections/immunisation.

Huang C, et al. Clinical features of patients infected with 2019 novel coronavirus in Wuhan, China. *Lancet*. 2020;395(10223):497-506.

Jones L. Health and rural access to healthcare. *J Public Ment Health*. 2018;17(2):50-53.

Mehta P, et al. COVID-19: consider cytokine storm syndromes and immunosuppression. *Lancet*. 2020;395(10229):1033-1034.

Seow J, et al. Longitudinal observation and decline of neutralizing antibody responses in the three months following SARS-CoV-2 infection in humans. *Nat Microbiol*. 2020;5(12):1598-1607.

Tan L, et al. Lymphopenia predicts disease severity of COVID-19: a descriptive and predictive study. *Signal Transduct Target Ther*. 2020;5(1):33.

Structure of the Lymphatic System

The lymphatic vessels begin as small capillary-sized, open-ended vessels in the peripheral circulation. These small vessels progressively join into larger and larger lymphatic vessels, and eventually empty into the circulation through two large lymphatic vessels called lymphatic ducts. As lymph is transported from the tissues to the circulation it passes through the lymph nodes. Lymph nodes are small, bean-shaped structures found scattered throughout the body. There are around 550 lymph nodes distributed throughout the human body. Unlike the circulatory system the lymphatic system has no central pump. Instead, lymph is forced through the system by the action of the muscle pump. As muscles (especially in the limbs) contract with movement the lymphatic vessels are squeezed. Like veins, lymphatic vessels have semilunar valves. These valves prevent the backflow of lymph and so the fluid is pumped in one direction only. Lymph flows from the tissues through the lymphatic system into progressively larger and larger vessels. Two large vessels, the right lymphatic duct and the thoracic duct, then empty the lymph into the circulation through large blood vessels in the chest.

Lymphatic Capillaries

The process of tissue fluid drainage begins at the lymphatic capillaries. These are tiny open-ended capillaries present in most tissues in the body. Lymphatic capillaries are interwoven between the arterioles and venules of the circulatory system in the soft connective tissues of the body. Lymphatic capillaries are not found in the central nervous system, bone marrow, bones, teeth and the cornea of the eye. The lymphatic capillaries are one cell thick and composed of endothelial cells (similar to the cells that line arteries and veins). They are open ended, meaning that fluid in the interstitial spaces can flow into the lymphatic capillaries. Increased pressure in the tissue forces fluid in and a cap at the end of the vessel closes if tissue pressure is low to prevent fluid flowing back out.

As well as collecting interstitial fluid lymphatic vessels also have an important role in the gut. As we absorb fats from our diet small lymphatic vessels, called lacteals, collect the absorbed fat. Once in the lymphatic system the fats combine with lymph to form a milky fluid called chyle. The chyle is mainly transported to the liver through a gut-specific lymphatic transport where the dietary fats are metabolised. The reason for this rather odd arrangement is thought to relate to the vulnerability of blood vessels walls to damage from high fat levels. The collection of fats in the chyle spares the blood vessel walls in the gut from potential damage due to carrying highly concentrated fats.

Lymphatic Tissues

As well as vessels the lymphatic system is also composed of several specialised tissues and organs. These tissues are scattered throughout the body and they serve as sites of communication between the innate and adaptive systems. The largest lymphatic organ is the spleen. The spleen sits in the left-hand side of the abdomen behind and under the stomach. The spleen has a rich lymphatic and blood supply. Lymphatic fluid and immune cells enter the spleen via lymph and blood. The spleen contains many Th cells of the adaptive immune system and it provides an environment where passing innate immune cells and B-cells from the bloodstream and lymph can communicate with these T cells. The lymph nodes scattered throughout the body have a similar function but work on a smaller scale. Lymph nodes also provide an environment for the T cells of the adaptive immune system and the cells of the innate immune system to communicate. Specialised lymphatic tissues also serve to protect the parts of the body exposed to the external environment. The tonsils and adenoids are important lymphatic system tissues that serve to protect the airways, again serving as communication sites for the innate and adaptive immune systems. In the gut, the appendix and the mucosal associated lymphatic tissue (MALT) also act as sites of communication between the innate and adaptive systems.

Lymphoedema

If lymphatic vessels or lymph nodes get blocked, then pressure in the lymphatic system can rise. In this case the local lymphatic vessel will not efficiently drain fluid from the tissues and instead that fluid will accumulate. The resulting swelling is termed lymphoedema and can occur after some surgeries where the local lymph nodes are removed (e.g. mastectomy). The result is a sustained oedema which can lead to ulceration and other tissue damage.

❖ Nursing Management and Health Promotion: Lymphoedema

Common Presenting Signs and Symptoms

As noted previously, lymphoedema presents as local, oedematous swelling of the tissues. Whole limbs can be involved. The condition can arise after some surgical procedures when the local lymph nodes are removed. The resulting scarring can block lymphatic vessels and therefore interfere with the drainage of fluid from the limb. If left unchecked lymphoedema leads to increased pressure on tissues and therefore tissue death and ulceration.

Diagnosis

Lymphoedema is usually diagnosed by simple clinical examination and history taking. The affected limb will be swollen and oedematous and may be warm to the touch. Ulceration may be present. In some cases, imaging is used to assess the condition. A lymphoscintigram may be carried out. Radioactive dye is injected and tracked through the lymphatic vessels to check for any blockages. Rarely, magnetic resonance imaging (MRI) may be used to assess local lymph drainage.

Treatment

The treatment for lymphoedema is decongestive lymphatic therapy (DLT). The aim of DLT is not to cure lymphoedema, but to control the symptoms. This can be a time-intensive process, but DLT can bring lymphoedema under control. There are four components to DLT.
- Compression bandaging is used to squeeze fluids from the tissues back into local blood vessels.
- Skin care is essential to keep the skin in good condition and reduce the chances of skin breakage and infection.
- Exercise is a cornerstone of the DLT approach. The National Institute for Health and Care Excellence (NICE) suggests patients should be encouraged to exercise their affected limbs (NICE 2017). Muscle contraction in exercise encourages lymph drainage.
- Specialised massage techniques known as manual lymphatic drainage (MLD) stimulate the flow of fluid through the lymphatic system and reduce swelling.

Throughout this phase of active treatment the affected area should be monitored for tissue integrity and for a reduction in swelling to make sure treatment is working.

Ongoing Care and Support

An important aspect of care for lymphoedema is self-care. As the swelling reduces, the patient should be taught exercise, massage and compression techniques as well as skin care to maintain or further improve the lymphoedema. Self-care will also give the patient a sense of control over their lymphoedema. Regular review, particularly for tissue integrity, is important.

INFORMATION 7.4

Aetiology and Pathogenesis of SLE

At least 50 antigen targets for autoantibody production are described in systemic lupus erythematosus (SLE). However, none of the diverse manifestations of SLE can be attributed to a single antigenic stimulus, and it is suggested that this broad spectrum of autoantibody production results from polyclonal B- and T-cell activation. Several autoantigens in SLE are components of the intracellular and intranuclear apparatus. In health, these antigens are 'hidden' from the immune system and will not aggravate an immune response. Whilst the triggers that lead to autoantibody production in SLE are unknown, one mechanism may be exposure of intracellular antigens on the cell surface during apoptosis. This premise is supported by the fact that environmental factors that are linked to flare-ups of lupus – for example, sunlight and artificial ultraviolet (UV) light, pregnancy and infection – increase oxidative stress and subsequent apoptosis.

Autoimmune Disease: A Failure of Self vs Non-Self Discrimination

Some diseases result from failure of the self/non-self discrimination system. These are known as autoimmune diseases. The pathology is caused by the immune system attacking the body. Common autoimmune diseases include rheumatoid arthritis (RA), Graves' disease, systemic lupus erythematosus (SLE) and motor neurone disease (see Information 7.4).

❖ Nursing Management and Health Promotion: Rheumatoid Arthritis

RA is an example of an autoimmune disease. RA disease usually affects women (3:1) and often arises between 40 and 50 years old. The actual causes are unknown but the end effect is immune system attack on the cartilage and synovial space in joints. The mechanisms include both innate and adaptive. In particular, antibodies against the cartilage in the joints arise and lead to immune system activity in the joints. Over time the joint damage in RA becomes crippling and there are often associated inflammatory changes in other organs as well. In addition to impacting the joints, rheumatoid arthritis (RA) can lead to anaemia associated with chronic conditions, cause fatigue, and potentially affect major organs. (Kadu et al. 2021). In RA, antibodies against the body's own antibodies also arise. These are termed 'rheumatoid factors'. Similarly, anticyclic citrullinated peptide (CCP) antibodies may also be present in some RA sufferers.

Common Presenting Signs and Symptoms

RA usually presents initially in the small, proximal joints of the fingers and toes, although larger joints can also be affected in the early stages. Synovitis and pain are early symptoms and movement of the joint is often difficult with a feeling of 'resistance'. This joint stiffness is usually worse in the morning and eases over the course of the day. The symptoms can often become suddenly worse – termed a 'disease flare' – for reasons that are unknown. RA sufferers can also present with fatigue and rheumatoid nodules may appear over the elbow or other joints. These nodules may initially be painful, but this pain usually recedes as time goes by.

Diagnosis

Diagnosis is based on clinical examination, blood tests (e.g. for rheumatoid factor, anti-CCP antibodies, C-reactive protein (CRP – elevated), erythrocyte sedimentation rate (ESR – elevated)). If persistent synovitis is present and RA suspected, then X-rays of the hands and feet are recommended along with a functional assessment of the joints to provide a baseline for treatment response (NICE 2020). Testing for rheumatoid factor and anti-CCP are not definitive, although most sufferers will test positive. Accordingly, even if these tests are negative, RA should be suspected if other signs and symptoms are present.

Treatment

RA cannot be cured but the disease course can be slowed by prompt intervention and frequent review. The aim of treatment is to get to a stage of remission or reduced disease activity, but symptom management remains important (NICE 2023). New RA patients should be offered first-line treatment with conventional disease-modifying antirheumatic drugs (cDMARDs), e.g. oral methotrexate, leflunomide or sulfasalazine, ideally within 3 months of onset of persistent symptoms. If required, initial doses should be escalated as tolerated (NICE 2020). Oral or intramuscular/intra-articular glucocorticoids may also be given if required to reduce inflammation. Glucocorticoids are usually used for flares or symptom control because these drugs have severe side-effects. Analgesia is important and current guidelines recommend nonsteroidal anti-inflammatory drugs (NSAIDs) such as ibuprofen along with a proton pump inhibitor to protect the gastric lining from the gastric erosion side-effect of NSAIDs (NICE 2020). The role of communication with new RA patients is emphasised to give them adequate opportunity to understand the treatment choices and make informed decisions (NICE 2020).

Associated Emergency Situations

The swelling associated with RA can cause pressure on nerves, including the cervical spine. This is more common late in the disease course but can occur at any time. Cervical compression can lead to a range of consequences from occipital headaches to rapid and severe neurological deterioration and death. Rapid recognition and management are essential. If cervical compression is suspected, the patient should be referred promptly for MRI and surgical assessment. Spinal fusion and/or immobilisation in a halo jacket may be required in extreme cases.

Partly because of the nature of the disease and partly because of the drug treatment, RA patients are more prone to infection and may present atypically with infections. Therefore if patients present feeling generally unwell but without fever or other typical signs, infection or sepsis should still be suspected.

Ongoing Care and Support

The multidisciplinary team (MDT) is important in RA. Adult sufferers should have access to MDT support and a named member of the MDT (e.g. a specialist nurse). This provides the opportunity for ongoing assessment of the effect of the disease on their lives and the effectiveness of symptom control, analgesia and strategies to manage fatigue and functional impairment (NICE 2020). Physiotherapy and occupational therapy are recommended. RA patients should be encouraged to exercise or continue exercising safely. Hand exercises in particular can be useful to maintain function and therefore independence. Training in self-care and self-management of flares is important.

The immune-suppressive nature of anti-RA drugs means that these patients should be encouraged to take immunisations for common infections such as influenza.

Transplant Rejection

Organ transplant is essentially the replacement of self tissue with non-self tissue so it should come as no surprise that this can provoke an immune reaction. Once the donor organ has been transplanted into the body, the host immune system recognises the donated tissue as non-self. This occurs partly because the donor organ carries different molecular markers on the surface of all the cells. These markers are termed major histocompatibility (MHC) molecules. The MHC molecules are important in the mechanisms that the immune system uses to differentiate self from non-self. In essence, every individual on the planet has a different MHC profile from the immune system's point of view. The MHC profile that a particular immune system developed in is the profile considered to mark 'self'. What this means in the context of transplant is that the donor organ or tissue does not look like 'self' to the immune system. The donor organ is therefore attacked by the host immune system and this can lead to graft rejection. In bone marrow transplant the situation is reversed. The donor immune system finds itself in a host it does not recognise. The donor immune system attacks and 'rejects' the host – graft versus host disease (GvHD). After transplant the host's immune system must be controlled by powerful immunosuppressive drugs. Unfortunately, these can leave people open to infections and increase the risk of developing cancer because they turn down the normal internal surveillance of the immune system.

Information 7.5 provides examples of some autoimmune disorders.

Viruses

Some pathogens, such as viruses, can hide inside the cells of the body and thus remain unseen by the phagocytes. Once infected by a virus body cells usually change the molecules they display on their surface. A specialised innate cell called a natural killer (NK) cell recognises these changes. The NK cell secretes chemicals that lead the virally infected cell to commit

---

INFORMATION 7.5

Examples of Autoimmune Disorders

- Addison's disease
- Anti-GBM disease (Goodpasture's syndrome, a type of glomerulonephritis)
- Autoimmune haemolytic anaemia
- Autoimmune hepatitis
- Bullous skin disorders (e.g. pemphigus, pemphigoid)
- Graves' disease hyperthyroidism
- Hypoparathyroidism
- Hypothyroidism
- Idiopathic thrombocytopenic purpura (ITP)
- Multiple sclerosis
- Myasthenia gravis
- Pernicious anaemia
- Rheumatoid arthritis
- Some types of male infertility
- Sympathetic ophthalmitis/ophthalmia
- Systemic lupus erythematosus (SLE)
- Thyroiditis hyperthyroidism
- Type 1 diabetes mellitus

apoptosis. Apoptosis is a controlled form of cell death that does not result in inflammation. As a result of apoptosis, both the virally infected cell and the virus it contains are destroyed. If the patient experiences prolonged or severe symptoms because of a virus, antiviral drugs may be prescribed to assist the immune system in fighting this.

Susceptibility to Flu, Salmonella and Herpes

Emerging findings in immunology have led to the discovery of an abnormality that lies somewhere in the communication between the innate and adaptive immune system. Abnormalities in this communication pathway can lead to people being more susceptible to contracting the flu, salmonella and herpes virus, amongst others. For now, testing for this abnormality is rare, but as an increasing number of people worldwide are being diagnosed with this abnormality, testing may become more common.

Immunodeficiency

Immunodeficiency describes a reduced function of the immune system and therefore compromised defence of the body. In addition to commonly known immunodeficiency diseases such as HIV, there are several genetic immune-deficiency disorders (primary immunodeficiencies) such as severe combined immunodeficiency (SCID).

Drug treatment for some conditions, such as cancer, transplants or some autoimmune diseases, can also lead to immunodeficiency. People taking immunosuppressive drugs for any reason are at risk of infection and should be regularly screened.

Immune Deficiency Disorders

Immune deficiency disorders can occur from birth. SCID is a rare genetic disorder with failure to develop functional T or B cells. The adaptive arm of the immune system therefore fails. The disease manifests very early in life with severe infections and requires extreme barrier nursing and care. The disease is currently treated by bone marrow transplantation to replace the patient's faulty haematopoietic stem cells with functional cells. Immune deficiency disorders occurring from birth are categorised by the part of the immune system they affect, e.g. the production of T cells or B cells or phagocytes. Chronic granulomatous disease (CGD) is an example of a primary immunodeficiency that affects phagocytes of the innate immune system. CGD is an umbrella term for a group of genetic mutations that lead to an inability of phagocytes to generate the reactive chemical species they use to kill phagocytosed bacteria. Whilst phagocytosis can take place, the bacteria cannot be properly killed and broken down. The bacteria-filled phagocytes are walled off behind fibrous granulomas in the organs of the body. CGD patients suffer recurrent infection with pneumonia being common, along with abscesses, septic arthritis and septicaemia. Education and prophylactic antibiotics are the cornerstones of treatment.

Secondary immunodeficiency is the term used to describe compromised immune function in response to illness or drug treatment. As noted previously, treatment for autoimmune diseases targets the immune system directly and therefore patients receiving treatment are inevitably immune compromised to some degree. Patient education is essential, and patients should especially be reminded that the classic signs and symptoms of infection may not be present and so they should be proactive in seeking help if they feel at all unwell.

Cancer

Although cancer is not strictly speaking caused by immunodeficiency, cancer does arise when immunosurveillance fails. Changes in cancerous cells mean that they are no longer recognised as self. The innate (natural killer) NK cells and the adaptive Tc cells patrol the body looking for cells that they do not recognise as self. If these immune cells are triggered, they instruct the cancerous cells to kill themselves via apoptosis. Apoptosis is a controlled, specific process (unlike necrosis) and involves the cancerous cell cutting up the DNA inside itself. As noted earlier the use of immunosuppressive drugs in e.g. transplant or autoimmune disease can increase the risk of cancer because this monitoring mechanism fails. Although the immune system sets out to kill these cancer cells, as cancer cells can multiply so quickly, they can overwhelm the immune system. Therefore treatments are primarily aimed at removing (e.g. surgery) or killing (e.g. radiotherapy) cancer cells. Additionally, a new line of controversial cancer treatments known as immunotherapies are designed to stimulate or target the immune system to fight the multiplying cancer cells. Many current anticancer drugs also affect cells of the immune system. These drugs can lead to a secondary immunodeficiency and can leave patients more vulnerable than normal to infection. Patients should therefore be educated to seek help if they begin to feel unwell even in the absence of classic signs of infection such as raised temperature or pulse.

Care of the Older Person

As people age, they become more susceptible to developing immune deficiency. Several factors contribute to this. For example, older people produce less T cells, their gut absorbs less calcium, they are more likely to be undernourished, and they are more susceptible to diseases that cause immune deficiency.

COVID-19

COVID-19, caused by the novel coronavirus SARS-CoV-2, has been found to significantly impact both the lymphatic and immune systems. In terms of the lymphatic system, COVID-19 can cause lymphopenia, which is a reduction in lymphocyte count, and this is common in patients who have a severe or critical condition (Huang et al. 2020). The exact mechanism of how SARS-CoV-2 induces lymphopenia is unclear, but it may be due to the virus causing lymphocyte apoptosis or the redistribution of lymphocytes in the body (Tan et al. 2020). Regarding the immune system, SARS-CoV-2 can trigger an intense and dysregulated immune response, which may lead to the 'cytokine storm syndrome'. This syndrome can lead to the hyperactivation of the immune system and can be severe enough to cause tissue damage, multiorgan failure and potentially death (Mehta et al. 2020). Moreover the immune response to SARS-CoV-2 can include both the innate and adaptive responses. The virus can stimulate the production of type I interferons (IFNs), cytokines which are crucial in the body's early antiviral response. However, SARS-CoV-2 has also evolved mechanisms to counteract the antiviral effects of type I IFNs, thereby evading the immune response and facilitating its replication and dissemination within the host (Blanco-Melo et al. 2020). In terms of the adaptive immune response, the development of antibodies against SARS-CoV-2 can aid in controlling the virus during the acute phase of infection and may provide protection against re-infection. However, it is still unclear how long this immunity lasts, and it seems to vary greatly between individuals (Seow et al. 2020).

Addressing Health Inequalities

Health inequalities represent a significant concern in the context of immune and lymphatic illnesses. These disparities typically exist due to social, economic and environmental factors which can influence people's ability to prevent, manage and seek treatment for such conditions. In the realm of immune and lymphatic illnesses, for instance, certain vulnerable groups such as low-income populations, ethnic minorities, the elderly and individuals with pre-existing conditions may have increased susceptibility due to a confluence of various factors. These can include inadequate access to nutritious food, higher stress levels, exposure to pollutants and limited access to healthcare, all of which can weaken the immune system. Financial constraints can make it difficult for individuals to afford necessary medications, immunisations or treatment protocols, effectively exacerbating health inequalities. In contrast, those in wealthier strata are more likely to afford preventative care, medical treatments and healthier lifestyles that can boost their immune and lymphatic systems. Furthermore, geographical disparities can impact healthcare access. Individuals residing in rural or underserved areas might face logistical challenges in accessing healthcare facilities, contributing to delayed or missed diagnoses and treatments (Jones 2018). Regarding care accessibility, the UK's National Health Service (NHS) provides free healthcare at the point of service to all UK residents, striving to mitigate these disparities. However, health inequality persists, reflecting the broader socioeconomic inequalities within society (Barr 2017). Efforts to reduce health inequalities and improve access to care include community-based health initiatives, public health campaigns promoting prevention and healthy behaviours and government policies aimed at addressing social determinants of health. Furthermore, initiatives like home health services, telemedicine and localised clinics aim to improve accessibility for those in remote locations.

Summary: Key Nursing Issues

- The three lines of body defence are: *first-line* natural, nonspecific barriers such as intact skin; *second-line* natural, nonspecific defences, such as inflammation and phagocytosis; and *third-line* adaptive, specific immune responses – humoral (antibody) and cell-mediated immunity.
- Although immunity is divided into innate and adaptive responses, numerous interactions and collaboration occur between different components of the immune system.
- Nurses in all areas of practice will care for people with disorders affecting the immune system – ranging from life-threatening allergies through to varying degrees of immunodeficiency and autoimmunity.
- Knowledge and understanding of the complexity of immunological processes and disorders are still incomplete and many exciting developments can be anticipated in the future. The use of immunological treatments for diseases such as cancer will expand over the next decade.

Reflection and Learning – What Next?

- Test your knowledge by visiting the Evolve website ⊕ and answering the multiple-choice questions and critical thinking questions.
- Consolidate your learning by looking at some of the further reading suggestions, references and specialist websites.
- Revisit some of the additional material on the website.
- Consider what you have learnt and how this will help your professional development.
- Reflect on how you can apply this knowledge to the care of your patients.
- Discuss your learning with your assessor/supervisor, lecturer and colleagues.

References

Barr B. The impact of NHS resource allocation policy on health inequalities in England 2001–11: longitudinal ecological study. *BMJ.* 2017;348:g3231.

Blanco-Melo, D. Nilsson-Payant B. Liu, W. et al. Imbalanced host response to SARS-CoV-2 drives development of COVID-19. *Cell.* 2020;181(5):1036–1045.e9.

Huang C, et al. Clinical features of patients infected with 2019 novel coronavirus in Wuhan, China. *Lancet.* 2020;395(10223):497–506. https://www.thelancet.com/article/S0140-6736(20)30183-5/fulltext#.

Jones L. Health and rural access to healthcare. *J Public Ment Health.* 2018;17(2):50–53.

Kadu, K. P., Kadu, S. K., Bhore, S. A. Prevalence of anaemia in patients of rheumatoid arthritis. *Int J Res.* 2021;8(3).

Mehta P, et al. COVID-19: consider cytokine storm syndromes and immunosuppression. *Lancet.* 2020;395(10229):1033–1034. https://www.thelancet.com/journals/lancet/article/PIIS0140-6736(20)30628-0/fulltext.

NICE (National Institute for Health and Care Excellence) 2017. Advanced breast cancer: diagnosis and treatment. Clinical guideline [CG81]. https://www.nice.org.uk/guidance/cg81/chapter/Recommendations#managing-complications.

NICE (National Institute for Health and Care Excellence) 2020. Rheumatoid arthritis in adults: Management. NICE guideline [NG100]. https://www.nice.org.uk/guidance/ng100.

NICE (2023). Rheumatoid arthritis. https://bnf.nice.org.uk/treatment-summaries/rheumatoid-arthritis/.

Resuscitation Council UK (RCUK). Emergency treatment of anaphylaxis; Guidelines for healthcare providers. 2021. https://www.resus.org.uk/sites/default/files/2021-05/Emergency%20Treatment%20of%20Anaphylaxis%20May%202021_0.pdf.

Seow J, et al. Longitudinal observation and decline of neutralizing antibody responses in the three months following SARS-CoV-2 infection in humans. *Nat Microbiol.* 2020;5(12):1598–1607. https://www.nature.com/articles/s41564-020-00813-8.

Tan L, et al. Lymphopenia predicts disease severity of COVID-19: a descriptive and predictive study. *Signal Transduct Target Ther.* 2020;5(1):33.

Further Reading

Colledge NR, Walker BR, Ralston SH. *Davidson's Principles and Practice of Medicine*. 24th ed. Edinburgh: Churchill Livingstone; 2022.

Peate I, Evens S. *Fundamentals of Anatomy and Physiology: For Nursing and Healthcare Students*. 3rd ed.. Wiley; 2020.

Rich R, Fleisher T, Shearer W, et al. *Clinical Immunology: Principles and Practice*. 5th ed. Edinburgh: Mosby; 2018.

Waugh A, Ross Grant A, Wilson. *Anatomy and Physiology in Health and Illness*. 13th ed. Edinburgh: Churchill Livingstone; 2018.

Useful Websites

Allergy UK (previously known as British Allergy Foundation), www. allergyuk.org

Arthritis Action, https://www.arthritisaction.org.uk/

Arthritis Research UK, www.arthritisresearchuk.org/

British National Formulary (BNF), www.bnf.org/

NHS National Patient Safety Agency, www.npsa.nhs.uk/

Primary Immunodeficiency Association, www.pia.org.uk/

Resuscitation Council (UK), www.resus.org.uk/

Severe Combined Immunodeficiency (SCID), www.ich.ucl.ac.uk/gosh_families/information_sheets/immunodeficiency_scid/immunodeficiency_scid_families.html

World Health Organisation, www.who.int/immunization/en/

8

Nursing Patients With Disorders of the Breast and Reproductive Systems

GEORGINA LEWIS

PART 1: NURSING PATIENTS WITH DISORDERS OF THE FEMALE REPRODUCTIVE SYSTEM

PART 2: NURSING PATIENTS WITH DISORDERS OF THE BREAST

PART 1: NURSING PATIENTS WITH DISORDERS OF THE FEMALE REPRODUCTIVE SYSTEM

Introduction

Any threat to an individual's reproductive capacity affects that person's body image, self-esteem and gender identity. Since these are influenced by personal attitudes, social customs and cultural background, people respond differently to such a threat. Attitudes towards sexual reproduction, underlying beliefs held and feelings experienced are influenced by cultural, social and religious values, background, lifestyle and parental and peer pressure.

Reproduction and the ability to procreate are important issues, evidenced by the incidence of subfertility in the UK and other parts of the world and the ongoing development of reproductive technologies. While the physiological aspects of reproduction are concerned with continuance of the species, the psychosocial aspects of reproduction are of significance to the feelings of health and well-being for people. For some people, having their own children and raising a family are key parts of their role in life. For others, these are inconsequential and for some this may be desirable but if not possible may cause unhappiness and remorse.

Disease prevention rather than disease control/treatment is an underpinning philosophy of healthcare. Healthcare professionals have an important role in advising and encouraging good health awareness and in facilitating and conducting screening and health monitoring. However, screening is not always possible and some conditions can be far advanced before a diagnosis is made.

When a person's quality of life is affected by the condition, intervention is required and developments in techniques and technology mean that recovery is often much faster. Minimally invasive techniques have the advantage of a shorter general anaesthetic, or the use of conscious sedation or local anaesthetic, thus allowing some treatments to be carried out in a community care setting, in outpatients, as a day case or a shorter inpatient stay in hospital. This has consequences for nursing and patient care after treatment to adapt to the dynamic nature of nursing in a changing society.

Anatomy and Physiology of the Female Reproductive System

The primary function of the reproductive system is the propagation of the human species. Sexual drive and anticipated pleasure help to meet the reproductive need. The female reproductive system produces gametes (secondary oocytes; strictly speaking these are not known as ova until penetration by a spermatozoon), receives the male penis during sexual intercourse and facilitates the passage of male gametes (spermatozoa). It supports the growth and development of the embryo/fetus during pregnancy and expels the fetus during labour (Figs 8.1 and 8.2). See Anatomy and Physiology of the Breast. The events occurring at the start and the end of a female's reproductive life, the menarche (the first menstruation) and the climacteric and menopause, are outlined.

The female reproductive system consists of:
- internal genitalia – ovaries (2)
- uterus
- uterine (fallopian) tubes (2)
- vagina
- external genitalia – vulva.

Ovaries

There are two ovaries, the size and shape of large almonds, one on either side of the uterus. The surface of the ovary consists of a single layer of germinal epithelium surrounding connective tissue that forms the stroma of the ovarian cortex and medulla. The ovarian follicles develop in the cortex. Female infants are born with approximately 100,000 primordial follicles, which may fall to approximately 30,000 by adolescence. Each follicle contains a

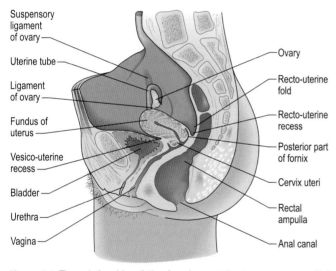

Figure 8.1 The relationship of the female reproductive organs: sagittal section.

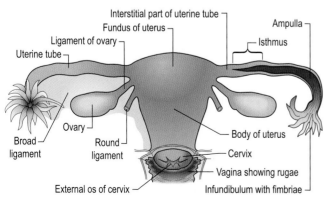

Figure 8.2 Organs of the female reproductive system and attachments.

secondary oocyte. The medulla consists of connective tissue, blood vessels and nerves.

The ovary has two functions:
- secondary oocyte production
- hormone secretion.

Oocyte (Ovum) Production

Ovarian cycles begin at puberty; a cycle lasts around 28 days (range 21–35 days) and has two phases, follicular (days 1–14) and luteal (days 14–28). Follicles begin to mature under the influence of the follicle-stimulating hormone (FSH) and luteinising hormone (LH), released by the anterior pituitary gland. During the cycle, follicles can pass through five stages (Fig. 8.3):
- primary follicle – each oocyte is surrounded by a thin layer of epithelial cells
- developing follicle – the follicular epithelium proliferates, the oocyte moves to a side position and a fluid-filled cavity develops within the epithelium
- mature (Graafian) follicle – the follicle reaches its maximum size
- corpus luteum – a yellow body forms in the ovarian follicle after ovulation
- corpus albicans – scar tissue on the surface of the ovary when the degenerated corpus luteum atrophies.

The maturing follicle is surrounded by a layer of ovarian tissue, known as the theca. Several follicles may develop together but usually only one will become the dominant follicle and mature fully. The mature (Graafian) follicle ruptures at the surface of the ovary and discharges the oocyte and fluid into the peritoneal cavity – a process called ovulation. Wafting movements of the fimbriated (finger-like) ends of the uterine tubes assist the transfer of the oocyte into the uterine tube. It is thought that fertilisation of the oocyte usually occurs in the ampulla of the uterine tube.

The ruptured follicle contracts around leaked blood after ovulation. The epithelial cells (granulosa) multiply and the corpus luteum is formed under the influence of LH. The corpus luteum synthesises sex hormones for at least 8–10 days. If the oocyte is not fertilised, the corpus luteum degenerates, hormone production ceases and a scar forms near the surface of the ovary. If the ovum is fertilised, the corpus luteum continues to develop, increasing its size and hormone production for about 2 months.

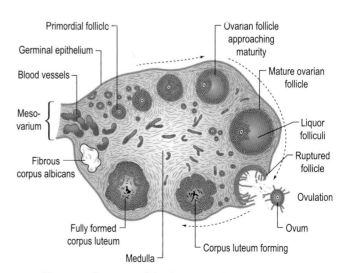

Figure 8.3 Sequence of development of the ovarian cycle.

Hormone Secretion

Ovarian sex hormone secretion is influenced by hypothalamic gonadotrophin-releasing hormone (GnRH), which stimulates the pituitary gland to release FSH and LH. FSH stimulates the initial development of ovarian follicles and their secretion of oestrogen; LH stimulates further follicular development, initiates ovulation and stimulates ovarian hormone production. FSH and LH control the secretion of two ovarian steroid hormones – oestrogens and progestogens.

Oestrogens. The effects of oestrogens include:
- development of female secondary sexual characteristics
- pubertal growth spurt
- development and functioning of female reproductive structures – oogenesis and maturation of follicles
- metabolic effects including protein anabolism, calcium homeostasis, lipid metabolism and fluid and electrolyte balance.

The oestrogen secreted by the theca interna cells of the developing follicle is oestradiol, and its metabolite (waste product) is oestriol. Many other oestrogens may be identified in the urine. Oestradiol is also produced by theca interna cells that invade the corpus luteum.

Progestogens. The main progestogen is progesterone (the 'gestation' hormone); it is produced by the luteinised cells of the corpus luteum. The metabolite of progesterone is pregnanediol, which is also excreted in the urine.

Uterus

The uterus is a hollow, muscular, pear-shaped organ approximately 7.5 cm long. It has three main parts (see Figs 8.1 and 8.2):
- fundus (top)
- body
- cervix (cervix uteri or uterine cervix).

The uterine tubes enter the uterus at its upper outer angles or cornua. The body of the uterus narrows towards the cervix, an area known as the isthmus. The cavity of the uterus connects with the cervical canal at the internal os. The cervical canal opens into the vagina via the external os. The cervix occupies the lower third of the uterus and half of the cervix projects into the vagina. The uterus normally lies in an anteverted position, almost at right angles to the vagina (see Fig. 8.1).

Structure

The uterus has three layers
- endometrium – specialised mucous lining
- myometrium – smooth muscle
- perimetrium – outer serous coat (parietal peritoneum).

Endometrium. The lining mucosa of the uterus is highly vascular and contains many tubular glands. The layers of the endometrium are the:
- outer layer – which is shed during menstruation (stratum functionalis)
- inner layer – permanent layer responsible for the regeneration of the endometrium after menstruation (stratum basale).

The thickness of the endometrium varies from 0.5 mm just after menstrual flow to about 5 mm near the end of the menstrual (uterine) cycle (see later).

Myometrium. The myometrium comprises three interlocking layers of smooth muscle fibres:
- an outer layer of longitudinal fibres
- an intermediate layer, in which fibres run irregularly, transversely and obliquely
- an inner layer of circular fibres.

Perimetrium. Parietal peritoneum forms the external coat of the uterus but does not cover the lower anterior quarter of the uterus and the cervix.

The cervix consists mainly of fibrous tissue. The endocervical canal is lined with columnar epithelium, but this changes to stratified squamous epithelium in the ectocervix (the part that protrudes into the vagina) (see Pre-I nvasive Cervical Cancer).

Blood Supply

The blood supply to the uterus is from the uterine artery, a branch of the internal iliac artery. Veins accompany the arteries and drain into the internal iliac veins. Tortuous arterial vessels enter the layers of the uterine wall and divide into capillaries between endometrial glands.

Nerve Supply

Innervation of the uterus and the uterine tubes comprises parasympathetic fibres from the sacral outflow and sympathetic fibres from the lumbar outflow.

Supporting Structures

The uterus is maintained in an anteverted and anteflexed position in the pelvis by fascia and muscle structures (Fig. 8.4). The uterine ligaments are the:
- broad ligament – a fold of peritoneum and fibromuscular tissue extending from the uterus to the pelvic side wall
- cardinal ligaments (transverse cervical or Mackenrodt's ligaments) – formed by dense fascia at the base of the broad ligaments, from the cervix to lateral walls of the pelvis
- round ligaments – extend from the anterior cornua of the uterus forwards and down through the inguinal canal to the subcutaneous fat of the labia majora
- uterosacral ligament – passes from the cervix and cardinal ligaments backwards to the sacrum, dividing to pass around the rectum
- pubocervical ligament – passes from the anterior cervix forwards to the pubic bone, dividing to pass around the urethra.

These ligaments support the position of the uterus within the pelvis. Paracervical tissue, fatty and connective tissue form a supportive

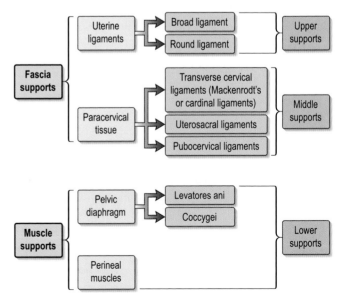

Figure 8.4 The supports of the uterus.

sling, allowing the uterus to pivot either backwards or forwards. This gives the uterus mobility anteriorly and posteriorly. Lateral and downward movements are limited by the muscles of the pelvic floor.

Functions

The functions of the uterus are:

- menstruation – sloughing off of the stratum functionalis layer of endometrium with loss of blood from torn vessels; an outline of the menstrual (uterine) cycle is provided later
- maintenance of pregnancy – implantation of the ovum in the uterine lining and retention of the embryo/fetus during growth and development
- initiation of labour – the uterine muscle develops powerful, rhythmic contractions which shorten and dilate the cervix and expel the infant.

Menstrual (Uterine) Cycle

The menstrual (uterine) cycle describes the changes in the endometrium caused by the ovarian hormones. It corresponds to the hormonal events of the ovarian cycle and can be divided into three phases:

- proliferative phase (follicular or preovulatory)
- secretory phase (luteal or postovulatory)
- menstrual phase.

Although the menstrual phase occurs at the end of the cycle, by convention the first day of menstruation is counted as day 1 of the cycle, as it provides an observable landmark (Fig. 8.5).

Menstrual Phase. Menstruation is believed to be caused by low levels of progesterone and oestrogens causing vasospasm of arteries to the endometrium. The menstrual phase usually lasts for 3–6 days and is characterised by bleeding from the uterus, with 50–60 mL of blood being lost at each menstrual period when necrotic parts of the stratum functionalis slough away, leaving a thin, bleeding area of tissue. By the third day of menstruation, new epithelial cell growth has begun to cover the disorganised stratum basale of the endometrium; by the fifth day, epithelium covers the whole surface.

Proliferative Phase. During this phase the stratum functionalis regrows, under the control of oestradiol from the maturing follicle. The growth of epithelium, glands, blood vessels and connective tissue produces thickening of the endometrium. This phase extends to the 14th or 15th day of the cycle, when ovulation occurs.

Secretory Phase. This commences after ovulation. Progesterone produced by the corpus luteum promotes the secretory phase. The endometrial glands become enlarged, the arteries coil, connective tissue hypertrophies and tissues rich in glycogen become oedematous. At 7–8 days following ovulation, the endometrium is 5–6 mm in depth and is in a state of readiness to implant a fertilised ovum.

If implantation occurs, the corpus luteum continues to produce progesterone and maintains the pregnancy until the placenta is sufficiently developed (fully functioning by 10 weeks). In the absence of implantation, the corpus luteum degenerates and production of oestrogen and progesterone declines. The endometrial stroma starts to disintegrate, oedema disappears and the endometrium shrinks. Vasoconstriction occurs. The endometrium begins to slough and menstruation begins again 14 (±1) days after ovulation. This time relationship is constant.

Fluctuations in the length of the cycle occur in the pre-ovulatory phase, as follicles may not mature at the same rate each month. Although this may result in variation in the time of onset of menstruation, most women establish a regular pattern.

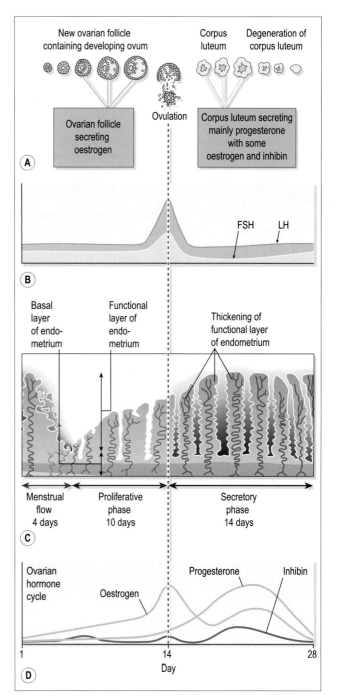

Figure 8.5 Summary of one menstrual cycle. (A) Ovarian cycle: maturation of follicle and development of corpus luteum. (B) Anterior pituitary: LH and FSH levels. (C) Menstrual cycle: menstrual, proliferative and secretory. (D) Ovarian cycle hormones: oestrogen and progesterone levels. *FSH,* Follicle-stimulating hormone; *LH,* luteinising hormone. (Reproduced from Waugh A, Grant A. Ross and Wilson: Anatomy and Physiology. 12th ed. Edinburgh: Churchill Livingstone; 2014 with permission.)

Uterine Tubes

The uterine tubes (10–14 cm long) turn posteriorly as they extend laterally from the cornua (or horns) of the uterus towards the lateral pelvic wall. The ends open as funnel-shaped structures with fimbriae (finger-like projections) (see Fig. 8.2). The broad ligament of peritoneum forms the outer serous layer of the tubes. The middle coat, of muscular tissue, is arranged in two layers: an outer longitudinal layer and an inner circular layer. The lining mucosa, comprised mainly of ciliated columnar epithelium and secretory cells, lies in folds. The lumen of the tube is narrow. The ends of the tubes are mobile, and at ovulation the fimbriae enfold the adjacent ovary to take up the released oocyte.

Functions

The uterine tubes convey oocytes from the ovary to the uterus. They are the site of fertilisation of the oocyte by a spermatozoon. Passage of the oocytes or ova along the tube is facilitated by the action of cilia and peristalsis.

Vagina

The vagina is a fibromuscular channel extending downwards and forwards from the cervix to the labia. The endocervix protrudes into the upper end of the vagina, known as the vault. This creates anterior, posterior and lateral fornices (see Fig. 8.1). The anterior wall of the vagina is approximately 7.5 cm and the posterior wall about 9 cm in length. The vagina is composed mainly of smooth muscle with a lining mucosa arranged in folds or rugae. Until first sexual intercourse, a fold of mucous membrane, the hymen, forms a border around the external opening of the vagina, partially closing the outlet. Normally the anterior and posterior walls lie in apposition but the vagina is capable of considerable distension during intercourse and childbirth.

The vagina is kept moist during the reproductive years by mucus from the cervix and transudation of fluid through the vaginal wall. Glycogen produced in the vagina is fermented by the bacterium *Lactobacillus* (Döderlein's bacillus) (part of the normal flora of the vagina) to produce lactic acid. This maintains a slightly acid environment in the vagina, inhibiting the growth of some other microorganisms.

Functions

The vagina:
- receives semen, deposited in the posterior fornix during sexual intercourse
- provides an outlet for menstrual flow, the fetus and other products of conception (POCs) and has an acid environment as part of the nonspecific (innate) defences against infection.

Vulva

The vulva comprises the external genitalia, consisting of:
- mons pubis
- labia majora
- labia minora
- clitoris
- fourchette
- urinary orifice
- vaginal orifice
- greater vestibular glands (Bartholin's glands)
- vestibule (Fig. 8.6).

Pelvic Floor

The pelvic floor is formed by tissues that fill the pelvic outlet and support the pelvic organs.
- The *levator ani muscles* form a broad muscular sheet extending from the pubic bone to the sacrum and coccyx and laterally to the pelvic walls. The urethra, vagina and rectum perforate this muscular sheet.
- The *superficial perineal muscles* lie under the levator ani muscles. They pass from the pelvic side walls, the pubis and the

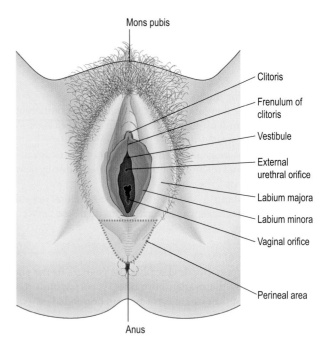

Figure 8.6 Female external genitalia. (Reproduced from Waugh A, Grant A. Ross and Wilson: Anatomy and Physiology. 12th ed. Edinburgh: Churchill Livingstone; 2014 with permission.)

sacrum to unite centrally between the vagina and the rectum, where they form the superficial part of the perineal body.
- The *perineal body* consists of wedge-shaped muscle and fibrous tissue lying between the lower vagina and lower rectum.

The Menarche

The menarche describes the first menstruation, it usually occurs between 9 and 16 years of age. Nutrition and body weight and composition affect menstruation and sexual development. The onset of menstruation may be delayed by excessive physical activity.

Some oestrogen synthesis stimulates early secondary sexual characteristics to occur some time before the menarche. There may be follicular growth and some oestrogen withdrawal bleeding to give the early periods of the first few months. These cycles are anovular (without ovulation) and such periods are painless. More discomfort can be experienced with menstruation following ovulation. A rise in basal temperature may be a guide to whether ovulation has occurred.

Variation in menstrual cycle length occurs in response to significant life events. Excitement, stress, anxiety or change of environment can delay the maturing of a follicle, ovulation and menstruation. Excessive exercise, as in athletes, can result in irregular periods, anovulatory cycles and amenorrhoea (Klein et al. 2019).

The Climacteric and Menopause

The climacteric describes the normal changes occurring in the lead up to the menopause (cessation of menstruation). The process of the climacteric is typically gradual and can extend over several years. Most women experience the climacteric or perimenopause over a period of 2–3 years, however, it may extend longer. During this time the body adjusts to less oestrogen.

The ovaries 'age', resulting in ripening of fewer follicles and decreased stimulation by the pituitary hormones. The ovaries atrophy and less oestrogen is released into the circulation. Initially this reduced oestrogen level in the blood causes excessive production of FSH from the anterior pituitary gland, and this feedback mechanism can continue for several years. The withdrawal of oestrogen and the increase in pituitary hormone add to the changes associated with the climacteric.

The menopause is marked specifically by the date of the last menstrual period so can only be identified in retrospect some months after the event. The menopause is only one effect of the climacteric. Events occurring after menstruation has stopped for at least a year are termed postmenopausal.

The menopause signifies the end of a woman's reproductive capacity. This normally occurs between 45 and 58 years of age; in the UK the average age when periods stop is 51 years.

A premature menopause is one that occurs before the age of 40 years. This can occur naturally or may be induced iatrogenically. The age of menarche, socioeconomic factors, ethnicity, use of oral contraceptives and number of pregnancies appear to have no effect on whether a woman has an early or a late menopause (British Menopause Society (BMS) 2017).

The fluctuations in oestrogen production, while following a gradual decline, alter the menstrual pattern in many women, showing considerable variation amongst women until the menopause.

After the menopause there is continued secretion of oestradiol and oestrone, although in varying and declining amounts. Oestrone becomes the predominant oestrogen. Small amounts of oestrogen can be found in the blood and urine of postmenopausal women.

Information about the disorders associated with oestrogen withdrawal and hormone replacement is outlined in a later section.

Uterine Bleeding Patterns

The climacteric is characterised by irregular menstruation. Periods may become scanty, or bleeding may be heavy. The menstrual cycle shortens, associated with a decrease in oestradiol secretion. As this continues, LH levels rise and then menstrual cycles lengthen. Anovulatory cycles result in oestrogen-withdrawal bleeding patterns, irregular cycles with intermittent and prolonged spotting (low oestrogen profile) or prolonged amenorrhoea followed by sudden, profuse bleeding (high oestrogen profile).

Somatic Changes

Somatic changes are caused by a decrease in oestrogen and an increase in gonadotrophins. As the diurnal secretion of oestrogen varies from woman to woman, changes experienced will vary in severity but they are progressive.

The ovaries atrophy and follicles disappear or fail to respond to gonadotrophins. Other internal reproductive organs become thinner and atrophy. Vaginal mucosa atrophies with a loss of rugae, elasticity and lubrication with an increase in pH. Vaginal dryness can result in pruritus and dyspareunia. Loss of the acidic environment permits microorganisms to multiply more easily. There is an increase in connective tissue, causing narrowing and shortening of the vagina. The vagina is more prone to ulceration and bleeds easily to touch. Vaginitis may occur in the older woman. The labia thin and lose their sexual responsiveness. Pubic hair growth decreases as age advances. The pelvic floor loses tone and elasticity, and becomes less effective in supporting the pelvic contents. The urethral mucosa may also show atrophic changes, resulting in symptoms of urethritis and cystitis, in the absence of bacteriuria.

Physiological changes, resulting in lack of lubrication, loss of libido and dyspareunia, can contribute to sexual problems for the woman. Hormone replacement therapy (HRT) may be a possible

treatment choice, and psychosexual counselling may be of benefit. Many factors contribute to a satisfying sex life – satisfaction in a relationship, psychological well-being and emotional security can all make an important contribution, demonstrating the need for a holistic approach.

Vasomotor Disturbances

Vasomotor disturbances often accompany the climacteric. The incidence and intensity of these vary between individuals. Hot flushes/flashes are the most common but perspiration, headache, fainting and palpitations may also be experienced. Hot flushes can start with a sensation of extreme warmth in the chest, quickly followed by flushing of the face and neck. The flush may be accompanied by sweating and palpitations. Dizziness and nausea may also be experienced. Shivering is often reported after the flush, probably due to compensatory constriction of the blood vessels. While vasomotor symptoms will eventually subside with no long-term effects, hot flushes and sweats are embarrassing, uncontrollable and can be distressing for many women. Randomised controlled trials (RCTs) have indicated the value of oestrogen in reducing the severity of vasomotor symptoms when compared with placebo.

In addition to oestrogen therapy, other treatments, such as vitamin E and/or B$_6$, clonidine, phytoestrogens, propranolol and oil of evening primrose (contains gamma linoleic acid), have been used. Progestogens have been shown to alleviate hot flushes. Phytoestrogens, found in soya products, have been suggested as a remedy for menopausal symptoms. While some women do find them valuable, there is controversy about advocating them as a therapy for menopausal symptoms.

Other Changes

These can include emotional changes. These can include anxiety, poor concentration, dizziness, a bloated feeling and depressive feelings after the menopause. In addition to hormonal changes occurring at the perimenopause, women may also be facing other psychosocial changes such as children leaving home, which can affect their emotional state.

Menstrual Disorders

Amenorrhoea

Amenorrhoea (absence of menstruation) is either primary or secondary. Primary amenorrhoea is the nonappearance of menstruation in a female by the age of 16 years. There may be an anatomical fault or some disturbance in hormonal secretions. Delayed puberty may be familial or constitutional. Secondary amenorrhoea is the absence of menstruation for a period of time which is twice the length of the normal menstrual cycle for a woman who has previously menstruated, i.e. missing two or more menstrual periods. This may result in the woman waiting some time before seeking investigation.

Amenorrhoea is physiological before puberty, during pregnancy and lactation and after the menopause. Inheritance, ethnicity, climate and general nutrition influence the menarche.

Before Puberty

A teenage girl may be seen by her practice nurse or GP because of delay in the onset of menstruation. The specialist nurse practitioner or doctor may undertake a general physical examination to determine if other secondary sex characteristics are present; if so, menstruation will follow in due course. If secondary sex characteristics or menstruation fail to develop, the patient is referred to a consultant gynaecologist and endocrinologist for investigation.

During Pregnancy

Following ovulation, cells of the ovarian follicle are stimulated by LH to develop the corpus luteum which produces progesterone. This hormone stimulates the endometrium and its secretory glands in readiness to receive the fertilised ovum from the uterine tube. When the fertilised ovum embeds in the lining of the uterus (known as the decidua), it produces the hormone human chorionic gonadotrophin (hCG). This hormone supports the corpus luteum to continue producing progesterone until the placenta is established and producing hormones. The presence of the growing fetus and the continued production of progesterone prevent the loss of endometrium and the menstrual flow.

Amenorrhoea is frequently one of the first symptoms that lead a woman to suspect that she is pregnant. Levels of hCG in the urine provide a positive diagnosis when undertaking a urinary pregnancy test. Confirmation is made by the presence of fetal heart pulsation seen on ultrasound scan (USS) from 5 to 6 weeks' gestation onwards.

During Lactation

Women who totally breast feed may not ovulate or menstruate during the first 6 months after childbirth or until weaning commences. As such, breast feeding exerts a measure of birth control, but must not be recommended as an effective contraceptive.

Total nipple stimulation is important for suppression of ovarian function. The suckling stimulus to the nipple leads to a neurohormonal reflex production of prolactin by the anterior pituitary gland which inhibits gonadotrophin hormone release, preventing ovulation and menstruation.

Suppression of the ovaries declines where supplements comprise more than 50% of the diet of the baby who is breast feeding. The incidence of ovulation and the risk of pregnancy then rise rapidly.

A poor state of nutrition in the woman can inhibit ovulation, particularly in developing countries. To ensure contraception during the period of lactation, the woman may be advised to use a barrier method. The progestogen-only pill is considered safe during lactation as it does not impact on the milk supply and only insignificant quantities will enter the milk. However, the combined oral contraceptive pill inhibits lactation.

After the Menopause

The menopause, the date of the final menstrual period, may not be fully acknowledged until a year without periods has passed.

Pathological Amenorrhoea

There are a several pathological causes of amenorrhoea.

Uterine Lesions, Congenital Abnormalities

● Pathophysiology

Examples include:
- congenital absence of uterus and vagina
- primary deficiency of endometrium – the endometrium may be absent, deficient or fail to be stimulated by oestrogen.

Ovarian Lesions

Failure of normal ovarian development is rare. Chromosomal abnormalities such as Turner's syndrome may occur (see Chapter 5, Nursing Patients With Endocrine Disorders).

● Pathophysiology

Turner's syndrome is a condition that results from the absence of one female sex chromosome. It is characterised by infantile development of the genitalia, absence of breasts, short stature and a webbed neck. There may be associated congenital cardiac lesions.

● Medical Management

Chromosomal studies confirm the diagnosis. Early diagnosis is important and investigations can usually be initiated before puberty, suspicion being aroused by the short stature of the child. Treatment, such as ethinyl oestradiol 0.01 mg twice daily, in 3-week cycles, given for several months, then norethisterone added for the last 10 days of each cycle, can be used to stimulate development of the breasts and uterus. Menstruation may occur with this treatment.

Pituitary Disorders

Disorders of the pituitary gland may result in the secretion of abnormal levels of hormones which affect the sensitive feedback mechanism ultimately affecting hormones of the menstrual cycle (see Chapter 5, Nursing Patients With Endocrine Disorders).

Other Endocrine Disorders

These include:
- congenital adrenal hyperplasia (also known as adrenogenital syndrome)
- Cushing's syndrome/disease
- Addison's disease
- Hypothyroidism
- hyperthyroidism
- diabetes mellitus.
  See Chapter 5 for further information.

Emotional Stress

Emotional disturbance is likely to affect menstrual function through the hypothalamic–pituitary axis. Emotional distress caused by some traumatic event may contribute to amenorrhoea.

● Medical Management

Discussion with a health professional will help the patient understand and be reassured about the effects of stress on menstruation. Physical and mental relaxation will help her deal with the stress and will promote a spontaneous return of menstruation.

Eating Disorders

Eating disorders such as anorexia nervosa can affect the menstrual cycle.

● Pathophysiology

Anorexia nervosa is associated with distortion of body image which results in disordered eating behaviour that includes dieting and extreme exercise routines and misuse of laxatives. There is extreme weight loss and dislike for foods, particularly carbohydrates. There is failure in hypothalamic stimulation of LH release and amenorrhoea occurs.

● Medical Management

Girls and women with anorexia nervosa are often reluctant to accept that they have a problem or to ask for help and there are many reasons for this. Their weight loss may be being investigated or they may present to the practice nurse or GP with another problem, but when a diagnosis is made, care is usually maintained by mental healthcare professionals. Positive physical and psychological changes can promote a return to menstruation.

Important Mental Health Illness
Psychotic illness may be a cause of amenorrhoea and the woman may not menstruate for many months or years.

Pathophysiology
A life crisis can contribute to disturbances in the activity of neurotransmitter catecholamines in the brain or the chemistry of the hypothalamic–pituitary axis may be disrupted.

Care and Management
It is essential to ascertain that the woman is not pregnant. A reliable source of information will be needed, either the patient herself or her partner. Once the acute symptoms of the patient's illness have been treated and the body chemistry becomes more stable, a return to normal menstruation would be expected.

Severe Systemic Illness
Pathophysiology
The stress of severe illness may induce ineffective functioning in multiple body organs and may temporarily suppress menstrual function. Stress, as experienced by prisoners of war or refugees, associated with malnutrition, minimal protein and vitamin intake, leads to amenorrhoea.

Medical Management
When amenorrhoea is secondary to general illness, the medical condition must be treated before the amenorrhoea can be relieved. The influences of emotional and physical stress are complex, and sometimes assisting the patient to relax and lower anxiety levels may promote menstruation before the general illness is fully relieved.

❖ Nursing Management and Health Promotion: Amenorrhoea
The nursing care for a patient with amenorrhoea is commonly undertaken in the community.

Assessment. As part of the routine assessment, the nurse should take a detailed history, including:
- the date of the last menstrual period
- any problems with menstruation
- knowledge from the person about the reason for amenorrhoea
- does the patient perceive amenorrhoea as a problem?

Assessment should take account of lifestyle, including nutrition, eating pattern, body weight, level of exercise and any stressful life events.

Planning Care. The nurse should discuss with the patient reasons for amenorrhoea and how these relate to the individual. The patient's level of anxiety should be noted and the nurse may recommend simple relaxation techniques or suggest relaxation audiotapes.

If, following a medical assessment, puberty is deemed to be delayed, reassurance and counselling are part of nursing care. Nurses can encourage optimism, provide general information about diet, exercise and lifestyle, and offer support, but in some cases skilled counselling may also be of value.

Evaluating Care. The patient's long-term goal of 'return of menstruation' may not be achievable within the early weeks of care and expectations should be realistic. This may include an evaluation of the level of the patient's anxiety. The patient should be asked to report menstruation. Achievement of such a long-term goal may occur as a result of medical treatment, particularly if hormonal or anxiolytic drugs have been prescribed.

Dysmenorrhoea
Dysmenorrhoea is pain associated with menstruation. Many women experience minor discomfort, but dysmenorrhoea is more disabling. Before the start of bleeding, the breasts may feel larger and ache; women may also experience abdominal distension and bloating, constipation and feeling generally unwell. The symptoms may persist for 1–2 days and be relieved or replaced by backache, urinary frequency and loose stools once menstruation occurs.

For some women, the first hours or the first day are most painful. Dragging sensations from the umbilical area down to the groins and thighs may be experienced, or the pain may be severe, colicky or spasmodic in nature across the abdomen and back. The pain may be so distracting as to interfere with the woman's usual daily activities. Prevalence rates vary widely in the literature and range from 16% to 91% in women of reproductive age being affected (National Institute for Health and Care Excellence (NICE) 2021). Absenteeism from work and school is common due to symptoms of dysmenorrhoea.

Two types of dysmenorrhoea are described:
- primary dysmenorrhoea (spasmodic) is due to physiological processes of menstruation, with muscle contraction
- secondary dysmenorrhoea (congestive) is associated with organic pelvic disease.

Primary Dysmenorrhoea
Primary dysmenorrhoea is seen in young women in their late teens and early 20s. At first they may have anovulatory pain-free menstruation. Later, when ovulation becomes established, they experience pain 24 hours before the flow begins. The pain is severe and colicky over the lower abdomen, often radiating to the thighs and back, and lasts for at least 12 hours. Nausea, fainting and diarrhoea may accompany the acute phase and the girl looks tense, pale and drawn.

Pathophysiology
Dysmenorrhoea is associated with an increased production of endometrial prostaglandins, resulting in intense uterine contractions. Uterine arterioles can go into spasm and the resulting muscle ischaemia produces uterine pain.

Misunderstandings about the physical changes of menstruation and the nature of dysmenorrhoea may underlie ineffective management. Information about the nature of dysmenorrhoea and its effective management should therefore be addressed with young girls and their parents as appropriate (Reflection 8.1).

Rarely, dysmenorrhoea may be due to an obstruction to the flow of blood as a result of a clot being lodged in the cervix. Other possible causes include pelvic inflammatory disease (PID), endometriosis (ectopic endometrium present in the muscle wall, ovaries or elsewhere in the pelvic cavity) and congenital abnormalities.

Medical Management
Detailed interviews may be carried out with the girl and her parent(s). In this way, shared and differing attitudes to the subject can be identified and problems defined. Vaginal examination may be carried out.

Efforts are made to offer information and advice to the girl and her parents, as necessary, about normal menstrual function. A period of rest and the application of warmth to the abdomen or back may be helpful. Regular exercise, the avoidance of constipation and the prevention of anxiety are emphasised. Exercise encourages the release of endogenous endorphins which have natural analgesic properties. A series of exercises to stretch the ligaments that support the uterus in the pelvis may relieve menstrual pain. Attention should be paid to maintaining good posture.

Treatment. Treatment for dysmenorrhoea aims to relieve pain or symptoms either by affecting the physiological mechanisms behind menstrual pain (such as prostaglandin production) or by relieving symptoms. Treatments using simple analgesics such as paracetamol, aspirin and nonsteroidal antiinflammatory drugs (NSAIDs) work by inhibiting prostaglandin production. An oral contraceptive may be indicated as these inhibit ovulation. A levonorgestrel-releasing intrauterine system may also be of use. Slow release of levonorgestrel into the uterine cavity prevents thickening of the endometrium. Women may experience amenorrhoea with resultant reduction in dysmenorrhoea. The levonorgestrel releasing intrauterine system has also been shown to be effective in reducing dysmenorrhoea in women with endometriosis (Kho and Shields 2020)

In some cases, hysteroscopy (endoscopic examination of the uterine cavity) may be necessary to exclude uterine pathology. A laparoscopy may be required to exclude endometriosis. A pregnancy and vaginal delivery may improve or cure primary dysmenorrhoea.

❖❖ Nursing Management and Health Promotion: Primary Dysmenorrhoea

Assessment. An assessment should be made of the patient's general health. The patient's description of the nature of her painful periods should be recorded along with any observations about her physical and emotional symptoms on particular days of the cycle. Any medication used for pain relief or contraception, and its effectiveness, should be noted. Dietary habits and exercise activities are also relevant. Sensitive questioning of the patient will reveal any anxieties or stressors which may be contributing to symptoms. A care plan is then formulated.

Planning Care. Care should be developed with the patient. Helping the girl/woman recognise signs of impending menstruation will allow her to take analgesics in time to prevent pain. A holistic approach to strategies to relieve pain should be discussed. Useful information includes:

- a simple explanation of how hormones function in the menstrual cycle and the effects of excessive prostaglandins
- discussion of the beneficial effects of a diet adequate in fibre, vitamins and polyunsaturated fats, and low in salt
- discussion of the patient's present level of physical exercise and the benefits of exercise and good posture in stimulating organs and the release of pain-relieving endorphins (see Chapter 19, Pain Management)
- teaching simple relaxation exercises with referral to massage and local heat application
- discussion about drugs that inhibit prostaglandin secretion.

Evaluating Care. A pain verbal rating scale could be used by the patient (see Chapter 20). If optimal pain relief is not achieved, it may be necessary to amend analgesic regimens. Relaxation exercises should be used while the effects of analgesics are awaited. The achievement of the patient's goals will be her first step in a change of lifestyle. Further support and encouragement may be given by her family, friend, partner, a school or practice nurse or the GP.

Secondary Dysmenorrhoea

Secondary dysmenorrhoea is experienced in later menstrual life by women in their mid-20s after years of painless menstruation.

● Pathophysiology

Women usually complain of a dragging pain in the lower abdomen, pelvic area and breasts, accompanied by headache. The pain occurs some days before the menstrual flow and may continue throughout bleeding.

The condition is usually associated with pelvic pathology, although anxiety or depression can be an aggravating factor:

- Adenomyosis (infiltration of the myometrium by endometrial cells) – increased tension in the uterine muscle, as blood accumulates in the cystic spaces.
- Fixed retroversion of the uterus can cause severe pain, especially if associated with a low-grade pelvic infection.
- Partial stenosis of the cervix, following cautery or surgery.
- Endometriosis interferes with normal rhythmic uterine contractions.
- Pelvic congestion, due to increased blood supply to the uterus, and menorrhagia (see later).
- Pelvic inflammation, particularly salpingitis, might contribute to pain.
- Fibromyomata ('fibroids') and polyps interfere with normal rhythmic uterine contractions and cause muscular spasms as the uterus attempts to empty itself of the abnormal tissue.

● Medical Management

History and Examination. A detailed history of the problem is recorded and a full physical examination including vaginal examination is performed to assess underlying causes. An accurate history regarding the pain is important, noting the age of onset, and the site, radiation, duration, character and time of onset in the menstrual cycle. Information about any related symptoms, possible abnormal uterine bleeding, pain on sexual intercourse (dyspareunia), pruritus and premenstrual tension is gathered.

Treatment. Investigations may involve hysteroscopy and endometrial biopsy. If endometriosis is suspected a laparoscopy may be performed. The presence of fibroids or polyps will be treated appropriately. Pelvic inflammation can be treated by antibiotics. An analgesic drug can be prescribed that is appropriate for inhibiting prostaglandin synthesis, for example mefenamic acid.

❖ Nursing Management and Health Promotion: Secondary Dysmenorrhoea

On assessment, pain will be identified as a problem. Goals and interventions will be similar to those described for primary dysmenorrhoea, particularly encouraging personal health messages. Additional problems will be identified and appropriate nursing interventions planned depending on the specific underlying pathology and the treatment interventions recommended.

Pre- and postoperative care planning will be needed if surgical procedures are planned (see Chapter 24, Nursing the Patient Undergoing Surgery). At the time of discharge the patient's future prospects for an improved pattern of menstrual cycles should be better.

Abnormal Uterine Bleeding

Abnormal uterine bleeding is described according to the rhythm or pattern of blood loss:
- menorrhagia – heavy or profuse menstrual bleeding; bleeding occurs at normal intervals but is increased in amount or duration
- polymenorrhoea – menstruation occurring with a frequency of less than 21 days
- polymenorrhagia – periods that are both heavy and frequent
- metrorrhagia – irregular or unusual uterine bleeding between periods
- dysfunctional uterine bleeding – abnormal uterine bleeding for which no organic cause is identified.

Abnormal uterine bleeding with the passing of blood clots is significant. The bleeding is greater than normal if the usual anticlotting agents released by the endometrium are unable to control the volume or rate of blood loss.

Menorrhagia

Menorrhagia may be ovarian or uterine in origin.

● Pathophysiology

Ovarian. There is hormonal imbalance (of oestrogen and progesterone secretion) usually due to the oversecretion of gonadotrophins. Emotional stress may contribute to this over secretion.

Ovarian lesions are of two types:
- Polycystic growths – may disturb the normal production of ovarian hormones and excessive endometrial growth occurs.
- Immature follicles – may fail to result in ovulation. The corpus luteum fails to form, so progesterone cannot be produced. Oestrogen levels continue to rise and there is a proliferation of the endometrium.

Uterine. Lesions include:
- Fibroids – increase the endometrial surface area, thereby increasing bleeding. Fibroids may prolong the flow by restricting or disturbing contractions.
- Polyps – increase endometrial surface area.

- Adenomyosis – interferes with muscle contractions.
- Multiparity – reduced tone in the uterine muscle fibres caused by replacement by fibrous tissue will interfere with normal contractions.
- Developmental anomalies, e.g. a bicornuate, septate or duplicated uterus – may impede contractions.
- Endometriosis – is accompanied by increased blood supply to the uterus.
- Tumour formation – increases blood supply and bleeding.
- Intrauterine contraceptive devices – cause endometrial irritation. Excessive bleeding may be problematic during the first 3 months after insertion.
- Tubal ligation – involves some alteration in the course of blood vessels that increases uterine blood supply.

● Medical Management

A physical examination will try to establish whether bleeding is a problem of quantity or rhythm, or both. Pelvic examination may reveal tenderness, masses or irregularities. If no pelvic abnormality is found, then a provisional diagnosis of dysfunctional uterine bleeding is made.

Investigations. A full blood count will identify anaemia. Other endocrine imbalances may be important so thyroid function tests may also be done. A USS will help identify the presence of fibroids or masses. Two types of USSs can be used to help diagnose fibroids:
- An abdominal USS – where the ultrasound probe is moved over the outside of the abdomen
- A transvaginal USS – where a small ultrasound probe is inserted into the vagina

Hysteroscopy and endometrial biopsy may also be undertaken based on results of examination and USS.

Treatment. Treatment will depend on the amount of blood lost. Any anaemia identified should be corrected as appropriate. Mefenamic acid 500 mg or tranexamic acid 1 g, three times daily on the first day of the period and on other days with a heavy flow is often helpful, for a period of 3 months, followed by review (NICE 2018c).

Hormone therapy may be given. Progesterone may be prescribed to balance oestrogen secretion and reduce excessive endometrial growth. This may be in the form of the levonorgestrell-releasing intrauterine system described under treatment of dysmenorrhoea. One of the combined contraceptive pills may be given to suppress hormone production. Progestogen administration will modify flow for patients with heavy but regular cycles.

Endometrial ablation is another treatment option for menorrhagia and is one of several minimally invasive procedures developed over recent years. It is undertaken as a day-case procedure and is increasingly done as an outpatient procedure (Clark and Gupta 2005). Although the work of Clarke and Gupta (2005) is now somewhat dated, the text is still recommended reading for hysteroscopists and still relevant to contemporary practice.

Endometrial ablation involves destroying the endometrium, preventing its cyclical regeneration. For many women the associated physical, social and psychological implications make it preferable to more extensive surgery such as hysterectomy. Different techniques have developed, but they are based on the same principle which involves the introduction of instruments to destroy the endometrium using heat via a hysteroscope. The first generation of this technique included freezing or lasering, both of which are now rarely used. The second generation of techniques include:
- Balloon endometrial ablation – a special catheter is introduced via the cervix into the endometrial cavity. Water distends the catheter

balloon so that it comes into direct contact with the endometrial lining. The water is then superheated to 87°C and left in situ for 8 minutes. The heat produced effectively destroys the endometrium.

• Electrical energy – The traditional form of this technique uses a resection device and or a 'rollerball' to resect or ablate the tissue and was one of the first generation of techniques used. Newer techniques involve uses a triangular heating device which is introduced to the uterine cavity and expands to conform to the endometrial lining. Electrical energy is then delivered to destroy the endometrium as earlier, but only takes 90 seconds instead of 8 minutes.

There are risks and benefits associated with each technique. Traditional resection techniques may be more beneficial for women with fibroids. Newer (second generation) treatment approaches are considered safer in terms of rate of fluid overload, cervical lacerations and haematometra, with similar rates of uterine perforation. They are generally quicker procedures and more likely to be done under local (rather than general) anaesthesia compared with first-generation approaches (Bofill Rodriguez et al. 2019)

Following the procedure, slight vaginal bleeding can be expected for a few days. Menstruation will become lighter or may cease, but dysmenorrhoea and premenstrual symptoms may continue. Procedures may need to be repeated at a later stage or a hysterectomy may eventually be necessary.

When a hysterectomy is deemed necessary, it may be possible to undertake this without major surgery by means of laparoscopic surgery or robotically assisted laparoscopic surgery. This requires insertion of a number of small trocars through the abdominal wall, providing entry sites for instruments. The viewing laparoscope is inserted below the umbilicus, two other insertion sites will be positioned just above the pubic hair line and accessory insertion sites will be used to insert instruments. This procedure can sometimes be undertaken as a day case, although the average inpatient stay is 1–2 days.

If large fibroids or endometriosis exist, an abdominal hysterectomy is required. Alternatively, in the case of fibroids, a myomectomy may be appropriate, particularly if the woman wants to retain her uterus. Here the fibroids are shelled out of the myometrium.

Metrorrhagia

Pathophysiology

• Lowered oestrogen level may occur just prior to the formation of the corpus luteum, resulting in vaginal blood spotting at the time of ovulation.
• Cervical pathology, e.g. inflammation, erosion, polyps or cancer, may cause slight bleeding, especially after intercourse or vaginal examination.
• Vaginal pathology, e.g. inflammation, infection, ulceration and atrophy, may cause bleeding.
• Endometrial cancer is a major cause of irregular bleeding.
• Complications of an early pregnancy – as a fertilised ovum embeds into the endometrium, slight bleeding may occur. This loss may be repeated during several months of the pregnancy. Haemorrhage might also occur in a pregnant woman due to placenta praevia (placenta implanted abnormally low in the uterus).

Medical Management

Investigations. The vulva, vagina and cervix should be inspected closely. Colposcopy examination, whereby the cervix is examined under magnification, will identify any abnormalities

including precancer or cancer. If abnormal cells are identified, biopsies of the cervix may be taken for histological examination.

Liquid-based cytology (LBC) smear tests have replaced Papanicolaou (Pap) smears as the routine investigation to evaluate changes in cells obtained from the cervix. A high vaginal swab (HVS) will allow the identification of infection (bacterial or fungal) or parasitic infestations. Where endometrial bleeding is suspected, it is important to perform a hysteroscopy and endometrial biopsy to rule out cancer.

Treatment. Treatment depends on the cause. Bacterial infections of the reproductive tract will be treated with the appropriate antibiotic, for example metronidazole or clindamycin for bacterial vaginosis. Vaginal candidiasis is treated with an antifungal, for example clotrimazole or nystatin pessaries. Trichomonal infections are treated with metronidazole or tinidazole.

In ovulation spotting, small quantities of oestrogen may be given for 6–7 days, 3 days before ovulation.

Any malignant changes identified will be treated appropriately by surgical excision, radiotherapy or cytotoxic medication.

Menstrual Considerations for Transgender and Nonbinary People

Transgender and nonbinary people may also experience issues related to menstruation and the menopause. For transgender males (and other gender-diverse individuals assigned female at birth), the approach of menarche may be met with worsening dysphoria, anxiety, depression and suicidal ideation (Weiselberg 2022).

Some individuals may choose to undergo gender affirmation, potentially including hysterectomy. However, one American study indicated that it was only a minority of transgender men who chose to undergo hysterectomy (14%) although considerably more (49%) had received gender affirming hormone treatment (GAHT) (Carbonnel et al. 2021).

Research based on menstruation and the menopause has been historically based on women and cannot be extrapolated to be the same for transgender males (Weiselberg 2022). This is an area of research which is expanding. In some instances, it would appear that even with GAHT, transgender men can still be prone to dysmenorrhea and endometriosis, with one study even suggesting that the prevalence of endometriosis in transgender men could be higher than in their female cisgendered counterparts (Okita et al. 2021).

Premenstrual Syndrome

Premenstrual syndrome (PMS) refers to physical and psychological symptoms occurring in the latter half of the cycle, 2–12 days prior to menstruation, subsiding once menstruation commences. There is a symptom-free week following menstruation. The symptoms vary between women but can also vary from cycle to cycle in individuals.

Most women will experience some symptoms during their reproductive life but 30%–40% of women are thought to experience true PMS, with 3%–8% experiencing symptoms of premenstrual dysphoric disorder (PMDD), which is a severe form which causes extreme mood shifts and can be particularly disruptive to daily life (Ryu and Kim 2015).

The symptoms of PMS frequently start after discontinuing the oral contraceptive pill or after a pregnancy and become progressively worse with age.

Signs and symptoms are varied but include:
- mood swings, feeling upset, irritability and anxiety
- fluid retention, weight gain, swollen extremities, breast tenderness, abdominal bloating and pelvic pain
- headache, food craving, increased appetite, palpitations, fatigue and dizziness or fainting
- depression, forgetfulness, confusion, crying and insomnia.

Pathophysiology

Numerous theories have been suggested to explain PMS, but the precise cause remains unknown.

Prostaglandins. These exert sedative effects on the central nervous system and affect both aldosterone and antidiuretic hormone (ADH) activity.

Fluid Retention or Redistribution. Redistribution of body fluids in intracellular and extracellular compartments.

Hypoglycaemia. Abnormalities of glucose metabolism in the luteal phase of the menstrual cycle that exaggerate blood glucose swings might account for premenstrual hypoglycaemic symptoms.

Vitamin B_6 (Pyridoxine) Deficiency. Vitamin B_6 increases inhibitory amines such as dopamine and 5-hydroxytryptamine (serotonin) and also acts as a coenzyme in converting excitatory amino acids to corresponding inhibitory amino acids, with sedative effects. Vitamin B_6 can reduce the excitatory amines.

Progesterone Withdrawal. PMS may be due to deficiency of progesterone production. Many PMS patients have been shown to have adequate corpus luteum functioning, suggesting that it may be the rate of fall of progesterone level during the late luteal phase causing PMS rather than a deficiency.

Endorphin Withdrawal. Endorphins appear to be important in the physiology of pain and mood change. It has been suggested that endorphin levels decrease in the week preceding menstruation, which may affect ovarian function.

Serotonin (5-Hydroxytryptamine). Serotonin acts as a neurotransmitter that influences mood, appetite and behaviour. In women with PMS, it can be significantly lower in the luteal phase of the menstrual cycle than in control subjects.

While researchers have been keen to find one reason for PMS, it is more likely that it is a combination of physical, psychological and social factors.

Medical Management

Recommended treatment focuses on identifying and controlling individual symptom clusters. Drug treatments are used cautiously. The patient–healthcare practitioner relationship is thought to be an important influence on some women, relieved that their condition is being taken seriously.

Investigations. A thorough examination is required to diagnose PMS accurately and identify any underlying pathology. Other medical, mental health and gynaecological conditions must be excluded or be identified as coexisting with PMS.

Estimations of oestrogen, progesterone, prolactin, gonadotrophin or electrolytes are not usually helpful in making a diagnosis of PMS.

Treatment. A complete cure does not yet exist but an integrated treatment programme can be adopted whereby women are asked to record, on a daily basis, personal experiences in mood, behaviour and physical discomforts for at least 3 months. This will identify symptom clusters and appropriate strategies to improve the severity of symptoms.

Women should be advised to:
- exercise regularly
- avoid coffee, tea and chocolate
- eat a diet low in sugar, fat and salt, and high in protein
- take supplements of vitamins B_6 and E_1 and magnesium
- limit fluid intake
- chart their weight daily
- avoid alcohol and smoking
- avoid stress.

It is important the woman understands that no single treatment will work for everyone and they may need to try a combination of treatments before they find one that suits them. Choice of treatment will depend on types and severity of symptoms and possible side-effects. All treatment options should be discussed fully with the practice nurse and GP.

General relaxation techniques may be helpful for some symptoms such as headache or fluid retention.

Drug treatments used in PMS will depend on the particular cluster of symptoms experienced.

Hormonal Treatment. Women may already have tried over-the-counter (OTC) remedies. There is limited evidence to support the use of complementary treatments and dietary supplements, including reflexology, acupuncture, calcium and vitamin D, ginkgo biloba, evening primrose oil, vitamin B_6 and magnesium, although some women may find them beneficial (NICE 2019a).

Hormonal treatment of PMS aims to interrupt the 'normal' menstrual cycle and associated hormone production by the body. Oral contraceptives will stop ovulation and help stabilise hormone levels but can cause side-effects. Progesterone or progestogen may also be used. In severe cases, analogues of GnRH, such as buserelin, will inhibit the release of gonadotrophins and so suppress follicular development, ovulation and the endocrine changes of the cycle. This creates a 'medical oophorectomy', but the woman may have unpleasant menopausal symptoms and this treatment should not be used on a long-term basis.

Diuretics. Women can now obtain these as OTC preparations at pharmacies. By reducing the excess fluid in the body, these can relieve feelings of bloatedness and sore breasts.

Analgesics. Abdominal cramps, sore breasts, headaches, muscular and joint pain can be relieved by NSAIDs but they can make fluid retention worse.

Selective Serotonin Reuptake Inhibitors (SSRIs). may be the most effective treatment for severe PMS. SSRIs such as fluoxetine and sertraline are antidepressants and can help relieve tiredness, sleep problems, food cravings and low mood. However, they may have negative side-effects which may outweigh their benefits.

Psychological Support. Having their symptoms taken seriously by a health professional can provide great support. Techniques to improve coping skills and stress management may also be helpful. Vitamin B_6 up to a dose of 100 mg/day can be helpful for premenstrual depression and other symptoms.

Surgery. In cases of severe PMS or those compounded by other gynaecological problems, hysterectomy with bilateral salpingo-oophorectomy (BSO) followed by HRT may be considered. Oophorectomy must be included to prevent the ovarian cycle; otherwise, the cyclical problems will persist.

❖ Nursing Management and Health Promotion: PMS

Assessment. Nurses may encounter women who experience PMS symptoms not discussed with their doctors. Nurses have opportunities to provide such women with information suggesting daily recording of physical changes, discomforts, emotional feelings and behaviour.

Planning Care. A supportive–educative approach combines the giving of information and advice, also allowing the woman to look at achieving the aims for her particular circumstances. Advice should be based on the areas previously outlined in treatment.

A counselling approach by the nurse can encourage the woman to verbalise her preferred choices. Information should be given to the patient about the nature of any drugs prescribed. The possible value of self-help groups can also be discussed with the woman, but the value of family support, emphasised in some cultures, should not be undermined. In recent years, there has been greater acknowledgement that cultural factors may have an influence on a woman's access to and their experiences of healthcare. These issues can be wide ranging and there is currently research ongoing as to how healthcare professionals can improve services related to women's health (Department of Health (DH) 2022).

Evaluating Care. It is important that the woman records the effect of treatment; keeping a diary may be advantageous to record these effects. Some symptoms may have greatly improved, whilst others have shown no improvement. The woman must appreciate that not all treatments suit everyone. Each planned action should be reviewed and alternative therapies tried. Evidence of a sustained low mood or other severe symptoms should be referred to the practice nurse, GP or PMS specialist.

Disorders of the Climacteric/Menopause

Physiological, psychological and social changes associated with the climacteric/menopause have been described earlier. This section outlines the long-term effects of oestrogen withdrawal on women's health.

Decreased oestrogen is associated with the development of osteoporosis and cardiovascular disease, resulting in an increased risk of fragility fractures, coronary heart disease (CHD) and stroke (see Chapter 2, Nursing Patients With Cardiovascular Disorders, Chapter 11, Nursing Patients With Disorders of the Nervous System, and Chapter 12, Nursing Patients With Musculoskeletal Disorders). Based on information from NICE (2017, 2023), the factors contributing to an increased risk of osteoporosis and cardiovascular disease include:

- inherited factors
- sedentary lifestyle
- low calcium intake/absorption
- low body mass index (BMI) – less than 22 kg/m² (there may be some variation with this risk factor depending on ethnicity) (Cauley and Nelson 2021)
- early menopause
- cigarette smoking
- excessive stress
- excessive salt intake
- high protein intake
- moderate to excessive alcohol intake
- caffeine intake
- pre-existing disorders of the kidney or thyroid, Crohn's disease, rheumatoid arthritis and diabetes.

Osteoporosis

Osteoporosis is a disease characterised by a decrease in bone density, predisposing to bone fragility and fractures. It is estimated that, annually, osteoporosis leads to nearly 9 million fractures worldwide, with over 300,000 patients presenting with fragility fractures each year in the UK (NICE 2017a).

The disease is age related but is more common in women due to the effects of reduced oestrogen levels. The World Health Organisation (WHO) defines osteoporosis as a bone mineral density (BMD) T-score of more than –2.5 standard deviations below the mean value for young adults (NICE 2017a). This definition has been used to diagnose osteoporosis based on BMD assessed at the hip and spine using dual-energy X-ray absorptiometry (DEXA).

Oestrogens play an important part in achieving maximum BMD. In early adult life, the rate of bone formation exceeds that of resorption, thus increasing BMD. When oestrogen levels decline, bone resorption increases and bone loss accelerates after the menopause.

Cardiovascular Disease

CHD is a leading cause of death in women. In the UK it accounts for 1 in 16 deaths in women (British Heart Foundation 2023). Conflicting study results have caused confusion over whether oestrogen helps prevent CHD. The latest evidence from the Women's Health Concern (2020) suggests that HRT does not increase cardiovascular disease when started under the age of 60 years, however, the risk of venous thromboembolism (VTE) is increased by the use of oral HRT compared with the baseline population risk. The risk of VTE associated with the use of transdermal HRT (given at a standard dose) is no greater than that of the baseline population (NICE 2019a).

The BMS has produced a guideline summary of the NICE guidance; they emphasised the importance of individualised treatment with considerations being based on symptoms, family history, diet and lifestyle and the preferences of the individual (BMS 2020). The timing of starting HRT is important and oestrogen may have a protective role in preventing CHD in women aged 50–59 years (BMS 2020). The Women's Health Concern (2020) notes that there have been concerns raised about HRT and the potential risks to various aspects of women's health; more recently published findings demonstrate that although not completely risk free, it is still the most effective solution for the relief of menopausal symptoms and is also effective for the prevention of osteoporosis. In certain age groups, it may provide protection against heart disease.

Medical Management: Menopause

Hormone Replacement Therapy (HRT). This is an area that has been extensively researched but the results of two major studies have provided additional information. The Million Women Study (MWS) was an observational study published back in 2005 that studied a range of HRT regimens for women (aged between 50 and 64 years) who attended the UK breast screening programme. Evidence from this study was developed into modern NICE guidance with contributions from the BMS.

Clinicians should discuss the risks and benefits with every woman on an individual basis before prescribing HRT. It effectively relieves vasomotor symptoms and can be effective in preventing osteoporosis. However, because of risks associated with long-term use, it is only recommended for prevention of osteoporosis for women unable to use other treatments such as bisphosphonates.

Unopposed oestrogen therapy for women with an intact uterus increases the risk of endometrial hyperplasia and cancer (Nees et al. 2022); for these reasons, systemic oestrogen-only HRT should not be used in women with a uterus.

Tibolone is a synthetic steroid with properties of oestrogens, progestogens and androgens; if taken continuously, it should not cause a withdrawal bleed although the use of tibolone is associated with an increased risk of endometrial cancer (Løkkegaard and Mørch 2018) (Evidence-Based Practice 8.1).

Short-term HRT may be prescribed for specific menopausal symptoms such as hot flushes and atrophic vaginitis, for as long as treatment is required. Long-term HRT may be prescribed for women under 40 years who have had a premature menopause occurring naturally, as a result of surgery or iatrogenically.

While HRT can provide benefits in easing the adverse effects of the menopause, it can also have side-effects, and there are risks particularly with long-term use. Treatment may be abandoned by women because of either the side-effects or the fear of the risks. Possible side-effects include:

- breast pain/tenderness
- leg cramps
- vaginal discharge/bleeding
- fluid retention/bloating
- mood changes
- increased appetite.

Such side-effects might be reduced or eliminated by changing to a different preparation. However, women are encouraged to persist with one form of therapy for at least 3 months as some of the early side-effects can be temporary. The link between HRT and breast cancer has been the subject of research for some time. Women's Health Concern (2019) found that unopposed oestrogen HRT (i.e. oestrogen only treatments) is associated with little to no change in the risk of breast cancer, but combined HRT (oestrogen with a progesterone) can be associated with a small increased risk when used for more than 5 years. After HRT is stopped the risk of a breast cancer diagnosis initially falls but may increase again after a few years' cessation. This can be explained by the action of HRT on the growth of undetectable, microscopic cancers already present in the breast. When HRT is stopped, the growth of any remaining undetectable cancers slows down, but they will continue to grow at a slower rate. Despite this, the risk of breast cancer with combined

HRT is less than that associated with being overweight or that associated with drinking two or more units of alcohol daily. It is thought that approximately 2% of breast cancer cases are attributed to the use of HRT (Women's Health Concern 2019).

NICE (2015) notes that women with a history of breast cancer are rarely offered hormonal treatment for menopausal symptoms however, the available alternatives are less effective. There is insufficient evidence on the efficacy and safety of nonpharmaceutical treatments in women with breast cancer and other hormone-sensitive conditions.

It is generally agreed that further research is required on this issue. Contraindications to HRT are usually described as absolute or relative. Absolute contraindications generally include:

- pregnancy
- undiagnosed endometrial bleeding
- endometrial or breast cancer
- severe active liver disease
- porphyria.

If individual women wish to take HRT for severe acute symptoms, they should be referred to a specialist centre for advice and monitoring.

Possible contraindications are identified to highlight potential complications, to ensure that underlying disorders are treated or monitored, and to monitor the appropriate therapy, which may differ from uncomplicated cases. Caution is therefore required in prescribing HRT for women with:

- endometrial hyperplasia, endometriosis or fibroids
- hypertension – treat prior to HRT
- coagulation problems – refer to a haematologist
- diabetes – liaise with diabetes team in case insulin requirements change
- gallstones – may increase the risk of disease, including cancers (Jackson et al. 2022)
- otosclerosis – referral to an ear, nose and throat (ENT) specialist may be indicated.

Over-the-Counter Treatments. As of 2022, it is possible to buy vaginal oestrogen (oestradiol) at a pharmacy over the counter. It is indicated for the treatment of vaginal atrophy due to oestrogen deficiency in postmenopausal women aged 50 years and above, who have not had a period for at least 1 year (Medicines & Healthcare Products Regulatory Agency 2022)

Menopause Clinics. HRT may be prescribed directly, whereas other women are referred to hospital menopause clinics staffed by nursing and medical staff.

❖ Nursing Management and Health Promotion: Postmenopausal Women

Women should be encouraged to make an informed choice about HRT. However, the media present reports on a regular basis with contradictory information on risks and benefits. The nurse is instrumental in providing up-to-date information enabling women to come to an informed decision on whether it is appropriate for them and reassuring them about risks.

It is important to warn about the early side-effects of the sudden rise in oestrogen levels when starting HRT. Women should understand that there are a range of medications, doses and types of HRT, so if one type is unacceptable, another regimen may be tried.

The following is a guide for nurses interviewing women facing the menopause:

- Provide information and advice according to individual needs/concerns and any ongoing postmenopausal symptoms.

EVIDENCE-BASED PRACTICE 8.1

Providing Information About HRT

Postmenopausal women with an intact uterus who use oestrogen-only HRT are at increased risk of endometrial cancer. Many women taking HRT who have an intact uterus use combined oestrogen–progestogen preparations. Limited information is available on the incidence of endometrial cancer in users of these therapies.

The MWS recruited from 1996 to 2001 over 700,000 postmenopausal women in the UK who had no previous history of cancer or hysterectomy. During the study, 1320 cases of endometrial cancer were diagnosed in this group.

The findings showed that oestrogens and tibolone increase the risk of endometrial cancer. Progestogens counteract the adverse effect of oestrogens on the endometrium and this effect is greater the more days each month that they are added to oestrogen and the more obese the woman is. However, combined oestrogen–progestogen HRT causes a greater increase in breast cancer than the other therapies do. Thus, when endometrial and breast cancers are added together, there is a greater increase in total cancer incidence with use of combined HRT, both continuous and cyclic, than with use of the other therapies. A woman's BMI significantly affected these associations, such that the adverse effects of tibolone and oestrogen-only HRT were greatest in nonobese women, and the beneficial effects of combined HRT were greatest in obese women.

Activities

- Access the study by Beral et al. (2005) and the MWS Collaborators and consider the results in full.
- Consider how you would convey the information in this study to a postmenopausal woman asking advice about starting HRT.

- Encourage healthy lifestyles and health awareness.
- Encourage the selection of low-fat, calcium-rich foods; explain links to cardiovascular conditions and the maintenance of BMD.
- Ask women about their usual physical exercise pattern; reinforce the need for regular weight-bearing exercise.
- Discuss the benefits and possible side-effects of HRT.
- Explain about breast awareness/self-examination and attending for routine screening.
- Check the woman's understanding of the information given by encouraging feedback.
- Provide information from unbiased organisations (see Useful Websites, e.g. the BMS) or booklets provided by health organisations.
- Provide contact details in the event of any problem occurring.

DISORDERS OF THE FEMALE REPRODUCTIVE SYSTEM

This section outlines some benign and malignant tumours, displacements of the reproductive organs, salpingitis, problems of early pregnancy (ectopic and miscarriage), family planning services, termination of pregnancy (TOP) and infertility.

Benign Ovarian Tumours

Most ovarian tumours are benign and many will resolve spontaneously (Kenny and Bickerstaff 2016). Management focuses on excluding malignancy or treating symptoms that may develop.

Dermoid Cyst (Benign Cystic Teratoma)

Dermoid cysts arise from embryonic tissue. They may develop at any age but are more common in young women.

● Pathophysiology

Dermoid cysts are usually unilocular cysts containing ectodermic structures. The cyst is thick walled, whitish-yellow in colour and lined with skin, hair follicles, hair and sweat glands. Teeth may be found emerging from primitive sockets, and bone, cartilage, lung and intestinal epithelium can be identified within the cyst.

● Medical Management

The majority of cysts are asymptomatic but sometimes the cyst may undergo torsion and the patient may present with abdominal pain. Patients are referred to a gynaecologist for further investigation and treatment.

Malignant change may occur in any of the primitive tissues of the cyst.

Investigations. A vaginal and abdominal examination will be undertaken. USS can identify the ovarian cyst and cervical cytology may also be checked. Any malignant cells present might be associated with an ovarian cancer.

Treatment. Surgery is by laparoscopy or laparotomy. The extent of surgery will vary according to the age of the woman. In women of reproductive age, the benign cyst alone may be shelled out, leaving the normal functioning ovarian tissue. Both ovaries will be assessed, as the cysts are often bilateral.

Women who have completed their family or are over 50 years of age would be advised to have the ovary removed (oophorectomy). In the event of malignancy of the dermoid cyst, both ovaries and the uterus would be removed. Metastatic spread to the peritoneum requires further management by an oncologist.

❖ Nursing Management and Health Promotion: Dermoid Cyst

General pre- and postoperative care is required (see Chapter 25, Nursing the Patient Undergoing Surgery). Specific nursing care will depend upon the extent of the surgery undertaken; for example patients may have day-case laparoscopic surgery, and those having an oophorectomy will usually have a very short hospital stay. Nurses must provide information and advice before discharge and support this with written material (Information 8.1 outlines discharge advice for day-case gynaecological surgery).

Benign Uterine Tumours

Endometrial Polyps

Polyps are benign growths of the endometrium. They may develop from an overgrowth of endometrial glands and stroma. The polyp may produce a stalk and may descend towards the vulva. Single or multiple polyps may occur commonly in women of any age group. Slight vaginal bleeding (metrorrhagia) occurs between menstrual

---

INFORMATION 8.1

Discharge Advice Following Day-Case Gynaecological Surgery

- The woman should have tolerated fluids and light diet before discharge.
- She must have passed urine prior to leaving the unit/ward.
- An explanation is given that the anaesthetic may take 24–48 hours to be cleared from the body.
- A responsible adult must accompany the woman home.
- A responsible adult must be present in the woman's home during the night after surgery in case she is taken ill during the night. She should not be alone with young children for this reason.
- The woman must have ready access to a phone overnight and contact numbers, should help or advice be needed, such as for increasing pain or heavy vaginal loss.
- She must be told that extra care should be taken for 24–48 hours after the operation, as the anaesthetic can affect coordination and reflexes and that she should not drive, drink alcohol or operate machinery.
- The woman should arrange to have some painkillers in the house such as paracetamol or ibuprofen.
- Women who have undergone laparoscopy must be warned of potential referred shoulder pain as well as abdominal pain. This is due to carbon dioxide used during the operation collecting under and irritating the diaphragm.
- Advice should be given about wound care, what type of skin closures have been used and, if they need removing, when she should visit her practice nurse for this.
- There is likely to be some vaginal loss and women should be advised not to use tampons initially because of the risk of infection. Increasing vaginal loss or discharge with an offensive odour should be reported to her practice nurse or GP. This is particularly relevant if she has had any surgery to the cervix. In this instance, she should be advised to refrain from sexual intercourse and using tampons for 6 weeks.
- She may be able to return to work after 2–3 days depending on the type of surgery carried out. Often women who have undergone laparoscopy require up to a week to recuperate fully and she should be warned that she might feel tired for a few days due to the anaesthetic.
- Women should be given information about when test results will be available and the date of any follow-up appointments.

Adapted from Cotton 2003; Quemby and Stocker 2014.

periods or following coitus. Polypectomy will be undertaken by twisting it off at its stalk either in an outpatient clinic or under anaesthetic depending on site and size. Any tissue removed must undergo histological examination to exclude malignant change.

Fibromyomata

Fibromyomata or fibroids are benign uterine tumours comprising fibrous and muscle tissue. They can occur in women between 35 years of age and the onset of the climacteric. The growth of fibroids is stimulated by ovarian hormones, particularly oestrogens. Women who have not had children are more prone to develop fibroids.

Pathophysiology

Fibroids are spherical in shape and firm in consistency. Some fibroids are small, while others may grow large enough to fill the abdominal cavity. They have a capsule which contains the blood vessels supplying the fibroid. As it grows, the centre of the fibroid becomes less vascular and liable to degenerative change.

Multiple fibroids may be present, giving the uterus an irregular shape (Fig. 8.7) or causing displacement of the uterus and uterine vessels.

Common Presenting Symptoms. Menorrhagia often occurs when there are fibroids in the uterus. If the fibroids are submucous then menstruation may become irregular and there may be metrorrhagia, but this is not common. Pain may result as the uterus strongly contracts to attempt expulsion of the fibroid. Pressure upon pelvic nerves may cause back or leg pain; pressure on pelvic organs may lead to:
- frequency of micturition
- retention of urine
- intestinal obstruction
- oedema of a leg.

A fibroid may become infected and necrotic, causing a purulent vaginal discharge.

The most noticeable change is that of increasing abdominal girth; rapid increase may indicate that malignant change has taken place in the fibroid. Fibroids can be a cause of infertility by interfering with spermatozoa transit or ova implantation.

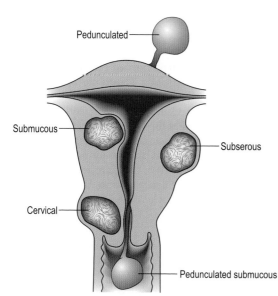

Figure 8.7 Common sites of fibromyomata in the uterus.

Medical Management

On pelvic examination, the uterus is usually found to be symmetrically enlarged. It feels harder than it does in pregnancy. The uterus may feel nodular due to the presence of multiple fibroids. The lower part of a fibroid may be felt through the cervix and the difference between fibroid and cervical cancer may be difficult to ascertain.

Investigations. Pelvic USS may assist with diagnosis of fibroids. Endometrial biopsy may be performed to exclude endometrial cancer.

Treatment. Small fibroids may not need treatment and any symptoms should disappear with the menopause. Medical treatment may be prescribed in the interim to relieve symptoms. A GnRH analogue may be prescribed which affects oestrogen secretion. In a woman whose family is not complete, it may be appropriate to shell out the fibroids from the myometrium (myomectomy) or resect the fibroids hysteroscopically (such as a transcervical resection of fibroids (TCRE)); an older woman may be treated by hysterectomy. If the fibroids are small, a vaginal hysterectomy or laparoscopic hysterectomy may be possible. Submucous fibroids can be removed hysteroscopically.

Embolisation of uterine arteries is an alternative treatment to hysterectomy (Rana et al. 2021). This involves cannulating the right femoral artery under local anaesthetic. Under screening control, a catheter is passed through the arterial system to the right and then left uterine arteries which are individually embolised with polyvinyl alcohol solution. Contrast medium is injected to ensure effective arterial occlusion. Women require effective opiate pain control following this procedure; but once pain is controlled, they can be discharged.

Nursing Management and Health Promotion: Fibromyomata

Nursing care will be prioritised depending upon the type of surgery completed. Observations of pulse, blood pressure and vaginal blood loss are recorded to monitor bleeding from the operation site. Pain assessment and administration of effective analgesia are required.

Care following hysterectomy will be similar to that described for invasive cervical cancer, but without the anxieties linked to cancer.

Trophoblastic Tumours

Trophoblastic tumours arise from the primitive tissues destined to develop into the placenta. They may be benign or malignant.

Hydatidiform Mole (Vesicular Mole)

A hydatidiform mole results in swelling of chorionic villous tissue, destined to become the placenta when the fertilised ovum implants. The uterus fills with grapelike vesicles which produce large quantities of hCG. No fetus develops.

Pathophysiology

A benign tumour mass of chorionic cells forms in the uterus and exists as though it were a developing pregnancy. Ovarian follicles are enlarged and there is an increase in blood and urine levels of hCG. The uterus increases in size, sometimes faster than in a pregnancy.

Common Presenting Symptoms. A woman may complain of loss of fresh or altered blood vaginally which does not seem like normal menstruation. She may be feeling unwell with some nausea and vomiting that resembles early pregnancy. It may be diagnosed if a woman has problems associated with early pregnancy.

🌑 Medical Management

A general physical and vaginal examination will be performed. The uterus may be increased in size. A 'blighted ovum' might be suspected but the watery vesicles of the mole, if identified or reported, will alert the doctor to the condition.

Investigations. Urinary pregnancy tests are positive, although there is no embryo/fetus present. The diagnosis is confirmed by USS and by the finding of high levels of hCG in urine or serum.

Treatment. Molar tissue must be removed either by surgical evacuation or medically by administering oxytocin. Thorough follow-up of the woman is necessary. In the UK, women are registered in a national follow-up programme. Blood and urine levels of hCG are monitored on a 2-weekly basis. The duration and type of follow-up depend on how quickly hCG levels fall.

Complications. A rising level of hCG with negative curettings of the uterine cavity suggests that the mole has invaded the myometrium and may even erode through the uterine wall. Deposits of molar tissue may be found in other parts of the body, in the peritoneum or in the lungs, and may cause death. Progression to malignant choriocarcinoma can occur following hydatidiform mole.

Choriocarcinoma

Choriocarcinoma is a malignant tumour of chorionic cells and occurs following a normal pregnancy, miscarriage or evacuation of a hydatidiform mole. Choriocarcinoma is a very rare neoplasm with varied incidence worldwide. In Europe and North America, about 1 in 40,000 pregnant patients and 1 in 40 patients with hydatidiform moles will develop choriocarcinoma. There appears to be an increased risk for the development of choriocarcinoma in Asian, American Indian and African American women, hence the varied incidence worldwide. Other risk factors include prior complete hydatidiform mole (a 100-fold increased risk), advanced age, long-term oral contraceptive use and blood type A (Bishop and Edemekong 2023).

🌑 Pathophysiology

The uterus becomes ulcerated, with invasion of the myometrium which can result in perforation. Metastatic spread of the cancer is speedy and extensive; the brain, lung, liver and other organs may be involved. Early deterioration is expected if the condition is not treated early.

Diagnosis is difficult but confirmed by hCG estimations in urine and plasma.

🌑 Medical Management

Follow-up arrangements after mole removal are usually stringent and take place in a specialist centre. There are greater risks of disease progression if a woman delays consultation.

Investigations. A choriocarcinoma produces large amounts of hCG, which is used as a tumour marker and also used to monitor the response to therapy.

Treatment. Choriocarcinoma is highly chemosensitive to single-agent chemotherapy, although women at high risk may require multiagent chemotherapy. Methotrexate is given intramuscularly, with oral folinic acid to protect the bone marrow, with almost 100% success.

If there is metastatic disease, methotrexate may be combined with other cytotoxic agents. Four per cent of patients may have cerebral metastases at the time of diagnosis (Bishop and Edemekong 2023).

For most women an appropriate regimen of intrathecal chemotherapy will be effective in treating cerebral metastases.

Women are advised not to become pregnant within 2 years of treatment. However, depending on the stage of disease, some women will require a hysterectomy.

❖ Nursing Management and Health Promotion: Hydatidiform Mole/Choriocarcinoma

Hydatidiform Mole

Nursing care following evacuation of hydatidiform mole will be similar to that following evacuation of the uterus. Patients should recover quickly from anaesthetic and the patient will become self-caring soon after returning to the ward. Postoperatively, the nurse should check the level of vaginal blood loss, which should be minimal within 24 hours.

Minimal abdominal discomfort should be experienced by the patient. A mild analgesic will be prescribed, if necessary. If a patient experiences more severe pain, she should be closely observed in case of uterine perforation. A series of postoperative urine and blood specimens will be required to estimate hCG levels. The patient must be registered with one of the specialised centres in the UK for appropriate follow-up.

Choriocarcinoma

In the event of persistently high levels of hCG, a diagnosis of choriocarcinoma would require the woman's transfer to a specialist centre for chemotherapy. The woman may be very anxious, having to face up to the seriousness of her illness and the urgency of treatment. The nurse should reassure and support her with information about future treatment.

The partner should be fully involved and can accompany the woman to the treatment centre.

Special facilities are available to protect her from infection as chemotherapy progresses and her immune system is compromised (see Chapter 18, Infection Prevention and Control). Physical, psychological and social aspects of nursing care will be of primary concern. Many weeks of treatment may be involved before recovery is achieved and the patient returns to normal life. Follow-up and further hCG monitoring are essential.

Gynaecological Cancer

The organs of the female reproductive system are susceptible to malignant tumours. Information about the characteristics and effects of benign and malignant tumours is provided in Chapter 31, Nursing the Patient With Cancer. The cervix, endometrium, ovary and vulva are potential sites for primary cancers. A rapid referral system whereby women suspected of having cancer are seen by specialists within 14 days of referral has been introduced and is recommended as best practice by NICE (2015, reviewed 2021).

Women with rarer cancers such as those of ovary or vulva must be treated in a cancer centre where specialist medical and nursing skills are available.

Cervical Cancer

In the UK, 3197 new cases of cervical cancer were diagnosed between 2016 and 2018, accounting for 2% of female cancers

(Cancer Research UK 2022a). There were 854 deaths from cervical cancer between 2016 and 2018 in the UK (Cancer Research UK 2022a). Women between 30 and 50 years of age are most at risk of cancer of the cervix, which is preceded by a pre-invasive condition that can be simply and effectively treated if identified by cervical cytological screening.

The main cancer linked with the human papillomavirus (HPV) is cervical cancer; high-risk subtypes include 16 and 18 (Ramakrishnan et al. 2015). This infection is acquired through sexual activity. Other risk factors include:

- age of first sexual intercourse
- number of sexual partners
- smoking
- less affluent lifestyle.

Since 2008, girls aged 11–13 years have been offered a vaccination against the two most common 'high-risk' types of HPV, HPV 16 and 18. Together, these two types cause about 7 out of 10 cervical cancers. Girls up to the age of 18 years may request vaccination through the National Health Service (NHS) if they were not routinely vaccinated. The HPV vaccine has been proven to be safe and effective.

From April 2018, the vaccine was rolled out for men who have sex with men in all sexual health and HIV clinics across the UK. In July 2018, the HPV vaccination was introduced for boys, in addition to the programme for girls.

Pre-invasive Cervical Cancer

Pathophysiology

The area where the columnar epithelium of the endocervix joins with the stratified squamous epithelium of the ectocervix is called the squamocolumnar junction (SCJ). Columnar cells migrate down to the ectocervix, moving the SCJ to a new position and causing a red area of columnar epithelium around the cervical os. The area where columnar cells are replaced with squamous cells is called the transformation zone and is most commonly where precancerous changes occur. Cells are removed from this area when a cervical smear is taken. Preinvasive changes identified early are curable.

In England, all women during their reproductive years should have a regular smear test from age 25 until 65 years (NHS Cervical Screening Programme 2018) (Information 8.2). If a woman has an abnormal result, the frequency is increased.

All women registered with a GP (and some trans men) are included in the screening programme. However, there are women from some hard-to-reach communities such as travellers or some immigrants who might not participate in the programme. These women must be encouraged to enter the screening programme and given appropriate information so they can appreciate the benefits of this.

Common Presenting Symptoms. The earliest knowledge of cervical changes may be from a report on a cervical smear test. In some cases, irregular vaginal bleeding may be associated with prolonged menstruation, occur between periods, follow sexual intercourse or be postmenopausal.

Medical Management

Investigations. These will include:

- cervical smear
- colposcopy and biopsy of cervical tissue.

Papanicolaou (Pap) Smear Test. Pap smears involve scraping a layer of cells from the SCJ using a wooden spatula which are then spread and fixed on a microscope slide before being examined

---

INFORMATION 8.2

NHS Cervical Screening Programme

- Failsafe recall system in place to encourage women to attend for screening and subsequent treatment if required.
- In England the current programme is:
  - age 25 years receive first invitation for screening
  - age 25–49 years smears repeated 3 yearly
  - age 50–64 years smears repeated 5 yearly
  - age 65 years or over – only women who have recently had abnormal cytology.
- Trans men who still have a cervix and are still registered as female with a GP will also be invited for cervical screening.
- Trans men who are registered as male will need to let a GP or practice nurse know so they can organise the test.

---

microscopically. This procedure has now been replaced across the UK by LBC which provides more accurate results and has reduced the number of smears showing borderline nuclear abnormality.

Liquid-Based Cytology. LBC is a newer method of preparing the sample. Samples are collected from the woman as for a Pap test but a brushlike device is used instead of a spatula. The head of the collecting device is rinsed or broken off into a small container of preservative fluid. In the laboratory the sample is prepared and a thin layer of cervical cells is placed on a microscope slide and stained for examination by a cytologist (NICE 2022). Advantages of LBC over the Pap smear are:

- improved slide preparation, allowing a more homogeneous sample for examination
- increased sensitivity and specificity
- improved handling procedures for laboratory samples.

Abnormalities in cervical cytology indicating pre-invasive disease are described as cervical intraepithelial neoplasia (CIN) – CIN1, CIN2 or CIN3 (Information 8.3).

A woman who has had a total hysterectomy performed for precancer or cancer will require subsequent vault smears. Routine cervical smears are required following a subtotal hysterectomy. Women may be asked to have a smear test repeated where there is an inconclusive diagnosis or if minor cytological abnormalities are detected.

Colposcopy and Biopsy. Colposcopy involves examining the cervix and surrounding tissue under binocular magnification. Women with abnormal cytology are referred either by the practice nurse, GP or by direct referral from cytology laboratories. Increasingly nurses are educated to perform colposcopy to diagnose and treat abnormalities.

INFORMATION 8.3

Histology of Cervical Intraepithelial Neoplasia (CIN)

The current terminology for CIN describes three grades of change as part of a continuum of pre-invasive disease:

- CIN1 corresponds to mild dysplasia – affects one-third thickness of cervical epithelium.
- CIN2 corresponds to moderate dysplasia – affects two-thirds thickness of cervical epithelium.
- CIN3 corresponds to severe dysplasia and carcinoma in situ (CIS) – affects two-thirds to full thickness of cervical epithelium.

Saline may be applied to the cervix to identify blood vessel patterns. Acetic acid is applied to the transformation zone, mucus is removed with a cotton wool ball or a swab and the area is carefully examined for abnormal epithelium. Iodine can be used to outline abnormalities. A diagnostic biopsy may be taken for histological examination to confirm pre-invasive disease. More commonly an excision biopsy is taken which also treats the abnormality.

Treatment Options

Conservative Treatment. In the early days of screening all instances of abnormal cervical cytology were treated. However, the majority of borderline abnormalities will revert to normal and so initially repeat smears will be used to monitor the woman.

Destructive Treatment. Several treatments have been developed that work on the same principle of destroying tissue either by heat or cold. However, the commonest treatment undertaken now is excision of the transformation zone. This procedure can be performed using laser or a diathermy loop. The latter method is easier to perform and more economical in terms of time. Large loop excision of the transformation zone (LLETZ) may be performed under colposcopic guidance by low-voltage diathermy. This is performed under local anaesthetic in the colposcopy department. A bloodstained vaginal discharge usually follows for 1–2 weeks. Secondary haemorrhage may occasionally occur. The patient should be advised against the use of tampons and intercourse for a month after the procedure as this may effect healing and/or cause bleeding.

❖ Nursing Management and Health Promotion: Pre-invasive Cervical Cancer

Treatment is provided as an outpatient or as a day patient under general anaesthetic if the patient is particularly anxious or the abnormal cells extend up the cervical canal and a large loop excision is required – for example if it is a repeat procedure.

This is a particularly anxious time for women and the nurse will need to ensure the patient understands the procedures planned and the expected outcome. Sensitive approaches are required to help the woman to express her feelings. Following the procedure, the woman must be given the following information:

- A bloodstained vaginal discharge should be expected for 1–2 weeks postprocedure.
- The woman should refrain from sexual intercourse or using tampons for 4–6 weeks to allow the cervix to heal.
- She should contact her practice nurse, GP or the colposcopy department if bleeding becomes heavy, bright red or offensive, which may indicate an infection.
- Details of when and how she will receive results of her tests.
- Future follow-up arrangements.

Information should also be given about the effects of lifestyle, and the woman should be encouraged to refrain from smoking and limit sexual partners.

🌐 **See Evolve website Critical thinking question 8.1**

Invasive Cervical Cancer

🔴 *Pathophysiology*

Squamous cell cancers account for 70%–80% of cervical cancer (Cancer Research UK 2022b). Adenocarcinomas account for 20% of cancers. Squamous cancers develop from the outer layer; adenocarcinomas develop from glandular cells, often in the cervical

---

INFORMATION 8.4

International Federation of Gynaecology and Obstetrics (FIGO) Staging of Cancer of the Cervix Uteri*

Stage	Description
I	The carcinoma is strictly confined to the cervix (extension to the uterine corpus should be disregarded)
II	The carcinoma invades beyond the uterus, but has not extended onto the lower third of the vagina or to the pelvic wall
III	The carcinoma involves the lower third of the vagina and/or extends to the pelvic wall and/or causes hydronephrosis or nonfunctioning kidney and/or involves pelvic and/or para-aortic lymph nodes
IV	The carcinoma has extended beyond the true pelvis or has involved (biopsy proven) the mucosa of the bladder or rectum

*There are also subdivisions of the four stages.
Based on Bhatla et al. 2018.

---

canal, and so can be more difficult to detect by screening. An ulcer may develop on the cervix, with tissues becoming eroded and infected producing an unpleasant vaginal discharge.

The cancer spreads by direct infiltration of surrounding tissues and via lymphatic vessels. The prognosis for cervical cancer relates to the extent of the growth at the time of diagnosis rather than to the histological type of the cancer. Information 8.4 outlines the International Federation of Gynecology and Obstetrics (FIGO) classification of cervical cancer.

Common Presenting Symptoms. A woman may have no particular symptoms, but a cervical smear result may confirm the presence of cervical cancer. However, she may have experienced postcoital bleeding. On vaginal examination, there may be an abnormal appearance to the cervix such as an ulcerated area or overgrowth of tissue.

As the disease progresses, vaginal discharge becomes more continuous; a thin bloodstained loss may change to a thicker, brown, offensive discharge or heavier bleeding episodes. Lower abdominal pain develops as the growth increases in size and exerts pressure on surrounding structures. Very severe lower back and sciatic pain may occur as lymphatic nodes adhere to the sacral plexus. Pressure on the pudendal nerve and blood vessels causes obstruction to the venous return and oedema of the legs.

Incontinence of urine and faeces may occur if there is spread of tumour to the bladder and rectum or as a later reaction to radiation side-effects. Ureters may become blocked and renal failure may ensue.

🔴 *Medical Management*

Investigations. Treatment depends on the stage of the disease so a number of investigations are required for staging. Radiological investigations will include a chest X-ray or computed tomography (CT) of the chest and magnetic resonance imaging (MRI) scan of the abdomen to determine the presence of any metastases.

A general physical and pelvic examination is undertaken. An examination under anaesthetic (EUA) is undertaken to assess the vagina, rectum and bladder to identify extent of spread and lymph node involvement.

Tumour-derived/associated markers in the plasma of patients with cervical cancer may be useful to support other clinical findings. Marker measurement values tend to increase with the stage of disease and decrease with effective treatment. However, histological examination provides a more definitive diagnosis on which to plan treatment.

Treatment

This depends on the extent of the disease and age of the woman. The woman will be cared for by a multidisciplinary team (MDT), including gynaecological and medical oncologists, radiologists, clinical nurse specialists (CNSs) and pathologists, in a gynaecology cancer centre.

Surgery. The extent of surgical excision will depend on the progression of the disease. When the cancer is confined to the cervix, cone biopsy of the endocervical tissue is appropriate, although if the woman has completed her family, a total abdominal hysterectomy (TAH) is performed. Where there is extension of the growth into the vagina, a trachelectomy (removal of the cervix and upper 2–3 cm of the vagina) or radical hysterectomy may be performed. Pelvic lymph nodes may be removed laparoscopically. A radical (Wertheim's) hysterectomy involves removal of cervix, uterus, upper third of vagina, parametrial tissue and bilateral pelvic lymph nodes. Concurrent radiotherapy and chemotherapy are indicated if lymph node involvement is confirmed.

Pelvic Exenteration. This is only undertaken where there is extensive recurrent disease. It involves removal of all the reproductive organs and the urinary bladder. If the rectum is also removed, a terminal colostomy is formed. This extremely radical surgery may be combined with cytotoxic drug therapy using cisplatin and other chemotherapeutic agents.

Radiotherapy. Radiotherapy is indicated in cases where lymph nodes removed surgically show involvement of disease or if the patient is unfit for surgery. It may also be used to reduce tumour size, inhibit its growth and reduce its blood supply before surgical removal by hysterectomy. Stages III and IV of cervical cancer are usually inoperable. Palliative irradiation therapy is then indicated. Radiotherapy will also affect healthy cells (see Chapter 31, Nursing the Patient With Cancer). The bladder and rectal tissue may become friable or fibrosed and a fistula may develop. The woman may become distressed by urinary problems or diarrhoea. Vaginal stricture may occur, which creates sexual dysfunction. Symptoms are relieved as they occur. The patient's general comfort is of prime importance.

❖ Nursing Management and Health Promotion: Hysterectomy for Cervical Cancer

Preoperatively, the assessment process will identify the patient's gynaecological details and her previous medical history will be documented to ensure she is fit for surgery and anaesthetic (general, epidural or spinal).

The woman's individual problems (actual or potential) and need for nursing assistance and support are identified. These include:

Anxiety. The woman may experience considerable anxiety related to the anaesthetic, surgery and her condition. She may be anxious about a change in body image and sexuality and its effect on her relationship with her partner. Anxiety may focus on family members at home as the woman is often the caring head of the family. She may be worried that her illness will affect her ability to work and support the family in the future. The nurse should be supportive and encourage her to express these concerns.

Information Needs. In preparation for surgery, the patient will need information about what to expect in both the lead-up to the operation and the recovery period. The benefits of planned information giving preoperatively are accepted (see Chapter 25, Nursing the Patient Undergoing Surgery). An information booklet explaining the operation and its resultant internal changes should be provided to support verbal advice given. This provides a record of discussions and reinforces her understanding.

It is usually recommended that sexual intercourse should not be resumed for about 6 weeks postoperatively to allow internal healing and reduce the incidence of infection. If appropriate the patient will benefit from knowing that sexual pleasure is achievable even though the uterus has been removed. Appropriate information at this stage will help recovery (Evidence-Based Practice 8.2).

Immobility

Patients will have limited mobility in the first 24 hours after a hysterectomy. There is a risk of VTE and possibly pressure ulcer development. They will be taught leg exercises preoperatively and encouraged to practise leg exercises pre- and postoperatively.

EVIDENCE-BASED PRACTICE 8.2

A Study of Self-concept and Social Support After Hysterectomy

Although a woman may be happy to have a hysterectomy to alleviate symptoms affecting her quality of life, it can affect her feelings of self-worth and sexuality. In Webb and Wilson-Barnett's (1983) seminal study, they considered depression, self-concept and sexual life in 128 women during recovery from hysterectomy as part of a nursing study. The women were interviewed 1 week and 4 months after the hysterectomy. The results showed that women felt physically and emotionally much better, were less tired and irritable, had gone back to work and had resumed leisure and social activities. Responses showed that:

- 94% were happy to have no more periods.
- 84% were glad they could no longer become pregnant.
- 90% of those who were sexually active said their sex life was now as good as, or even better than, previously.
- 92% were glad they had the operation.

The small numbers who gave 'negative' replies to these questions were still not completely recovered and gave this as the reason for their answers. They referred to physical complications of wound, urinary or vaginal infections which delayed recuperation rather than the psychological problems suggested in medical studies.

The greatest area of dissatisfaction was in the lack of information from medical and nursing staff. Women would have liked guidance on what they could do, how they might feel as they progressed and what symptoms or complications could occur.

Activities

- Access the research by Webb and Wilson-Barnett and think about how their findings have influenced the nature of information provided to women having a hysterectomy.
- Consider the information that a woman having a hysterectomy will require under the following headings:
  - procedure/consent
  - preparation for admission
  - nursing procedures preoperatively
  - nursing procedures postoperatively
  - information on recovery period to return to normal lifestyle.
- Reflect on the most appropriate timing of the information, e.g. in outpatient clinic before being booked for hysterectomy, at preadmission assessment, preoperatively on the ward or prior to discharge, and the format, e.g. verbal, written, telephone help line, web based.
- Thinking about Webb and Wilson-Barnett's work that was conducted over 30 years ago, do you consider it has relevance for contemporary practice?

Reference

Webb C, Wilson-Barnett J. Self concept, social support and hysterectomy. *Int J Nurs Stud.* 1983;20(2):97-107.

Women will be provided with antiembolic hosiery/stockings and subcutaneous heparin is prescribed prophylactically unless contraindicated. Patients will also benefit from being offered information about deep-breathing and coughing exercises and how to move effectively with minimal assistance postoperatively.

Protection From Hazards

Whilst the doctor is responsible for obtaining written informed consent from the patient, the nurse also checks that the woman has consented and confirms her identity before she leaves the ward for surgery. The perioperative team will transfer the patient safely to the operating theatre where the checks on identity and consent are repeated.

Postoperative Care

The patient's individual needs and actual problems will be identified in her postoperative care plan. This focuses on monitoring the patient's condition to identify complications at an early stage (see Chapter 25 for general care of a patient following major abdominal surgery). These could include haemorrhage, urinary retention and fluid imbalance.

The nurse has a vital role in providing the woman with advice prior to discharge 3–4 days following surgery (Information 8.5).

Endometrial Cancer

Most uterine cancer arises from the endometrium. Uterine (womb) cancer is the sixth most common cancer worldwide for females, and the 14th most common cancer overall, with over 380,000 new cases diagnosed in 2018 (British Gynaecological Cancer Society (BGCS) 2021). Uterine cancer is now the fourth most common cancer in females in the UK. The incidence of endometrial cancer increases with age and was highest in females aged 75 to 79 in the UK (2015–2017) (BGCS 2021). Risk factors for developing the disease include obesity, nulliparity, late menopause and unopposed oestrogen therapy. An excess of oestrogen is common to all the risk factors. As women are living longer, the present rate is expected to increase.

🔹 Pathophysiology

The cancer arises in the columnar epithelium lining the endometrial glands; the growth is usually an adenocarcinoma. The cancer penetrates the endometrium, spreads laterally and grows slowly. With time, it penetrates the myometrium, reaching the perimetrium, and the lymph nodes become involved. Secondary deposits may affect pelvic and aortic lymph nodes and the ovary. Blood-borne metastatic spread to the lung, bone, liver or brain may occur. The FIGO has developed a classification of the different stages (Information 8.6).

Common Presenting Symptoms. From the age of 45 years, women expect changes in the menstrual cycle. The early signs of endometrial cancer may be difficult to distinguish from the changes of the climacteric. Postmenopausal bleeding (PMB), any unexpected or irregular vaginal bleeding, is a significant sign. The majority of women presenting with PMB will have benign endometrial pathology (Clark and Gupta 2005). However, as 75%–80% of women with endometrial cancer present with PMB (BGCS 2021), investigations must be undertaken urgently to obtain a differential diagnosis.

🔹 Medical Management

Investigations. Sometimes a routine cervical smear test may yield the first evidence of malignant endometrial cells. Initial

---

INFORMATION 8.5

Discharge Advice Following Major Gynaecological Surgery

The advice and information given to women being discharged after major surgery such as hysterectomy or vaginal repairs will depend on the type and extent of surgery, but will include:

- That she will be reviewed either in the outpatient clinic or, increasingly, at her own general practice 6 weeks after her operation to ensure healing is complete. This appointment should be arranged before she leaves.
- Any drugs she needs to continue at home, such as a course of antibiotics, should be prescribed and given to the woman with a full explanation about how she should take them. Any of her own drugs she has brought in with her should be returned to her.
- Advice about the care of her wound is important, and in clean, healing wounds, there is usually no need to wear a dressing. However, the area should be carefully dried after bathing. She should be warned that the wound may itch for several months and if she is worried to contact the practice nurse. Arrangements should be made for removing sutures if there are any still in situ.
- Alteration to diet, reduction in normal pattern of exercise and analgesia containing codeine increase the risks of the woman becoming constipated. It may be painful if she has to strain at stool and can cause damage to surgery such as posterior vaginal repairs. Advice should be given about drinking sufficient water, taking a high-fibre diet and being alert for the development of constipation.
- It is important that the woman does not return home and become an invalid. She should continue abdominal/pelvic floor exercises as advised by the physiotherapist. Exercise should be encouraged in small amounts, increasing on a regular basis, as she feels stronger. Walking is an excellent mode of exercise but the woman should be advised not to walk too far at first, as she will have to walk back home when she may feel extremely tired. If she participates in regular exercise such as aerobics or tennis, she will be able to return to these by 6 weeks. Swimming should be avoided until the wound has healed completely because of the risk of infection.
- Driving a motor vehicle should not be attempted until the woman is able to sit comfortably in the driver's seat and undertake an emergency stop, at least 2–3 weeks after she has gone home. However, her gynaecologist may give her a specific time period before she should drive. The woman should check with her insurance company whether there are any restrictions on her policy whilst she is convalescing.
- After 6 weeks, most major surgical sites have healed completely. However, after a hysterectomy, some women will still feel tired and, if they have a physically demanding job, may require up to 10–12 weeks away from work to convalesce fully.
- Sexual intercourse should be avoided for 6 weeks if there has been vaginal surgery, particularly to the vaginal vault as in TAH. When the woman does resume sexual relations, she should be encouraged to take the lead and feel in control, as she may be apprehensive about discomfort.
- It is important that she returns to normal life as soon as possible. However, she should be advised against any heavy lifting or vacuuming for at least a month, but can then start to increase the activities as she is able.

Adapted from Cotton (2003) with permission.

---

investigations include a transvaginal scan (TVS) and endometrial biopsy. If the endometrial biopsy is insufficient for histological identification of malignancy or if there is thickening of the endometrium shown on the TVS (indicative of pathology), the diagnosis can be confirmed by a hysteroscopy with endometrial biopsy.

INFORMATION 8.6

International Federation of Gynecology and Obstetrics (FIGO) Classification of Cancer of the Corpus Uteri (Endometrial Cancer)*

Stage	Description
Stage I	Stage IA: Tumour limited to the endometrium or less than one-half the myometrium
	Stage IB: Invasion equal to or more than one-half the myometrium (middle layer of the uterine wall)
Stage II	Cervical stromal invasion but not beyond the uterus
Stage III	Local and/or regional spread of the tumour
	Stage IIIA: Invasion of the serosa (outermost layer of the myometrium) and/or the adnexa (the ovaries or fallopian tubes)
	Stage IIIB: Invasion of the vagina and/or parametrial involvement
	Stage IIIC1: Cancer has spread to the pelvic lymph nodes but not to distant organs
	Stage IIIC2: Cancer has spread to the paraaortic lymph nodes with or without positive pelvic lymph nodes but not to distant organs
Stage IV	Tumour invades the bladder and/or bowel mucosa and/or distant metastases
	Stage IV: The cancer has spread to the inside (mucosa) of the bladder or the rectum (lower part of the large intestine) and/or to the inguinal lymph nodes and/or to the bones or distant organs outside the pelvis, such as the lungs.
	Stage IVA: Tumour invasion of the bladder, the bowel mucosa or both
	Stage IVB: Metastasis to distant organs, including intraabdominal metastasis, and/or inguinal lymph nodes

*There are also subdivisions of the four stages.
Based on Abdelrahman 2017.

Treatment

Total Abdominal Hysterectomy and Bilateral Salpingo-Oophorectomy (TAH and BSO). Endometrial cancer usually requires the removal of the uterus, cervix, uterine tubes and ovaries. Radiotherapy may be necessary if there has been invasion through the myometrium.

Radical Hysterectomy. A radical hysterectomy also includes removal of pelvic lymph nodes. Surgical treatment may be combined with radiotherapy to the pelvic wall. Alternatively, the uterine tumour may be irradiated to shrink it and deplete its blood supply before surgery or if the patient is unfit for surgery.

Hormonal Treatments. Although there is a lack of randomised studies, it is felt by some that progestogens may prevent recurrence of early stage disease. When diagnosed at its earliest stage more than 90% of women with uterine cancer will survive their disease for 5 years or more, compared with approximately 15% of (Cancer Research UK 2022c).

❖ Nursing Management and Health Promotion: Endometrial Cancer

The nursing care of the patient with endometrial cancer involves general pre- and postoperative care and specific care for hysterectomy. Care will be individualised but will be similar to that outlined for a woman with cervical cancer.

Following TAH and BSO, most women will have normal bladder function postoperatively. Sometimes, however, a self-retaining urethral catheter may be used initially, to avoid distending the urinary bladder and exerting pressure on the posterior urethral wall, which may be swollen and bruised.

The woman will need information about her progress at regular intervals in the postoperative period. Of particular concern may be the need to have radiotherapy at an early, vulnerable stage after major surgery (see Chapter 31, Nursing the Patient With Cancer). Psychological support from the nurse should help the patient to view the radiotherapy as the final safety net in the treatment process. Positive improvements should be seen within 3 months of treatment being completed. Medical follow-up is essential to monitor progress and identify early signs of recurrent disease.

Ovarian Cancer

In the UK ovarian cancer is the sixth most common cancer in women. Between 2014 and 2016, 7495 women were diagnosed with ovarian cancer in the UK, and between 2016 and 2018 the disease caused the deaths of 4182 women (Cancer Research UK 2022d).

Ovarian cancer is more common in developed countries (Kenny and Bickerstaff 2016). A relationship is said to exist between multiple ovulation in women in well-nourished communities and the incidence of ovarian cancer. Pregnancy and the oral contraceptive pill have a protective effect. The condition is more common in infertile and nulliparous women and in women who are celibate. Increased risks for cancers of the ovary, fallopian tube and peritoneum are observed in carriers of a pathogenic BRCA1/2 variant. In the setting of an invasive ovarian cancer diagnosis, a pathogenic BRCA1 variant has been found in 3.8%–14.5% of women, and a pathogenic BRCA2 variant has been found in 4.2%–5.7% of women. Carriers of a pathogenic BRCA1 variant have an estimated 48.3% cumulative risk of ovarian cancer by age 70, whereas the cumulative risk by age 70 is 20.0% for carriers of a pathogenic BRCA2 variant (Daly et al. 2021). However, Daly et al. (2021) also identifies several studies which reported more favourable survival outcomes among carriers of a pathogenic BRCA1/2 variant in patients with ovarian cancer compared with noncarrier patients. This may be due to different treatment options such as PARP inhibitors (Mirza et al. 2020).

In the UK there is no national screening programme for ovarian cancer as there is no test that will reliably pick up ovarian cancer at an early stage.

The tumour is often widespread before symptoms appear. As a result, late detection of the condition prohibits effective treatment and the mortality rate is higher than for other genital malignancies.

🔴 Pathophysiology

Ovarian tumours may occur unilaterally or bilaterally. Occasionally, they arise from metastatic spread from a cancer in adjacent organs. However, more commonly, they develop as a primary tumour and are divided into epithelial, sex chord stromal tumour or germ cell tumours. Ovarian cancer spreads via lymph and blood vessels. Information 8.7 outlines the FIGO staging classification of ovarian cancer.

Ovarian cancer is histologically classified according to the type of cell from which it originates, the most common source being

INFORMATION 8.7

International Federation of Gynecology and Obstetrics (FIGO) Classification of Ovarian Cancer*

Stage	Description
I	Tumour confined to ovaries or fallopian tube(s)
II	Tumour involves one or both ovaries or fallopian tubes with pelvic extension (below the pelvic brim) or primary peritoneal cancer
III	Tumour involves one or both ovaries or fallopian tubes, or primary peritoneal cancer, with cytologically or histologically confirmed spread to the peritoneum outside the pelvis and/or metastasis to the retroperitoneal lymph nodes
IV	Distant metastasis excluding peritoneal metastases

*There are also subdivisions of the four stages.
Based on Prat 2014.

surface epithelium (formed from embryonic mesothelium). The three commonest types of tumour are:

- serous (tubal)
- endometrioid (endometrial)
- mucinous (endocervical).

Serous Papilliferous Cancer. The malignant serous tumour is the commonest type of primary ovarian cancer and often affects both ovaries. Tumour cells are disseminated into the peritoneal cavity to form multiple seedling metastases. In most cases, there is rapid spread in the peritoneal cavity with ascites (fluid in the peritoneal cavity).

Mucinous Cancer. Approximately 10% of ovarian tumours are classified as mucinous (Kenny and Bickerstaff 2016). Many of these tumours are identified at an early stage of growth, which gives a better prognosis for the patient. These are amongst the largest of ovarian tumours, often reaching up to 25 cm in diameter. Mucinous tumours of the ovary represent a spectrum of neoplastic disorders including benign, mucinous tumours of low malignant potential (borderline), and invasive mucinous ovarian carcinoma (Alves et al. 2021).

Endometrioid Cancer. This type of ovarian cancer resembles an endometrial adenocarcinoma. The tumour consists of endometrial tubular gland cells. It may be secondary to uterine disease or a primary ovarian growth that coexists with endometrial cancer.

Germ Cell Tumours. Similar tumours may arise in the germ cells of either gender and may be benign or malignant. Benign conditions are very common; malignancy is rare. The commonest type of germ cell tumour is the dermoid cyst or cystic teratoma. Dermoid cysts usually occur in the ovary but are very rare in the testes; malignant teratoma is more common in the testes.

Malignant germ cell tumours include dysgerminoma and choriocarcinoma. The former is highly malignant and metastasis via the blood and lymphatics.

Medical Management

Ovarian cancer is insidious in its growth and the woman may have no discomfort or suspicion of disease until an advanced stage. Almost half of ovarian cancers are diagnosed at a late stage (stage 3 and 4) due frequently to vague and late-onset any symptoms. In England in 2014, 49% of ovarian cancers were diagnosed at stage 3–4, with 31% diagnosed at stage 1 (Athey et al. 2021). Late symptoms are related to increased pressure in the abdominal

venous channels, causing oedema in the legs and pain from pressure on nerves to the legs. Metastatic growth in the peritoneum will contribute to extensive ascites, abdominal pain, urinary frequency, nausea, vomiting, emaciation and breathlessness. A thrombosis may form in an iliac vein or in the inferior vena cava. If growth has spread to other organs there may be symptoms, such as intestinal obstruction.

Investigations. A full pelvic examination is necessary, with palpation of the ovaries. Ultrasound and CT scanning of the abdomen and pelvis are indicated. Further CT or MRI scans are performed to assess the extent of lymph node involvement and other metastatic spread. Prediction models derived from CT findings have been extensively researched, with limited success. Fortunately, several articles reported that MRI has a good diagnostic performance for detecting peritoneal metastases using surgical scoring systems. Currently, two large trials (MISSION and MROC) are ongoing to confirm whether MRI can accurately select patients for whom a complete/optimal cancer resection surgery is feasible. If these trials show that MRI can accurately predict the extent of disease in the abdomen, current imaging guidelines will need to change to implement MRI as a noninvasive triaging tool in females with advanced ovarian cancer (Engbersen et al. 2021).

A chest X-ray may identify metastatic spread to the lungs, or pleural effusion.

An intravenous urogram (IVU) may be performed if obstruction of a ureter is suspected.

A full blood count, serum biochemistry and serum Ca-125 tumour markers are required. Ovarian tumours are always surgically removed and the final diagnosis is confirmed histologically. It is important that the ovary and peritoneal cavity should be fully assessed to define the spread of the disease.

Treatment. This will depend on the extent of the disease. When ovarian cancer is diagnosed, laparotomy is undertaken with a TAH, BSO, pelvic lymph node removal and omentectomy (removal of the omentum, part of the peritoneum) as it is important to achieve macroscopic clearance. As much malignant tissue as possible will be removed. Adjuvant chemotherapy is normally given except in early stages of the disease. Radiation is generally confined to palliation. In advanced stages, palliative treatment only may be possible (see Chapter 31, Nursing the Patient With Cancer, and Chapter 32, Nursing Patients Who Need Palliative Care), for example, abdominal paracentesis to drain ascites to relieve the pain and breathlessness.

❖❖ Nursing Management and Health Promotion: Ovarian Cancer

In addition to physical care, the patient with ovarian cancer and their family will need much psychological support from the nurse. Anxieties associated with investigations, diagnosis and the effects of hysterectomy and chemotherapy will need to be anticipated and managed in all aspects (see Chapter 31). The patient may make a full recovery quite quickly or, if metastatic disease remains, may be debilitated for longer. Oncology nurse specialists perform a pivotal role in supporting patients at this time.

The nurse will work towards helping the patient make physical and emotional adjustments. Attention will be given to the relief of pain, nausea and vomiting after surgery and chemotherapy. As physical problems are relieved, the patient may cope better emotionally, but when the prognosis is poor, time is needed to adjust to the sad news. Cancer nurse specialists have been shown to play a vital role in supporting the patient's physical, emotional and holistic needs and tailoring care to the individual (Kerr et al. 2021).

Chapter 32 provides detailed information about palliative care, symptom relief, end-of-life care and bereavement care.

Uterine Displacement and Prolapse

Cervicovaginal Prolapse

The cervix can become prolapsed and elongated by the opposing forces of pull of the transverse cervical and uterosacral ligaments against prolapsed vaginal walls. Importantly, in this situation the cervix prolapses but the uterus stays in the pelvis.

Types of Prolapse

Anterior Vaginal Wall Prolapse
- *Cystocele* – a prolapse of the bladder and upper anterior vaginal wall (Fig. 8.8A).
- *Urethrocele* – a lower vaginal wall prolapse with urethral descent.

Posterior Vaginal Wall Prolapse
- *Rectocele* – a prolapse of the rectum and the middle third of the posterior vaginal wall. If the lowest part of the vaginal wall prolapses, the perineal body is involved rather than the rectum (Fig. 8.8B).
- *Enterocele* – if the upper part of the posterior vaginal wall prolapses, the rectouterine recess/pouch is elongated and a loop of small bowel or omentum may descend.

Both anterior and posterior vaginal walls may be involved in the prolapse. When a large cystocele is present, bladder emptying tends to be incomplete, causing bladder hypertrophy. There

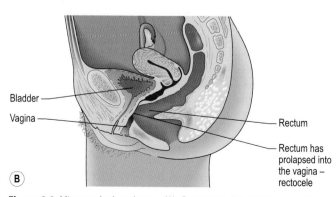

Figure 8.8 Uterovaginal prolapse. (A) Cystocele. (B) Rectocele. (Reproduced from Cotton 2003 with permission.)

is a lump, urinary frequency, dysuria and stress incontinence (see Chapter 24, Maintaining Continence). The uterus may become distorted, leading to reflux of urine and, ultimately, renal damage. Urinary tract infection is common.

A woman with a rectocele may notice a lump and experience difficulty during defecation.

Uterovaginal Prolapse

When the structures supporting the uterus and vagina become ineffective, the genital tract descends, prolapses or herniates through the gap between the muscles of the pelvic floor.

The uterus descends in the axis of the vagina taking the vaginal wall with it. This prolapse is essentially but not exclusively a post-menopausal condition.

Three degrees of uterine prolapse are described:
- *first degree* – the cervix is still within the vagina
- *second degree* – the cervix appears at the introitus
- *third degree* – the uterus and vagina are completely prolapsed and lie outside the vulva.

Rectal prolapse may also occur. This is sometimes called complete procidentia.

Contributing factors are:
- stretching of tissues from repeated child-bearing
- injury to the pelvic floor during childbirth
- the long-term maintenance of an upright, erect body position that strains the transverse ligaments (the chief support of the uterus)
- increased intra-abdominal pressure associated with obesity, chronic cough or heavy lifting work.

Medical Management

History. The woman may be overweight, complains of backache and describes a feeling of 'something coming down' when she is in an upright position. There is urinary frequency, incomplete bladder emptying and the residual urine is a focus for infection. Stress incontinence may be a major problem for some women (see Chapter 24, Maintaining Continence). There may be difficulty in voiding urine and in defecation. The cystocele or rectocele may have to be supported or pushed upwards vaginally before urine can be passed or the bowel evacuated.

Examination. Severe prolapse may be diagnosed by inspecting the vulva with the patient lying on her back and straining downwards. A vaginal speculum is used to allow direct vision of a prolapsed anterior vaginal wall and any rectocele or enterocele formed by a prolapsed posterior vaginal wall. A rectal examination is needed to confirm the latter type of displacement. The degree of uterine prolapse is usually assessed before surgery when the patient is anaesthetised.

Investigations. A diagnosis of uterine displacement can be made on examination. Preoperative assessment will involve investigations to assess the woman's general health prior to general anaesthetic.

Treatment. Surgical treatment is curative for prolapse but is not suitable for all women. Some may be unfit for surgery due to poor physical condition or may not have completed their family. The uterus may be supported by the use of a polyethylene or flexible vinyl ring pessary. Such pessaries can cause local inflammation and are changed every 4–6 months when the vaginal walls can be examined for inflammation or ulceration. A course of vaginal oestrogen may be prescribed to diminish atrophic changes, inflammation, infection and discharge.

Surgical Repair of Uterine Displacement and Prolapse. This may involve removal of the uterus vaginally and reconstruction of the supporting pelvic floor muscles between the anus, vagina and bladder, and approximating the medial borders of the pubococcygeus muscles. Childbirth can result in supporting structures being torn, separated and overstretched. Repair of cystocele is known as anterior colporrhaphy supporting the urethra and urethrovesical junction. A rectocele is repaired by a posterior colpoperineorrhaphy, the repair of the perineal body. Bladder, perineum and vulva have an excellent capacity for repair, related to a rich blood supply and good venous drainage. Surgery is usually very successful.

❖ Nursing Management and Health Promotion: Uterine Displacement

Preoperative Care

Preoperative assessment and care of women for major gynaecological operations have been discussed earlier in the chapter. Care is always individualised according to needs, but some problems and interventions are similar.

Information. Information about procedures before and after surgery will increase patient understanding and cooperation and reduce anxiety.

Potential Embarrassment. A woman admitted for repair of prolapse may experience embarrassment due to stress incontinence and the need for some type of protection. The nurse will ensure that her special requirements are met discreetly.

Evacuating the Lower Bowel Before Surgery. The woman's lower bowel may be emptied before surgery and an oral laxative, or suppositories or evacuant microenema, may be prescribed; local policy and procedure must be adhered to.

Identification of Sexual Activity. Whilst embarrassing for some women, it is important to identify if the woman is still sexually active. This will influence the amount of vaginal tissue removed during surgery.

Postoperative Care

Risk of Strain on Internal Suture Lines From a Full Bladder. An indwelling catheter on continuous drainage is required. Precautions are taken to prevent the introduction of infection when the closed urinary drainage system is breached when collecting specimens or changing drainage bags.

Loss of Bladder Tone. This is possible after catheter removal. Residual amounts of urine retained in the bladder after voiding should be assessed. This can be done by a noninvasive bladder scan or by catheterisation. A residual urine of less than 60 mL is satisfactory.

Risk of Wound Infection. Regular perineal cleansing can minimise the risk of infection.

Constipation. This will potentially strain the repaired posterior vaginal wall. A stool-softener laxative can be prescribed to promote easy defecation.

Predischarge Counselling. An opportunity is created for the patient to discuss her feelings and worries about the level of recovery from surgery, bladder functioning, future return to sexual activity and work. In particular, the woman is advised to avoid jarring or lifting activities for 2 months to prevent straining the healing tissues. Contact numbers should be given if problems arise once home (Information 8.5).

Infections of the Female Reproductive Tract

Infections of the female reproductive tract include vaginitis, cervicitis, endometritis, salpingitis and PID, oophoritis and toxic shock syndrome (TSS), some of which are sexually transmitted. This chapter concentrates on salpingitis and PID.

Salpingitis and Pelvic Inflammatory Disease

Inflammation/infection of the uterine tubes, salpingitis, usually affects both tubes simultaneously. It may result from ascending infection from the vagina, cervix or uterus or it can occur directly from appendicitis, a pelvic abscess or other site of inflammation such as diverticulitis. The ovaries may also be involved in the inflammatory process. Salpingitis may therefore be part of generalised PID.

Acute salpingitis may follow childbirth, miscarriage or termination, diagnostic or operative procedures involving the uterus or the insertion of intrauterine devices.

🩸 Pathophysiology

Ascending salpingitis is most commonly caused by the organism *Chlamydia trachomatis*. Gonococcal infection, which is sexually transmitted, may also be the cause. Streptococcal and staphylococcal salpingitis may follow miscarriage or termination, childbirth or the insertion of an intrauterine device. These causes may reflect reactivation of pre-existing disease. Intestinal tract commensals, *Escherichia coli* or *Streptococcus faecalis*, may be involved if the infection is linked to appendicitis or bowel infection. The blood-borne *Mycobacterium tuberculosis* may unobtrusively inflame the reproductive organs.

The uterine tubes become engorged and swollen, possibly filled with pus (pyosalpinx). The ciliated epithelial lining is damaged, thus reducing the ability to move oocytes/ova and spermatozoa within the tubes.

Common Presenting Symptoms. The patient feels generally unwell, with:
- pyrexia, sweating
- nausea, vomiting
- aching joints
- severe pelvic and abdominal pain.

🩸 Medical Management

Women usually present with symptoms of generalised PID, or salpingitis may be identified for the first time during laparoscopy where the tubes are inflamed, distended and blocked. Adhesions may form between the tubes and other pelvic structures and peritonitis may be evident.

On pelvic examination, tenderness will be felt over the uterine cornua. There may not be obvious vaginal discharge so this cannot be relied upon for diagnosis. Infection spread via the genital tract will affect the lumen of the uterine tube, creating a purulent, foul discharge that is drained through the vagina. Scar tissue may form, causing narrowing or closure of the tube which will affect fertility. Adhesions may form between the inflamed tubes and the peritoneum. Peritonitis may occur if pus leaks out of the tubes into the peritoneal cavity. Rarely, an abscess may form in the pelvis or on the ovaries.

Investigations. High vaginal or cervical swabs are taken and sent for microbiological culture and sensitivity to antibiotics. During surgery, samples for microbiological samples may be obtained.

Laparoscopy is not indicated in the acute phase as this may cause further spread of infection unless an abscess requires drainage or ectopic pregnancy is suspected.

Treatment. Antibiotic therapy is prescribed along with analgesia.

❖ Nursing Management and Health Promotion: Salpingitis/PID

Nursing care will be planned to relieve symptoms, particularly pain, nausea, vomiting and potential fluid and electrolyte imbalance (see Chapter 20, Pain Management, and Chapter 21, Maintaining Fluid, Electrolyte and Acid–Base Balance). Analgesics and antibiotic drugs are administered often intravenously for 24 hours. Information will need to be shared with the woman about the prevention of infection, the risk of infertility and the possibility of an ectopic pregnancy following salpingitis/PID.

Disorders of Early Pregnancy

Ectopic Pregnancy

An ectopic pregnancy occurs when the fertilised ovum implants and develops outside the uterus. In the UK 1200 ectopic pregnancies are diagnosed each year, although there is anecdotal evidence that the actual incidence rate may be higher. It has been estimated that 1 in 90 pregnancies are ectopic and that ectopic pregnancy remains the most frequent cause of maternal death in early pregnancy (MBRRACE 2022).

Pathophysiology

A delay occurs in the passage of the fertilised ovum through the uterine tube. This may be due to ciliary damage, obstruction in the tube or adhesions from an earlier infection. The pregnancy implants in the muscle wall of the tube and erodes into blood vessels. Increased tension in the tube will cause pelvic pain and may lead to rupture which can result in massive intraperitoneal haemorrhage.

Common Presenting Symptoms. The woman experiences the early signs of pregnancy.

The trophoblast slowly erodes the tubal wall, which results in gradual or sudden rupture of the tube. The woman experiences abdominal pain. Urgent attention should be paid if the woman complains of shoulder pain due to referred pain from the diaphragm, which is irritated by blood in the abdomen.

Tubal rupture causes severe localised pain, which is followed by intense, more generalised abdominal pain. The POCs are expelled into the peritoneal cavity and there is haemorrhage from the tubal placental site. This leads to hypovolaemic shock (Chapter 19, Recognising and Managing Shock), with rapid, feeble pulse rate, hypotension and pallor – an acute abdominal emergency exists and the woman must be treated as a gynaecological emergency. Despite medical advances in the past decade, there has been no decrease in the number of women dying from an ectopic pregnancy. The 2022 MBRRACE Report which reviewed the years 2018–20 shows that ectopic pregnancy remains the most frequent cause of maternal death in early pregnancy. The latest report shows that the death rate from ectopic pregnancy devastatingly has increased from five women dying to eight and all died within 48 hours of presentation with their ectopic pregnancy (MBRRACE 2022).

Medical Management

Investigations

Pregnancy Tests. Standard immunological pregnancy tests are unhelpful as a tubal pregnancy may not produce enough hCG to give a positive result. Estimation of the β subunit of hCG (β-hCG) is undertaken, which is accurate 2 weeks after conception. Absence of β-hCG excludes pregnancy. In ectopic pregnancy the levels are lower than those at a comparable gestation in a normal intrauterine pregnancy. At a titre of 1000–1500 IU/L, it should be able to detect an intrauterine sac on a TVS, but levels above 1500 IU/L in the presence of an empty uterus may indicate an ectopic pregnancy.

Repeat blood tests may be required after 48 hours to assess both the amount and rate of increase of β-hCG levels.

USS. By the 6th or 7th week of pregnancy, a gestational sac can be identified within the uterus on USS. A pregnancy outside the uterus often cannot be identified on scan. Consequently, the presence of a raised β-hCG level combined with the lack of an identifiable intrauterine pregnancy indicates an ectopic pregnancy.

Treatment

Surgical. An ectopic pregnancy always requires urgent surgery by laparoscopy or laparotomy. During laparoscopy under general anaesthetic, an incision is made into the tube and the pregnancy removed – the tube then heals spontaneously or the damaged tube is removed (salpingectomy). A laparotomy may be required if the tube has ruptured. Recovery after salpingectomy is usually rapid and uncomplicated.

Medical. Nonsurgical techniques have been developed. These include the puncture and aspiration of the ectopic sac or the local injection of embryotoxic drugs, such as methotrexate or potassium chloride (Kenny and Bickerstaff 2016). The need for a general anaesthetic with its associated risks is removed but careful follow-up is required to monitor the effects on the woman and the pregnancy.

A ruptured ectopic pregnancy quickly results in hypovolaemia and intravenous fluids are essential. The patient may need resuscitation but immediate surgery and treatment of the cause of bleeding are essential.

Women who are rhesus negative and are not sensitised should be given anti-D immunoglobulin following an ectopic pregnancy (NICE 2019b).

A woman who has had one ectopic pregnancy is at risk of developing a similar pregnancy in the second tube. However, the woman should be reassured she may be able to have a normal pregnancy via the remaining tube.

❖❖ Nursing Management and Health Promotion: Ectopic Pregnancy

Preoperative Care

Risk of Hypovolaemia. The nurse assesses and monitors the patient's physical state intensively from the time of admission to the ward. If the tubal pregnancy ruptures, the patient may experience hypovolaemic shock and cardiac arrest. Vital signs are recorded every 15 minutes. Tachycardia, hypotension and increasing pain are indications that urgent medical intervention is required.

Pain. The patient will experience pain which may be moderate, but may become intense and intolerable if the pregnancy ruptures. Analgesia is given as prescribed.

Preparation for General Anaesthesia. Emergency surgery will be required and fasting for an appropriate time may not be possible (see Chapter 25, Nursing the Patient Undergoing Surgery). Therefore it is important for the anaesthetist to know when the patient last ate or drank and any history of vomiting. It may be necessary to introduce a nasogastric tube prior to surgery to reduce the risk of regurgitation and inhalation of gastric contents when the patient is anaesthetised.

Anxiety and the Need for Information. The patient may be anxious about the operation and distressed about losing a pregnancy. She will need information about the surgery and postoperative care, and needs to be encouraged to talk about any worries she may have. The nurse must show empathy and understanding of the patient's feelings and concerns.

Postoperative Care. Postoperative care will be individualised according to patient need (see Chapter 25). Her condition will begin to stabilise as soon as the ectopic pregnancy is removed, bleeding controlled and blood volume restored. Her main problems will be similar to those of other patients who have had open abdominal surgery, plus those associated with pregnancy loss as follows:

- *Change in vital signs.* The nurse monitors pulse rate, blood pressure, respiration rate and body temperature. Wound site and vaginal blood loss are observed for more than minimal drainage. Primary and secondary haemorrhages are risks.
- *Postoperative pain.* The level of pain can be assessed using a verbal rating scale (see Chapter 20, Pain Management). Analgesics are prescribed and administered to control pain.
- *Postanaesthetic nausea.* This problem may be prevented or treated by giving an antiemetic medication with analgesics as prescribed.
- *Fluid and electrolyte imbalance.* Intravenous fluid and electrolyte replacement therapy is administered as prescribed, until oral intake is resumed. Fluid intake and output are recorded.
- *Risk of VTE.* The patient is actively encouraged to exercise her legs hourly whilst confined to bed. Antiembolism hosiery/stockings will be fitted preoperatively and worn until discharge. Early mobilisation is usual and encouraged.
- *Personal care.* Whilst intravenous therapy is in situ, assistance will be given to maintain the patient's preferred standard of personal care until fully mobile.
- *Loss and grieving.* It must be acknowledged that the woman has lost a pregnancy and she must be given opportunities to talk about her feelings and emotions freely. Information should be shared about the possibility of future pregnancies. Details of local support groups for those who experience loss should be given. The effect on future fertility should be acknowledged and the nurse should give the woman and her partner appropriate support and information about assisted conception services as required.

Miscarriage and Termination of Pregnancy

The legal definition of the term 'abortion' refers to the premature delivery of a nonviable fetus, spontaneously or by induction. The term 'miscarriage' is recommended when the pregnancy loss is spontaneous and is generally more acceptable to women who lose a wanted pregnancy (NICE 2019b). Currently, in the UK, a fetus is considered viable from the 24th week of pregnancy. This viability is recognised and safeguarded in the Infant Life (Preservation) Act 1929 and its amendment under the Human Fertilisation and Embryology Act 1990. However, debate is ongoing around reducing the gestational age of viable pregnancies due to the technological developments increasingly available to support very premature infants. Spontaneous miscarriage refers to all types of naturally occurring miscarriages. Induced 'abortion' refers to interventional TOP.

A spontaneous miscarriage is a response to a naturally occurring phenomenon such as hormonal problems, uterine abnormality, cervical problems, a genetic malformation in the embryo/fetus or psychological factors. An estimated one in five pregnancies ended in miscarriage (one in six if we only count women who realised/reported the miscarriage) (Tommy's Pregnancy Hub 2022).

Miscarriages in the early weeks of the second trimester of pregnancy may be due to a cervix that dilates in response to the increasing weight of the fetus. The cervical os dilates, the membranes rupture and the pregnancy is lost. The woman will be distressed by the loss of the pregnancy and will need psychological support from the nurse, encouraging her and her partner to express their feelings.

To counteract recurrence of miscarriage, it is necessary to identify the pregnancy and any incompetence of the cervix at an early stage. In the case of cervical incompetence, a purse-string (Shirodkar's) suture can be inserted surgically, closing the internal os. The suture is removed at 38 weeks' gestation or when labour commences, to enable delivery to occur.

Miscarriage may be categorised by the:
- level of certainty of the miscarriage occurring
  - threatened
  - inevitable
  - missed
  - induced
- degree of expulsion of the POC
  - incomplete
  - complete.

See Fig. 8.9.

The care of women having a miscarriage is increasingly undertaken in outpatient settings or in the community.

Threatened Miscarriage

Pathophysiology

A threatened miscarriage is when a woman known to be pregnant develops vaginal bleeding during the first 24 weeks of gestation. Some lower abdominal pain related to uterine muscle contractions may be experienced at the time of bleeding, but there may be no uterine contractions and no pain. The blood loss may be brown or red.

It is not unusual for a show of blood to coincide with the woman's regular date of menstruation. This type of bleeding is due to the fertilised ovum becoming more deeply implanted in the uterine wall. There is little risk of loss of the pregnancy if the bleeding settles quickly (Fig. 8.9A).

Medical Management

The presence of bleeding, slight uterine contractions and a closed cervical os established by examination assist in identifying threatened miscarriage; 70%–80% of women can be expected to continue to full-term pregnancies.

Treatment. While the woman is continuing to lose blood vaginally, it is recommended that she does not undertake strenuous activities. Bed rest is unlikely to influence the outcome but the woman may blame herself if she goes on to miscarry following strenuous activity.

Women who are rhesus negative and are not sensitised should be given anti-D immunoglobulin if they have a threatened miscarriage:
- over 12 weeks' gestation or
- with heavy vaginal bleeding or associated with pain before 12 weeks' gestation (NICE 2019b).

❖ Nursing Management and Health Promotion: Threatened Miscarriage

The woman and her partner will be very concerned about the possible loss of the pregnancy. This may result in tearfulness, anxiety, irritability and feelings of frustration. The woman may be apprehensive of pain and uncertain of what to expect.

Nursing care aims to reduce anxiety by providing accurate information about likely outcomes and support and reassurance for the couple. Vaginal bleeding will be monitored closely and abdominal discomfort or pain will be assessed. The supportive, counselling contact time with the nurse will be appreciated by the woman and her partner.

Figure 8.9 The types of miscarriage. (A) Threatened miscarriage. (B) Inevitable miscarriage. (C) Missed miscarriage. (D) Incomplete miscarriage.

Inevitable Miscarriage

Pathophysiology

A threatened miscarriage can become inevitable if vaginal bleeding continues. A miscarriage becomes inevitable, with no possibility of saving the pregnancy, when the following are present:
- heavy vaginal blood loss often with clots
- strong uterine contractions
- pain
- dilatation of the cervix.

Contractions will increase, the fetal sac membranes rupture and the uterine contents move through the cervical os. Part or all of the POC will be voided from the uterus (Fig. 8.9B). An inevitable miscarriage may be complete if all POCs are voided, or incomplete if some products are retained.

Medical Management

Estimation of blood loss and assessment of pulse, blood pressure, respiration and appearance of the patient will indicate whether hypovolaemic shock is developing. Intravenous fluids may be required and analgesics are administered as necessary.

Fetal tissue that has been expelled is retained and examined to assess whether the fetal sac and contents are intact or whether remnants have been retained. USS can be useful to determine the type of miscarriage and, based on this, appropriate information can be given to the woman about the likely outcome and therapeutic options. Following a complete miscarriage, the uterus will

contract and the complex interlocking layers of smooth muscle fibres of the myometrium will exert pressure on blood vessels to restrict blood loss. If any of the POCs are thought to have been retained, the uterus cannot contract fully and bleeding will continue. Retained POC may also provide a locus for infection. Several treatment options are available and the woman must be involved in the choice of approach. They are:
- evacuation of the retained products of conception (ERPC) from the uterus, an invasive procedure; in the UK a general anaesthetic is usual, but in many countries, local anaesthetic or sedation is used (NICE 2019b)
- medical management with the use of a prostaglandin analogue such as misoprostol
- expectant management ('wait and see'), but women must be aware that it may take several weeks for complete resolution.

Women who are rhesus negative and are not sensitised should be given anti-D immunoglobulin if they have a miscarriage over 12 weeks' gestation, or have an ERPC or medical management (NICE 2019b).

❖ Nursing Management and Health Promotion: Inevitable Miscarriage

The nurse must monitor vaginal blood loss extremely closely whichever form of management is undertaken. The patient may be distressed by the blood loss, pain and the anguish of losing a pregnancy, particularly if planned. The nurse has an important role to provide support for both the woman and her partner at this time, encouraging them to talk through their feelings of loss. In this respect, time and empathy from the nurse will be appreciated. If a fetus has been passed, the woman should be supported in viewing the fetus if she wishes and photographs should be taken to provide a record which the woman may want either at the time or later. Information about support groups, such as the Miscarriage Association, can be helpful.

Missed Miscarriage

Pathophysiology

A missed miscarriage is one in which the embryo/fetus dies, but is not expelled. The size of the uterus fails to increase during the first trimester, the fetus does not develop and the expected signs of a normally developing pregnancy will be missing. In some cases a fertilised ovum fails to develop further than embryonic stages. The death of the embryo/fetus may occur at any week of gestation. Some placental tissue survives to produce progesterone and prevent expulsion (Fig. 8.9C).

Medical Management

Following a positive pregnancy test, the woman may have stopped feeling pregnant. She may experience a brown vaginal discharge. Some hCG may still be present but levels fall.

Investigations. USS of the uterus will indicate a gestational sac smaller than that expected for the gestational age and the absence of a fetal heart.

Treatment. Once a missed miscarriage has been diagnosed, treatment options should be discussed with the woman. These include:
- ERPC (see earlier).
- Medical management with the administration of mifepristone (an antiprogesterone) orally then misoprostol vaginally 24–48 hours later. This induces the uterine muscles to contract and the woman experiences labour.

- Expectant/conservative management where nature is allowed to take its course; however, this can take several weeks and some women cannot cope with the thought of carrying their dead baby in utero during this time. The woman must also be provided with 24-hour contact details in case of haemorrhage following expulsion of the POC.

As discussed earlier, the administration of anti-D immunoglobulin may be needed for unsensitised women who are rhesus negative.

❖ Nursing Management and Health Promotion: Missed Miscarriage

If ERPC is planned, the woman will need the usual preparation to undergo anaesthesia safely (see Chapter 25, Nursing the Patient Undergoing Surgery). Following treatment, observations of vital signs and vaginal blood loss will be required to assess recovery.

If medical management is planned, the nurse must be available to observe the patient's vital signs and need for pain relief and provide support during the 'labour' phase. The patient should be nursed in a single room but must not feel isolated during this time. Patients and their partners cope emotionally in different ways but the nurse can anticipate that couples may feel sad and angry about the lost pregnancy. They must be given opportunities to express their needs and feelings freely.

Incomplete Miscarriage

An incomplete miscarriage is one in which only part of the POC is expelled from the uterus (Fig. 8.9D).

● *Pathophysiology*

Portions of placenta and membranes are retained; some bleeding continues and could possibly be heavy. Retained products can become infected so the aim should be to remove them.

● *Medical Management*

The residual products may be voided spontaneously by the woman but otherwise they will need to be removed either by surgical evacuation using vacuum aspiration or by the administration of misoprostol, previously described for inevitable miscarriage.

Women who are rhesus negative and are not sensitised should be given anti-D immunoglobulin if they have a miscarriage over 12 weeks' gestation, or have an ERPC or medical management (NICE 2019b).

❖ Nursing Management and Health Promotion: Incomplete Miscarriage

The patient's symptoms will depend on the amount of tissue retained. She may experience moderate to severe abdominal pain while the uterus contracts trying to expel the retained POCs. Nursing care involves administering analgesics and monitoring their effect. Vaginal blood loss must be monitored, as heavy, continuous blood loss may reduce circulating blood volume, resulting in hypovolaemic shock. Observations of vital signs will facilitate early recognition of shock and prompt correction of the condition by intravenous fluid replacement. A supportive approach must be used as for other forms of miscarriage (Reflection 8.2).

Recurrent Miscarriage

Recurrent miscarriage refers to spontaneous miscarriage that occurs in three or more successive pregnancies at a similar gestational age. Many factors may contribute to recurrent miscarriage.

● *Pathophysiology*

Genetic, hormonal, anatomical, infectious and immunological factors have been implicated in the causation of recurrent miscarriage. However, the underlying mechanisms are poorly explained, largely speculative and require further investigation.

● *Medical Management*

This depends on the reason for recurrent miscarriage. There is insufficient evidence for many treatments previously thought to have been useful, for example leucocyte transfusions (Royal College of Obstetricians and Gynaecologists (RCOG) 2011). Surgery to correct uterine abnormalities should be considered carefully as postoperative scarring may affect future fertility.

❖ Nursing Management and Health Promotion: Recurrent Miscarriage

Physical and psychological care are paramount at the time that the miscarriage occurs. Referral to a specialist unit where further chromosomal testing can be undertaken should be offered to the couple.

Termination of Pregnancy

An unwanted pregnancy creates emotional anguish for a woman. She may experience feelings of conflict about both wanting and rejecting the pregnancy. She may fear having to explain it to others. Family standards of behaviour, cultural norms and religious beliefs may appear to be violated both by the pregnancy and by the possibility of termination. The woman may feel very alone, indecisive and under pressure from a partner who may reject the pregnancy. The conditions of the Abortion Act require decision-making to be completed early in the pregnancy.

The Abortion Act 1967 and 1990 Amendments

In the UK, the Abortion Act 1967 became law in 1968 and applies to England, Wales and Scotland but not Northern Ireland. The Act states that the TOP by a registered practitioner is not illegal

---

REFLECTION 8.2

Pregnancy Loss

Failure of a fertilised embryo to develop into a successful pregnancy resulting in a live baby can occur at many different stages of the pregnancy.

Activity

- Think about the different types of pregnancy loss that can happen.
- Reflect on how the woman and her partner may be feeling after the loss of a pregnancy and what you might say to the couple to support them.

under certain conditions. Notification of a termination must be given on a prescribed form to the Chief Medical Officer of the DH within 7 days of the termination. The Abortion Act 1967 was amended by the Human Fertilisation and Embryology Act 1990, recognising viability of the fetus at 24 weeks' gestation.

Conditions of the Act and Statutory Grounds
A legally induced termination must be:
- performed by a registered medical practitioner
- performed, except in an emergency, in an NHS hospital or in a place for the time being approved for the purpose of the Act
- certified by two registered medical practitioners as necessary on any of the following grounds:
  - the continuance of the pregnancy would involve risk to the life of the pregnant woman greater than if the pregnancy were terminated
  - the continuance of the pregnancy would involve risk of injury to the physical or mental health of the pregnant woman greater than if the pregnancy were terminated
  - the continuance of the pregnancy would involve risk of injury to the physical or mental health of any existing child(ren) in the family of the pregnant woman greater than if the pregnancy were terminated
  - there is a substantial risk that if the child were born it would suffer from such physical or mental abnormalities as to be seriously handicapped
- in emergency, certified by the operating practitioner as immediately necessary:
  - to save the life of the pregnant woman
  - to prevent grave permanent injury to the physical or mental health of the pregnant woman.

Conscientious Objection and the Abortion Act 1967
The Act states that no one shall be under any legal obligation to participate in any treatment authorised by the Act to which he or she has a conscientious objection unless the treatment is necessary to save the life or prevent grave permanent injury to the physical or mental health of a pregnant woman. The conscience clause does not only apply to members of a particular religion or faith and the objector must participate in emergency care of the patient should it be necessary. This is affirmed in The Code: Professional standards of practice and behaviour for nurses, midwives and nursing associates (Nursing and Midwifery Council (NMC) 2018).

Counselling of the Pregnant Woman Requesting Termination
A woman who requests a TOP will be referred for counselling to discuss any contraindications to termination and provide evidence for the final decision making. If possible, she should be seen with her partner, although the partner may not want to be involved. All women/girls, even those under the age of 16 years, are entitled to complete confidentiality when requesting termination and partners or parents are not informed without the woman's consent. However, those under 16 years of age are encouraged to speak to their parents. Adolescent girls may be accompanied by parents who are angry and there is a risk the girl passively acts in accordance with her parents' wishes.

The counselling service ensures that adequate assessment and advice are provided for the woman who seeks a termination. It is suggested that in this way she will experience less regret, guilt or long-term psychological problems.

Medical Management
All nonsensitised rhesus-negative women having a TOP should have anti-D immunoglobulin (NICE 2019b).

Methods Used for Termination
Suction Termination. This is the most commonly used method for early TOP. It may be performed with a local or general anaesthetic, or conscious sedation. Preoperatively, the patient may have vaginal misoprostol to soften the cervix. The cervix is dilated, a flexible cannula is inserted and the contents of the uterus are aspirated by suction. The uterus is then curetted to ensure total removal of the POC.

Surgical Dilatation and Evacuation. This can be used in the second trimester of pregnancy. The cervix is dilated and the POCs are removed using forceps and suction, usually under general anaesthetic. Preoperatively the patient may have vaginal misoprostol to soften the cervix and facilitate easier dilatation.

Medical Termination (Unlicensed Regimens). The specific regimen depends on the period of gestation, but is based for example on oral mifepristone 200 mg followed by vaginal misoprostol 800 μg after a period of time (1–3 days for pregnancies up to 9 weeks' gestation; 36–48 hours for 9–24 weeks' gestation).

Following administration of misoprostol, the patient remains under observation for a further 6 hours. Before discharge, arrangements are made for the patient to return in 5–9 days to assess the outcome.

If the POCs have not been expelled 4 hours following the misoprostol in pregnancies over 7 weeks' gestation up to 9 weeks, a second dose of misoprostol 400 μg (oral or vaginal) may be administered.

For pregnancies of 9–13 weeks' gestation, a further four doses of misoprostol 400 μg (oral or vaginal) can be given at intervals 3 hours apart if needed. In later terminations of 13–24 weeks' gestation, should further doses of misoprostol 400 μg be needed, it is administered orally.

While this method of terminating a pregnancy has its advantages – not least that there is no anaesthetic or surgical intervention – there are also potential problems of which the woman should be made aware. These include:
- a chance that the termination will be unsuccessful/incomplete, resulting in the need for surgical intervention; excessive vaginal bleeding may occur
- the possibility of pain, necessitating powerful analgesics
- possible psychological distress for the woman seeing the expelled fetus.

Other methods involving the administration of prostaglandins, for example intravenously, extra-amniotically or intra-amniotically, are now rarely performed.

Complications of Pregnancy Termination
- Pelvic infection – inflammation of the endometrium (endometritis) and salpingitis.
- Perforation of the uterus – caused accidentally during cannula insertion or use of the curette.
- Haemorrhage – bleeding should not be more than a normal menstruation.

- Laceration of cervix, cervical incompetence and recurrent miscarriage.
- Ectopic pregnancy – related to previous salpingitis.
- Incomplete removal of uterine contents.
- Hydatidiform mole.
- Delayed menstruation.
- A live fetus at the time of delivery.
- Possible susceptibility to subsequent pregnancy loss and premature births.
- Infertility.

With improved services, the numbers of complications associated with TOP can be greatly reduced.

❖ Nursing Management and Health Promotion: Termination of Pregnancy

Care Before the Procedure
The procedure is generally completed on an outpatient basis or as a day patient in hospital. The nurse must demonstrate a non-judgemental attitude and provide support and information for the woman. Blood tests such as ABO grouping and the rhesus factor are necessary precautions prior to the procedure.

Care Following the Procedure
Vital signs related to bleeding, i.e. pulse and blood pressure, and abdominal cramping pain must be observed by the nurse. Vaginal loss must be monitored closely. Pyrexia may indicate the onset of infection. Mild analgesics may be ordered to relieve cramping pain and also for their antipyretic properties. Nurses should be aware of those women who require anti-D immunoglobulin.

Women are advised to avoid the use of tampons, strenuous activities or sexual intercourse for 2 weeks to reduce the risk of infection and aid healing. Appropriate contraception must be discussed to prevent a further unwanted pregnancy. However, the nurse must be sensitive to the fact that some couples decide to terminate a wanted pregnancy due to serious fetal abnormalities.

Family Planning Services

Free contraceptive services are now available from GPs, family planning clinics in hospitals and the community, and voluntary organisations such as the FPA and Brook Advisory Centres, who receive grants from central government or from purchasing commissioners. Male and female sterilisations are available in NHS facilities but must be considered permanent. Vasectomies may be performed in some large family planning clinics and by some GPs in the surgery.

Postnatally, community midwives, health visitors and GPs routinely discuss birth control methods with the new mother. This is invaluable in reminding women of their fertility and the possibility of another early pregnancy if precautions are not taken when resuming sexual activities.

The Contraceptive Needs of Young People
Provision of extra contraceptive services for young people after puberty, under 16 years and up to 20 years of age, is controversial and, in the past, was given a low priority. With more recent concern about sexually transmitted infections and teenage pregnancy rates, young people have been specially targeted for health education and advice about their sexual behaviour. Specialist services are now delivered through many health and voluntary services such as

Brook, which specifically aim at reaching and meeting the needs of teenagers.

Infertility

While some couples choose not to have children, for many people this is an important role, and when childlessness is a reality it brings disappointment. In addition, many other feelings, associated with social and cultural expectations and religious beliefs, may be experienced.

Some couples choose to delay having children but later may experience difficulty in conceiving. One in six couples will seek specialist help for a fertility problem. In one-third of couples experiencing subfertility, the problem lies with the woman, in one-third with the man, and in the remaining third both the man and the woman contribute some causative factor.

A couple is said to be subfertile if they have been having unprotected sexual intercourse for 12 months without conception occurring. Primary subfertility describes cases where a pregnancy has never occurred, and secondary subfertility those cases where there has been a previous pregnancy, irrespective of the outcome.

● Medical Management
The diagnosis and management of subfertility are complex. The couple may be required to undergo a variety of tests and investigations, which can cause embarrassment and stress.

Female Subfertility
Female subfertility may be due to failure to produce oocytes or a patent system for a fertilised ovum to travel to and implant in the endometrium. This may be due to failure to ovulate, irregular ovulation, tubal obstruction, hostile cervical mucus, endometriosis or uterine conditions that inhibit implantation. Fertility declines with the age of the female and sharply so after 37 years. This is becoming more important as many couples are deferring starting families until later in life due to careers and personal choice. They may then encounter difficulties which need investigating and treating, providing extra pressure due to time constraints.

Ovulation Disorders
These are among the commonest causes of subfertility. Failure to ovulate is linked with the functioning of hormones from the hypothalamus, pituitary and ovary (HPO axis).
- Hypothalamic disorders – abnormal levels of GnRH. There may be over- or underproduction resulting in anovulation.
- Pituitary disorders – abnormal secretion of prolactin resulting in anovulation and amenorrhoea.
- Ovarian causes – in polycystic ovary syndrome (PCOS), multiple small follicles partly develop but none reaches maturity, resulting in small cysts on the ovary. Often associated with obesity and hirsutism (see Chapter 5, Nursing Patients with Endocrine Disorders).

Treatment. seeks to remedy problems from imbalances in the HPO axis. Ovulation induction is aimed at encouraging development of more than one follicle. Clomiphene citrate stimulates gonadotrophin release. It can be prescribed for up to six cycles. This is also often effective for women with PCOS.

For women who do not respond to clomiphene therapy, human menopausal gonadotrophin (hMG) may be used for direct ovarian stimulation. Careful monitoring of the dose is required to reduce the risk of multiple pregnancy and ovarian hyperstimulation syndrome.

If a woman has hyperprolactinaemia, bromocriptine, a powerful dopamine agonist, inhibits prolactin release and may be an appropriate therapy.

Tubal Disorders

A tubal disorder may prevent spermatozoa reaching the oocyte or, if fertilisation does occur, the ovum may not reach the uterine cavity for implantation. Tubal surgery may be advised to attempt to restore normal anatomy and function. However, the risks of further adhesions developing must be balanced against proposed benefits. Diagnostic procedures will include laparoscopy and hysterosalpingography for full assessment of the condition.

Treatment. Surgical procedures used to treat tubal infertility include fimbrioplasty, salpingostomy and tubal cannulation. However, a successful outcome of such surgery depends on the degree of tubal damage and the adequacy of the surgery performed. Many patients will decide to opt for assisted conception techniques such as in vitro fertilisation (IVF), embryo transfer (ET) and gamete intrafallopian transfer (GIFT) rather than undergo further surgery.

Endometriosis

The association between endometriosis and infertility is complex. Many women with the condition conceive successfully without intervention.

Treatment. There is controversy over the treatment of infertile women with endometriosis without distortion of the pelvic viscera. Treatment using minimal access surgical techniques is usually only indicated for women with other symptoms such as pelvic pain.

Male Subfertility

Please refer to Chapter 9, Nursing Patients With Disorders of the Male Reproductive System.

Treatment. should be aimed at achieving natural conception. When natural conception is not possible, assisted conception techniques are offered. IVF involves fertilisation using male and female gametes under laboratory conditions. The fertilised embryo is then transferred into the uterus – a procedure known as embryo transfer (ET). This procedure is carried out in cycles of ovarian stimulations to produce several mature follicles at the same time. This principle has now been developed for other assisted conception techniques. These include:

- GIFT – gametes are introduced into the uterine tube for fertilisation in vivo
- donor insemination (DI) – donor spermatozoa used in cases of azoospermia
- subzonal insemination (SUZI) – used in cases of oligozoospermia or tetratozoospermia
- intracytoplasmic sperm injection (ICSI) – small amounts of viable sperm required
- testicular sperm aspiration (TESA) – percutaneous sperm aspiration (PESA) – used in cases where an obstruction prevents spermatozoa travelling along the deferent duct; spermatozoa are aspirated from the testes through the scrotum
  - microsurgical epididymal sperm aspiration (MESA) – as for PESA.

Chromosomal screening is required to exclude conditions such as cystic fibrosis and check karyotyping.

Provision of Information and Counselling

Investigations and treatments for subfertility can be intrusive and stressful for couples already anxious about not being able to conceive. It is essential that couples are given appropriate information about risks, benefits and alternatives of investigations and proposed treatments. Emotional support and counselling must be available to support the couple through the roller coaster of emotions they will experience. The importance of this is recognised by most assisted conception units, who employ specialist counsellors to provide this service.

In Vitro Fertilisation and Embryo Transfer

The success rate of IVF has improved as a result of advances in ovulation induction regimens, oocyte retrieval, embryo culture, ET and improved facilities of cryopreservation. IVF is now widely accepted as a form of treatment for unexplained subfertility. However, certain inclusion factors must be considered (Information 8.8).

Data from the Human Fertilization and Embryology Authority (HFEA) showed that in 2019 birth rates for patients under 35 were 32% per embryo transferred, compared to below 5% for patients aged 43+ when using their own eggs. Patients aged 35–37 and 38–39 had a live birth rate per embryo transferred of 6% in 1991, this increased to 25% and 19%, respectively, in 2019 (HFEA 2021).

In the UK the HFEA licenses and regulates assisted conception centres. The HFEA was established by the Human Fertilisation and Embryology Act 1990 (DH 1990). There have been recent changes to these rules specifically regarding storage and consent. In most cases a consent period is 10 years from date of first storage for gametes and embryos (although there are some exceptions) (HFEA 2019). The full HFEA code of practice is due to be updated in the coming year to fully reflect all the changes related to the new rules

The Human Fertilisation and Embryology Act has a conscientious objection clause. Consequently anyone who can show a conscientious objection to any of the activities governed by the Act is not obliged to participate in them. Nurses must make known any conscientious objection to the appropriate person as soon as possible (NMC 2018).

Ovarian Stimulation. Various protocols are in use to achieve controlled hyperstimulation of the ovaries. Agents used include clomiphene citrate, purified FSH, exogenous gonadotrophin and GnRH agonists (GnRHAs). Modifications to protocols depend on the patient's response.

INFORMATION 8.8

Information Concerning IVF

- The chances of success reduce with increasing age of the woman.
- There is a trend of increasing demand for IVF in same-sex female couples.
- Ovarian stimulation is advised prior to IVF with ultrasound monitoring of the ovarian response.
- Progesterone is used after ET for luteal phase support.
- Women aged under 40 years should be offered three cycles.
- Those women who reach 40 years during treatment should not be offered further cycles.
- Women aged over 40 years should be offered one cycle of IVF as long as these women:
  - Have never had IVF in the past.
  - Have no evidence of low ovarian reserve.
  - Have had a discussion of the additional implications of IVF and pregnancy at this age.

Commonly, daily injections of FSH or hMG are used until dominant follicles have reached 18–20 mm in diameter. The ovaries are scanned regularly to monitor the size of follicles. A condition known as ovarian hyperstimulation syndrome can develop whereby the ovaries are overstimulated and additional symptoms develop. In severe cases, fluid passes out of the circulatory system resulting in ascites and haemoconcentration. It can be life-threatening and if signs are detected during treatment cycle, that cycle should be abandoned.

Once follicles have developed to an appropriate size, hCG is administered and oocyte collection is undertaken 24–36 hours later. The timing is important; if left too long the woman may ovulate spontaneously, but if undertaken too soon it may be difficult to harvest follicles that are mature enough.

Oocyte Harvesting. Oocytes for fertilisation can be recovered from mature ovarian follicles by:
- ultrasound-guided follicle needle puncture and aspiration; can be performed under light general anaesthetic or sedation
- laparoscopy and needle aspiration; requires a general anaesthetic.

Each mature follicle is carefully aspirated and the oocytes are collected in the culture tube.

Laboratory Procedures. The aspirate is immediately passed to the embryologist for examination and identification of oocytes. Once sufficient suitable oocytes have been identified, they are placed in an incubator.

Close coordination between the embryology and surgical services is essential for treatments to be effective.

Fertilisation. A fresh specimen of semen is required and this is often produced in the department, which can be embarrassing and stressful for the man. The sample is centrifuged to separate spermatozoa from seminal fluid. In IVF, the spermatozoa and oocytes are mixed together. Between 16 and 20 hours later, the oocytes are examined for fertilisation and once fertilisation has been established the embryos are returned to culture in fresh medium for another 24 hours. In GIFT the oocytes and prepared spermatozoa are placed into a catheter to be inserted into the fimbrial end of the uterine tube, where the gametes are deposited for fertilisation. In ICSI, a spermatozoon is injected into the oocyte.

Embryo Transfer. This occurs 2–3 days after oocyte retrieval when the embryos are at the two- or four-cell stage. ET into the uterus is a delicate procedure that does not necessarily result in successful implantation and pregnancy. The incidence of pregnancy increases with the number of embryos replaced; the HFEA Code of Practice (2019) provides guidance on reducing the risk of multiple pregnancy. (Please note that this code of practice is due to be updated shortly to reflect updates to the rules regarding storage of embryos and gametes.)

If menstruation does not occur, the woman will undergo a urinary pregnancy test to confirm if a pregnancy has been achieved.

Pre-implantation Diagnosis of Genetic Disease (PGD). This technique has been developed for embryos produced through IVF. A single cell is removed for genetic testing. This is particularly useful for couples who carry genetic defects that can affect the well-being of the child. However, the benefits must be weighed against the potential damage removal of the cell may cause to the developing embryo.

Gamete Intrafallopian Transfer

GIFT offers an alternative treatment to IVF when women have at least one patent tube. It is primarily used in patients who have unexplained subfertility and cervical hostility. It is contraindicated in women with severe endometriosis, active infection and intrauterine abnormalities.

The technique involves ovarian stimulation and harvesting of oocytes as in IVF. The oocytes are then mixed with the freshly donated spermatozoa and transferred into the fimbriated ends of the tube(s) (Fig. 8.10). GIFT is normally performed laparoscopically.

Zygote Intrafallopian Transfer (ZIFT)

The oocytes are fertilised in vitro before transfer to the uterine tube. In this treatment, therefore, fertilisation is known to have occurred and embryos have the opportunity to benefit from the tubal environment and to enter the uterine cavity naturally.

❖ Nursing Management and Health Promotion: IVF

The couple may have experienced many investigations and surgical interventions before being offered the opportunity to seek pregnancy by IVF, and, although always hopeful for success, must recognise that this is not guaranteed.

Prelaparoscopy Care

Reducing Anxiety
Pretreatment counselling provides a realistic picture of the chances of cumulative success rather than encouraging the couple to focus on success of the first cycle. The British Infertility Counselling Association provides information (www.bica.net). The Royal College of Nursing (RCN) notes that counselling must be provided by specialist fertility counsellors who have in-depth understanding of contemporary issues in fertility (RCN 2020b).

The nurse must ensure that couples have appropriate information about the various stages of treatment and procedures to provide reassurance during a highly stressful time.

Self-Care in the Follicular Stage
The woman's role in maintaining self-care can be explained – collecting her urine for laboratory testing, and administering injections at specified times crucial to her ovarian stimulation. The woman should understand that there are differences in need between individual women and the nurse's explanations can alleviate concerns.

Preparation for Oocyte Recovery
Explanation should be given about USS monitoring of follicular development. Once proposed ovulation has been estimated, preparation should be made for harvesting of oocytes. If this is to be done laparoscopically, the woman will be starved for a minimum of 6 hours before general anaesthetic and will be prepared as for any other surgery (according to local policy and procedure). Some healthcare providers will permit drinking clear fluids up until 2 hours before to reduce the risk of dehydration. However, it can also be done under sedation vaginally with ultrasound guidance.

Postlaparoscopy Care
Recovery from the laparoscopy is rapid and the woman will be ready for discharge a few hours after the procedure. Mild analgesics such as paracetamol may be prescribed for relief of pain. The couple will be keen to know whether the laparoscopy was successful and how many oocytes were recovered.

Sometimes the time of ovulation has been misjudged and the follicles have already ruptured prior to laparoscopy or the

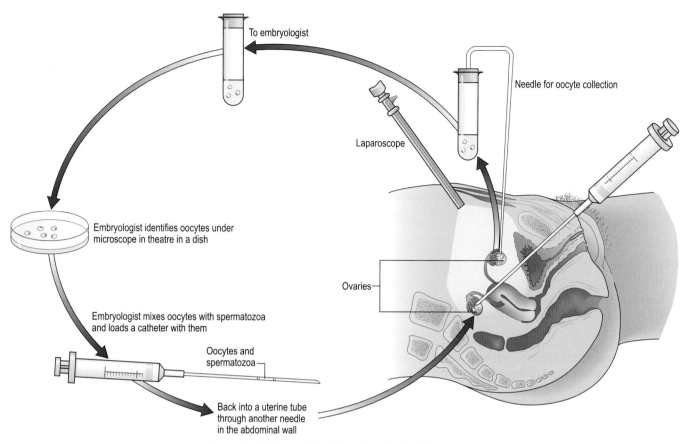

To embryologist

Needle for oocyte collection

Laparoscope

Embryologist identifies oocytes under
microscope in theatre in a dish

Ovaries

Embryologist mixes oocytes with spermatozoa
and loads a catheter with them

Oocytes and
spermatozoa

Back into a uterine tube
through another needle
in the abdominal wall

Figure 8.10 Gamete intrafallopian transfer (GIFT) treatment.

recovered oocytes are too immature to be viable. Adhesions may obscure the ovarian tissue, thus negating the procedure.

The nurse should adopt a sensitive approach when informing the couple of the outcome of the procedure, particularly if suitable oocytes have not been successfully collected. In this case, details of possible reentry to another treatment cycle may be required by the couple.

Preparation for Embryo Transfer

As described earlier, the oocytes are matured in the laboratory for up to 2–3 days. The embryos are observed in the laboratory as they develop to a two- or four-cell stage prior to transfer. Failures may also occur at this delicate laboratory stage and this is a further worrying time for the couple.

Once it is confirmed there are suitable embryos for transfer, the woman attends the unit. In theatre, the woman is positioned in a modified lithotomy (Trendelenburg) position for the procedure of ET. Following ET the woman can resume her normal activities.

Continuing Need for Support and Counselling

Nurses working in all settings will be required to utilise their counselling skills with couples who are involved in subfertility treatment. Treatment may not be successful or the resulting pregnancy may result in a miscarriage. Couples may continue to need to talk about their feelings of inadequacy or failure and to be allowed to grieve for their losses.

Some couples may have to accept that they will not have children of their own. Other possibilities such as adoption should be sensitively discussed.

CULTURAL AWARENESS IN REPRODUCTIVE HEALTH

Socioeconomic factors and liberal attitudes to expression of beliefs and values have encouraged people from all over the world to settle in the UK. Whilst this has resulted in vibrant multicultural societies, people moving between cultures will inevitably bring aspects of their own culture with them, including practices and beliefs that shape their approach to their way of life. It is important that nurses are aware of how the attitudes of people from different cultural backgrounds influence their approach to sexuality and reproductive health.

Communication can be a challenge if English is not the patient's first language. Although family members may be able to speak English as their mother tongue, it is not appropriate to use them as interpreters. Previously children have often been used when discussing reproductive health issues or intimate problems however, it can be intensely embarrassing for the patient to reveal these details to their offspring during a consultation. In addition, if there are any tensions between a couple, the nurse cannot be sure that all appropriate information is communicated. Consequently accredited interpreters should be used who have an understanding of health and treatments.

Physical examination of a patient's reproductive system can involve intimate procedures such as vaginal or testicular examination which can be intensely embarrassing. Often, a same-gender health professional will be requested and clinicians should respect these wishes and do their utmost to support these requests. Sometimes, due to pressures on available medical staff, this may not be possible and this should be explained to the patient.

Although illegal in the UK, female circumcision and female genital mutilation (FGM) are widely practised in some groups in Africa and Egypt, in parts of the Middle East and in South East Asia. Health professionals who encounter women who have undergone this must be able to provide appropriate support or refer to other agencies, and reporting of FGM cases has been mandatory since 2015 (Home Office 2015). It could be the first time the woman may present is in pregnancy and a care plan must be developed with the woman, a midwife and consultant obstetrician to ensure safe delivery for both mother and child.

Nurses and other healthcare professionals must ensure that they adopt an open and nonjudgemental attitude towards all patients/clients. They need to develop a rapport quickly during relatively brief interactions in order to provide reassurance and support putting into practice the 6 Cs. Whilst this is important for all patients, it is particularly relevant for men and women from different cultural backgrounds. The nurse should have a good awareness of cultural aspects and, whilst they may not have an in-depth knowledge of particular cultural beliefs, they should know what resources they can access when required.

Providing information, advising and counselling people who have different beliefs, values and attitudes concerning health issues from those of the health professionals providing help and support require care and sensitivity. Understanding and empathy can help nurses to appreciate what others consider to be important. A balance is required between giving sound advice and respecting the social, cultural and religious views of others.

Summary: Key Nursing Issues

- Reproductive structures and function are very closely linked to an individual's feelings of self-worth, attractiveness and sexuality.
- Reproductive tract conditions and subsequent examination and investigation can be acutely embarrassing. Embarrassment may cause the individual to delay seeking help.
- People may present in a very emotional state. The nurse must adopt a sensitive and nonjudgemental attitude at all times. Often, the nurse will have to discuss intimate details with the person at the first meeting and so must be able to establish a rapport and trust quickly, thereby ensuring that patients feel comfortable and able to discuss their issues and anxieties.
- The nurse is required to have a good level of knowledge underpinning their practice so that they are able to give explanations in a way the patient understands but also to provide answers to any queries the patient may have. It is unrealistic to expect the nurse to be able to deal fully with all queries but they must know how to access further information and be able to direct the patient to recognised websites providing accurate up-to-date information.
- Privacy and dignity of the patient are particularly key whilst carrying out nursing procedures. Procedures should be conducted in a private area where there will be no interruptions as this will help the patient to relax, reducing the discomfort of any procedures.
- Nursing patients with reproductive system disorders can be challenging but is extremely rewarding, particularly when the nurse has contributed to improving the patient's quality of life.

Reflection and Learning – What Next?

- **Test** your knowledge by visiting the Evolve website ⊕ and answering the multiple-choice questions and critical thinking questions.
- **Consolidate** your learning by looking at some of the further reading suggestions, references and specialist websites.
- **Revisit** some of the additional material on the Evolve website.
- **Consider** what you have learnt and how this will help your professional development.
- **Reflect** on how you can apply this knowledge to the care of your patients.
- **Discuss** your learning with your mentor/supervisor, lecturer and colleagues.

PART 2: NURSING PATIENTS WITH DISORDERS OF THE BREAST

Introduction

Breast disease can affect females and males. The majority of people diagnosed with a breast disease are female. Breast tissue (mammary glands) fulfils different functions and can mean different things to an individual throughout their lifetime. Physiologically, for women, breasts are organs of lactation, developing in puberty to enable a mother to feed her offspring, but in psychological and social terms, they can symbolise femininity and sexuality.

Physiologically, for men, the breast tissue sits on the chest wall and has no function with lactation. It is not surprising therefore that breast disease and the treatments provided can impact not only on an individual's physical health but also on their social and psychological well-being.

This chapter outlines the anatomy and physiology of the breast before considering disorders of the breast. In addition, the role of the nurse to influence health promotion, disease prevention, physical, psychological and social well-being is summarised. All nurses who care for these patients will be working within the NMC (2018) Code of Professional Standards of Practice and Behaviour for Nurses, Midwives and Nursing Associates (The Code) at all times.

Anatomy and Physiology

Structure of the Breast

The composition of the breast is glandular, fatty and fibrous tissue which is covered by skin. Medially, the breasts reach the sternal edge and laterally the midaxillary line and extend up into the axilla forming the triangular shaped axillary tail. The breast lies on a thick layer of fascia, underneath which are the pectoralis major and the serratus anterior muscles. Behind the pectoralis major is the pectoralis minor muscle. Its function is to stabilise the shoulder girdle, serratus anterior and the latissimus dorsi muscles from the base and back of the axilla, respectively. These structures and their nerve supply are important considerations when axillary lymph node surgery is required for the treatment of breast cancer (Fig. 8.11).

The nipple and areolar complex are situated centrally but actual positioning varies with the size of the breast. The nipple can project above the areolar skin and is constructed of smooth muscle. This becomes erect when stimulated, allowing the baby to suckle more easily during breast feeding. The pigmented skin of the areola has a number of small protuberances (Montgomery's tubercles), which lubricate the areolar skin during breast feeding.

The glandular tissue of the breast is divided into 12–20 lobes or segments (Fig. 8.12). Each segment is made up of hundreds of lobules or alveoli which are activated during pregnancy to produce milk. They are connected by terminal ducts which join to form lactiferous ducts before ending in approximately 10 openings in the nipple. These tree-like structures are lined with ductal and alveolar (lobular) epithelium and are surrounded by contractile myoepithelial cells. These cells contract in response to the hormone oxytocin to facilitate the ejection of milk during breast feeding.

Breast tissue is supported by Cooper's ligaments, fibrous bands which connect the skin of the breast to the underlying fascia. These

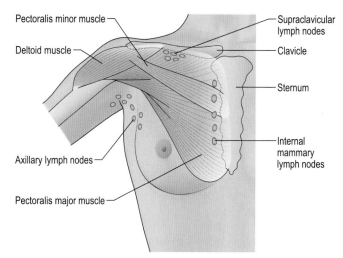

Figure 8.11 The breast and associated structures.

ligaments may contract when affected by cancer, causing peau d'orange (dimpling of the skin). With increasing age and weight, these ligaments stretch, causing ptosis of the breasts (droop).

Blood and Lymph Vessels

The breast is highly vascularised. It receives arterial blood from the thoracic branches of the axillary artery, branches of the internal mammary artery (from the subclavian artery) and branches from the internal thoracic artery.

Venous drainage is from the subareolar complex draining to the intercostal, axillary and internal thoracic veins.

The lymphatic drainage is of great significance in the potential spread of breast cancer. Most lymph drainage of the breast comes from the breast parenchyma and the subareolar region which then drains to the axillary lymph nodes. Further drainage occurs in the subcapsular and interpectoral node groups. Drainage from the medial part of the breast is via the internal mammary nodes which lie beneath the ribs and lateral to the sternum.

Nerve Supply

Most of the breast innervation is via the sensory and autonomic nerves accompanying the blood vessels. Branches of three thoracic nerves containing sympathetic fibres innervate the breast parenchyma. The area around the nipple has many sensory nerve endings. When touched, these cause reflex erection and, during breast feeding, milk release.

Normal Breast Changes

Physiological changes in females occur at puberty, during the menstrual cycle, pregnancy and lactation and with normal ageing and the menopause.

Puberty

Breast development begins at puberty. Under the control of the hypothalamus, the pituitary gland produces the gonadotrophins, FSH and LH. These hormones stimulate ovarian follicles and the

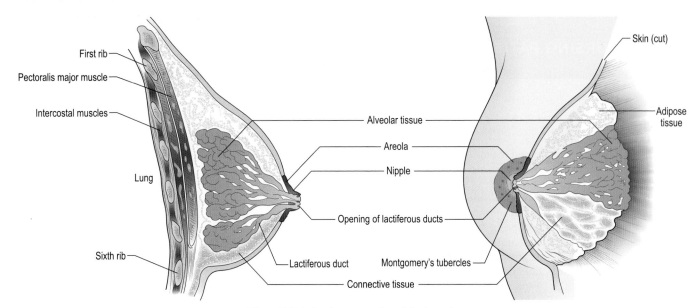

First rib
Pectoralis major muscle
Intercostal muscles
Lung
Sixth rib

Alveolar tissue
Areola
Nipple
Opening of lactiferous ducts
Lactiferous duct
Montgomery's tubercles
Connective tissue

Skin (cut)
Adipose tissue

Figure 8.12 Lateral cross-section of the breast.

release of oestrogens, which in turn cause the increase in the breast connective tissue, a lengthening of the ducts in the breast and the formation of the breast lobules. Complete development of the lobules is achieved only with adult levels of progesterone.

Menstrual Cycle

At the start of each menstrual cycle, rising oestrogen levels cause breast ducts and lobules to enlarge. After ovulation, the corpus luteum produces progesterone which causes further breast changes. At this time, some women experience breast tenderness and heaviness. This can also be experienced whilst taking contraceptive medications or in the presence of some intrauterine devices. If pregnancy does not occur, hormone levels fall, ducts and lobules regress, and the breasts lose their tenderness and swollen feeling. This usually precedes the onset of menstruation.

Pregnancy

If pregnancy does occur, the levels of oestrogen and progesterone continue to rise, causing the ducts and lobules to increase in size and number in preparation for lactation. The enzymes necessary for milk production are stimulated by prolactin (see Chapter 5, Nursing Patients With Endocrine Disorders) and by placental lactogen, but milk production is suppressed during pregnancy by high progesterone levels. Further information about lactation is provided on the companion website.

Menopause

As a woman approaches the menopause, changes in ovarian function and a subsequent drop in hormone levels cause breast glandular epithelium and adjacent connective tissue to regress and be replaced by fat. This process of involution causes the breasts to become softer and less dense.

Benign Breast Disorders

Benign breast disorders account for approximately 90% of all breast problems. The most prominent group of benign disorders results from 'anomalies of normal development and involution'

(ANDIs). The largest group of ANDI disorders is developmental and can occur before birth and during prepubertal and pubertal breast development.

Developmental Disorders

It is estimated that about 1% of men and 5% of women are born with one or more extra nipples (polythelia). The most common site for the location of extra nipples is along the milk line or the ectodermal ridge. Extra breasts can also develop and mostly occur in the lower axilla.

Abnormalities of breast development include the absence (amastia) or underdevelopment (hypoplasia) of one breast.

There is usually some difference between breasts in size and shape for a woman but the difference should not be extreme. If it is, then surgical intervention involving augmentation of one breast and reduction of the other breast may be offered. Prepubertal breast enlargement is quite common and only requires investigation if it is associated with other signs of premature sexual development. Otherwise known as juvenile hypertrophy, the overgrowth of breast tissue can occur in adolescent girls whose breasts develop normally during puberty but then continue to grow. Usually, no hormone abnormality can be detected. Treatment if required is usually a reduction mammoplasty (removal of tissue from each breast).

Fibroadenomas

A fibroadenoma can be considered as an aberration of normal breast tissue growth. It usually presents as a dense mass comprising both fibrous and glandular breast tissue. It grows as a centrifugal nodule that is usually well circumscribed and freely movable within the surrounding breast tissue. Fibroadenomas are very common (in young women, they account for 68% of breast masses, Lee et al. 2015) (Reflection 8.3). Fibroadenomas in men are very rare. Juvenile or giant fibroadenomas, which occur in adolescence, are also rare. They are often a fast-growing lesion that can grow up to 5 cm in size and will distort the breast. For individuals who present with a presumed fibroadenoma, a biopsy will be performed to confirm the diagnosis.

 See Evolve website Fig. 8.1

Aasiya is 18 and has found a palpable, smooth breast lump in her right breast. Although very worried that it is breast cancer, it was 6 weeks before she plucked up courage to see her GP. She is given an appointment to be seen at her local breast unit for a definitive diagnosis.

Activities

- Reflect on the feelings that may have influenced her delay in seeking help.
- Which tests and investigations will Aasiya undergo?
- The results confirm the lump to be a fibroadenoma. How can this be explained to Aasiya to give her reassurance?
- Discuss with your mentor how you would introduce the topic of breast awareness with Aasiya.

Cysts and Nodularity

Diffuse lumpiness or thickening of breast tissue can occur, due to single or multiple cysts. Cysts are distended, fluid-filled sacs, confirmed when examined under ultrasound. They may increase in size, stay the same or disperse over time.

Duct Ectasia

Duct ectasia occurs during breast involution when the major subareolar ducts dilate and shorten (Breast Cancer Care 2018a). Women have duct dilatation or duct ectasia around and sometimes after the menopause. Normal breast secretions can be retained behind these blocked ducts. Presentation of duct ectasia includes nipple discharge, nipple retraction, inflammation or a palpable mass. Indications for surgery are problems with discharge.

Epithelial Hyperplasia

This is a common condition. Histologically, the cells show hyperplasia (an increase in the number of cells in an area of breast tissue) but with unaltered individual cellular appearance. However, if atypical hyperplasia is present, the cells have an altered shape and the risk of cancer developing in the breast is raised; regular screening may be advised (Breast Cancer Care 2019a).

Other Disorders of Breast Structure

Some other disorders of breast structure are outlined in Information 8.9.

Management of Breast Conditions

Investigations

Assessment of an individual who presents with a lump or lumpiness within their breast/s usually require a referral to a Breast (or Chest) Assessment Clinic. This will involve a clinical examination which may proceed to mammography, USS, core biopsy and sometimes a fine-needle aspiration (FNA), or a vacuum-assisted biopsy, depending on their age and the clinical findings. The investigations are referred to as 'triple assessment'. Cystic fluid is usually sent for examination if it is bloodstained, as this may indicate cancer.

Follow-up examinations are not usually required unless histology reveals atypical hyperplasia. If there is a significant family history of breast cancer, the options for surveillance will be discussed with the individual.

Duct Papillomas

These are benign wart-like lesions in the lactiferous duct wall. Most occur beneath the areola. Papillomas present with pain or bloody discharge and are usually soft and difficult to locate. They are usually surgically resected.

Lipomas

When examined, these fatty lumps can be mistaken for cysts within the breast tissue. They do not cause major problems and diagnosis by ultrasound and cytology should be all that is needed.

Mondor's Disease

This is caused by a superficial thrombosis of a breast vein. It is usually very painful, requiring analgesics. Malignancy should always be excluded, but no other treatment should be necessary and the condition usually resolves in 6 months.

Galactocele

This cystic breast lesion occurs during pregnancy or lactation. Once diagnosed, treatment is by aspiration. This may have to be performed on several occasions to allow the walls of the cyst to adhere.

Fat Necrosis

Presenting as a painful mass, fat necrosis can imitate breast cancer and should be diagnosed with care. About half of the cases of fat necrosis are caused by breast trauma, although the other cases have no history of trauma. The mass is usually excised to ensure that it is not cancerous.

Assessment

Fibroadenomas are not usually removed unless they are large or increasing in size.

A nursing assessment at this time will incorporate asking the individual relevant questions to determine their understanding of their condition, investigations and any treatments they are undergoing. The nurse will also ask questions to explore their fears, concerns and the impact it is having on their life.

For general pre- and postoperative care, see Chapter 25. Surgery is frequently performed on a day-case basis or may require an overnight stay in hospital. Postoperatively, the nursing priorities are wound management and pain control. Because the breast is very vascular, there may be bruising even though the surgery is minor. A wound drain is rarely needed, but, if used, is usually removed the following morning.

The breast is likely to be painful for several days. Paracetamol or a nonsteroidal anti-inflammatory drug (NSAID) is usually sufficient for pain relief, but if bruising and oedema are very extensive, a stronger analgesic may be required. Wearing a supportive bra shortly after surgery is usually advised and for at several weeks postoperatively to improve comfort and avoid strain being placed on the wound.

Breast Pain

Breast pain (mastalgia) has been reported by approximately two-thirds of women who develop this pain during their reproductive life and seek medical attention either because it adversely affects their daily life or out of the fear of any serious underlying pathology like breast cancer (Tahir and Shamsudeen 2022). For most women, some breast discomfort is accepted as a part of the normal breast changes of the menstrual cycle. However, some women suffer more intense pain affecting quality of life, usually from midcycle onwards and often relieved by menstruation. The pain can differ from cycle to cycle and can continue for many years. Noncyclical breast pain is usually unilateral and a specific area of the breast is affected. The causes can be cysts, mastitis and stretching of Coopers ligaments. For both cyclical and noncyclical mastalgia, wearing a firm, well-fitted bra can help with NSAIDs either in tablet form or gel applied to the breast (Breast Cancer Care 2019b). Some women anecdotally report that a reduction in caffeine has been helpful. The benefit of gamma linolenic acid (GLA) is individual, with mixed evidence regarding the benefit (Breast Cancer Care 2019b).

Chest pain can be caused by costochondritis, pain at the rib joining the breast bone. Anti-inflammatories can help along with muscle relaxants and heat pads (London Pain Clinic 2018).

Breast Infections
Pathophysiology

Breast infections, such as mastitis, are relatively common, and present with swelling, redness, tenderness and pain, which may be associated with a breast abscess or nipple discharge. Breast abscesses are commonly seen during or following lactation. Infection may arise from a cracked nipple, but often there is no apparent cause. Staphylococcal infections are common.

Medical Management

Pus is aspirated from a palpable breast abscess with a wide-gauge needle following local anaesthesia. The pus is sent for microscopy, culture and sensitivity, and antibiotics are prescribed. A persistent abscess may require surgical drainage and excision of the surrounding capsule. A persistent nipple discharge may be treated by a microdochectomy (removal of a major duct behind the nipple), or a duct clearance (removal of the major duct system behind the nipple). The surgery can usually be performed on a day-case basis.
- An explanation of the nature and possible cause of infection will help to reassure the individual, particularly as recurrent infections with pain are quite common and may cause distress.
- A supportive bra, applications of heat or cold 'packs' and padding to protect a sore nipple may all reduce discomfort. Mild to moderate analgesia is also usually needed to control pain.

Gynaecomastia (Overdevelopment of Male Breast Tissue)
Pathophysiology

Gynaecomastia is a rare benign disorder resulting from oestrogen production. This is often seen at puberty but may occur at any age. Gynaecomastia is thought to be caused by an imbalance between the sex hormones testosterone and oestrogen, although why this occurs is still often unknown (NHS Choices 2018).

As men get older, they produce less testosterone and may have more fat, which contains oestrogen. Other causes can be linked to testicular lumps or cancers, liver disease, decreased testosterone, Klinefelter's syndrome, extra X chromosome or to some drugs.

Medical Management

Surgery is not usually recommended. If the condition has arisen as a side-effect of drug administration, medication review can be considered. Hormonal manipulation may be needed where gynaecomastia is due to the oversecretion of oestrogen.

Overdevelopment of breast tissue in a boy or man may cause an altered body image and emotional distress. Some men with gynaecomastia believe they have lost their masculinity and experience anxiety and depression as a result. When gynaecomastia occurs in adolescence, such feelings may be particularly acute. A clear explanation of why the breast tissue has developed and of any treatment that may be given is usually helpful to all age groups.

Nursing Management and Health Promotion: Benign Breast Disorders

Patients who detect a breast lump or a change to their breast can fear this will lead to a diagnosis of breast cancer. Until a benign disorder is diagnosed, the patient may require psychological support. Verbal information should be provided throughout the process of confirming a diagnosis. Once the diagnosis is confirmed, written information should be offered about the benign condition and helpful advice to deal with symptoms, either provided in the clinical area or recommending the patient access the website for Breast Cancer Care (see Useful Websites). The patient should be reminded of the importance of continuing to be breast aware and report any new breast changes.

Breast Cancer and Potential Sequelae

Incidence and Mortality

Incidence
- There are around 55,920 new breast cancer cases in the UK every year – more than 150 every day (2016–2018).
- 1 in 8 women and 1 in 870 men will be diagnosed with breast cancer during their lifetime.
- Breast cancer is the most common cancer in the UK, accounting for 15% of all new cancer cases (2016–2018).
- In females in the UK, breast cancer is the most common cancer, with around 55,500 new cases every year (2016–2018).
- In males in the UK, breast cancer is not among the 20 most common cancers, with around 370 new cases every year (2016–2018).
- Over the last decade, breast cancer incidence rates have increased by less than a twentieth (3%) in the UK. Rates in females have increased by a twentieth (5%), and rates in males have remained stable (2016–2018).
- Most invasive breast cancers occur in the upper-outer quadrant of the breast.
- Breast cancer incidence rates in England in females are 14% lower in the most deprived quintile compared with the least, and in males are similar in the most deprived quintile compared with the least (2015–2017).
- Around 3000 cases of breast cancer each year in England in females are linked with lower deprivation.
- Incidence rates for breast cancer are lower in the Asian and Black ethnic groups, and in people of mixed or multiple ethnicity, compared with the White ethnic group, in females in England (2015–2017) (Cancer Research UK 2022e).

Mortality
- There are around 11,500 breast cancer deaths in the UK every year; that's 32 every day (2017–2019).

- Breast cancer is the fourth most common cause of cancer death in the UK, accounting for 7% of all cancer deaths (2017–2019).
- In females in the UK, breast cancer is the second most common cause of cancer death, with around 11,400 deaths every year (2017–2019).
- In males in the UK, breast cancer is not among the 20 most common causes of cancer death, with around 85 deaths every year (2017–2019).
- Mortality rates for breast cancer in the UK are highest in people aged 90+ (2017–2019).
- Each year, almost half of all breast cancer deaths (48%) in the UK are in people aged 75 and over (2017–2019).
- Since the early 1970s, breast cancer mortality rates have decreased by around two-fifths (41%) in the UK. Rates in females have decreased by almost two-fifths (37%), and rates in males have decreased by more than two-fifths (44%) (2017–2019).
- Over the last decade, breast cancer mortality rates have decreased by around a sixth (18%) in the UK. Rates in females have decreased by almost a sixth (16%), and rates in males have remained stable (2017–2019).
- Mortality rates for breast cancer are generally lower in females of non-White minority ethnicity, compared with the White ethnic group, in England and Wales (2017–2019) (Cancer Research UK 2022e).

Risk Factors (Information 8.10)

- Age – breast cancer in women is very rare below the age of 35 years; 80% of cases occur in women aged 50 years or over (NHS Choices 2018). Age is the most significant risk factor for breast cancer (Breast Cancer Care 2018c).
- Previous breast cancer – those already diagnosed with breast cancer are at an increased risk of developing another one.
  - Family history – if several members of an individual's family have had a cancer diagnosis, this may indicate an increased genetic predisposition. The National Institute for Health and Care Excellence has categorised the specific risk of familial breast cancer and procedures to influence risk reduction in the form of medication and surgery (NICE 2017b).

Hormone-Related Factors. Women who have children have a slightly lower risk of breast cancer than those who do not have children. The risk reduces further the more children a woman has.

In addition, the younger a woman is when having her first child also reduces the risk (Cancer Research UK 2022e).

Levels of oestrogen and testosterone can affect the risk of breast cancer. After the menopause, women with higher levels of oestrogen and testosterone in their blood have a higher risk of breast cancer compared to women with the lowest levels. Women with higher levels of testosterone in their blood before menopause have a higher risk of breast cancer (Cancer Research UK 2018b).

There is an increased risk of breast cancer in women with higher levels of a hormone called insulin-like growth factor 1 (IGF-1). It is not clear what controls levels of IGF-1 in the bloodstream. It is probably related to genes, body weight and how much exercise is undertaken (Cancer Research UK 2018b).

There is also a link with an increase in breast cancer if a woman's periods started before the age of 12 or stopped after the age of 55. This may be linked to hormone levels (Cancer Research UK 2018b).

Hormone Replacement Therapy. It has been shown that HRT increases the risk of breast cancer while taking it and for some time afterwards (Cancer Research UK 2018a). Researchers have found that women using combined HRT (for a median duration of 5.4 years) were 2.7 times more likely to develop breast cancer (Breast Cancer Now 2018a, Institute of Cancer Research 2018). The decision to take HRT is a personal one and one that needs to be discussed in detail with the woman's GP, considering the risks and benefits to that individual.

Weight. Overweight, postmenopausal women and men have an increased risk of breast cancer (Cancer Research UK 2018a).

Alcohol Intake. An increased risk of breast cancer correlates with the amount of alcohol consumed (Table 8.1).

Exposure to Radiation. Being exposed to large amounts of radiation to the chest wall such as a radiation accident can cause breast cancer. Traditionally, treatment for Hodgkin's lymphoma (see Chapter 13, Nursing Patients With Blood Disorders) included radiation to the chest and this may be a contributory factor to an increased risk of breast cancer for those young women who were treated in puberty or their early 20s. Most people are not exposed to enough radiation to affect their risk. The amount of radiation used within a breast screening examination is very small.

Smoking. There is some evidence that smoking may increase the risk of developing breast cancer (Cancer Research UK 2018d).

Having Dense Breast Tissue. Breasts are described as being dense if they have less fatty tissue and more glandular and fibrous

---

INFORMATION 8.10

Factors Increasing the Risk of Early Breast Cancer

- Increasing age
- Previous breast cancer
- Family history
- Some benign breast disease
- Hormone-related factors and HRT use (particularly oestrogen combined with a progestogen)
- Weight
- Alcohol intake
- Radiation exposure

TABLE 8.1	Number of Breast Cancer Cases in Relation to Alcohol Consumption, per 1000 Women
Alcohol Consumed	**Number Diagnosed With Breast Cancer**
No alcohol	116
Up to 3 units a day	121
3–6 units a day	143
More than 6 units a day	186

Data from Cancer Research UK. Science blog: alcohol and breast cancer – how big is the risk? 2017. http://scienceblog.cancerresearchuk.org/2017/05/25/alcohol-and-breast-cancer-how-big-is-the-risk/.

tissue. Women with dense breasts have a higher risk of developing breast cancer (Breast Cancer Care 2018d). These also tend to more invasive forms of breast cancer (Cancer Research UK 2008).

Prevention and Early Detection

The focus of primary prevention is on the identification of risk factors and at-risk individuals (see Chapter 29, Nursing the Patient With Cancer). Survival rates for breast cancer have doubled in the last 40 years to the current overall 10-year survival rate of 78% (Cancer Research UK 2018b). However, this survival rate varies according to the stage of the cancer at diagnosis: nearly 100% 5-year survival rate for stage I down to 15% for stage IV cancers (Cancer Research UK 2018c). Therefore, taking measures to detect breast cancer earlier is important in reducing breast cancer mortality.

Breast Awareness

Patient Education

The nurse should take the opportunity to promote breast health by discussing breast screening with women and breast awareness for all adults.

An individual who is aware of any changes that occur in their breast tissue and practises self-examination is more likely to notice any changes. This may aid diagnosis when a cancer is small, so enabling a wider choice of treatment options to be offered. It also encourages an individual to participate in their own healthcare.

Breast awareness is about the individual knowing what is normal for them and detecting the following changes such as:

- change in breast size, noticeably smaller or larger
- newly inverted nipple or a nipple that has changed its shape
- discharge from one or both nipples
- change in colour of the breast skin
- a new lump or thickening in the breast or axilla that feels different from the rest of the breast tissue
- a rash or eczema-like changes around the nipple
- pain in one part of the breast or in the axilla
- puckering dimpling or indentation of the skin of the breast.

If any changes are noticed, the individual should contact their GP immediately for an examination and advice.

Breast Cancer Screening

The UK NHS Breast Screening Programme invites women aged between 50 and 70 years (73+ age group can self refer) to attend for screening using two-view digital mammography (X-ray of the breast). There is an expansion of the service in some areas which offers a mammogram at age 47 and a mammogram at age 73. The results of this change in screening will be evaluated and any learning/action from this implemented in due course.

The aim of screening is to detect breast cancer at an earlier stage than is possible by clinical or self-examination. In addition, it is hoped that pre-invasive disease (in situ) cancer will be detected before the cancer cells have shown any evidence of spread. It is most effective in postmenopausal women in whom breast tissue has been largely replaced by fat. For young women, in whom breast tissue is dense, and detection of abnormalities is therefore more difficult, mammography is usually used in conjunction with breast ultrasound.

The national screening programme depends on a high uptake of the service. If fewer women attend, the cost per life saved increases and, although some women will clearly benefit, the cost-effectiveness of the programme will be called into question (Reflection 8.4).

REFLECTION 8.4

Breast Screening Uptake

Poor attendance for breast screening may result from various factors, such as GP registers not being up to date, fear of cancer, fears of discomfort or radiation exposure, lack of awareness of screening (perhaps because the publicity is not provided in the woman's language or poor literacy skills) or a lack of understanding of the value of mammography, so it is essential that women fully understand what breast screening is about.

To further explain breast screening, all women invited into the programme are sent a leaflet entitled *NHS Breast Screening – Helping You Decide* (NHS 2019).

However, in 2017–18 the uptake continues to result in a decade-low level and may result in the minimum standard of 70% not being achieved (Breast Cancer Now 2018b). This has been further impacted by the COVID-19 pandemic, with estimates that around 986,000 women missed their mammograms when breast screening programmes were paused in March 2020 (Breast Cancer Now, 2020), potentially resulting in delays and a backlog of those awaiting treatment.

Activities

- Access the *NHS Breast Screening – Helping You Decide* and reflect on why 3 in 10 women choose to ignore the invitation for screening.
- Find out if leaflets are available in a variety of languages and font sizes.
- Discuss with your mentor how well known it is that women older than the screening age range can request screening and consider how awareness could be increased.

References

Breast Cancer Now. Breast screening uptake in England remains at a decade low. 2018. https://breastcancernow.org/news-and-blogs/news/breast-cancer-now-responds-to-new-figures-showing-uptake-of-nhs-breast-screening-falls-to-decade-low.
NHS. Breast Screening – helping you decide (BSP01). 2019. www.gov.uk/government/publications/breast-screening-helping-women-decide.

Screening may take place in static or mobile units. Screening involves taking two X-ray views of each compressed breast. Mammograms are repeated every 3 years. The woman is notified of her result by letter. If an abnormality is detected, the letter will ask her to attend for an appointment at an assessment centre (Fig. 8.13).

Most women who present for breast screening are asymptomatic: people who come to be reassured that all is well. Inevitably, screening reminds the individual that breast cancer is a potential threat. It is therefore important that a Breast Care Specialist Nurse is available to communicate with women participating in the programme and available during the assessment clinic appointment if recalled. It is particularly important that results are sent quickly. If the first screening is a positive experience, the woman will be more likely to attend 3 years later and may urge her friends to do likewise. If a woman is recalled to assessment, it is important to encourage her to return for the next screen if it is determined not to require further treatment (false-positive) (Mottram et al. 2021).

Screening for Trans Patients

Breast or chest cancer screening is for anyone between the ages of 50 and 70 who has breasts, due to either naturally occurring oestrogen or oestrogen hormone therapy. There is currently limited research into the risks of breast cancer in trans people however, one study showed an increased risk of breast cancer in trans women compared with cisgender men, and a lower risk in trans

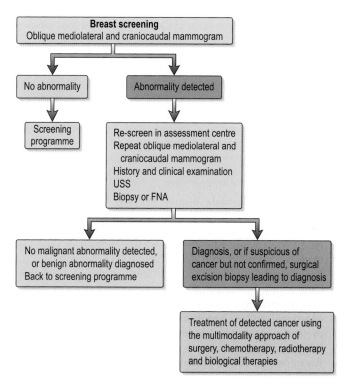

Figure 8.13 Flow diagram of the breast cancer screening procedure. *FNA,* Fine-needle aspiration; *USS,* ultrasound scan.

men compared with cisgender women. In trans women, the risk of breast cancer increased during a relatively short duration of hormone treatment and the characteristics of the breast cancer resembled a more female pattern. These results suggest that breast cancer screening guidelines for cisgender people are sufficient for transgender people using hormone treatment (De Blok et al. 2019).

A National LGBT survey demonstrated that trans people are at a high risk of having negative experiences when accessing public healthcare and many fear a negative reaction (Government Equalities Office 2018). As healthcare professionals, it is vital to reduce inequality and promote gender affirming care, including using inclusive language.

Pathophysiology

Breast cancers are classified according to the type of tissue from which they arise and their appearance under the microscope. The histological type of a cancer is often relevant to the choice of treatment. Ductal carcinomas arise from the epithelial cells of the ducts. Medullary, colloidal and tubular carcinomas are all types of breast cancer arising from ductal tissue. They are usually localised, but can be multifocal. Cancers arising from cells of the breast lobules are known as lobular carcinomas. These account for up to 15% of breast cancers (Breast Cancer Care 2018b). This type can develop in women of any age, but it is most common in women between 45 and 55 years old. It is very unusual for a man to develop an invasive lobular breast cancer. They are more commonly multifocal, often presenting as an area of thickening or swelling, a change in the nipple or a change in the skin (Breast Cancer Care 2018b).

In Paget's disease of the nipple, malignant cells are found in the epidermis of the nipple and are usually associated with small multifocal areas of ductal carcinoma behind the nipple and deep in the breast. Other breast cancer types, such as squamous cell

or inflammatory carcinomas, are less common. Sarcomas and lymphomas may also arise in the breast, as may metastatic cancer tumours, although these are rare.

Breast cancers are classified as noninvasive or in situ (confined to the ducts or lobules) or invasive (able to invade the basement membrane of the duct or lobule). This distinction has a bearing on prognosis and treatment. Ductal carcinoma in situ (DCIS) represents a very early stage of breast cancer, although clinical opinion is divided at this time and trial data are awaited regarding the disease trajectory and therefore the appropriate treatment. DCIS is often seen as microcalcifications on a mammogram and the cellular changes are categorised as low, intermediate and high grade. It currently cannot be predicted when, or if, a noninvasive breast cancer will become invasive.

Cellular differentiation, i.e. the degree to which cancer cells for invasive cancer resemble their tissue of origin, is another important prognostic factor: cells are described as well differentiated, moderately differentiated or poorly differentiated, or grades I, II or III. Poorly differentiated cancers tend to be more aggressive, with the ability to metastasise at an earlier stage, and hence carry a poorer prognosis.

Common Presenting Signs and Symptoms

A change in breast size or shape may be noticed. Signs of inflammation and tissue oedema may also be present, and superficial veins can dilate and become more visible if partially obstructed by tumour. If the tumour is advanced at the time of presentation, it may be fixed to the muscles beneath the breast. There may also be large palpable axillary lymph nodes or ulceration of the tumour through the skin, causing an infected, weeping, malodorous wound. Oedema of the arm may result if the cancer in the axilla is blocking the drainage of blood and lymph from the arm.

Clinical Management

The individual is assessed using a triple assessment.

FNA Cytology. A syringe with a small-bore needle is inserted into the axillary lymph node if it is palpable on clinical examination or if the cortex of the node is enlarged on ultrasound. Pathology results are graded C1–C5 if cytology is the method and B1–B5 if a biopsy is the method:

- C1 or B1 – insufficient specimen or if a biopsy is undertaken for microcalcification and there is no microcalcification in the specimen
- C2 or B2 – benign cells
- C3 or B3 – indeterminant
- C4 or B4 – cells suspicious of carcinoma
- C5 or B5 – carcinoma.
- B5a – carcinoma in situ
- B5b – invasive cancer.

Biopsy. The information obtained from a biopsy, including the type of cancer, is very important when planning treatment.

- Core biopsy – removal of a core of tissue using a special large-bore needle. When guided by ultrasound, it can accurately obtain good specimens of the suspicious lesion.
- Vacuum-assisted biopsy – an X-ray-guided outpatient biopsy, useful for the investigation of breast calcifications. Tissue samples can be taken from a defined area.
- Excision biopsy – excision of the lump in its entirety, usually under general anaesthesia, as a day case.
- Localisation biopsy – where a mammographic abnormality has been detected but there is no associated palpable mass. A wire may be inserted into the abnormal area under X-ray or

ultrasound control. This tissue, once surgically excised from the breast, will be X-rayed to ensure that the surgeon has removed the area of abnormality. On occasions, a wire is not inserted but the skin is marked by the radiologist preoperatively.

The tissue obtained is sent for a histological diagnosis.

Overview of Treatment

Once a histological diagnosis has been confirmed then treatment is decided at an MDT meeting. The MDT provides a broad base of expert knowledge to manage the patient with breast cancer, and should comprise core personnel who meet weekly. The core members should include consultant radiologist, surgeon, pathologist, clinical oncologist, medical oncologist, MDT coordinator and clinical specialist nurse. Other professionals may also join the MDT, including a reconstructive/plastic surgeon, physiotherapist, radiographer, geneticist/genetics counsellor, psychologist and social worker. The MDT reviews the pathology, radiology, patient history including performance status, holistic needs assessment and presentation, which formulates a treatment plan for the individual patient. Decisions are based on several factors, including:

- the size, position and type of tumour
- whether the axillary lymph node is positive with a diagnosis of invasive breast cancer
- spread of the disease
- patient's general health
- patient's priorities and wishes.

Staging of the cancer is determined (see Chapter 29, Nursing the Patient With Cancer). There are two ways of staging breast cancer: stages 1–4 or the tumour, nodes, metastasis (TNM) classification (see Useful Websites, e.g. Cancer Research UK). The purpose of staging breast cancer is to:

- inform treatment planning
- act as a prognostic indicator
- evaluate the results of treatment.

Once the patient has been discussed at the MDM, a treatment plan based on national policy and best practice (NICE guidelines) will be discussed with the patient. The patient may have a choice of treatment options and entry into a relevant clinical trial may also be a possibility. These therefore may form components of the treatment discussion. In addition, if the patient wishes to seek a second opinion, this should be supported.

Treatments for breast cancer can be divided into two categories – *local* and *systemic*.

Local treatments are surgery and radiotherapy. Systemic treatments include chemotherapy, hormonal therapy (endocrine) and targeted therapies. Systemic treatments can be given before surgery (neoadjuvant) and/or after surgery (adjuvant). Radiotherapy may be offered after surgery.

Surgical Interventions

The extent and nature of the surgery are dependent on the type, size and position of the cancer. An accurate pathological diagnosis is obtained before the definitive surgical procedure is decided.

Surgical procedures are as follows:

- **Lumpectomy** or **termed wide local excision** – removal of the breast lump with a margin of surrounding normal tissue.
- **Re-excision** – may be recommended if, after pathological examination, the margins around the cancer are not clear.
- **Mastectomy** – complete removal of all the breast tissue, overlying skin and sometimes the nipple. The pectoralis major

and minor muscles remain and the axillary skin fold remains intact.

- **Axillary dissection** – usually performed if the patient has a confirmed positive axillary lymph node preoperatively or following a positive sentinel lymph node biopsy (SLNB). The presence of cancer cells in the lymph nodes indicates that there may be a risk of further spread of disease and that additional adjuvant drug therapy maybe indicated. Where possible, axillary dissection (removal of some or all of the axillary lymph nodes) may be undertaken through the same incision as that made for the breast surgery. Axillary dissection can lead to chronic swelling, or lymphoedema, of the affected arm.
- **Sentinel lymph node biopsy (SLNB)** – to determine if there are cancer cells within the lymph nodes. This procedure has been developed to reduce the risk of compromising the lymphatic system. SLNB requires the removal of only one to three sentinel lymph nodes (those draining closest to the breast) and the nodes are usually analysed during surgery for close review by the pathologist. If the sentinel nodes do not demonstrate cancer cells, this eliminates the need to dissect additional axillary lymph nodes. However, if cancer cells are present in the sentinel nodes the patient will undergo an axillary dissection.

Breast reconstruction procedures are discussed later.

❖ Nursing Management and Health Promotion: Breast Cancer Surgery

All patients have an individual response to their cancer diagnosis and planned treatment. A breast care CNS is integral in the short- and long-term well-being of the patient and their loved ones. The CNS should be present when the patient receives their cancer diagnosis and treatment plan. Nursing intervention at this time will include a holistic assessment. This assessment will inform the care plan which will identify the services required to meet the social and psychological needs of the patient.

The CNS will identify:

- the patient's reaction, and that of the family, to the diagnosis
- any major fears and concerns of the patient and their family
- the patient's feelings about body changes
- knowledge of breast cancer and cancer generally
- information, understanding and the amount of information required at each interaction
- previous experience of family or friends having breast cancer or any other kind of cancer; the support available to the patient through family and friends and work colleagues (Evidence-Based Practice 8.3)
- any concurrent stressors, e.g. bereavement
- previous anxiety/depression episodes. Pitman et al. (2018) states that for patients with a cancer diagnosis 'depression affects up to 20%, and anxiety 10% of cancer respectively compared with figures of 5% and 7% for past year prevalence in the general population'.

Ongoing assessment is key to providing psychological and emotional support which is responsive to each patient's needs

Patients who undergo surgery for breast cancer may initially experience euphoria that the cancer has 'gone'. Others deny the removal of their breast or are unable to discuss it or to look at the scar. Following diagnosis and surgery, a period of adjustment occurs with fluctuating emotions. This period of adjustment may last some considerable time. For the majority of patients who have undergone breast surgery, anxiety usually begins to reduce after

EVIDENCE-BASED PRACTICE 8.3

Early Psychological Adjustment in Breast Cancer Patients: A Prospective Study

In a study by Nosartis et al. (2002), the presence of social support was cited as a predictor for a more successful adjustment to a diagnosis of breast cancer.

Many patients will suffer significant psychological morbidity in the first year after their diagnosis of breast cancer. This study aimed to identify and understand the risk factors for developing this morbidity. Eighty-seven patients aged 40–75 years were assessed psychologically prior to their diagnosis of breast cancer, 8 weeks after the beginning of their breast cancer treatment and again 9 months after their first follow-up. Assessments included standard psychological instruments for measuring morbidity and coping, symptom attribution, beliefs about breast cancer, social support, sociodemographic and clinical variables and the General Health Questionnaire (GHQ-12) and Mental Adjustment to Cancer (MAC) questionnaire.

A total of 85.1% of patients completed both follow-ups. Results showed that a significant proportion of patients had considerable psychological morbidity before they received their definitive diagnosis of breast cancer, especially those who thought they had breast cancer. At first follow-up, those who had significant psychological morbidity included those with prediagnostic morbidity as well as a lack of social support and feelings of 'personal responsibility/avoidance'. Those at second follow-up with considerable psychological morbidity could be predicted by their lack of social support alone.

Conclusions were that psychological morbidity is higher before, rather than following, a definitive diagnosis of breast cancer. Early reactions of this kind are predictive of posttreatment adjustment. Only the presence of social support in this study seems to be associated with successful adjustment in the first year after a breast cancer diagnosis. Women who have poor social support can thus be identified and cared for with this in mind.

Activities

- Access the study by Nosartis et al. (2002) and think about how you could use their findings in the assessment of women undergoing surgery for breast cancer.
- Discuss with your mentor how a lack of social support might be strengthened for women, for example a lone mother with two primary school-aged children newly moved to an area away from family, or a single woman in her late 70s with no family.

Reference

Nosartis C, Roberts JV, Crayford T, et al. Early psychological adjustment in breast cancer patients: a prospective study. *J Psychosom Res.* 2002;53(6):1123-1130.

several months. Some patients, however, will continue to experience great anxiety, show signs of depression, withdraw from social contact or have sexual problems (Breidenbach et al. 2022).

Some patients have significant depression at the end of the initial adjustment phase and this is not diagnosed. These patients are likely to benefit from more in-depth psychological support. Nurses, particularly those in the community and in outpatient departments, should recognise emotional problems and, where necessary, suggest referral to a counsellor, psychiatrist or psychologist via the CNS, GP or hospital medical staff.

Living with the diagnosis of breast cancer (Survivorship) can be difficult for the patient and their family. Consequences of treatment including the effects of long-term hormone therapy or chemotherapy, resources of the patient and their family and the

meaning of illness to the family were all found to have an effect on the experience of living with the diagnosis of breast cancer (Schmidt et al. 2018). Being diagnosed with breast cancer is for many a life-changing event, and the changed future this represents for the individual must be taken into account when caring for them.

Supporting Information Needs

Research has shown that many patients find that information helps them to make sense of their situation, and hence to feel more in control, less vulnerable and less anxious. Most patients have some knowledge of breast cancer, but may not be familiar with the details of the tests or treatments being discussed. Many may have misconceptions about breast cancer and its prognosis (Jassim et al. 2023). Different groups of patients receive differing amounts of information from the available sources. For example younger women may prefer to use online resources (White et al. 2018).

Surgical Admission

On the patient's admission to hospital, the nurse should review the preoperative assessments and update any changes with the patient. In particular, the factors relevant in the pretreatment phase should be reassessed to determine if the patient's needs and concerns have changed. It is important to assess preoperative shoulder function if axillary surgery is planned; early involvement of the physiotherapist will improve postoperative function. Good communication between the patient, ward nurses and the CNS will help to identify any particular issues important to the patient that may affect coping abilities and recovery from the surgery. See Chapter 25, Nursing the Patient Undergoing Surgery, for a detailed discussion of general preoperative care.

See Evolve website Critical thinking question 8.3

Patient Education

The preoperative routine should be explained, including the approximate time of surgery and the timing of any medication to be administered.

The patient is advised that they may have drainage tubes in situ on return from theatre, sometimes in the breast wound and/or in the axilla to prevent the collection of blood and serous fluid beneath the suture line. Mobility is not compromised and the patient can be reassured that it is difficult to dislodge the tubing as it is sutured in place. Sutures to the breast and axillary wound are usually subcutaneous and dissolvable; surgical glue is often used. It is worth telling the patient that they may not have a dressing, and so the breast wound may be exposed on return from theatre.

A patient undergoing axillary dissection is warned that they may experience discomfort on moving their arm for a few weeks postoperatively (Ammitzbøll et al. 2020). The nurse should stress the importance of postoperative exercises and work with the physiotherapist who will teach exercises. Written information about arm exercises is provided so that the patient can refer to the information following discharge. Because surgery may compromise the axillary lymphatics, nurses should provide information about the risk of lymphoedema and preventative measures (Information 8.11).

Anxiety arises in response to diagnostic evaluation, diagnosis and adjunctive treatment and is particularly elevated prior to breast cancer surgery (Grocott et al. 2023). Patients often find it helpful to be told of the expected appearance of the wound and

---

INFORMATION 8.11

Practical Advice on Avoiding the Complications of Lymphoedema

The British Lymphology Society recommends the following advice:

- Take care not to develop infection in the affected arm by avoiding injections and vein puncture in that arm. An infection in the arm could further compromise the lymphatic system by causing localised swelling and inflammation.
- Avoid using the affected arm when blood pressure is manually recorded.
- Try to avoid cuts and scratches in the arm. If damage to the arm does occur, wash the area carefully with soap and apply an antiseptic cream to the wound.
- Report any signs of infection to the GP or the hospital.
- Wear protective gloves when gardening.
- Avoid insect bites by using insect repellent.
- Use a thimble for sewing.
- Avoid the use of a wet-shave razor for removal of underarm hair by using depilatory cream or an electric razor instead.
- Take care not to burn in the sun and use protective sun cream.
- Use the arm as normally as possible as regular movement will help lymph drainage.

Resources

The British Lymphoedema Society (BLS)
The Lymphoedema Support Network. http://www.lymphoedema.org.

---

scar. Wound size and position, and wound closure to be used can be mentioned. Drawings, photographs and DVDs/videos may be helpful aids.

It is important to warn the patient that, because the breast is so vascular, bruising and swelling are expected postoperatively. The patient should be reminded of this when first looking at the scar. Women who are not having immediate reconstruction should be informed about the availability of prostheses.

Information given verbally may be reinforced with printed material or various web-based sources of reliable information, such as Breast Cancer Care and Macmillan Cancer Support (see Useful Websites).

Postoperative Care

For general postoperative nursing care see Chapter 25, Nursing the Patient Undergoing Surgery. The following discussion focuses on considerations that are particularly relevant to breast surgery.

Wound Management (see Chapter 23, Tissue Viability and Managing Chronic Wounds). The size and position of the wound will depend on the operation performed. A low-suction drain may be placed beneath the breast wound and in some cases another in the axillary region to reduce the likelihood of a collection of serous fluid (seroma) forming. Initially, any drains and the wound dressing should be observed frequently for signs of excessive blood loss. Undue blood loss should be reported to medical staff immediately.

The wound drains will remain in situ until the wound drainage is minimal, usually less than 50 mL/day. The nurse should ensure that the drains are patent and that, unless informed otherwise, suction is maintained; drainage volume should be recorded. Removal of the drains can be painful; this should be explained to the patient and removal should be preceded by the administration of oral analgesics. Patients may go home with the drain still in situ. The patient is given instructions about managing the wound

and drain. Community nurses/practice nurses may be involved in the patient's discharge, and may empty and finally remove the drains at home. Close contact is usually maintained with the hospital and patients are asked to notify the hospital should the drain become loose, blocked or cause pain. Research shows that, with good support, early discharge with axillary drains in situ is safe and does not cause any greater psychological distress for patients (Soteropulos et al. 2019).

The wound should also be observed for signs of infection, i.e. redness, swelling, pain and discharge. Temperature, pulse and respiration should be monitored 4–6-hourly initially and a raised temperature brought to the attention of the medical staff.

Wound dressings should be changed only if they are saturated by wound exudate. Unnecessary dressing changes slow wound healing and increase the risk of infection. The patient can have a shower or bath providing the dressing does not get wet or the wound is not soaked. If there is no dressing the patient should carefully pat the area dry with a clean towel.

The nurse must also consider other factors, such as nutritional intake, medication, stress and concurrent illness (e.g. diabetes mellitus), which may affect wound healing and resistance to infection (see Chapter 23).

Managing Pain. Pain from the wound will always be experienced to some degree, but pain on shoulder movement is often more of a problem. Pain is sometimes more intense a day or so after the operation, when the initial numbness has faded. Patients should be encouraged to take analgesics regularly for the first 48 hours, but many patients find that the wound is less painful than they had expected and require oral analgesics infrequently beyond this period. It should be stressed that it is preferable to take analgesics and continue arm exercises than to take no analgesics and avoid the exercises.

The experience of pain is influenced by many factors, such as anxiety and emotional distress (see Chapter 20, Pain Management), and must be considered by the nurse when promoting comfort postoperatively.

Patients who have had a mastectomy may experience phantom breast and nipple sensations at some point. This may be very distressing and requires the nurse to reassure. Nerve damage may occur during surgery, causing numbness and altered sensation which for some can be distressing (Kokosis et al. 2019). If the nerve has only been bruised, patients may complain of an uncomfortable tenderness (neuropraxia) but this sensation should fade over a period of weeks to months. Referral to a physiotherapist is needed if the patient has long-term discomfort, cording (fibrosis which looks and feels like a tight cord running from the axilla down the arm) or altered range of arm movement.

Preparing the Patient for Discharge. As with other specialties, there has recently been a move towards enhanced recovery after surgery (ERAS) in breast surgery (Offodile et al. 2019) which are designed to reduce length of stay without compromising overall quality of care.

Looking at a breast scar for the first time can be very difficult and may confirm a patient's fears about breast loss and intensify grief. However, others find the scar neater and less distressing than they had imagined. The patient must never be forced to look at the wound and it may not be until the first outpatient visit that the patient is able to take this step.

Rehabilitation proceeds at different rates (Ribeiro 2019), but the nurse should explain to each patient that it may take several months before their energy returns to normal. Persistent fatigue may cause frustration and may give rise to anxiety that the cancer has returned. Fatigue is more likely if chemotherapy or radiotherapy is given postoperatively, but where it is profound, depression should also be considered as a possible contributing factor.

Most patients can begin driving again in 2–3 weeks, providing they feel confident, their arm movement is not too uncomfortable and the seat belt is not pressing on the scar line. They must be confident enough to perform an emergency stop if necessary. Patients should check with their insurance regarding cover. Light household duties can be undertaken when they feel well enough, usually 2–3 weeks postoperatively. Return to work is dependent on the type of work and the treatment plan.

If a patient develops a persistent seroma, it may be aspirated. Many specialist breast care nurses and nurse practitioners have been trained to carry out aspiration and patients should be informed whom to contact should this problem arise.

Lymphoedema is a possible long-term complication that can occur in anyone who has axillary surgery or radiotherapy. Patients should have access to a breast care nurse to provide information (verbal and written) before or at the time of cancer treatment. This includes advice regarding care of a potentially swollen limb or other area and to contact the breast care nurse if swelling occurs, so that they can then refer to the appropriate service. Some units in the UK require patients to attend their GP for a referral to the local lymphoedema service. Lymphoedema following breast surgery is discussed later.

Prior to discharge, any woman who has had a mastectomy or a significantly wide local excision without immediate breast reconstruction should be given a temporary prosthesis, shown how to position it in her bra and alter its shape and advised how to wash it (Information 8.12).

Adjuvant Therapy

Adjuvant Local Treatments

Radiotherapy (see Chapter 31, Nursing the Patient With Cancer)
After breast-conserving surgery, radiotherapy to the conserved breast halves the rate at which the disease recurs and reduces the breast cancer death rates considerably. There have also been recent developments in targeted radiotherapy options (Haussmann et al. 2020).

Radiotherapy is offered to all patients following breast-conserving surgery and to selected patients after mastectomy, depending on grade and stage (NICE 2018a).

In the UK, most radiotherapy is administered by external beam or intensity modulated radiotherapy (IMRT) using linear accelerator machines (linac). IMRT is a multileaf collimator (tube of overlapping metal leaves) that focuses the radiation beam and is part of the newer linear accelerators. This allows the shape of the beam to be adjusted, thus reducing the exposure of healthy tissue to radiation. In addition, the dose intensity can be modulated across the beam in such a way as to remove localised overdosage (hot spots), which was common in traditional techniques (Haussmann et al. 2020).

A course of radiotherapy is given in daily doses, known as fractions; a course is usually given in 15 fractions. Radiotherapy is usually given to the breast/chest wall over a period of 3 weeks, five times a week. In most units, radiotherapy is planned using a non-diagnostic CT scan to enable more accurate delivery of radiation and avoidance of the underlying organs such as lung and heart (for left-sided tumours).

There have been several technological advances in the delivery of radiotherapy over the last decade. These aim to increase accuracy and reduce the side-effects from radiation.

INFORMATION 8.12

Breast Prostheses

The fitting of a breast prosthesis is an integral part of the rehabilitation following mastectomy or partial mastectomy without immediate breast reconstruction. The aim of the prosthesis is to match as closely as possible the woman's other breast in terms of size, shape, weight and feel, so that she may look normal and feel confident in clothing. This is important in helping her to resume her normal social activities and regain a healthy body image.

Temporary Prostheses

A temporary prosthesis (sometimes known as a 'cumfie') is fitted as soon as the wound drains from the mastectomy scar have been removed and is worn until a permanent prosthesis can be fitted. It is soft, light and washable, and can be pinned securely into the cup of a bra. If a bra cannot be worn because of discomfort, the prosthesis can be pinned into a camisole or slip. The woman may find that wearing loose clothing helps to achieve an even appearance. However, it is important that the nurse spends time fitting this prosthesis well, as it is with this that the woman will first face the outside world again.

Permanent Prostheses

A permanent prosthesis is usually fitted 5–6 weeks after surgery or 2 weeks after the completion of radiotherapy, when the wound is well healed. Every woman should be given a fitting appointment prior to leaving hospital. The fitting may be undertaken by a specialist nurse, surgical appliance officer or visiting prosthesis company fitter. A private room with a full-length mirror is necessary and it is essential that each woman is treated with respect and sensitivity.

Today most permanent prostheses are made of silicone gel which feels soft and comfortable next to the skin and takes on the body's temperature. Many shapes and sizes are available; it should be possible for all women to be fitted with a prosthesis that gives a balanced appearance in a bra. Partial prostheses are available for women who have breast conservation. Silicone prostheses generally last for 2–3 years, but a woman is entitled to a replacement whenever it begins to show signs of wear and tear or if she loses or gains weight or changes shape.

Special 'mastectomy bras' are not necessary, but the bra does need to be supportive and of the correct cup size, covering all of the tissue of the remaining breast. It is helpful if the nurse can give basic advice about bras and instruct a woman where she may be fitted for a bra locally, if her previous bras are now inappropriate. Volunteer organisations give helpful advice about bras, swimwear and other clothing (see Useful Websites, e.g. Breast Cancer Care).

- **The breath-hold technique**, with the patient using goggles to guide their breathing during treatment, has been proven to protect the heart if the patient is requiring radiotherapy for the left side (Bergom et al. 2018).
- **Intra-operative radiotherapy (IORT)**: radiotherapy is delivered during surgery for certain size single tumours and node negative disease. The tissue is removed and a sphere inserted in to the cavity to deliver the radiotherapy for up to 50 minutes. If the margins are clear and the lymph node status does not change, no further radiotherapy is required. If this changes, external beam radiotherapy is then administered. There has been a clinical trial, TargitA, and TargitB is at present ongoing and a registry to continue to follow the long-term benefits and side-effects (NICE 2018b).

Side-effects of Radiotherapy. Side-effects are classified as early and late onset (see Chapter 31 for a detailed account). Early effects of radiotherapy can include erythema, swelling and soreness of the skin over the treated area. Aches, twinges or sharp pains in the breast/chest area can also be experience. Stiffness and discomfort around the shoulder and chest area can occur. Hair loss in the armpit or chest area can also occur and may be permanent. Fatigue towards the end of the treatment period is common.

Photosensitivity of the skin can occur and the skin should be protected by covering it, staying in the shade and using products with high sun protection factor (SPF).

Rarely, moist desquamation of the skin may occur.

Late-onset effects of radiotherapy include lymphoedema, which can occur as a result of damage to the lymphatic system.

Other rare long-term effects include:
- Radiation pneumonitis, which presents with a cough, fever and dyspnoea.
- Damage to the myocardium and the coronary arteries as a side-effect of radiotherapy to the left side of the chest. Every effort is made to individualise treatment plans to reduce the amount of cardiac tissue subjected to radiation to minimise this toxicity and with the advancement of radiotherapy the number of people affected by this is reducing.
- Late skin effects can include the development of telangiectasia (dilatation of small blood vessels), which has no physical effects but the permanent mark on the skin is an enduring reminder of the radiotherapy that the person has been given.

Systemic Treatments

Systemic therapy has become increasingly important in the management of breast cancer as women with breast cancer often develop disseminated disease from undetectable micrometastases present at diagnosis (Pondé et al. 2019). The aim is to destroy micrometastases before they become clinically apparent and this is achieved by using treatments that treat the whole body and not just the primary cancer. Treatments include chemotherapy (using cytotoxic drugs), hormone manipulation therapy and therapies that target cancer cells.

Neoadjuvant (Primary) Chemotherapy

For women presenting with a tumour greater than 2–3 cm in size, many UK breast units will offer neoadjuvant chemotherapy in order to shrink the tumour with the intention of making surgery possible or allowing more conservative surgery. Giving systemic treatment preoperatively leads to improved overall survival in patients with locally advanced cancers, who are at higher risk of having distant disease. Any micrometastases that may have spread from the original tumour are also systemically treated by chemotherapy. However, recent studies are questioning the effectiveness of this approach against improved outcomes using newer drugs (Vaidya 2018).

In some circumstances, endocrine therapy is used to achieve the same result.

Throughout the chemotherapy (up to eight courses), the tumour size will be assessed clinically. However, this can be very subjective, so a more accurate assessment can be undertaken using ultrasound or MRI. When the optimum response to the medication has been achieved, surgery is performed and in some cases breast conservation can be achieved. Sometimes, at the end of the chemotherapy, the tumour is no longer detectable radiologically, but surgery in the previous location of the tumour is always recommended as small lesions are not always seen radiologically. Radiotherapy may then be given to the breast or the chest wall to complete the local treatment.

Adjuvant Chemotherapy

Chemotherapy in addition to surgery has now become the standard treatment in many early breast cancers and has resulted in

significant survival benefit. The use of chemotherapy drugs is regularly changing and the addition of targeted therapies and monoclonal antibodies plays an important role in breast cancer management. Therefore these have not been detailed. These treatments are referred to as systemic anticancer treatments (SACTs).

Further information on current chemotherapy, targeted therapies and monoclonal antibody regimes can be found on the Cancer Research website: http://www.cancerresearchuk.org/about-cancer/breast-cancer/treatment/chemotherapy/drugs.

The patient can usually have adjuvant SACT administered intravenously over a 4–12-month period as an outpatient.

Hormonal Therapies

Adjuvant hormonal therapies are used to prevent breast cancer cells from receiving stimulation from endogenous oestrogen. Many breast cancers are thought to be stimulated by female sex hormones, particularly oestrogen, and are known as oestrogen receptor-positive, or ER-positive. Hormonal therapies act by inhibiting oestrogen synthesis, or blocking its effect on cells. They include:

- **Ovarian suppression** – is particularly relevant for premenopausal women who have an oestrogen-positive tumour. Suppression may be achieved by bilateral oophorectomy. For younger women who have not had a child, luteinising hormone-releasing hormone (LHRH) agonists such as goserelin can be used. Goserelin given as a subcutaneous (SC) bolus injection every 28 days prevents ovarian oestrogen production. Once goserelin is discontinued, the effect is usually reversed.
- **Tamoxifen** – a selective oestrogen receptor modulator (SERM) that inhibits the growth of breast cancer cells by competitive antagonism of oestrogen at the ER receptor site. Tamoxifen also exhibits partial oestrogen agonist activity which can be both beneficial and detrimental. Tamoxifen prevents bone demineralisation but does increase the risk of endometrial cancer and VTE. In addition to reducing rates of disease relapse and death, tamoxifen also reduces the risk of developing a contralateral breast cancer. Tamoxifen is given orally and can be used for both pre- and postmenopausal women. Women should be informed about the side-effects that include menopausal signs and symptoms with hot flushes, night sweats, vaginal dryness/discharge and increased risk of VTE. However, these effects are usually outweighed by the benefits of treatment.
- **Aromatase inhibitors (AIs)** – drugs that markedly reduce the concentration of circulating oestrogen levels in postmenopausal women. They work by inhibiting or inactivating aromatase, the enzyme required to synthesise oestrogens from androgenic substrates. In contrast to tamoxifen, these drugs lack agonist activity. Initially, AI's were used only in postmenopausal patients to prevent disease recurrence, but together with LHRH agonists LHRH analogs, they can sometimes be used in premenopausal patients to produce better oestrogen suppression than can be achieved with tamoxifen plus an LHRH analogue (Pistelli et al. 2018). AIs may be nonsteroidal or steroidal. Anastrozole and letrozole are in the nonsteroidal group and exemestane in the steroidal group.

These are treatments directed against specific molecular targets considered to be involved in the development of cancer cells (Simmons et al. 2022), that is, therapies that target specific characteristics of cancer cells that allow them to grow in a rapid or abnormal way. The main targets are the human epidermal growth factor receptor-2 (HER2), tyrosine kinases and angiogenesis (formation of new blood vessels). Targeted therapies aim to limit toxicities whilst selectively acting against cancer cells. Cancers that are HER2-positive have been found to be more aggressive, which leads to a poor prognosis. Overexpression of HER2 can result in inappropriate cellular responses such as deactivation of normal apoptosis (cell death) involved in cellular migration, which can lead to distant metastases. Two methods for evaluating the level of HER2 have evolved to discover whether cancer cells overexpress these receptors: immunohistochemistry, which is used to determine HER2 overexpression, and fluorescence in situ hybridisation (FISH), which is used to determine the HER2 copy number.

One of the most successful targeted therapies for breast cancer has been trastuzumab, a humanised monoclonal antibody specifically able to block the function of HER2 (Simmons et al. 2022).

❖ Nursing Management and Health Promotion: Adjuvant Therapy

Postoperatively, the patient will attend a surgical outpatient clinic where their wound healing will be assessed, advice given on recovery and their psychological and social needs addressed. They will be advised of the pathology results of their surgery, i.e. number of lymph nodes involved with cancer, the size and grade of the tumour and its oestrogen status, all factors that will determine the need for adjuvant treatment. These results are discussed at an MDM where decisions will be made about an appropriate treatment plan prior to the patient being seen. The options are then discussed with the patient. The addition of a test to determine the value of chemotherapy will be offered if indicated – for example Oncotype DX (NICE 2018d).

Information about radiotherapy and SACT will be given, as relevant, both verbally and in writing. The patient should understand why adjuvant treatment has been advised, time period, intervals and side-effects. At any point the patient may be invited to join a research study.

Radiotherapy

All patients should be given clear advice about skin care before, during and after their radiotherapy treatment. They should be encouraged to use a cream, for example diprobase, to moisturise the area that is receiving the radiotherapy and should wash or shower the area during the treatment period using tepid water and a very mild soap. Patients should wear loose-fitting, cotton clothing next to their skin and avoid wearing underwired bras (Ramseier et al. 2020).

🌐 **See Evolve website Critical thinking question 8.4**

Chemotherapy

Several different chemotherapy regimens are used and the patient may have already received chemotherapy preoperatively. Chemotherapy may be administered through a temporary venous cannula or a central venous access device (CVAD) of some type (see Chapter 31, Nursing the Patient With Cancer).

Vascular access in patients receiving chemotherapy can be difficult due to the multiple cannulations required to administer a course of adjuvant chemotherapy. Regular venepuncture and cannulation can lead to thrombophlebitis, particularly as the chemotherapy practitioner will be advised to use only one arm to avoid compromising the skin and lymphatics of the arm affected by the breast surgery. Infusion thrombophlebitis can occur at any stage during the lifetime of a short peripheral cannula (Lv and Zhang

2020); it is essential therefore that nurses are aware of the importance of assessing the vein and adhering to local policies and good practice on venous assessment.

The alternative to temporary venous cannulation is to use a semipermanent venous access device. CVADs are used mainly to overcome poor peripheral venous access, or for prolonged courses of intravenous chemotherapy.

Outline of Side-Effects

See Chapter 13, Nursing the Patient With Blood Disorders, and Chapter 31, Nursing the Patient With Cancer. The patient should be reassured that adjuvant chemotherapy regimens used in breast cancer can usually be managed by the outpatient department.

Nausea is commonly experienced but usually can be controlled by oral antiemetics if significant. Vomiting should be rare.

Breast cancer chemotherapy regimens containing an anthracycline such as adriamycin or epirubicin will cause total alopecia, which can be very stressful for some patients. Scalp cooling caps can restrict the amount of chemotherapy reaching the hair follicles and so may prevent complete hair loss, although the hair may thin and become drier and of poorer quality. Gentle shampoos should be used, and perms, colourants and the use of heated tongs should be avoided.

Myelosuppression (bone marrow suppression) occurs with all cytotoxic drugs, but it is rare for neutropenia to be severe or for septic shock to result (Amjad et al. 2020). The avoidance of obvious risks of infection should be discussed and if the patient's temperature rises above normal or they feel unwell. they should be advised to contact the hospital immediately using the emergency number they have been given (see Chapter 13, Nursing Patients With Blood Disorders, and Chapter 31, Nursing the Patient With Cancer). Some treatments may now be administered on a weekly basis to help reduce side-effects.

Fatigue is a common problem and can be quite debilitating for some patients.

Stomatitis/mucositis and a susceptibility to mouth ulcers can be helped by pain relief, using a soft toothbrush, bactericidal mouthwashes and antifungal drugs. Some patients find certain foods soothing, for example yogurt, and pineapple assists with keeping the tongue clean. Some foods can be an irritant, for example hot, spicy food. Taste does change as a result of the treatments.

Menstrual cycle disruption is usual, with menstruation becoming irregular or stopping. Menopausal symptoms, such as hot flushes, may be experienced. In younger women, there is a chance of menstrual cycles returning after chemotherapy finishes. Women in their early 40s are much more likely to have an early climacteric/menopause.

Endocrine Therapy

For most of the endocrine therapies, pre- and postmenopausal women will usually experience menopausal symptoms, which can be very distressing. These symptoms are also experienced by men. These may include fatigue, hot flushes, night sweats, joint pain, headaches and insomnia. Some patients find that preparations containing gamma-linolenic acid can help with such symptoms; otherwise, the patient's consultant or GP can prescribe medication to reduce the hot flushes or recommend complementary therapies/acupuncture. Unfortunately, these remedies are not without side-effects and many patients prefer to manage without such intervention.

Gastric upsets are uncommon but may occur, particularly if the tamoxifen tablets are not taken with food. A small increase in

VTE is associated with tamoxifen use and patients must inform their clinician of any new pain and swelling in their calves or sudden and unusual shortness of breath. Many patients complain about an increase in weight, particularly around the abdomen, soon after starting the tablets. This may be due in part to fluid retention and in part to a reduction in physical activity following surgery. Other rare and more serious side-effects include endometrial cancer and cataract formation. Any abnormal vaginal bleeding should be investigated as well as any rapid deterioration in eyesight.

As AIs lower endogenous circulating oestrogen levels, a consequence for some patients is osteoporosis. Patients receiving an AI should be assessed for risk factors for osteoporosis, including a family history, fragility fractures, calcium intake, smoking and alcohol use, BMI and exercise. Bone density should be measured at baseline, and women with T-scores higher than –2.5 SD (osteoporosis) should receive calcium/vitamin D, and a bisphosphonate (see Chapter 11, Nursing Patients With Musculoskeletal Disorders). They should also be advised on weight-bearing exercise. Patients with bone densities between –1.5 and –2.5 SD (osteopenia) should have an adequate intake of calcium and vitamin D with regular bone density measurements as an essential, ongoing assessment.

Targeted Therapies

The biological therapy trastuzumab can cause several side-effects for some, but not all, patients. These include fatigue, which certainly occurs during the treatment but can continue for up to a year, a flu-like reaction of fever, chills, rash and nausea, headache, breathlessness, wheezing, diarrhoea and myalgia. Side-effects occur in a significant number of patients after the first treatment but usually decrease after the first few treatments. Diarrhoea can affect about a third of the people who receive this treatment but is usually mild and can be helped with antidiarrhoeal tablets. Congestive cardiac failure is a rare side-effect but the drug should not be given to a patient with cardiac conditions without prior review. Patients have a baseline echocardiogram and at 3-monthly intervals (NICE 2018a).

Follow-Up for Asymptomatic Patients

The aims of follow-up should be to detect and treat local recurrence and the adverse effects of treatment (NICE 2018a). Intensive follow-up, designed to detect metastatic disease before symptoms develop, is not beneficial and routine tests to detect metastatic cancer are not necessary because they do not improve quality of life or survival.

Many breast units within the UK have developed systems for patient-led follow-up where patients no longer attend an outpatient breast clinic but have access to breast care nurses who will arrange an appointment if there is any cause for concern. These are called rapid access clinics (NICE 2018a).

Breast Cancer Subgroups

Breast cancer can affect both sexes and all ages, although it is predominantly a disease of women over 50 years of age. This section outlines the needs of men, older patients, young women and patients from Black and ethnic minority groups.

Male Breast Cancer

Male breast cancer (MBC) is rare and accounts for less than 1% of all breast cancers (Breast Cancer Care 2018d). Male breast anatomy is the same as that of the female breast; it is the absence of hormonal stimulation which accounts for the developmental and physiological differences. However, the disease is similar in both male and female. It is generally accepted that male and female breast cancers are the same disease. All histological types reported among women also occur among men, and *BRCA2* gene mutations have been reported with the same frequency in the tumour tissue of both men and women. Increasing age remains relevant, as Simmons et al. (2022) demonstrate the median age at diagnosis is 64.

Diagnosis of MBC is made by triple assessment, as in symptomatic women. The majority of MBCs are invasive ductal carcinomas which are ER-positive, and treatment for MBC is similar to that of females. Surgery is the mainstay of treatment, and mastectomy is the treatment of choice due to the small quantity of breast tissue in males. Diagnosis is often at a later stage where the skin and underlying fascia are involved (Simmons et al. 2022). Adjuvant radiotherapy, chemotherapy, endocrine therapy and targeted therapies are also used.

It is important that nurses recognise the particular needs that men may have when they are diagnosed and treated for breast cancer. Information about breast cancer is often aimed at women, which can make it difficult for men to talk about. Hormone therapy causes similar side-effects such as hot flushes or reduced libido. This can impact on a man's sexuality and may require support from the nurses who care for him.

Breast Cancer in Trans People

Both trans women and trans men can be affected by breast cancer. Although there hasn't been much research in this area, one study by De Blok et al. (2019) suggested that transgender women (people assigned male at birth but who identify and live as women) undergoing hormone treatment have an increased risk of breast cancer compared with cisgender men (people assigned male at birth who identify and live as men). Over the course of the study, 15 cases of invasive breast cancer (breast cancer that has the potential to spread to other areas of the body) were detected in 2260 transgender women that the researchers were following. In cisgender men, over the same period of time, only 0.32 cases of breast cancer would be expected to be detected. This is why scientists suggest transgender women are 47 times more likely to develop breast cancer. However, 15 out of 2260 is still a very small number of cases and more research is needed.

The conclusion from these statistics is that both trans women and trans men need to be breast or chest aware, as both groups are at risk of breast cancer.

Breast Cancer in Older Women

Breast cancer is a major health problem in older women. The biology of breast cancers in women aged 70 years is similar to the 50–69 age group in terms of grade, HER2 and ER status. This indicates that breast cancer survival in the older woman is similar to survival rates for the general population (Healthcare Quality Improvement Partnership (HQIP) 2020).

Moodley et al. (2018) identify that this patient group presented with more advanced breast cancers and was more likely to have positive lymph nodes. This has been exacerbated by delays with mammograms during the COVID-19 outbreak and patients being more cautious about attending healthcare settings due to COVID-19 (Prodhan et al. 2023).

However, chronic comorbidities increase with age and breast cancer is not always the most significant threat to life in this age group (Biganzoli et al. 2021); it is therefore necessary to evaluate comorbidities and tumour biology prior to making treatment decisions. As a result, breast cancer treatments in older women show reduced rates in surgery, radiotherapy and chemotherapy as well as targeted therapies. Chronological age should not determine treatment decisions. Surgery is the mainstay of treatment, but for older women with comorbidities and ER-positive tumours, it may provide little benefit for those who have had a good response to endocrine therapy alone. However, women who are fit and healthy should be offered standard surgical therapies.

Breast Cancer in Young Women

Despite the increase of breast cancer incidence with age, approximately 7% to 10% of women diagnosed with breast cancer are younger than the age 40 (Rossi et al. 2019). There are very few women diagnosed in their teens or early 20s (Cancer Research UK 2018b). Young women tend to have larger tumours at diagnosis than older women. This is in part because they have denser breast tissue, which makes it difficult to detect a lump, and also because breast tissue is influenced by cyclical hormonal changes making diagnosis more difficult. Younger women are not within a national screening programme, and compared with older women, breast cancer in young women is usually more aggressive, often of a higher grade and tending to be ER, PR and HER2-negative, defined as triple-negative. The incidence of DCIS is lower in the younger women age group. Younger women of African origin are more likely to have a basal phenotype and be oestrogen-negative. Treatment for breast cancer in younger women includes the multimodality treatments of surgery, chemotherapy, radiotherapy, endocrine and targeted therapies. Due to the adverse prognostic features displayed by these tumours, young women are much more likely to be treated with chemotherapy, which has significantly contributed to improved survival in younger women but is also associated with acute and long-term side-effects such as a chemically induced menopause and infertility (Sobota and Ozakinci 2021). Prior to treatment the woman should be offered a referral to discuss egg preservation if she wishes to have children in the future. Reduced bone density caused by loss of circulating oestrogen needs also to be considered. Young women can have a significantly poor prognosis, in part due to the more aggressive tumour. All younger women should be offered genetic testing. Premature menopause, sexual dysfunction, infertility, mental health issues and adverse body image are well-documented effects of cancer therapy. Therefore holistic assessment, good information, communication, counselling and support are essential interventions for young women treated for triple-negative breast cancer (Reflection 8.5).

Breast Cancer in Black and Ethnic Minority Women

A study by Gathani et al. (2021) demonstrated that ethnic minority women are at greater risk of breast cancers with less favourable characteristics, even after allowing for age and other potential confounders. These differences are greater in older than younger women, and in the Black rather than South Asian ethnic groups.

There have also been several studies evaluating health inequalities between different demographics of patients which indicate that Black and ethnic minority women are more likely to experience delays with treatment and poorer outcomes (Blazek et al. 2021, Gehlert et al. 2021, Martins et al. 2022).

Evidence-Based Practice 8.4 provides readers with an opportunity to consider these differences and reflect on how the care of Black and ethnic minority women can be improved.

REFLECTION 8.5

A Young Woman With Breast Cancer

Lucy is a 33-year-old single woman in a long-term relationship. She has just been diagnosed with breast cancer and will require adjuvant chemotherapy after her surgery. Adjuvant chemotherapy has contributed to the overall survival in women with early breast cancer, but it is also associated with long-term side-effects, often causing temporary (and for some, permanent) menopause.

Activities

- Think about the symptoms of a temporary menopause and how you could explain them to Lucy.
- Reflect on how nurses might help Lucy and her partner to deal with a breast cancer diagnosis and treatment and its effects as well as her recovery.

Breast Reconstruction

Following loss of breast tissue due to a risk of breast cancer or treatment for breast cancer, reconstruction surgery will be offered to the patient. It is a very personal decision as to whether a woman has breast reconstruction and will only be undertaken as a fully informed decision. Many women prefer not to have further surgery.

All women who undergo a mastectomy will be offered reconstruction surgery. As part of the discussion the different choices of reconstruction techniques available will be explained and offered to the woman, irrespective of whether the surgery is available locally (NICE 2018a). Reconstruction may be undertaken when a woman has a bilateral prophylactic mastectomy due to a high genetic predisposition to breast cancer, or following breast cancer surgery in which a significant part, or all, of a breast or both breasts were removed.

Reconstruction surgery can sometimes be undertaken at the time of initial surgery (mastectomy) or as a delayed reconstructive procedure. Reconstruction following breast cancer surgery aims to

---

EVIDENCE-BASED PRACTICE 8.4

Breast Cancer in Black and Ethnic Minority Women

Martins et al. (2022) report that Black and Asian women are significantly more likely than White women to be diagnosed with breast cancer at a stage where cancer cells have spread to other areas of the body.

Activities

- Access the study by Martins et al. (2022) and consider the reasons why Black and Asian women are more likely to present with more advanced breast cancer.
- What differences in the type of breast cancer and age at presentation between groups are identified in the study?
- Consider with your mentor how you would raise awareness of breast cancer symptoms in Black and Asian women and increase the uptake of screening.

Reference

Martins T, Abel G, Ukoumunne OC, et al. Ethnic inequalities in routes to diagnosis of cancer: a population-based UK cohort study. *Br J Cancer.* 2022;127(5):863–871.

create a breast form which resembles the woman's other breast as closely as possible in size, shape and consistency. Complete symmetry when the woman is naked is not possible to achieve but the aim of the surgery should be that any differences are slight when she is wearing a bra.

Breast reconstruction surgery can be undertaken using different surgical techniques (for further information, see Useful Websites, Breast Cancer Care). Surgery may involve a prosthetic implant or moving tissue from another part of the body (e.g. abdomen) to form a breast mound. The transplantation of tissue can result in a major surgical procedure with a significant stay in hospital and recovery period.

Breast reconstruction may help to reduce the psychological or emotional problems experienced by women after surgery. The presence of bone metastases should not prohibit a woman from having reconstructive surgery if she perceives that this will improve her quality of life and she is generally well enough to undergo surgery.

Fungating Breast Tumours

For a small number of patients, a fungating breast tumour is diagnosed, either at time of presentation, which is usually due to the patient seeking assistance at a late stage, or a recurrence near the original site of the cancer which has been treated. The patient presents with a cancer that has invaded the skin surface to cause ulceration. The resulting wound may be deep or superficial and can be distressing for the patient. As the cancer outgrows its blood supply, there is central tissue necrosis and possible infection with excessive wound exudate, bleeding and unpleasant odour. Nerve involvement can cause pain and itching, again very distressing for the patient and presenting a care challenge.

Medical management would consider any previous surgery and radiotherapy but both can be used again, often with great success to control the disease locally. Hormone treatment and chemotherapy can also be used for systemic disease control and to control the active tumour (see Useful websites, e.g. Macmillan Cancer Support).

Breast Cancer-Related Lymphoedema

Lymphoedema is the excessive accumulation of protein-rich fluid (lymph) in the interstitial spaces in the tissue of a limb or other body area causing swelling, discomfort and sometimes reduced movement.

Lymphoedema related to breast cancer can occur at any time of a patient's breast cancer pathway. Occasionally, it can be a presenting symptom before diagnosis or very shortly after diagnosis. It can also present during or after treatment of breast cancer. The lymphoedema may be related to the presence of tumour or subsequent surgery or/and radiotherapy. It is caused by a structural defect causing a reduction of inhibition of the free flow of the lymphatic fluid around the limb. The reported prevalence of lymphoedema for patients diagnosed with breast cancer varies. Cancer Research UK (2020) states it is one-fifth (20%) of all patients treated for a breast cancer.

It is worth considering it in some depth as it is a condition that has been greatly improved by better understanding and nursing intervention.

Pathophysiology

Lymphoedema results from defective lymph drainage due to tissue fibrosis, disease or a congenital disorder. Those affected may have an uncomfortable, unsightly and functionally impaired arm, sometimes with some swelling of the adjacent chest and pain. Those patients with a greater number of lymphoedema symptoms or specific symptoms, including burning pain, tension, heaviness, and warmth/redness, have poorer quality of life, particularly in the domains of perceived physical health and stress (Togawa et al. 2021).

The aetiology of breast cancer-related lymphoedema (BCRL) is still not fully understood and multifactorial, although it is thought that BCRL is caused by surgical damage to the axilla that leads to interruption of lymph vessels draining the arm.

Axillary surgery to remove some or all of the axillary lymph nodes, or axillary radiotherapy, increases the risk of lymphoedema of the limb on the affected side (Johnson et al. 2019). Scarring from these treatments may occlude or narrow many lymph vessels, thereby reducing lymph drainage from the arm. For most women the drainage remains adequate and collateral vessels may develop to increase drainage. However, lymphoedema may develop weeks, months or years after surgery or radiotherapy, sometimes following a wound complication, cording, infection or injury, but often without an obvious reason. It may remain mild or gradually progress until the arm is so heavy that it is difficult to lift and to use. Over time, fibrosis within the tissue of the arm may occur, causing hardness. There is also a higher risk of infection and cellulitis, as the protein-rich fluid is an ideal culture for bacteria.

Disease within the axillary region which obstructs lymph flow may also cause lymphoedema, such as recurrent cancer or late presentation with advanced cancer of the breast. Signs of venous obstruction are sometimes seen, commonly as colour changes of the arm and distended veins visible on the upper arm and chest wall.

Brachial plexus nerve damage is rarely seen but may also result from radiation fibrosis or cancer infiltration of the nerve plexus, causing weakness, paraesthesia or nerve pain.

Medical Management

Treatment options are limited and depend on whether the lymphoedema has been caused by fibrosis or by axillary disease. Assessment may include scanning to determine the amount of scarring, venous obstruction or disease.

Where venous obstruction is due to a thrombosis, anticoagulation therapy should be initiated.

In the case of axillary disease, surgery to remove as much of the cancer as possible may be of use by reducing the obstruction of lymph and venous flow. However, chemotherapy or endocrine therapies, which cause less disruption to normal structures than surgery, are more likely to be used. Analgesics will be used as required. If, however, the pain is due to brachial plexus damage, it is unlikely to respond adequately to opiates since nerve pain is only partly opiate-responsive. Other drug groups may be required (e.g. anticonvulsants, antidepressants, corticosteroids and NSAIDs) for nerve pain (see Chapter 19, Pain Management).

The risk of infection in a swollen limb is high and can result in cellulitis. A small cut or insect bite may provide an entry point for infection and potentially severe cellulitis requiring intravenous antibiotics (Information 8.11). If cellulitis is recurrent, patients are often given a prescription or a supply of antibiotics to ensure treatment as soon as infection occurs.

❖ Nursing Management and Health Promotion: Lymphoedema

Specialist nurses have an important role to play in the prevention of lymphoedema for breast cancer patients. Explaining to patients what lymphoedema is, the risk factors and how risk can be mitigated (Cancer Research UK 2018e) is important for the patient's long-term welfare. Informing patients as to how they can self-monitor their limbs for signs of lymphoedema and self-refer should there be a concern ensures timely intervention, which improves outcomes. The earlier a lymphoedema is diagnosed and the earlier it can be treated, the better the results/outcomes, including the less impact it can have on a patient's life.

Treatment effectiveness is measured in terms of the reduction in size and weight of the arm, and for most patients this is possible. However, sometimes all that can be done is to increase the softness and movement of the arm and to reduce the discomfort, but these improvements can represent a substantial increase in the quality of life for the patient.

All interventions will be preceded by an assessment to identify the physical and psychosocial needs of the individual patient.

Nursing Interventions

Nursing interventions aim to:
- improve the use of the arm
- improve the comfort of the arm
- improve the shape of the arm.

There are now four recognised elements to the management of lymphoedema:
- skin care
- exercise and movement
- lymph drainage
- external containment.

It is very important to explain clearly the aim of treatment and to promote a realistic expectation of outcome. Although therapy is aimed at control rather than cure, the patient who is given sufficient information and is encouraged to participate in treatment is likely to adopt a more positive attitude towards her situation and compliance can therefore be maintained.

Skin Care

The emphasis is on the importance of skin hygiene and care. Advice given at the time of the axillary surgery should be reemphasised. The skin of the arm should be moisturised, as dry skin is less supple and tiny breaks in the skin occur through which bacteria can enter, increasing the risk of infection.

Exercise and Movement. Skin protection when undertaking some tasks should be worn, for example gardening gloves. Some tasks at a higher risk of skin penetration and therefore infection may be avoided, for example pruning roses.

Lymph Drainage. Lymph drainage can be promoted through massage, movement and appropriate exercise as muscle contraction enhances lymph drainage.

Manual lymph drainage (MLD) is a specialised massage technique carried out by trained MLD therapists. Simple lymphatic drainage (SLD) has been developed from MLD for use by patients and their relatives. However, recent evidence supporting its use is mixed (Liang et al. 2020, Lin et al. 2022).

The aims of SLD as with MLD are to:
- stimulate normal lymph drainage
- 'milk' fluid away from the congested areas
- improve superficial lymph drainage

SLD massage is light, aiming to stimulate the lymphatic vessels in the skin. Deeper massage increases blood flow to the muscles, causing more fluid to accumulate in the tissues, and would thus be counterproductive.

Lymph tape is another form of lymph drainage whereby a special tape is applied to the affected area. A thin, porous cotton fabric tape applied correctly will lift the skin to increase the space between the skin and muscle. Muscle contraction and relaxation promote lymph flow and decrease pain. The tape is left on for 3–5 days and is helpful in decreasing swelling of difficult and stubborn areas, especially the breast following radiotherapy. The therapist initially applies the tape and then teaches the woman to do this independently. However, some studies have questioned the effectiveness of the use of lymph tape for patients post breast surgery (Ergin et al. 2019).

Compression hosiery assists with the flow of lymphatic fluid. It supports muscles to maximise the pump action and thereby increases lymphatic drainage. It has been shown to be beneficial for the reduction of lymphoedema particularly in the first year post treatment (Paramanandam et al. 2022).

For people with severe lymphoedema, lymphorrhoea (leakage of lymph), skin problems or difficulty using a sleeve, compression bandaging is the treatment of choice.

Low-stretch bandages are used to bandage the fingers and hand before the arm is encased. The pressure applied should be graduated, greater pressure being applied at the lower end of the limb. The bandages should be reapplied daily. Community nurses experienced in this technique can undertake compression bandaging in the patient's home. This is particularly helpful for patients with advanced disease and those who feel unwell. Bandaging of a large arm may provide great comfort and relief from pain even if it is unlikely to reduce arm size.

Several ready-made compression sleeves are available for lymphoedema management. Compression must be fairly strong if it is to be effective. Supports such as Tubigrip are not adequate for this purpose. Sleeves may be difficult to put on but once fitted are supportive and comfortable. They should be worn during the day when the patient is most active. The sleeves should not be allowed to form creases, as this will cause ridging in the swollen tissue. The sleeve may need to be worn for several weeks. It is easily laundered. If the oedema is modest, it may be possible for the arm to return to its normal size. Regular monitoring of the arm will need to be undertaken by both the patient and their care provider.

Previously, attempts to reduce the size and weight of the arm by surgical removal of tissue have had very little success and have frequently caused further problems with infection, swelling and pain as well as extensive scarring. Suction of lymphatic fluid has been used for limb lymphoedema with very limited success. It is important to note that suction does not correct the lymphatic failure and patients will still require compression hosiery. The benefits of suction can be short, with the risk of infection and further scarring increased.

The Lymphoedema Support Network (see Useful Websites) may be a useful resource to signpost patients to for further information and support.

Metastatic Breast Cancer

Approximately 10% of patients diagnosed with breast cancer have metastatic disease at clinical presentation, but metastasis can also occur months or years after presentation (Macmillan Cancer Support 2018).

The majority of patients who relapse do so within the first 2 years of diagnosis (Macmillan Cancer Support 2018). In the UK we have chosen not to screen for metastatic disease at the time of diagnosis or at subsequent follow-up visits unless there are clinical indications.

If there is suspicion of metastatic disease, positron emission tomography (PET) and CT scanning are recommended if plain X-rays and ultrasound are not diagnostic (Jafari et al. 2018)

Once breast cancer has metastasised systemically, the disease is no longer considered curable and the aim of treatment is to increase the patient's survival whilst providing the best quality of life possible.

Pathophysiology

Breast cancer appears to spread by direct invasion into the surrounding tissue and via the lymphatic and arteriovenous systems to distant areas. If untreated, local invasion of the breast cancer will cause ulceration, fixation to the chest wall and oedema of the arm. It may also, in extreme circumstances, erode blood vessels, causing haemorrhage, and invade the ribs or lungs and pleura, causing pleural effusion. Invasion of the brachial plexus can cause severe pain with functional and sensory loss in the arm. Invasion of the cutaneous nerves causes irritation and burning pain in the affected area. Because such aggressive local disease is not necessarily accompanied by metastatic spread, a woman may survive for many years with these problems.

Spread to distant sites is common but may not become apparent for months or many years after the initial diagnosis and treatment. The most common sites of distant metastases are bone, lungs, liver and brain. Less frequently, metastases occur in the ovaries and mediastinum and, rarely, in the oesophagus, stomach, intestine and pericardium. Breast cancer has a predilection for spreading to bone, and bone metastasis is one of the major causes of increased morbidity and eventual mortality in breast cancer patients. Table 8.2 outlines some common problems associated with metastatic breast cancer (see Chapter 32, Nursing Patients Who Need Palliative Care).

Medical Management

Management involves the use of both local and systemic measures that control and/or palliate symptoms and improve quality of life (see Chapter 32). The first choice of treatment is one that is the least toxic but has the highest response rate. This strategy aims to achieve optimal disease control and maintain remission for as long as possible.

Local treatments include surgery and radiotherapy, and systemic treatments include endocrine therapy, chemotherapy, targeted therapies and the use of bisphosphonates.

Local Treatments

Surgery. Surgery is rarely used in the management of metastatic breast cancer but can help with locally recurrent disease. If the disease occurs locally following breast conserving surgery and radiotherapy, then mastectomy may be undertaken. If there is a large area to be excised a tissue flap may be used to enable the wound to be closed.

Radiotherapy. Radiotherapy is sometimes used to relieve bone pain and in the oncological emergencies such as metastatic spinal cord compression (referred to as MSCC), cerebral oedema and superior vena cava obstruction, where tumour pressure must be reduced quickly. Corticosteroids, usually dexamethasone, are used with radiotherapy to reduce the oedema in tissues surrounding the tumour and hence relieve pressure further.

Systemic Treatments

Hormonal Therapies. Women who have ER-positive breast cancer survive longer after recurrence than women with ER-negative

TABLE 8.2	Common Problems Associated With Metastatic Breast Cancer
Site of Distant Spread	**Problems**
Bone	Bone pain Pathological fractures *Hypercalcaemia *Spinal cord compression (SCC)
Bone marrow	Pancytopenia – neutropenia (infection), anaemia and thrombocytopenia (bleeding, bruising)
Lung/pleura	Pleural effusion Reduced lung expansion/dyspnoea with persistent cough
Liver	Right upper quadrant abdominal pain 'Squashed stomach' syndrome Nausea and vomiting Ascites
Skin	Ulceration/fungation Pain/irritation
Central nervous system – cerebral metastases	Confusion, headaches, nausea, vomiting, altered behaviour, seizures, altered consciousness *Cerebral oedema, raised intracranial pressure
Mediastinum	*Superior vena cava (SVC) obstruction
Axilla/supraclavicular fossa	Lymphoedema Brachial plexus pain and paraesthesia/paralysis of arm

*Oncological emergencies.

breast cancer. Tissue from the recurrent tumour should be tested for ER and HER2 status where possible; ER and HER2 can be a different result than found in the original tumour. Hormonal therapies that may be used include those also used as adjuvant treatment for early stage breast cancer. The use of endocrine therapies for this group of patients is strongly indicated in receptor-positive disease.

There are many different systemic anticancer therapy (SACT) drugs used to treat metastatic breast cancer, which can either be used as single therapy or as combination therapy.

Treatment is given as outpatient infusions in a series of treatments known as cycles. The frequency of administration varies. Treatment response is measured, for example, by CT scan, bone scan or X-ray. The decision to continue, change or stop treatment is based on response and the patients tolerance to treatment.

Chemotherapy can cause unpleasant side-effects (see Chapter 29, Nursing the Patient With Cancer), but for patients with metastatic breast cancer, it can also relieve the cancer symptoms thereby improving quality of life.

Bisphosphonates. Bone is commonly the site for metastatic breast cancer. Once metastatic spread to bone occurs, the disease is no longer curable. It can cause weakening of bone structure, pain and pathological fractures with potential disability.

Bisphosphonates are a group of synthetic analogues of pyrophosphate which bind to calcium. Bisphosphonates help to strengthen bone and reduce the risk of fractures. They can also help to relieve bone pain and have reduced the need for radiotherapy in managing bone pain. Often, such pain is poorly localised and is described as a burning, aching, gnawing or stabbing which is unrelieved by rest. Other sequelae of metastatic bone disease (MBD) are SCC caused by pathological fractures of the vertebrae and hypercalcaemia, both of which are oncological emergencies.

The bisphosphonates usually prescribed for MBD in breast cancer are zoledronic acid and ibandronic acid.

Zoledronic acid is given by intravenous infusion, once a month or so. However, this is given on an outpatient basis and careful monitoring of renal function is required prior to administration.

Ibandronic acid can be given orally, or by intravenous infusion. Patients are advised that they should sit or stand upright to take the tablet, which should be swallowed whole with ample water. The tablet is taken on an empty stomach before breakfast. The patient needs to be in an upright position (standing or sitting) and fast for at least 30 minutes or 60 minutes depending on the dose (British National Formulary (BNF) 2022).

Patients need to be advised that there might be a temporary increase in bone pain, known as tumour flare, following intravenous administration and they may require analgesics until this subsides. Very rarely, bisphosphonates can cause jaw necrosis and patients are advised to inform their dentist that they are being treated with bisphosphonates. There are several other side-effects associated with bisphosphonates and readers are directed to the BNF or their own national formulary.

Bisphosphonates are usually given for as long as they are working. If the bisphosphonate is given to reduce high levels of calcium in hypercalcaemia it may only be given when required.

❖ Nursing Management and Health Promotion: Metastatic Breast Cancer

Nurses are paramount to the care of patients with metastatic breast cancer and should be involved in a holistic assessment which should address the physical, psychological, social and spiritual impact of the disease, with particular consideration of the patient's own perception of these problems. The difficulties faced by the patient are likely to be determined in part by the site(s) of cancer spread. It should be remembered that medical priorities will not necessarily match the personal priorities of the patient, and the decision to treat should be discussed carefully.

The reaction of the patient and their family to the news of progressive disease should be sensitively explored, and the nurse should assess how well they are coping. For many, the discovery of metastatic disease is more devastating than the original diagnosis of breast cancer, as the realisation dawns that treatment is now aimed at controlling rather than curing the illness. The patient and their family may once again experience shock, anger, denial, depression and despair as they try to come to terms with the implications of the diagnosis. They may feel that they completed the recommended treatment at the time of their original diagnosis and struggle to understand why they now have a diagnosis of metastatic breast cancer.

Even where cure is no longer possible, the philosophy of rehabilitation and health promotion will remain at the centre of care, so that the highest quality of life can be maintained for as long as possible.

Palliative Care

Despite remarkable advances in screening, early detection, diagnosis and treatment of breast cancer, it remains a disease with significant mortality. There were 11,563 deaths from breast cancer in the UK in 2016 (Cancer Research UK 2018b). Nursing and medical staff have a responsibility for the provision of individual care for patients with a palliative diagnosis and those approaching the end of life and their families (see Chapter 32, Nursing Patients Who Need Palliative Care).

Secondary breast cancer is when the cancer cells have spread from the breast to other parts of the body and when it can be treated but is no longer curable. The earlier people with secondary breast cancer are introduced to palliative care, the better their quality of life, according to research (Mutebi et al. 2020).

Patients with a palliative breast cancer may live for many years with the knowledge and effects of their progressive disease. The need for holistic assessment and care from those with the expertise and skill set remains paramount for this group of patients. Breast Cancer Care (2019c) has developed standards of care for secondary (metastatic) breast cancer patients.

The Role of the Clinical Nurse Specialist in Breast Care

The role of the CNS in breast care has developed largely in response to the recognition that patients with breast cancer benefit from the support and expertise of nurses specialising in this area (Brown et al. 2021). It must be stressed that the CNS provides an additional service to that provided by hospital and community nursing staff, and not an alternative to that service. The CNS functions as a resource for patients, their families and other nurses.

Ideally, the clinical involvement of the CNS with the patient will begin at the time of diagnosis and prior to hospital admission. This may involve meeting patients in screening assessment units. All patients should be offered a holistic assessment and, where problems arise, referral for more in-depth psychological support can be made, but the nurse will continue their involvement with the patient and their family. The patient should be offered a care plan that can be shared with other agencies and be signposted to services to meet their identified needs. Because of the increasing complexity of the treatments available, the larger centres may employ more than one nurse specialist, and each is then able to focus their expertise on different aspects of the patient's care.

The CNS also provides a contact point for patients and their family should they require advice or support at any time. The CNS should facilitate communication between the community care team and the hospital but should also be able to use discretion on the patient's behalf if a large number of carers become involved. They will resume contact with patients should metastatic breast cancer develop. Many breast care nurse specialists also provide breast prosthetic and lymphoedema services.

In some breast units across the UK the traditional role of the breast care nurse, which was firmly based in the psychological care of patient with breast cancer, has developed into the nurse practitioner. This newer role incorporates the psychological care of the patient with some physical care of the patient, including the physical assessment and examination of new patients and the follow-up assessment of patients who have finished their initial treatment for breast cancer. The role of the CNS in breast care will continue to develop and respond to the changes in the care and treatment of patients diagnosed and treated for breast cancer.

Summary: Key Nursing Issues

- Nurses need to be aware that breasts have physical, social and emotional aspects and these need to be recognised when caring for a person with breast disease.
- Breasts are organs of lactation that develop in puberty under the influence of hormones. They can be subject to benign and malignant disease.
- The gold standard treatment for breast cancer incorporates a multidisciplinary approach involving surgery, radiotherapy, chemotherapy, hormonal and targeted biological therapies.
- Breast surgery and specifically breast reconstruction are continually developing areas of breast cancer treatment.

- The medical treatments for breast cancer aim to treat the local disease and act systemically for any cancer cells that have spread. These treatments are constantly under review, being researched and developed to improve their efficacy and to reduce their side-effects.
- Being diagnosed with breast cancer is a profound experience that affects individuals in different ways, taking into account that individual's context. It is a complex disease and a condition that the individual should, with good nursing care, learn to adapt their life style.

Reflection and Learning – What Next?

- **Test** your knowledge by visiting the Evolve website 🌐 and answering the multiple-choice questions and critical thinking questions.
- **Consolidate** your learning by looking at some of the further reading suggestions, references and specialist websites.
- **Revisit** some of the additional material on the Evolve website.

- **Consider** what you have learnt and how this will help your professional development.
- **Reflect** on how you can apply this knowledge to the care of your patients.
- **Discuss** your learning with your mentor/supervisor, lecturer and colleagues.

References

Alves A, Félix A, Cunha TM. Clues to the diagnosis of borderline ovarian tumours: An imaging guide. *Eur J Radiol*. 2021;143 Accessed Clues to the diagnosis of borderline ovarian tumours: an imaging guide – ScienceDirect. 25 February 23.

Amjad MT, Chidharla A, Kasi A. *Cancer chemotherapy*. Treasure Island (FL): Study Guide from StatPearls Publishing; 2020. Available at Cancer Chemotherapy – Abstract – Europe PMC.

Ammitzbøll G, Andersen KG, Bidstrup PE, et al. Effect of progressive resistance training on persistent pain after axillary dissection in breast cancer: a randomized controlled trial. *Breast Cancer Res Treat*. 2020;179:173–183.

Athey RA, Macdonald MC, Jha S. Stage of ovarian cancer at diagnosis. Does presentation as an emergency make a difference? *Eur J Obstet Gynecol Reprod Biol*. 2021;216:7–11.

Bergom C, Currey A, Desai N, Tai A, Strauss JB. Deep inspiration breath hold: techniques and advantages for cardiac sparing during breast cancer irradiation. *Front Oncol*. 2018;8:87.

Biganzoli L, Battisti NML, Wildiers H, et al. Updated recommendations regarding the management of older patients with breast cancer: a joint paper from the European Society of Breast Cancer Specialists (EUSOMA) and the International Society of Geriatric Oncology (SIOG). *Lancet Oncol*. 2021;22(7):e327–e340.

Bishop BN, Edemekong PF. Choriocarcinoma. *StatPearls*. Treasure Island (FL); StatPearls Publishing; 2023. https://www.ncbi.nlm.nih.gov/books/NBK535434/.

Blazek A, O'Donoghue C, Terranella S, et al. Impact of inequities on delay in breast cancer management in women undergoing second opinions. *J Surg Res*. 2021;268:445–451.

Bofill Rodriguez M, Lethaby A, Grigore M, Brown J, Hickey M, Farquhar C. Endometrial resection and ablation techniques for heavy menstrual bleeding. *Cochrane Database Syst Rev*. 2019;1:CD001501. doi:10.1002/14651858.CD001501.pub5.

Breast Cancer Now. Duct ectasia. 2018a. https://breastcancernow.org/about-breast-cancer/breast-lumps-and-benign-not-cancer-breast-conditions/duct-ectasia/.

Breast Cancer Now. Invasive lobular breast cancer. 2018b. https://breast-cancernow.org/about-breast-cancer/diagnosis/types-of-breast-cancer/invasive-lobular-breast-cancer/.

Breast Cancer Now. Breast cancer causes. 2018c. https://breastcancer-now.org/about-breast-cancer/awareness/breast-cancer-causes/.

Breast Cancer Now. Information and support for men with breast cancer. 2018d. https://breastcancernow.org/information-support-men-breast-cancer.

Breast Cancer Now. Hyperplasia and atypical hyperplasia. 2019a. https://breastcancernow.org/about-breast-cancer/breast-lumps-and-benign-not-cancer-breast-conditions/hyperplasia-and-atypical-hyperplasia/

Breast Cancer Now. Breast pain. 2019b. https://breastcancernow.org/about-breast-cancer/breast-lumps-and-benign-not-cancer-breast-conditions/breast-pain/.

Breast Cancer Care. Secondary breast cancer standards of care. 2019c. https://www.breastcancercare.org.uk/information-support/secondary-metastatic-breast-cancer/standards-care-secondary-breast-cancer-patients.

Breast Cancer Now. Breast Cancer Now Generations Study. 2018. https://breastcancernow.org/breast-cancer-research/research-projects/our-research-projects/breast-cancer-now-generations-study.

Breast Cancer Now. 2020. Almost one million women in UK miss vital breast screening due to COVID-19 [Press Release, September 2020]. https://breastcancernow.org/about-us/media/press-releases/almost-one-million-women-in-uk-miss-vital-breast-screening-due-covid-19.

Breidenbach C, Heidkamp P, Hiltrop K, Pfaff H, Enders A, Ernstmann N, Kowalski C. Prevalence and determinants of anxiety and depression in long-term breast cancer survivors. *BMC Psychiatry*. 2022;22(1):101.

British Gynaecological Cancer Society (BGCS). Uterine Cancer Guidelines: Recommendations for Practice, 2021. https://www.bgcs.org.uk/wp-content/uploads/2021/11/British-Gynaecological-Cancer-Society-v13-for-website-with-figure1.pdf

British Heart Foundation. UK factsheet; 2022. BHF UK CVD Factsheet. 2023. https://www.bhf.org.uk/-/media/files/for-professionals/research/heart-statistics/bhf-cvd-statistics-uk-factsheet.pdf?rev=b88610e2495b4564821ab365bd8e1b2e&hash=294E7519486335830B73739235600CE7.

British Menopause Society (BMS). Management of Menopause. 6th ed. 2017.

British Menopause Society (BMS). British Menopause Society Tool for Clinicians: NICE menopause, diagnosis and management – from guide to practice. Guideline summary. Women's health concern. 2020. https://thebms.org.uk/wp-content/uploads/2022/12/09-BMS-TfC-NICE-Menopause-Diagnosis-and-Management-from-Guideline-to-Practice-Guideline-Summary-NOV2022-A.pdf

Brown T, Cruickshank S, Noblet M. Specialist breast care nurses for support of women with breast cancer. *Cochrane Database Syst Rev.* 2021(2).

Cancer Research UK. Research may explain link between dense breast tissue and aggressive cancer. 2008. https://www.cancerresearchuk.org/about-us/cancer-news/news-report/2008-08-27-research-may-explain-link-between-dense-breast-tissue-and-aggressive-cancer.

Cancer Research UK. Risks and causes of breast cancer. 2018a. https://www.cancerresearchuk.org/about-cancer/breast-cancer/risks-causes.

Cancer Research UK. Incidence and mortality. 2018b. https://www.cancerresearchuk.org/health-professional/cancer-statistics/statistics-by-cancer-type/breast-cancer.

Cancer Research UK. Stages and grades of breast cancer. 2018c. https://www.cancerresearchuk.org/about-cancer/breast-cancer/stages-grades.

Cancer Research UK. How does smoking cause cancer? 2018d. http://www.cancerresearchuk.org/about-cancer/causes-of-cancer/smoking-and-cancer/smoking-facts-and-evidence#smoking_facts.

Cancer Research UK. Lowering your risk of lymphoedema. 2018e. Available at: https://www.cancerresearchuk.org/about-cancer/coping/physically/lymphoedema-and-cancer/lowering-your-risk.

Cancer Research UK. Lymphoedema after breast cancer treatment. 2020. https://www.cancerresearchuk.org/about-cancer/breast-cancer/living-with/lymphoedema-after-treatment.

Cancer Research UK. Cervical cancer statistics. 2022a. https://www.cancerresearchuk.org/health-professional/cancer-statistics/statistics-by-cancer-type/cervical-cancer#heading-Zero. Accessed May 2022.

Cancer Research UK. Cervix cancer: types and grades. 2022b. https://www.cancerresearchuk.org/about-cancer/cervical-cancer/stages-types-grades/types-and-grades.

Cancer Research UK. Womb cancer survival. 2022c. https://www.cancerresearchuk.org/about-cancer/womb-cancer/survival.

Cancer Research UK. Ovarian cancer mortality. 2022d. https://www.cancerresearchuk.org/health-professional/cancer-statistics/statistics-by-cancer-type/ovarian-cancer#heading-One.

Cancer Research UK. Breast cancer mortality. 2022e. https://www.cancerresearchuk.org/health-professional/cancer-statistics/statistics-by-cancer-type/breast-cancer#heading-Two. Accessed June 2022.

Carbonnel M, Karpel L, Cordier B, Pirtea P, Ayoubi JM. The uterus in transgender men. *Fertil Steril.* 2021;106(4):931–935.

Cauley JA, Nelson DA. Race, ethnicity, and osteoporosis. In: Dempster Cauley, Bouxsein, Cosman, eds. *Marcus and Feldman's Osteoporosis.* Fifth Edition. Academic Press; 2021:453–475.

Clark TJ, Gupta JK. *Handbook of Outpatient Hysteroscopy.* London: Hodder; 2005.

Daly MB, Pal T, Berry MP, et al. Genetic/familial high-risk assessment: breast, ovarian, and pancreatic, version 2.2021. NCCN Clinical Practice Guidelines in Oncology. *J Natl Compr Canc Netw.* 2021;19(1):77–102.

De Blok CJM, Wiepjes CM, Nota NM, et al. Breast cancer risk in transgender people receiving hormone treatment: nationwide cohort study in the Netherlands. *BMJ.* 2019;365:l1652.

Department of Health, 2022. 'Results of the Women's Health – lets talk about it' survey. https://www.gov.uk/government/calls-for-evidence/womens-health-strategy-call-for-evidence/outcome/results-of-the-womens-health-lets-talk-about-it-survey#:~:text=girls%20(30%25).-,Women's%20voices,mental%20health%20conditions%20(59%25).

Engbersen MP, Van Driel W, Lambregts D, Lahaye M. The role of CT, PET-CT, and MRI in ovarian cancer. *Br J Radiol.* 2021;94:1125.

Ergin G, Şahinoğlu E, Karadibak D, Yavuzşen T. Effectiveness of Kinesio Taping on anastomotic regions in patients with breast cancer-related lymphedema: a randomized controlled pilot study. *Lymphat Res Biol.* 2019;17(6):655–660.

Gathani T, Reeves G, Broggio J, Barnes I. Ethnicity and the tumour characteristics of invasive breast cancer in over 116,500 women in England. *Br J Cancer.* 2021;125(4):611–617.

Gehlert S, Hudson D, Sacks T. A critical theoretical approach to cancer disparities: breast cancer and the social determinants of health. *Front Public Health.* 2021;9:674736.

Government Equalities Office. National LGBT survey research report. 2018. https://www.gov.uk/government/publications/national-lgbt-survey-summary-report.

Grocott B, Reynolds K, Logan G, Hebbard P, El-Gabalawy R. Breast cancer patient experiences of perioperative distress and anxiety: a qualitative study. *Eur J Oncol Nurs.* 2023:102299. ISSN 1462-3889. https://doi.org/10.1016/j.ejon.2023.102299.

Haussmann J, Corradini S, Nestle-Kraemling C, et al. Recent advances in radiotherapy of breast cancer. *Radiat Oncol.* 2020;15:1–10.

Healthcare Quality Improvement Partnership (HQIP). National Audit of Breast Cancer in Older Patients. Royal College of Surgeons. 2020. https://www.hqip.org.uk/wp-content/uploads/2020/07/REF212_NABCOP-2020-Annual-Report-V1_high-res_20200702.pdf.

Home Office. Mandatory reporting of female genital mutilation: procedural information. 2015. Updated 2021. https://www.gov.uk/government/publications/mandatory-reporting-of-female-genital-mutilation-procedural-information.

Human Fertilisation and Embryology Authority (HFEA). Fertility treatment 2019: trends and figures. UK statistics for IVF and DI treatment, storage, and donation. 2021. https://www.hfea.gov.uk/about-us/publications/ . research-and-data/fertility-treatment-2019-trends-and-figures/.

Institute of Cancer Research. Effect of combined HRT on breast cancer risk likely to have been underestimated, new study finds. 2018. https://www.icr.ac.uk/news-archive/effect-of-combined-hrt-on-breast-cancer-risk-likely-to-have-been-underestimated-new-study-finds.

Jackson SS, Pfeiffer RM, Gabbi C, Anderson L, Gadalla SM, Koshiol J. Menopausal hormone therapy and risk of biliary tract cancers. *Hepatology.* 2022;75(2):309–321.

Jafari SH, Saadatpour Z, Salmaninejad A, et al. Breast cancer diagnosis: imaging techniques and biochemical markers. *J Cell Physiol.* 2018;233(7):5200–5213.

Jassim GA, Doherty S, Whitford DL, Khashan. Psychological interventions for women with non-metastatic breast cancer. *Cochrane Database Syst Rev.* 2023. https://doi.org/10.1002/14651858.CD008729.pub3.

Johnson AR, Kimball S, Epstein S, et al. Lymphedema incidence after axillary lymph node dissection: quantifying the impact of radiation and the lymphatic microsurgical preventive healing approach. *Ann Plast Surg.* 2019;82(4S):S234–S241.

Kenny L, Bickerstaff H. *Gynaecology by Ten Teachers.* 20th ed. Boca Raton: CRC Press; 2016.

Kerr H, Donovan M, McSorley O. Evaluation of the role of the clinical nurse specialist in cancer care: an integrative literature review. *Eur J Cancer Care.* 2021;30:e13415. https://doi.org/10.1111/ecc.13415.

Kho K, Shields J. Diagnosis and management of primary dysmenorrhea. *JAMA Network.* 2020;323(3):268–269. www.jamanetwork.com.

Klein DA, Paradise SL, Reeder RM. Amenorrhea: a systematic approach to diagnosis and management. *Am Fam Physician.* 2019;100(1):39–48.

Kokosis G, Chopra K, Darrach H, Dellon AL, Williams EH. Re-visiting post-breast surgery pain syndrome: risk factors, peripheral nerve associations and clinical implications. *Gland Surgery.* 2019;8(4):407.

Lee M, Soltanian HT. Breast fibroadenomas in adolescents: current perspectives. *Adolescent Health Medicine and Therapeutics.* 2015;6:159–63.

Løkkegaard ECL, Mørch LS. Tibolone and risk of gynecological hormone sensitive cancer. *Int J Cancer.* 2018;142(12):2435–2440. doi:10.1002/ijc.31267 PMID: 29349823.

Lin Y, Yang Y, Zhang X, Li W, Li H, Mu D. Manual lymphatic drainage for breast cancer-related lymphedema: a systematic review and meta-analysis of randomized controlled trials. *Clinical Breast Cancer.* 2022;22(5):e664–e673.

Liang M, Chen Q, Peng K, et al. Manual lymphatic drainage for lymphedema in patients after breast cancer surgery: a systematic review and meta-analysis of randomized controlled trials. *Medicine (Baltimore).* 2020;99(49).

London Pain Clinic. Costochondritis. 2018. https://www.londonpainclinic.com/conditions/costochondritis.

Lv L, Zhang J. The incidence and risk of infusion phlebitis with peripheral intravenous catheters: a meta-analysis. *J Vasc Access.* 2020;21(3):342–349.

Macmillan Cancer Support. 2018. Understanding secondary breast cancer booklet. https://www.macmillan.org.uk/cancer-information-and-support/stories-and-media/booklets#search-result-stories-and-media_q=Understanding%20secondary%20breast%20cancer&search-result-stories-and-media_e=0.

Martins T, Abel G, Ukoumunne OC, et al. Ethnic inequalities in routes to diagnosis of cancer: a population-based UK cohort study. *Br J Cancer*. 2022;127(5):863–871.

MBRRACE. Confidential Enquiries Into Maternal Deaths and Morbidity. Saving lives, improving mothers' care. Lessons learned to inform maternity care from the UK and Ireland Confidential Enquiries into Maternal Deaths and Morbidity 2018–20. 2022. https://www.npeu.ox.ac.uk/assets/downloads/mbrrace-uk/reports/maternal-report-2022/MBRRACE-UK_Maternal_CORE_Report_2022_v10.pdf.

Mirza M, Coleman R, González-Martín A, et al. The forefront of ovarian cancer therapy: update on PARP inhibitors. *Ann Oncol*. 2020;31(9):1148–1159.

Moodley J, Cairncross L, Naiker T, Constant D. From symptom discovery to treatment-women's pathways to breast cancer care: a cross-sectional study. *BMC Cancer*. 2018;18(1):1–11.

Mottram R, Knerr WL, Gallacher D, et al. Factors associated with attendance at screening for breast cancer: a systematic review and meta-analysis. *BMJ Open*. 2021;11:e046660. doi:10.1136/bmjopen-2020-046660.

Mutebi M, Anderson BO, Duggan C, et al. Breast cancer treatment: a phased approach to implementation. *Cancer*. 2020;126:2365–2378.

Nees LK, Heublein S, Steinmacher S, et al. Endometrial hyperplasia as a risk factor of endometrial cancer. *Arch Gynecol Obstet*. 2022;306(12); 1–15.

NHS. Breast screening: helping women decide (BSP01). 2019. www.gov.uk/government/publications/breast-screening-helping-women-decide.

NHS Choices. What is gynaecomastia? 2018. https://www.nhs.uk/common-health-questions/mens-health/what-is-gynaecomastia/.

NHS Cervical Screening Programme. Cervical screening. 2018. https://www.nhs.uk/conditions/cervical-screening/.

NICE (National Institute for Health and Care Excellence). *Menopause diagnosis and management*; 2015. https://www.nice.org.uk/guidance/ng23/resources/menopause-diagnosis-and-management-pdf-1837330217413.

NICE (National Institute for Health and Care Excellence). Osteoporosis: assessing the risk of fragility fracture clinical guidance [CG146]. 2017a. https://www.nice.org.uk/guidance/cg146.

NICE (National Institute for Health and Care Excellence). Familial breast cancer: classification, care and managing breast cancer and related risks in people with a family history of breast cancer. Clinical guideline [CG164]; 2017b. https://www.nice.org.uk/guidance/cg164.

NICE (National Institute for Health and Care Excellence). *Early and locally advanced breast cancer: diagnosis and management*. NICE guideline [NG101]; 2018a. https://www.nice.org.uk/guidance/ng101.

NICE (National Institute for Health and Care Excellence). *Intrabeam radiotherapy system for adjuvant treatment for breast cancer*. Technology appraisal guidance [TA501]; 2018b. https://www.nice.org.uk/guidance/ta501.

NICE (National Institute for Health and Care Excellence). Menopause diagnosis and management. 2018c. https://cks.nice.org.uk/topics/dysmenorrhoea/.

NICE (National Institute for Health and Care Excellence). Tumour profiling tests to guide adjuvant chemotherapy decisions in early breast cancer. Diagnostics guidance [DG34] 2018d. https://www.nice.org.uk/guidance/dg34.

NICE (National Institute for Health and Care Excellence). Menopause, diagnosis and management. NICE Guideline [NG23]. 2019a. https://www.nice.org.uk/guidance/ng23.

NICE (National Institute for Health and Care Excellence). Ectopic pregnancy and miscarriage: diagnosis and initial management NICE guideline [NG126]. 2019b. https://www.nice.org.uk/guidance/ng126.

NICE (National Institute for Health and Clinical Excellence). Heavy menstrual bleeding: assessment and management. *NICE guideline* [NG88]. 2021. https://www.nice.org.uk/guidance/ng88.

NICE (National Institute for Health and Clinical Excellence). *CKS cervical screening*; 2022. https://cks.nice.org.uk/topics/cervical-screening/.

NICE (National Institute for Health and Clinical Excellence). Cardiovascular disease: risk assessment and reduction, including lipid modification. Clinical guideline [CG181]. 2023. https://www.nice.org.uk/guidance/cg181.

Nosartis C, Roberts JV, Crayford T, et al. Early psychological adjustment in breast cancer patients: a prospective study. *J Psychosom Res*. 2002;53(6):1123–1130.

Nursing and Midwifery Council (NMC). The code: professional standards of practice and behaviour for nurses, midwives and nursing associates. 2018. https://www.nmc.org.uk/globalassets/sitedocuments/nmc-publications/nmc-code.pdf.

Offodile AC, Gu C, Boukovalas S, et al. Enhanced recovery after surgery (ERAS) pathways in breast reconstruction: systematic review and meta-analysis of the literature. *Breast Cancer Res Treat*. 2019;173:65–77.

Okita F, Abra M, Lara LAS, Andres MP, Cunha C, Oliviera Brito LG. Endometriosis in transgender men – a systematic review with meta-analysis. *J Minim Invasive Gynecol*. 2021;28(11):S103–S104.

Paramanandam VS, Dylke E, Clark GM, et al. Prophylactic Use of Compression Sleeves Reduces the Incidence of Arm Swelling in Women at High Risk of Breast Cancer-Related Lymphedema: A Randomized Controlled Trial. *Journal of Clinical Oncology: Official Journal of the American Society of Clinical Oncology*. 2022;40(18):2004–2012.

Pistelli M, Della Mora A., Ballatore Z., Berardi R. Aromatase inhibitors in premenopausal women with breast cancer: the state of the art and future prospects. *Current Oncology* 2018;25(2);168–175.

Pitman A, Suleman S, Hyde N, Hodgkiss A. Depression and anxiety in patients with cancer. *BMJ*. 2018;361:k1415.

Pondé NF, Zardavas D., Piccart M. Progress in adjuvant systemic therapy for breast cancer. *Nat. Rev. Clin. Oncol*.2019;16(1);.27–44.

Prodhan ASU, Islam DZ, Khandker SS, Jamiruddin MR, Abdullah A, Godman B, Opanga S, Kumar S, Sharma P, Adnan N, Pisana A. Breast cancer management in the era of Covid-19; key issues, contemporary strategies, and future implications. *Breast Cancer: Targets and Therapy* 2023;51–89.

Ramakrishnan S, Partricia S, Matahn G. Overview of high-risk HPVs 16 and 18 infected cervical cancer: pathogenesis to prevention. *Biomed Pharmacother*. 2015;70:103–110.

Ramseier JY, Ferreira MN, Leventhal JS. Dermatologic toxicities associated with radiation therapy in women with breast cancer. *Int J Womens Dermatol*. 2020;6(5):349–356.

Rana D, Wu O, Cheed V, et al. Uterine artery embolisation or myomectomy for women with uterine fibroids wishing to avoid hysterectomy: a cost–utility analysis of the FEMME trial. *BJOG*. 2021;128(11):1793–1802.

Ribeiro IL, Moreira RFC, Ferrari AV, Alburquerque-Sendín F, Camargo PR, Salvini TF. Effectiveness of early rehabilitation on range of motion, muscle strength and arm function after breast cancer surgery: a systematic review of randomized controlled trials. *Clinical Rehabilitation*. 2019;33(12):1876–1886.

Rossi L, Mazzara C, Pagani O. Diagnosis and Treatment of Breast Cancer in Young Women. *Curr Treat Options Oncol*. 2019;20(12):86.

Royal College of Nursing. *Female Genital Mutilation. RCN Guidance for Sexual Health Care*. London: RCN; 2020a. https://www.rcn.org.uk/-/media/Royal-College-Of-Nursing/Documents/Publications/2020/October/009-376.pdf.

Royal College of Nursing (RCN). *Women's Health Pocket Guide. Accessible via Women's Health Pocket Guide*. Royal College of Nursing; 2020b. https://www.rcn.org.uk/Professional-Development/publications/womens-health-pocket-guide-uk-pub-010-898.

Royal College of Obstetricians and Gynaecologists (RCOG). The investigation and treatment of couples with recurrent first-trimester and second-trimester miscarriage. Green-top guideline no. 17. 2011. https://www.rcog.org.uk/globalassets/documents/guidelines/gtg_17.pdf.

Ryu A, Kim T H. Premenstrual syndrome: a mini review. *Naturitas*. 2015;82(4):436–440.

Schmidt ME, Wiskemann J, Steindorf K. Quality of life, problems, and needs of disease-free breast cancer survivors 5 years after diagnosis. *Qual Life Res*. 2018;27:2077–2086.

Sobota A, Ozakinci G. "Will It Affect Our Chances of Having Children?" and Feeling "Like a Ticking Bomb" -The Fertility Concerns and Fears of Cancer Progression and Recurrence in Cancer Treatment Decision-Making Among Young Women Diagnosed With Gynaecological or Breast Cancer. *Front Psychol.* 2021;12:632162.

Simmons C., Rayson D., Joy AA, Henning JW, Lemieux J, McArthur H, Card PB, Dent R, Brezden-Masley C. Current and future landscape of targeted therapy in HER2-positive advanced breast cancer: redrawing the lines. *Therapeutic Advances in Medical Oncology.* 2022;14; p.17588359211066677.

Soteropulos CE., Tang SY, Poore SO. Enhanced recovery after surgery in breast reconstruction: a systematic review. *J. Reconstr. Microsurg.* 2019;35(09):695–704.

Tahir MT, Shamsudeen S. Mastalgia. *StatPearls [Internet].* Treasure Island (FL); 2022 Jan. Updated 1 November 2022. https://www.ncbi.nlm.nih.gov/books/NBK562195/.

Tommy's Pregnancy Hub. Baby loss statistics. 2022. https://www.tommys.org/baby-loss-support/pregnancy-loss-statistics#:~:text=Estimates%20suggest%20there%20are%20250%2C000%20miscarriages%20every%20year,pregnancy%20in%20the%20UK%20and%20Ireland%20in%202018.

Vaidya JS. Rethinking neoadjuvant chemotherapy for breast cancer. *BMJ.* 2018;360:j5913.

Weiselberg E. Menstrual considerations for transgender male and gender diverse adolescents who were assigned female at birth. *Curr Probl Pediatr Adolesc Health Care.* 2022;52(8).

White V, Farrelly A, Pitcher M, Hill D. Does access to an information-based, breast cancer specific website help to reduce distress in young women with breast cancer? Results from a randomised trial. *Eur J Cancer Care.* 2018;27:e12897. https://doi.org/10.1111/ecc.12897.

Further Reading

Alexander I, Johnson-Mallard V, Kostas-Polston E, et al. *Women's Health Care in Advanced Practice Nursing.* New York: Springer Publishing Company; 2017.

Arulkumaran S, Ledger W, Denny L, Doumouchtsis S, eds. *Oxford Textbook of Obstetrics and Gynaecology.* Oxford University Press; 2019.

Boakes E, Woods A, Johnson N, Kadoglou N. Breast infection: a review of diagnosis and management practices. *Eur J Breast Health..* 2018;14(3):136.

Chan RJ, Teleni L, McDonald S, et al. Breast cancer nursing interventions and clinical effectiveness: a systematic review. *BMJ Support Palliat Care.* 2020;10(3):276–286.

Fahad Ullah M. Breast cancer: current perspectives on the disease status. *Breast Cancer Metastasis and Drug Resistance: Challenges and Progress.* 2019:51–64.

Guillebaud J, Macgregor A, eds. *Contraception: Your Questions Answered.* Amsterdam: Elsevier; 2017.

Joe BN, Lee AY. *Breast Imaging: The Core Requisites.* 4th Edition. Elsevier; 2022.

Royal College of Nursing (2019). A Competency Framework for Nurses Providing Care to People With Breast Cancer. https://breastcancernow.org/sites/default/files/rcn_framework.pdf

Togawa K, Ma H, Smith AW, Neuhouse ML, George SM, Baumgartner KB, McTiernan A, Baumgartner R, Ballard RM, Berstein L. Self-reported symptoms of arm lymphedema and health-related quality of life among female breast cancer survivors. *Sci Rep.* 2021. https://doi.org/10.1038/s41598-021-89055-0.

Waks AG, Winer EP. Breast cancer treatment: a review. *JAMA.* 2019;321(3):288–300.

Williams N, Griffin G, Farrell V, Hauck YL. Gaining insight into the supportive care needs of women experiencing gynaecological cancer: a qualitative study. *J Clin Nurs.* 2020;29(9-10):1684–1694.

Useful Websites

Adjuvant Online, www.adjuvantonline.com, 2023
Breast Cancer Care, www.breastcancercare.org.uk, 2023
Breast Cancer Now, https://breastcancernow.org/, 2023
British Menopause Society, www.thebms.org.uk/index.php, 2023
British Gynaecological Cancer Society, www.bgcs.org.uk, 2023
Brook Advisory Services, www.brook.org.uk, 2023
Cancer Counselling, www.cancercounselling.org.uk, 2023
CoppaFeel, https://coppafeel.org/, 2023
Cancer Research UK, www.cancerresearchuk.org.uk, 2023
Cancer Research UK – About cancer, www.cancerresearchuk.org/about-cancer, 2023
ESMO clinical guidelines for gynaecological cancers, www.esmo.org/guidelines/guidelines-by-topic/gynaecological-cancers, 2023
Family Planning Association, https://www.fpa.org.uk/, 2023
Human Fertilisation and Embryology Authority (HFEA), www.hfea.gov.uk, 2023
Lymphoedema Support Network (UK), www.lymphoedema.org, 2023
Macmillan Cancer Support, www.macmillan.org.uk, 2023
Miscarriage Association, www.miscarriageassociation.org.uk, 2023
Newson LR, My menopause doctor, www.menopausedoctor.co.uk, 2023
NHS Breast Screening Programme, www.cancerscreening.nhs.uk/breast-screen/, 2023
Royal College of Obstetricians and Gynaecologists, www.rcog.org.uk, 2023
Royal Marsden NHS UK, www.royalmarsden.nhs.uk/, 2023
Women's Health Concern, www.womens-health-concern.org, 2023

9

Nursing Patients With Disorders of the Male Reproductive Systems

MARTIN STEGGALL, ANTHONY SHANAHAN

CHAPTER OUTLINE

Introduction

Any threat to an individual's reproductive capacity affects that person's body image, self-esteem and gender identity. Since these are influenced by personal attitudes, social customs and cultural background, people respond differently to such a threat. Attitudes towards sexual reproduction, underlying beliefs held and feelings experienced are influenced by cultural, social and religious values, background, lifestyle, parental and peer pressure.

Reproduction and the ability to procreate are important issues, evidenced by the incidence of subfertility in the UK and other parts of the world and the ongoing development of reproductive technologies. While the physiological aspects of reproduction are concerned with continuance of the species, the psychosocial aspects of reproduction are of significance to the feelings of health and well-being for men and women. For some people, having their own children and raising a family are key parts of their role in life. For others, these are inconsequential and for some this may be desirable but if not possible may cause unhappiness and remorse.

Disease prevention rather than disease control/treatment is an underpinning philosophy of health care. Healthcare professionals have an important role in advising and encouraging good health awareness and in facilitating and conducting screening and health monitoring. However, screening is not always possible and some conditions can be far advanced before a diagnosis is made.

When a person's quality of life (QoL) is affected by the condition, intervention is required and developments in techniques and technology mean that recovery is often much faster. Minimally invasive techniques have the advantage of a shorter general anaesthetic, or the use of conscious sedation or local anaesthetic, thus allowing some treatments to be carried out in a community care setting, in outpatients, as a day case or a shorter inpatient stay in hospital. This has consequences for nursing and patient care after treatment to adapt to the dynamic nature of nursing in a changing society.

This chapter explores areas of men's health and infertility along with disorders/conditions that can affect the testes, the penis, and sexual function (Fig. 9.1).

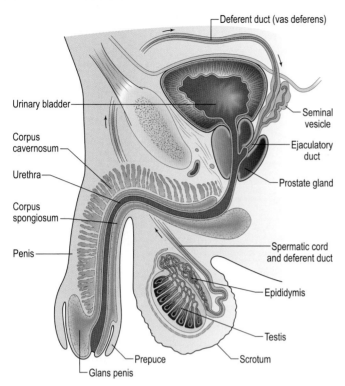

Figure 9.1 Anatomy of the male reproductive system.

Testicular Disorders

The testes (or testicles) are a pair of sperm-producing glands that maintain the health of the male reproductive system (Fig. 9.2). They are usually situated within the scrotum however, certain conditions can prevent this from occurring. There are two functions of the testes, to produce sperm for reproduction and also produce testosterone. Testosterone is an important androgenic hormone for male maturation such as growth and development of muscle mass and body hair, as well as initiating and maintaining sexual development and reproduction such as libido/sex drive and initiating erections (Fig. 9.1).

The following section will consider diseases, conditions and injuries that affect testicular function.

Undescended Testes (Cryptorchidism)

● Pathophysiology

This is a condition in which one or both testes have not descended into the scrotum within 12 months of birth. About 3% of full-term and 30% of premature male infants are born with one or both testicles undescended, and commonly the right testis is affected (Leslie et al. 2022). It may be self-correcting or require surgery in the form of orchidopexy. Normal descent keeps the testes cooler in the scrotum, which is important as this avoids germ cell degeneration caused by the higher temperature in the abdomen, which carries a risk of malignancy.

Common Signs and Symptoms. The most common sign for undescended testes is the asymmetry of the scrotum with the absence of one of the testicles. This is usually asymptomatic. The types of undescended testis are:
- a mobile testis that is normally in the scrotum but can move up and down

- an ectopic testis that does not descend from the inguinal canal into the scrotum
- an undescended testis (possibly abnormal): remains in the abdomen and fails to enter the inguinal canal and pass into the scrotum.

● Medical Management

Treatment aims to promote normal testicular function. Treatment should be completed by the boy's second year, ideally between 6 and 18 months of age before the testis starts functioning (Radmayr et al. 2023). Untreated cryptorchidism results in sterility (especially if both testes are undescended), since the cells involved in the initial development of sperm cells are destroyed by the higher temperature within the body. The testis may migrate spontaneously, or require surgical intervention in the form of an orchidopexy to bring the testis into the scrotum. During orchidopexy, the testis is fixed in the scrotum with nonabsorbable sutures to prevent the testes from migrating back into the inguinal canal (Radmayr et al. 2023).

More extensive surgery may be needed with removal of the abnormal testis (orchidectomy) and repair of an inguinal hernia if present. In addition to the risk of infertility, there is also a high risk of malignancy if the testes are left in the abdomen.

Nursing Management

Nursing assessment is required through history taking and physical examination. If the testes can be palpated within the high scrotum or inguinal canal, then surgical intervention would be recommended. Appropriately, information on the risks and benefits of the procedure can be obtained and given the patient or family. These information leaflets can be sourced from the British Association of Urological Surgeons (BAUS) or the EIDO Healthcare websites. Alternatively, if the testes cannot be palpated, then radiology imaging may be required to identify where the testes is located prior to any treatment.

Wound management advice and support would be essential to reduce chances of wound infection post procedures. This would entail conservative measures such as daily hygiene, wound dressings, skin care advice and the need for supportive underwear for promoting comfort and protection, to further advanced support such as antibiotics or topical creams if required. N.B., remember to check from the surgeons, whether the wound sutures are dissolvable or the need to be removed at a later date.

If orchidectomy procedure was performed, then providing psychological or emotional support would be required in light of the patient's body image, especially if the patient is within their adolescence years and are more aware of their body image. Some patients may benefit from insertion of a testicular prosthesis to improve their cosmetic appearance; however, this would not improve testicular function such as improve fertility.

Testicular Torsion

This is an acutely painful condition caused by the twisting of the testis on its spermatic cord resulting in obstruction to the blood supply. It may occur spontaneously or as the result of strenuous exertion. It commonly occurs in adolescents aged 10–16 years and is uncommon in men over 30 years. This condition is a surgical emergency requiring immediate treatment in accordance with the recommendation guidelines by the European Association of Urology (EAU) (Radmayr et al. 2023) for management of testicular torsion.

Figure 9.2 Anatomy of the testes. (Source: Waugh A, Grant A. Ross & Wilson Anatomy and Physiology in Health and Illness, 14th Edition. 2023. Elsevier.)

Pathophysiology

Testicular torsion results when an abnormality of the tunica vaginalis (outer, double membrane around a testis) allows increased mobility of the testis and axial rotation of the spermatic cord above. The resulting ischaemia can lead to cell damage and infection within approximately 6 hours.

Common Signs and Symptoms. There will be sudden onset of acute pain in the groin, often radiating to the scrotum and abdomen. The scrotum is swollen and red. Exercise may be the precipitating factor, but the onset of pain can also occur at rest. Nausea and vomiting are very common.

Medical Management

The patient may give a history of previous, less severe episodes which resolved spontaneously. Testicular examination may be hampered by the severity of the pain. The affected testis will be elevated, but abnormal mobility may be present in the other testis.

Immediate surgical intervention is required to relieve the torsion and secure testicular fixation. However, if the torsion is detected at an earlier stage, it may be possible by gentle external manipulation to rotate the twisted testis in the appropriate direction. This may immediately resolve the emergency, but the testis should later be surgically secured to prevent recurrence.

Nursing Management and Health Promotion: Testicular Torsion

The patient will normally be young and fit and his stay in hospital brief. Although the surgery is not considered major, the acute onset of pain and the nature of the problem may cause considerable anxiety and embarrassment. Giving the patient adequate information will help to relieve anxiety and promote recovery. He should be informed that analgesics can be given immediately and that the acute pain will cease once the operation has been performed.

Postoperatively, the patient will have a small inguinal wound and perhaps some scrotal swelling. He will normally be able to return to school or to work in about 2 weeks, at which point he should feel comfortable walking and sitting. Lifting, heavy work and sports involving running, jumping or stretching should be avoided for about 6 weeks. An athletic support should always be worn when sports activities are resumed.

The patient who has received treatment in good time should also be reassured that no impairment to sexual function or fertility will result.

Hydrocele

Pathophysiology

A hydrocele is a collection of serous fluid in the tunica vaginalis surrounding the testes. It may occur spontaneously or it may be secondary to an inflammatory condition of the testis or epididymis. The hydrocele usually occurs on one side only (although it can be bilateral), is painless and can swell to a considerable size. It may accompany a condition that causes oedema, such as congestive heart failure or nephrotic syndrome.

Common Signs and Symptoms. Hydrocele is usually asymptomatic, but an increase in scrotal size and associated discomfort will often prompt the man to seek advice. The embarrassment caused by the swelling may be such that the individual curtails or impedes social activities, swimming, sunshine holidays and sexual relations.

Medical Management

The presence of fluid within the scrotal sac makes it dull to percussion and provides a red glow on transillumination. As a hydrocele can form around a testicular cancer, the possibility of cancer should be excluded usually with an ultrasound scan (USS).

The condition may be reducible by the wearing of a scrotal support and managing this conservatively and analgesia for symptom control as and when needed. Intervention maybe required such as an aspiration under local anaesthetic, to reduce the size, although patients need to be aware that fluid can reaccumulate. Bleeding and infection are common complications, and recurrence at 6–15 weeks is also common.

For definitive treatment, surgery in the form of a hydrocele repair can be performed to ensure that the fluid cannot reaccumulate. This procedure would be done under a general anaesthetic along with its anaesthetic risks, but also surgical risks of pain (chronic and acute), swelling, bleeding and injury to testicle.

Nursing Management

Nursing assessment is required through history taking and physical examination. As mentioned earlier, the need for USS is essential to rule out any other pathology.

Appropriate information leaflets on the risks and benefits of the procedure can be obtained and given the patient or family. The benefits of surgery could consist of improved comfort, especially during activities, a boost in self-esteem and body image. Some of the risks would consist of anaesthetic complications, bleeding/bruising, infection/healing problems, swelling and recurrence.

Following surgery, there will be a wound on the scrotum with reduced scrotal size.

Wound management advice and support would be essential to reduce chances of wound infection post procedures. This would entail conservative measures such as daily hygiene, wound dressings, skin care advice and the need for supportive underwear for promoting comfort and protection.

Postoperative antibiotics is not usually required however, in some patients who are immunocompromised, such as those with uncontrolled diabetes, with transplanted organs or on chemotherapy treatments, then these patients are higher risk of infections and delayed wound healing and may benefit from prophylactic antibiotics. This could consist of antibiotics either in a tablet or topical cream. N.B., remember to check with the surgeons, whether the wound sutures are dissolvable or the need to be removed at a later date.

Varicocele

Pathophysiology

A varicocele occurs when the veins draining the testes become distended and tortuous. This may cause enlargement of the spermatic

cord. Varicoceles occur in 20% of men in the general population, with 90% of all varicoceles diagnosed occurring on the left (National Institute for Health and Care Excellence [NICE] 2023). This is caused by the draining of the right and left spermatic veins, more so the angulation that the left drains into the renal vein and the right drain directly at a less angulation into the main vena cava.

Common Signs and Symptoms. Varicoceles can be asymptomatic, but when symptomatic, the patient will describe persistent unilateral scrotal pain, where the pain is usually exacerbated after physical activities.

Palpation of the scrotum reveals a mass of enlarged varicose veins. Varicoceles are classified as (EAU 2023a):
- Subclinical – detectable only using Doppler ultrasound
- Grade 1 – (small) palpable only with Valsalva manoeuvre
- Grade 2 – (moderate) palpable without Valsalva manoeuvre
- Grade 3 – (large) visible scrotal swelling and palpable when lying down.

A persistent varicocele may raise the temperature within the scrotum due to the increased blood supply and contribute to a subfertile state (refer to Undescended Testes).

Medical Management

The dragging discomfort felt in the scrotum may be relieved by the wearing of a scrotal support and analgesia as and when required for symptom control.

If the condition is more severe or pain is not managed, then further intervention may be required such as radiological embolisation of a varicocele (BAUS) or surgery in the form of an open and microscopic repair/ligation of a varicocele (BAUS).

Nursing Management

Prior to any of these two procedures, if fertility is an issue, then semen analysis is required to check that there is sperm prior to procedure, as one of the complications of treatments is injury to the testicle.

Following radiological embolisation, there will be a small wound in the groin or neck and following open ligation, there will be a small wound at the high scrotal area. Wound management advice and support would be essential to reduce chances of wound infection post procedures. This would entail conservative measures such as daily hygiene, wound dressings, skin care advice and the need for supportive underwear for promoting comfort and protection. On the rare occurrence, further support such as antibiotics or topical creams may be required, especially in high-risk patients or immunocompromised patients. N.B., remember to check from the surgeons, whether the wound sutures are dissolvable or the need to be removed at a later date.

Epididymitis (Inflammation of Epididymis)

Pathophysiology

A bacterial infection causes acute inflammation of the epididymis. The microorganisms responsible include *Chlamydia trachomatis* and *Neisseria gonorrhoeae*, which are sexually transmitted, and *Escherichia coli*; rarely, it may be caused by *Mycobacterium tuberculosis*.

Common Signs and Symptoms. The testes are swollen, tender and painful. The man is pyrexial and may complain of general aches and pains. He may experience nausea and vomiting.

Medical Management

It is vital to rule out testicular cancer or torsion of the testes as this requires urgent surgery. Doppler ultrasound can be used to differentiate between epididymitis and testicular torsion. Conservative treatment would include bed rest, extra oral fluids, analgesia, scrotal support or elevation and possibly cold packs applied locally.

Antibiotics would be recommended for possible complications of epididymitis such as abscess development and chronic epididymitis. Other possible complications are infarction of the testis and reduced fertility.

Nursing Management

Nursing support and advice for the conservative treatments earlier would improve patient recovery and prevent any complications. No sport or overexertion activities should be performed for at least 6 weeks, but discomfort can be persistent for up to 2 to 3 months.

Orchitis (Inflammation of the Testes)

Pathophysiology

Orchitis is an inflammation of one or both testicles. It is usually caused by a bacterial and/or viral infection, especially mumps occurring after puberty.

Common Signs and Symptoms. Orchitis is usually unilateral and the testis is painful and swollen. Nausea and vomiting can occur. The complications include atrophy of the testes, and if both testes are affected, it can cause reduced fertility.

Medical Management

The inflammation usually resolves without treatment in about 10 days, but men will need the same supportive measures outlined previously for epididymitis.

Nursing Management

Conservative advice and support as previously outlined for epididymitis.

Testicular Cancer

Testicular cancer is relatively rare, with around 2400 men diagnosed within the UK each year (less than 1% of all cancers in the UK), but is the most common cancer in males aged 15–49 years, with almost 50% of those diagnosed being under 35 years of age (Cancer Research UK 2022).

It is unusual in prepubertal boys and commonly occurs in the mid-20s.

The mortality from testicular cancer has steadily declined, with over 98% of men with testicular cancer in the UK are presently cured (Cancer Research UK 2022).

Improvements in survival for men with testicular cancer have been ascribed to effective diagnosis, use of improved tumour markers, changes in surgical procedures and highly effective chemotherapy.

Pathophysiology

The risk factors implicated in the development of testicular cancer include:
- undescended testes
- orchidopexy
- inguinal hernia
- carcinoma in situ (CIS)
- testicular torsion, although trauma has not been proven to cause testicular cancer
- mumps-associated orchitis (inflammation of a testis) after puberty.

These risk factors are themselves influenced by:
- Age (see earlier) – different types of tumours occur in different age groups. For example, germ cell tumours (GCTs) are common in the 20–45-year age group and seminomas occur in men aged 35–45 years. Yolk sac tumours have been diagnosed in boys under the age of 10 years, and lymphomas are diagnosed in older men.

Common Signs and Symptoms. There is usually a lump or painless swelling in a testis, which is discovered incidentally or during testicular self-examination (TSE) (Reflection 9.1). Presentation may include:
- a lump, swelling or area of hardness in the testis
- a heavy dragging sensation or dull ache felt in the lower abdomen, anal or scrotal area
- for around 10% of men, pain is the main symptom
- present with infertility, with 6%–24% azoospermic (no sperm) and 50% oligiozospermic (low sperm count) (Moody et al. 2019).

Types of Testicular Tumours

There are several cell types in the testes, any of which may develop one or more tumour types. It is vital to differentiate between these tumour types as their prognosis and treatment differ. Testicular cancers are grouped as follows.

Germ Cell Tumours. The majority of testicular cancers (95%) develop in the germ cells (Cheng et al. 2018). There are two main types of GCTs in men – seminomas and nonseminomas – but many testicular tumours contain features of both types. The growth, spread and response to treatment of these 'mixed tumours' are such that they are regarded as being nonseminomas.

Invasive testicular germ cell cancers generally start as noninvasive CIS or intratubular germ cell neoplasia.
- **Seminoma.** Some 50% germ cell cancers of the testis are seminomas, which develop from the spermatozoa-producing germ cells of the testis. These tumours are classified as either typical (or classic) seminomas or spermatocytic seminomas. The majority of seminomas are typical. Most spermatocytic tumours grow very slowly and usually do not spread (see Chapter 31, Nursing the Patient With Cancer).
- **Nonseminoma germ cell cancer.** These tumours generally occur at an earlier age than seminomas, usually affecting young men in their 20s. Nonseminoma germ cell cancers include embryonal carcinoma, yolk sac carcinoma, choriocarcinoma and teratoma. These tumours may be mixed and involve various cell types, but all nonseminomatous germ cell cancers are treated the same way, i.e. orchidectomy followed by chemotherapy, which means that the exact histological type of this form of testicular cancer is not always important.
  - **Embryonal carcinoma.** About 20% of testicular tumours are embryonal tumours. Microscopically, these tumours can resemble tissues of very early embryos. This type of nonseminoma tends to be aggressive, increasing the likelihood of metastatic spread.
  - **Yolk sac carcinomas** (also known as endodermal sinus tumours, infantile embryonal carcinoma or orchidoblastoma). Yolk sac carcinoma is the most common form of testicular cancer in infants and young boys. When these tumours occur in young children, they are often successfully treated, but in adults, they are more dangerous, especially if they are 'pure', i.e. they do not contain other types of non-seminoma cells.
  - **Choriocarcinoma.** This is a very rare and aggressive type of adult testicular cancer. Such cancers are likely to spread rapidly to distant organs of the body.

- **Teratomas.** There are three main types: mature teratoma, immature teratoma and teratoma with malignant transformation. Mature teratomas are benign tumours formed by cells similar to cells of adult tissues. Immature teratomas are cancers that may spread to other organs.

Stromal Tumours. Cancers occurring in the stroma of the testes (supportive and hormone-producing tissues) are described as gonadal stromal tumours. The cancer can affect the Sertoli cells or the Leydig (interstitial) cells. They are uncommon cancers accounting for 4% of adult testicular cancer and 20% of childhood testicular tumours (Kapoor and Leslie 2022).

- **Sertoli cell tumours.** Sertoli cells support and nourish the spermatozoa-producing germ cells. These tumours are usually benign but once spread occurs, they are likely to be resistant to radiotherapy and chemotherapy.

- **Leydig cell tumours.** These tumours develop from the normal Leydig cells of the testis. These are the cells that normally produce androgen hormones (such as testosterone). Leydig cell tumours may develop in adults (75% of cases) or children (25% of cases). They frequently produce androgen hormones and sometimes the cancers produce oestrogens (female sex hormones). Most Leydig cell cancers do not metastasise and are cured by orchidectomy, but a small proportion do spread from the testis. Metastatic cancers have a poor prognosis, as they are not very responsive to chemotherapy or radiotherapy.

Secondary testicular cancer can result from, for example, lymphoma, colon and prostate cancers, which can metastasise to the testis. Among men over 50 years of age, testicular lymphoma is more common than primary testicular tumours, and prognosis depends on the type and stage of lymphoma (see Chapter 13). Treatment, like other forms of testicular cancer, is orchidectomy, supported by radiotherapy and/or chemotherapy.

Other cancers, for example melanoma and those of the lung and kidney, can metastasise to the testes. Prognosis is usually poor because these cancers can metastasise widely to other organs.

Disease Progression. A summary of disease progression is as follows:

- Rarely there is spontaneous regression.
- GCTs should be considered malignant.
- Lymphatic spread can occur in all types of testicular cancer.
- Local spread from the testis to the epididymis or spermatic cord can occur. This increases the chances of metastasis via the lymph or blood.
- Distant metastasis occurs from either direct blood vessel invasion or cancer cell emboli from lymphatic metastasis.

With the exception of seminoma, the growth rate among GCTs tends to be high.

🔹 Medical Management

General physical examination is undertaken along with a thorough examination of the testes. During palpation, a 'normal' testis has a smooth consistency, is mobile and is separate from the epididymis. A hard, firm or fixed area within the testis should raise suspicions and should be further investigated as a matter of urgency.

These investigations include blood assay, USS, computed tomography (CT) scan and surgical exploration. USS can exclude other testicular problems, for example hydrocele or epididymitis (inflammation of the epididymis), and should be used in all men with suspect signs/symptoms. A CT scan may be used to identify metastatic spread to lymph nodes and lung, although many patients will undergo chest X-ray to identify metastases.

Blood tests for testicular tumour markers are routinely used and they are:

- alpha fetoprotein (AFP) – produced by yolk sac cells
- lactate dehydrogenase (LDH) – a marker of tissue destruction
- β human chorionic gonadotrophin (β-hCG) – secreted by yolk-sac cells and trophoblastic cells.

The overall sensitivity of any test or marker will vary with the degree of tumour burden. Determinations of AFP and β-hCG, along with other staging modalities, help to achieve accurate staging of the tumour.

Treatment of primary tumour will involve surgery with a radical orchidectomy to remove the tumour, testicle and the spermatic cord (Cheng et al. 2018). This will be done under a general anaesthetic as a day-case procedure. Future treatment may be required such as radiotherapy and/or chemotherapy however, this is dependent on the staging and risk factors from histology, tumour markers and radiological staging.

The staging of a cancer is needed to determine the extent of spread and inform treatment choices.

There are different ways of staging testicular cancer – the number system and the tumour, nodes, metastasis (TNM) classification.

Tumour, Nodes, Metastasis (TNM) Staging. This is based on the three criteria: tumour size (T), lymph node involvement (N) and metastasis to distant sites (M). In common with the number system, each of the three TNM criteria has several stages.

- T stage – The T stage is determined after histological examination of the entire testis following orchidectomy and has five incremental stages ranging from CIS up to spread of the cancer within the scrotum:

pTis – Intratubular germ cell neoplasia (CIS)

pT1 – Tumour limited to the testis and epididymis without vascular/lymphatic invasion

pT2 – Tumour limited to the testis and epididymis with vascular/lymphatic invasion

pT3 – Tumour invades the spermatic cord with or without vascular/lymphatic invasion

pT4 – Tumour invades the scrotum with or without vascular/lymphatic invasion.

- N stage – has four stages ranging from no lymph node involvement to the presence of a lymph node >5 cm in diameter. Lymphatic spread occurs via the testicular vessels that drain to the para-aortic (close to the aorta) lymph nodes; CT scanning can be used to assess lymph node involvement:

N0 – No regional lymph node metastasis

N1 – Metastasis with lymph nodes 2 cm or less

N2 – Metastasis with lymph nodes more than 2 cm, but less than 5 cm

N3 – Metastasis with lymph nodes more than 5 cm.

- M stage – has two stages ranging from no metastasis up to spread to organs such as the liver. Early venous spread occurs, for example to the liver, lungs and bone, if early embryonic cells (trophoblasts) are present:

M0 – No distant metastasis

M1 – Distant metastasis

    M1a – Nonregional lymph node(s) or lung metastasis

    M1b – Distant metastasis other than nonregional lymph node or lung.

Treatments. Treatment modalities are:

- Surgery – partial or radical (total) orchidectomy
- Radiotherapy.
- Chemotherapy.

The cryopreservation (using extreme cold) of spermatozoa should be discussed as it must be undertaken before surgery, even if the man is expected to have unilateral orchidectomy, because subsequent chemotherapy or radiotherapy can affect his fertility. The availability of testicular prostheses must also be discussed preoperatively.

🌐 **See Evolve website Critical thinking question 9.2**

Surgical orchidectomy may be curative in early-stage testicular cancer, but the addition of chemotherapy or radiotherapy is curative in over 95% of men (Macmillan 2018).

Chemotherapy and radiotherapy can be used alone or in combination. Tumours discovered to be benign tumours need no further treatment following orchidectomy.

Usually, the survival of men with GCTs depends on the stage at presentation and therefore the quantity of tumour burden and the efficacy of later treatment choices.

A characteristic of testicular cancers that influences the usefulness of treatment is that they originate from germ cells, which are generally sensitive to radiotherapy and a variety of chemotherapeutic agents.

Decisions about treatment options will be informed by the relative advantages and disadvantages of different regimens. Successful outcomes have been ascribed to combination therapy, but accurate cancer staging and the ability to know that treatment is ineffective by using 'simple' investigations such as USS and AFP/β-hCG mean that the man's progress can be monitored and new therapy commenced quickly if necessary.

Since more than half the men with testicular tumours already have metastatic disease on presentation, it is usual for other treatment modalities to be used after orchidectomy.

Post orchidectomy, treatment is determined by tumour histology, risk factors associated with the cancer stage and the prognosis for advanced disease.

Cure rates are exceptionally good for stage 1 and 2 cancer, whatever treatment is used. However, for metastatic disease, survival is dependent on individual clinical factors and treatment choices (EAU 2023b).

Chemotherapeutic regimens frequently used in testicular cancer include a combination of bleomycin, etoposide and the platinum-based cisplatin (PEP). The use of these drugs is associated with risks, for example dose-related side-effects with bleomycin, which must be considered against the high cure rate (see Chapter 31, Nursing the Patient With Cancer). The durations of chemotherapeutic regimens depend on the class of drug prescribed.

Radiotherapy to para-aortic lymph nodes can be used in metastatic seminoma.

❖ Nursing Management and Health Promotion: Testicular Cancer

All men will have a unilateral orchidectomy, but some will need chemotherapy or radiotherapy depending on the stage of the cancer.

Nurses have an important role in the early diagnostic stages because staging of this cancer can only be made once the testis has been removed. Nurses should anticipate that men will experience major anxieties about their prognosis and recovery that will not be answered until the histology is known. Many men will experience disbelief and find it difficult to absorb and retain information

given during consultation. Consequently, nurses should plan time with these men after they have had their histology report explained to them. This allows for clarification and reiteration of points explained by their consultant/doctor. This contact can be within a clinic or by telephone. Nurse/patient conversations are best supported with literature (pamphlets).

Many men now access web-based information on a variety of health problems. This can be overwhelming and confusing, as there is a mix of semiprofessional and research literature. The nurse can recommend appropriate and reputable websites that provide more detailed information than pamphlets, for example Macmillan Cancer Support. The nurse should also explain that whilst statistics summarise populations of men, every case is unique and their treatment and care will also be unique to them. Examples of men's experiences of testicular cancer diagnosis and treatment are available at http://www.checkemlads.com/.

Nursing care comprises several phases, which include preoperative preparation, managing pain, prevention of postoperative complications such as wound infection (see Chapter 25, Nursing Patients Undergoing Surgery), and longer-term aspects including the cancer diagnosis, changes to sexual function and fertility, altered body image and health promotion (by encouraging regular TSE of the unaffected testis, see Reflection 9.1).

Postoperatively, men will need the opportunity to express feelings about having cancer and the treatment, particularly their perception of body image changes. Where appropriate, the man's sexual partner may also benefit from an opportunity to ask questions about treatment and changes to body image. The word cancer still 'strikes fear', so any cancer diagnosis will provoke fears of death, disfigurement and ability. Therefore the man experiences loss attached to the psychological self. Testicular cancer can also be coupled to fear of embarrassment because the cancer involves the genitalia and sexual function.

Surgery will not inevitably lead to reduced sexual function or fertility but there is evidence that points to changes in fertility. Moody et al. (2019) reported that men with testicular cancer had reduced fertility before and after diagnosis.

Men should understand the importance of attending follow-up appointments aimed at early diagnosis of recurrence or spread of the cancer and prompt reporting if they have signs or symptoms. If further treatment, such as chemo/radiotherapy, is required, the man and his family should be informed of the risks and side-effects. Many men will benefit from the long-term support provided by patient support groups, and information should be provided; some men may need referral to a professional counsellor.

Vasectomy

Couples who have used a range of birth control methods over the years may decide that permanent surgical sterilisation would now be preferable. Vasectomy is one of the most reliable and cost-effective permanent methods of contraception.

Preoperative Counselling

Before such a decision is taken, the couple should meet with their GP or family planning counsellor to discuss their needs and circumstances and their reasons for considering permanent sterilisation. The counsellor should provide information about both female and male sterilisation and the risks, side-effects and failure rates of the procedures available. From the patient information leaflet on vasectomy provided from the BAUS, they list some of the risk, such as swelling, bruising, blood in the semen initially, a 5% (1:20) risk of chronic testicular pain and a 0.4% risk (1:250) of an early failure rate. The long-term effects and prospects for reversal of the sterilisation should be explained. The couple should also be encouraged to consider the implications of a breakdown of their marriage or partnership, or the loss by death of one of the couple or of any existing children.

A man contemplating vasectomy may have particular anxieties about the effect of the procedure on his masculinity and sex drive. He must be assured that, as the testes will not be removed, his hormone production, virility and sex drive will be unaffected. The nature of the operation should be described with the aid of a simple diagram. He can be reassured that vasectomy is usually performed under local anaesthetic as a day case and there should be little disruption to his usual routine. Men are advised to avoid strenuous exercise for 48 hours post procedure. Initially, there may be swelling and bruising but this should soon subside. Simple analgesics such as paracetamol are usually sufficient for any mild pain/discomfort experienced. If scrotal swelling increases, pain becomes prolonged or severe or there is discharge from the incision site, the man should contact his GP or out-of-hours service.

It should be explained that eventually the ejaculate will contain no spermatozoa and that spermatozoa are still produced but are broken down and reabsorbed. However, it is essential that the man must be aware that:

- Vasectomy may be irreversible.
- There is a small risk of spontaneous late recanalisation of the deferent duct, i.e. a new canal forms, potentially resulting in unexpected conception.
- Spermatozoa may appear in ejaculate up to 3 months after vasectomy, so an alternative barrier contraception must be considered until two semen analyses have shown no spermatozoa.
- If spermatozoa persist in ejaculate, the procedure may need to be redone.

Disorders of the Penis

The penis is another organ within the male reproductive system. Its anatomy consists of three tubular muscles. There are two corpus cavernosal muscles that fill up with blood to achieve an erection for use with sexual intercourse. Below these structures is another muscle called corpus spongiosum that surrounds the urethra. The corpus spongiosum then extends distally to form the glans penis.

Surrounding these three muscles is a strong thin membrane fascia called tunica albuginea.

Superficially to tunica albuginea is the dartos layer that consists of connective tissue, nerves, dorsal veins and arteries.

These structures are then surrounded by skin which covers all of the shaft of the penis, but also retractable excess skin over the glans penis called the prepuce (foreskin).

The other function of the penis is for urination, where the bladder empties via the urethra (Fig. 9.3).

The following section will look at diseases, conditions and injuries that affect penile function.

Phimosis and Paraphimosis

Pathophysiology

Phimosis refers to a condition where tightness of the prepuce (foreskin) of the penis prevents it being retracted over the glans penis. There may be problems in passing urine or can cause discomfort on erections. Phimosis may be present at birth, but much more commonly, it is associated with repeated balanitis (see later) which leads to scarring.

Paraphimosis occurs when the prepuce can be retracted behind the glans penis but cannot be easily returned. In this situation the circulation to the glans penis is compromised, and there is pain and swelling. This requires urgent treatment as it could lead to ischaemia to tissues that can lead to necrosis and gangrene.

Importantly, paraphimosis most commonly occurs if the prepuce is not returned after patient/client hygiene or urinary catheterisation (Information 9.1).

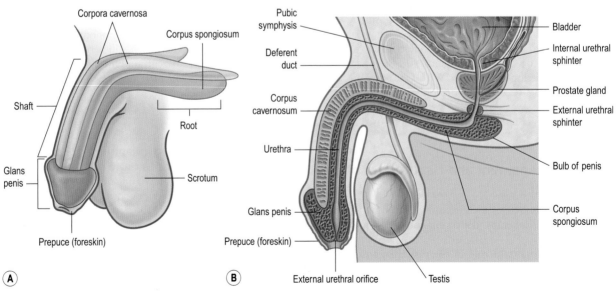

Figure 9.3 (A, B) Anatomical diagram of the penis. (Source: Waugh A, Grant A. Ross & Wilson Anatomy and Physiology in Health and Illness, 14th Edition. 2023. Elsevier.)

INFORMATION 9.1

Preventing Paraphimosis

The prepuce is routinely retracted to allow cleansing of the glans penis, limiting the chance of irritation and infection, but if it is not returned to its normal position during bed bathing or following catheterisation, paraphimosis easily occurs. Nurses must ensure that self-caring patients, healthcare assistants and other carers are aware of the importance of repositioning the prepuce after retracting it to facilitate washing and drying of the glans penis.

Nurses need to observe for signs of inflammation such as redness or swelling and report any difficulty in repositioning the prepuce.

INFORMATION 9.2

Complications of Circumcision

- Pain – requires a local anaesthetic, such as lidocaine-based gel, or systemic analgesia.
- Erection – may require a benzodiazepine to limit the likelihood of erection, e.g. diazepam.
- Oedema – the penis should remain upright; the man should wear close-fitting underwear with a nonabsorbent dressing.
- Bleeding – frequent wound checks for blood loss; excessive blood loss may require a return to theatre.
- Wound infection – observation of wound site; nature and colour of any discharge and raised temperature should be considered suspicious and reported immediately.

Medical Management

It may be possible to reduce a paraphimosis manually under local anaesthetic or light general anaesthesia. However, if this is not successful the man will need an emergency circumcision. An elective circumcision may be necessary for men with phimosis, paraphimosis or recurrent episodes of balanitis. The complications associated with circumcision include bleeding, pain and oedema (Information 9.2). Further information about phimosis, paraphimosis and circumcision is provided in Chapter 10.

Nursing Management

Skin care advice is recommended to prevent further skin breakages causing further scarring leading to progression of the tightness to the foreskin. These include daily hygiene and use of topical skin emollients to keep skin integrity and hydrated.

If the male is of sexual age, then using lubrication for any sexual activity is recommended to prevent further trauma to the foreskin.

Balanitis

The term balanitis refers to inflammation of the glans penis; if the prepuce is also involved, it is known as balanoposthitis.

Pathophysiology

The causes/contributing factors of balanitis include:
- inadequate hygiene
- bacterial infection – including some sexually transmitted infections (STIs), e.g. chlamydia, gonorrhoea
- fungal infection – candidiasis, which can be associated with diabetes (see Chapter 6, Nursing Patients With Diabetes Mellitus)

- allergy
- skin conditions
- phimosis.

Common Signs and Symptoms. There is inflammation with redness, soreness, irritation and sometimes a discharge. Balanitis associated with an STI may be accompanied by dysuria.

Medical Management

It is important to differentiate between balanitis and penile cancer (refer to later section). Treatment includes advice about hygiene – retracting the foreskin and washing the glans penis at least daily. A swab of any discharge is sent for microscopy, culture and sensitivity and the appropriate antibacterial or antifungal drug is prescribed.

If phimosis is a problem, it may be that circumcision will be needed or in severe cases, such as a buried and trapped penis, then excision of the skin with skin graft reconstruction may be required.

Further investigations should be considered if diabetes, allergy or other skin condition is suspected.

Nursing Management

Balanitis is a chronic skin condition, just like other conditions such as eczema or psoriasis, and can be managed topically to prevent the condition deteriorating. Topical creams, such as coconut oil or Bio oil, help hydrate skin and reinforce its natural barrier, but also have anti-inflammatory properties that help with any flare-up of the skin condition. Also note that topical creams will only prevent the condition from deteriorating and not reverse the skin condition.

Penile Cancer

Penile cancer is an uncommon but potentially devastating tumour for the individual, where radical treatments may have significant psychological and physical impacts on the patient's body-image, self-esteem, QoL and also their sexual function (Audenet and Sfakianos 2017).

In the UK, around 699 men during 2016 and 2018 were diagnosed with penile cancer each year (Cancer Research UK 2022). Risk factors for penile cancer include the absence of childhood circumcision, phimosis, chronic inflammation, poor penile hygiene, smoking, immunosuppression and infection with human papillomavirus (HPV) (Thomas et al. 2021).

Prevention of Penile Cancer

Prevention of penile cancer is achieved through neonatal circumcision or good personal hygiene. Circumcision needs to be performed in early childhood for the benefits of avoiding penile cancer in later life. Although circumcision is a relatively common operation, there are very few medical indications that require it. The surgery is often performed for cultural/religious reasons or because parents believe that it is more hygienic, will reduce the (already very low) risk of cancer or avoid the prospect of having to perform the surgery later.

At birth the foreskin normally adheres to the surface of the glans penis. The adhesion spontaneously separates over time, allowing mobility and retraction of the foreskin therefore circumcision is rarely required unless a phimosis is present. The foreskin should never be forcibly retracted; once the foreskin is mobile and retractile, boys should be taught how to clean the foreskin. This will further reduce the chances of developing penile cancer.

Pathophysiology

Cancer of the penis has been attributed to chronic irritation of the glans penis caused by smegma, to phimosis (see previous discussion), which makes washing difficult if the prepuce is not easy to retract, and HPV.

The incidence of penile cancer is higher where neonatal circumcision is not routinely performed. However, this is not a recommendation that all male babies be circumcised to prevent penile cancer.

Men who present with penile growths may have high anxiety about the prospect of having cancer; however, not all growths will be cancerous. Some penile tumours (usually squamous cell carcinoma) are strictly benign, whereas others have the potential to become malignant. Penile cancer is more common in men over 60 years of age, but it can affect younger men.

Most cancers develop on the glans penis or the prepuce.

Risk factors for penile cancer include:
- **Age** – penile cancer is rare below the age of 40 (Brouwer et al. 2023).
- **Premalignant lesions** – lesions appearing on the glans penis as chronic painless red or pale patches are premalignant.
- **Prepuce present** – penile cancer is rare in men circumcised at a young age. Chronic irritation with smegma and balanitis in men with inadequate hygiene are contributory.
- **HPV** – HPV wart infection. Men with HPV are more likely to develop cancer of the penis (Brouwer et al. 2023).
- **Tobacco use** – has been found to significantly and independently increase the incidence of penile cancer (as well as lung cancer).

There are several types of penile lesions. However, a key element in determining whether penile cancer is present or not is to determine the normal colours/features of the penis and what are benign lesions. This is usually achieved by referring the man to his GP, urologist or uro-oncology nurse specialist.

Types of lesions include:
- **Benign lesions** – benign tumours include linear, curved or irregular rows of conical or globular excrescences, varying from white to yellow to red, arranged along the coronal sulcus

Premalignant lesions, or more commonly known as 'Penile intraepithelial Neoplasia (PeIN)' of the glans penis or prepuce, spread locally before attacking the corpus cavernosum of the penis and the urethra (Table 9.1). There will eventually be spread into the perineum

TABLE 9.1 Premalignant Lesions of the Penis

Lesion	Incidence
Cutaneous horn of the penis	Lesions infrequently linked with squamous cell carcinoma of the penis
Bowden papulosis of the penis	
Lichen sclerosis (balanitis xerotica obliterans)	
Intraepithelial neoplasia grade III	Premalignant lesions (up to one-third will transform to invasive squamous cell carcinoma
Giant condylomata (Buschke–Löwenstein)	
Erythroplasia of Queyrat	
Bowen's disease	
Paget's disease intradermal Actinic Keratosis (ADK)	

Adapted from Hakenberg OW, Compérat EM, Minhas S, Necchi A, Protzel C, Watkin N. EAU guidelines on penile cancer: 2014 update. *Eur Urol.* 2015;67(1):142–150.

and pelvic cavity. Spread to the inguinal lymph nodes is slow, and distant spread to the liver or lungs via the blood is uncommon.

- **Viral-related lesions** – some penile lesions have been related to the HPV. Other viral-related lesions include classic Kaposi's sarcoma.
- **Squamous cell carcinoma** – squamous cell carcinoma is the most common tumour of the penis (Thomas et al. 2021) account for 95% of penile malignancies.

Medical Management

Investigations and Diagnosis. Penile cancers often present as a hard painless lump on the glans penis. The lump can be large because it may have been ignored or gone unnoticed, particularly if it is underneath the prepuce. A chronic red or pale patch on the glans warrants further investigation by a urologist.

Usually there is little doubt of the diagnosis of penile lesions, since individuals often delay seeking treatment and the lesions are clearly visible. Phimosis, or a tight prepuce, can mask colour changes in the glans penis, although other signs, such as odour, discharge and bleeding, may be present and therefore provide an indicator that a lesion exists. Delaying diagnosis allows the tumour to spread into the local lymph nodes, worsening the clinical picture due to metastasis of the tumour.

A biopsy of the affected area will confirm diagnosis and indicate the degree of invasion and spread. Most penile tumours are squamous cell carcinomas, and imaging of the inguinal lymph nodes is required to establish the degree of any metastasis, particularly if inguinal lymph nodes are palpable. The man will have, unless contraindicated, a magnetic resonance imaging (MRI) scan of the prostate and pelvis along with CT of the chest abdomen and pelvis to further investigate any lymph nodal or metastatic spread.

Staging. It is important to assess tumour grade, depth of invasion and tumour configuration since these relate to prognosis and subsequent treatment. There is no universally accepted staging of penile cancer therefore the TNM system is most commonly used.

Tumours of the penis are given a grade based on histopathological features:
- GX – grade of differentiation cannot be assessed
- G1 – well differentiated
- G2 – moderately differentiated
- G3–4 – poorly differentiated/undifferentiated.

The grade is used when determining the extent of additional treatment required; growth patterns are particularly useful in determining the 'aggressiveness' of a tumour (Brouwer et al. 2023).

Further staging can be assessed from radiological imaging, including MRI of penis, ultrasound of inguinal lymph nodes with fine-needle aspiration (FNA) and finally a CT of chest abdomen and pelvis:
- Tx – Primary tumour cannot be assessed.
- T0 – No evidence of primary tumour.
- Tis – CIS.
- Ta – Noninvasive verrucous carcinoma.
- T1 – Tumour invades subepithelial connective tissue.
    - T1a – Tumour invades without lymphovascular invasion and is not poorly differentiated.
    - T1b – Tumour invades with lymphovascular invasion or is poorly differentiated.
- T2 – Tumour invades corpus spongiosum with or without invasion of urethra.
- T3 – Tumour invades corpus cavernosum with or without invasion of urethra.

- T4 – Tumour invades other adjacent structures.
- Nx – Regional lymph nodes cannot be assessed.
- N0 – No palpable or visibly enlarged inguinal lymph nodes.
- N1 – Palpable mobile unilateral inguinal lymph node.
- N2 – Palpable mobile, multiple or bilateral inguinal lymph nodes.
- N3 – Fixed inguinal nodal mass or pelvic lymphadenopathy, unilateral or bilateral.
- M0 – No distant metastasis.
- M1 – Distant metastasis.

Treatment. Treatment options of penile cancer are dependent on the grading, the stage and also the overall fitness of the patient. The aim is removal of the tumour without loss of function.

For treatment of PeIN or premaligant tumours, chemotherapeutic agents, for example topical 5-fluorouracil or imiquimod, have been used for superficial disease, and can be applied to the glans penis and/or the penile skin.

Surgery is the gold standard treatment of penile cancer, with a better 5-year survival prognosis. There are numerous surgical procedures that are tailored to the patients staging and patient's needs/well-being. The procedures are:

- Circumcision – to treat preputial cancers.
- Excisional biopsies – to remove cancerous lesions with clear margins.
- Wide local excision – similar to an excisional biopsy but with a wide margin of clearance.
- Glans-resurfacing – to remove superficial skin layer along with the cancer and use a split skin graft reconstruction for added protection and improve wound healing.
- Glansectomy with or without neo-glans reconstruction – removal of the glans penis, but preserving the penile shaft and urethra.
- Partial or total penectomy and perineal urethrostomy – removal of part or all of the penis and urethra, with diversion of the urethra down to the perineal space between the scrotum and anus (Brouwer et al. 2023).

Radiotherapy may be considered in individuals who refuse surgery or are not fit for surgery and/or those men with metastasis who do not wish to undergo a disfiguring penectomy (amputation of the penis).

Once the primary tumour has been treated, depending on the risk factors, further investigations of the inguinal lymph nodes may be required. Penile cancer progression has a predictive pattern of metastasis, and very rarely deviates from this pathway. Penile vessels drain to the superficial inguinal lymph nodes and any cancerous spread is usually identified here first. From here, the spread will occur in the deep inguinal lymph nodes, then the pelvic lymph nodes and from there metastasis is very high to sites such as lung, liver or bones.

If lymph nodes are seen, then USS with FNA is required to confirm nodal disease. If nodal disease is confirmed, further surgery in the form of radical inguinal lymph node dissection can be performed (and/or pelvic lymph node dissection), or radiotherapy depending on the patient's input, to treat lymph nodes disease.

With some patients who have no evidence of lymph node disease, following the primary treatment, they will be categorised into low, medium and high risk or cancer recurrence. All patients within the high-risk category will be offered dynamic sentinel lymph node biopsies (DSLNBs) to ensure that there is no nodal disease, that has not been seen on radiological imaging. Patients in the medium risk will have the option of DSLNB or close surveillance with USS FNA.

Reconstructive surgery of the penis, using tissue from the forearm and an implant, is possible once there is confirmation that there is no residual cancer. The forearm site is used because it is comparatively sensitive, has little hair and is well vascularised.

If the tumour has not invaded the lymph nodes, 5-year survival rates are between 65% and 90%; however, if there is metastatic squamous cell carcinoma, 5-year survival rates fall to less than 10%.

❖ Nursing Management and Health Promotion: Penile Cancer

Changes to the colouration of the glans penis may be an incidental finding on urethral catheterisation or during routine teaching of catheter care. Discolouration should be noted and the relevant medical team informed for further advice. As the commonest presentation of penile cancer is as a painless lump, nurses should be aware that even an interview question about men's genitalia and urinary symptoms could lead to an early detection of penile cancer.

Partial or total penectomy will result in a profound change in the man's body image. The man will need time to accept the diagnosis of cancer, its implications in terms of treatment and the long-term changes that will occur in his relationship. The nurse should ensure that the man is in contact with a psychosexual counsellor and the erectile dysfunction (ED) team who will help him to cope with issues surrounding body image and sexual function that accompany penectomy. It is vital that this referral occurs as soon as possible in order to reduce the level of anxiety he and his partner will experience.

After a penectomy, men will require time to express feelings and thoughts regarding their diagnosis and treatment, especially their change in body image and sexual function.

Nurses need to be aware of the specific postoperative complications of partial/total penectomy and the nursing actions required. The complications include

- Haemorrhage – check the wound dressing and bedding for blood loss; regular vital signs observations and colour until stable.
- Infection – assess the wound for signs of infection (e.g. redness, discharge, pain) and record regular temperature measurement; ensure that urinary meatus and catheter are cleaned daily during usual hygiene.
- Oedema – a supportive dressing is used for at least 24 hours; the wound is checked daily for swelling EAU-ASCO Collaborative Guidelines on Penile Cancer (Brouwer et al. 2023)

Information 9.2 outlines the complications following circumcision.

Sexual Dysfunction

Erectile Dysfunction

ED is a common male sexual dysfunction, with an estimated incidence of 20%–40% of men in their 60s, increasing to 50%–100% of men in their 70s (Lewis et al. 2010). ED is defined as the inability of a man to get and maintain an erection that is sufficient for sexual intercourse. ED commonly has a profound negative impact on QoL in the patient and his partner, which may also impact compliance with other prescribed medications where it is known that side effects can cause ED (Steggall et al. 2021).

● Pathophysiology

The common causes of ED have traditionally been classified as either 'organic' or 'psychogenic'. Organic causes include some antihypertensive drugs, diabetes mellitus with associated acceleration of atherosclerosis, postsurgical intervention, for example following prostate surgery or radiotherapy, etc. Psychological or 'psychogenic' causes include change in body image following illness/surgery, relationship difficulty or breakdown, etc. The evidence linking ED and cardiovascular disease is incontrovertible, with risk factors for both problems including hypertension, dyslipidaemia, physical inactivity, obesity and tobacco consumption (Sarma et al. 2019).

ED can be an early manifestation of coronary artery and peripheral vascular disease and should not be regarded only as a QoL issue, but as a potential warning sign of cardiovascular disease (Pozzi et al. 2020, Zhao et al. 2019).

The introduction of phosphodiesterase type-5 inhibitors (PDE5Is), particularly sildenafil (Viagra) in 1998, encouraged some men to raise their concerns of their sexual function. Since then, sildenafil and other PDE5Is can be bought over the counter, without prescription in the UK, which may result in failure to identify the underlying cause of the problem.

Epidemiology and Aetiology. The prevalence of ED is more common as men age but is also affected by the presence of comorbidities, for example diabetes, obesity, dyslipidaemia, hypertension, depression and cardiovascular disease (Pellegrino et al. 2023). The exact effects of lifestyle and medical factors on ED still need further clarification. Potential risk factors such as smoking, hypertension, abnormal blood lipids, vascular disease and diabetes mellitus have been proposed given their effects on the cardiovascular system (Table 9.2).

A number of common medical conditions, for example diabetes mellitus and treatment for hypertension, are known to cause ED. Treatment for hypertension lowers blood pressure, therefore making it more difficult to gain an erection. Diabetes mellitus accelerates atherosclerosis, thereby narrowing arteries. Since the

corpus cavernosum of the penis is made up of small arteries, these are more likely to become blocked due to atheroma, resulting in ED.

The precise relationship between blood supply and nerve supply is unknown, but an additional key element is that of desire.

Medical Management

Currently, opinion and treatment options focus on improving penile blood flow. Clearly, any medication or medical conditions that affect arterial tone or diameter can affect the strength of the erection. Drugs implicated in the development of ED (Farmakis et al. 2022) include:

- cardiovascular – angiotensin-converting enzyme (ACE) inhibitors
  - β-blockers
  - calcium antagonists
  - centrally acting agents, e.g. methyldopa
  - digoxin
  - lipid-lowering drugs
  - thiazide diuretics
- endocrine – antiandrogens
  - luteinising hormone-releasing hormone (LHRH)
  - oestrogens
  - testosterone
- psychoactive – anxiolytics, hypnotics
  - selective serotonin reuptake inhibitors (SSRIs)
  - tricyclic antidepressants (TCAs)
- miscellaneous – carbamazepine
  - H_2-receptor antagonists
  - metoclopramide
  - all recreational drugs.

Investigations and Diagnosis. The diagnosis of ED is often determined by the patient himself although careful questioning is needed to differentiate between premature ejaculation (PE) and ED or other forms of sexual dysfunction. For example, a man who ejaculates very early may describe loss of erection rather than PE. Although treatment for PE can include PDE5Is, these tend to shorten post-ejaculatory recovery time (PERT) rather than manage the underlying problem. The inability to penetrate is frequently the main precipitating factor, but it needs to be elicited whether this is because the penis is not firm or because the man has already ejaculated. If the former, then it is likely to be ED; if the latter, it is likely to be PE. Some practitioners may find that completing one of the erectile function assessment scores – for example the 5-item International Index of Erectile Function (IIEF) (Rosen et al. 1999) – can help in establishing the severity of ED, and this is a recommendation in both the British Society of Sexual Medicine (BSSM) (Hackett et al. 2018) and EAU guidelines (EAU 2023c).

A thorough organic and psychogenic assessment is required to determine the type of ED and inform subsequent treatment choices (Table 9.3). Both the BSSM 2017 and EAU 2023 guidelines recommend laboratory testing of serum lipids, fasting plasma glucose and haemoglobin A1c (HbA1c), unless there is already a clinical diagnosis of cardiovascular disease and/or diabetes mellitus, as well as a focused clinical examination (EAU 2023c). Serum testosterone, taken between 08:00 and 11:00 (because this is when testosterone 'peaks'), and prostate-specific antigen (PSA) (if clinically indicated) also form part of the guidance notes. Depending on results, treatment can be commenced. If low testosterone is detected, referral to secondary care (endocrinology or urology) for further investigation or commencement of testosterone supplementation should be considered.

TABLE 9.2	Organic and Psychogenic Risk Factors for Erectile Dysfunction
Examples of Organic Factors	**Examples of Psychogenic Factors**
• Diabetes mellitus • Smoking • Excessive alcohol consumption • Hypertension • Antihypertensive and other drugs (SSRIs, NSAIDs, finasteride, antiepileptics) • Post myocardial infarction • Following urological treatment, e.g. radical prostate surgery • Chronic renal failure • Renal dialysis and following renal transplant • Neurogenic causes/diseases (e.g. multiple sclerosis, Parkinson's disease) • Hypogonadism (with reduced libido) • Spinal injury • Pelvic injury • Arterial insufficiency	• Stress • Depression • Low mood • Anxiety • Bereavement • Relationship difficulties • Negative sexual experiences • Pressure to perform • Fear of failure • Iatrogenic • Personality

Adapted from Dick B, Reddy A, Gabrielson AT, Hellstrom WJ. Organic and psychogenic causes of sexual dysfunction in young men. *Int J Med Rev.* 2017;4(4):102–111. https://doi.org/10.29252/IJMR-04040.

TABLE 9.3	Assessment for ED	
Assessment	**Rationale**	**Implication for Treatment**
Surgical history	Clues to organic causes of ED, i.e. damage to nerves or blood supply, or altered body image	Changes to blood supply or nerve damage
Changes to blood supply or nerve damage	Clues to organic causes of ED, i.e. specifically assessing whether there is known physiological dysfunction	Changes to blood or nerve damage
Current medication	Clues to organic causes of ED, i.e. antihypertensives commonly worsen the quality of an erection	Check for contraindications to any treatment for ED
Allergies	Interaction with treatment	Interaction with treatment
Tobacco	Assess vascular damage	Give lifestyle advice as needed
Alcohol (and/or illicit drugs)	Desensitises the individual to stimulation	Potential to effect success of treatment
Specific History		
Description of the problem	Is it erection failure, loss of desire or premature ejaculation? What is the duration of problem?	Guides management and treatment
Gradual or sudden onset?	Organic or psychogenic causes?	Gradual suggests organic causes whereas sudden onset suggests psychogenic causes
Early morning or nocturnal tumescence	Functionality of blood and nerve supply	If tumescence is present, this suggests that the blood flow/nerve supply is intact, and point to potential psychology causation
Libido	Assess desire for sexual activity	Often absent in long-term ED; can be endocrine related
Is penetration possible?	Assess strength of erection	Assesses blood flow; may indicate 'strength' of medication required
Current sexual relationship	Need to know if there is some sexual activity	Absence of intimacy is important – for the medication to work, some type of sexual stimulation is required
Psychological Factors		
Social problems (particularly prior to onset of problem)	Anxieties inhibit function	Feelings of 'impotence' in other areas will be reflected in sexuality – need to resolve underlying problem
Performance anxiety	Maintains problem	Break cycle of failure/restore confidence
Does the partner know of their visit?	Status of relationship	Address unresolved issues with both partners

ED, Erectile dysfunction.
Adapted from Steggall M, Mohammed I, Jones K, et al. Management pathways for erectile dysfunction in primary care. *Pract Nurs.* 2021;32(1):2-6.

Treatment. The common treatment options are summarised in Table 9.4. The efficacy can be variable and dependent on frequency of dosing and the strength of the medication.

The estimated efficacy is approximately:
- 70% for PDE5Is (there is some variation in efficacy between the PDE5Is)
- up to 50% for medicated urethral system for erections (MUSE) (pellets)
- 90% for intracavernosal injections
- 90% for vacuum devices
- 40% for alprostadil cream.

Evidence suggests that 8%–12% of treatment failures respond to a second or third PDE5I (NICE 2019); thus, swapping to alternative PDE5Is may be beneficial.

❖ Nursing Management and Health Promotion: Erectile Dysfunction

ED is a common problem for men. There is a strong association between vascular disease and erection failure, and therefore, all men with cardiovascular risk factors are at risk of ED. The key to treatment is that of communication; men do not know which words to use to broach the subject, and are therefore hopeful that it will be discussed at some point during their care. An excellent opportunity for raising the profile of ED is simply to have a poster in the waiting/clinical area, with advice to talk to a GP or clinical nurse specialist about the problems. To facilitate conversation, perhaps during a medication review or when giving patients tablets to take away (TTAs), it is useful to make a comment such as 'Some men who are taking blood pressure/diabetic medication, or who have had a recent stay in hospital, can have trouble with their sex lives. If you find that you experience problems, talk to your GP or ask to be referred to a clinical nurse specialist who deals with this problem.'

Priapism

Priapism is a rare urological emergency characterised by an abnormal and often painful erection that persists beyond, or is unrelated to, sexual stimulation, for which prompt recognition and management are fundamental to preventing long-term complications (Bullock et al. 2018). Detumescence is achieved by aspirating one of the corpora with a butterfly cannula. For further information, refer to EAU (2023c) Sexual and Reproductive Health.

Ejaculation Dysfunction

This section outlines PE and retrograde, delayed or absent ejaculation.

TABLE 9.4	Summary of Treatments Available for Erectile Dysfunction		
Treatment	Dosage Guide	Contraindications	Mode of Action
Avanafil	100 mg initially, then dose adjust depending on response. Range is 50–200 mg as needed.	Concurrent use of nitrates; recent myocardial infarction, unstable angina or stroke; ischaemic optic neuropathy, hypotension; do not use with nicorandil (lowers BP), some antibiotics and grapefruit juice	Phosphodiesterase type 5 inhibitor, increases blood flow to the penis
Sildenafil citrate (Viagra)/sildenafil	25–100 mg, need 6–10 doses before benefits seen; regular dosing helps to reduce performance anxiety	As above	As above
Tadalafil (Cialis)	10–20 mg, need 6–10 doses before benefits seen; regular dosing helps to reduce performance anxiety; Tadalafil 2.5–5 mg daily dosing	As above	As above
Vardenafil (Levitra)	5–20 mg, need 6–10 doses before benefits seen; regular dosing helps to reduce performance anxiety	As above	As above
Medicated urethral system for erections (MUSE): intraurethral alprostadil (prostaglandin E₁)	250–1000 μg, essential to massage the intraurethral medication for up to 10 minutes	Sickle cell disease, or bleeding disorders	Increases blood flow to the penis
Vitaros (contains alprostadil)	3 mg/g applied to the tip of the penis. Takes 5 to 30 minutes to work	As above	As above
Intracavernosal injection of alprostadil (prostaglandin E₁) – Caverject, Caverject dual chamber or Viridal Duo	2.5–60 μg, essential to provide full teaching of injection technique and support/discuss patient anxieties	Warfarin, bleeding disorders	Increases blood flow to the penis
Vacuum devices	Important to teach correct technique and reinforce that the vacuum needs to be inflated slowly	None, but must be competent to remember to remove the constriction ring within 30 minutes	Nonpharmacological, drawing blood into the corpus cavernosum under pressure. Blood held in place by constriction band
Surgery (prostheses)	Various prostheses available	Depends on fitness for surgery	Prosthesis – artificial implants replace the corpus cavernosum. Erection then possible 'on demand'
Psychosexual therapy (behavioural programme with counselling of underlying issues)	Weekly or regular attendance with 'homework'	Lack of acceptance, culturally unacceptable	Breaks pattern of failure, removes anxiety and restores confidence

BP, Blood pressure.
Adapted from Steggall M, Mohammed I, Jones K, et al. Management pathways for erectile dysfunction in primary care. *Pract Nurs.* 2021;32(1):2-6; see also NICE (National Institute for Health and Care Excellence). Erectile dysfunction: alprostadil cream. 2014a. https://www.nice.org.uk/guidance/esnm50 (alprostadil) and NICE (National Institute for Health and Care Excellence). Erectile dysfunction: avanafil. 2014b. https://www.nice.org.uk/guidance/esnm45 (avanafil).

Premature Ejaculation

PE is usually defined according to the International Society of Sexual Medicine (ISSM) (Althof et al. 2014, American Psychiatric Association 2013) and American Psychiatric Association (APA), which both require the three criteria of (i) short ejaculatory latency (called 'intravaginal ejaculatory latency time', or IELT), (ii) perceived lack of control over ejaculation and (iii) presence of distress due to the condition (Colonnello et al. 2022). Recent definitions have sought a more inclusive definition. For example, Sansone et al. (2021) suggest definitions that include (i) a persistent and recurrent subjective perception of loss of control over the mechanism of ejaculation in the presence of proper erotic stimuli; (ii) a subjective, PE-related, distress induced in the patient and in the partner; and (iii) a short IELT, subjectively perceived and partner perceived (PIELT and PPIELT, respectively), or objectively (SIELT) measured as being lower than 180s, that could also be

applied to other sexual stimuli, such as masturbation (evaluating MELT) or oral (valuating OELT) and anal (evaluating AELT) intercourses, as well to nonheterosexual settings.

Medical Management

Diagnosis. The features considered in a diagnosis of PE are:
- When PE started (onset) or how long it has been happening (duration) – has the man always had PE (lifelong) or did it start sometime after he became sexually active (acquired)? Is it secondary to an infection in the prostate (e.g. prostatitis)?
- When does it happen – is it a generalised occurrence (in every situation) or situational (occurs in some situations but not in all)?

The normal estimated ejaculatory latency time (ELT) range is from 6.9 minutes to 13.6 minutes after vaginal penetration.

Treatment. The treatment options for PE are behavioural therapies (after Masters and Johnson 1970), lidocaine or lidocaine-based creams or sprays, constriction devices that compress the urethra, desensitising bands (Jan Wise and Watson 2000), SSRIs or atypical antidepressants or TCAs (Martin-Tuite and Shindel 2020, Qin et al. 2019).

Behavioural therapies involve solitary and/or mutual masturbation, which can present the participant with particular religious/cultural problems; therefore, behavioural therapy programmes can be unsuccessful. The use of SSRIs has been extensively reported to markedly delay ejaculation from baseline levels (EAU 2023c). However, they do not produce long-term benefit in all men: often, the individual returns to pretreatment ELT levels on cessation of medication.

Delayed, Retrograde or Absent Ejaculation

Delayed or anejaculation may be lifelong or acquired, situational or persistent (Gray et al. 2018). Men with lifelong delayed ejaculation have always had difficulty, whereas men with acquired anejaculation previously had little or no trouble. Situational means that the circumstance influences whether the man can ejaculate, which may be linked with pressure to perform or other factors. Causes of delayed ejaculation have been suggested as inadequate sexual stimulation or a decreased sensation linked with penile neuropathy.

Anything that interferes with the mechanisms of ejaculation, for example damage to the peripheral sympathetic nerve supply, can cause delayed ejaculation. Pharmacological delays can be a result of using SSRIs, for depression as an example, although other medicines such as alpha blockers, opioids and benzodiazepines are also thought to have an impact on ejaculation (Gray et al. 2018).

Retrograde ejaculation, where semen is discharged into the bladder, can occur following prostate, bladder or testicular surgery and is associated with diabetic neuropathy (see Chapter 6, Nursing Patients With Diabetes Mellitus).

Treatment for delayed ejaculation includes behavioural therapy and psychotherapy. Alternative strategies include the use of vibro-tactile stimuli to bombard the pudendal nerve increasing the amount of stimulation, which may also allow ejaculation. Irrespective of cause, however, treatment is difficult. If fertility becomes the main issue, alternative methods of semen harvest are possible (see Infertility). Individuals are not always necessarily infertile.

CULTURAL AWARENESS IN REPRODUCTIVE HEALTH

Socioeconomic factors and liberal attitudes to expression of beliefs and values have encouraged people from all over the world to settle in the UK. Whilst this has resulted in vibrant multicultural societies, people moving between cultures will inevitably bring aspects of their own culture with them, including practices and beliefs that shape their approach to their way of life. It is important that nurses are aware of how the attitudes of people from different cultural backgrounds influence their approach to sexuality and reproductive health.

Communication can be a challenge if English is not the patient's first language. Although family members may be able to speak English as their mother tongue, it is not appropriate to use them as interpreters. Previously, children have often been used when discussing reproductive health issues or intimate problems however, it can be intensely embarrassing for the patient to reveal these details to their offspring during a consultation. In addition, if there are any tensions between a couple, the nurse cannot be sure that all appropriate information is communicated. Consequently accredited interpreters should be used who have an understanding of health and treatments.

Physical examination of a patient's reproductive system can involve intimate procedures such as rectal or testicular examination which can be intensely embarrassing. Often a same-gender health professional will be requested and clinicians should respect these wishes and do their utmost to support these requests. Sometimes, due to pressures on available medical staff, this may not be possible and this should be explained to the patient.

Nurses and other healthcare professionals must ensure that they adopt an open and nonjudgemental attitude towards all patients/clients. They need to develop a rapport quickly during relatively brief interactions in order to provide reassurance and support. Whilst this is important for all patients, it is particularly relevant for men and women from different cultural backgrounds. The nurse should have a good awareness of cultural aspects and, whilst they may not have an in-depth knowledge of particular cultural beliefs, they should know what resources they can access when required.

Providing information, advising and counselling people who have different beliefs, values and attitudes concerning health issues from those of the health professionals providing help and support require care and sensitivity. Understanding and empathy can help nurses to appreciate what others consider to be important. A balance is required between giving sound advice and respecting the social, cultural and religious views of others.

Summary: Key Nursing Issues

- Reproductive structures and function are very closely linked to an individual's feelings of self-worth, attractiveness and sexuality.
- Reproductive tract conditions and subsequent examination and investigation can be acutely embarrassing. Embarrassment may cause the individual to delay seeking help.
- People may present in a very emotional state. The nurse must adopt a sensitive and nonjudgemental attitude at all times. Often, the nurse will have to discuss intimate details with the person at the first meeting and so must be able to establish a rapport and trust quickly, thereby ensuring that patients feel comfortable and able to discuss their issues and anxieties.
- The nurse is required to have a good level of knowledge underpinning their practice so that they are able to give explanations in a way the patient understands but also to provide answers to any queries the patient may have. It is unrealistic to expect the nurse to be able to deal fully with all queries but they must know how to access further information and be able to direct the patient to recognised websites providing accurate up-to-date information.
- Privacy and dignity of the patient are particularly key whilst carrying out nursing procedures. Procedures should be conducted in a private area where there will be no interruptions as this will help the patient to relax, reducing the discomfort of any procedures.
- Nursing patients with reproductive system disorders can be challenging but is extremely rewarding, particularly when the nurse has contributed to improving the patient's QoL.

Reflection and Learning – What Next?

- **Test** your knowledge by visiting the Evolve website 🌐 and answering the multiple-choice questions and critical thinking questions.
- **Consolidate** your learning by looking at some of the further reading suggestions, references and specialist websites.
- **Revisit** some of the additional material on the Evolve website.

- **Consider** what you have learnt and how this will help your professional development.
- **Reflect** on how you can apply this knowledge to the care of your patients.
- **Discuss** your learning with your assessor/supervisor, lecturer and colleagues.

References

Althof SE, McMahon CG, Waldinger MD, et al. An update of the International Society of Sexual Medicine's guidelines for the diagnosis and treatment of premature ejaculation (PE). *J Sex Med.* 2014;11(6):1392–1422.

American Psychiatric Association. *Diagnostic Criteria From DSM-V.* Washington, DC: American Psychiatric Association; 2013.

Audenet F, Sfakianos J. Psychosocial impact of penile carcinoma. *Transl Androl Urol.* 2017;6(5):874–878.

Brouwer OR, Albersen M, Parnham A, et al. European Association of Urology-American Society of Clinical Oncology collaborative guideline on penile cancer: 2023 update. *Eur Urol.* 2023;83:548–560.

Bullock N, Steggall M, Brown G. Emergency management of priapism in the United Kingdom: a survey of current practice. *J Sex Med.* 2018;15(4):476–479.

Cancer Research UK, Testicular Cancer; 2022. http://www.cancerresearchuk.org.

Cheng L, Albers P, Berney DM, et al. Testicular cancer. *Nat Rev Dis Primers.* 2018;4(1):29.

Colonnello E, Sansone A, Zhang H, Zhang Y, Jannini EA. Towards a universal definition of premature ejaculation. *J Sex Med.* 2022;19(12):1717–1720.

Dick B, Reddy A, Gabrielson AT, Hellstrom WJ. Organic and psychogenic causes of sexual dysfunction in young men. *Int J Med Rev.* 2017;4(4):102–111.

European Association of Urology. Kitrey ND, Djakovic N, Hallscheidt P, et al. Urological Trauma. *Eur Accoc Urol.* 2021. https://uroweb.org.

European Association of Urology. Paediatric Urology. Eur Accoc Urol. 2023a. http://www.uroweb.org.

European Association of Urology. *Guidelines on Testicular Cancer.* European Association of Urology. EAU Guidelines – Uroweb; 2023b.

European Association of Urology. Guidelines on Sexual and Reproductive Health; 2023c. http://www.uroweb.org.

Farmakis IT, Pyrgidis N, Doundoulakis I, Mykoniatis I, Akrivos E, Giannakoulas G. Effects of major antihypertensive drug classes on erectile function: a network meta-analysis. *Cardiovasc Drugs Ther.* 2022;36(5):903–914.

Gray M, Zillioux J, Khourdaji I, Smith RP. Contemporary management of ejaculatory dysfunction. *Transl Androl Urol.* 2018;7(4):686–702.

Hackett G, Kirby M, Wylie K, et al. British Society for Sexual Medicine guidelines on the management of erectile dysfunction in men—2017. *J Sex Med.* 2018;15(4):430–457.

Jan Wise ME, Watson JP. A new treatment for premature ejaculation: case series for a desensitising band. *Sex Relation Ther.* 2000;15(4):345–350.

Kapoor M, Leslie SW. Sex cord stromal testicular tumor. Updated 28 November 2022. *StatPearls [Internet].* Treasure Island (FL): StatPearls Publishing; 2022 Jan. https://www.ncbi.nlm.nih.gov/books/NBK558916/.

Leslie SW, Sajjad H, Villanueva CA. Cryptorchidism. *StatPearls [Internet].* StatPearls Publishing; 2022.

Lewis RW, Fugl-Meyer KS, Corona G, et al. Definitions/epidemiology/risk factors for sexual dysfunction. *J Sex Med.* 2010;7(4 pt 2):1598–1607.

Macmillan. Treatment for testicular cancer. 2018. https://www.macmillan.org.uk/information-and-support/testicular-cancer.

Martin-Tuite P, Shindel AW. Management options for premature ejaculation and delayed ejaculation in men. *Sex Med Rev.* 2020;8:473.

Masters WH, Johnson VE. *Human Sexual Inadequacy.* Boston, MA: Little Brown; 1970.

Moody JA, Ahemd K, Yap T, Minhas S, Majid S. Fertility management in testicular cancer: the need to establish a standardized and evidence-based patient-centric pathway. *BJU Int.* 2019;123(1):160–172.

NICE (National Institute for Health and Care Excellence). Erectile dysfunction: alprostadil cream. 2014a. https://www.nice.org.uk/guidance/esnm50.

NICE (National Institute for Health and Care Excellence). Erectile dysfunction: avanafil; 2014b. https://www.nice.org.uk/guidance/esnm45.

National Institute for Health and Care Excellence. Scenario: Management of erectile dysfunction. 2019. https://cks.nice.org.uk/erectile-dysfunction#!scenario.

NICE (National Institute for Health and Care Excellence). Varicocele. 2023. Health topics A to Z. CKS. NICE. https://cks.nice.org.uk/topics/varicocele

Pellegrino F, Sjoberg DD, Tin AL, et al. Relationship between age, co-morbidity, and the prevalence of erectile dysfunction. *Eur Urol Focus.* 2023;9(1):162–167.

Pozzi E, Capogrosso P, Boeri L, et al. Longitudinal risk of developing cardiovascular diseases in patients with erectile dysfunction-which patients deserve more attention? *J Sex Med.* 2020;17:1489.

Qin Z, Wang Y, Zhu J, et al. Safety and efficacy characteristics of oral drugs in patients with premature ejaculation: a Bayesian network meta-analysis of randomized controlled trials. *Int J Impot Res.* 2019.

Radmayr C, Bogaert G, Dogan HS, et al. *Paediatric urology.* European Association of Urology; 2023. https://uroweb.org.

Rosen RC, Cappelleri JC, Smith MD, Lipsky J, Peña BM. Development and evaluation of an abridged, 5-item version of the International Index of Erectile Function (IIEF-5) as a diagnostic tool for erectile dysfunction. *Int J Impot Res.* 1999;11(6):319–326.

Sansone A, Aversa A, Corona G, et al. Management of premature ejaculation: a clinical guideline from the Italian Society of Andrology and Sexual Medicine (SIAMS). *J Endocrinol Invest.* 2021;44:1103–1118.

Sarma AV, Hotaling JM, de Boer IH, et al. Blood pressure, antihypertensive medication use, and risk of erectile dysfunction in men with type I diabetes. *J Hypertens.* 2019;37(5):1070–1076.

Steggall M, Mohammed I, Jones K, et al. Management pathways for erectile dysfunction in primary care. *Pract Nurs.* 2021;32(1):2–6.

Thomas A, Necchi A, Muneer A, et al. Penile cancer. *Nat Rev Dis Primers.* 2021;7(1):11.

Zhao B, et al. Erectile dysfunction predicts cardiovascular events as an independent risk factor: a systematic review and meta-analysis. *J Sex Med.* 2019;16:1005.

Further Reading/Information Sites

European Association of Urology (EAU), https://uroweb.org/
British Association of Urological Surgeons (BAUS), https://www.baus.org.uk/
British Association of Urology Nurses (BAUN), https://www.baun.co.uk/
NHS Health A-Z Topics, https://www.england.nhs.uk/ourwork/a-to-z/
Testicular Cancer UK, https://www.testicularcanceruk.com

10

Nursing Patients With Urinary Disorders

ANTHONY SHANAHAN, MARTIN STEGGALL

CHAPTER OUTLINE

Introduction

This chapter begins with a brief overview of the anatomy and physiology of the urinary system and of the male reproductive organs. With respect to the latter, this chapter complements the anatomy and physiology described in Chapter 9 on the reproductive systems. Common disorders of the kidneys and the rest of the urinary tract and their treatment and nursing care are then described, including infections, significant renal disorders, obstructive disorders and disorders of the bladder. With regard to the male urinary system and reproductive organs, only prostatic disorders and conditions primarily affecting the urethra are considered here. Conditions more directly affecting reproductive and sexual function, such as erectile dysfunction (ED) and testicular cancer, are discussed in Chapter 9.

Anatomy and Physiology

The urinary system comprises the kidneys, the ureters, the urinary bladder and the urethra. Its function is to excrete the waste products of metabolism in the form of urine.

The Urinary Tract

The Kidneys

The kidneys are paired organs that lie on the posterior abdominal wall, extending from the 12th thoracic vertebra to the 3rd

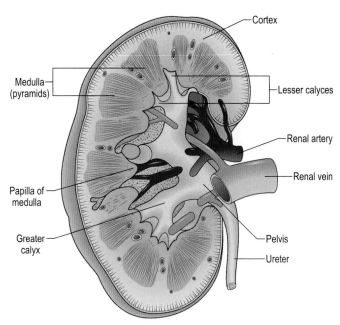

Figure 10.1 Longitudinal section of the right kidney.

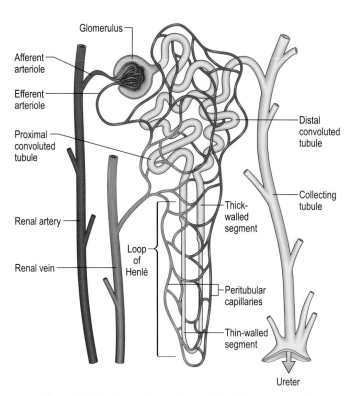

Figure 10.2 Nephron with long loop of Henlé (deep nephron).

lumbar vertebra. Because of the position of the liver, the right kidney is normally slightly lower than the left. Three layers of supportive tissue surround each kidney: an inner fibrous capsule, a middle fatty layer and an outer fascia. This fatty encasement is necessary for maintaining the kidneys in their normal position. Beneath this, a dark outer cortex surrounds a paler medulla, which consists of pale conical striations called the renal pyramids (Fig. 10.1).

At the hilus, i.e. the concave medial border of the kidney, blood vessels, lymph vessels and nerves enter and leave the organ. Medial to the hilus is the flat, funnel-shaped renal pelvis, which is continuous with the ureter leaving the hilus. Extending from the pelvis into the medulla are the cup-shaped calyces; these receive from the renal papillae the urine that has been formed in the nephrons and has passed through the collecting tubules. From the calyces the urine passes into the renal pelvis, which acts as a reservoir.

Each kidney receives approximately 625 mL of blood per minute from branches of the renal artery (the two kidneys receive around 25% of cardiac output) and are a key organ in maintaining homeostasis with the functions of:

- production of urine by glomerular filtration, reabsorption (selective) of substances needed by the body, such as glucose, and tubular secretion of waste products and other substances in order to maintain fluid, electrolyte and acid–base balance
- control and maintenance of fluid balance (see Chapter 21, Maintaining Fluid, Electrolyte and Acid–Base Balance)
- maintenance of acid–base balance (see Chapter 21)
- control and maintenance of electrolyte balance (see Chapter 21)
- renin production – initiates the renin–angiotensin–aldosterone system concerned in the control of blood pressure (see Chapter 21)
- erythropoietin production, a hormone that stimulates red blood cell production in the bone marrow (erythropoiesis)
- control of calcium reabsorption and vitamin D hydroxylation.

The Nephron

The functioning units of the kidneys are the nephrons, of which there are two types: cortical and juxtamedullary. The cortical nephrons have their glomeruli in the cortex and have short loops of Henlé, and the juxtamedullary nephrons, with long loops of Henlé, are located in the medulla. Eighty-five per cent of the nephrons are cortical.

A nephron comprises a convoluted tubular system and a tuft of capillaries known as the glomerulus (Fig. 10.2). The glomerulus is enclosed in the cup-shaped upper end of the tubule (glomerular or Bowman's capsule). The tubule has three sections: the proximal convoluted tubule (PCT), the loop of Henlé and the distal convoluted tubule (DCT). The DCTs merge to form straight collecting tubules; these ultimately terminate at the renal papillae.

Blood Supply

The renal arteries (see earlier) branch into smaller and smaller vessels, ultimately becoming wide-bore afferent arterioles which lead into the glomeruli. These capillaries then merge again to form a narrower-bore efferent arteriole which leaves the capsule and subdivides into a second network of peritubular capillaries which supply the renal tubule, and a specialised capillary network (the vasa recta) associated with the loop of Henlé. The capillaries merge into venules and then veins, eventually joining the renal vein, which in turn flows into the vena cava.

Formation of Urine

The first process in the production of urine is *filtration*. Arterial blood arriving in the wide-bore afferent arteriole enters the glomerulus within the Bowman's capsule, where substances that are between 3 and 7 nanometres can pass through holes in the capsule endothelium called fenestrations. Note that in health, blood cells and large molecules such as proteins with a molecular weight of 69,000 or above do not pass through the glomerular filtration barrier into the tubule. Once inside the body of Bowman's capsule, the material that has been filtered, which is called filtrate, enters the first section of the PCT, which is the main site of *reabsorption* in the nephron. To maintain a flow of blood into the glomerulus, and therefore to maintain filtration, blood must enter at a constant pressure and constant volume. This is achieved by two structures that line the afferent arteriole, the macula densa and the juxtaglomerular apparatus (JGA). When the blood volume and pressure fall, perhaps as a result of blood loss during surgery, the diameter of the arteriole is reduced, thereby maintaining perfusion pressure. This situation cannot last, i.e. the arteriole cannot continue to get smaller because this would limit the kidney's ability to remove waste products and maintain fluid balance. The constriction of the arteriole is achieved by release of renin. Renin combines with angiotensinogen to form angiotensin I, which is converted by angiotensin-converting enzyme (ACE) into angiotensin II, which is a strong vasoconstrictor. In addition, it stimulates the release of aldosterone (a hormone from the adrenal cortex), which promotes sodium reabsorption, which therefore enhances water reabsorption (see Chapter 21). This, in conjunction with antidiuretic hormone (ADH; also known as arginine vasopressin (AVP) or vasopressin), helps to increase water reabsorption and water intake, and accounts for the fact that urine would normally be expected to be concentrated, i.e. have a specific gravity towards 1.035, in states where fluid loss and dehydration had occurred (see Chapter 21).

Further material covering kidney function – glomerular filtration, selective reabsorption and tubular secretion – is available on the companion website.

See also Patton (2018) in Further Reading.

The functions occurring in the nephron have been summarised in Table 10.1.

TABLE 10.1	Summary of Processes Occurring in the Nephron
Location in the Nephron	**Processes**
Proximal convoluted tubule (PCT)	The PCT is the site of most selective reabsorption – the vast majority of filtrate is reabsorbed in the PCT. Specifically, specialised cells that line the PCT reabsorb water (H_2O), electrolytes including bicarbonate ($HCO3-$), glucose and other substances, returning them to the circulation via the vasa recta. Substances such as the waste products urea and creatinine are not reabsorbed as they need to be excreted. At the end of the PCT the filtrate contains water, waste and some electrolytes.
Loop of Henlé	The cells change their structure in the loop of Henlé, allowing selective reabsorption of water and sodium (Na^+).
Distal tubule (DCT)	Sodium and chloride (Cl^-) can be reabsorbed here. The hormone aldosterone facilitates the reabsorption of sodium (and with it water) and chloride, but the hormone ADH is required for any reabsorption of water. The cells of the DCT are also concerned with the reabsorption and/or secretion of hydrogen (H^+) and potassium (K^+) ions into the filtrate. This last process, known as tubular secretion, is vital in the maintenance of acid–base balance.
Collecting duct	Once the filtered fluid gets to the collecting ducts, only in exceptional circumstances can water and sodium chloride (NaCl) be reabsorbed. ADH is required to make the collecting ducts more permeable to water in order to produce concentrated urine.

The Ureters

Urine is conveyed from the pelvis of each kidney to the bladder via the ureters (Fig. 10.3). The ureters are tubular structures approximately 25–30 cm long, ranging in diameter from 2 to 8 mm at various points along their length.

Each ureter descends behind the peritoneum from the kidney to the bladder and comes obliquely through the bladder wall before opening into the bladder cavity on its posterior inner surface. This arrangement is such that, when the bladder fills or empties, it is compressed, closing the distal ends of the ureters; in this way, there is no backflow into the ureters.

Each ureter is composed of three layers of tissue:
- an outer fibrous layer
- a middle layer of smooth muscle; contraction of the muscle layer produces peristaltic movement of urine along the ureter into the bladder
- an inner mucosa of transitional epithelium (urothelium).

The Bladder

The bladder is a muscular sac which acts as a reservoir for urine before it is expelled from the body. It lies behind the peritoneum in the pelvic cavity, with its anterior surface located just behind the symphysis pubis. In males, the bladder lies in front of the rectum and is superior to the prostate gland and the urethra. In

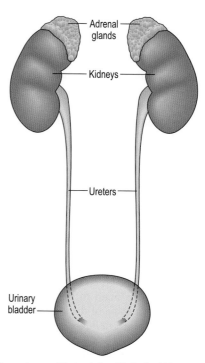

Figure 10.3 The ureters and their relationship to the kidneys and the bladder.

Ureters

Opening
of ureters

Trigone of
bladder

Urethral orifice

Figure 10.4 The trigone of the bladder.

females, it lies just anterior to the uterus and the superior section of the vagina.

The bladder is composed of four layers:

- an outer fibrous adventitia (except where the peritoneum covers the superior surface)
- a muscular layer consisting of smooth muscle arranged in inner and outer longitudinal layers and a middle circular layer
- a submucosal layer of connective tissue
- a mucosal layer of specialised transitional epithelium.

The muscle layer is called the *detrusor* and is an exceptionally strong muscle that contracts during micturition (passing urine). The interior of the bladder has three orifices, two for the ureters and one for the opening of the urethra. This forms a triangle called the trigone (Fig. 10.4).

The nerve supply to the bladder is both sensory and motor. Sympathetic nerves arise from T9 to L2 and parasympathetic and somatic nerves from S2 to S4. The motor innervation involves the parasympathetic supply to the detrusor muscle and the sympathetic supply to the trigone. Pudendal nerves under voluntary control supply the external sphincter and muscles of the perineum.

In adults the normal bladder holds around 200–400 mL of urine before the urge to pass urine becomes too great. However, in some patients this volume can be more than 1 L. This is often caused by a blockage in the urinary system or some nerve damage to the spinal cord that controls the bladder. If patients are unable to control the bladder, renal failure can ensue if pressure (i.e. volume) is allowed to build in the bladder.

Micturition is a complex process that involves exchange of nerve information from the brain to the detrusor, coordinating muscle contraction and opening of the internal and external urinary sphincters, so that urine can flow down the urethra.

Babies are incontinent because the nerve supply from the bladder to the spinal cord is incomplete until the age of around 2 years. This is referred to as the spinal reflex arch.

The Urethra

The urethra is the tube that carries the urine from the bladder to the outside world. It has an outer layer of smooth muscle continuous with that of the bladder. Beneath this lies a thin, spongy layer supplied with blood vessels, lymph vessels and nerves. The innermost layer is a lining of mucous membrane continuous with that of the bladder.

In males, the urethra is around 20–25 cm long, has several curves and must pass through the prostate gland. In addition to carrying urine, the male urethra also carries semen. It has an internal sphincter composed of smooth muscle which responds to parasympathetic and sympathetic stimulation. The external urethral sphincter lies at the point where the urethra leaves the prostate; this sphincter is composed of skeletal muscle and is hence under voluntary control.

The female urethra is approximately 3–4 cm in length, is straight and is not involved in reproduction. It runs behind the symphysis pubis, opening at the external urethral orifice (the meatus) located between the clitoris and vagina. The passage of urine from the bladder through the urethra is governed by two sphincter muscles. At the opening from the bladder is an internal sphincter composed mainly of elastic tissue and smooth muscle and controlled by autonomic nerves. Near the external urethral orifice, the smooth muscle is replaced by striated muscle to form an external sphincter under voluntary control.

The Male Reproductive Organs

The male reproductive organs are those structures responsible for the production, maturation and delivery into the female reproductive tract of spermatozoa necessary for the fertilisation of secondary oocytes (immature ova). The essential organs of this system are the two testes, in which spermatogenesis (spermatozoa production and maturation) occurs (Fig. 10.5). The accessory organs which support the reproductive process include:

- ducts – the epididymis, deferent ducts (vas deferens), ejaculatory ducts and urethra, which convey spermatozoa to the exterior
- glands – the seminal vesicles, the prostate gland and the bulbo-urethral (Cowper's) glands, which produce fluid as a vehicle for sperm
- supporting structures – the scrotum, penis and spermatic cords (see Fig. 10.5).

The Testes

The testes are paired oval organs suspended in the scrotum by the spermatic cords and are encased in three layers of tissue. The complex two-stage process of spermatogenesis (*spermatocytogenesis* – production of haploid spermatids, and *spermiogenesis* – a maturation stage) required to produce mature viable spermatozoa takes place in the testes. The testes also produce androgens (masculinising hormones), the most important of which is testosterone, which is produced by interstitial cells (Leydig's cells). Testosterone promotes:

- maleness and male sexual behaviour
- the development and maintenance of male secondary sex characteristics and the functions of the accessory structures
- protein anabolism
- growth of bone and skeletal muscle and closure of the bony epiphyses
- a mild stimulant effect on the kidney tubule, with reabsorption of sodium and water and excretion of potassium

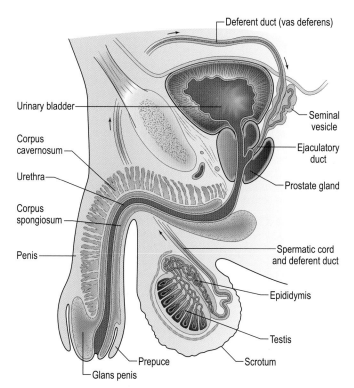

Figure 10.5 Section of male reproductive structures. *Arrows* show the structures through which the spermatozoa pass.

- inhibition of anterior pituitary secretion of the gonadotrophins follicle-stimulating hormone (FSH) and interstitial cell-stimulating hormone (ICSH). FSH stimulates the seminiferous tubules of the testes to produce spermatozoa. A negative feedback mechanism operates whereby when testosterone levels are high, FSH and ICSH production is inhibited.

The Ductal System

The epididymis is the first part of the ductal system and forms a collection of tubules arising from the testis. The deferent duct (vas deferens), which is continuous with the epididymis, loops through the inguinal canal and joins the ejaculatory ducts, which pass through the prostate gland and lead into the urethra. Spermatozoa undergo further maturation as they pass through the ductal system before ejaculation. They remain in the deferent duct (vas deferens) for varying periods of time, depending upon the frequency of ejaculation.

The Accessory Glands

The seminal vesicles secrete a thick, nutritive alkaline fluid that mixes with sperm on ejaculation. This fluid accounts for 30% of the volume of the seminal fluid and contains fructose and protein, which are essential to sperm motility and metabolism.

The prostate gland is a lobulated structure which lies in the pelvic cavity in front of the rectum and behind the symphysis pubis, surrounding the uppermost part of the urethra. It is palpable on rectal examination. The prostate gland secretes a thin, milky, alkaline fluid that makes up 60% of the seminal fluid; this fluid creates an environment more hospitable to sperm by giving protection from the normally acidic environment of the male urethra and female vagina. A neutral or slightly alkaline medium also increases sperm motility.

The prostate begins to enlarge after the age of 40 years, which, because the urethra passes through it, can lead to obstructive urinary symptoms, such as difficulty passing urine (poor flow), getting up at night to pass urine and emptying the bladder.

The bulbourethral glands are two pea-sized glands opening onto either side of the urethra. They produce a lubricating alkaline mucus that is expressed into the urethra during ejaculation, further reducing its typically acidic state, and contribute less than 5% to the volume of seminal fluid.

The Supporting Structures

The penis is a pendulous, soft tissue structure with a root and a body. There is erectile tissue supported by fibrous tissue and covered with skin. The three elongated masses include the corpus spongiosum containing the urethra, and two parallel columns, the corpora cavernosa, which provide the organ's main structural support.

The expanded distal end of the penis, the glans penis, surrounds the urethral meatus. The covering of skin folds upon itself at the glans penis to form a movable double layer called the prepuce.

The scrotum is divided into two compartments and each contains one testis, one epididymis and the testicular end of the spermatic cord. The temperature of the testes is 2–3°C below body temperature, which helps to preserve sperm viability.

Spermatic cords Leading from each testis is a spermatic cord consisting of a testicular artery, a testicular venous plexus, lymph vessels, a deferent duct (vas deferens) and nerves.

DISORDERS OF THE URINARY SYSTEM

This section covers a range of investigations and disorders of the kidney and other parts of the urinary system. The nursing management is discussed along with an outline of the medical and surgical treatment. Readers who require more detail about treatment are directed to Further Reading suggestions, for example National Institute for Health and Care Excellence (NICE), Renal or Ureteric Colic (2020); NICE Urinary Tract Infection (Lower) Men (2023); and NICE Urinary Tract Infection (Lower) Women (2023).

General Investigations of the Renal and Urinary Tract

Disorders of the renal and urinary system can be detected using various tests and investigations. Some pathologies, for example prostate enlargement and prostate cancer, have similar signs and symptoms, and therefore in practice, multiple tests and investigations can be used to aid diagnosis. The common tests and investigations have been divided into those testing urine (Table 10.2), those testing blood (Table 10.3) and those that examine the structure of the urinary tract (Table 10.4). Other investigations used include computed tomography (CT) scan, magnetic resonance imaging (MRI) scan and radionuclide studies.

Urinary Tract Infections (UTIs)

UTIs are a common problem across the lifespan; they are more common in females than males, except in the neonatal period. For most patients with a normal urinary tract, UTIs are easily treated

TABLE 10.2	Urine Tests	
Type of Test/Investigation	Indication/Associated Pathology	Significance of Findings
Urinalysis a. Specific gravity (SG) b. Glucose c. Blood d. Protein e. Nitrites and/or leucocytes f. Ketones	All	a. Range 1.001–1.035 indicates degree of hydration b. Glycosuria may indicate diabetes mellitus, use of corticosteroids. If positive result, need fasting blood glucose c. Haematuria indicates infection, calculi, renal damage, tumour. A positive result for blood warrants further (specific) investigation. d. Proteinuria or albuminuria indicates infection or renal damage; further investigation, e.g. MSU, needed e. Indicates urinary tract infection (UTI) f. Ketonuria indicates breakdown of fats and suggests starvation or possibly uncontrolled diabetes mellitus; further (specific) investigations needed
Midstream urine (MSU) or catheter specimen of urine (CSU)	UTI – cystitis, acute pyelonephritis and chronic pyelonephritis (reflux nephropathy) Prostatic enlargement Renal failure	Detects presence of infection; ensure aseptic technique to avoid contaminants and false-positive results. Microbiological examination of the specimen will indicate the presence of and the types of infective organism
24-hour urine analysis, e.g. calcium, phosphate, oxalate	Urinary calculi	Measures the substances excreted in the urine in different types of urinary calculi
Urine cytology	Bladder cancer	Detects presence of tumour cells. Not diagnostic but used in combination with other tests
Urinary flow rate	Prostatic enlargement/cancer	Determines the speed of bladder emptying, volume voided and time taken to empty the bladder. Used to determine the extent of prostate/urethral compression
Postvoid residual volume	Urinary retention/prostatic enlargement	Determines the volume of urine in the bladder

TABLE 10.3	Blood Tests	
Type of Test/Investigation	Indication/Associated Pathology	Significance of Findings
Urea and electrolytes (U/Es)	All	Elevations in urea and creatinine indicate decreased renal function
Full blood count (FBC)	All	Low haemoglobin may indicate blood loss; anaemia. Increase in white cell count may indicate infection
Serum creatinine clearance (used to estimate glomerular filtration rate) 🌐 See Evolve website Fig. 10.1	Renal failure and conditions affecting renal function, e.g. diabetic nephropathy	Estimate of renal function. Monitoring patients with reduced renal function
Erythrocyte sedimentation rate (ESR)	Nephritis	Nonspecific test that detects inflammation/infection Erythrocytes sediment more quickly in individuals in whom disease is present
Prostate-specific antigen (PSA) (a screening test, also used to monitor response to treatment of prostatic cancer)	Prostatic cancer	PSA result <4 ng/mL is within normal range; PSA result 4–10 ng/mL indicates an intermediate risk of prostate cancer; PSA >10 ng/mL indicates a high risk of prostate cancer

by antibiotic therapy, although early identification and treatment of patients with complicated infections are essential.

UTIs are defined as an inflammatory response of the urothelium (cells lining the urinary tract) to bacterial invasion that is usually associated with bacteriuria and pyuria, and can be divided into complicated and uncomplicated infections (European Association of Urology (EAU) 2023).

Normally, the urine does not contain bacteria; the presence of bacteria in the urine is termed bacteriuria. Bacteriuria can be symptomatic or asymptomatic. Pyuria is the presence of pus (white blood cells [WBCs]) in the urine, indicating an inflammatory response of the urothelium to bacterial invasion. Bacteriuria without pyuria suggests bacterial colonisation not infection. Pyuria without bacteriuria warrants evaluation for renal

TABLE 10.4	Tests of Urinary Tract Structure/Function	
Type of Test/ Investigation	Indication/ Associated Pathology	Significance of Findings
Intravenous urogram/ pyelogram (IVU/IVP)	Renal failure, calculi, recurrent urinary tract infection (UTI), trauma	Indication of structural abnormality or obstruction
Urethrogram; endoscopy: urethroscopy, cystoscopy, nephroscopy	Calculi, obstruction	Indication of presence of calculi or mass
X-ray or ultrasound (U/S, USS) of kidneys, ureter and bladder (KUB)	Prostate, calculi, UTI	Imaging of renal tract may indicate presence of calculi
Biopsy	Kidney, prostate, bladder	Diagnostic for pathology, e.g. cancers, causes of renal failure, types of glomerular disease, etc. Determines the stage of the disease

TABLE 10.5	Classification of Common Urinary Tract Infections by Site	
Site	Type of Infection	Causes/Signs
Kidney	a. Acute pyelonephritis b. Chronic pyelonephritis (reflux nephropathy)	a. Chills, fever, flank pain; accompanied by bacteriuria and pyuria b. Chronic bacterial infection of the kidney associated with vesicoureteric reflux (VUR) (reflux of infected urine from the bladder into the ureters); causes scarring on the kidney
Bladder	Cystitis	Dysuria (pain on passing urine), frequency, urgency, cloudy urine that may have a strong odour and sometimes haematuria, suprapubic or back pain. There is inflammation of the bladder which can be bacterial or non-bacterial
Urethra	Urethritis	As cystitis but it is inflammation of the urethra

tuberculosis, stones or cancer. Infections are generally defined clinically by their presumed site of origin.

Most bacteria enter the urinary tract through the urethra into the bladder (NICE 2018). This is enhanced in individuals with significant soilage of the perineum with faeces and patients with intermittent or indwelling catheters. Depending on the location of the infection, there are further classifications of UTI (Table 10.5).

Recurrent UTIs are commonly due to reinfection or bacterial persistence; reinfection is especially common in women.

Pathogens

Most UTIs are caused by facultative anaerobes (bacteria that can grow in the presence or absence of oxygen) that generally come from bowel flora.

The most common cause of UTIs is the bacterium *Escherichia coli*, accounting for 85% of community-acquired and 50% of hospital-acquired infections. Other gram-negative Enterobacteriaceae include *Proteus mirabilis* and *Klebsiella* and gram-positive *Enterococcus faecalis* and *Staphylococcus epidermidis*.

Hospital-acquired infections are frequently caused by *E. coli* and *E. faecalis* as well as by *Enterobacter*, *Klebsiella* and *P. aeruginosa*.

In patients with diabetes mellitus, the most common infection is by *Klebsiella* spp.; less common organisms such as *Gardnerella vaginalis*, *Mycoplasma* spp. and *Ureaplasma urealyticum* may infect patients with intermittent or indwelling catheters.

Defences Against UTI

The main defences against infection are the flow of urine and the acidity of urine. Normally, urine is acidic, which inhibits bacterial growth. In addition, the urine contains urea and organic acids that make the conditions less favourable for bacterial survival. Other factors that protect against UTI include the antibacterial effects of bladder mucosa, as well as neutrophils and the cytokines interleukin IL-6 and IL-8.

For women, the vaginal flora is an important host defence against UTI since it is an acidic environment. Lactobacilli make up the majority of the vaginal flora in healthy, premenopausal women; sexual intercourse, use of antibiotics and intravaginal antimicrobials can reduce the normal lactobacillus-dominant vaginal flora, increasing susceptibility to UTI. One way in which to reduce the likelihood of getting a UTI after sexual activity is to pass urine after intercourse.

Pyelonephritis

Pyelonephritis, or inflammation of the renal pelvis and renal tissue, may occur in one or both kidneys. Bacteria may enter the urinary tract, especially the kidneys, via the bloodstream or, more commonly, the bladder. Most organisms causing UTI – *E. coli*, *Klebsiella* spp., *Proteus*, *Pseudomonas*, *E. faecalis* and *S. epidermidis* (*S. albus*) – are found in the bowel and the perineum. There are two types of pyelonephritis, acute and chronic (often called reflux nephropathy as it can result from vesicoureteric reflux (VUR)), but the presenting features are different (see Table 10.5).

Investigations for Acute Pyelonephritis

- Determine whether a pyrexia is present and/or loin pain.
- Collect a midstream specimen of urine (MSU) for microscopy examination, culture for evidence of a causative organism and antibiotic sensitivity (a dipstick urine test is not needed and

should not be undertaken in people with an indwelling urinary catheter or who are over 65 years of age (NICE 2023).

If symptoms are very severe, admission to hospital may be required.

Treatment of Acute Pyelonephritis

The main aim of treatment is to eradicate the infection by means of antibiotic therapy. This may be commenced even before organism sensitivities are known but should only be commenced *after* the MSU has been taken. A more specific antibiotic can then be used following urine culture results. The selection of the antibiotic will be determined by the prescriber, although as a guide, in women who are *not* pregnant, men and people with an indwelling urinary catheter, suitable antibiotics include ciprofloxacin, co-trimoxazole, trimethoprim, co-amoxiclav or cefalexin. Pregnant women cannot take trimethoprim as it a folate antagonist and therefore cefalexin is currently recommended (refer to Clinical Knowledge Summary, https://cks.nice.org.uk/topics/pyelonephritis-acute/). In addition, analgesics, antiemetics and antipyretics may also be prescribed. Oral fluids are recommended, up to 3 L/24 h.

Further investigations may be needed to identify the underlying cause of the condition. Where inflammation persists, renal impairment may progress to end-stage renal failure requiring treatment by dialysis.

Investigations for Chronic Pyelonephritis (Reflux Nephropathy)

- Collect an MSU for microscopy examination, culture for evidence of a causative organism and antibiotic sensitivity. A full blood count, C-reactive protein (CRP) and urea and electrolyte estimation are needed. A raised WBC count and erythrocyte sedimentation rate (ESR) may be revealed in response to *E. faecalis* and *S. epidermidis* infection. CRP may be raised.
- An ultrasound scan (U/S, USS) or CT urography (CTU) is performed to exclude any obstruction or abscess formation in the urinary tract (Information 10.1).
- Specific investigations to demonstrate the presence of VUR, for example a micturating cystogram.

Cystitis

Cystitis may be chronic or acute and is characterised by severe inflammation of the bladder walls. More commonly affecting women, cystitis may also result from predisposing factors such as the presence of foreign bodies or stones, obstruction, tuberculosis, carcinoma in situ, chronic urinary infection and schistosomiasis (disease caused by trematodes or flukes). Features of cystitis include burning on micturition, urinary frequency and urgency, and possibly incontinence. The results of MSU may be needed to treat any infection, although there is no need to wait for the results before commencing antibiotic therapy. Persistent infections warrant further investigations, for example renal tract USS, flexible cystoscopy, uroflow studies and postvoid residual volume scan, and may be treated with long-term antibiotic therapy or intravesical therapy. A key feature in treatment should be increased fluid intake to help 'flush' the urinary system. In addition to increasing fluid intake, there is a range of self-help measures available to women who suffer from recurrent cystitis, for example attention to personal hygiene, passing urine frequently during the day and not 'holding on', emptying their bladder just before going to bed, etc. (Reflection 10.1, Evidence-Based Practice 10.1). Nurses providing information to patients should

---

INFORMATION 10.1

Intravenous Urogram or Pyelogram (IVU/IVP)

This investigation, which involves the intravenous injection of an iodine-based contrast agent which is then excreted by the kidneys, allows a series of X-ray images of the kidneys, ureters and bladder to be taken.

The IVU radiograph may demonstrate a variety of pathologies:
- absence of kidney
- congenital abnormalities affecting the urinary tract, e.g. duplex ureter, horseshoe kidney
- renal trauma
- obstruction of the kidney, e.g. a large calculus in the renal pelvis, or scarring from repeated UTIs caused by VUR
- obstruction of the ureter – within the lumen, in the wall or arising from outside the ureter, such as late-stage cervical cancer
- irregularities of the bladder wall – causes include bladder cancer, calculi, diverticulum (an abnormal pouch in the wall) or a foreign body.

Before, During and Following an IVU

Where there are no contraindications, the patient is given a laxative to clear the bowel and thus ensure a clear image of the contrast agent on the X-ray. The patient may be requested to abstain from food and fluids for a period of time before the start of the X-ray examination. The patient should void beforehand to make sure that the contrast agent remains concentrated as it is excreted into the ureter and bladder, thus providing high-quality images. Voiding just beforehand is also important for patient comfort as the examination can take 40–60 minutes. Prior to the intravenous injection of the contrast agent, a control X-ray of the kidneys, ureters and bladder (KUB) is taken. Patients should be informed that some people experience a warm feeling and some may be aware of a metallic taste in their mouth following the administration of contrast agent; they can be reassured that it is short-lived. Rarely patients have an allergic reaction to the iodine-based contrast agents; they should tell the radiographer at once if they have difficulty breathing or their skin feels itchy. Following the investigation, the patient is allowed to eat and drink again. The contrast medium will be passed when the patient voids urine, with no after-effects or change in the colour of the urine.

Note: In some situations such as an emergency (e.g. suspected kidney trauma), the examination can be undertaken without withholding fluid.

---

be aware that cranberry juice may possibly increase the action of coumarin anticoagulants, for example warfarin.

Obstructive Disorders of the Urinary Tract

There are many disorders that cause obstruction to the flow of urine, for example prostate enlargement, strictures, stones/calculi or tumours (Fig. 10.6). Although the early stages may cause only mild symptoms that are easily ignored, the progressive damage caused by abnormal pressure, infection and stone formation can lead to renal failure. The importance of early detection and intervention cannot be overemphasised.

Urinary Stones (Renal Calculi)

The formation of stones or calculi in the urinary tract can be as a consequence of increased salt and protein consumption and there is an association between stone formation and a number of common conditions such as diabetes, hypertension, cardiovascular disease and chronic renal trouble (Stamatelou and Goldfarb 2023). In addition, malnutrition and dehydration can also cause stone formation as concentrated urine can enable particles in the urine to clump together. Renal stones are more common in men than in women (M:F = 3:1).

Pathophysiology
Urinary calculi are generally formed by more than one substance fusing together from mineral crystal deposits in the urine (Wang et al. 2021) and the main types of stone are calcium oxalate,

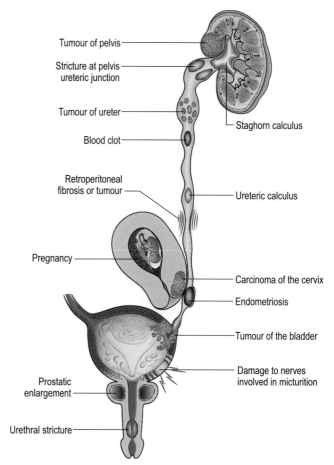

Figure 10.6 Conditions causing obstruction to the urinary tract.

although other compositions of stone occur. The risk factors for developing calculi are stasis of urine, chronic urinary infection and excess excretion of stone-forming substances. The most common presenting feature is pain and haematuria, caused by movement of the calculi, although this is not a universal symptom. Stones lodged in the renal pelvis (e.g. 'staghorn' calculus) tend to be immobile and so the presenting features are UTI and pyrexia.

See Evolve website Fig. 10.2

Medical Management and Treatment
Stones less than 10 mm in diameter may pass unobstructed through the urinary tract and be excreted in the urine. In some cases an alpha-blocker (e.g. tamsulosin) can be used to aid the passing of a stone. Increasing fluid intake to increase fluid output is not recommended in the acute phase of management because it will result in further distension of the urinary system; a normal fluid intake should be encouraged. For further information see Further Reading (e.g. NICE 2020, Reynard et al. 2019, Stamatelou and Goldfarb 2023).

Management of Acute Renal Colic
Information about investigations is provided in Tables 10.2, 10.3 and 10.4.
The patient with renal stones may be acutely ill, suffering from excruciating pain arising in the loin and radiating to the groin (and the testis or labium), which can last 5–6 hours. Pain is caused by small calculi being moved along the ureter by peristaltic

INFORMATION 10.2

Stenting

The stents used by most surgeons are called 'double-J' or 'pigtail' stents and have small holes down most of the length of their tubing. These stents are self-retaining and must be removed endoscopically.

Some surgeons use an infant feeding tube as a stent following pyeloplasty (reconstructive surgery on the renal pelvis), pyelolithotomy or ureterolithotomy (removal of a stone from the renal pelvis and ureter respectively). Infant feeding tubes are self-retaining to a degree, but the patient will need a urethral catheter in situ to keep the tube in place.

When the catheter is removed, the patient may pass the feeding tube without intervention. If this does not happen within 24 hours, endoscopic removal will be required.

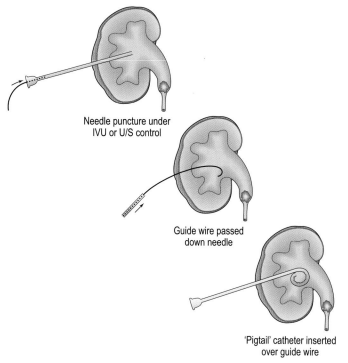

Needle puncture under IVU or U/S control

Guide wire passed down needle

'Pigtail' catheter inserted over guide wire

Figure 10.7 Percutaneous nephrostomy.

movements, by impaction and by obstruction of urine. Bed rest, warmth to the site of pain (Conway et al. 2018) and analgesics are the first line of treatment.

Nonsteroidal anti-inflammatory drugs (NSAIDs), if not contraindicated, by any route should be offered as first-line treatment, possibly with an alpha-blocker to aid the passing of the stone. If NSAIDs are contraindicated, intravenous paracetamol should be offered. Opioids should only be offered if NSAIDs and intravenous paracetamol are contraindicated or have not been effective. Muscle relaxants should not be offered. Nausea may be relieved by an antiemetic such as intramuscular (IM) prochlorperazine.

Flush-Back of Calculi and Stenting (Information 10.2). This procedure affords temporary relief when a calculus causes obstruction and pain in the ureter. The stone is flushed back to the pelvis of the kidney. A small silicone tube called a stent is positioned in the ureter from the pelviureteric junction (PUJ) to the bladder. This stent is left in position to hold the stone in place. Further treatment to remove the stone can now be planned. The stent should not be left for more than 12 weeks. If the planned treatment cannot be carried out by the end of this period, the stent should be changed. Patients who have a ureteric stent inserted may need further symptom control caused by the stent. These symptoms can consist of urinary frequency, haematuria and discomfort in your kidneys/bladder/urethra and genitals especially after urinating or physical exercise.

Insertion of a Nephrostomy Tube. is indicated when obstruction in the kidney or the ureter cannot be relieved by flush-back and stenting (Fig. 10.7). This is carried out under X-ray control, usually with a local anaesthetic. A small silicone tube is placed percutaneously into the collecting system of the kidney. The tube is held in place by a suture and connected to a closed-system drainage bag.

Ureteroscopic Removal of Calculi. This procedure is suitable in the treatment of small calculi in the ureter. The ureteric orifice is dilated cystoscopically and a ureteroscope, to which a 'stone basket' is attached, is introduced into the ureter. The basket is opened out to ensnare the stone. The basket and stone are then withdrawn.

Rigid ureteroscopes can be inserted under direct vision and the stone can be disintegrated in situ (using mechanical means or laser) before removing the smaller fragments in a 'basket' (EAU 2018).

Shock Wave Lithotripsy (SWL). This is a noninvasive treatment that focuses shock waves on the stone and breaks it into smaller fragments that can be passed spontaneously. Large calculi are broken up by means of this technique before percutaneous removal.

Depending on the density of the stone, more than one treatment may be required. The patient lies on a special table which allows shock waves produced by the lithotriptor machine to pass through it.

🌐 **See Evolve website Fig. 10.3**

The position of the patient on the table is dependent on the location of the stone. The whole procedure is performed under specialised X-ray and ultrasonic control. The disintegrated or powdered calculus is then allowed to pass down the ureter over the next few days.

Percutaneous Nephrolithotomy (PCNL). This procedure is used to remove calculi lying within the kidney. Large staghorn calculi may need to be broken up first, using SWL. PCNL is performed under X-ray and ultrasound control. The patient will normally have a general anaesthetic. The kidney is punctured and the tract into the kidney is dilated to allow the nephroscope and a variety of grasping instruments to be inserted (Fig. 10.8). The stone can then be removed or broken down into fine powder by ultrasonic probes. This powder can be aspirated through the centre of the probe.

Sometimes, an electrohydraulic probe is used. This produces shock waves in the irrigating fluid to the kidney and results in the stone splitting into several fragments.

At the end of the procedure, a large nephrostomy tube with a smaller tube running down its centre is left in position to allow drainage and to prevent haematoma formation. This also allows access for a nephrogram 24–48 hours postoperatively to assess the effectiveness of treatment.

No anaesthetic is required for a nephrogram X-ray. A contrast agent is injected down the smaller inner tube of a nephrostomy

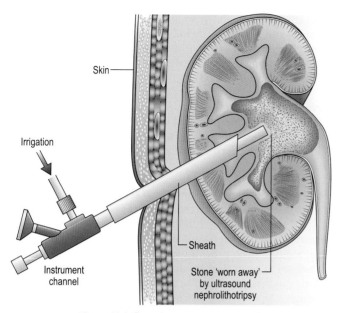

Figure 10.8 Percutaneous stone removal.

tube into the kidney. X-rays can then be taken and any fragments of calculi identified. Provided that there are no fragments left, the tubes can be removed.

Ureterolithotomy. This open surgery (rarely used) is appropriate in the treatment of calculi occurring midureter and causing obstruction that cannot be dealt with in any other way. An X-ray to identify the position of the stone will determine the incision to be made. The ureter is exposed and opened and the stone removed. The ureter is repaired either by removing a small section or by suturing the opening. A stent is usually left in place, positioned along the length of the ureter. This allows the ureter to heal and prevents leakage. A wound drain will be left in position to prevent haematoma formation. The stent will normally be removed after 7 days.

Pyelolithotomy. This open surgery (rarely used) can be used for the removal of calculi in the renal pelvis or kidney which are causing an obstruction that cannot be removed by SWL or PCNL. The procedure involves first exposing the affected kidney and then opening the renal pelvis to remove the stone. Sometimes it is not possible to remove all of a staghorn calculus in this way, in which case further incisions into the surrounding renal tissue (nephrolithotomy) are necessary. A stent will be left in place for 7 days.

❖ Nursing Management and Health Promotion: Acute Renal Colic

Major Nursing Considerations

A patient admitted with renal colic can often do little more than cope with the excruciating pain, and is often unable to answer questions or to follow advice and instructions until the pain is relieved.

🌐 **See Evolve website Critical thinking question 10.1**

Once the acute attack has subsided, the patient should be allowed to rest since only then will it be possible to absorb all the necessary explanations relating to investigations and treatment.

Priorities in postoperative nursing care depend on the procedure undertaken, but care following interventions to remove renal or ureteric calculi includes (and see Chapter 25, Nursing the Patient Undergoing Surgery, for general perioperative care):

- Record observations, temperature, pulse, respirations and blood pressure and observe for signs/symptoms of infection, such as dark coloured, cloudy urine with an abnormal odour or deterioration in National Early Warning Score 2 (NEWS2).
- Monitor fluid intake and urine output and record the volume and colour of urine on the fluid chart. A decrease in volume may indicate obstruction. Haematuria may indicate trauma, but some haematuria is to be expected (but it should reduce, becoming less red).
- Encourage a fluid intake of 3 L daily to prevent infection.
- Administer analgesics if the patient is in pain. Severe pain must be reported to medical staff as this may indicate trauma, a misplaced stent or return of obstruction.

Discharge Advice

The patient should be advised:

- to continue to drink 3 L daily
- to take mild analgesics such as paracetamol or co-proxamol if in pain
- to seek help from the GP if urine output is bloodstained or they experience discomfort or a burning sensation on voiding urine.

The patient should also be advised when follow-up treatment will take place and what this will entail. If treatment is not within 12 weeks, it must be impressed upon the patient that it is very important to have the stent changed. If it is not changed, sediment and crystals will build up around it and form more calculi.

Renal Disorders

This section of the chapter outlines a range of conditions that affect the kidney, including glomerulonephritis, nephrotic syndrome, acute kidney injury (AKI) and chronic renal failure (CRF).

Glomerulonephritis

Glomerulonephritis is a group of disorders usually characterised by inflammation of the glomeruli or filtration units of the kidney, but some are not associated with inflammation. The disorder may be primary to the glomeruli (e.g. minimal change nephropathy, IgA nephropathy), post infection (an immune response to streptococcal infection), autoimmune (e.g. anti-glomerular basement membrane (GBM) disease or Goodpasture's syndrome) or secondary to a systemic disorder (e.g. systemic lupus erythematosus, amyloidosis). There are acute and chronic types with varying prognosis.

Proteinuria, haematuria, hypertension, nephrotic syndrome (see later) and renal impairment characterise this disorder, but the severity of these effects will vary between individuals. Presentation is usually described in terms of a range of clinical syndromes, but accurate diagnosis requires histological investigation. (For further information, see Anders et al. 2023).

🔬 Pathophysiology

Histological examination of renal tissue will demonstrate inflammation in the majority of cases, but it is also possible to have minimal change and no evidence of an inflammatory process. The disease process results from a defect in the immune response, such as a hypersensitivity to an exogenous antigen. The antigen–antibody reaction results in the formation of insoluble immune complexes that circulate in the blood and, instead of being ingested by macrophages, reach the kidney, where they become 'trapped' and set up a damaging inflammatory reaction in the delicate filtration structure. As a result of this:

- large molecules such as proteins and red blood cells are able to pass through the filtration fenestrations into the PCT
- the osmotic pressure of the blood plasma falls, leading to oedema
- sodium and water are retained, as are waste products and potentially toxic substances.

Many cases of acute glomerulonephritis occur 1–3 weeks after a streptococcal infection such as tonsillitis or otitis media, most commonly in children or adolescents; however, only 5% of these infections lead to glomerulonephritis. It is rare in developed countries as a result of better hygiene and the appropriate use of antibiotics. The disease can range from a mild, transitory, asymptomatic condition to a very severe form that precipitates AKI, cardiac failure and seizures.

Medical Management
Tests and Investigations
Investigations include:
- urinalysis
- MSU
- full blood count and urea and electrolyte estimation
- antistreptolysin O (ASO) titre
- throat swab
- chest X-ray
- electrocardiogram (ECG)
- ultrasound scan
- renal biopsy.

Treatment
Treatment will vary according to the type of glomerulonephritis, but broadly the aim of treatment is to reduce renal workload, restore and maintain fluid and electrolyte status and prevent uraemia. Thus management aims to prevent serious complications from occurring.

Nursing Management and Health Promotion: Glomerulonephritis

Major Nursing Considerations
Promoting Rest
Bed rest is a necessity, especially in the early period, to reduce the workload of both the kidneys and the heart. This can pose quite a challenge in the care of younger patients. Time needs to be spent with the patient, explaining why rest is so important.

Maintaining Fluid and Electrolyte Balance (See Chapter 21)
While renal function is impaired and fluid overload poses a very real problem, fluid and sodium intake must be restricted. Potassium levels in the blood must be closely monitored and, if necessary, dietary modification made or ion exchange resins given. If hypertension is marked, antihypertensive medication may be required.

Preventing Uraemia
While renal function is impaired, the waste products of metabolism will build up in the blood. To prevent this, a protein-restricted diet will be necessary. Calorie intake can be maintained

with carbohydrates, and vitamin supplements can be given. This diet must also be low in salt and many patients find meals unpalatable. The dietitian can contribute greatly to the patient's well-being by ensuring that the restricted diet includes at least some of the patient's favourite foods.

Preventing Infection
If a link to a recent streptococcal infection is confirmed, penicillin may be prescribed. All patients with renal impairment are prone to infection. All infection prevention and control measures must be adhered to.

Promoting Convalescence and the Maintenance of Health
Most patients make a full recovery, but convalescence may take as long as 2 years. The acute condition can resolve fairly rapidly, and the majority of people recover normal renal function within a couple of months. Such patients often feel better quite quickly and it can be hard to persuade them that restrictions are still needed. Proteinuria can persist and regular monitoring will be necessary. After discharge, support for the patient and family will ensure that necessary lifestyle adjustments are made for the initial months. Exercise should be gentle and energetic sports activities avoided. Any infection should be treated seriously and medical advice sought.

Incomplete resolution and permanent glomerular damage can result in chronic glomerulonephritis and all the associated symptoms of renal impairment. Decreasing renal function may require renal replacement therapy such as dialysis.

Nephrotic Syndrome

The nephrotic syndrome encompasses a group of signs and symptoms including proteinuria, hypoalbuminaemia (low serum albumin), oedema and lipidaemia. It can be a manifestation of certain forms of glomerulonephritis but may also occur as a complication of diabetes mellitus or amyloidosis, whereby insoluble starch-like deposits occur in kidney tissue. Often no cause can be found.

Pathophysiology and Clinical Features
The glomerular filtration membrane is normally impermeable to blood cells and macromolecules such as proteins with a molecular weight of 70,000 or above. In the nephrotic syndrome, increased glomerular permeability occurs, and protein molecules such as albumin enter the filtrate within the tubules. When the capacity of the tubule to reabsorb protein is exceeded, protein is lost in the urine. A low plasma albumin reduces plasma osmotic pressure and fluid leaks into the extracellular compartment. The resultant oedema occurs in dependent areas and may give rise to ascites (free fluid in the peritoneal cavity) in severe cases. Intravascular volume is maintained in many cases. How this occurs is not fully understood, but activation of the renin–angiotensin–aldosterone mechanism is thought likely.

This syndrome is characterised by heavy proteinuria (especially albumin) and hypoalbuminaemia leading to oedema. These patients generally have a low urine output and low urine sodium. Derangement of lipoproteins is evident and loss of fibrinogen in the urine can occur. Infection and thrombosis are common complications.

Medical Management
Treatment
The main aim of treatment is to reduce oedema. Diuretic therapy can be adjusted according to the severity of the oedema and small

maintenance doses can be administered when the oedema is under control. Severe oedema may also be treated by the administration of salt-poor albumin to temporarily increase plasma osmotic pressure. Patients are advised to adhere to a diet free from added salt.

Identification of the underlying disease process, possibly by renal biopsy and histological examination, will dictate the nature of ongoing treatment. In many patients, CRF will eventually develop.

Acute Kidney Injury

AKI, a sudden and severe reduction in normal renal function, may result from primary renal disease but is more frequently associated with other organ failure. To maintain renal perfusion, a mean arterial pressure (MAP) (systolic pressure minus diastolic pressure, divided by 3 plus diastolic pressure or 2 × diastolic plus systolic divided by 3) of >60 mmHg is needed (Chapter 2 of this text discusses cardiovascular disorders). Failure is often reversible, but should the kidneys fail to recover, permanent replacement treatment will be required with either dialysis or transplant.

AKI is associated with an increased risk of mortality, and those who do recover are at risk of developing chronic kidney disease (CKD) (Dainton 2019).

⬤ Pathophysiology
Causes
The causes of AKI may be classified into three categories – prerenal, intrarenal and postrenal – each having a different physiological location.

Prerenal causes are those in which a loss or decrease in renal perfusion results in renal ischaemia. They include:
- Extracellular depletion, resulting from large gastrointestinal tract loss such as vomiting, diarrhoea, drainage or nasogastric aspiration; urinary loss due to polyuria or diuresis; loss from the skin, e.g. sweating or burn injury (see Chapter 21, Maintaining Fluid, Electrolyte and Acid–Base Balance, and Chapter 29, Nursing the Patient With Burn Injury)
- Circulating volume loss, as in haemorrhage or hypoalbuminaemia
- Reduced cardiac output, as in cardiac arrest, valvular disease, cardiac tamponade
- Vascular disease, e.g. renal artery thrombosis or embolism

Intrarenal causes include conditions that impair renal function by damaging the structure of the kidney (tubules, interstitium, glomeruli or capillaries). If tubular damage occurs, this is termed acute tubular necrosis (ATN). ATN is often caused by prolonged pre- and postrenal events.

Nephrotoxic substances can also result in acute failure. These include:
- medications – aminoglycoside antibacterial drugs (e.g. gentamicin) and NSAIDs
- exogenous chemicals, e.g. heavy metals, phenols, carbon tetrachloride, chlorates, ethyl glycol
- bacterial toxins, particularly those released by gram-negative microorganisms responsible for septicaemia (see Chapter 19, Recognising and Managing Shock).

Postrenal causes are mainly attributed to obstruction. The most common of these is bladder output obstruction which may be due to prostatic hypertrophy, tumours, strictures or calculi.

Clinical Features
AKI proceeds through four phases or stages: onset or initiating, oliguric, diuretic and recovery. The onset or initiating phase is

the time from the initial renal insult to the onset of oliguria. The oliguric phase is characterised by a urine output of less than 400 mL/24 h; however, some patients may be anuric. The oliguria is accompanied by abnormal plasma levels of creatinine, urea and electrolytes. The effects of acute fluid overload and hyperkalaemia (K^+ >6 mmol/L) can result in sudden death. The patient may complain of anorexia, nausea and vomiting. Increased respiration due to pulmonary oedema and acidosis can occur. Drowsiness, confusion and coma may follow. The diuretic phase indicates that the kidney is re-establishing functionality and can result in a period of polyuria. The recovery stage can last many months and is characterised by a return to normal function. There may be scarring from the initial injury, but may not be clinically significant.

⬤ Medical Management
Tests and Investigations
These will depend on the suspected cause and on the immediacy of the presentation but may include:
- full blood count, urea and electrolyte estimation, serum creatinine clearance (used to estimate glomerular filtration rate [GFR])
- urinalysis, MSU, 24-hour collections of urine for creatinine clearance
- X-ray of kidneys, ureters and bladder
- ultrasound
- renal biopsy.

Treatment
The goal is to restore biochemical balance and prevent AKI progressing. The onset of renal failure must be identified early to minimise damage and, if possible, prevent the necessity for dialysis. The priorities of treatment are as follows.

Treating the Cause. Examples are correcting hypovolaemia and increasing renal perfusion, managing sepsis and relieving any urinary obstruction.

Reversing, Restoring and Maintaining Fluid and Electrolyte Status (see Chapter 21).
- *Hyperkalaemia.* Immediate measures may be required to correct hyperkalaemia, which could cause fatal dysrhythmias. Cardiac monitoring is essential, in particular observing for any changes in cardiac rhythm. Hyperkalaemia can be corrected in the short term by intravenous (IV) insulin-glucose infusion or sodium bicarbonate, either of which will shift potassium into the cells. Other measures include the administration of ion exchange resins, which when administered orally or rectally remove potassium ions.
- *Hyponatraemia and hypernatraemia.* In the oliguric state, there is a danger of hyponatraemia, due to the risk of fluid overload and to the failure of the damaged tubules to reabsorb sodium. However, hypernatraemia can also be a problem in prerenal AKI, as mechanisms instituted retain sodium in order to restore blood volume. Fluid intake must be restricted to the equivalent of insensible loss plus the previous day's urinary output. Sodium intake must be monitored closely.
- *Uraemia.* The inability to excrete the nitrogenous waste products of metabolism is managed by dietary restrictions, but ensuring adequate calorie intake to prevent the patient becoming catabolic (see Chapter 22). Parenteral nutrition may be necessary and potassium intake will be restricted.
- *Metabolic acidosis.* The loss of the kidneys' buffering function, the electrolyte imbalance and the increased anaerobic

respiration by damaged renal cells all result in acidosis. In the short term, this is managed by IV sodium bicarbonate.

If AKI is very severe, persists or worsens, dialysis will be necessary.

❖ Nursing Management and Health Promotion: Acute Kidney Injury

Major Nursing Considerations

The care of patients with AKI will involve a large multidisciplinary team and may be carried out either in an intensive care setting or on a ward, depending on the condition of the patient. Priorities of nursing intervention are to:

- Reduce the patient's anxieties and recognise the risk of altered consciousness due to uraemia and electrolyte imbalance.
- Control fluid and electrolyte balance by:
  - monitoring cardiac status for signs of dysrhythmias
  - monitoring pulse, respiration and blood pressure for signs of overload and hypertension
  - restricting fluid intake and ensuring the accurate measuring and recording of urine output and other losses; daily weighing may be required
  - administering prescribed medication and carrying out urinary assays as required.
- Assess and maintain nutritional status within the necessary limitations by the oral, enteral or parenteral route and monitor the nutritional status of the patient.
- Prevent infection due to uraemia by strict asepsis with regard to infusion sites and catheter management and by close monitoring of temperature and the patient's reported symptoms.
- Manage anaemia by the safe administration of blood transfusions, if required.
- Promote comfort at all times.

The Diuretic and Recovery Phases

The oliguric phase of renal failure may last 1–2 weeks and is followed by the diuretic phase, which indicates that renal function is returning. This is often a time of relief, but because the kidneys will not yet have regained their capacity for selective reabsorption, urine output can be as much as 4 L/day. This, in itself, could potentiate dehydration and electrolyte imbalances. Close monitoring must therefore continue. The recovery phase that follows can last several months and will require close medical follow-up of renal function. Convalescence in the form of rest, restricted activity, the avoidance of infections and alertness to any symptoms that might indicate renal problems may be a source of considerable stress to the patient, who may also be concerned about fulfilling family and work responsibilities (Thomas 2019).

Chronic Kidney Disease/Renal Failure

CKD or CRF is the gradual and progressive reduction in renal function. CKD is defined as the presence of kidney damage or an estimated glomerular filtration rate (eGFR) less than 60 mL/min per 1.73 square meters, persisting for 3 months or more (Vaidya and Aeddula 2022).

There are five stages of CKD:
- Stage 1, with normal eGFR (>90 mL/min)
- Stage 2, with mild CKD (eGFR 60–89 mL/min)
- Stage 3, with moderate CKD (eGFR 30–59 mL/min)
- Stage 4, with severe CKD (eGFR 15–29 mL/min)
- Stage 5, with end-stage CKD (eGFR <15 mL/min)

INFORMATION 10.3

Common Causes of Chronic Renal Failure

Congenital and inherited: 5%, e.g. polycystic kidney disease
Renal artery stenosis: 5%
Hypertension: 5%–25% (see Chapter 2, Nursing Patients With Cardiovascular Disorders)
Glomerular disease: 10%–20%, IgA nephropathy is the most common
Interstitial diseases of the kidney: 5%–15%, e.g. chronic interstitial nephritis caused by a variety of conditions that include analgesic nephropathy, systemic lupus erythematosus (SLE), amyloidosis, etc.
Systemic inflammatory disease: 5%, e.g. vasculitis, SLE
Diabetes mellitus: 20%–40% (see Chapter 5, Nursing Patients With Endocrine Disorders)
Unknown: 5%–20%

Adapted from Conway B, Phelan PJ, Stewart GD. Nephrology and urology. In: Ralston SH, Penman ID, Strachan MWJ, Hobson RP, eds. *Davidson's Principles and Practice of Medicine.* 23rd ed. Edinburgh: Churchill Livingstone; 2018.

The available treatments are changes to lifestyle, antihypertensives and statins, dialysis – haemodialysis, peritoneal dialysis (PD) – or transplantation, which may be from cadaveric, living related donors or linked unrelated donors (i.e. a 'swop').

Pathophysiology

Any disorder that damages kidney function can result in renal failure. Common causes are outlined in Information 10.3.

Clinical Features

In the initial stages of CRF, the patient may be asymptomatic. Proteinuria, haematuria, hypertension, anaemia or an elevated blood urea are, however, common presenting features.

As renal failure progresses the GFR declines and the patient may complain of fatigue, lethargy, pruritus, nausea, vomiting and indigestion. Breathlessness on exertion, headaches, visual disturbances, pallor and loss of libido may also be noted. A reduced immune response occurs, making the patient prone to infection, particularly of the urinary tract (see Chapter 18, Infection Prevention and Control).

Metabolic bone disease, generalised myopathy, neuropathy and metabolic acidosis can occur in advanced stages of renal impairment. Atherosclerosis due to altered lipid and carbohydrate metabolism and hypertension may also occur. Vascular calcification and pericarditis may also be identified.

Medical Management

Treatment

Treatment aims to identify the cause, extent and complications of the renal failure and to preserve useful renal function for as long as possible.

Where hypertension is evident, antihypertensive drugs may be used to reduce and control blood pressure gradually. Lifestyle advice should also be given to assist with reducing blood pressure, for example stopping smoking, losing weight or maintaining normal weight and regular exercise.

Fluid restriction may be required if the GFR is less than 5 mL/min as fluid overload can exacerbate problems with hypertension. Poor urine concentration can, however, result in a urine output of more than 2.5 L/24 h, in which case an intake of about 3 L/day is required.

Dietary measures are likely to include potassium and phosphate restrictions. Sodium restriction is not indicated unless there is evidence of oedema, hypertension or cardiac failure. In the case of sodium-losing conditions, sodium supplements may be required. A diet with no added salt may be appropriate in some cases.

Regular monitoring of biochemistry, GFR, creatinine clearance and assessment of symptoms allow treatment to be readjusted and progression of the disease to be assessed.

Renal replacement therapy, in the form of haemodialysis or PD, is the treatment available to replace the excretory functions of the kidneys (Information 10.4, Fig. 10.9). At present, transplantation (Fig. 10.9D) is restricted by a lack of available cadaver donor kidneys. However, for some patients, it may be possible to consider a matched family member as a live donor. Recently there have been donations from live unrelated donors. Some are linked (two donors/two recipients) in which the unrelated but matched donors donate a kidney to the unknown recipients (i.e. a 'swop').

❖ Nursing Management and Health Promotion: Chronic Renal Failure

Nursing management requires a strategy to help the patient and family come to terms with an illness for which there is no cure and in which sudden death can occur. Nursing intervention should aim to help the patient maintain a good quality of life by developing ways to cope with the constraints of the treatments and the possibility of complications occurring.

Adherence With Treatment

Patient beliefs about the value and benefit of a treatment may differ markedly when compared with the priority given to the same treatment by the nurse. Failure to adhere to diet and fluid restrictions may indicate that the patient has an underlying problem, or is not coping with some aspect of the treatment; alternatively, there may be a lack of understanding of the importance of the treatment regimen. Knowing the patient and having an understanding of the patient's social and cultural background, especially their health beliefs, can give insight into behaviour with regard to a particular treatment.

Major Problems Experienced by Patients

Fatigue and lethargy characteristic of CKD/CRF can reduce both ability and performance at work. Absence from work due to sickness or attendance at hospital may result in unemployment or reduction of income. Feelings of helplessness, hopelessness and depression are often expressed by patients with a long-term condition (see Chapter 30, Care and Rehabilitation of People with Long term Conditions). Loss of control over many aspects of life and low self-esteem are likely to influence family relationships. Transplantation is acknowledged as the treatment of choice for a person with CKD stage 5, end-stage renal disease (ESRD). A successful transplant offers the patient freedom and independence as well as an enhanced quality of life.

Living With Peritoneal Dialysis

PD is performed either as continuous ambulatory peritoneal dialysis (CAPD) or automated peritoneal dialysis (APD) (Fig. 10.9C). CAPD is a continuous treatment, generally performed four times a day; APD is achieved by machine, generally overnight in the patient's own home. PD offers patients a greater degree of control

INFORMATION 10.4

Renal Replacement Therapy: Dialysis

Dialysis requires a semipermeable membrane to combine three principles – diffusion, osmosis and filtration – in order to permit the removal of solutes (metabolic wastes, excess electrolytes) and fluids from patients with renal failure. A favourable solute gradient is required.

Diffusion is the movement of molecules from an area of high concentration, across a semipermeable membrane, to an area of low concentration. This process continues until the concentrations in each compartment are the same.

Osmosis is the movement of a fluid or solvent from a lower concentration to a higher one.

Filtration is the movement of both solvent and solute across a semipermeable membrane under pressure.

Haemodialysis (Fig. 10.9A)

Haemodialysis requires a means of vascular access, e.g.:
- *Percutaneous access* including subclavian, femoral and jugular lines which are either temporary or permanent.
- *Arteriovenous fistula and arteriovenous grafts (synthetic).* Forming a fistula involves the anastomosis of an artery and a vein. The increased blood flow causes increased pressure on the vein walls which leads to thickening and dilatation (arterialisation); this allows the repeated insertion of needles for dialysis. This developmental stage takes about 12 weeks. The fistula can be seen as well as felt.

The blood is pumped from the patient to an artificial kidney (the dialyser – comprising blood and dialysate compartments separated by a semipermeable membrane) and back to the patient, having now been 'cleansed' as unwanted solutes and fluid pass through the membrane into the dialysate (fluid formulated to promote diffusion and removal of waste). The dialyser is normally a disposable hollow fibre or flat plate dialyser; different dialysers consist of different membranes. The type of membrane used is important as part of the patient's individualised dialysis prescription. Issues to consider are desired clearance, fluid removal and biocompatibility.

Peritoneal Dialysis (Fig. 10.9C)

The patient's peritoneal membrane serves as the semipermeable membrane for dialysis. A temporary or permanent Tenckhoff catheter is placed into the peritoneal cavity. The dialysate is instilled into the abdomen (usually 2 L at each session). A set time ('dwell time') elapses and the dialysate is drained out.
- Continuous ambulatory peritoneal dialysis (CAPD) – 2 L of dialysate are instilled into the peritoneal cavity and left in place, usually for 6 hours, when the fluid is exchanged. Once patients have been instructed in and are competent in this method, they can be more independent, visiting the hospital only for clinic appointments or when any problems arise; the main potential problems are peritonitis, dehydration and constipation.

Other Methods

Other methods of renal replacement therapy are often used in intensive care, including:
- continuous arteriovenous haemofiltration (CAVH)
- continuous arteriovenous haemodiafiltration (CAVHD)
- continuous venovenous haemofiltration (CVVH) 🌐 **See Evolve website Fig. 10.4**
- continuous venovenous haemodiafiltration (CVVHD).

Note: In haemofiltration the person's blood is passed through a filter allowing separation of an ultrafiltrate containing fluid and solutes. The ultrafiltrate is discarded and replaced with an isotonic solution (Fig. 10.9B). The process is usually continuous as in continuous venovenous haemofiltration. Haemodiafiltration is similar, but with the addition of dialysate. Diffusion occurs and the removal of unwanted solutes is enhanced (Brooker 2010).

(A) **Haemodialysis**

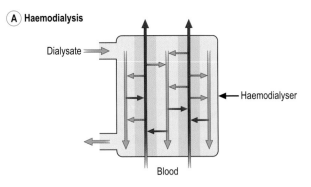

- Typical small solute clearance 160 mL/min
- Used in both acute and chronic renal failure

(B) **Haemofiltration**

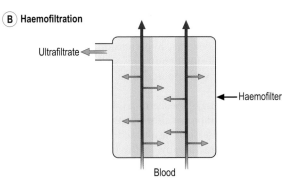

- Typical small solute clearance (2 L/h exchanges) 33 mL/min
- ? Less circulatory instability than haemodialysis
- Used mostly in acute renal failure

> • **Access to the circulation** for haemodialysis or filtration is required.
> Arteriovenous fistulae, temporary or semi-permanent tunnelled central
> venous lines or arteriovenous shunts (e.g. Scribner shunt) may be used.
> The extracorporeal circuit requires anticoagulation, typically with heparin

(C) **Peritoneal dialysis**

- **Access to the peritoneal cavity** via 'Tenckhoff' catheter
- **Continuous ambulatory peritoneal dialysis** (CAPD):
  typically 4 exchanges of 2 L of fluid a day 4–6 h apart
- **Automated peritoneal dialysis** (APD): uses a machine to perform
  exchanges overnight (8–10 h). Used mostly in chronic renal failure

(D) **Transplantation**

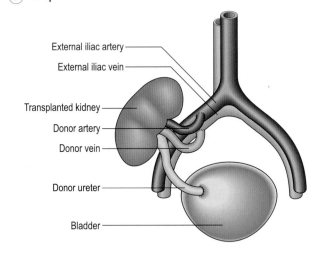

- Successful transplantation extends the life expectancy
  of patients with end-stage CRF
- Requires long-term use of immunosuppressives with attendant risks

Figure 10.9 Renal replacement therapy. (A) Haemodialysis. (B) Haemofiltration. (C) Peritoneal dialysis (PD). (D) Renal transplantation.

over their treatment and lifestyle. While the number of fluid exchanges per day will be prescribed by the doctor, the timing of each exchange can be decided by the patient, to fit in with family life or work commitments. In addition, freedom to be away from home for visits or holidays is possible. For travel abroad, the dialysate manufacturer may be able to deliver fluid requirements to the destination.

The need for regular fluid exchanges and aseptic technique can be limiting for some patients. Performing the exchange in a designated area at home can give confidence and reassure patients that they have done all they can to reduce the risk of peritonitis. There may be a reluctance to perform exchanges in the homes of friends and relatives, particularly if the patient's illness is poorly understood and a source of embarrassment.

The insertion of a tube and presence of fluid in the abdomen can alter body image and sexuality, thus discouraging those

who are conscious of their appearance. A further disadvantage of CAPD is that it presents a constant reminder to the patient of their illness (for further information, see Thomas 2019 and Further Reading).

Nursing Support During Haemodialysis

Assessments to be performed before haemodialysis include:

- Weigh the patient – compare with weight after last dialysis and the patient's recognised dry weight, i.e. the weight at which there is no clinical evidence of oedema, increased jugular venous pressure (JVP), shortness of breath or hyper/hypotension.
- Record temperature, pulse and blood pressure – compare these with values after the last dialysis. Any temperature increase could indicate an infected dialysis site. Raised blood pressure may indicate fluid overloading.

- Enquire how the patient has been feeling, i.e. well or unwell.
- Assess any known specific medical problem, e.g. blood glucose in patients with diabetes mellitus.
- Once a month, take blood for urea and electrolyte levels pre- and postdialysis; a full blood count should be checked every month.

During dialysis, the nurse should record the pulse and blood pressure. A drop in blood pressure may mean that the patient needs extra fluid. If necessary, the nurse should check the patient's weight halfway through the session.

At the end of dialysis, the patient's temperature, pulse, blood pressure and weight should be recorded in order to assess the effectiveness of the treatment. Any prescribed medications should be administered and the patient should be given the opportunity to raise any further concerns.

Disorders of the Bladder

This section of the chapter deals with bladder cancer.

Bladder Cancer

Bladder cancer occurs more commonly in men than in women and is the seventh most common cancer diagnosed in males worldwide. Seventy-five per cent of patients present with a tumour in the mucosa (stage Ta or CIS), that will be treated with resection of the tumour or transurethral resection of a bladder tumour, or TURBT, with or without additional treatment, for example intravesical installations.

There are geographical variations in incidence: tumours are more common in industrialised regions than in underdeveloped regions. The possible causative agents or factors include:

- cigarette smoking/tobacco use (accounting for circa 50% of cases)
- occupational exposure (industrial dyes, solvents) (accounting for circa 10% of cases)
- dietary habits (a westernised diet has been associated with an increased risk of developing bladder cancer when compared with a Mediterranean diet)
- schistosomiasis.

There is little or no evidence for family history increasing the chances of developing bladder cancer.

There are three types of bladder cancer. Urothelial, more commonly known as transitional cell carcinoma (TCC), accounts for about 90% of all bladder tumours diagnosed, with 5% squamous cell carcinomas, 2% adenocarcinomas, and the rest consisting of rarer types of tumours such as small cell cancer and sarcomas of the bladder (Cancer Research UK 2023b)

Histopathology grading for bladder cancer follows:

Grade 1	Well differentiated. Cancer cells look close to normal cells. Low grade and tends to grow slowly.
Grade 2	Moderately differentiated. Cancer cells look less normal (abnormal).
Grade 3	Poorly differentiated. Cancer cells look very abnormal. High grade and tends to grow more quickly.

Along with histology grading, full staging of bladder cancers are classified according to the tumour, node, metastasis (TNM) system.

Tumour
TX Primary tumour cannot be assessed
T0 No evidence of primary tumour
Ta Noninvasive papillary carcinoma
Tis carcinoma in situ: 'flat tumour'
T1 Tumour invades subepithelial connective tissue (Lamina Propria)
T2 Tumour invades muscle
T2a Tumour invades superficial muscle (inner half)
T2b Tumour invades deep muscle (outer half)
T3 Tumour invades perivesical tissue
T3a Microscopically
T3b Macroscopically (extravesical mass)
T4 Tumour invades any of the following: prostate stroma, seminal vesicles, uterus, vagina pelvic wall, abdominal wall
T4a Tumour invades prostate stroma, seminal vesicles, uterus or vagina
T4b Tumour invades pelvic wall or abdominal wall
Nodes (N) – Regional lymph nodes
NX Regional lymph nodes cannot be assessed
N0 No regional lymph node metastasis
N1 Metastasis in a single lymph node in the true pelvis (hypogastric, obturator, external iliac, or presacral)
N2 Metastasis in multiple regional lymph nodes in the true pelvis (hypogastric, obturator, external iliac, or presacral)
N3 Metastasis in common iliac lymph node(s)
M – Distant metastasis
M0 No distant metastasis
M1a Nonregional lymph nodes
M1b Other distant metastases

Otto et al. (2017) in European Association of Urology (2023).

Pathophysiology

Tumour growth usually commences in the transitional cell epithelium (urothelium) lining the bladder, often as a papillary growth (papillae are minute nipple-shaped projections). Benign growth will, without treatment, usually progress to malignancy and then, by stages, from superficial to deep muscle tissue involvement, eventually spreading locally into surrounding tissue and other parts of the urinary tract or organs.

Common Presenting Symptoms

Approximately 80% of people with bladder cancer will notice haematuria (often painless). This may be the only presenting feature of the disease. Dysuria, frequency, symptoms of obstruction and cystitis may also be noticed, but embarrassment may prevent the individual from visiting their GP. Symptoms may not persist following initial presentation, for example if associated infection is resolved by a course of antibiotics. Investigations should, however, be undertaken if the cause of haematuria is unclear.

Medical Management
Investigations

Diagnosis may be aided by physical examination, a full blood count, urea and electrolyte estimation and other biochemical assays. Examination of an MSU specimen will exclude evidence of infection. If the patient has microscopic or macroscopic hae-maturia and an infection has been excluded, the patient's upper urinary tract and bladder must be investigated. A renal USS will be performed, and CTU if the patient has experienced visible haematuria or persistent microscopic haematuria. Cystoscopy is essential so that biopsies of suspicious lesions can be examined for abnormal cells. CT of the chest, abdomen and pelvis is performed ± MRI of the pelvis if local spread of cancer is suspected. In situa-tions where secondary (metastatic) spread of cancer is a possibility the patient will have a chest X-ray, a bone scan and liver function tests (LFTs). Intravenous urography and multiparametric MRI (mpMRI) may also be used to aid diagnosis.

The staging of bladder tumours is important for selecting the appropriate treatment modality (see Chapter 31, Nursing the Patient With Cancer).

For more on diagnosis and management see EAU Non-Muscle-Invasive Bladder Cancer (TaT1 and CIS) (EAU 2023) for further reading.

Treatment

The choice of treatment will depend on the type of tumour and the degree of invasion of local tissue, as determined by cystoscopy. Superficial lesions without muscle invasion can be treated by:

- excision of the tumour through the urethra – transurethral resection (TUR) or cystodiathermy (using an electrocautery) during cystoscopy.

Single instillation with mitomycin C (MMC), epirubicin or pirarubicin, as well as gemcitabine, has shown to lower the intra-vesical recurrence rates.

For invasive bladder tumours, a combination of surgery (i.e. total cystectomy), external beam radiotherapy and chemotherapy, for example cisplatin may be used.

Total cystectomy involves removing the lower ureters, bladder, pros-tate, urethra and lymphatics in men, and also, in women, the repro-ductive organs. Urinary diversion is required, most commonly by ileal

conduit and stoma formation. With this type of diversion, the ureters are anastomosed to an isolated section of the bowel, usually ileum with blood supply (in an operation known as ureteroileostomy or ileoure-terostomy) and the loop brought to the abdominal surface as a stoma (Fig. 10.10). This is a major procedure which will fundamentally affect the lifestyle of both the patient and family members. The complica-tions (including those that occur later) must be discussed with the patient and their family to ensure that the patient is able to give fully informed consent for radical surgery (Information 10.5). Information about preoperative and postoperative care, including a care plan for the first 24 hours following surgery, is provided on the companion website.

INFORMATION 10.5

Complications Following Total Cystectomy

Specific Complications Post Cystectomy

- Breakdown of anastomosis
- Breakdown of blood supply to stoma leading to necrosis
- Pelvic abscess
- Urinary infection
- Poor wound healing postradiotherapy
- Prolapse of stoma
- Retraction of stoma
- Renal failure

Later Complications

- Depression
- Recurrence of tumour
- Prolapse of stoma
- Retraction of stoma
- Stenosis of stoma
- Stone formation
- Urinary infection
- Urinary reflux

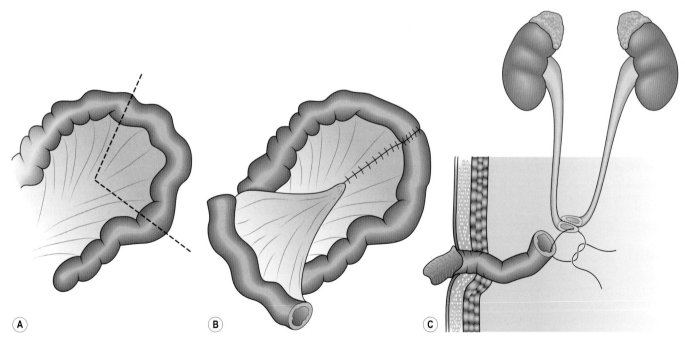

Figure 10.10 Ileal conduit urinary diversion. (A, B) Isolation of segment of terminal ileum. (C). Fashioning of the anastomosis between the ureters and ileum. The stoma is made to protrude from the skin to minimise skin contact with urine and so reduce irritation.

Radiotherapy is normally given as an external treatment for bladder carcinoma over a 6-week period. It may be used as a palliative measure or in conjunction with surgery and/or chemotherapy, pre- or posttreatment. The age and general condition of the patient will determine whether treatment is given on an outpatient or inpatient basis. Sometimes, the severity of the patient's symptoms leads to conversion from outpatient to inpatient care and a short period of respite from the treatment plan to allow the patient to recuperate before progressing to the next treatment.

Chemotherapy. Treatment of invasive bladder cancer with systemic chemotherapy is under investigation. Regimens of treatment vary. Some patients receive care on a day-care basis, receiving IV injections, while others attend for inpatient hospital care involving 2–3 days in hospital for each cycle of treatment (see Chapter 31, Nursing the Patient With Cancer).

Intravesical chemotherapy may be offered in some cases. The recurrence of superficial bladder tumours resected endoscopically is approximately 65%. Recurrent tumours are usually of the same type and stage as those resected. Further endoscopic resection may be the treatment of choice, but intravesical chemotherapy is also given. A urethral catheter is inserted and the chosen medication is instilled via the catheter. Treatment may be weekly, monthly or bimonthly, depending upon the type of tumour and the medication used.

Once the medication is instilled, the catheter can be removed. The patient is asked to try to avoid passing urine for an hour and is asked to turn from back to front to sides every 15 minutes, in order to wash the medication around the bladder. The nurse administering the treatment should bear in mind that this patient may have difficulty in postponing the voiding of urine for up to 1 hour because of frequency and bladder irritability. The patient should be reassured that an inability to comply with this request is not a sign of 'failure'. After the treatment has been completed, the patient should be advised that urine passed will contain chemical substances that will irritate the skin and that leakages or dribbles should be washed off immediately.

The side-effects of the medications used in this treatment vary, but chemical cystitis leading to inflammation and bladder irritability, urgency and frequency is common. Sensitivity rashes are seen less commonly, as are more severe effects such as systemic toxicity and bone marrow suppression.

Effectiveness of treatment with intravesical chemotherapy varies considerably from individual to individual.

Disorders of the Prostate

This section of the chapter outlines two important conditions affecting the prostate gland: benign enlargement and cancer.

Benign Prostatic Enlargement (BPE)

After the age of 40 years, the prostate begins to enlarge and will gradually narrow the diameter of the urethra, leading to urinary symptoms. The most bothersome symptoms can be nocturia (having to get up at night-time to empty the bladder), urinary frequency and urgency. Bladder outflow obstruction can occur for a number of reasons, but the most common cause is BPE (Information 10.6). Note: BPE is also known as benign prostatic hyperplasia (BPH).

🔵 Pathophysiology

The precise cause of prostate enlargement has yet to be fully explained, but it is thought to be related to changes in androgen hormone (e.g. testosterone) levels.

INFORMATION 10.6
Bladder Outflow Obstruction

Causes
- BPE (also known as benign prostatic hyperplasia)
- Bladder calculi
- Bladder tumour
- Phimosis
- Prostatic carcinoma
- Urethral strictures, stenosis, trauma
- Diuretic drugs
- Neurological disturbances

Common Symptoms
- Diminished force of urine flow/stream
- Double voiding
- Dribbling postvoiding
- Dysuria
- Frequency
- Haematuria (occasional)
- Hesitancy
- Interrupted stream
- Loss of urinary continence
- Nocturia
- Urgency
- Urinary retention
  Inadequate emptying of the bladder can result in an increased residual urine, increasing the risk of UTI and the incidence of bladder calculi formation.

Diagnosis
Diagnosis of bladder flow obstruction may be assisted by:
- History of symptoms
- Physical examination
- Routine urinalysis
- MSU for microscopy, culture and sensitivity
- Blood screen of urea, electrolytes and creatinine
- Urethroscopy and cystoscopy
- Ultrasound scan – residual urine volume and upper urinary tract
- Urodynamic evaluation
- Voiding cystometrogram (a record of the changes in pressure within the bladder during voiding)

Common Presenting Symptoms
Symptoms of BPE include:
- urinary frequency
- hesitancy
- poor urinary flow
- incomplete bladder emptying, i.e. feeling the bladder retains urine
- having to strain to empty the bladder
- terminal dribbling
- urgency
- nocturia (specifically, having to get up from sleep to empty the urinary bladder.

🔵 Medical Management
Investigations
The diagnosis of prostate enlargement is made by digital rectal examination and urinary flow rate studies. However, more specific investigations are required to ascertain the nature of the enlargement and its effects:
- ultrasound scan (abdominal and transrectal)
- assessment of postvoid residual urine
- blood for renal function tests

- full blood count
- symptom score to quantify symptoms and measure how 'bothersome' they are, for example International Prostatic Symptom Score (IPSS)
- estimation of prostate-specific antigen (PSA) in the blood to eliminate diagnosis of cancer in men over 40 years of age
- MSU.

Treatment

Treatment options include:
- watchful waiting
- medication – alpha-blockers, e.g. alfuzosin, tamsulosin, or 5-alpha reductase inhibitors, e.g. dutasteride or finasteride to reduce prostate size, or a combination of both, e.g. Combodart.
- catheterisation, both indwelling urethra catheter and patient intermittent self-catheterisation
- surgery, e.g. transurethral resection of the prostate (TURP), or variations of this (see Further Reading, e.g. Reynard et al. 2019).

🌐 **See Evolve website for Critical thinking question 10.2**

TURP is commonly used to treat prostate enlargement, although other interventions, for example Rezum, Green Light Laser and prostatic artery embolisation, are also used in some centres. A resectoscope is passed up the urethra to the prostate gland and small sections are trimmed away from the prostatic lobes, removing the material that had been intruding into the urethra and bladder neck. Irrigation fluid (a nonelectrolyte solution, glycine) constantly flushes out the bladder during the procedure. Most commonly, irrigation continues postoperatively, as the operative bed can give rise to considerable bleeding and clots could lead to obstruction of the urinary catheter. Information 10.7 outlines postoperative complications of TURP.

❖ Nursing Management and Health Promotion: BPE

Caring for Men With Acute Retention

Most men presenting with acute retention as a result of BPE will be discharged home with a catheter in situ and will return for either a trial without catheter or planned surgery at a later date. Once the obstruction is relieved, there is no urgency to perform surgery, which allows the treatment of any associated medical conditions and, when appropriate, the man can be admitted for surgery. However, the presence of a urinary catheter for any reason poses an infection risk.

Caring for Men With Chronic Retention

Chronic urinary retention is usually the result of a crescendo of symptoms of 'prostatism'. These men do not always complain of symptoms of bladder outflow obstruction, but mainly of urge incontinence, dribbling urine or wet beds at night. They usually have no pain and, although they have a large amount of residual urine, their bladder distension is not always obvious to the eye or palpable on physical examination.

Because of the large volume of residual urine, these men are at risk of developing upper urinary tract dilatation and impaired renal function. It is urgent to make a diagnosis so that the level of hydration and renal function can be returned to normal. However, if there is no renal impairment, it is not essential that these individuals are catheterised. Catheterisation will permit bladder drainage and allow renal function recovery.

The use of urinary catheters is outlined in Information 10.8 and the principles of catheter management for both men and women are outlined in Information 10.9.

INFORMATION 10.7

Postoperative Complications of TURP

Potential Postoperative Complications

- Haemorrhage – evident as haematuria
- Clot retention
- Infection – UTI, epididymis or testis
- Extravasation – escape of urine into surrounding tissue due to bladder or urethral damage
- TUR syndrome – absorption of irrigant into the bloodstream, resulting in dilutional hyponatraemia (see Chapter 21)
- Venous thromboembolism – deep vein thrombosis and pulmonary embolism

Possible Late Complications

- Urethral stricture
- Loss of urinary continence
- ED
- Retrograde ejaculation of semen into the bladder
- Bladder neck stenosis

INFORMATION 10.8

The Use of Catheters

Indications for Catheterisation

- Acute or chronic retention of urine
- Diagnostic investigations of the bladder function
- Specific pre- and postoperative needs
- Following trauma, burns, road traffic accidents or any trauma to the lower urinary tract
- Therapeutic instillations of medication, e.g. chemotherapy
- Intractable incontinence where all other methods have failed
- Protracted loss of consciousness.

Choice of Catheter

Points to consider when choosing a catheter include:
- Purpose of the catheterisation
- Length of time the catheter must remain in situ
- Whether a self-retaining catheter is necessary
- Presence of latex allergy
- Age and gender.

Features of the Catheter

- The smallest catheter that will adequately drain the bladder should be used: size 12–16 FG for adults with clear urine; size 18–22 FG for adults with haematuria.
- The lumen of the catheter will vary depending on the material used.
- Balloon size: the larger the balloon, the higher the drainage eye lies in the bladder. This can impair drainage and cause more irritation to the sensitive trigone of the bladder (Fig. 10.4,). The balloon should be just large enough to stop the catheter from falling out or being pushed out if the patient bears down. The recommended balloon size for routine use is 5–10 mL. A 30-mL balloon should be used only following surgery on the prostate gland.
  Note that underinflation of a large-capacity balloon causes distortion of the tip of the catheter and occlusion of the drainage eye. Therefore, a large balloon should be filled with at least 20 mL of water. A smaller-ballooned catheter, because the water must reach the balloon, should be filled with at least 10 mL.
- Catheters for short-term use are made of a latex material that can cause irritation of the urethra and build-up of crystals in the bladder. Therefore, it is not recommended to use this type of catheter for longer than 2 or 3 weeks.
- Catheters for long-term use are made of 100% silicone material; they are less irritating, are softer and cause less build-up of crystals.

INFORMATION 10.9

Principles of Catheter Management: For Men and Women

Performing Catheterisation

The nurse performing catheterisation must introduce the catheter into the bladder using aseptic technique, without causing trauma and with minimum discomfort to the person. The following considerations are essential:

- Providing sufficient information to allow the person to give informed consent to the procedure.
- Positioning the person correctly.
- Adequate cleaning of the genital area.
- Working under good light, especially when catheterising women.
- Ensuring the person's privacy.
- Ensuring adequate anaesthesia of the urethra for both men and women. A local anaesthetic-containing antiseptic should be instilled and left to take effect for a minimum of 5 minutes.

Management of the Indwelling Catheter

The main priorities of catheter care are to prevent infection and to safeguard the person's dignity. To minimise the risk of infection the nurse should:

- Establish and maintain a closed system of drainage.
- Promote good personal hygiene – meatal hygiene can be achieved by washing with soap and water daily (NICE 2017). More recently, evidence-based guidelines indicate that a daily bath or shower is sufficient (Loveday et al. 2014).
- Encourage a fluid intake of 2–4 L daily, according to the individual's needs.
- Encourage maximum mobility.
- Avoid causing trauma to the urethra and bladder neck.
- Give bladder washouts only when absolutely necessary, i.e. when the catheter is blocked or when washouts have been prescribed as a treatment (Shepherd et al. 2018). Bladder washouts should not be employed as a prophylactic treatment for urine infections.

Maintaining the Person's Dignity

The following measures will help to preserve the person's dignity and self-esteem by:

- Providing education and promoting self-care where possible in meatal hygiene, emptying and changing bags.
- Using the correct length catheter for gender and the use of leg bags which allows people to conceal the bag more easily and have a choice of clothing, for example a woman may wish to wear a skirt.
- Encouraging maximum mobility to promote confidence and give better drainage.

Changes, Problems and Possible Interventions

The nurse should be prepared for the following changes or potential problems:

An Increase in Urethral Discharge

- Urethral secretion is increased with the presence of a foreign body, i.e. the catheter. To prevent this becoming troublesome, the person is advised that daily meatal hygiene (see above) should be instituted from the first day of catheterisation.

Bypassing

- Check to see if the catheter or drainage tube is blocked, kinked or looped.
- Consider changing to a smaller-gauge catheter. It is a misconception that if the catheter bypasses, a larger catheter is required.
- Check whether or not medication which can cause spasm has been prescribed.
- Exclude constipation – relieve constipation immediately and emphasise the importance of a high-fibre diet.
- Check with the doctor or other prescriber about the possibility of prescribing anticholinergic drugs if the bypassing still persists.

Balloon Not Deflating

- Attach a syringe to the valve in position without aspiration. It may self-deflate.
- The balloon may be burst by injecting 2–5 mL of dilute ether via the balloon inflating channel.
- A fine sterile wire may be passed up the inflating channel and the balloon burst.
- Never cut off the end of the inflation channel of the catheter.

Blockage

- May be caused by medication, e.g. aperients causing phosphate debris in the urine – change or stop the drug, encourage the person to take a high-fibre diet and encourage more exercise.
- Infection must be treated with the correct antibiotic. Check the amount of fluid intake and where possible try to increase this. Check the standard of personal hygiene.
- If clots occur, carry out a bladder washout with 0.9% sodium chloride solution.

Once the man has been catheterised, his renal function restored and any anaemia corrected, there is no urgency to proceed to surgery. The individual may in fact benefit from a period of recuperation and bladder rest with the catheter in situ. Depending upon the ability of the individual to care for the catheter and upon community resources, ideally care will be given in the man's home.

A trial without the catheter should not be made, as this would again lead to chronic retention followed by renal failure. If the patient is able, intermittent self-catheterisation may be taught.

For those with milder symptoms, it is a matter of discussion between the man and his clinician as to whether symptoms are interfering with the individual's lifestyle sufficiently to warrant an operation and whether he stands a good chance of improvement from surgery. In rare cases where there is poor life expectancy or the man is too unfit for surgery, operative treatment may not be offered and a permanent indwelling catheter may be considered the best management.

Caring for Men Undergoing TURP

The man must be given a clear explanation of the after-effects of TURP, so that he can give his informed consent prior to the procedure. The surgery and the complications (outlined in Information 10.7) should be discussed with all men and their questions honestly answered. It should never be presumed that any specific groups of men are not sexually active. Apart from the general anxieties associated with the prospect of surgery and an anaesthetic (see Chapter 25, Nursing the Patient Undergoing Surgery), many men will worry about loss of continence, ED, retrograde ejaculation and a decrease in fertility (Reflection 10.2). Since many men have retrograde ejaculation (ejaculation of semen into the bladder) after prostate surgery, it is essential that they are counselled adequately beforehand. Retrograde ejaculation does not cause ED, but a man who has not been given adequate reassurance on this point could suffer psychological effects resulting in difficulty in achieving or maintaining an erection. Retrograde ejaculation will not render the man sterile, but neither will it necessarily permit him to father children easily.

Specific Nursing Considerations

Risk of Haemorrhage. Since haemorrhage is a major risk after prostate surgery, preoperative care should involve determining baseline haematological values. Careful consideration must be given to those individuals receiving oral anticoagulants for any other disease, since the risk of haemorrhage is considerable. It may be necessary to discontinue oral therapy preoperatively and to use heparin or clexane until the oral regimen can be recommenced and stabilised postoperatively. This may take some weeks to achieve and will require the patient to make additional visits to the hospital or GP surgery.

Fluid and Electrolyte Balance (see Chapter 21). Preoperative determination of urea and electrolyte levels will provide baseline measurements and permit correction before surgery if required. This may involve urethral catheterisation to enable adequate bladder drainage and the use of IV fluids to achieve hydration.

During TURP, the bladder is irrigated with a fluid that contains glycine (saline cannot be used as it is electrolytic and can't be used with diathermy) to provide a clear view for the surgeon. Some of this fluid is usually absorbed, and if there is an interruption in the venous system during the resection, the fluid absorbed can be excessive, leading to TUR syndrome. Excessive absorption of irrigant (usually glycine) will cause the patient to become hyponatraemic. This can lead to confusion, a restless mental state and, in some cases, altered consciousness. This imbalance can be corrected by restricting fluid intake and encouraging diuresis but medical assistance will be required in respect of the electrolyte balance (Frede and Rassweiler 2017).

In most hospital centres, the risk of TUR syndrome has been further minimised with using bipolar diathermy resectoscopes, giving the clinician the option of using normal saline during the surgery. Nurses caring for postoperative TURP patients should be aware of which method was used during surgery to manage postoperative accordingly.

Urinary Infection. The presence of an indwelling urethral catheter preoperatively is associated with a high risk of infective complications. The effectiveness of prophylactic antibiotics is uncertain, but it would seem that those who do not receive systemic therapy at the time of operation, followed by a postoperative course, will be likely to develop bacteraemia and become unwell.

Management of Irrigation

An irrigation set with a Y-connection will be used to allow two 3 L bags of 0.9% sodium chloride solution to be in place at any one time, with one bag running at a time. The irrigation runs into the bladder via the irrigating channel of the catheter, diluting the urine, which then drains out through the outlet channel of the catheter into a drainage bag. Irrigation prevents blood clots forming and obstructing the catheter. The irrigation is regulated, via a clamp, to run at a speed sufficient to keep the bladder clear of blood clots. The bags are numbered and the amount of irrigation fluid recorded on a fluid chart. The patient's total output, i.e. urine and irrigation fluid, should be measured and recorded. The amount of irrigation fluid used should be subtracted from the measured output to give an approximate urine output volume (note that the urine will initially contain blood).

The nurse should:

- Observe and palpate the man's lower abdomen. Abdominal distension may indicate clot retention or extravasation. Clot retention is a common complication in the first 12–24 hours. Bladder washout or deflation and reinflation of the catheter balloon may be required.
- Note the colour of the irrigation fluid: a bright red colour may indicate fresh bleeding; a dark red colour would suggest old blood.
- In an uncircumcised man, check that the prepuce (foreskin) is over the glans penis to prevent paraphimosis.

The morning following surgery, the irrigation will usually be discontinued, provided the man is able to drink sufficient fluid to help flush the prostatic bed of any further bleeding or clots.

Pain relief should be adequate to allow the man to rest and feel comfortable.

Catheter Care. A common problem while the catheter is in situ is the bypassing of urine around it. This is sometimes difficult to resolve, and the nurse should take the following preventive measures:

- Check that the catheter is not blocked by clots or debris and that it is in the bladder.
- Check the amount of water in the balloon. If it is 30 mL, then reduce it to approximately 20 mL or so, but not less than 15 mL.
- Give anticholinergic medication as prescribed, e.g. oxybutynin.
- Encourage the man to continue to drink sufficient fluids.

The catheter will remain in situ for 1–2 days following surgery or until the urine output is clear. Before removing it, the nurse should ensure that the man has had a bowel movement, as straining following catheter removal can lead to further urethral bleeding. Following removal, the man may experience urgency and frequency as before. He should be reassured that this is normal and that it may take up to 8 weeks for a normal voiding pattern to be established. The man should be educated to tighten the sphincter muscle and to hold on as long as possible before passing urine.

Men who had chronic retention before surgery often fail to void postoperatively. A long-term catheter will normally be inserted in such cases, and the patient allowed home for several weeks (usually 6). This time period allows the bladder to rest and regain its elasticity.

Discharge From Hospital

Once the man's urine is clear, the catheter can normally be removed. This is usually done in the morning to allow him to establish a normal voiding pattern before retiring to bed. Provided the man is able to pass a normal volume of urine (e.g. >150 mL in one void) without difficulty, on at least two occasions with low postvoid residual scan volumes, he may be discharged from hospital.

Many men feel, after the operation, that they have gained no relief from their problems. It must be understood that it will take about 6 weeks for the prostatic bed to heal, such that full urinary control is possible. During the early postoperative weeks, the man should refrain from vigorous exercise/heavy lifting. He should drink sufficient fluids and avoid becoming constipated. The practice nurse or community nurse will give advice and support should urinary problems occur.

It should be noted that at about 14 days postoperatively, when desiccated tissue has sloughed off the prostatic bed, secondary haemorrhage can occur (see Chapter 25, Nursing the Patient Undergoing Surgery).

Occasionally, urethral stricture occurs as the urethral mucosa in the prostatic region heals.

Prostate Cancer

Prostate cancer is the most commonly diagnosed malignancy in men in the United Kingdom. According to Cancer Research UK (2023a), there were over 52,000 new cases of prostate cancer diagnosed in the UK each year during 2016–2018, and prostatic cancer accounted for 27% of new cancer diagnoses. Incidence rates are lower in the Asian ethnic group and in people of mixed or multiple ethnicity, but higher in the Black ethnic group, compared with the White ethnic group, in males in England (2013–2017). Furthermore, incidence increases with age and postmortem studies have shown that approximately 30% of asymptomatic men over the age of 50, and 90% over the age of 90, have microscopic foci, evident only on histological examination. About 10% of men thought to have benign prostate disease on examination are later found by histological examination to have prostatic cancer. Prostate cancer is the second most common cause of cancer death in males in the UK, accounting for 14% of all cancer deaths in males in the UK (2017–2019).

Pathophysiology

The cause of prostate cancer is not clear, but there is some evidence to show that hormonal activity plays a part in the transformation of certain normal cells into cancerous ones. Benign enlargement (due to hypertrophy and or hyperplasia) and cancer arise in different parts of the gland. Cancer occurs in the peripheral gland. Metastases (secondary spread) often occur in bone, where they are associated with severe pain. In cases of extreme bony destruction, pathological fractures may occur. It has been known for vertebral destruction to cause spinal cord compression (SCC) which without urgent treatment can lead to paraplegia.

Common Presenting Symptoms

The diagnosis of prostate cancer is difficult because the man is often asymptomatic, with the majority of prostate cancers being identified via abnormalities in PSA level or findings on digital rectal examination. Men with locally advanced disease are likely to complain of symptoms associated with bladder outflow obstruction (see Information 10.6), a sudden onset of urgency to void urine and possibly haematuria or haematospermia (blood in semen).

Chronic urinary retention secondary to bladder outflow obstruction may cause renal damage by dilating the upper renal tracts. The man may present with a palpable bladder or with renal failure; he is likely to be generally unwell and losing weight. Renal failure may also be caused by ureteric infiltration of tumour or by para-aortic lymph node enlargement causing ureteric obstruction. Those who feel unwell and are anaemic are likely to have suffered bone marrow infiltration and/or renal failure. A complaint of persistent backache may suggest bone metastases.

An irregular, enlarged, hard prostate gland does not prove the diagnosis, although most advanced carcinomas will be felt as such on rectal examination. However, prostatitis or prostatic stone disease may feel similar on rectal examination. Moreover, if there is a cancer within the anterior part of the gland, rectal examination will reveal no abnormality.

Medical Management

Investigations

PSA blood test is used in combination with digital rectal examination to determine if the man may have prostate cancer. Neither is completely accurate, with PSA having a false-positive test result of 30% and only tumours that occur in the peripheral zone of the prostate are commonly palpable.

The NICE (2019) Prostate Cancer: Diagnosis and Management Guidance recommends that patients with two elevated PSA bloods tests, or a single elevated PSA with an abnormal digital rectal examination, should have mpMRI of the prostate for further investigations. These MRIs are reported using either a PIRADS scoring or Likert scale identifying any abnormalities. If abnormalities are found, then targeted biopsies can be done to reduce the chances of false-negative results.

The only certain means of making a diagnosis is by histological examination. Fine-needle transrectal ultrasonographic prostatic biopsy can be done with or without local anaesthetic for this purpose.

mpMRI should be undertaken in men who are going to have active treatment but is not needed in men who have elected not to have radical treatment. Additional investigations to provide evidence of metastatic spread include CT scan if MRI is contraindicated and bone scan.

Prostatic cancer is graded histologically to assess malignant potential, such as by using the one-to-five-stage Gleason grading system.

Treatment

The nature of the treatment offered and whether it is given on an outpatient or an inpatient basis will depend upon the extent of the disease and on how the man presents symptomatically and clinically.

Active Surveillance. Active surveillance is an option to men with low-risk localised prostate cancer or for those with intermediate-risk localised prostate cancer who do not wish to have immediate radical prostatectomy or radiotherapy. These patients should have their PSA checked at regular intervals (see NICE 2019).

Surgery. TURP can be carried out to relieve urinary symptoms and retention. This does not, however, afford a cure. Radical prostatectomy and clearance of any pelvic lymphatic involvement are performed in the hope of achieving a cure. This treatment is restricted to those with disease localised to the prostate, a life expectancy of greater than 10 years and no significant comorbidity. The man should be counselled preoperatively about his disease and the almost certain complication of urinary incontinence and ED.

Radiotherapy. This is given as either external beam or interstitial seed implantation (brachytherapy). For external beam radiotherapy, if the man is generally fit, he will probably attend for daily treatment as an outpatient. In some cases, the side-effects will necessitate hospitalisation, for example when nausea, vomiting and diarrhoea cause dehydration, or when urinary frequency or incontinence causes severe physical and psychological distress.

Cryotherapy. Cryotherapy is being used more commonly to treat prostate cancer, but is not recommended in men with localised prostate cancer. The procedure involves freezing the prostate gland in order to destroy it, and is achieved by inserting probes into the prostate gland via the perineum.

High-Intensity Focused Ultrasound (HIFU). HIFU uses ultrasound energy to kill cancer cells in the prostate with minimal damage to the surrounding tissue. Like cryotherapy, it is not recommended in men with localised prostate cancer.

Treating Advanced Disease

The aims of treatment in advanced disease are to provide symptomatic relief and to preserve an acceptable quality of life for the individual. Current recommendations from NICE (2019) suggest combined forms of radiotherapy with androgen deprivation therapy. Other forms of treatment offered include interventions that lower or remove testosterone such as bilateral orchidectomy (surgical removal of the testes) or antiandrogen tablets (see NICE 2019).

Chemotherapy with docetaxel is recommended for patients with advanced prostate cancer who do not have significant comorbidities.

Radiotherapy is sometimes beneficial in the relief of bony pain caused by metastases. Vertebral collapse caused by metastatic disease leading to SCC requires emergency radiotherapy or laminectomy and hormonal manipulation. If effective, these measures may prevent neurological manifestations including paraplegia from developing.

Pain control by means of opiate analgesics may cause constipation; this in turn can cause urinary retention. It may be more appropriate to administer NSAIDs to avoid this side-effect. Should analgesics be required, they should be given in doses that prevent pain occurring (see Chapter 20, Pain Management, and Chapter 31, Nursing the Patient With Cancer). Sustained- or slow-release medication is often very useful.

❖ Nursing Management and Health Promotion: Prostate Cancer

The nursing management of the man with prostatic cancer is very much influenced by the particular presentation and the stage of the disease in each individual. The nurse should take a problem-solving approach to care and promote independence and self-care for as long as possible. The nurse should bear in mind that constipation and urinary retention or urinary incontinence are commonly encountered and can be very distressing both for the individual and for his family. Ongoing liaison between hospital and community teams will help to ensure that care is effective and genuinely responsive to the man's unique situation (see Chapter 31, Nursing the Patient With Cancer, and Chapter 32, Nursing Patients Who Need Palliative Care).

A range of medical interventions may be necessary at different stages in the disease process. Nursing involvement will then include assisting with procedures such as:
- correction of anaemia by blood transfusion
- TURP to relieve retention

- bilateral subcapsular orchidectomy to reduce the androgen hormone level, help prevent the spread of metastases and reduce pain.

In some cases, medical intervention can offer only temporary improvement, and the emphasis of care will turn to palliation. Treatment of advanced disease is usually shared between hospital and home, and the patient and his family will need a great deal of moral and practical support in both settings. It is important to convey a sense of optimism so that life can continue to be enjoyed to the fullest degree possible. Once the end-of-life stage of the illness has been reached, however, it should not be seen as a defeat or failure to help the man and his family to let go of life and face death with dignity (see Chapter 32).

Urethral Stricture and Disorders of the Male Urethra and Penis

This section of the chapter outlines a range of conditions including urethral stricture and those affecting the male urethra and penis: phimosis, paraphimosis and congenital conditions.

Urethral Stricture

A stricture is a narrowing within the lumen of the urethra, which may be congenital or acquired.

● Pathophysiology

Urethral strictures can be congenital, caused by trauma (as in pelvic fracture), occur as a consequence of instrumentation of the urethra (e.g. cystoscopy) or result from the presence of an indwelling urethral catheter. Inflammation caused by infections such as nongonococcal urethritis (previously known as nonspecific urethritis) and gonorrhoea may also result in stricture formation. It is a condition that more commonly affects men because of the length and structure of the male urethra. A stricture may also result from muscular spasm or from occlusion of the urethra by a cancerous growth.

Common Presenting Symptoms

Symptoms can prove to be both distressing and frustrating. They include poor urinary flow, a feeling of incomplete bladder emptying, frequency, dysuria or haematuria, and dribbling incontinence, secondary to chronic urinary retention.

● Medical Management

Tests and investigations required are flow-rate studies, retrograde urethrogram, urethroscopy and full blood screening.

The treatment options include the following:

Urethral Dilatation/Urethrotomy. The use of meatal or urethral dilators to stretch the narrowing or an optical urethrotome allows the surgeon, under direct vision, to divide the urethral stricture. A silicone catheter will normally be left in place for a specified period to allow healing. However, the length of time it will be left in situ is variable.

Self-dilatation. This is often used in conjunction with urethral dilatation or urethrotomy. The technique involves the person using a self-lubricating urethral catheter on a regular basis to increase the urethral diameter and keep the urethral passage open.

Urethroplasty. This reconstructive procedure is usually performed in two stages, involving excision of the stricture and anastomosis. In some cases a graft is required to replace the excised urethral tissue. This surgery requires a longer stay in hospital and is normally performed only after other treatments have failed.

Phimosis

In this condition, the foreskin or prepuce of the penis is too tight to be retracted over the glans penis. It may be caused by balanitis xerotica obliterans (BXO)/lichen sclerosus et atrophicus (Csillag's disease), a group of chronic disorders that cause soreness and irritation. Other causes include infection, trauma as a result of early attempts to draw back the foreskin before it has naturally separated or developed fully in size or a poorly performed circumcision operation.

Pathophysiology

The natural separation of the two layers of skin from the glans penis normally occurs by about the age of 2 years. Following separation, daily bathing is necessary to ensure hygiene is maintained. Poor personal hygiene can give rise to inflammation and infection and has been implicated as a cause of penile cancer.

Common Presenting Symptoms

Phimosis often causes balanoposthitis (inflammation of glans penis (balanitis) and the prepuce (posthitis)). Presenting features include itching, a white discharge, pain, discomfort and bleeding during sexual intercourse and sometimes urinary retention.

Medical Management

The initial treatment may be with antibacterial or anticandidal agents. If the individual is sexually active, he and his partner will both require treatment to prevent the infection being passed back and forth. Circumcision is the treatment of choice and may have to be performed as an emergency if urinary retention has occurred (Information 10.10).

❖ Nursing Management and Health Promotion: Phimosis

Prevention

Health promotion is important for prevention, and information should be available to parents/carers in the early years. They should be advised that retraction of the foreskin for cleansing should not be attempted before natural separation around 2 years of age. During childhood, older boys should be taught to retract the foreskin to wash the glans penis (during bathing or showering), dry the area and reposition the foreskin.

INFORMATION 10.10

Male Circumcision

Circumcision, the surgical removal of the prepuce (foreskin), may be indicated for penile carcinoma, balanitis (inflammation of the glans penis), candidal infection, phimosis or adherent prepuce. These conditions generally affect adults. Circumcision may also be performed in accordance with religious practices, in which case the procedure is usually performed in infancy or childhood.

The main complications of circumcision are infection and bleeding. Painful erections in the immediate postoperative period can usually be relieved by the application of a local anaesthetic gel. Postoperative swelling or oedema may make micturition difficult. Dribbling or urinary leakage to the wound area can delay or prevent wound healing and cause secondary infection. The insertion of a urethral catheter may be necessary to relieve this problem in order that wound healing may take place.

Promoting Wound Healing After Circumcision

The nurse can promote wound healing by:
- Teaching good personal hygiene to the newly circumcised man.
- Washing the wound area daily with soap and water and applying a protective, nonadherent dressing to prevent clothing disturbing wound healing.
- Providing more frequent washing and dressing changes should urine leakage occur onto the wound or dressing.
- Counselling the man to refrain from sexual intercourse until the wound is well healed.

Further information about phimosis and circumcision is provided in Chapter 9.

Paraphimosis

Paraphimosis is a condition in which a foreskin that has been retracted over the glans penis cannot be returned to its usual position. The swollen band of foreskin obstructs the circulation to the glans, which in turn becomes swollen and painful. It is a medical emergency as delayed action may lead to gangrene of the glans.

Cold compresses applied to the penis may help to relieve the swelling and pain. The health professional may be able to manipulate the glans back under the foreskin with or without anaesthesia. Because of extreme pain, men may require a penile nerve block, topical analgesic or oral opioids. If manipulation is unsuccessful, a dorsal slit may be made in the foreskin. There remains a risk of recurrence of the paraphimosis and circumcision may be advisable at a later date. Further information about the prevention of paraphimosis is provided in Chapter 9.

Congenital Disorders of the Urethra and Penis

At birth, an infant is examined to confirm its sex and to make sure that expected bodily structures are present. In boys, the urethral meatus is normally seen at the anterior tip of the glans penis. Occasionally, a malformation of the urethra is identified as a congenital defect.

Hypospadias

Hypospadias is a condition where the urethral meatus is positioned on the undersurface of the glans penis and is the second most common congenital abnormality after undescended testes (Van der Horst and De Wall 2017). The condition is usually treated quite effectively by enlargement of the meatus by plastic surgery. In some cases the urethral orifice is positioned further back on the lower surface of the penis, and this will complicate treatment. Surgical reconstruction should take place before the age of 2 years, as this avoids cosmetic and fertility problems in later life. The position of the meatus, distal urethra and presence or absence of chordee (downward curvature of the penis) will influence the surgical approach adopted.

Epispadias

In epispadias the urethra opens onto the upper surface, or dorsum, of the penis. The meatus of the urethra may be positioned anywhere along the length of the penile surface. Epispadias may coexist with other serious congenital abnormalities involving a poorly developed anterior section of the urinary bladder and abdominal wall. Surgical reconstruction is likely to be complex and may involve transplantation of ureters.

Summary: Key Nursing Issues

- Nursing people with disorders of the urinary system is a challenging and rapidly developing area of practice in which to work, one in which the role of the nurse is constantly developing.
- Caring for people who have problems within the urinary system is complex and demanding.
- Conditions that affect the urinary tract can be either acute or chronic and it is important that the nurse recognises that the person's needs are often multifactorial.

- In order to provide high-quality nursing care, when caring for people with urinary problems, the nurse must demonstrate not only a good understanding of anatomy and physiology, the disease process and the potential complications but also good interpersonal skills and sensitivity in the experience of illness.

Reflection and Learning – What Next?

- **Test** your knowledge by visiting the Evolve website 🌐 and answering the multiple-choice questions and critical thinking questions.
- **Consolidate** your learning by looking at some of the further reading suggestions, references and specialist websites.
- **Revisit** some of the additional material on the Evolve website.

- **Consider** what you have learnt and how this will help your professional development.
- **Reflect** on how you can apply this knowledge to the care of your patients.
- **Discuss** your learning with your assessor/supervisor, lecturer and colleagues.

References

Anders HJ, Kitching AR, Leung N, Romagnani P. Glomerulonephritis: immunopathogenesis and immunotherapy. *Nat Rev Immunol.* 2023:1–19.

Brooker C, ed. *Mosby's Dictionary of Medicine, Nursing and Health Professions.* UK ed. Edinburgh: Mosby; 2010.

Cancer Research UK (2023a), Prostate Cancer Statistics, Cancer Research UK.

Cancer Research UK. *Bladder Cancer Statistics, Cancer Research UK, Types of Bladder Cancer.* Cancer Research UK; 2023.

Conway B, Phelan PJ, Stewart GD. Nephrology and urology. In: Ralston SH, Penman ID, Strachan MWJ, Hobson RP, eds. *Davidson's Principles and Practice of Medicine.* 23rd ed. Edinburgh: Churchill Livingstone; 2018.

Cooper TE, Tene C, Howell M, Teixeria-Pinto A, Jaure A, Wong G. D-Mannose for preventing and treating urinary tract infections. *Cochrane Database Syst Rev.* 2022;8(8):CD013608.

Dainton M. Acute kidney injury. In: Thomas N, ed. *Renal Nursing: Care and Management of People with Kidney Disease.* 5th ed. John Wiley and Sons Ltd.; 2019:105–126.

European Association of Urology (2018). Urolithiasis. http://uroweb.org.

European Association of Urology (2023). Urological infections. EAU Guidelines – Uroweb. https://uroweb.org/guidelines/urological-infections.

Frede T, Rassweiler JJ. Management of postoperative complications following TURP. In: Rané A, Turna B, Autorino R, Rassweiler J, eds. *Practical Tips in Urology.* London: Springer; 2017;493–502.

Loveday HP, Wilson JA, Pratt RJ, et al. epic3: National evidence-based guidelines for preventing healthcare-associated infections in NHS hospitals in England. *J Hosp Infect.* 2014;86S1. https://improvement.nhs.uk/documents/847/epic3_National_Evidence-Based_Guidelines_for_Preventing_HCAI_in_NHSE.pdf.

National Institute for Health and Care Excellence (NICE). *Healthcare-associated infections: prevention and control in primary and community care.* Clinical guideline [CG139]; 2017. http://www.nice.org.uk.

National Institute for Health and Care Excellence (NICE). Urinary tract infection (lower): antimicrobial prescribing [NG109]. 2018. http://www.nice.org.uk/guidance/ng109.

National Institute of Health and Care Excellence (NICE). *Prostate cancer: diagnosis and management.* NICE guideline [NG131]; 2019. http://www.nice.org.uk/guidance/ng131.

National Institute for Health and Care Excellence (NICE). Clinical knowledge summary, pyelonephritis – acute. 2023. https://cks.nice.org.uk/topics/pyelonephritis-acute/.

Otto W, Breyer J, Herdegen S, et al. WHO 1973 grade 3 and infiltrative growth pattern proved, aberrant E-cadherin expression tends to be of predictive value for progression in a series of stage T1 high-grade bladder cancer after organ-sparing approach. *Int Urol Nephrol.* 2017;49:431. https://pubmed.ncbi.nlm.nih.gov/28035618/ In: European Association of Urology Non-muscle invasive bladder cancer (TaT1 and CIS) 2023.

Shepherd A, Mackay WG, Hagen S. Catheter washout solutions for long-term urinary catheterisation in adults: a Cochrane review summary. *Int J Nurs Stud.* 2018;82:167–170.

Thomas N, ed. *Renal Nursing: Care and Management of People With Kidney Disease.* 5th ed. John Wiley and Sons Ltd.; 2019.

Vaidya SR, Aeddula NR. Chronic Renal Failure. *StatPearls [Internet].* Treasure Island (FL): StatPearls Publishing; 2022. Updated 24 October 2022. https://www.ncbi.nlm.nih.gov/books/NBK535404/.

Van der Horst HJR, De Wall LL. Hypospadias, all there is to know. *Eur J Pediatr.* 2017;176:435–441.

Wang P, Zhang H, Zhou J, et al. Study of risk factor of urinary calculi according to the association between stone composition with urine component. *Sci Rep.* 2021;11(1):8723.

Williams G, Hahn D, Stephens J, Craig J, Modson E. Cranberries for preventing urinary tract infections. *Cochrane Database Syst Rev.* 2023. https://doi.org/10.1002/14651858.CD001321.pub6.

Further Reading

National Institute for Health and Care Excellence (NICE). Urinary tract infection (lower): antimicrobial prescribing. NG109. 2018. www.nice.org.uk/guidance/ng109.

National Institute for Health and Care Excellence (NICE). Renal or Ureteric Colic. 2020. https://cks.nice.org.uk/topics/renal-or-ureteric-colic-acute/.

National Institute for Health and Care Excellence (NICE). Clinical knowledge summary renal or ureteric colic – acute. 2020. https://cks.nice.org.uk/topics/renal or ureteric colic acute.

National Institute for Health and Care Excellence (NICE). Urinary Tract Infection (Lower) Men. 2023 https://cks.nice.org.uk/topics/urinary-tract-infection-lower-men/.

National Institute for Health and Care Excellence (NICE). Urinary Tract Infection (Lower) Women. 2023. https://cks.nice.org.uk/topics/urinary-tract-infection-lower-women/.

National Institute for Health and Clinical Excellence (NICE). Bladder cancer: diagnosis and management. NICE guideline [NG2]. 2015. https://www.nice.org.uk/guidance/ng2.

Patton KT. *Anatomy and Physiology*. 10th ed. St. Louis, MO: Mosby Elsevier; 2018.

Reynard J, Brewster S, Biers S. *Oxford Handbook of Urology*. 4th ed. Oxford: Oxfordhandbooks; 2019.

Stamatelou K, Goldfarb DS. Epidemiology of kidney stones. *Healthcare*. 2023;11(3):424. https://doi.org/10.3390/healthcare11030424.

Useful Websites

British Association of Urological Nursing (links to other sites), www.baun.co.uk

Kidney patient guide, www.kidneypatientguide.org.uk

Kidney Research UK, www.kidneyresearchuk.org

National Institute for Health and Care Excellence (NICE) – improving outcomes in urological cancers, www.nice.org.uk/Guidance/CSGUC

Prostate Cancer Charity, https://prostatecanceruk.org/

The Renal Association, https://renal.org/

The Urology Foundation, www.theurologyfoundation.org/

UK Prostate Link, www.prostate-link.org.uk

11

Nursing Patients With Disorders of the Nervous System

SUE WOODWARD

CHAPTER OUTLINE

Introduction

Many nurses may have contact with patients living with neurological disorders. Community nursing staff are increasingly involved in the care of patients recovering at home following acute neurosurgical interventions or with long-term neurological conditions. This chapter considers the more common neurological and neurosurgical disorders and, where appropriate, makes reference to some less common disorders. The further reading suggestions at the end of the chapter provide more detailed information. It is hoped that the information contained here will raise awareness of this specialised field of nursing and stimulate further reflection on how best to meet the needs of the person with a neurological condition and of their family (Evidence-Based Practice 11.1).

EVIDENCE-BASED PRACTICE 11.1

Living With a Lifelong or Long-Term Illness

Purpose

The study by Sixsmith et al. (2014) explored the experiences of service users and providers. The authors conducted 50 qualitative semistructured interviews with both patients and health professionals who cared for people with long-term neurological conditions about their experiences of health, well-being and quality of life in relation to service provision. Three major themes emerged: 'Diagnosis and treatment', 'Better connected services' and 'On-going rehabilitation'. Patients reported that effective care was provided within hospital settings, but that this often changed on return home even though they had ongoing needs. In both hospital and community settings, health professionals reported that they lacked the support and resources to provide continuous care, with patients often reaching a crisis point before being referred to specialist care.

Activity

- Access the study by Sixsmith et al. (2014) and read about the three themes that emerged.
- Discuss with your practice assessor how you can use the experiences of people with lifelong or long-term illness to enhance person-centred care.

Reference

Sixsmith J, Callender M, Hobbs G, et al. Implementing the National Service Framework for long-term (neurological) conditions: service user and service provider experiences. *Disabil Rehabil.* 2014;36(7):563-572.

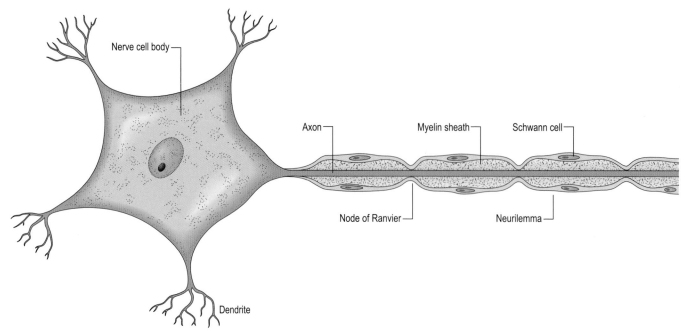

Figure. 11.1 Structure of a multipolar neurone. It consists of three parts: (1) The nerve cell body, which is grey in colour. Each cell body is enclosed in a selectively permeable membrane, which also extends along the cell processes. The cell body contains a nucleus surrounded by cytoplasm which also contains other structures called organelles. (2) The dendrites are thread-like extensions of the cell body which increase the surface area available to receive signals from other neurones. (3) The axon is a single long process that conducts impulses away from the cell body. In many large peripheral axons, the axolemma is surrounded by another covering called the myelin sheath. This is a multiple-layered covering of fatty material which is white in colour. Its function is to insulate the neurone electrically and thus speed up the conduction of the nerve impulse, by segmentation. Each interruption of the sheath is known as a node of Ranvier and the speed of the impulse is increased by its 'jumping' from node to node. The axon and its collaterals branch into axon terminals, the ends of which form a bulb-like structure. These help to transmit an impulse from one neurone to another across the gap (synapse) between them or at the junctions with effector cells.

Anatomy and Physiology

The nervous system is a complex, interrelated body system responsible for many functions, including communication, coordination, behaviour and intelligence. It constantly receives data from the external and internal environments, interprets these, and then responds by adapting appropriately to demands.

The nervous system has two main divisions: the central nervous system (CNS), comprising the brain and spinal cord, and the peripheral nervous system (PNS), consisting of the cranial and spinal nerves. The PNS has two functional parts, the somatic (sensory and motor) and autonomic divisions.

Basic Tissue Structure

Nervous tissue consists of neuroglia (glial cells) and neurones (nerve cells). The neuroglia markedly outnumber the neurones and form a supportive, nutritive and protective network for the nervous system. In the PNS, supporting cells, called Schwann cells, form the myelin sheath as well as having a phagocytic role, whereas in the CNS oligodendrocytes secrete myelin.

Myelin protects and electrically insulates nerve fibres from one another and speeds up nerve impulse transmission. Myelinated nerve impulses are transmitted by saltatory conduction, whereby the impulse jumps from one node of Ranvier to the next (Fig. 11.1). Impulses in myelinated nerves are therefore transmitted very much faster than in unmyelinated nerves and require much less energy.

Neurones

Neurones are the structural and functional unit of the nervous system. They are capable of conducting impulses throughout the nervous system and to other excitable tissues, including muscles and glands. The structure of a typical multipolar neurone is shown in Fig. 11.1.

The axons of sensory and motor neurones constitute the nerve fibres. They are bundled together in the PNS by connective tissue to form the peripheral nerves.

🌐 **See Evolve website Fig. 11.1**

Sensory (Afferent) Neurones transmit impulses from receptors in the skin, sense organs and viscera to the brain and spinal cord. These are usually unipolar (cells with processes projecting from one pole) or bipolar (processes project from two poles at opposite ends of the cell body). Bipolar neurones are found only in special sense organs, for example, the retina of the eye.

Motor (Efferent) Neurones transmit impulses from the brain and spinal cord to muscles and glands in the body (the effectors) (see Fig. 11.1).

Interneurones convey impulses from one neurone to another within the CNS.

The Nerve Impulse

A nerve impulse can be initiated by a stimulus such as a change in temperature, pressure or the chemical environment, or impulses can be generated spontaneously by pacemaker cells. The impulse is a self-propagating wave of electrical charge along the neuronal membrane.

At rest, the neurone has an unequal distribution of potassium and sodium ions on either side of the plasma membrane, which are necessary to maintain the chemical difference that produces an electrical difference: the inside of the cell is negatively charged in relation to the outside. This has been measured at −70 mV and is termed the resting membrane potential. This state is maintained by an exchange of ions between the intracellular and extracellular fluids. A property of all neurones is their ability to produce an impulse when a stimulus is sufficient to initiate certain electrical and chemical changes within the cell membrane. These positive–negative changes occur in rapid succession, spreading to the end of the axon (See Further Reading, e.g. Marieb and Hoehn 2020).

Generally, the larger the diameter of the axon, the quicker the nerve impulse travels, but the alternative process of saltatory conduction is found in myelinated neurones (Fig. 11.2).

Neurotransmitters

The junctions between one neurone and another, and between neurones and muscles or glands, are known as synapses. Nerve impulses are transmitted across the gap at most synapses by chemical transmitters (neurotransmitters). The chemical is stored in vesicles in the expanded end of the axon and is released when the nerve impulse reaches this point. Several neurotransmitters have been identified, the most common ones being acetylcholine and noradrenaline. Many neurotransmitters are excitatory, resulting in the nerve impulse producing an effect such as contraction of muscle cells. Some, however, have an inhibiting effect and prevent the onward transmission of impulses, allowing, for example, muscle cells to relax. The effect of the neurotransmitter is terminated when it is destroyed by enzymes or reabsorbed into the neurone.

The Central Nervous System

The CNS consists of the brain and spinal cord.

The Brain

The Cerebrum

The cerebrum forms the bulk of the brain. The outer surface, the cortex (grey matter), consists of neuronal cell bodies. The surface area of the cerebral cortex is increased by folding into a series of grooves (sulci) and ridges (gyri). The deeper grooves are termed fissures and some form landmarks, for example, the longitudinal fissure which almost splits the brain into left and right hemispheres (Fig. 11.3).

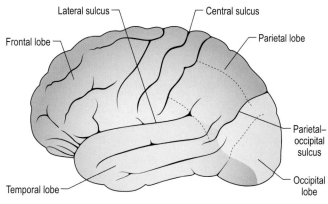

Figure 11.3 The lobes and sulci of the cerebrum. Each of the lobes is bounded by 'landmark' fissures: the frontal lobe is separated from the parietal lobe by the central sulcus; the temporal lobe is separated from the frontal and parietal lobes by the lateral sulcus; and the occipital lobe is separated from the temporal and parietal lobes by the parietal–occipital sulcus.

Each hemisphere is subdivided into lobes, and each lobe is named according to the skull bones it underlies:

- frontal
- temporal
- parietal
- occipital.

The cerebral cortex is responsible for three main functions:

- receiving and interpreting sensory information from the internal and external environments
- initiating and controlling voluntary movement in response to the sensory information received
- integrating crucial functions such as memory and consciousness.

Certain areas of the cerebral cortex have been identified as being responsible for specific functions, and can be mapped (Fig. 11.4).

Relative Size. The thumbs, fingers, lips, tongue and vocal cords are more sensitive than the trunk, due to the greater number of receptors found in them. The homunculus (Fig. 11.5) illustrates how the various parts of the body are represented in the corresponding motor and sensory areas of the cerebral hemispheres, i.e. representation is proportional not to the relative size

Figure 11.2 Saltatory conduction in a myelinated nerve.

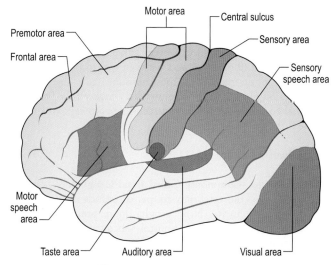

Figure 11.4 The cerebrum showing the functional areas.

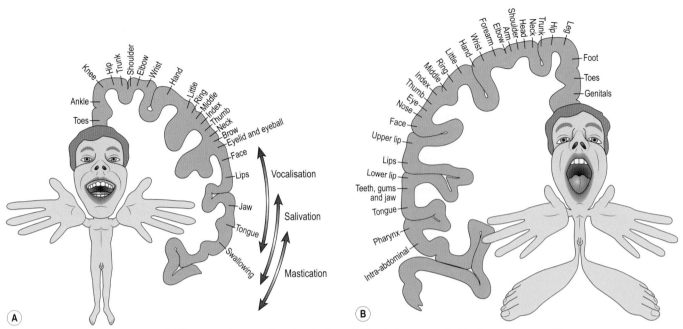

Figure 11.5 (A) The motor homunculus showing how the body is represented in the motor area of the cerebrum. (B) The sensory homunculus showing how the body is represented in the sensory area of the cerebrum. (Reproduced with permission from Montague SE, Watson R, Herbert R. Physiology for Nursing Practice. 3rd ed. London: Baillière Tindall; 2005.)

of the body parts, but to each part's complexity of movement or the extent of its sensory innervation.

Cerebral Dominance. Some functions (e.g. speech) are controlled from only one hemisphere, i.e. they are lateralised. Motor control is usually more highly developed in one cerebral hemisphere than in the other. This is referred to as dominance. Approximately 95% of the population are dominant in the left hemisphere and are right-handed. If the dominant hemisphere is damaged, the opposite hemisphere is capable of taking over and assuming a dominant role.

Association Areas. Association areas are less well defined and are thought to be responsible for complex functions such as integration of the senses, memory, learning, thought processes, behaviour and emotion.

Connecting Pathways. White matter containing myelinated axons lies below the outer cortical layer and forms connections between the cerebral cortex and other areas of grey matter in the CNS. Three types of connecting pathways have been identified:

- association fibres – connect between gyri in the same hemisphere
- commissural fibres – connect between gyri in different hemispheres, for example, the corpus callosum
- projection fibres – provide connections between the brain and spinal cord in ascending and descending pathways; one example is the internal capsule.

🌐 **See Evolve website Fig. 11.2**

Basal Nuclei (Commonly Called Basal Ganglia). Within the white matter of the cerebrum are paired islands of grey matter called the basal nuclei (N.B. 'ganglia' more properly describes structures in the PNS). They control subconscious movements, such as swinging the arms while walking, and regulating muscle tone for specific body movements, a function that is lost in Parkinson's disease (PD).

Cerebellum

The cerebellum is located below the posterior part of the cerebrum and is separated from it by a fold of dura mater. It consists of two hemispheres separated by a narrow strip called the vermis. The cortex of the cerebellum consists of grey matter, folded to increase its surface area. The interior comprises white matter presented in a branching configuration termed the arbor vitae (tree of life). Links to the rest of the brain and spinal cord allow the cerebellum to receive sensory information and thereby to maintain equilibrium and modify voluntary movement, making it smooth and coordinated.

Pituitary Gland

The pituitary gland is situated at the base of the brain in a depression or fossa in the sphenoid bone called the 'sella turcica'. It is attached to the brain via a stalk which is continuous with the hypothalamus, and communication is by means of nerve fibres and blood vessels (see Chapter 5 Part 1, Nursing Patients With Endocrine Disorders).

Diencephalon

Three bilaterally symmetrical structures comprise the diencephalon:

- the thalamus
- the hypothalamus
- the epithalamus.

The Thalamus consists of two oval-shaped masses, mainly consisting of grey matter, situated within the cerebral hemispheres just below the corpus callosum. Sensory impulses associated with pain, temperature, pressure and touch are conveyed to the thalamus, which acts as a 'gateway'. Chaos would reign if all sensory information were allowed to reach the sensory cortex.

The Hypothalamus is situated below the thalamus and forms the walls and floor of the third ventricle. It controls the output of the hormones from the pituitary gland. Other functions include the regulation of hunger, thirst and body temperature (see Chapter 21, Maintaining Fluid, Electrolyte and Acid–Base balance, and Chapter 22, Nutrition and Health).

The Epithalamus forms the roof of the third ventricle. Extending from its posterior border is the pineal gland that contains high concentrations of melatonin and is thought to influence circadian rhythms, for example, the sleep/wake cycle.

Brain Stem

This comprises three structures: the medulla, the pons and the midbrain. Inferiorly the medulla is continuous with the spinal cord and connects with the pons above. The pons is continuous with the midbrain, which connects with the lower portion of the diencephalon.

The Medulla. All the spinal pathways pass through the medulla. Descending motor pathways (corticospinal and corticobulbar) cross to the opposite side in triangular-shaped structures called the pyramids, a process known as decussation. The medulla:

- contains the reticular formation, a diffuse area of grey and white matter that connects with the rest of the brain stem and cerebral cortex, within which is the reticular activating system (RAS), responsible for consciousness and arousal
- accommodates the reflex centres that control vital functions:
  - the cardiac centre – regulates heartbeat and force of contraction
  - the medullary rhythmicity area – adjusts the rhythm of breathing

- the vasomotor centre (VMC) – regulates the diameter of blood vessels
- contains other nonvital centres, including those responsible for coordinating swallowing, vomiting, coughing, sneezing and hiccupping
- contains the nuclei of cranial nerves VIII to XII (Table 11.1).

The Pons. The pons is a bridge between the medulla and the midbrain. It comprises fibres that connect with the cerebellum and fibres that link between the spinal cord and the brain. It contains the nuclei of cranial nerves V to VIII inclusive (see Table 11.1). Other important nuclei also exert an influence on respiration.

The Midbrain. The midbrain contains the centres for visual, auditory and postural reflexes. It is located above the pons and contains the nuclei of cranial nerves III and IV (see Table 11.1). Cranial nerves I and II originate in the cerebrum.

The Limbic System

A diffuse collection of nuclei, the limbic system, comprises an interconnected complex of structures, with links to the hypothalamus, cerebral cortex and the olfactory system. These are thought to be responsible for behaviour associated with emotions, subconscious motor and sensory drives and feelings of pain and pleasure.

TABLE 11.1	Outline of the Cranial Nerves	
Cranial Nerve Name and Number	**Type**	**Functions**
Olfactory (I)	Sensory	Smell (olfaction)
Optic (II)	Sensory	Vision
Oculomotor (III)	Motor Sensory	Controls four of the extrinsic (external) muscles that move the eyeball, and the muscle that raises the upper eyelid. Some fibres control the iris muscle that constricts the pupil, and the ciliary muscle, which changes lens shape. Proprioception
Trochlear (IV)	Motor Sensory	Controls the external muscle that moves the eyeball down and outwards. Proprioception
Trigeminal (V) (three branches: ophthalmic, maxillary, mandibular)	Motor Sensory	Motor to the muscles of chewing (mastication). Sensory to the face, mouth, teeth and the nose
Abducens (VI)	Motor Sensory	Controls the extrinsic (external) muscle that moves the eyeball outwards. Proprioception
Facial (VII)	Motor Sensory	Controls the facial, scalp and some neck muscles – facial expression. Autonomic fibres to the lacrimal (tear), nasal and some salivary glands – lacrimation and salivation. Also controls the tiny stapedius muscle in the middle ear. Taste
Vestibulocochlear (VIII)	Sensory	Hearing (audition) and balance
Glossopharyngeal (IX)	Motor Sensory	Controls the pharyngeal muscles involved in swallowing. Autonomic fibres to some salivary glands – salivation. Taste. Carotid sinus – regulation of blood pressure. Proprioception
Vagus (X)	Motor Sensory	Supplies external ear, heart, larynx, trachea, bronchi, lungs, pharynx, oesophagus, stomach, small intestine and proximal part of large intestine, the liver, gallbladder and pancreas – swallowing, digestive secretions and movement, etc. Taste and other sensory inputs from structures innervated
Accessory (XI)	Motor Sensory	Controls muscles of the neck and shoulders – head movement, shoulder shrugging. The pharynx, soft palate and larynx – swallowing. Proprioception
Hypoglossal (XII)	Motor Sensory	Tongue movements during speech and swallowing. Proprioception

Adapted from Bowie I, Woodward S. Nursing patients with neurological problems. In: Woodward S, Mestecky AM, eds. *Neuroscience Nursing – Evidence Based Practice*. Oxford: Wiley–Blackwell; 2011.

The Meninges

The brain and spinal cord are surrounded and protected by three meninges. From inside working out they are:

- pia mater
- arachnoid mater
- dura mater.

Pia Mater has its own blood supply and is a delicate layer that closely follows and adheres to the contours of the brain and spinal cord.

Arachnoid Mater is a fibrous layer between the pia and dura maters. It is separated from the pia mater by the subarachnoid space which contains cerebrospinal fluid (CSF). The arachnoid mater projects villi into the venous sinuses, which are responsible for the absorption of CSF.

Dura Mater is a double layer of dense fibrous tissue. It is separated from the arachnoid mater by the subdural space. The outer layer adheres closely to the underside of the cranial bones, whilst the inner, meningeal layer is much thinner. The spinal dura mater has only one layer, which corresponds to the meningeal layer of the cranium. The two layers of the dura mater separate at several locations and these spaces contain the venous sinuses, for example, the falx cerebri and the tentorium cerebelli. The former forms an incomplete division dipping down between the two cerebral hemispheres (Fig. 11.6). The tentorium cerebelli forms a division between the occipital lobes of the cerebrum and the cerebellum.

The Ventricular System

The ventricular system of the brain comprises four fluid-filled irregular cavities (ventricles) interconnected by narrow pathways (Fig. 11.7) and connected with the central canal of the spinal cord and the subarachnoid space. There are two lateral ventricles, one in each cerebral hemisphere, one ventricle (the

Fig. 11.6 The meninges.

Figure 11.7 The ventricular system.

third) located in the diencephalic region and the fourth located in the medulla.

Cerebrospinal Fluid circulates within the closed ventricular system. The normal features of CSF are:

- colour – crystal clear
- cells – <5 × 10^6/L (all mononuclear)
- protein (total) – 100–400 mg/L
- glucose – 2.5–4.0 mmol/L.

The CSF production–absorption cycle is continuous and a fairly constant volume of 120–150 mL is maintained. When this process is interrupted and the volume is increased beyond normal limits, hydrocephalus occurs.

Most CSF is produced by the choroid plexus, a collection of specialised capillaries located within the lining of the ventricles, the largest amount being produced in the lateral ventricles. From here, the CSF passes through two interventricular foramina (foramen of Monro) to the third ventricle, then via the single cerebral aqueduct (aqueduct of Sylvius) to the fourth ventricle. Some CSF passes down into the central canal of the spinal cord but most passes up through the two lateral and one medial foramina in the roof of the fourth ventricle, to circulate round the brain and spinal cord in the subarachnoid space before being reabsorbed into the blood via the arachnoid villi.

The functions of CSF are to:

- protect and cushion the brain and spinal cord
- provide nourishment
- maintain a uniform intracranial pressure (ICP)
- remove waste products.

Blood Supply and Drainage

The brain cannot survive without a constant supply of oxygen and glucose and receives 850 mL of oxygenated blood per minute. The blood supply to the head arises from the left and right common carotid arteries, which divide to form the internal and external carotid arteries. These supply blood to the anterior part of the brain, and the vertebral arteries supply the posterior part.

The greater part of the brain is supplied with blood by the arteries branching from the circulus arteriosus (circle of Willis), a ring of blood vessels located at the base of the brain (Fig. 11.8).

Venous drainage is by small veins in the brain stem and cerebellum, and external and internal veins draining the cerebrum. Some of the external and internal veins empty into one large vein called the vein of Galen (great cerebral vein). Unlike other parts of the body, these veins do not correspond with their arterial supply. All these veins empty directly into a system of venous sinuses, including the superior and inferior sagittal, the straight, transverse, sigmoid and cavernous sinuses.

⊕ **See Evolve website Fig. 11.3**

The Blood–Brain Barrier

This selective barrier normally prevents many harmful substances crossing from the blood to the brain, for example, microorganisms. The blood–brain barrier (BBB) is formed by the capillary endothelial cells that form 'tight junctions' in the presence of astrocytes (a type of neuroglial cell) to ensure that the capillary wall is relatively impermeable. The barrier allows the passage of oxygen, nutrients and metabolic waste, and some drugs, alcohol and other toxic substances.

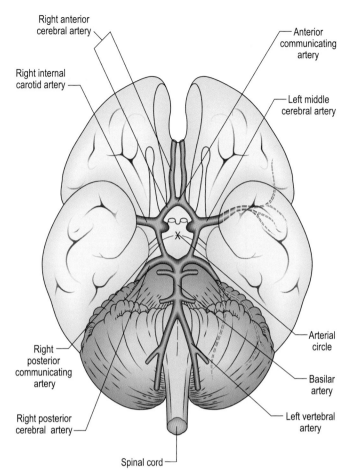

Figure 11.8 The blood supply to the brain.

The Spinal Cord

The spinal cord is an oval cylinder that lies within the spinal cavity of the vertebral column. In adults, it is approximately 45 cm long and extends from the medulla to the first or second lumbar vertebrae. Beyond this, the spinal nerves from the lumbar and sacral segments of the cord form the cauda equina, or 'horse's tail'. The lower part of the cord is attached to the coccyx by the filum terminale and is tapered in shape (Fig. 11.9).

The cord is segmented into five parts or regions, each corresponding to the specific vertebrae:

- cervical (C1–7)
- thoracic (T1–12)
- lumbar (L1–5)
- sacral (S1–5 fused bones)
- coccygeal (C1 fused bones).

A labelling system identifies different levels within the spinal cord and vertebrae; the third cervical vertebra becomes C3, the fourth lumbar vertebra becomes L4 and so on.

Two enlargements of the spinal cord are seen: (1) from C4 to T1 containing the nerve supply for the upper limbs; and (2) from L2 to S3 which supplies innervation to the lower limbs. Paired spinal nerves, part of the PNS, are attached by two short roots to the cord.

The structure of the spinal cord is illustrated in cross-section in Fig. 11.10.

The spinal pathways are described as:

- sensory – ascending from the body and transmitting impulses to the sensory cerebral cortex for interpretation

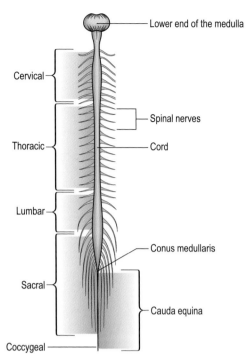

Figure 11.9 The spinal cord.

- motor – descending from the brain to skeletal muscles, where they initiate a motor response.

Each pathway has a name, derived from the spinal column in which it travels, the origin of the cell bodies and the termination of the axon.

Sensory Pathways

These consist of the:

- posterior column pathway
- spinothalamic pathway
- cerebellar pathway.

Posterior Column Pathway. Each pathway comprises a chain of three neurones which transmit information such as discriminative touch and vibration sense from the appropriate receptors to the sensory cortex.

● See Evolve website Fig. 11.4

Spinothalamic Pathways are the lateral and anterior spinothalamic tracts. The first-order neurone in both pathways connects the receptor with the spinal cord where it synapses with the second-order neurone in the posterior grey horn. The pathway crosses over to the opposite side of the cord and ascends in either the lateral or anterior spinothalamic tract to the thalamus. The second-order neurone synapses with the third-order neurone, which then continues, terminating in the sensory cortex. Between them the spinothalamic tracts are responsible for conveying information about pain (see Chapter 20, Pain Management) and temperature, light touch and pressure.

Cerebellar Pathways are the posterior spinocerebellar and anterior spinocerebellar tracts. Both tracts convey impulses about joint position sense (proprioception) from muscles and joints, terminating in the cerebellum instead of the cerebral cortex. This time there are only two neurones involved, synapsing in the posterior grey horn.

● See Evolve website Fig. 11.5

Motor Pathways

Once a motor process is initiated within the cerebral cortex, the impulses descend via two main motor pathways:

- pyramidal tracts that pass through the internal capsule and form the main pathway for impulses to voluntary muscles

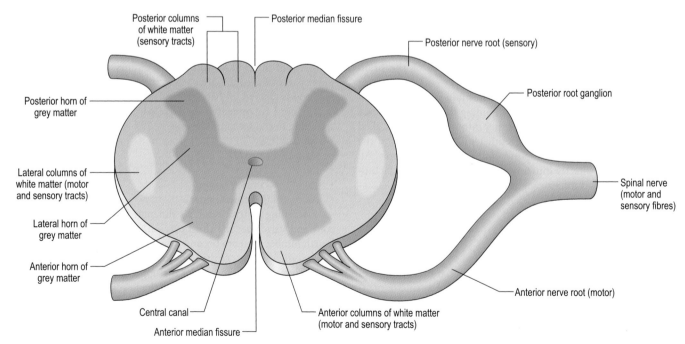

Figure 11.10 Cross-section of the spinal cord. The cord is incompletely divided into right and left halves by the posterior and anterior median fissures. In the centre is the central canal which contains CSF originating from the fourth ventricle. Extending the entire length of the cord, this is located within an H-shaped area of grey matter with posterior and anterior and, at some levels, lateral horns. The remainder of the cord is made up of white matter organised in columns in the posterior, lateral and anterior segments.

extrapyramidal tracts consisting of all the descending motor pathways that do not pass through the pyramids; extrapyramidal tracts collectively assist in maintaining muscle tone, posture and balance and gross automatic skeletal muscle movements.

Upper and Lower Motor Neurones

These are the functional units of the motor system and convey motor impulses. Damage to one or the other will result in very different functional impairment. Damage to an upper motor neurone results in spasticity, while damage to a lower motor neurone results in flaccid paralysis.

Upper motor neurones extend from the motor cortex to either the cranial nerve nuclei in the brain stem or the anterior horn of the spinal cord. The upper motor neurone is contained entirely within the CNS.

Lower Motor Neurones start within the brain stem or anterior horn of the spinal cord and pass via cranial or spinal nerves respectively to the motor end-plate of muscles.

The Peripheral Nervous System

The PNS has two functional parts:
- somatic nervous system, which is further subdivided into motor and sensory divisions
- autonomic nervous system (ANS), which conducts impulses from the CNS to smooth muscle, cardiac muscle and glands.

The Cranial Nerves

The 12 pairs of cranial nerves pass from their origin, principally within the brain stem, out via small openings in the skull to innervate structures around the head and neck, and beyond (see Table 11.1). Cranial nerves were formerly described as either motor or sensory, or mixed nerves; however, most motor nerves are now considered to be mixed, but with a dominance of motor or sensory fibres. (See Further Reading, e.g. Tortora and Derrickson 2017.)

Spinal Nerves

There are 31 pairs of spinal nerves, named and grouped according to the vertebrae they are associated with. There are:
- 8 cervical
- 12 thoracic
- 5 lumbar
- 5 sacral
- 1 coccygeal.

It should be noted that there is one more pair of cervical spinal nerves than there are vertebrae. This is because the first pair leave the vertebral canal between the occipital bone and the atlas, i.e. above C1, and the eighth pair leave below C7. Thereafter, the spinal nerves are named according to the vertebra immediately above.

Each spinal nerve has an anterior (motor nerve fibres) and a posterior root (sensory) (see Fig. 11.10). The posterior root can be distinguished by its root ganglion, a cluster of nerve cell bodies.

Shortly after leaving the intervertebral foramina, both roots join together to form a mixed nerve. From here the spinal nerves continue to form a complex network all over the body, carrying motor signals to effectors, such as the skeletal muscles, and conveying sensory information such as touch to the CNS for interpretation. (See Further Reading, e.g. Tortora and Derrickson 2017).

The Autonomic Nervous System

The ANS comprises the nerves carrying motor impulses to the internal organs; thus it is exclusively peripheral and motor. Its activity is influenced by many factors, including sensory information from the internal organs, numerous peptides and hormones, and signals from higher control centres such as the hypothalamus. It is described as having two divisions, the sympathetic and parasympathetic, each imposing different effects (Figs 11.11 and 11.12). (See Further Reading, e.g. Tortora and Derrickson 2017).

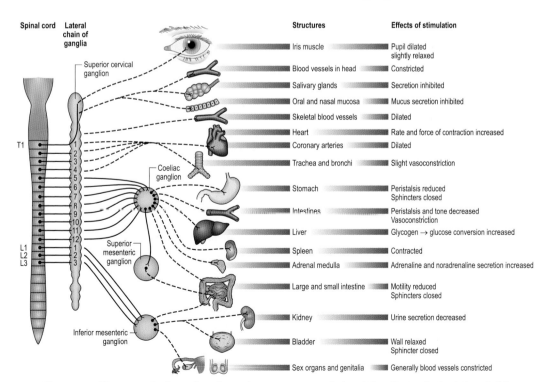

Figure 11.11 The sympathetic outflow, the main structures supplied and the effects of stimulation. *Solid lines*, preganglionic fibres; *broken lines*, postganglionic fibres.

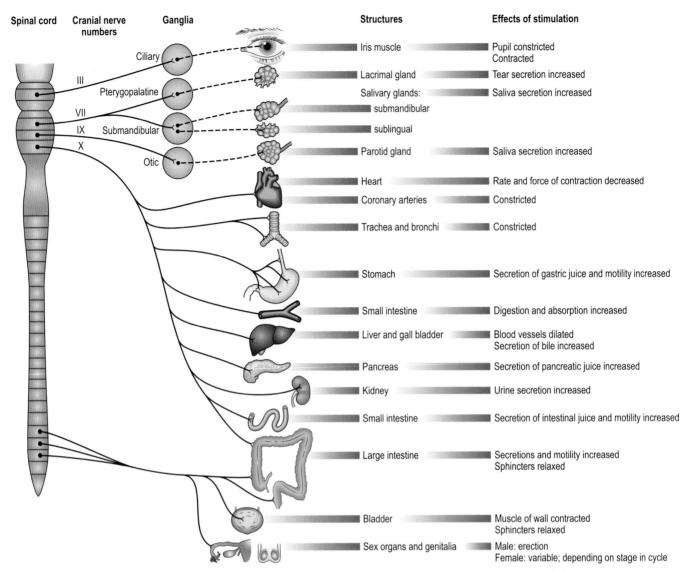

Spinal cord	Cranial nerve numbers	Ganglia		Structures	Effects of stimulation
		Ciliary		Iris muscle	Pupil constricted Contracted
	III				
		Pterygopalatine		Lacrimal gland	Tear secretion increased
				Salivary glands:	Saliva secretion increased
	VII			submandibular	
	IX	Submandibular		sublingual	
	X			Parotid gland	Saliva secretion increased
		Otic		Heart	Rate and force of contraction decreased
				Coronary arteries	Constricted
				Trachea and bronchi	Constricted
				Stomach	Secretion of gastric juice and motility increased
				Small intestine	Digestion and absorption increased
				Liver and gall bladder	Blood vessels dilated Secretion of bile increased
				Pancreas	Secretion of pancreatic juice increased
				Kidney	Urine secretion increased
				Small intestine	Secretion of intestinal juice and motility increased
				Large intestine	Secretions and motility increased Sphincters relaxed
				Bladder	Muscle of wall contracted Sphincters relaxed
				Sex organs and genitalia	Male: erection Female: variable; depending on stage in cycle

Figure 11.12 The parasympathetic outflow, the main structures supplied and the effects of stimulation. *Solid lines*, preganglionic fibres; *broken lines*, postganglionic fibres. Where there are no broken lines, the second neurone is in the wall of the structure.

Neurological Investigations

Patients may undergo a range of neurological investigations depending on their condition. Preprocedure preparation and postprocedure care are identified in Table 11.2. The specific investigations performed for each condition are detailed throughout the chapter.

Head Injury and Raised Intracranial Pressure

Around 1.4 million people attend hospital in England and Wales as a result of head injury every year (NICE 2019) and 200,000 are admitted. The majority are young males, although the incidence in females is increasing. These figures have risen significantly since the implementation of the National Institute for Health and Care Excellence (NICE) head injury guidelines in 2003, which were last updated in 2019. The majority of head injuries are mild (Glasgow Coma Scale (GCS 13–15) but moderate (GCS 9–12)

or severe injuries (GCS 3–8) are more likely to result in morbidity and mortality.

Falls (24%–43%) and assaults (30%–50%) are the most common causes of mild head injury in the UK, followed by road traffic collisions (RTCs) (25%), although these account for a far greater proportion of moderate to severe head injuries. Alcohol may be implicated in up to 65% of all adult head injuries (NICE 2019). Younger people are more likely to sustain injury through assault or RTC, while in older people falls are a more common mechanism of injury.

Pathophysiology

The adult skull can be considered as a rigid box divided into two major compartments, containing noncompressible components. A uniform pressure, called intracranial pressure (ICP), is maintained, defined as the pressure exerted within the cerebral ventricular system. When an individual sustains a head injury or there is some abnormal pathology, for example, a tumour, it can cause ICP to rise.

TABLE 11.2	Neurological Investigations		
Investigation	Description	Preprocedure Care	Postprocedure Care
Computed tomography (CT) scan	Specialised X-ray in which multiple X-rays are taken at different slices through the brain. These are then reconstructed by computer. The scan reveals different densities of tissue	No specific care is required. Any allergies, particularly to iodine-based contrast media, should be noted	No specific postprocedure care is required
Magnetic resonance imaging (MRI) scan	A patient is bombarded by radio waves as they lie inside a large magnet. This affects the atoms within the body and as the atoms move back to their original alignment, an energy signal is emitted. This is picked up by the scanner and a computer is then able to produce detailed images of body tissues	Completion of a checklist is vital as some patients are unable to enter an MRI scanner (e.g. those with pacemakers, metal fragments in the eye or some other metal prostheses) All jewellery and watches should be removed and no mobile phones, credit cards or other devices with magnetic information should be taken into the scan room Patients should be warned of possible claustrophobia and the need to lie still Some patients may require mild sedation or a general anaesthetic	No specific postprocedure care is required, unless the patient has undergone a general anaesthetic
Lumbar puncture (LP)	A lumbar puncture involves passing a fine needle through the space between two vertebrae (normally L4/5 or L5/S1 in an adult) to obtain a specimen of CSF	Explain the procedure and the need to lie still in a 'fetal position' on their side During the procedure the nurse should remain with the patient and reassure them throughout, but may also be required to assist the doctor to collect specimens of CSF	A small plaster will be placed over the puncture site. Check the wound site for signs of a CSF leak over the first few hours Encourage the patient to rest on their bed for a while and take oral fluids as they feel able Some patients will develop a post-LP headache. Administer simple analgesia if this occurs
Electroencephalogram (EEG)	An EEG involves placing small electrodes onto the patient's scalp in order to record the electrical activity within the brain	No specific preprocedure care is required	The patient may require assistance to wash their hair and remove the electrode gel and glue that have been used
Angiography	Angiography involves the injection of contrast media into the arterial system and X-ray images are taken as the contrast media circulates round the cerebral circulation. This has been superseded by MR angiography in most cases as this is noninvasive	Patients normally undergo sedation or a general anaesthetic, so all the normal preparation for this is required	Half-hourly systemic and neurological observations are required – patients are at risk of neurological deterioration and developing signs of stroke, as well as bleeding from the puncture site Check the puncture site regularly for signs of bleeding or haematoma Report any haemorrhage immediately and apply pressure Ensure the patient remains on bed rest for at least 4 h
Evoked potentials	Visual, auditory and somatosensory evoked potentials record the conduction velocities along nerve pathways	No specific preprocedure preparation is required	No specific postprocedure care is required

CSF, Cerebrospinal fluid.
Data from Woodward S, Waterhouse C. Oxford Handbook of Neuroscience Nursing. 2nd ed. Oxford: Oxford University Press; 2021.

Three intracranial components contribute to maintaining ICP:
- brain tissue
- CSF
- blood.

The brain tissue contributes 80% of the content. The remaining 20% is taken up in equal proportion by the CSF and the blood. Under normal circumstances, ICP is maintained within normal limits (0–15 mmHg), but when there is an increase in the volume of one of these components within the confined space of the skull a rise in ICP may occur. Transient rises in pressure occur with activities such as coughing or sneezing and this is a normal physiological response.

Changes to the brain and its associated structures following trauma may cause ICP to rise to a dangerous level, resulting in coma and leading to permanent brain damage or even death.

The Causes and Presenting Symptoms of Raised ICP

A raised ICP can be due to intracerebral or extracerebral causes (Information 11.1).

A rise in ICP can develop over a number of months in a slow-growing brain tumour, with the patient hardly noticing any symptoms, or it can occur in a matter of minutes following severe head injury, when the patient becomes immediately unconscious. A distinct correlation exists between ICP and conscious level; as ICP rises, conscious level deteriorates.

A relationship exists between the volume of a lesion inside the head and ICP, represented by the pressure–volume curve (Fig. 11.13).

During the initial rise in ICP, compensatory mechanisms come into play. The cerebral ventricular system can reduce the volume of CSF by displacing it into a distensible spinal dural sac. A reduction in cerebral blood volume also occurs as a result of autoregulation, the ability of blood vessels to constrict according to local conditions. This is represented by the flattened part of the curve. However, this is only a temporary measure and, as the volume of the expanding lesion increases, compensation is overcome and the steep part of the curve is entered. Then for every small increase in volume, the corresponding rise in ICP is dramatic. This process has four identifiable stages (Information 11.2).

Other factors which have an influence on this complex process include cerebral blood flow and cerebral oedema. (See Further Reading, e.g. Woodward and Mestecky 2011.)

Herniation

The skull has two compartments:
- the supratentorial compartment above the tentorium
- the infratentorial compartment below the tentorium.

Herniation is the process by which tissue in a high-pressure compartment is compressed and forced through an available opening into an adjoining low-pressure compartment. Such a situation can exist in the patient with raised ICP.

The opening that permits transtentorial herniation is the tentorial notch, and that which permits tonsillar herniation is the foramen magnum.

Subfalcine Herniation involves the herniation of brain tissue across the midline from one side of the head to the other, under the falx cerebri.

Transtentorial Herniation involves the downward displacement of the cerebral hemispheres, diencephalon and midbrain

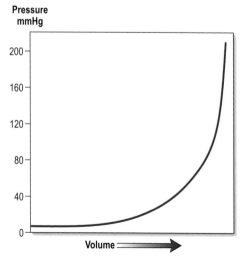

Figure 11.13 Volume–pressure curve.

INFORMATION 11.1

Causes of Raised Intracranial pressure

Intracerebral Causes
- Tumours
- Haematomas
- Cerebral oedema
- Cerebral abscess
- Hydrocephalus (due to increased production, decreased absorption or blockage to the flow of CSF)
- Idiopathic intracranial hypertension

Extracerebral Causes
- Hepatic encephalopathy
- Hypercarbia (hypercapnia) – raised CO_2 tension in arterial blood
- Anoxia leading to cerebral oedema

INFORMATION 11.2

Stages of Volume–Pressure Relationship in Raised Intracranial Pressure

Stage 1 Compensation phase: there is no rise in ICP and conscious level remains unaltered.
Stage 2 Early phase of reversible decompensation: a slight increase in ICP. Early signs of deterioration in conscious level are noted and focal neurological deficits.
Stage 3 Late phase of reversible decompensation: ICP is very high and conscious level deteriorates rapidly accompanied by pupil changes. Detrimental changes occur in the respiratory rate and pattern. ICP will soon equal mean arterial blood pressure (MABP) with, ultimately, cessation of cerebral blood flow.
Stage 4 Irreversible decompensation phase: brain herniation leads to 'coning' and death.

(central herniation). The nerves and posterior cerebral arteries are stretched and compression of the oculomotor nerve (IIIrd cranial nerve) occurs, resulting in a nonreactive pupil that may also be dilated. These and other structures are displaced into the posterior fossa.

Lateral transtentorial herniation occurs in the presence of an expanding lesion located close to the temporal lobe. The medial part of the temporal lobe (the uncus) is forced downwards and can subsequently develop into a central herniation (Fig. 11.14).

Tonsillar Herniation is the downward displacement of the lower part of the cerebellum (the cerebellar tonsils) through the foramen magnum, where compression of the medulla results.

Medical/Surgical Management

Common Presenting Symptoms

The head-injured patient with raised ICP may be fully alert and orientated, but consciousness is usually impaired. Neurological deficits can be found, for example, limb weakness or occurrence of a seizure. Answers to the questions listed should be obtained as they have an influence on the management and outcome:

- *How long has the patient been unconscious?* The period of unconsciousness relates to the severity of brain damage, i.e. the longer the patient is unconscious, the more severe the damage.

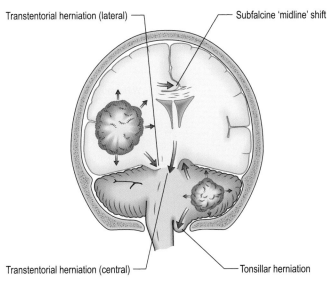

Figure 11.14 Types of herniation.

- *Does post-traumatic amnesia (PTA) exist and for how long?* The patient's memory for events following injury is an indicator of the severity of brain damage, i.e. the longer the period of PTA, the worse the brain damage.
- *What were the cause and circumstances of the injury?* This may indicate if other extracranial injuries exist.
- *Does the patient have any headache or vomiting?*

Early signs and symptoms of raised ICP include reduction in level of consciousness and focal neurological deficits (e.g. limb weakness or speech deficits), followed by pupil changes and finally systemic changes (Cushing's triad – bradycardia, hypertension and reduced/irregular respiratory rate). Hyperthermia may also occur due to compression of the hypothalamus and loss of the ability to autoregulate temperature.

Investigations. In the head-injured patient, computed tomography (CT) scanning has replaced skull X-ray as the primary method of assessment (NICE 2019) and may reveal skull fractures, cerebral contusions or lacerations and/or an intracranial haematoma (Information 11.3).

ICP Monitoring. One of the most important diagnostic measures is the monitoring of ICP. This is an invasive technique involving direct measurement of ICP. A typical system comprises a fibreoptic transducer-tipped catheter, which can be placed in the lateral ventricle, subdural or extradural space. The level of ICP is then transmitted to a digital data display as a waveform. A pulsatile waveform will be demonstrated along with a pressure level indicating if the patient's ICP is within normal limits (≤15 mmHg) (Fig. 11.15).

Treatment. In 2012 a network of trauma centres was established in the UK and treating people in these specialist centres reduces mortality after severe head injury (Vali et al. 2017). In the past, the treatment of head injury focused primarily on the interventions required to reduce ICP. However, greater emphasis is now placed on maintaining cerebral perfusion pressure (CPP), which is the pressure needed to perfuse the brain with blood, at more than 70 mmHg (Reflection 11.1). Those patients with a high ICP, low blood pressure and low CPP make a poorer recovery. The means by which this is achieved are varied according to circumstances.

Hyperosmolar Agents. An intravenous infusion of 100 mL of 20% mannitol over 15 minutes will reduce ICP by establishing an osmotic gradient between the plasma and brain tissue, thus

INFORMATION 11.3

Brain Injuries

Contusions

Contusions are bruising of the cerebral tissue, most commonly affecting the frontal, occipital and undersurface of the temporal lobes.
There are two types:
- coup – indicates haemorrhage and oedema immediately under the injury site
- contrecoup – damage occurs directly opposite the injury site. This is caused by the rapid acceleration or deceleration movement of the brain within the skull following severe trauma, resulting in cerebral oedema and raised ICP.

Lacerations

Brain tissue is lacerated as a result of, for example, a skull fracture, resulting in disruption to cellular activity which will produce focal neurological deficits such as hemiparesis (weakness on one side of the body).
Contusions and cerebral oedema may also occur.

Haematoma

A localised collection of blood, named according to its location:
- extradural – between the skull and the dura mater
- subdural – between the dura mater and the arachnoid mater
- intracerebral – within the brain substance.

Diffuse Brain Injury

Here, there is no specific focal pathology. Shearing of the white matter occurs, causing disruption and tearing of the axons.

removing water from the oedematous brain tissue to the blood. This will 'buy' time to allow the patient to be prepared for transfer to a specialist unit or for surgery. Repeated boluses may be administered over 24 hours, but may lead to a rebound increase in ICP.

Controlled Ventilation. In the past it was recommended that the reduction of $PaCO_2$ would reduce ICP. However, it also causes vasoconstriction, thus reducing cerebral blood volume. The resultant reduction in cerebral blood flow may itself cause ischaemic brain damage (El Hussein et al. 2017) so patients are ventilated to keep $PaCO_2$ within normal limits. Maintaining the blood pressure and CPP appears to be as important, if not more important, than lowering ICP. Recent evidence has also shown that prolonged prehospital hypoxia is associated with increased mortality so early intubation and ventilation is important (Butterfield et al. 2023).

Fluid Management. Dextrose infusions should not be given to patients with head injuries. Due to disruption to the BBB, administration of dextrose could exacerbate cerebral oedema; 0.9% sodium chloride is the fluid of choice.

Sedatives. If ICP fails to respond to standard measures then sedation, under carefully controlled conditions, may help by reducing cerebral metabolism and thus offering a degree of protection for the brain (Schizodimos et al. 2020).

Surgical Intervention. Surgery may be performed to remove a focal lesion such as an expanding haematoma and this may be combined with decompression. Withdrawal of small amounts of CSF via a ventricular catheter results in a reduction of ICP, but this provides only temporary relief. To be effective, drainage would require to be continuous, but this is often impractical.

Figure 11.15 The fibreoptic transducer-tipped catheter system for monitoring intracranial pressure (Camino system). (Adapted from Hickey JV. The Clinical Practice of Neurological and Neurosurgical Nursing. 8th ed. Philadelphia: Lippincott; 2019.)

REFLECTION 11.1

Relationship Between Cerebral Perfusion Pressure (CPP), ICP and MABP

CPP is equal to the mean arterial blood pressure MABP − ICP (i.e. CPP = MABP − ICP)

Activity

- Reflect on what might happen to the CPP of a patient whose ICP rose significantly or who became hypotensive. What effects might these changes have on brain function? Discuss your conclusions with your practice assessor.

❖ Nursing Management and Health Promotion: Head Injury

Head injury is preventable. This is an area in which nurses should exercise their health promotion skills, for example, by emphasising the dangers associated with head injury and its detrimental effects when communicating with patients who have experience of minor head injury with good recovery, and with their families. This may include consideration of driver behaviour or unsafe work practices. The use of seatbelts for the driver and all car passengers has led to a reduction in head injuries, as has the use of protective headgear for motorcyclists, cyclists and horse riders (Connor et al. 2019). Protective headgear is now also being investigated to reduce concussion injuries in other sports such as rugby and soccer, although there is little evidence

of effectiveness. Because a common contributing factor in head injury is alcohol intake, where appropriate, the patient can be encouraged to consider personal lifestyle and the consumption of alcohol.

Head-injured patients with raised ICP can present in different ways on admission to hospital. The person may initially appear not to have sustained an injury but can progress to become drowsy or confused, or develop speech problems or limb deficits. Seizures may occur.

Immediate Priorities

The immediate nursing aim is to prevent further damaging rises in ICP, and the first priority is to identify any alteration in respiratory function due to an inability to maintain an airway (Information 11.4). The nurse should be aware of the presence of other injuries, especially spinal injuries, for example, if the patient has been in a RTC (see Chapter 19, The Deteriorating Patient: Recognising and Managing Shock, and Chapter 26, Nursing the Patient Who Experiences Trauma, for detail of assessment and interventions).

Assessment of Neurological Status

This is performed in order to:
- identify any immediate action that needs to be taken
- record a baseline to detect any changes in neurological condition.

Any deterioration in neurological status may be an early indication that ICP is rising further, thus increasing the likelihood of herniation (de Sousa and Woodward 2016). Neurological assessment is important, as this may be the only indication that the patient's condition is deteriorating and a standardised method of

Respiratory Care Priorities in a Patient With Raised Intracranial Pressure

- Assess the rate, depth and pattern of respirations to indicate the patency of the airway. Report if the rate is less than 12 and more than 20, and any irregularities in rate or rhythm, as these may indicate a rise in ICP.
- Monitor O_2 saturations and assess the skin/mucosae for cyanosis, which would indicate inadequate respiration as a late sign.
- Apply oropharyngeal and tracheal suctioning only as required to remove secretions. Suction for no more than 15 seconds and consider preoxygenation prior to suctioning with 100% oxygen to prevent a build-up of carbon dioxide in the blood, resulting in further elevation of ICP.
- Institute measures to achieve optimal respiratory status including insertion of a Guedel airway, positioning the patient on their side with a 30-degree head-up tilt, and administer oxygen as prescribed.
- Assist with monitoring arterial blood gases and mechanical ventilation as required.

Caring for a Patient With Raised Intracranial Pressure

A range of signs and symptoms may become apparent in a patient with raised ICP (see Information 11.2).

Activity

- Reflect on what sequence of events/changes in neurological observations might occur. Discuss these with your practice assessor.

monitoring neurological status enhances this process. The gold standard method is the GCS (NICE 2019) (see Chapter 27, Nursing the Unconscious Patient).

The frequency of observations is determined by the patient's condition, ranging from intervals of 15 minutes to 2 hours. Conducting serial assessments is more important than a one-off set of observations. Medical staff should be promptly informed of any pertinent changes in the patient's neurological status, i.e. if there is a sustained drop of one point on GCS over 30 minutes or a drop of two points at any time (NICE 2019).

The nurse, as the healthcare professional who normally spends most time with the patient, should learn to observe changes in the patient's behaviour which may herald an impending change in neurological status, for example, the patient who does not answer questions so readily or who is becoming agitated and restless (Reflection 11.2).

Cardiovascular Assessment

The final life-threatening concern in a patient with a rising ICP is the effect of alterations to systemic and cerebral circulation, due to shock and cardiovascular instability. Unless requested by medical staff to do otherwise, the nurse should always report if:
- systolic pressure is less than 90 or more than 170 mmHg

- diastolic pressure is less than 50 or more than 100 mmHg
- the pulse rate is less than 50 or more than 100 beats per minute.
  Readings that are outside of these parameters will make the patient more susceptible to secondary brain damage as a result of raised ICP and lowered CPP. The recognition of the vulnerable patient has been greatly facilitated by the use of early warning system charts.

Surgery

Preoperative Care. Urgent surgery (e.g. craniotomy) may be indicated on admission or in response to subsequent deterioration. The nurse may need to prepare the patient in a very short time and also provide adequate explanation and reassurance (see Chapter 25, Nursing Patients Undergoing Surgery).

Postoperative Care. The overall priorities for patients following neurosurgery are:
- continuous assessment of neurological status (see Chapter 27, Nursing the Unconscious Patient)
- instituting measures to avoid secondary brain damage (El Hussein et al. 2017)
- administration of appropriate therapies.
  Table 11.3 outlines the main complications of neurosurgery.

As the patient progresses, their needs will require to be reassessed and the nursing interventions adjusted accordingly. The aim of care is to ensure optimal function and the early detection of complications.

Subsequent Considerations

All of the nursing interventions identified in Chapter 25 will apply. Only those interventions specific to the patient who is unconscious due to raised ICP are included here. The main aim of care remains that of preventing further rises in ICP.

TABLE 11.3 Complications of Neurosurgery

Complications	Cause	Interventions
Altered conscious level	Increased ICP due to cerebral haemorrhage/oedema	Frequent assessment of neurological status
Onset of seizures	Cerebral irritation	Observation of seizures. Appropriate interventions if they occur (see section on Epilepsy)
Limb weakness	Increased ICP due to cerebral haemorrhage/oedema	Frequent assessment of limb movements
Speech problems	Increased ICP due to cerebral haemorrhage/oedema	Frequent assessment of verbal responses
Respiratory problems	Increased ICP due to cerebral haemorrhage/oedema	Frequent assessment of respiratory status
Loss of swallowing reflex	Increased ICP due to cerebral haemorrhage/oedema	Assessment of swallowing and keep nil by mouth
Loss of corneal reflex	Increased ICP due to cerebral haemorrhage/oedema	Eye care. Keep eyes closed to protect cornea
Periorbital oedema	Direct result of surgery	Observe for swollen/bruised periorbital tissues

ICP, Intracranial pressure.

The patient care outlined in the following sections uses the Roper et al. (1980) framework of activities of living.

Communicating

Unpleasant stimuli are known to increase ICP, so the nurse should take a calm, reassuring approach. Relatives should be encouraged to talk to the patient and, although they may feel rather foolish at first, they will be encouraged if they see the nurse doing this. They should, however, be warned to avoid discussing potentially upsetting topics as the unconscious patient may still be able to hear (El Hussein et al. 2017) and this may cause their ICP to rise.

Nonverbal communication, particularly touch, has been shown to decrease ICP, so relatives should be encouraged to touch the patient, for example, holding hands, despite the extensive equipment which may surround them.

Any investigations or care to be performed should be explained to the patient and their family who will be anxious and distressed at this time, particularly as outcomes may be uncertain.

Breathing

Respiratory assessment and appropriate intervention will continue as long as the ICP remains elevated. The patient's position should be changed every 2 hours or as the need arises, and chest physiotherapy should be instituted to help prevent pooling of secretions in the lungs and atelectasis. The patient, if able, should be encouraged to undertake deep-breathing exercises. There is evidence to demonstrate the benefits of adopting the prone position to improve respiratory status and CPP in brain-injured patients in intensive therapy unit (ITU), but it may lead to a further rise in ICP (Nekludov et al. 2006) (see Chapter 28, Nursing the Critically Ill Patient).

Maintaining a Safe Environment

The patient's bed should be positioned where they can be easily observed. If the patient is restless or agitated, the nurse should attempt to find out why. Adequate non-narcotic analgesics, such as codeine phosphate and tramadol, may relieve a headache, but patients suffer significant pain following craniotomy, which is often unrelieved by these analgesics, or patients experience side-effects (nausea and vomiting). Opioids have been avoided in these patients due to fears of masking neurological signs, but there is now mounting evidence that morphine is safe and effective following cranial surgery (Vadivelu et al. 2016). Increasingly neurosurgical units are using enhanced recovery strategies, including effective pain management, following craniotomy (Stumpo et al. 2021). If the patient is confused, they may attempt to climb out of bed and may not appreciate a limb deficit and attempt to walk, thus endangering themselves. If appropriate, relatives can help persuade the patient to stay in bed. Any form of restraint (e.g. sedation, bed rails) should always be a last resort and only used following risk assessment, discussion with the family, in accordance with local policy and after all conservative methods of managing challenging behaviour have been exhausted. If the patient's behaviour proves very difficult to manage safely, it may be necessary to replace the bed with a mattress on the floor. (See Further Reading, e.g. Mortimer and Berg 2017, and Useful Websites, e.g. National Neuroscience Benchmarking Group.)

Controlling Body Temperature

Each 1°C rise in body temperature increases the metabolic demand of the brain by 10% (Hickey 2019). This increases blood pressure and encourages vasodilatation, which will increase ICP. Body temperature should be recorded at least 4-hourly, as an increase may indicate hypothalamic damage or infection. Any source of potential infection, such as leakage of CSF from the patient's ears (otorrhoea) or nose (rhinorrhoea) from a base-of-skull or anterior-fossa fracture, must be identified and reported. Confirmation of this is obtained by testing the fluid for the presence of glucose, using a reagent strip. A positive result, although not conclusive, is indicative of the presence of CSF.

Mobility

The patient will require frequent positional changes to avoid developing pressure ulcers. Semi-prone and lateral positions are both suitable. Moving the patient also encourages expansion of the lungs and prevents pooling of secretions. A head-up tilt of 30 degrees will reduce ICP, aid lung expansion and prevent chest infection. The patient's body should be maintained in neutral alignment, avoiding neck flexion and rotation. The hips should be carefully positioned, avoiding flexion over 90 degrees. These positions aid venous drainage as they minimise intra-abdominal and intrathoracic pressure, which will help to decrease ICP.

Passive exercises should be performed to prevent muscle wasting and limb contractures, but isometric exercising should be avoided as this raises ICP. Anti-embolism stockings or intermittent pneumatic compression should be used to minimise the risk of deep venous thrombosis and continued for 30 days or until discharge, whichever is sooner, but anticoagulation should not be given or should be used with caution in neurosurgical patients (NICE 2018).

As the patient's condition improves, further movement should be encouraged. Sitting out of bed in a chair will help to reduce respiratory complications and encourage limb movements. It may also act as an important psychological boost for the patient and their family as they will view this as progress and referral to physiotherapy is indicated.

Eating and Drinking

As soon as the patient is able, oral food and fluid intake should be encouraged. Intravenous fluids may be required, however, and fluid restrictions should be carefully monitored and recorded to avoid inadvertent increases in ICP due to worsening cerebral oedema. Some patients may require enteral feeding, and the nurse should observe all the usual precautions (see Chapter 4, Nursing Patients With Gastrointestinal, Liver and Biliary Disorders, and Chapter 22, Nutrition and Health). The patient with a basal skull fracture must not have the tube passed nasally as there is a danger of further damage and infection; the tube should be passed orally.

Eliminating

Urinary output should be monitored and some patients require urinary catheterisation (see Chapter 10, Nursing Patients With Urinary disorders). As the level of consciousness improves, the patient may attempt to remove the catheter. Constipation should be avoided to minimise rises in ICP caused by straining at stool (see Chapter 4, Nursing Patients With Gastrointestinal, Liver and Biliary Disorders).

Rehabilitation

This forms a crucial part of the recovery process and the principles are outlined in Chapter 30 (Care and Rehabilitation of People

With Long-Term Conditions). The aim is to maintain and promote function, and prevent further deterioration and occurrence of complications. The neurological deficits which can impede progress during rehabilitation include:

- motor impairment, e.g. spasticity or ataxia
- sensory impairment, e.g. loss of sense of pain or touch
- communication disability, e.g. dysphasia
- psychological disability:
  - cognitive impairment, e.g. memory loss
  - perceptual, e.g. eye–hand coordination
  - emotional, e.g. irritability
  - behaviour or personality, e.g. poor self-image
- social disability, e.g. social withdrawal
- educational or vocational disability.

All the above have an effect on the patient's ability to resume employment and educational or vocational activities.

The multidisciplinary team (MDT), in partnership with the patient and their family, should aim to assess the patient's needs and provide optimal care and support. Realistic goals should be set as rehabilitation may take months or years to achieve. Some patients may remain in a persistent vegetative state requiring constant nursing in a care facility (see Chapter 27, Nursing the Unconscious Patient).

In some circumstances, the patient's role within the family changes. They may previously have been the provider within a family and may now be dependent on others. Employment prospects may alter and, for some, a return to work is impossible. This can affect both the family's short- and long-term plans and may also have financial implications. An alteration to the patient's personality may affect relationships within a family, resulting in stress and discord. Indeed, some families will report that the person has completely changed and is now different from the person they knew before (see Chapter 30) and need additional support, for example, information and emotional support.

Preparation for Discharge

Many patients and their families will be particularly anxious as the time for discharge approaches. Much of this anxiety can be allayed by appropriate preparation and reassurance and an effective plan for discharge. The residual problems that may persist vary widely, ranging from headache to major behavioural changes. A home assessment may be performed jointly by the occupational therapist (OT) and community nurse. Predischarge visits home may be considered and will help to identify potential problems. If appropriate, referral to the primary healthcare team should be made to enable optimal assessment and support within the community setting.

Despite these preparations, it is not usually until the patient is at home that the family members fully appreciate the difficulties that may be before them. Home routines may need to be adjusted, and whilst this may be easy in the early stages, it becomes more difficult to accept in the long term. Other members of the family will often view the disruption to their personal lives negatively and much of the early support gradually disappears. The patient's partner may be left to shoulder the burden alone, and in this situation a support group, for example, Headway (see Useful Websites), may help. Some families report a sense of failure should the patient require to be admitted for long-term care. They may feel that they have let their loved one down and do not like to admit that they are unable to cope.

Cerebrovascular Disease

Cerebrovascular disease occurs as a result of a disorder of the blood vessels or the blood supply to the brain. This section considers:

- stroke – the most common cerebrovascular disorder
- subarachnoid haemorrhage (SAH) – an uncommon but major life-threatening situation that demands acute neurosurgical intervention.

Stroke

A stroke can occur at any time during adult life. In the UK, 100,000 strokes occur annually, with someone having a stroke somewhere in the UK every 5 minutes. Age increases the risk. Most strokes occur in the 65–75 year age group and are more common in men. It is a leading cause of disability, with over 250,000 people living in the UK with disability as a result of stroke. Stroke is the third most common cause of death in developed countries and in the UK stroke accounts for around 38,000 deaths per annum (NICE 2022a).

Subarachnoid Haemorrhage

Subarachnoid haemorrhage (SAH) is bleeding into the subarachnoid space, but is often wrongly referred to as 'cerebral' or 'brain haemorrhage'. It affects 6–12 people per 100,000 in the UK per year (NICE, 2022a), with 15% dying before they reach hospital. It has a male bias in the under-40s, but this changes to a female bias in the over-40s.

Pathophysiology

The three main causes of stroke are:

- cerebral thrombosis
- cerebral embolus
- cerebral haemorrhage.

As a result of the rise in substance misuse, an increasing cause of stroke in the under-45s is the detrimental effects of illegal drugs such as crack cocaine.

Cerebral Thrombosis

This is the most common cause of stroke, in which atherosclerosis causes narrowing of the lumen of the affected blood vessels (see Chapter 2, Nursing Patients With Cardiovascular Disorders). As the atheroma builds up, it initially only partially occludes the blood vessel until the blood supply is suddenly disrupted. During the 24–48 hours following this, neurological deficits frequently worsen.

Cerebral Embolus. An embolus may lodge in the narrowed lumen of a bifurcation in the cerebral circulation. The usual origin of the embolus is a cardiac thrombus, in the presence of cardiac disease such as myocardial infarction. Air or fat, the latter for example from a fractured femur (see Chapter 12, Nursing Patients With Musculoskeletal Disorders), can also act as an embolus.

Cerebral Haemorrhage. Haemorrhage can occur into the cerebral tissues – intracerebral haemorrhage, or the subarachnoid space – SAH.

Approximately 85% of SAHs are caused by a weakness in the wall of a cerebral blood vessel, which causes a dilatation (aneurysm) (NICE 2022b). Other causes include arteriovenous malformations (AVMs), but in some patients no cause is identified. Hypertension may be present, but damage caused by arteriosclerotic changes is common. Most aneurysms form on the anterior part of the circulus arteriosus (circle of Willis) and some patients have multiple aneurysms.

The exact cause of aneurysm formation remains unknown and some remain silent, causing no symptoms. Some bleeding can occur through the very thin aneurysmal wall and produce mild signs and symptoms of SAH without rupture occurring.

Risk Factors

Certain predisposing factors increase the likelihood of cerebrovascular disease, such as raised serum cholesterol, hypertension and tobacco smoking (see Chapter 2, Nursing Patients With Cardiovascular Disorders).

Classification of Stroke

A classification system for stroke is outlined in Information 11.5.

The Effects of a Stroke

A stroke results in an interruption to the cerebral blood supply, reducing the supply of oxygen and glucose reaching the brain. Within hours, oedema occurs at the site of the main lesion as a result of the changes to the cell membranes, allowing fluid to leak into the extracellular space. This gradually worsens, peaking between the fifth and seventh day and then gradually resolving.

The damage caused by a stroke is due largely to the extent of ischaemia that occurs. It has been established that there is a reduction in global cerebral blood flow following stroke. In and around the immediate area of the infarction, more subtle changes are detected in regional cerebral blood flow. Progression from reversible ischaemia to infarction depends on the degree and duration of the reduced blood flow. The affected area of the brain loses its ability to carry out its function, for example:

- controlling movement in a specific part of the body
- controlling cognitive or emotional processes, speech or language.

Cerebral oedema also occurs and as the oedema subsides, cells begin to function again, explaining the rapid progress potentially made in the first 2–3 weeks.

After the initial period, recovery is slower, partly due to other cells taking over the functions of permanently damaged cells. At this stage, the patient begins to learn ways of handling their disability.

Generally speaking, if a patient shows a marked improvement within the first week, then minimal deficit will result. Conversely, if little or no improvement is made during this time, the outcome is likely to be poorer. Information 11.6 lists the most common types of residual disability.

Common Presenting Symptoms/Signs

The onset of cerebrovascular disease can be difficult to pinpoint. In thrombotic and embolic stroke, minor symptoms are often dismissed by patients and it is not until a significant symptom presents that the patient seeks medical help. Earlier symptoms, for example, tingling and weakness of a limb, are the result of mild transient interruptions of neurological function. Major symptoms include loss of consciousness, speech difficulties and hemiplegia, which may be accompanied by loss of vision on the affected side. Stroke needs to be recognised early and treated as a medical emergency because 'time is brain' (English 2016). The **FAST** test (**F**acial weakness, **A**rm and leg weakness, **S**peech problems, **T**ime to call 999) is used by paramedics, GPs and the public and has been encouraged by the government and the Stroke Association.

INFORMATION 11.6

Common Types of Disability Caused by Stroke

Motor Deficits

- Movement deficits
  - loss of movement in the limbs on one side of the body (hemiplegia)
  - weakness in the arms and legs (hemiparesis)
- Speech difficulties
  - dysarthria, where the patient has distorted and indistinct speech but is able to understand what is said and can still read and write
  - dysphasia, i.e. loss of the ability to talk, read and write
- Facial paralysis on the affected side, causing drooling, indistinct speech and difficulty in chewing and swallowing

Sensory Deficits

- Visual deficits
  - partial loss of the visual field
  - double vision (diplopia)
  - poorer vision than previously
- Poor response to superficial sensation, e.g. heat and cold
- Perceptual deficits, such as incorrect perception of the environment or loss of sense of smell
- Lack of awareness of the disabled part of the body

Loss of Consciousness

- From mild impairment to coma
- Loss of memory or shortened attention span

Emotional Deficits

- Emotional disturbances, e.g. change of personality, from quiet and pleasant to surly and aggressive, or vice versa
- Loss of self-control or inhibitions
- Confusion
- Depression

Bladder/Bowel Dysfunction

- Loss of bladder and/or bowel control (incontinence)
- Urinary frequency and urgency
- Constipation

INFORMATION 11.5

Classification of Stroke

Transient Ischaemic Attack (TIA)

- Onset and disappearance of a neurological deficit within 24 hours due to temporary disturbance of blood supply to the brain
- No residual neurological deficit
- Symptoms last from several minutes up to 24 hours

Reversible Ischaemic Neurological Deficit

- Neurological deficit persists longer than 12–24 hours
- Symptoms may last days or weeks
- Minimal, partial or no residual neurological deficit

Stroke in Evolution

- Symptoms persist beyond 24 hours with an associated progressive deterioration of neurological status
- Residual neurological deficits
- Probably due to a failure of collateral circulation

Completed Stroke

- Condition stabilises and neurological deficit remains

SAH typically causes sudden, severe headache, often accompanied by vomiting. The patient may be alert and orientated and may feel intense fear at what they are experiencing. Alternatively, there may be loss of consciousness, seizures and evidence of neurological deficits such as IIIrd cranial nerve palsy, hemiplegia or hemiparesis (Hickey 2019). Many of these symptoms/signs are related to the effects of raised ICP (see p. 293).

The patient may still have a residual headache and neck stiffness which may be confirmed by passive neck flexion. This indicates meningism, caused by the presence of blood in the subarachnoid space irritating the meninges. Other findings may include hypertension and pyrexia. Signs and symptoms will depend on a variety of factors, including the area of the brain affected (see Fig. 11.4).

🜢 Medical/Surgical Management

The Intercollegiate Stroke Working Party (ISWP) (National Clinical Guideline for Stroke for the UK and Ireland 2023) and NICE (2022b) have published guidelines for the management of stroke. People suspected of acute stroke should be managed in a hyperacute stroke unit with minimum staffing recommended (ISWP 2023) as there is clear evidence that patients cared for outside of such centres have worse clinical outcomes.

Investigations

CT Scan. must be performed urgently on arrival at hospital (ISWP 2023) to determine the location and type of stroke and to ensure that there is no other lesion to account for the symptoms. Thrombolysis may then be considered up to 9 hours as part of hyperacute care. CT may also reveal subarachnoid or other haemorrhagic stroke. If the diagnosis is uncertain, but if stroke is suspected magnetic resonance imaging (MRI) is performed.

Lumbar Puncture. If an SAH is suspected, but not evident on CT, and the patient is alert, obeying commands and has no focal neurological deficits, a lumbar puncture may be performed. Examination of the CSF reveals uniform bloodstaining or, if 6 hours have elapsed since the original bleed, straw-coloured CSF (xanthochromia) is apparent due to the breakdown of haemoglobin.

If the patient is displaying signs of raised ICP, for example, altered consciousness or has a neurological deficit, lumbar puncture is contraindicated because of the risk of brain herniation (see p. 284).

Angiography/Magnetic Resonance Angiography (MRA). If blood is detected, either by lumbar puncture or CT scan, angiography is indicated. The presence and location of aneurysms and other blood vessel anomalies such as stenosis will be demonstrated. Angiography is not without risk and MRA is more commonly used as this is noninvasive.

Treatment

Approaches to stroke management vary widely because of the variety of presentations. The aims are to prevent further brain damage, reduce the risk factors, provide supportive care and regain functional independence.

Hyperacute Care, Thrombolysis and Thrombectomy. There is clear evidence to support the use of thrombolysis with recombinant tissue plasminogen activator (rTPA), alteplase or tenecteplase (ISWP 2023) after haemorrhagic stroke has been excluded.

Antiplatelet Agents. The use of aspirin as an antiplatelet agent in secondary prevention is now well-established practice, but there is no evidence that it can prevent stroke in patients who have never had a stroke or transient ischaemic attack (TIA). Dual antiplatelet therapy, for example, aspirin/clopidogrel or aspirin/ticagrelor, should be considered in patients presenting within 24 hours of TIA.

Surgical Management for Stroke. Treatment with thrombectomy after stroke is becoming more widely available (ISWP 2023) and is recommended.

Aims of Treatment in SAH

The main aims of treatment are to avoid ischaemia and potentially fatal recurrence of bleeding. Of untreated patients, 30% will re-bleed within 28 days, and 70% of these will die.

Interventional Radiology. Most patients with SAH are treated with endovascular coiling by the insertion of helical platinum coils into the aneurysmal sac to induce thrombosis. The evidence is clear supporting this technique over more invasive surgical interventions (Lee et al 2022).

Surgery. An aneurysm may also be treated by placing a metal clip across the neck of the aneurysm via a craniotomy. This prevents blood flowing into the aneurysm and therefore prevents re-bleeding. Clipping may not be possible due to the size or location of the aneurysm; it may then be treated by wrapping in muslin gauze.

Pharmacological Management. Calcium antagonists, for example, nimodipine, are recommended to reduce the incidence of cerebral infarction due to vasospasm following SAH. Triple-H therapy (hypervolaemia, hypertension and haemodilution) to treat vasospasm aggressively with fluid administration is now controversial (Chan et al. 2021).

Other Complications of SAH

Hydrocephalus. The normal drainage of CSF may be impaired by the presence of a haematoma pressing on the narrow pathways or by haemorrhage into the CSF impeding the flow and blocking the arachnoid villi (Information 11.7).

Intracerebral Haematoma. The haemorrhage may result in a haematoma, which will raise ICP.

Epilepsy. Seizures may occur, necessitating treatment with anticonvulsants (see p. 295).

❖ Nursing Management and Health Promotion: Stroke

Prevention

One of the most important aspects of stroke management is prevention, by identifying at-risk individuals and dealing with early predisposing factors such as hypertension.

INFORMATION 11.7

Hydrocephalus

Hydrocephalus is a progressive dilatation of the cerebral ventricular system due to a production of CSF which exceeds the absorption rate. This may be brought about by an obstruction to the flow of CSF, overproduction or reduced absorption. It can occur at all ages; it may be congenital in the newborn or secondary to some other intracranial pathology in the older child and adult.

Treatment is by insertion of a ventriculoperitoneal shunt. This is a long narrow plastic tubing, valve and reservoir device. One end is inserted into the lateral cerebral ventricle and the other end is sutured into the patient's peritoneal cavity via a subcutaneous route. The excess CSF is now 'shunted' from the ventricles into the peritoneal cavity, from where it then returns to the bloodstream. In the acute stages of hydrocephalus an external ventricular drain may be inserted (Thompson 2017).

Reference

Thompson SD. An introduction to hydrocephalus: types, treatment and management. Br J Neurosci Nurs. 2017;13(1):36-40.

TABLE 11.4	Risk Factors for Stroke and TIA	
Factors That Can Be Changed (Modifiable)	**Factors That Cannot Be Changed**
Hypertension	Age
Heart disease	Sex
Peripheral vascular disease	Race
Smoking	Family history of TIA and stroke
Obesity	Past medical history of TIA and stroke
Diabetes	
Sedentary lifestyle	
High cholesterol	
Excess alcohol intake	
Other rare factors, e.g. clotting disorders, oral contraceptive pill	

TIA, Transient ischaemic attack.

Transient Ischaemic attack (TIA) and Secondary Prevention

A TIA is caused by insufficient blood reaching the brain, for a brief period (see Reflection 11.2). If an individual or their relative notices the symptoms of a mild TIA, they should dial 999. Patients will often be seen in a nurse-led TIA clinic and secondary prevention to reduce risk factors (Table 11.4) will be instituted.

Nursing Care Following a Stroke

Often the immediate priorities and follow-up care overlap, and they are separated here for the purposes of explanation only. An optimal outcome is more likely when appropriate techniques and resources are utilised, encompassing every member of the MDT, and when the rehabilitation process commences as soon as possible. The Stroke Specific Education Framework provides a framework of core competencies for all healthcare professionals involved in the care of individuals with or at risk of a stroke, in acute and primary care settings.

Immediate Priorities

Breathing

Techniques for maintaining a patent airway and adequate ventilation (see Information 11.4) are a priority (see Chapter 27, Nursing the Unconscious Patient). Patients are particularly at risk of aspiration (silent or otherwise) and may develop chest infections. Nurses need to be alert for wet, gurgling voice or respiratory difficulty and swallow screening should be performed within 4 hours of admission to hospital.

Safety and Comfort

Hemiplegia often results from stroke, so the care of paralysed limbs and avoiding the hazards of immobility are vital. Similarly the patient with a decreased level of consciousness will require their safety needs to be met (see Chapter 27, Nursing the Unconscious Patient). ICP may be raised due to cerebral oedema (see interventions for care of a patient with a head injury).

The patient who has experienced a haemorrhage will be assessed for headache and an analgesic prescribed. An antiemetic may also be prescribed for nausea and vomiting.

Patient safety and comfort are greatly enhanced when consideration is given to the patient's ability to communicate and to their emotional well-being, as well as that of their family.

Communicating

Speech impairment or loss can be a frightening experience for the patient and their family. Early referral to a speech and language therapist (SLT) is important, so that an expert assessment can be performed and an appropriate strategy identified. It is crucial to ascertain the type and nature of the speech deficit.

Powerful emotions are often apparent and patients may become emotionally labile due to the damage to the brain or become depressed (Wijeratne and Sales 2021). Patients who are unable to communicate their feelings verbally may feel trapped inside a body that refuses to do as they want. Some patients are convinced that their words are properly formed and fail to realise that what the nurse or family is hearing is indistinct or jumbled. Patients and their friends and family can become very distressed when they meet and this needs to be handled with sensitivity.

(See Further Reading, e.g. Woodward and Mestecky 2011.)

Mobility

Early mobilising is recommended if possible (ISWP 2023). The nurse should ensure that any obstacles are removed and that the patient is wearing appropriate clothing and footwear, i.e. outdoor shoes rather than loose-fitting slippers.

Visual impairment, such as diplopia, may also be dangerous for the patient. Simple interventions that may help include providing an eye patch to eliminate double vision and approaching the patient with homonymous hemianopia, i.e. loss of vision in the same half (right or left) of the visual field in both eyes, from the unaffected side. These interventions should also be explained to the patient's family, who should be advised about similar safety precautions at home. Patients should also be referred for physiotherapy and should be positioned to prevent spasticity and contractures (neutral alignment and support of affected limbs). The patient's affected shoulder is at risk of subluxation and should be moved carefully. Pressure area risk assessment and care are also vital (see Chapter 23, Tissue Viability and Managing Chronic Wounds).

Differences of opinion exist with regard to mobility following SAH. Patients are often kept on bedrest or reduced mobilising due to fears of exacerbating cerebral vasospasm, but a study has shown that early rehabilitation does not increase the risk of this complication (Karic et al. 2017). The patient with a neurological deficit or alteration in conscious level should be nursed in an easily observable bed.

Eating and Drinking

Fluid intake via an intravenous infusion may be required and the nurse will be responsible for maintaining this accurately. Oral diet may be introduced after detailed swallowing assessment (often in conjunction with the SLT) has been performed and shown to be safe. The patient may need help with eating or may be given adapted utensils allowing them to feed themselves. Being fed can be embarrassing and sensitivity is required to preserve the patient's dignity and self-esteem. The nurse should determine the patient's capability; for example, hemiplegia may prevent them from cutting up their own food but, once this is done, they can feed themselves.

Dysphagia. may put patients at risk of aspiration and they may need to be kept nil orally. Recommendations may include the use of nasogastric feeding with a prescribed proprietary liquid diet (see Chapter 22, Nutrition and Health) and the use of specialised exercises and techniques to aid swallowing. Increased oral hygiene is important in both instances. The patient with dysphagia receiving nasogastric feeding will be more prone to a dry mouth and the patient who is managing to take an oral diet may leave food debris in the affected side of their mouth. Regular oral inspection and oral hygiene are essential.

Eliminating. Incontinence of urine may occur due to the damage to the brain (urge urinary incontinence) or due to loss of consciousness and enforced immobility. Urge urinary incontinence can be treated by bladder retraining or administering antimuscarinic drugs. Urinary incontinence may also be helped by using bedpans or urinals at specified intervals, rather than resorting to catheterisation. Urinary sheaths may be suitable for male patients, but these are not without practical problems (see Chapter 24, Maintaining Continence).

Constipation may also be a problem and bowel habit must be monitored and treated as necessary.

Rehabilitation

The overall aim of rehabilitation (see Chapter 30, Care and Rehabilitation of People With Long-Term Conditions) is the active promotion and restoration of independence, and this applies equally to all patients following a stroke, whether they are at home, in hospital or in a rehabilitation centre (Reflection 11.3).

Therapy

Clear evidence exists of the value of an MDT approach to managing the patient.

Physiotherapists. can assist people with mobility and suggest suitable aids. They can also help the patient to regain movement in paralysed arms, improve balance and advise on managing spasticity.

OTs (occupational therapists). can help patients learn adaptive ways to dress and cook for themselves, and can suggest suitable home aids. They can also advise on emotional and cognitive care.

SLTs (speech and language therapists). help patients to overcome problems with speech and swallowing.

Nursing interventions identified during the acute period will be continued during rehabilitation. Attention to speech difficulties and sensory deficits and preparing the patient for discharge home with adequate support and advice within a well-constructed

---

REFLECTION 11.3

Individualised Discharge Advice

Farida had a haemorrhagic stroke, leaving her completely paralysed on the right side and unable to speak. A CT scan showed a large area of ischaemic damage on the left side. Within 12 days her speech was normal, but she still could not walk at all or use her right arm. She took her first steps after another 3 weeks, and 1 month later was walking alone using a tripod. A little movement returned in her right arm 6 weeks after her stroke. She was discharged following in-patient neurorehabilitation 2 months after the stroke, and after 5 months she was walking to the local shops, talking normally and was able to use her right hand and arm for holding cans.

Activity

- Reflect on Farida's recovery and consider the specific advice she might need to be given prior to discharge.

REFLECTION 11.4

Advice for Home Carers of Individuals Recovering From Stroke

- Do not overprotect the individual.
- Do encourage them to exercise.
- Do not accuse them of 'not trying'.
- Do not pull their weak arm.
- Do encourage friends to visit.
- Do not become gloomy and pessimistic.
- Do think twice before selling the double bed.
- Do continue a normal sex life.
- Do continue to position and support limbs as shown in hospital.

Activity

- Reflect on the points above and concentrate on two or three points.
- Discuss with your mentor how easy it will be for carers to follow the advice.

---

care package will be required. Involvement of the patient's family in the recovery phase is crucial as their cooperation can result in the increased likelihood of success (Reflection 11.4, Evidence-Based Practice 11.2).

The patient will have been referred to the local primary healthcare team for assessment and support. Once home, the patient's ability to live independently can be enhanced by aids such as hand rails in the bathroom. Information from the Stroke Association

---

EVIDENCE-BASED PRACTICE 11.2

Long-Term Caregivers

'During the first few months after a stroke, family caregivers must learn how to care for the stroke survivor in the home setting. Although there are some studies that address the needs and concerns of stroke caregivers during the early poststroke period, there are very few caregiver studies that report strategies used by caregivers to deal with their needs and concerns. Studies are also lacking that report the advice that caregivers would offer to others. The purpose of this study was to determine the self-reported needs, concerns, strategies and advice of family caregivers of stroke survivors during the first 6 months after hospital discharge. Using open-ended questions, 14 female family caregivers of stroke survivors were interviewed to identify their needs and concerns, strategies they used to deal with stroke and advice they would offer to other stroke caregivers. Findings revealed five major categories of caregiver needs and concerns: information, emotions and behaviours, physical care, instrumental care and personal responses to caregiving. Based on the findings, an initial needs and concerns checklist was developed. This checklist, as well as the list of strategies and advice, may help to identify relevant areas for caregiver intervention.'

Activities

- Access the study by Bakas et al. (2002) and identify the items on the checklist.
- Consider how the experiences of longer-term caregivers could be used to assist family members caring for relatives with other chronic conditions.

Reference

Bakas T, Austin JK, Okonkwo KF, et al. Needs, concerns, strategies and advice of stroke caregivers the first 6 months after discharge. *J Neurosci Nurs.* 2002;34(5):242-251.

(see Useful Websites) should be considered along with help and support from appropriate community groups.

🌐 **See Evolve website Critical thinking question 11.2**

Intracranial Tumours

Approximately 5200 people in the UK die from a brain tumour (or other CNS tumour) every year (Cancer Research UK 2018). The cause of primary brain tumours is unknown. Astrocytoma, a malignant tumour of astrocytes (neuroglia), occurs twice as often in males as in females and is most common in the 40–60-year age group. There are two age peaks for intracranial tumours: the first decade of life, and the 50s and 60s.

🔵 *Pathophysiology*

Intracranial tumours can be classified according to their pathology. Primary brain tumours arise from the neuroglial cells within the brain (glioma is the umbrella term), whereas secondary tumours metastasise to the brain from elsewhere in the body. Primary brain tumours are named after the cell from which they arise, for example, astrocytomas from astrocytes, but this can only be determined when a biopsy is taken and examined.

Brain tumours may be benign or malignant, but even benign tumours (e.g. meningioma) can cause a life-threatening rise in ICP. Cerebral oedema is common due to disruption of the BBB.

Common Presenting Symptoms

Presentation will be determined by the location, type, size and speed of growth of the tumour and its effect on surrounding structures.

The neurological symptoms of brain tumours include epilepsy, focal symptoms such as hemiparesis or cranial nerve deficits and signs of raised ICP such as headache.

Patients with pituitary tumours will often present with visual field defects.

🔵 *Medical/Surgical Management*

Investigations

CT or MRI scanning are likely to be the investigations of choice. Additional investigations include measuring the erythrocyte sedimentation rate (ESR) and taking a chest X-ray to establish the possible presence of metastases. If a pituitary tumour is suspected, endocrine studies and visual field testing will be performed. If acoustic neuroma is suspected, audiometric studies will be performed.

Exploratory Surgical Procedure

Burr hole biopsy, in which a small piece of tissue is removed for pathological examination, may confirm the diagnosis.

Treatment

This may be with surgery, radiotherapy and/or chemotherapy with newer treatments such as stereotactic radiosurgery and carmustine wafers being used for localised delivery of irradiation and chemotherapy. High energy proton beam therapy, a new form of radiotherapy, was used for the first time in the UK in 2018. Patients are also usually prescribed dexamethasone (steroid) to reduce the cerebral oedema around the tumour.

Surgery

The tumour is removed (if possible) using an approach that depends on the type and location of the tumour, for example, craniotomy, posterior fossa craniectomy or transsphenoidal, and a combination of radiotherapy and surgery may be indicated where surgery alone cannot remove all of the tumour.

A tumour may be inoperable due to inaccessibility or because of its type and size. This situation poses a considerable challenge to all members of the MDT to be able to communicate effectively and offer adequate support (see Chapter 31, Nursing the Patient With Cancer, and Chapter 32, Nursing Patients Who Need Palliative Care).

Chemotherapy

Use of chemotherapy is limited due to difficulty in getting the drugs across the BBB. Chemotherapy treatment is usually palliative.

(See Further Reading Woodward and Mestecky 2011.)

❖ Nursing Management and Health Promotion: Intracranial Tumours

Assessment should be made of the patient's and family's understanding of the reason for admission. Someone with an intracranial tumour can usually carry out their normal daily activities, unless there is a rise in ICP caused by swelling or by tumour enlargement.

Immediate Priorities

The patient should be assessed for increasing ICP, primarily through the use of neurological observations, and the nurse should observe for any deterioration in the patient's condition. If the patient has experienced seizures before admission, this should be carefully noted and the nurse should be prepared should a seizure occur.

If the patient has speech problems, for example, dysphasia, time should be taken to ensure they have communicated their needs, possibly drawing on information from relatives.

Subsequent Considerations

After physical and neurological assessment, the SLT, physiotherapist and OT should be involved in assessing the patient, offering advice and assistance.

Psychological Support

The patient will be anxious to know the results of investigations and worried about the diagnosis. The investigations can confirm the diagnosis and/or identify the type of tumour, and the patient should be encouraged to discuss their fears and anxieties. An excellent account of the problems encountered by patients can be found in this new study of the experience of living with a brain tumour (Zanotto et al. 2023). The nurse should be aware of the reality of a grieving process should the diagnosis be life limiting and accept the patient's reactions. Some fears and anxieties may be unfounded and can be alleviated by sensitive nursing interactions.

Ongoing Care

Preparation for Discharge

Many patients have a good neurological recovery, with no residual deficits and no recurrence of tumour growth. Others may have only slight deficits, such as limb weakness. If this is so, they should be encouraged to maintain their previous lifestyle.

If the patient has severe neurological deficits and requires considerable assistance with daily living, the situation should be discussed with both patient and family.

If the family members are anxious to have the patient at home, their wishes should be discussed with the ward team, community nurses and the patient's GP in order to ensure adequate support is available and in place prior to the patient's discharge.

It may be necessary to discuss issues around end of life and the patient's preferred place of care. Most people will wish to go home, but may be fearful of discussing palliative care through beliefs that this is directly linked to dying, rather than symptom management.

Epilepsy

Epilepsy affects 1 in 100 of the population and can be a symptom of an underlying pathology, but more commonly it is a disorder with no identifiable cause (idiopathic). Five per cent of the population will have a seizure in their lifetime, but the occurrence of an isolated seizure does not mean that the person has epilepsy. Epileptic seizures can occur at any age, although the age of onset can often provide a clue as to the cause, such as pyrexia in infants, trauma in adults or vascular disease in later life.

Pathophysiology

An intermittent, uncontrolled discharge of neurones within the CNS results in a seizure. It can range from a major motor convulsion to a brief period of lack of awareness and can occur in any individual at any time.

Common Presenting Symptoms

Presenting symptoms will depend on when the person is examined. During certain types of seizure, the patient may be unconscious, apnoeic and incontinent of urine, whilst in others, changes are barely noticeable. Between seizures, the patient may show no neurological impairment or deficit. Seizures have been classified by the International League Against Epilepsy (ILAE) and the classification was last updated in 2017 (ILAE 2017).

Medical/Surgical Management

Investigations
Electroencephalography (EEG) will be performed. Other investigations such as CT and MRI may also be considered in order to identify possible organic causes.

The most dependable diagnostic tool is a reliable eyewitness account of the seizure.

Treatment
The mainstay of therapy is medication, which is effective in keeping many people seizure-free. A range of antiepileptic (anticonvulsant) medications is available (e.g. carbamazepine, lamotrigine, etc.) and guidance is provided by NICE (2021) on their use.

Epilepsy Surgery. For those patients who have intractable epilepsy with frequent seizures that impact on quality of life and an identifiable focus, surgery may be considered. This may involve resection of the specific cortical area, for example, temporal resection, hemispherectomy, corpus callosotomy, or more recently vagal nerve stimulation.

Nursing Management and Health Promotion: Epileptic Seizures

Most individuals with seizures live independently, with regular monitoring by the primary care team, but NICE recommends annual review by a specialist (NICE 2021).

Immediate Priorities
Once notification is received that a patient is to be admitted with seizures, the following essential equipment should be readily available:
- oxygen and suction in working order
- a selection of various sizes of artificial airways
- charts for recording neurological status, vital signs and seizures
- side rails in place and possibly padded for additional safety
- antiepileptic medication, particularly in parenteral preparations.
  If the patient is having a seizure, the following actions must always be carried out:
- Ensure privacy for the patient if at all possible.
- Ensure side rails are in place, using pillows as padding if required.
- Ensure safety by removing any objects or furniture likely to cause harm.
- Loosen any restrictive clothing.
- Insert an airway *only* when teeth have unclenched (after the tonic stage); any attempts to insert objects into the patient's mouth prior to this serve no purpose and may cause harm to the nurse (bitten fingers) or to the patient (broken teeth).
  Immediately following a seizure, the nurse should:
- Place the patient in the recovery position, to facilitate the drainage of secretions.
- Use suction if necessary to prevent aspiration of secretions.
- Administer oxygen as prescribed.
- Allow the patient to recover with minimal disturbance.
- Allow time for the patient to wake up and provide gentle reassurance and assistance to encourage reorientation.
- Record a description of what happened on the seizure observation chart (Information 11.8).

Prescribed antiepileptic medication should be administered and, where appropriate, medical staff informed.

(See Further Reading, e.g. Woodward and Mestecky 2011).

Further Considerations
The patient should be allowed to express their feelings and fears and they and their family should be given adequate explanations and support. Discussion about the medication, its effects and side-effects, will promote the patient's concordance with prescribed regimens. Monitoring of medication serum levels should be carried out, as this test will indicate if there is an adequate or inadequate dosage of the medication, or if the blood levels are too high. If too high, the patient may experience side-effects; if too low, seizures may recur. Common side-effects of antiepileptic drugs are:
- drowsiness
- dizziness
- gastric upset
- diplopia
- ataxia.

Overdose or sudden withdrawal of medication can also lead to a rebound rise in seizure frequency.

The patient must be allowed time to come to terms with the diagnosis of epilepsy. They may experience feelings of anger,

---

INFORMATION 11.8

Documentation of Seizure Activity

- Time at which seizures occurred
- What the patient was doing at the time
- Any aura or crying out prior to the seizure
- Any loss of consciousness
- Which parts of the body were affected and any sequence to this
- Any stiffening or jerky movements
- Urinary or faecal incontinence
- The duration of the seizure (ictal phase)
- The duration of the (postictal) recovery period
- Patient's behaviour after the seizure
- Pupil reactions

---

grief and/or disbelief, and the nurse should discuss with both the patient and family the realities of epilepsy, but encourage a positive outlook.

The patient may experience an aura (warning) prior to a seizure and the nurse can advise how to use the time available to ensure personal safety. Advice should be given prior to discharge about safety in the home and the involvement of the primary care team.

⊕ **See Evolve website Critical thinking question 11.1**

Equally, 'triggers' that may induce a seizure should be discussed, such as:
- lack of food and sleep
- excessive heat
- constipation
- menstruation
- alcohol
- anxiety or stress.

Medical opinion varies as to whether someone with epilepsy should drink alcohol, as it can interact with antiepileptic medications, preventing them from achieving optimal seizure control. Large amounts of any liquid are known to trigger a seizure, but significant alcohol intake is also often associated with late-night, irregular eating habits and forgotten tablets. The decision to drink alcohol is an individual one, but patients should bear in mind the medical advice.

Patients may be encouraged to wear a MedicAlert; bracelet to inform others about their condition should a seizure occur.

Employment

Most people with epilepsy work, but the safety of the individual and others is paramount. Employment should be discussed, especially if it entails driving or operating machinery. The patient must be told that they have to inform the Driver and Vehicle Licensing Agency (DVLA) of their liability to have seizures and should be advised to stop driving in the meantime, otherwise their motor insurance will be invalid. The healthcare professional is responsible for telling the patient that informing the DVLA is their responsibility and this conversation must be documented in the medical records. This may present major problems to the patient, who may have to look for alternative employment; this may affect self-esteem or outlook for the future.

It is illegal not to employ someone simply because they have epilepsy; people living with epilepsy are covered by the Equality Act (2010) and employers must make reasonable adjustments.

However, some careers are restricted by law to people with epilepsy, for example, pilot, diver, fire fighter, train driver.

Physical Activity

The patient should be encouraged to continue normal physical activities, with some emphasis being placed on the need to take adequate precautions, for example, when swimming the patient should let someone know or take a friend who could deal with a potential seizure.

Involving the Patient's Family

The patient's family should be given time and the opportunity to express their concerns, and the nurse should be prepared to provide advice and explanations. The nurse should explain about the type of seizure the patient is experiencing and family members should be told what to expect if a seizure occurs, for example, that the patient will have sudden uncontrolled movements and will appear to be holding their breath. They should know exactly what to do and why they are doing it. Epilepsy Action provides helpful advice through their website (see Useful Websites). Consideration must be given to meeting the needs of children whose parents have epilepsy. Advice should include the following:
- Ensure the safety of the individual, which can involve removing harmful objects and loosening all restrictive clothing.
- After the seizure, place them in the recovery position, and allow them to sleep, giving them adequate time to wake up and reorientate to time and place.
- Seek medical advice if a seizure lasts longer than usual or if seizures continue without the individual regaining consciousness in between.
- Ensure that the family is aware that the individual may have feelings of shock, anger and lack of self-esteem and that time should be allowed for them to come to terms with these feelings.

Women and Epilepsy

Seizure frequency may increase during menstruation. Some anticonvulsants may reduce the effectiveness of the oral contraceptive pill.

Preconceptual counselling may be required as some anticonvulsants, such as sodium valproate, can lead to fetal abnormalities and are not to be used in pregnancy (NICE 2021).

Multiple Sclerosis

Multiple sclerosis (MS) is a chronic, progressive, demyelinating neurological disorder and is one of the most common neurological causes of long-term disability. The age of onset is 20–50 years and it is slightly more common in females. The aetiology is unknown but is suggested to be an interaction between a number of environmental and genetic factors. MS most commonly follows a remitting and relapsing course, but the disease has several forms.

The prevalence of MS varies significantly in different parts of the world. It is described as a disorder of temperate climates. However, those who move from an area of high risk to one of low risk before the age of 7 reduce the chance of the disease occurring. MS is not hereditary, but the risk of a child developing MS where a parent is afflicted is approximately 15 times greater than in the unaffected population.

A definitive diagnosis may be difficult initially because demyelination develops over a varying period of time. To be conclusive, attacks must occur on multiple occasions and at multiple sites throughout the CNS. New MRI diagnostic criteria were developed and revised to be used with clinical examination (Thompson et al. 2017).

Pathophysiology

MS is thought to be an autoimmune disorder, whereby the body's own myelin within the CNS is recognised as 'foreign' and attacked by the immune system, possibly as an abnormal response to a virus. The demyelination results in scarring or sclerotic patches, and the remission, typical in MS, is the result of healing of these areas. However, in time, these lesions degenerate to a point where recovery is unlikely and the resultant disruption of function becomes permanent.

Common Presenting Symptoms

Clinical features vary considerably, depending on which nerves are affected, but may include:

- blurred or double vision – a common early symptom due to optic neuritis
- weakness and dragging of limbs
- slurred speech
- nystagmus – a disturbance in eye movement in which a slow drift in one direction is followed by a fast corrective movement
- loss of sensation in a specific area of the body or loss of proprioception
- extreme fatigue
- stiff limbs
- intention tremor
- clumsiness/difficulty with movement
- urge urinary incontinence/retention of urine.

Medical Management

Investigations

MRI. identifies areas of demyelination, particularly in the white matter around the ventricles and within the brain stem, and is the primary investigation conducted.

Lumbar Puncture. Examination of the CSF may reveal changes in protein levels and the presence of oligoclonal bands.

Evoked Potentials. A delay in conduction velocity may be seen in visual, auditory or somatosensory pathways.

Treatment

There is no curative treatment. There is evidence that beta-interferons and other disease-modifying treatments can reduce the number of relapses and NICE (2022c) recommends their use for patients with minimal disability and who have remitting–relapsing disease. Tools exist to help patients choose which treatment is right for them (see Useful Websites, MS Trust).

Corticosteroid therapy may be helpful in acute exacerbations to manage symptoms and physiotherapy is helpful in the rehabilitation of numb, affected limbs. Many people with MS will access complementary therapies for symptomatic relief, for example, special diets, reflexology and hyperbaric oxygen, and some may use cannabis for pain relief.

Essentially, care consists of supporting the patient and their family and alleviating symptoms.

❖ Nursing Management and Health Promotion: Multiple Sclerosis

Many patients with MS lead a productive life at home, requiring admission to hospital only if they experience deterioration in their condition. Comprehensive guidelines on the management of patients in both primary and secondary care, including the management of relapses, have been issued by NICE (2022c).

Immediate Priorities

Communicating

The patient undergoing investigations is likely to be anxious and will require adequate explanation about the procedures to be carried out. Frequently, the nurse is asked about these tests and should be prepared to answer questions or, if unable to do so, should find the answer for the patient (see Table 11.2, p. 292). It is important that there is an awareness of the patient's knowledge regarding the condition, as the patient will either fear the worst, often with only a partial understanding of what the diagnosis may be, or may not be aware of the possibility of having MS until the diagnosis is confirmed. Increasingly, patients are well informed from use of the internet.

It is advisable for the nurse to be present when the doctor is speaking to the patient, so that the nurse knows what information the patient has received. Often, the patient wishes to discuss certain points and will find it reassuring to seek supporting advice and information from the nurse after the doctor has left.

The patient will need time to consider the condition and what effects it will have on their outlook for the future. Patients often experience a range of feelings and emotions related to the loss of self-esteem and body image and may worry about how the condition will eventually affect them. Normally, the patient's family will be included, with the patient's consent, and they will require explanations about their relative's condition. They too should be provided with opportunities to discuss their feelings and fears. Providing information about support groups, for example, the MS Society (see Useful Websites) is often helpful.

Admission to hospital during the course of the disease progression can cause considerable stress, especially for the patient who has a set routine at home that allows maintenance of independence. The nurse should encourage the patient to continue to be independent and to follow their daily routine as far as possible when in hospital.

Subsequent Considerations

Communication

Communication impairment in the patient with MS can include difficulties in pronouncing words, slow and/or slurred speech and poor concentration.

The SLT should be involved and can give advice on how to improve the patient's ability to communicate. Useful techniques to help the patient include:

- ensuring that an erect posture is maintained, as this aids breathing and assists with speech
- reducing background noise as much as possible
- encouraging the patient to express the most important points at the beginning of a sentence, when energy and concentration are greatest
- using communication aids such as picture boards or computer.

Maintaining a Safe Environment

The patient with MS can experience difficulties with:

- movement, e.g. ataxia or spasticity
- vision, e.g. diplopia
- sensory disturbance, e.g. detection of pain and temperature.

When in hospital, an accurate assessment of the patient's condition, level of understanding and, if necessary, home conditions should be made. This will involve assessments by the community team as adaptations to the home may be required in order to maintain safety.

In hospital, the nurse should involve the patient in making any necessary changes to their new surroundings, as they will know best what suits them, for example, the height of the bed, depending on their mobility. Ensure there is adequate space to manoeuvre a wheelchair properly if necessary. The nurse-call system should be within easy reach and the patient should be instructed in its use. The patient with clumsiness of movement or tremor may require assistance with some activities, for example, at mealtimes.

Mobility

Maintaining mobility is vital for being independent. A problem for the patient with MS is the uncertainty of the rate at which deterioration in mobility will occur.

The attitude of the ward team is very important; the members should work together to encourage a positive outlook for the patient, while making time to understand the patient's and family's feelings and fears.

If the patient uses mobility aids at home, they should also be used when hospitalised. This enables the patient to maintain independence and also allows the physiotherapist to assess the effectiveness of any aids. Common problems may include ataxia, limb weakness and spasticity. Techniques that may be useful in helping these problems are:
- maintaining good posture
- making contact with the ground with the heel of the foot first
- taking care to place feet firmly in the direction of travel
- looking straight ahead rather than down at the ground
- relaxing and trying not to feel self-conscious.

The physiotherapist may suggest exercises to maintain a good functional position and range of limb movements. Edwards and Pilutti (2017), in a systematic review of exercise therapy, concluded that exercise can be beneficial for people with MS, including those with severe mobility disability.

Skin Care

The patient and family should be taught the importance of regular skin inspection, for example, to observe the sacrum and heels closely and to look for redness or blanching of the skin (see Chapter 23, Tissue Viability and Managing Chronic Wounds). If this occurs, the patient should be aware of the importance of relieving the pressure from the problem area, for example, by lying on their side.

Using a Wheelchair

The physiotherapist and OT may advise that the patient requires a wheelchair in order to maintain mobility. It can be very distressing for the patient to realise that this stage has been reached. It must be emphasised that this does not mean that the patient becomes totally reliant on the wheelchair and is unable to maintain independence.

If the patient requires physiotherapy when at home, advice and support can be obtained from the community physiotherapist. Some local MS Society branches also offer a physiotherapy service.

Advice should be given to the patient about when to use the wheelchair, in particular:
- The wheelchair should be used only when necessary.
- Emphasise the importance of relieving pressure.

- Careful positioning of limbs should be ensured.
- The footrest on the wheelchair should always be used.
- The legs should be placed in proper alignment and the patient should check regularly that the limbs are safely in position on the footrest.

Balance of Rest and Exercise

Fatigue is a common feature of MS. The patient should be advised about the importance of rest periods to avoid becoming overtired or overstressed, which will exacerbate the condition. Relaxation techniques and a specific rest/exercise programme may be beneficial and should be discussed with the patient and their family.

Although rest is very important, exercise is also vital to maintain muscle strength and help reduce the risk of spasticity. It will also improve circulation and prevent pressure ulcers and joint stiffness. Exercise will contribute to maintaining the patient's independence.

Temperature Control

Fatigue and MS symptoms are also exacerbated by heat, which slows conduction velocities. Patients should be advised to avoid hot baths, hot climates and infections if at all possible.

Employment

If the patient's current employment involves physical exertion, this may prove problematic with regard to returning to work. The patient may have to consider how their disorder will affect current employment and think about finding alternative work, although in many cases this may prove impossible. Patients with MS are protected by the Equality Act (2010) and employers have to make reasonable adjustments or consider redeployment.

Eliminating

The patient may experience bladder dysfunction, which can vary in severity and include incontinence, urinary frequency or urine retention. Problems with constipation and/or faecal incontinence are also of concern (Evidence-Based Practice 11.3). The urinary problems are due to the reflex action of the bladder having been disturbed due to sites of demyelination in the lower spinal cord, particularly the sacral segments.

The social implications of incontinence can be enormous and some patients will avoid going out for fear of embarrassment (see Chapter 24, Maintaining Continence). If a urine infection is suspected, a specimen should be sent to bacteriology for culture and sensitivity. Bladder retraining and antimuscarinic drugs (e.g. oxybutynin) may help, but it may be necessary to use aids such as protective clothing and pads (see Chapter 24).

Urinary catheterisation may be required if persistent urinary retention is experienced. Intermittent self-catheterisation is preferable and many become very competent at performing this procedure. Advice from a continence advisor may also be useful (see Chapter 24).

The importance of an adequate fluid intake of 2.5–3 L/day should be stressed. Many patients mistakenly think that if they stop drinking they will no longer be incontinent.

The immobile patient will be especially prone to constipation, which will aggravate coexisting urinary problems. The patient and the family should be advised as to how constipation can be avoided by taking an appropriate diet, an adequate fluid intake and maintaining as much mobility as possible. Regular oral laxatives may be required and the occasional use of enemas and suppositories may be indicated.

Expressing Sexuality

The patient may experience a change in body image. Sexual counselling may be beneficial for both partners.

Men may experience erectile dysfunction and women diminished libido, due to neurological damage. The patient may be too embarrassed or worried to discuss such difficulties with a health professional, and support groups and relationship guidance services may be helpful. A free booklet published by the MS Society is available online (https://www.mssociety.org.uk/about-ms/signs-and-symptoms/sex-and-relationships).

Advice on contraception may be required, especially by women, as some oral contraceptives may interfere with existing medication. Pregnancy should be avoided during active stages of the disease as this may exacerbate the symptoms, although successful pregnancy may be achieved.

Eating and Drinking

There has been some research into the link between diet and MS, and a number of specialised diets have been identified. It has been demonstrated that people with MS have higher levels of saturated fats and lower levels of polyunsaturated fats in the myelin sheath and the patient should take a healthy diet and reduce the intake of saturated fats (see Chapter 22, Nutrition and Health).

The SLT and dietitian may be able to offer assistance and advice if the patient has swallowing difficulties. The nurse can assist by encouraging the patient to:

- Sit up straight with the head supported, if necessary.
- Eat in a quiet, relaxed atmosphere and not speak while eating.
- Take time when eating, to avoid choking.

- Eat foods that are easier to swallow, e.g. semi-solid or liquidised foods, following advice from SLT.

Personal Cleansing and Dressing

The patient should be encouraged to maintain independence with regard to washing and dressing. It may seem to the patient, and at times to the nurse or to the patient's family, that it would be quicker and easier for the nurse to perform these activities for the patient. The patient may feel under stress to hurry in order to release the nurse to go and attend to other patients. The nurse should explain that there is no hurry to have everything finished for a set time.

The OT can assess the patient and give advice regarding washing and dressing, offer a range of dressing aids and suggest specially adapted clothing, for example, with Velcro instead of buttons and zips.

Education

The patient and the family should be as well informed as possible about the diagnosis of MS and should be aware of the most successful methods of maintaining independence. They should also be aware of the possibility of the occurrence of behavioural and mood changes. Euphoria, depression, apathy and emotional lability are common. Many MS nurse specialists run courses for newly diagnosed patients or an expert patient programme may be available.

Preparation for Discharge

Episodic hospitalisation may become necessary as the disease progresses and the patient and family should be given the opportunity to voice any worries or fears to allow adequate preparation for discharge. Some adjustments may be required in the house, for example, bath aids and rearrangement of furniture. If the patient depends on a wheelchair for mobility, the doorways may have to be widened, cupboards lowered, and a shower may be required instead of a bath.

Rehousing to ground floor accommodation may be needed to allow wheelchair access. This involves major changes not only for the patient but also for the family and can be very traumatic.

Advice regarding income and benefits available, for example, Disability Living Allowance (DLA), can be given by the social worker. Outpatient appointments can be arranged for physiotherapy, occupational or speech therapy, if necessary.

Some doctors advocate discussing the possibility of relapse so that the patient is better prepared when it occurs. On the other hand, some patients may not have a period of relapse for up to 20 years and may worry unnecessarily if the subject is broached too soon. Some patients may benefit from being informed of the availability of support groups,

Parkinson's Disease

Parkinson's disease (PD) is a chronic neurodegenerative disorder of the basal nuclei, with a slow onset that progresses gradually. It has an annual incidence of approximately 0.2/1000 and a prevalence of 1.5/1000 in the UK (Parkinson's UK 2018). Both incidence and prevalence increase with age and the prevalence has doubled in the last 25 years, with the majority of those diagnosed aged over 60, but 1 in 20 will be under 40 years.

Progressive supranuclear palsy and multisystem atrophy, known as Parkinson's plus syndromes, both present with parkinsonian features and patients are often misdiagnosed with PD.

Pathophysiology

PD is characterised by degenerative changes in the substantia nigra within the basal nuclei. Depletion of the dopaminergic neurones in the substantia nigra results in a decrease in the levels of the neurotransmitter, dopamine, essential for the control of movement, coordination and posture. As a result, the balance between dopamine and acetylcholine is lost and the acetylcholine effects are exaggerated. Parkinsonism may also be seen as a side-effect of some drugs. Although genetic and environmental factors have been implicated, the cause of the degenerative changes is unknown.

Common Presenting Signs/Symptoms

PD was once thought to be purely a movement disorder, but is now understood to be a multiple system disorder. The diagnostic features of PD are a triad of features: tremor, muscle rigidity and bradykinesia (slowness in initiating or repeating movements) with impairment of fine movements.

Other clinical features include:

- expressionless face
- disturbance in free-flowing movement, stooped posture and festinating gait, recurrent falls
- micrographia (tiny handwriting)
- loss of postural reflexes
- autonomic manifestations, e.g. excessive perspiration, drooling and excess salivation
- constipation and urge urinary incontinence
- microphonia (weak voice).
  (See Further Reading, e.g. Woodward and Mestecky 2011).

Medical/Surgical Management

Investigations

Investigations such as CT scanning may be considered in order to eliminate other disorders. There is no specific diagnostic test for PD. Diagnosis is usually based on clinical presentation.

Treatment

Medication is the mainstay of treatment. Treatment is symptomatic, does not halt the pathological process and requires careful management and monitoring (see Further Reading, e.g. British National Formulary).

Dopaminergic preparations such as levodopa are administered to replace the depleted dopamine. In older people, levodopa with a dopa-decarboxylase inhibitor is often used (e.g. co-beneldopa), but it is only used once the symptoms of the disease compromise the individual's normal functioning. In younger patients, dopamine agonists are given to stimulate the surviving dopamine receptors. The enzymes monoamine oxidase A and B play a key role in the breakdown of dopamine. Selegiline is a medication that inhibits this process and appears to have a symptomatic effect. Amantadine acts by allowing the dopamine to stay longer at its site of action without being used up by other cells. It may be useful in the control of tremor but helps only a small proportion of patients. Catechol-*O*-methyltransferase (COMT) inhibitors (e.g. entacapone) block the action of an enzyme that breaks down levodopa and, given in combination, may prolong the action of levodopa.

Patients who experience sudden fluctuations in their symptoms in spite of careful management of their medications may be prescribed apomorphine. This is a potent dopa agonist and is sometimes given as a 'rescue' medicine in advanced states. It produces a direct effect at the sites where dopamine is active in the brain.

Many of the medications have variable side-effects and accurate titration may necessitate admission to hospital. Another drug effect is an 'on–off' phenomenon, whereby the patient loses the benefit of the dopamine and becomes rigid and immobile for a period of time. Surgery, for example, deep brain stimulation (Hitti et al. 2019), may be indicated for some patients and provides long-term symptomatic relief.

❖ Nursing Management and Health Promotion: Parkinson's Disease

The support of the patient's family or carer and of the primary healthcare team is important. The family's/carer's ability to cope with the mobility and other problems, such as impulse control disorders, associated with PD can make the difference between a level of independence, with the patient living in their own home, and total dependence in long-term care.

Immediate Priorities

Many of the early symptoms of PD may be treated by the family doctor, with the patient and their family making necessary adjustments to their home, for example, removal of rugs and other obstacles, but early referral to a specialist centre is warranted.

The progress of the disease can vary, but should the patient's condition worsen, admission to hospital may become necessary. This provides an opportunity for nursing staff, physiotherapist, SLT and OT, to advise the patient and the family on how to deal with the problems which are interfering with the patient's daily life.

The most important priority is to ensure medication is given on time, especially before meals, to promote maximal functional abilities and independence.

Mobility

Problems can include difficulty in starting to walk or stopping, shuffling, tottering, impaired balance when turning and ongoing stiffness, interrupted by a 'freezing' of movement. Falls are also common. Passive and active range of movement exercises are a good starting point. Relatives should be advised to continue this activity at home. Effort should also be directed towards improving the patient's gait, with the assistance of the physiotherapist. Useful tips are given in Information 11.9.

Moving and handling assessment is required as well as falls risk assessment. If the patient experiences difficulty in rolling over in bed or getting in and out of bed, they can be advised to use a low bed with a firm mattress or to place a board under their existing mattress (see Information 11.9). (See Useful Websites, e.g. Parkinson's UK, where additional suggestions inspired by patients themselves can be accessed.) It is vital that medicine administration times are adhered to.

Exercise

Some patients may benefit from an exercise programme to assist mobility and improve posture. It is important that this programme is performed under supervision initially, until the patient and their helper are conversant with the techniques. Again, the importance of continuing these at home should be stressed to both patient and family.

Eating and Drinking

The person with PD may have difficulty with eating and drinking due to abnormal posture, tremor, poor swallowing and excessive

INFORMATION 11.9

Useful Tips for the Nurse/Carer to Encourage a Frail Older Person With Parkinson's Disease to Move

General Tips

- Advise the person to consciously lift each foot as he is walking and to place his heel on the ground first. To encourage this, ask the person to think that he has a series of imaginary steps to climb.
- Teach the person to broaden his stance to provide a more stable base.
- Remind the person to think about his posture and to stand erect.
- If the person starts to shuffle, ask him to stop and start again.
- Ask the person to adopt the habit of taking small steps when he is turning and to turn only in a forward direction.

Rolling Over in Bed

The person is advised to bend her knees so that her feet are flat on the mattress and then swing the knees in the direction that she wishes to turn.

The person then clasps her hands and lifts them straight up, straightening the elbows, then turns the head and swings the arms in the same direction as the legs.

The person then grips the edge of the mattress and adjusts her position until comfortable.

Getting Into and Out of Bed Independently

- To get into bed, the person sits on the edge of the bed near the pillow.
- The person then only has to lift his legs onto the bed and then adjust himself into a comfortable position.
N.B. Getting out of bed is more complicated and several techniques can be suggested by a physiotherapist.

Rising From a Chair

- The person should avoid low chairs, choosing instead firm, high-backed chairs. In the home, the height of a low chair can be increased with blocks under the legs.
- Cushions or a spring-ejector seat will also help.

---

saliva, resulting in malnutrition. There may be embarrassment about their untidiness when eating, and the length of time it takes to eat often results in food going cold. People will often choose to eat alone rather than endure the social embarrassment of seeing others watching them eat. Nutrition risk assessment should be undertaken (see Chapter 22, Nutrition and Health) and eating small amounts at frequent intervals is preferable.

The SLT may do a swallowing assessment and prepare a programme of swallowing management. This could include techniques to encourage swallowing, for example, taking a sip of iced water to stimulate the swallowing reflex

The dietitian's advice should also be sought. It is usual to establish what kind of foods the patient likes best. A review of their current dietary intake will alert the nurse to any deficiencies. If tremor is a problem, the patient can be taught to hold their arm close into their body, using their elbow as a pivot. Bendable straws could be used and cups containing hot liquids should only be filled halfway to avoid spillage or scalding.

It is important for the patient's self-esteem to resist the temptation to feed them before this is absolutely necessary. Many patients may still be able to feed themselves if their food is cut up for them. Feeding the patient for the convenience of speed is unacceptable.

Some signs/symptoms of dysphagia are:

- coughing within a few seconds of swallowing
- food sticking in the throat
- nasal regurgitation
- fear of swallowing
- drooling
- food remaining in the mouth after the meal.

If the patient wears dentures, these should be checked frequently to ensure a proper fit. The importance of good oral hygiene should be emphasised. Patients should check and record their body weight weekly, as weight loss may occur.

Communication

The communication impairment seen in the patient with PD includes loss of facial expression, which may lead to the assumption that the patient is cognitively impaired. Loss of normal eye contact and body language may occur due to the stooping posture. Facial exercises encourage the patient to pronounce sounds more clearly, for example, by mouthing words slowly and clearly. There are also exercises for breathing, strengthening the voice and controlling the speed of speech, many of which can be continued in the patient's home.

Eventually the voice may become so weak that meaningful communication is impossible and an alternative means of communication becomes necessary. Communication aids must be appropriate to the patient's needs, and advice regarding their use should be taken from the SLT.

It may be possible for the patient to write down messages using pen and paper. However, the ability to write also deteriorates progressively and the writing becomes smaller and smaller (micrographia) as muscle stiffness increases. The progressive difficulties with communications are frustrating for both patient and their family (Reflection 11.5).

Elimination

The impairment of mobility in conjunction with urinary frequency or hesitancy can lead to embarrassing episodes of incontinence and increases the risk of falls. Urge incontinence may occur and bladder retraining and continence aids may be indicated (see Chapter 24, Maintaining Continence). It is important that patients are encouraged to maintain an adequate fluid intake. Eventually urinary catheterisation may be unavoidable.

Constipation is a common problem in PD, so the patient and family should be taught preventive action. A high-fibre diet and plenty of fluids will encourage regular bowel motions. Failing this,

REFLECTION 11.5

Parkinson's Disease: the Family's Perspective

We are 7 years into living with Father's PD. There have been so many challenges for him and for us over the years, and the challenges keep changing as the disease progresses. With each new admission to care, we are having to work harder to make sure that staff understand that the painfully slow speech from an expressionless face still conveys humour, awareness of world events, kindness and insight.

Activity

- Reflect on how nurses can assist patients with progressive PD to communicate effectively.
- Discuss with your practice assessor how nurses and other members of the healthcare team could support the family in the scenario.

it will be necessary to administer oral faecal softeners or bulking agents regularly and, when required, an enema.

Personal Cleansing and Dressing

The oily skin and excessive perspiration seen in patients with PD demand more frequent washing and bathing. If tremor is present, men will find an electric or battery-operated shaver safer and easier to use.

Slowness in performing voluntary movement (bradykinesia) can make daily activities such as dressing difficult. Adaptations to clothing style or fastenings without loss of dignity, for example, wearing tracksuit trousers or replacing buttons and zips with Velcro, and the use of appropriate aids will allow the patient to continue to dress independently for as long as possible.

Preparation for Discharge

Every opportunity should be taken to advise the patient and family about the best way to manage the disorder at home. Each of the areas already outlined should be included in the discharge plan.

Additional points to consider following discharge from hospital are as follows:

- The names and times of the medicines to be taken should be written down. The importance of maintaining the correct dosage is emphasised and some indication of the medicine's action and possible side-effects should be given.
- A daily exercise programme should be devised for the patient.
- Contact should be established with the appropriate community services, who may be providing the patient and family with support at home.
- Advice on dietary intake along with sample menus should be provided.
- Advice on safety, for example, removal of loose rugs and other obstacles, should be given.

The patient should be encouraged to remain as active as possible for as long as possible, but should also be warned to pace their activity. Each individual will approach this situation in their own unique way and this has to be taken into account when proffering advice.

Infections of the Central Nervous System

This section outlines three infections of the CNS – meningitis, encephalitis and cerebral abscess.

Meningitis

Meningitis is inflammation of the meninges; it may be bacterial, viral, fungal or protozoal. The most serious infective organism that causes meningitis is the *Neisseria meningitidis* (meningococcus) bacterium (group B causes most cases in the UK as group C has declined since vaccination was introduced), which causes a characteristic nonblanching rash and can rapidly result in septicaemia and death. Other bacteria include:

- *Haemophilus influenzae* type B (Hib)
- *Streptococcus pneumoniae* (pneumococcus)
- and, less commonly, *Mycobacterium tuberculosis*.

Most people with meningococcal meningitis are young children, teenagers and university students who work in close proximity. Meningitis and meningococcal septicaemia are notifiable in the UK. Vaccines against Hib (introduced 1992), group C meningococcal disease (1999) and pneumococcal disease (2007) are part of the routine immunisation programme in the UK (see Health Protection Agency www.hpa.org.uk/ for up-to-date epidemiological data on cases of meningococcal meningitis). Other strains have

been identified and an ACWY vaccine is now offered to teenagers at 14 years and young people (up to age 25) going to university (NHS 2022). Since these vaccines were introduced there has been a significant reduction in cases – Hib infection in general reduced by 99%, deaths from group C meningococcal disease have reduced from an average of 79 per year to less than 1 death on average, and for further information, including patient stories, see http://vk.ovg.ox.ac.uk/meningococcal-disease.

Approximately 10,000 people contract viral meningitis annually (also known as aseptic/chemical meningitis) but rarely require hospitalisation. Patients present with headache, which resolves spontaneously. Fungal meningitis is rare and usually seen in immunosuppressed patients, for example, in HIV disease, and may be caused by *Cryptococcus neoformans* or *Candida* infections.

Encephalitis

This much rarer infection affects 2–4 people per 100,000 per annum. The most common infective organism is the herpes simplex virus.

Cerebral Abscess

Cerebral abscess is a focal collection of pus within the white/grey matter of the brain, caused by pyogenic bacteria such as staphylococci and streptococci (Sonneville et al. 2017).

● *Pathophysiology of CNS Infections*

Meningitis. In bacterial meningitis, purulent exudate is found in the subarachnoid space. The most likely route of entry is via the bloodstream, which can carry microorganisms from, for example, an infected middle ear. Other routes of entry include direct extension from a skull or facial fracture, via the CSF, and extensions along cranial and spinal nerves. The circulating CSF acts as an effective means of spreading the microorganisms.

Encephalitis. Herpes simplex encephalitis produces swelling and necrosis of the temporal lobes, accompanied by inflammation and haemorrhage.

Cerebral Abscess. most commonly occurs following middle ear and mastoid infections or dental abscess. Pus accumulates in the cerebral tissue and becomes encapsulated. Other related conditions are extradural abscess, where pus accumulates in the extradural space, and subdural empyema, where pus accumulates in the subdural space. Cerebral abscess is highly irritant with many patients developing epilepsy and/or raised ICP.

Common Presenting Symptoms

Infections of the CNS affect all age groups. Common signs and symptoms are described in Information 11.10. Admission to hospital will be necessary and, if the patient's condition is serious, referral to a neurosurgeon will be made as the condition can become fatal, especially in children. Complications include deafness, seizures, personality changes, fatigue and death.

● *Medical/Surgical Management*

Investigations

The patient with any focal neurological signs, or presenting with a GCS <7, should have a CT scan performed to exclude an intracranial mass, such as an abscess. A lumbar puncture is usually performed to identify the offending organism in meningitis. The changes seen in the CSF are outlined in Table 11.5.

Other investigations may include blood cultures and X-rays to detect the source of infection. Brain biopsy guided by CT scan

INFORMATION 11.10

Features in the Presentation of CNS Infections

Bacterial meningitis **(Abrupt Onset*)**

*N.B. except in meningitis caused by Mycobacterium tuberculosis, when it is insidious.

Nonspecific Features

- Vague 'flu-like' symptoms
- Vomiting
- Fever, although the person may have cold extremities
- Back, muscle or joint pains
- Headache
- Drowsiness

More Specific Features

- Neck stiffness
- Photophobia
- Phonophobia
- Confusion
- Altered consciousness
- Seizures
- Purpuric or petechial rash that does not blanch under pressure
  N.B. Infants may exhibit some of the following:
- Pallor
- Irritability
- Decreased responses
- A high-pitched cry
- Refusing feeds
- Floppiness – reduced muscle tone
- Bulging fontanelle ('soft spot')

Late Features

- Coma
- Neck retraction (in severe cases this, in combination with spasm, causing the heels to bend backwards, produces opisthotonos)
- Shock due to septicaemia
- Widespread haemorrhagic rash

Viral Encephalitis (Insidious Onset)

- Headache
- Fever
- Conscious level deteriorates gradually
- Confusion is common
- Moderate neck stiffness
- Seizures can occur
- ICP may be elevated as a result of cerebral oedema
- Cranial nerve deficits and focal neurological signs may be present

Cerebral Abscess (Insidious Onset, 2–3 weeks or More)

- Headache is recurrent
- Fever is usually present
- Confusion
- Drowsiness
- Neck stiffness (indicative of circulating CSF infection)
- Partial or generalised seizures may occur
- ICP is elevated as abscess expands
- Cranial nerve deficits occur and focal neurological signs include speech disorders, motor and sensory deficits and ataxia

TABLE 11.5	Cerebrospinal Fluid in Bacterial Meningitis and Viral Encephalitis	
CSF Parameters	**Acute Bacterial Meningitis**	**Viral Encephalitis**
Appearance	Yellow	Clear
Cells	Polymorphonuclear $1000–5000 \times 10^6$/L	Mononuclear $50–1500 \times 10^6$/L
Protein	Elevated	Mildly elevated
Glucose	Low	Normal
Organisms	Present on culture	Absent on culture. Require specialist virological testing to identify
Pressure	Increased	Increased

CSF, Cerebrospinal fluid.

Treatment

The patient with bacterial meningitis or a cerebral abscess should commence antibiotics as soon as possible (before admission to hospital in suspected bacterial meningitis). Penicillin is the antibiotic of choice and is usually given intravenously in high doses; alternative antibiotics are used if the person has an allergy to penicillin (see Chapter 7, Nursing Patients With Disorders of the Lymphatic and Immune System).

Surgery will be performed to drain a cerebral abscess and adequate explanations should be given to the patient and family of what is involved in this course of treatment. This may involve burr hole aspiration, primary excision of the whole abscess or evacuation of the abscess contents leaving the capsule intact. This avoids damaging the surrounding brain.

Patients with encephalitis will be prescribed intravenous aciclovir (antiviral) and anticonvulsants.

❖ Nursing Management and Health Promotion: CNS Infections

For those patients who require surgery, the general pre- and postoperative care is as given in Chapter 25. The nurse should observe the patient for signs of raised ICP postoperatively. The patient's family will require explanations, support and comfort.

Immediate Priorities

Neurological Status and Vital Signs

The patient with an intracranial infection may have a decreased conscious level and may deteriorate rapidly, therefore observations should be recorded and any change in condition reported immediately. Vital signs are important as the patient may be pyrexial. Pulse, temperature, blood pressure and respirations may be high when recorded, owing to infection: any changes in these observations should be reported. There may be signs of raised ICP.

Breathing

The respiratory pattern should be observed for rate, depth and frequency. Any respiratory distress should be reported immediately. Oxygen may be prescribed and the nurse should encourage the patient to tolerate it, giving explanations when necessary. Nursing the patient with a head-up tilt of 30 degrees will not only help to decrease ICP, but also encourage lung expansion. The nurse should be aware of the risk of a chest infection developing.

may be helpful. When an abscess is suspected, the CT scan should be enhanced with contrast medium to highlight small lesions (daughter loculi) which may otherwise be missed. The abscess will be enhanced with a ring surrounding the pus-filled centre on CT scan.

Controlling Body Temperature

In order to detect and reduce pyrexia, the patient's temperature should be recorded frequently and any further rise reported immediately, as this may indicate that the antibiotics are not controlling the infection and that the patient's condition could deteriorate. Each 1°C increase in temperature increases the body's demand for oxygen by 10%, which encourages vasodilatation and increases ICP.

Observe Seizure Activity

Seizures are common with abscess and encephalitis. Seizures should be recorded, noting the type of seizure, its duration and exactly what happened. An airway, oxygen and suction should be available.

Communication

Communication can be difficult, as the patient may be experiencing severe headache, nausea and vomiting, have photophobia and be disorientated and drowsy. A calm darkened environment will comfort the patient, who will be distressed about their condition and what is happening to them. Patients may become aggressive and behaviour becomes challenging (see Further Reading, e.g. Woodward and Mestecky 2011).

Explanations should be given to the patient about what is happening and why, and the patient should be given time to ask questions and express their feelings.

The family will also require reassurance and explanations, but they should be advised not to overstimulate the patient.

Maintaining a Safe Environment

Side rails may be in position to prevent the patient falling out of bed due to restlessness or confusion following risk assessment. In extreme circumstances the patient may be nursed on a mattress on the floor.

Medication and Fluid Balance

Patients will have headache and analgesics should be administered.

The nurse should ensure that prescribed antibiotics are given or taken at the correct time by the patient, to ensure maintenance of the medication at a therapeutic level in the bloodstream. People who have been in close contact with patients with meningococcal meningitis will need to be traced and prescribed prophylactic antibiotics, for example, rifampicin, ciprofloxacin or ceftriaxone.

An accurate fluid balance chart should be maintained as the patient can become dehydrated due to pyrexia, nausea and vomiting. Intravenous fluids will be prescribed until the patient is able to tolerate adequate oral fluids (see Chapter 21, Maintaining Fluid, Electrolyte and Acid–Base Balance).

Personal Cleansing and Dressing

If the patient has a decreased conscious level, care should be exercised in meeting their needs and, as their condition improves, independence should be encouraged.

Mobility

Initially, bed rest may be necessary and all care should be taken to ensure that the patient's position is changed 2-hourly. Examination of the skin should be carried out at frequent intervals in order to detect signs of pressure, such as redness.

Preparation for Discharge

If the source of the infection has been treated successfully, for example, in sinusitis or an ear infection, the patient should be advised to contact their GP if there is a recurrence of the infection. The need to continue medication on discharge should be fully explained, with emphasis on the importance of completion of the course of antibiotics.

While rehabilitating in the ward, the patient will have been assessed by the ward team. Maintenance of optimal function (both physically and psychologically) is vital and outpatient appointments may be required, for example, for physiotherapy. The patient's family should be involved in the patient's planned discharge and rehabilitation programme at home. Advice should also be given about employment, driving and other activities, especially if the patient has experienced seizures.

Both the Meningitis Trust and the Encephalitis Society (see Useful Websites) offer a comprehensive support system for those affected. Complete recovery takes time and they provide guidance on how to deal with a range of minor after-effects, for example, general tiredness, headaches and difficulty in concentration.

Huntington's Disease

Huntington's disease is an autosomal dominant inherited neurological condition, therefore affecting males and females equally. Signs and symptoms, which may vary, usually start during middle age but they can occur earlier. Signs and symptoms include:
- involuntary movements (chorea)
- poor concentration and memory problems
- mood changes, depression
- cognitive and behavioural changes
- later dementia
- weight loss
- dysarthria and dysphagia.

Patients progressively deteriorate until they are totally dependent and require full nursing care. They will eventually die from secondary infections, for example, pneumonia. There is currently no cure and treatment is symptomatic only, such as drugs to control involuntary movements. Family members should be offered presymptomatic testing, genetic counselling and ongoing support. A detailed discussion of this and other inherited neurological diseases is beyond the scope of this book and readers can find information from the appropriate support group, for example, Huntington's Disease Association (see Useful Websites).

Summary: Key Nursing Issues

- Patients with neurological conditions have complex needs.
- Detailed assessment of consciousness, neurological function and other vital systems is essential.
- Treatment of patients with many long-term neurological conditions is often symptomatic and nurses play a vital role at the centre of an MDT in helping patients maintain function and independence as far as possible.
- Nurses caring for such patients require excellent communication skills and to be able to provide psychological and emotional support to patients and their families.

Reflection and Learning – What Next?

- **Test** your knowledge by visiting the Evolve website 🌐 and answering the multiple choice questions and critical thinking questions.
- **Consolidate** your learning by looking at some of the further reading suggestions, references and specialist websites.
- **Revisit** some of the additional material on the Evolve website.

- **Consider** what you have learnt and how this will help your professional development.
- **Reflect** on how you can apply this knowledge to the care of your patients.
- **Discuss** your learning with your mentor/supervisor, lecturer and colleagues.

References

Bakas T, Austin JK, Okonkwo KF, et al. Needs, concerns, strategies and advice of stroke caregivers the first 6 months after discharge. *J Neurosci Nurs*. 2002;34(5):242–251.

Butterfield M, Bodnar D, Williamson F, Parker L, Ryan G. Prevalence of secondary insults and outcomes of patients with traumatic brain injury intubated in the prehospital setting: a retrospective cohort study. *Emerg Med J*. 2023;40:167–174.

Cancer Research UK. Brain, other CNS and intracranial tumours mortality; 2018. https://www.cancerresearchuk.org/health-professional/cancer-statistics/statistics-by-cancer-type/brain-other-cns-and-intra-cranial-tumours#heading-One.

Chan AY, Choi EH, Yuki I, et al. Cerebral vasospasm after subarachnoid hemorrhage: developing treatments. *Brain Hemorrhages*. 2021;2(1):15–23.

Connor TA, Clark JM, Jayamohan J, et al. Do equestrian helmets prevent concussion? A retrospective analysis of head injuries and helmet damage from real-world equestrian accidents. *Sports Med Open*. 2019;5:19.

Dibley L, Coggrave M, McClurg D, et al. 'It's just horrible': a qualitative study of patients' and carers' experiences of bowel dysfunction in multiple sclerosis. *J Urol*. 2017;264(7):1354–1361.

Edwards T, Pilutti LA. The effect of exercise training in adults with multiple sclerosis with sever mobility disability: a systematic review and future research directions. *Mult Scler Relat Disord*. 2017;16:31–39.

English V. Time is brain: the role of the nurse in acute ischaemic stroke. *Nurs Crit Care*. 2016;11(5):43–46.

El Hussein M, Zettel S, Suykens AM. The ABCs of managing increased intracranial pressure. *J Nurs Educ Pract*. 2017;7(4):6–14.

Hickey JV. *The Clinical Practice of Neurological and Neurosurgical Nursing*. 8th ed. Philadelphia: Lippincott; 2019.

Hitti FL, Ramayya AG, McShane BJ, Yang AI, Vaughan KA, Baltuch GH. Long-term outcomes following deep brain stimulation for Parkinson's disease. *J Neurosurg*. 2019;132(1):205–210.

International League Against Epilepsy (ILAE). Operational classification of seizure types by the International League Against Epilepsy; 2017. https://www.ilae.org/guidelines/definition-and-classification/operational-classification-2017/ilae-2017-classification-of-seizure-types-checklist.

Karic T, Røe C, Nordenmark TH. Effect of early mobilization and rehabilitation on complications in aneurysmal subarachnoid haemorrhage. *J Neurosurg*. 2017;126(2):518–526.

Lee KS, Zhang JJY, Nguyen V, et al. The evolution of intracranial aneurysm treatment techniques and future directions. *Neurosurg Rev*. 2022;45:1–25.

Marieb EN, Hoehn KN. *Human anatomy and Physiology, Global Edition*. 11th ed.. Pearson; 2020.

NHS. Vaccination: Meningitis; 2022. https://www.nhs.uk/conditions/meningitis/vaccination/.

National Institute for Health and Care Excellence (NICE). *Venous thromboembolism in over 16s: reducing the risk of hospital-acquired deep vein thrombosis or pulmonary embolism*. NICE guideline [NG89]; 2018. https://www.nice.org.uk/guidance/ng89.

National Institute for Health and Care Excellence (NICE). *Head injury: triage, assessment, investigation and early management of head injury in children, young people and adults*. Clinical guideline [CG176]; 2019. https://www.nice.org.uk/guidance/cg176.

National Institute for Health and Care Excellence (NICE). *Epilepsies: diagnosis and management*; 2021. Clinical guideline [CG137]. https://www.nice.org.uk/guidance/cg137.

National Institute for Health and Care Excellence (NICE). What is the prevalence of stroke and TIA in the UK? 2022a. https://cks.nice.org.uk/topics/stroke-tia/background-information/prevalence/

National Institute for Health and Care Excellence (NICE). *Stroke and transient ischaemic attack in over 16s: diagnosis and initial management*. Clinical guideline [CG 128]; 2022. https://www.nice.org.uk/guidance/ng128.

National Institute for Health and Care Excellence (NICE). Multiple sclerosis in adults: management. *Clinical guideline CG220*. 2022. https://www.nice.org.uk/guidance/ng220.

Nekludov M, Bellander BM, Mure M. Oxygenation and cerebral perfusion pressure improved in the prone position. *Acta Anaesthesiol Scand*. 2006;50(8):932–936.

Parkinson's UK. The incidence and prevalence of Parkinson's in the UK Report; 2018. https://www.parkinsons.org.uk/professionals/resources/incidence-and-prevalence-parkinsons-uk-report.

Roper N, Logan W, Tierney AJ. *The Roper–Logan–Tierney Model of Nursing. The Activities of Living Model*. Edinburgh: Churchill Livingstone; 1980.

Schizodimos T, Soulountsi V, Iasonidou C, et al. An overview of management of intracranial hypertension in the intensive care unit. *J Anesth*. 2020;34:741–757.

de Sousa I, Woodward S. The Glasgow Coma Scale in adults: doing it right. *Emerg Nurse*. 2016;24(8):33–38.

Sonneville R, Ruimy R, Benzonana NESCMID Study Group for Infectious Diseases of the Brain (ESGIB). An update on bacterial brain abscess in immunocompetent patients. *Clin Microbiol Infect*. 2017;23(9):614–620.

Stumpo V, Staartjes VE, Quddusi A, et al. Enhanced Recovery After Surgery strategies for elective craniotomy: a systematic review. *J Neurosurg*. 2021;135(6):1857–1881.

Thompson SD. An introduction to hydrocephalus: types, treatment and management. *Br J Neurosci Nurs*. 2017;13(1):36–40.

Thompson AJ, Banwell BL, Barkhof F, et al. Diagnosis of multiple sclerosis: 2017 revisions of the McDonald criteria. *Lancet*. 2017;17(2):162–173.

Vadivelu N, Kai AM, Tran D, et al. Options for perioperative pain management in neurosurgery. *J Pain Res*. 2016;9:37–47

Vali Y, Rashidian A, Jalili M, et al. Effectiveness of regionalization of trauma care services: a systematic review. *Public Health*. 2017;146:92–107.

Wijeratne T, Sales C. Understanding why post-stroke depression may be the norm rather than the exception: the anatomical and neuroinflammatory correlates of post-stroke depression. *J Clin Med*. 2021;10(8):1674.

Woodward S, Waterhouse C. *Oxford Handbook of Neuroscience Nursing*. 2nd Ed Oxford: Oxford University Press; 2021.

Zanotto A, Goodall K, Ellison M, McVittie C. 'Make them wonder how you are still smiling': the lived experience of coping with a brain tumour. *Qual Health Res*. 2023;33(7):601–612.

Further Reading

Braine M. Assessment and management of challenging behaviour. In: Woodward NS, Mestecky AM, eds. *Neuroscience Nursing – Evidence Based Practice*. Oxford: Wiley–Blackwell; 2011.

Burnol L, Payen JF, Francony G, et al. Impact of head-of-bed posture on brain oxygenation in patients with acute brain injury: a prospective cohort study. *Neurocrit Care*. 2021;35:662–668.

Finlayson M, Van Denend T, Hudson E. Aging with multiple sclerosis. *J Neurosci Nurs*. 2004;36(5):245–251.

Gimenez R. My experience with a second brain aneurysm. *Clin Nurse Spec*. 2000;14(6):253–255.

Kelly MJ, Baig F, Hu MT, Okai D. Spectrum of impulse control behaviours in Parkinson's disease: pathophysiology and management. *J Neurol Neurosurg Psychiatry*. 2020;91:703–711.

Meehan M, Doody O. The role of the clinical nurse specialist multiple sclerosis, the patients' and families' and carers' perspective: an integrative review. *Mult Scler Relat Disord*. 2020;39:101918.

Mortimer DS, Berg W. Agitation in patients recovering from traumatic brain injury: nursing management. *J Neurosci Nurs*. 2017;49(1):25–30.

National Clinical Guideline for Stroke for the UK and Ireland. London: Intercollegiate Stroke Working Party. 2023. http://www.strokeguideline.org.

NHS Education for Scotland. Stroke: core competencies for healthcare staff; 2018. http://www.strokecorecompetencies.org/node.asp?id=home.

Price AM, Collins TJ, Gallacher A. Nursing care of the acute head injury: a review of the evidence. *Nurs Crit Care*. 2003;8(3):126–133.

Sarhan F, Sarhan K. The needs of family and friends as caregivers of individuals with a spinal cord injury. *Br J Neurosci Nurs*. 2023;19(1):25–30.

Stephen LJ, Harden C, Tomson T, Brodie MJ. Management of epilepsy in women. *Lancet Neurol*. 2019;18(5):481–491.

Tortora G, Derrickson B. *Principles of Anatomy and Physiology*. Global edition Hoboken, NJ: Wiley; 2017.

Waterhouse C. Development of a tool for risk assessment to facilitate safety and appropriate restraint. *Br J Neurosci Nurs*. 2007;3(9):421–426.

Woodward S, Mestecky AM. *Neuroscience Nursing – Evidence Based Practice*. Oxford: Wiley–Blackwell; 2011.

Yang J, Wang K, Chiang Y, et al. Effects of head elevation on cerebral blood flow velocity in post-cerebral operation patients. *J Nurs Res*. 2003;11(2):129–136.

Useful Websites

British Association of Neuroscience Nurses, www.bann.org.uk
Encephalitis Society, www.encephalitis.info
Epilepsy Action, www.epilepsy.org.uk
Headway – the Brain Injury Association, www.headway.org.uk
Huntington's Disease Association, www.hda.org.uk
Meningitis Trust, www.meningitis-trust.org
MS Trust, www.mstrust.org.uk
Multiple Sclerosis Society, www.mssociety.org.uk
National Neuroscience Benchmarking Group, www.nnbg.org.uk
National Society for Epilepsy, www.epilepsynse.org.uk
Stroke Specific Education Framework
(https://stroke-education.org.uk/)
Parkinson's UK, www.parkinsons.org.uk
Scottish Huntington's Association, www.hdscotland.org
Stroke Association, www.stroke.org.uk

12

Nursing Patients With Musculoskeletal Disorders

JULIE SANTY-TOMLINSON

CHAPTER OUTLINE

Introduction

A fully functioning musculoskeletal system is fundamental to optimal health and well-being. Injury or disease involving this system can have a profound effect on an individual's mobility and, therefore, their ability to perform activities of daily living and can result in temporary or permanent disability.

This chapter outlines the relevant anatomy and physiology and describes some of the more common disorders of the musculoskeletal system caused by trauma or disease along with the principles of nursing management and health promotion. The main causes of musculoskeletal trauma or disease in the UK include road traffic collisions (RTCs), industrial and other work-related accidents, sporting/leisure activity injuries and damage due to underlying disease such as osteoarthritis (OA) and osteoporosis. The overall aim of nursing care is to prevent further injury, reduce the risk of and recognise complications, promote healing and recovery, maximise independence and promote optimal rehabilitation.

Anatomy and Physiology of the Musculoskeletal System

This section provides a brief overview of the anatomy and physiology of the musculoskeletal system (see Further Reading, e.g. Marieb and Hoehn 2019).

The Skeletal System

The skeletal system consists of approximately 206 bones, each of which articulates with another at joints.

The main functions of the skeleton are:
- a support framework
- protection for internal organs
- movement – bones and muscles act as levers to produce movement at the joints
- mineral storage – particularly calcium and phosphorus
- blood cell formation – red bone marrow produces red and white blood cells (WBCs) and platelets.

Structurally, the skeletal system comprises two types of connective tissue: bone and cartilage.

Bone

Bone contains large amounts of calcium which provides its structure and strength. There are two types of bone tissue: compact and cancellous.

The hard, outer layer of a bone consists of compact (or cortical) bone, while cancellous bone fills the inside. Cancellous bone tissue is spongier and more open in appearance and its larger spaces contain highly vascular red bone marrow and fatty yellow bone marrow. The thickness of each type of tissue varies depending on the type and function of the bone. In long bones, such as the femur, the shaft (diaphysis) is enclosed by a thick layer of cortical bone, providing strength for weight-bearing. At each end (epiphysis), the cortical bone is thinner and encloses a greater mass of cancellous tissue which is lighter. Bone tissue is constantly being renewed and replaced due to the actions of three types of bone cell: osteoblasts, osteocytes and osteoclasts. Osteoblasts are involved in bone production, osteoclasts in bone resorption and osteocytes maintain bone tissue structure.

Cartilage

Another form of connective tissue; cartilage is tough, flexible, avascular and devoid of nerve fibres. It provides flexibility to the musculoskeletal system.

There are three types of cartilage:
- Hyaline cartilage – firm and pliable, the articular cartilage that covers the surfaces of synovial joints.
- Fibrocartilage – strong, compressible and tension-resistant; found in areas such as the intervertebral discs.
- Elastic cartilage – contains more elastin fibres so has greater ability to stretch while retaining its strength; found in the external ear and the epiglottis.

The Axial Skeletal System

The skull, vertebral (spinal) column and the sternum/ribcage form the central axis of the skeletal system to which the rest of the skeleton is attached. The spinal column is a strong, flexible pillar of 33/34 bones, 24 of which are 'true' vertebrae; 7 cervical (C1–7), 12 thoracic (T1–12) and 5 lumbar (L1–5) vertebrae – the remainder being 9/10 fused bones that form the sacrum (S1–10) and coccyx (Fig. 12.1). Between each of the vertebrae from C2 to S1 are spaces, each filled with fibrocartilaginous intervertebral discs that provide flexibility for the spine and act as shock absorbers when the spine is subjected to vertical forces.

The vertebral (spinal) column protects the spinal cord, supports the skull and acts as a point of attachment for the ribs and the muscles, tendons and ligaments of the back.

The Appendicular Skeletal System

The bones of the upper and lower limbs and their girdles (the upper, pectoral, girdle and the lower, pelvic, girdle) form the appendicular skeletal system. They are characterised by the presence of synovial

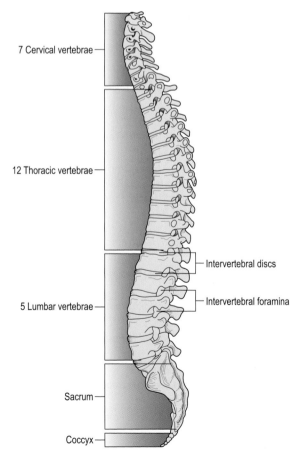

Figure 12.1 The vertebral (spinal) column – lateral view.

7 Cervical vertebrae

12 Thoracic vertebrae

Intervertebral discs

Intervertebral foramina

5 Lumbar vertebrae

Sacrum

Coccyx

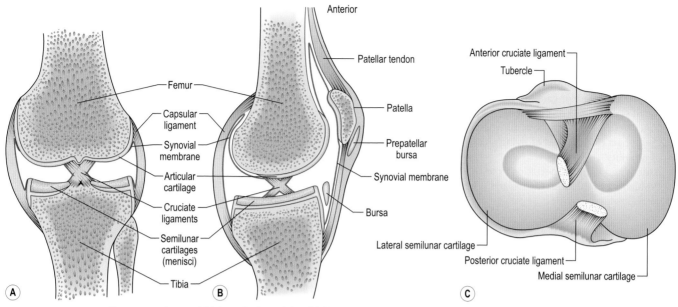

Figure 12.2 A synovial joint – the knee joint. (A) Section viewed from front. (B) Section viewed from side. (C) Superior surface of the tibia showing the semilunar cartilages and cruciate ligaments.

joints which connect the articular surfaces of adjoining bones (Fig. 12.2). The bone ends that make up the joint are held within a fibrous capsule consisting of two layers:

- an outer layer of dense connective tissue that allows movement but resists dislocation,
- an inner layer lined with synovial membrane that secretes synovial fluid, providing nourishment and lubrication.

The articular surfaces of the bones are covered in hyaline (articular) cartilage.

Ligaments

Ligaments attach bone to bone and maintain joint stability. They are made of dense connective tissue and have a poor blood supply. A joint may have many ligaments. The knee, for example, has cruciate ligaments to prevent the femur and tibia moving forwards on each other and medial and lateral collateral ligaments to prevent side-to-side movement (see Fig. 12.2). Damage to ligaments can result in an unstable and painful joint, common in sports injuries.

The Muscular System

Skeletal muscle (voluntary, or striated, muscle) provides the power for movement. Skeletal muscle tissue is composed of long, cylindrical multinucleated muscle cells. Each muscle is comprised of muscle fibres and connective tissue. A good blood and nerve supply are essential for muscle function.

Tendons

Tendons attach muscle to bone and allow movement to take place at joints. They also have poor blood supply. Damage to tendons can, therefore, be as serious as bony injury and significantly affect movement and mobility.

❖ Nursing Management and Health Promotion: Nursing Assessment

Effective nursing management necessitates holistic assessment of the patient, as musculoskeletal disorders can have profound physical, psychological and social effects. Visual inspection,

palpation, measurement and other investigations such as radiological (X-ray) and other imaging studies (Information 12.1) and blood tests (in rheumatoid arthritis (RA), for example) may also be necessary.

INFORMATION 12.1

Investigations for Musculoskeletal Abnormalities

Radiological and Imaging Studies

- Radiograph (X-ray) – to detect abnormal position, fractures, arthritis and presence of fluid or abnormalities in joint capsules.
- CT scan – makes use of the fact that different tissues have varying radiodensities. A series of radiographs are made at different angles and planes and the computer integrates the information to produce pictorial slices (sometimes 3D) which can be used to detect soft tissue injuries or tumours and inflammatory or metastatic skeletal disease or fracture.
- MRI – magnetic fields are used to show the difference in hydrogen density of various muscle and soft tissues, indicating the presence of abnormalities especially of the back and knee.
- DEXA scan – scan for bone density, e.g. to detect osteoporosis.

Joint Examination

- Arthroscopy – endoscopic visualisation of structures inside a joint undertaken under general or spinal anaesthetic. May also involve withdrawal of synovial fluid for analysis, and treatments such as washout of the joint to remove debris or the trimming of any damaged structures, e.g. the menisci in the knee joint.

Muscle and Nerve Studies

- Electromyography (EMG) – measures electrical potential of muscle during rest and activity.
- Nerve conduction velocities (NCVs) – measure speed of nerve impulse conduction.

Other Tests

- These include bone biopsy, total body calcium and various blood tests (biochemical haematological studies) that include full blood count (FBC), erythrocyte sedimentation rate (ESR), rheumatoid factor, C-reactive protein (CRP), hormone and mineral levels, blood culture, etc.

The nurse should assess the patient's:

- perception of the primary problem
- knowledge and understanding of their condition
- description of pain and other symptoms
- abnormal position or appearance of limbs or affected area, with loss of function (compare with contralateral side)
- abnormal posture or gait
- use of walking aids or prostheses
- concurrent health problems, allergies and medications
- the impact on activities of living (ALs), especially impairment of mobility
- patient and family expectations and coping strategies.

Problems and solutions (actual and potential) will be identified in the following categories:

- life-threatening problems such as shock and other emergency health threats
- pain
- impaired mobility
- knowledge deficit
- potential for further injury/complications – physical safety and neurovascular complications, especially; compartment syndrome (CS), venous thromboembolism (VTE) and fat embolus (see later)
- psychosocial consequences
- patient and family strengths and coping strategies – identified and supported constructively
- rehabilitation.

Nursing Interventions

These will include:

- Treating life-threatening problems – ABC of resuscitation (see Chapter 2, Nursing Patients With Cardiovascular Disorders, and Chapter 26, Nursing the Patient Who Experiences Trauma) to ensure early recognition, and treatment, of shock (see Chapter 19, Recognising and Managing Shock) and other emergencies
- Managing pain
- Maintaining a balance between rest/restricted movement and mobility/activity
- Constantly monitoring and reducing the risk of neurovascular complications such as CS and VTE
- Maintaining a safe environment
- Exploring patient and family understanding of the condition and provide support and education based on individual needs
- Coordinating multidisciplinary intervention for psychosocial problems
- Facilitating rehabilitation

❖ Nursing Management and Health Promotion: Core Potential Complications

The three potentially life- and/or limb-threatening complications – acute limb compartment syndrome (ALCS), VTE and fat embolus – can occur following musculoskeletal injuries or after orthopaedic surgery. They are vital considerations when caring for patients with any acute musculoskeletal injury/condition or following orthopaedic surgery.

Acute Limb Compartment Syndrome (ALCS)

Compartments are areas where muscles, nerves and blood vessels are enclosed within inelastic structures composed of skin, fascia and/or bone. ALCS occurs when there is increased tissue pressure (usually due to increased contents of the compartment due to swelling or bleeding) within the compartment leading to compromised circulation and function of associated tissues (Cone and Inaba 2017). Within 6–8 hours of onset, this will result in tissue death (necrosis) and permanent loss of function. Increased pressure can also result from the application of a cast or other immobilisation aid which becomes too tight. Examination of the limb for colour, warmth, sensation and movement (CWSM) in the foot or hand distal to the injury, surgery site or constricting device such as a cast is an essential element of care for any patient following limb injury or surgery.

The most important signs of ALCS are:

- pain – increasing or out of proportion to the injury and despite analgesia.

Late signs might also include:

- paraesthesia – altered sensation such as 'pins and needles' or numbness
- paralysis
- pallor (it is important to remember that darker skin tones make skin colour more difficult to assess)
- pulselessness (a very late sign).

To reduce the risk of ALCS developing, the affected limb should be elevated (unless ALCS is suspected to have occurred, when elevation can exacerbate the condition and should be avoided). ALCS is an emergency and patients require surgery immediately. A fasciotomy is performed: the inelastic tissue surrounding the compartment is cut and left open to release the pressure (Cone and Inaba 2017).

Venous Thromboembolism (VTE)

VTE is the collective name for two related conditions: deep vein thrombosis (DVT) which can lead to pulmonary embolism (PE). DVT can occur due to:

- venous stasis (e.g. due to reduced mobility after musculoskeletal trauma or surgery)
- damage to veins due to trauma
- hypercoagulability of the blood after injury.

It is usually a combination of these factors that causes a DVT – a clot in a deep vein, most commonly of the lower leg. Signs and symptoms may include pain/tenderness in the limb, calf pain when the foot is dorsiflexed, redness, heat, swelling and hardness of the affected areas. There may, however, be no physical signs. Nursing management and health promotion include educating patients about the signs and symptoms so that they can inform staff if they occur and the use of preventative measures to reduce the risk (see Chapter 25, Nursing the Patient Undergoing Surgery). These measures may be pharmacological (e.g. low-molecular-weight heparin injections) or nonpharmacological such as properly fitted antiembolism stockings, foot impulse device and early mobilisation (Santy-Tomlinson et al. 2022).

A DVT can dislodge and travel through the heart to the pulmonary circulation, resulting in a PE. This is an emergency as it can lead to respiratory arrest and death. The clinical presentation depends on severity, but nurses should watch carefully for sudden sharp chest pain, tachycardia, dyspnoea, cough, cyanosis, fainting, sometimes haemoptysis and restlessness/confusion in previously orientated patients. There will also be characteristic electrocardiogram changes. (For more about VTE see Further Reading, National Institute for Health and Care Excellence (NICE) 2020).

Fat Embolus

Fat emboli can occur following fracture of any long bone or after orthopaedic surgery where a long bone is incised, such as in a joint replacement. There are two theories relating to the cause: (1) fat cells from damaged tissue migrate into ruptured veins; (2) catecholamines are released in response to the physiological stress of trauma, and lipids are mobilised from fatty tissue. In the lung, these droplets are converted into free fatty acids which are toxic to lung tissue and disrupt alveolar function. The droplets may also become enmeshed in the capillary network of the alveoli and disrupt gas exchange. This can lead to cerebral hypoxia and, if large vessels in the pulmonary system are involved, to respiratory failure and death. Early signs of fat emboli are increased respiratory rate, anxiety, confusion and transient petechial haemorrhage (broken tiny capillary blood vessels) on the head, neck and face.

The nurse must be alert for early signs of altered mental status: anxiety, irritability and, especially, confusion. This should be reported to senior medical staff immediately, preparations made to deal with respiratory failure and arrest and to transfer the patient to intensive care. Equipment should be ready for immediate blood gas analysis.

SKELETAL DISORDERS

This section of the chapter outlines a range of common skeletal injuries and conditions, including fractures, spinal injury, osteoporosis, tumours and infections.

Fractures

A fracture or 'broken bone' is a break in the continuity of a bone due to direct or indirect trauma, underlying disease (pathological fracture) or repeated stress on a bone (stress fracture) (Craig et al. 2023a). 'Closed' fractures occur when there is no communication between the external environment and the fracture site, and 'open' when communication occurs through a wound or blister. 'Stable' fractures occur where the bone ends are lying in a position from which they are unlikely to move. In 'unstable' fractures the bone ends are displaced or have the potential to be displaced. The edges of fractured bones may damage soft tissues or blood vessels/nerves at the time of the injury or later through poor handling of the limb.

🔵 Medical/Surgical Management

All fractures, regardless of their position or the bone involved, are managed according to three principles: reduction, maintenance of position and rehabilitation. The aim is to allow bone healing to take place. The stages of bone healing are explained in Fig. 12.3.

Reduction of Fractures
Reduction of fractures involves pulling displaced bone fragments back into their normal anatomical position. In many cases, a general anaesthetic will be necessary to overcome the protective muscle spasm and severe pain caused by the procedure.

Maintenance of Position
The fracture needs to be held in the correct position until bone healing takes place, which can take from 6 to 12 weeks, depending on the fracture site and age and health of the patient. Position can be maintained by external splintage using an orthosis – a

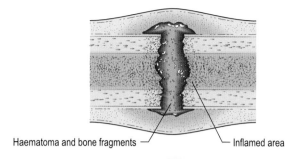

Haematoma and bone fragments ———   ——— Inflamed area

Phagocytosis of clot and debris.
Growth of granulation tissue begins

Osteoblasts begin to form new bone

Gradual spread of new bone to bridge gap

Bone healed. Osteoclasts reshape bone

Figure 12.3 Stages in bone healing.

removable splint, plaster of Paris (POP) or synthetic (resin/plastic based) cast, skin or skeletal traction or an external fixator frame. Surgical reduction of the fracture with internal fixation using metal pins, plates, screws or nails may also be used to hold the bone fragments in position. When the blood supply is significantly disrupted by the fracture, it may be necessary to implant a prosthesis to replace the affected bone, as in some cases of hip fracture. Without adequate maintenance of position and the optimum conditions for healing, the fracture may heal with the bone ends not properly aligned (malunion), may take longer to heal (delayed union) or may not unite at all (nonunion).

Restoration of Function

Joints and muscles close to the fracture can become stiff and weak and exercise and physiotherapy are essential.

Patients require varying degrees of rehabilitation, involving a multidisciplinary team approach (see Chapter 30, Care and Rehabilitation of People With Long-term Conditions). Even when the physical damage is slight, the psychosocial impact may be considerable and this needs to be considered in nursing care.

Traction

Orthopaedic traction involves applying a pulling force to a part or parts of the body, including counter-traction, a pulling force in the opposite direction (Duperouzel et al. 2018). Counter-traction is usually supplied by the body weight of the patient. Traction is used to:

- reduce and immobilise fractures/dislocations
- maintain normal alignment of injured tissues
- prevent and correct deformity
- reduce muscle spasm
- relieve pain
- immobilise an injured or inflamed joint
- keep joint surfaces apart.

Traction is less used than in the past as alternative methods such as internal fixation enable patients to become mobile more quickly and, therefore, avoid the problems of immobility. However, it still has a place in treatment and nurses must know the principles of its use.

Types of Traction

Balanced or Sliding Traction. This relies on the patient's own body weight to produce the necessary counter-traction, usually by tilting of the bed. Skeletal pins may be used to provide a firm point of attachment (Fig. 12.4), but the most common type of balanced traction uses skin traction; Buck's traction (Fig. 12.5) is sometimes used as a temporary measure for pain relief in patients awaiting surgical fixation of a fracture of the lower limb.

Fixed Traction. This is the application of counter-traction acting through an appliance which obtains purchase on a part of the body (Fig. 12.6). The most common is a Thomas' splint, usually used for immobilising a fractured shaft of femur while definitive surgical management is planned or for transferring a patient, for example between hospitals. It is most used in the treatment of fractures of the shaft of femur in children (Gray and Santy-Tomlinson 2018).

❖ Nursing Management and Health Promotion: Traction

In addition to the general principles outlined earlier for management of musculoskeletal disorders, the following are specific to the care of a patient in traction:

Health Promotion

Patients need to understand the reasons for their traction and how to position themselves and move safely within the bed. They also need to understand the risk of complications and their own role in prevention.

Management of Equipment

All parts of splints, frames, pulleys, ropes and slings should be inspected at least every day to ensure they are correctly positioned

Figure 12.4 Skeletal traction may be applied by (A) a Kirschner wire and traction stirrup; (B) a Steinmann pin and traction stirrup; or (C) a Steinmann pin and Böhler stirrup.

and in good working order; this is especially important when the patient has been moved, for example after using a bedpan.

Reducing the Risk of Complications

- Observation of CWSM of the injured limb is essential throughout the patient's stay in hospital for early detection of neurovascular problems.
- Potential skin breakdown in vulnerable areas such as the sacrum and under splints should be monitored and appropriate skin care provided.

Figure 12.5 Buck's traction sometimes used as a temporary measure for pain relief for patients awaiting surgical fixation of a lower limb fracture or hip fractures.

Figure 12.6 (A) Fixed traction using skin traction and Thomas' splint. (B) Fixed traction using skeletal pin and Thomas' splint.

- Observation for dropped-foot caused by excessive pressure on the common peroneal nerve at the head of the fibula.
- Work with physiotherapists to ensure that patients are aware of the importance of deep breathing exercises and exercise of limbs to prevent chest infection, DVT, joint stiffness and muscle wasting.

Care of Skeletal Pin Sites

Skeletal traction and external fixation involve the insertion of pins or wires through soft tissue into/through bone. This creates a percutaneous wound that can be in place for several weeks with a subsequent risk of site infection (Santy-Tomlinson et al. 2011). There is little reliable and valid evidence confirming which pin site care regimen best reduces infection rates but there are best practice guidelines based on the available literature and expert opinion (Timms and Pugh 2012). These indicate that:

- Once-weekly pin site care is enough if no exudate is present; wound care should be conducted after a shower (but bathing should not be allowed), drying of the fixator and skin with a freshly laundered towel.
- Pin sites should be gently cleaned using nonshedding gauze and chlorhexidine and alcohol solution unless the patient's skin is sensitive to alcohol/chlorhexidine (in which case 0.9% saline should be used).
- Pin site crusts and scabs should be left in place, although some crusts/scabs will be removed during the gentle cleansing process.
- Pin sites should always be kept covered with a nonshedding key-hole dressing secured with nonallergenic tape.
- Gentle compression of each pin site should be applied using a clip or bung.
- The patient should be taught to conduct their own pin site care and to observe for signs of infection.
- Severe pain around the wound, increased discharge, purulent discharge and/or redness (redness is more difficult to assess in darker toned skin) suggest infection and appropriate antibiotics should be commenced and the earlier cleaning regime conducted daily if discharge is evident on the dressing.

Fundamental Aspects of Care

Patients with traction have limited mobility and may be on bed rest for several weeks. Fundamental nursing care should include:

- maintaining adequate fluid and dietary intake to facilitate healing and prevent constipation and urinary tract infection
- maintaining patient dignity when meeting hygiene and toileting needs
- helping patients to maintain contact with partners, family and friends, providing privacy
- helping patients to find ways of alleviating the boredom of prolonged bed rest (Reflection 12.1).

Casts

A cast is a splinting device comprising layers of bandages impregnated with POP, fibreglass or resin, some of which are applied wet and solidify as they dry out. These are used to immobilise the limb and hold bone fragments in place while healing takes place. POP moulds more easily but it takes 48 hours to dry, and it is heavy. Synthetic casts set within 20 minutes and allow early weight-bearing but do not accommodate swelling and are not usually used in the initial stages of treatment, when a POP 'back-slab' is usually used. Other types of casts include adjustable focused rigidity primary casts which can be adjusted as swelling reduces (Large 2001) and cast braces, which have hinges at the joints to allow restricted amounts of bending of a joint to facilitate mobilisation.

Dealing With Boredom

Ahmed may be on bed rest for many weeks while on traction. He is worried about the long period of immobility and not being able to attend his university course or continue with his active social life.

Activity

- Think about times when you were bored and reflect on having to be on traction for several weeks.
- Discuss with your practice supervisor/assessor ways in which you can help Ahmed to relieve the boredom.
- Which other health professionals and other people could you call upon to help in this respect?

Figure 12.7 An example of external fixation – Ilizarov frame. (Courtesy of Barts and the London NHS Trust.)

INFORMATION 12.2

Advice to a Patient With a Hand-to-Elbow Plaster Cast

The plaster cast holds all the broken bones firmly in place to allow them to heal in the correct position.

To prevent your fingers swelling, support your arm in the sling provided during the day and on pillows at night.

It is important that you exercise the finger, elbow and shoulder joints of your injured arm at regular intervals, otherwise they will become stiff and painful to move.

The following exercises should be carried out at least four times each day:

- Make a firm fist then stretch the fingers as wide as possible.
- Try to touch each fingertip with the thumb of that hand.
- Bend and stretch the elbow joint.
- Lift your arm high above your head – use the other arm to help.
- Move your arm behind your back as if you wanted to scratch between your shoulder blades.

Do not wet, heat or otherwise interfere with the plaster and do not insert objects between the plaster and the skin to scratch – this could cause skin damage and infection.

Report to a doctor or emergency department AT ONCE if:

- The plaster cracks, becomes loose or uncomfortable.
- There is pain.
- The fingers become numb or difficult to move.
- The fingers become more swollen, blue or very pale.
- There is discharge of fluid into the cast or from it.
- You have any other problems.

❖ Nursing Management and Health Promotion: Casts

In addition to the general principles of nursing management for musculoskeletal disorders, the following also apply:

Care of Casts

POP casts should be handled carefully while drying, using the palms of the hands rather than the fingers to prevent indentations which may cause pressure points inside the cast. Patients should understand that a cast must not get wet; synthetic protective covers can be used to allow them to take a shower. Patients should be taught how to protect the cast when washing and using bedpans and urinals.

Many patients will go home wearing casts and need clear verbal and written instructions specific to their cast (Information 12.2 outlines advice for a patient with a hand to elbow cast).

Potential for Neurovascular Impairment

Swelling within the cast or a cast that is too tight may lead to neurovascular impairment and/or CS. CWSM observations should be carried out for early identification of problems. If CS or neurovascular impairment is suspected, the cast needs to be split or bivalved down to the skin. If a local pressure injury develops beneath a cast, usually identifiable by specifically located pain, an inspection window can be cut, and the injury dressed before the window is taped or bandaged back into place.

Removal of Casts

Removal of a cast is a skilled activity and should only be carried out by staff who have been trained and assessed as competent in this role. Plaster shears can be used for POP casts or an electric oscillating saw for POP and/or synthetic casts.

External Fixation

Bone fragments are held in position by skeletal pins or wires inserted into or through the bone on either side of the fracture and held in alignment by a metal frame (Fig. 12.7). They are used for the treatment of open fractures and closed fractures with extensive soft tissue damage until the soft tissue has healed, for fractures that have not united by other methods and following reconstructive surgery or limb lengthening. Depending on the reason for their use, they can be in place for a few weeks or up to 1 year, for example in nonunion of a tibial fracture.

❖ Nursing Management and Health Promotion: External Fixation

The general principles relating to potential neurovascular impairment, positioning and potential for pin site infection that have already been discussed are important in the care of patients with an external fixator. In addition, it is important that the patient, carers, and community staff are confident in caring for the fixator when the patient is discharged from hospital, including managing psychosocial issues including altered body image (Newton-Triggs et al. 2022). Care of skeletal pin sites is discussed in the nursing management and health promotion: traction section.

Internal Fixation

Fractures may also be stabilised by surgical intervention where nails, plates, wires, screws or rods are inserted to hold the bone fragments in place (Fig. 12.8). This permits earlier mobilisation and reduces the potential for complications. The general principles of nursing management and health promotion of musculoskeletal disorders including core potential complications (nursing management and health promotion: core potential complications section) and the perioperative principles of nursing management are all relevant (see Chapter 25, Nursing the Patient Undergoing Surgery).

Fragility Fractures

Fragility fractures are those which occur in bone that is weakened by osteoporosis, a common preventable condition in which bone mineral density (BMD) is depleted due to the ageing processes. Fragility fractures most commonly occur in older people following a fall or other relatively minor trauma event. Most fragility fractures occur in the spine, humerus, wrist and hip. Fractures of the hip, however, are the most severe fractures because hospitalisation is always necessary, and rates of complications (morbidity) and death (mortality) are very high.

Hip Fractures

Over 75,000 hip fractures occur each year in the UK alone (NHFD 2022). Global incidence continues to rise, especially in developing countries where populations are ageing at the greatest rate. There is increasing evidence that a coordinated approach to care of this patient group, known as orthogeriatric care (Marsh et al. 2021), can significantly improve their outcomes and quality of care (Evidence-Based Practice 12.1, Reflection 12.2, Table 12.1).

🔴 Surgical Management

History and Examination

The patient will be admitted to the emergency department (ED) complaining of pain in the hip or knee and there may be visible shortening and external rotation of the affected leg. Diagnosis will be confirmed by X-ray. A history of the fall is important as it may identify underlying conditions such as hypotension and indicate how long the patient may have been lying on the floor before receiving help.

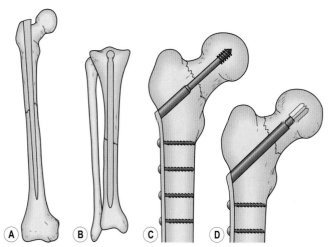

Figure 12.8 Types of internal fixation. (A, B) Intramedullary nails. (C) Compression nail for fixation of femoral neck. (D) Sliding nail fixation of the femoral neck.

TABLE 12.1	Extract From the Integrated Care Pathway of a Patient Following Surgery for a Hip Fracture – Postoperative Day 1 (Nursing Part Only)	
Patient Problem/Need	Nursing Intervention	Expected Outcome
Recovery from anaesthetic	At least 4-hourly monitoring of vital signs	Vital signs within patient's normal limits
Wound care	Check wound site dressing Check and record wound drainage	Dressing dry and intact Drain to be removed at 24 hours after surgery as further drainage minimal
Neurovascular status of limb	Monitor neurovascular status of affected limb	No neurovascular deficit
Pain management	Assess pain using pain score at least 4-hourly Administer and evaluate effect of analgesics as prescribed	Pain relief at level acceptable to patient
Risk of deep vein thrombosis (DVT)	Ensure antiembolism stocking in situ and remove at least daily to care for and check skin/circulation Administer thromboprophylaxis medication as prescribed Monitor for signs of DVT	Reduction in risk and early detection of problem
Reduced mobility	Begin to remobilise as soon as possible – preferably postoperative day 1 Ensure patient understands correct way to transfer and mobilise	Patient to sit in chair Patient to walk to end of bed with aid of Zimmer frame
Nutrition and hydration	Maintain IV fluids as prescribed until drinking normally Monitor fluid intake and output Support return to normal eating and drinking as soon as possible Support calorie and protein intake with dietary supplements	High-protein, high-calorie diet and adequate fluid intake to support recovery and healing
Risk of postoperative delirium	Observe closely for signs of unusual behaviour, confusion or excessive drowsiness Orientation (to time/place) Early mobilisation (maintaining function/normal routine) Involve family	Avoidance of or early resolution of delirium

From Murphy C, Mullen E, Hogan K, O'Toole R, Teeling S. Streamlining an existing hip fracture patient pathway in an acute tertiary adult Irish hospital to improve patient experience and outcomes. *Int J Qual Health Care*. 2019;31(Suppl 1):45-51; Tarling M, Aitken E, Lahoti O, et al. Closing the audit loop: the role of a pilot in the development of a fractured neck of femur integrated care pathway. *J Orthop Nurs*. 2002;6(3):130–134.

Treatment

Treatment is almost always surgical to enable the patient to remobilise as soon as possible. Depending on the site of the fracture, surgery will either involve internal fixation with plates and/or screws or replacement of the head of femur with a metal prosthesis if the fracture is within the joint capsule and there is a risk of damage to the blood supply of the femoral head (Fig. 12.9). The underlying osteoporosis and reason for the fall need to be managed (van Oostwaard 2018).

❖ Nursing Management and Health Promotion: Hip Fracture

Sustaining a hip fracture is very frightening and patients need highly skilled, age-sensitive nursing care. In addition to the general principles relating to musculoskeletal injury and fractures, the following priorities need to be addressed.

Potential Complications

Most patients are elderly, and many are frail due to comorbidities and declining physical and cognitive function. Consequently, complication rates are high, including delirium, dehydration, malnutrition, respiratory tract infection, urinary tract infection, pressure injuries and wound infection. Assessment of the patient for risk and evidence of these complications must lead to prompt prevention and management and measures taken to reverse any hypothermia and/or dehydration (see Chapter 25, Nursing the

Figure 12.9 Blood supply of the femoral head via the capsule, intramedullary vessels and ligamentum teres.

Patient Undergoing Surgery, and Chapter 33, Nursing Older Patients).

Pain

Hip fracture and subsequent surgery cause severe pain. Without effective pain assessment and age-sensitive pain management (see Chapter 20, Pain Management) early mobilisation, prevention of complications and rehabilitation are impossible, and outcomes are much poorer. The use of femoral nerve blocks is increasingly common in this patient group (Myhre Jensen et al. 2018).

Rehabilitation

Expert multidisciplinary orthogeriatric care of the patient from injury to beyond discharge is the most effective way to ensure good patient outcomes (Falaschi and Marsh 2021). This includes:

- the involvement of a geriatrician in the daily care of the patient so that frailty and comorbidities can be effectively managed
- expert nursing care provided by those with skills in the care of older people as well as the trauma patient
- management of osteoporosis and prevention of further falls
- a multidisciplinary rehabilitation and discharge programme involving the patient and their family.

For further reading see Hertz and Santy-Tomlinson (2023) and Santy-Tomlinson and Hertz (2023).

Fractures of Specific Sites – Lower Limb

Any of the bones in all limbs are commonly fractured due to trauma, and the principles of reduction, maintenance of position and restoration of function apply to all. The specific treatment and associated nursing care and health promotion depend on the exact nature and position of the fracture and the health status of the patient. Fractures of the tibia and fibula are one of the most common in the lower limb and are discussed here in more detail.

Fracture of the Tibia and Fibula

Fracture of the tibia and fibula a common injury, usually occurring due to from direct trauma following road traffic trauma and sports injuries. There is frequently extensive skin and soft tissue damage and fractures heal slowly due to the less effective circulation to the lower leg.

 Management

Treatment

There are three choices of treatment.

- *Cast immobilisation* – for closed, stable injuries and the patient may remain in a cast for 12–16 weeks.
- *Internal fixation* – closed but unstable fractures are usually internally fixed with a nail; routine postoperative care will be required (see Chapter 25, Nursing the Patient Undergoing Surgery), with a focus on limb observation and elevation. The patient will be able to mobilise using crutches once fully recovered from the effects of surgery. Information about the correct use of crutches/sticks is provided on the companion website.
- *External fixation* – if there is skin loss or a contaminated wound at the fracture site, an external fixator may be applied under a general anaesthesia; the patient will often begin to mobilise partially weight bearing, depending on the stability of the fixation, as this enhances bone healing (Reflection 12.3).

REFLECTION 12.3

External Fixation: Ken

Ken is a 40-year-old man who lives alone. He sustained an open (compound) fracture to his left tibia and fibula while skiing with friends.

Confirmation of the diagnosis was made by radiography and it was decided to take Ken to the operating theatre for application of an external fixator to his left leg. This was explained to him and a picture of an external fixator in position was shown to him and the two friends who had accompanied him.

After an uneventful postoperative period, Ken was allowed to sit in an armchair on day 1 with his leg elevated on a stool to reduce the swelling. The wound had been dressed in theatre following the local wound dressing policy of the hospital. The physiotherapist gradually assisted Ken to walk with the help of crutches and showed him how to manage the awkward appliance to avoid injuring himself. He was helped to widen two pairs of trousers below the knee so that he could cover the external fixator.

Ken was discharged home 6 days after his accident with a return appointment for 2 weeks later.

Activity

- Reflect on the discharge needs of Ken. Discuss with your practice supervisor/assessor how these can be managed.

 Nursing Management and Health Promotion: Fractures of the Tibia and Fibula

The principles of nursing management for each type of treatment: casts, internal fixation and external fixation, have been discussed in this chapter.

Fractures of Specific Sites – Upper Limb

As with the lower limb, there are many different fractures of the upper limb. The two commonest are those of the distal humerus (the upper arm) and a Colles' fracture (the wrist), both of which commonly occur due to a fall on an outstretched hand in older adults with osteoporosis, so are often fragility fractures.

Fracture of the Distal Humerus

 Management

This injury is very painful and is associated with significant bruising but can usually be treated at home following the initial visit to the ED, providing there is no major displacement or neurovascular complications (when internal fixation will be required) and pain is well controlled. The arm is supported in a broad arm sling or collar and cuff with the weight of the arm acting as a form of traction. Movement is gradually introduced, supported by outpatient physiotherapy, to prevent stiffness in the shoulder joint. Because of bone fragility, the fracture may heal slowly but, if it fails to heal, internal fixation may be required.

Nursing Management and Health Promotion: Fracture of the Neck of Humerus

As well as general principles of nursing management, including core potential complications, the following also apply.

Assessment of Function

An immobilised arm, especially if it is the dominant arm and the patient is elderly, can have a significant impact on function. Assessment of ability to carry out ALs and support available at home should be carried out before discharge from the ED. A home care package should be put in place (Reflections 12.4 and 12.5).

Skin Care of Injured Arm

It may be necessary to arrange for community nursing to attend to wash the injured arm two or three times a week, with particular

Figure 12.10 The 'dinner fork' deformity of Colles' fracture.

attention to care of the axilla to avoid skin breakdown. The sling should be checked and reapplied and neurovascular status and degree of mobility monitored.

Colles' Fracture

This is one of the most common injuries seen in the ED and involves the lower end of the radius within 2.5 cm of the wrist joint, with a classic 'dinner fork' deformity (see Fig. 12.10) and is often classified as a fragility fracture.

⚙ Management

Diagnosis is confirmed by examination and X-rays. The fracture usually requires reduction under local or general anaesthesia followed by application of a back-slab (a half POP cast) until any swelling has reduced and then a full below-elbow cast for 6 weeks. Internal or external fixation may be necessary if this is unsuccessful.

❖ Nursing Management and Health Promotion: Colles' Fracture

As well as the management principles already discussed which relate to musculoskeletal trauma, fractures and casts, the following priorities should be considered.

Health Promotion

A Colles' fracture is often the first sign of osteoporosis (an 'index' fragility fracture) and patients should be investigated and treated for this with referral to a fracture liaison service if available. Advice should be given on how to prevent future falls and referral may be made to a falls clinic.

Removal of Rings

Severe swelling of the fingers occurs in any arm injury, but particularly of the wrist and hand, so it is important to immediately remove all rings and bracelets from the injured hand/wrist.

Prevention of Complications of Fractures – Summary

The prevention of some general complications of fractures, such as neurovascular compromise, malunion, infection, etc., is summarised in Table 12.2.

Spinal Injuries

Injury or damage to the vertebral (spinal) column which protects the spinal cord may be confined to bony and/or ligament injury or may be accompanied by damage to the cord itself. This spinal cord damage can happen at the time of injury or be the result of poor handling of the patient by healthcare professionals. It is

---

REFLECTION 12.4

Shoulder Immobilisation

Support for a humeral fracture, or other arm fractures, can be achieved by a broad arm sling, a high arm sling or a collar and cuff.

Activities

- Think about the appropriate choice of sling for patients and discuss these with your practice supervisor/assessor.
- After initial instruction from your tutor or practice supervisor/assessor, and with a fellow student, practice applying a broad arm sling, a high sling and a collar and cuff. Put the sling on your dominant arm and attempt to carry out an ordinary task, such as combing your hair or, cutting up food or going to the toilet.
- How difficult was it to undertake the task? Reflect on the potential difficulties for patients who may well be considerably older than yourself.

REFLECTION 12.5

Fracture of the Humerus: Mrs Ojo

Mrs Ojo is a 78-year-old lady living alone in sheltered housing. She was admitted to the emergency department following a fracture of the neck of humerus after a fall, which was treated with a sling. The supported discharge scheme Sister undertook a multidisciplinary assessment of Mrs Ojo, who was discharged home after a stay of 2 hours in the emergency department. The social worker from the supported discharge team arranged a suitable social care package to provide the support Mrs Ojo would require.

The supported discharge scheme staff nurse visited Mrs Ojo at home to wash and dry the skin around her injured shoulder (particularly the axilla), inspecting it for any signs of friction or pressure. Extensive bruising was noted over the shoulder region. The sling was reapplied. The nurse checked that she was moving her joints as advised and that no joint stiffness was present. It was established that no neurovascular deficit was present and Mrs Ojo was provided with information that would help her to identify any developing signs of tingling or numbness of the fingers, change in finger colour, sensation or warmth and/or reduced ability to move the arm.

The team's occupational therapist carried out an assessment and suggested changes to the environment, such as removing the bath mat on which Mrs Ojo had slipped and replacing it with a non-slip one. She attended the hospital outpatient department 10 days later where she was seen by an orthopaedic specialist. The supported discharge team completed their package of care at this point, but social services continued to provide social care, including help with hygiene needs.

Activity

- Think about the psychological needs Mrs Ojo might have after her fall and fracture, and how the primary care nursing staff might help her to meet these needs.

TABLE 12.2 **Prevention of Complications of Fractures**

Complication	Cause	Prevention
Damage to soft tissue – neurovascular compromise	Trauma Sharp fragments/edge of bone	Monitor neurovascular function regularly – report abnormalities
Complications associated with immobility: Diminished function of all body systems Muscle atrophy – decreased range of movement – contractures	Decreased physical stimulation Lack of normal exercise	Encourage active and passive exercise Coordinate physiotherapy programme
Altered psychological processes	Decreased social stimulation	Provide social and mental stimulation
Pressure injuries	Immobility Casts – prolonged pressure	Regular pressure area care and position change
Infection	Surgical site Open fracture wound Skeletal pin sites	Apply standard principles of infection prevention and control
Malunion	Mal-apposition of bony fragments Inadequate cast fit (e.g. when swelling subsides – cast becomes loose)	Meticulous and regular monitoring of cast fit and traction alignment
Delayed union	Unstable fracture Poor blood supply	Support adequate circulation, e.g. limb elevation Maintain splintage
Nonunion	Infection Soft tissue intrusion	Infection prevention and control
Fat embolus – emergency	Fat globules released into circulation from bone marrow at fracture site – usually associated with fractured femur or multiple fractures	Early reduction and splintage Ensure early diagnosis and treatment by reporting confusion, petechial haemorrhages, chest pain, dyspnoea immediately

estimated that there are more than 50,000 people in the UK living with spinal cord injury (Rodger 2022), although many more sustain vertebral fractures or ligament damage with no spinal cord damage. Common reasons for spinal cord injury are:
- RTCs
- falls, such as falling downstairs
- industrial injuries, e.g. building site falls
- sports injuries, e.g. rugby, skiing and diving.

🟦 Pathophysiology

The resultant damage can involve transection, compression, contusion or interference to the spinal cord, accompanied by varying degrees of paralysis and sensory deficit below the level of the damage (Fig. 12.11). Damage to the ligaments supporting the spinal column may result in a dangerously unstable spine.

🟦 Medical/Surgical Management

The three principles of management (Smith 2004) are:
- *Preserving existing neurological function* – involving correct moving and handling of the patient. Every patient with spinal trauma should be treated as having a potential spinal cord injury until investigations such as magnetic resonance imaging (MRI) provide a clear diagnosis. Vertebral fractures may be stabilised by surgery or with halo vest traction (Fig. 12.12) to facilitate early mobilisation in patients with intact neurological function. Some stable fractures, especially lower thoracic and lumbar fractures, can be treated by firm-base bed rest.
- *Physiological resuscitation* – attending to the potential life-threatening respiratory and cardiovascular effects of neurological damage, including:
  - ineffective airway clearance
  - ineffective breathing pattern
  - hypotension

- bradycardia
- hypothermia.

The last three are caused by spinal shock – the temporary cessation of conduction within the spinal cord neurones – resulting in loss of voluntary movement and sensation below the level of the injury and progressive loss of sympathetic and parasympathetic activity which can last for up to 6 weeks.
- *Prevention of secondary complications* – physical or psychological. Patients will usually be transferred to a spinal injuries unit (SIU), although transfer may not happen for a few days and patients may initially be treated in a general hospital.

✦ Nursing Management and Health Promotion: Spinal Injury

Basic Principles of Positioning and Movement

It is essential to maintain the anatomical alignment of the vertebral (spinal) column in patients with suspected, potential and actual spinal cord injury both before patients reach hospital and once they are admitted, to avoid scenarios such as that outlined in Reflection 12.6. Manoeuvres such as log rolling the patient (see Chapter 26, Nursing the Patient Who Experiences Trauma) (for thoracolumbar injuries), pelvic twists (for cervical injuries) and using special beds (e.g. an electric turning bed) are carried out under the guidance of an experienced practitioner (MASCIP 2009). The level of neurological functioning must be constantly monitored and recorded to detect any deterioration.

Respiratory and Cardiovascular Monitoring

Detecting deterioration in the functioning of these systems is an essential nursing responsibility. Depending on the level of injury patients may be mechanically ventilated. VTE is also a potential

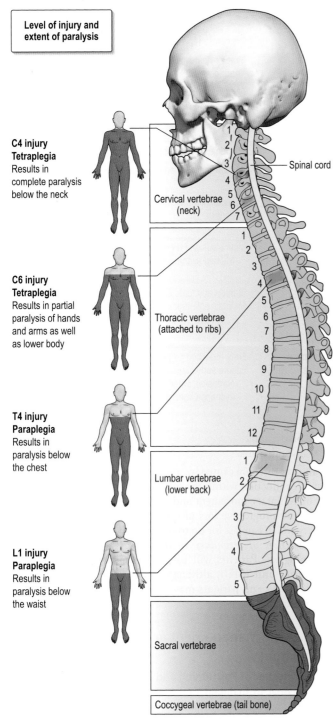

Level of injury and
extent of paralysis

C4 injury
Tetraplegia
Results in
complete paralysis
below the neck

C6 injury
Tetraplegia
Results in partial
paralysis of hands
and arms as well
as lower body

T4 injury
Paraplegia
Results in
paralysis below
the chest

L1 injury
Paraplegia
Results in
paralysis below
the waist

Spinal cord

Cervical vertebrae
(neck)

Thoracic vertebrae
(attached to ribs)

Lumbar vertebrae
(lower back)

Sacral vertebrae

Coccygeal vertebrae (tail bone)

Figure 12.11 Level of injury and extent of paralysis. (Reproduced from Harrison P. *Managing Spinal Injury: Critical Care*. London: Spinal Injuries Association; 2000, with permission from the Spinal Injuries Association and Claire MacDonald.)

complication and prophylaxis should be carried out according to local policy.

Additional Physical Care

Patients with a spinal cord injury have the potential to develop several additional physical problems, in particular paralytic ileus, gastric ulceration and pressure injuries. During the acute stage of spinal cord injury, the patient will have a flaccid bowel and

Figure 12.12 'Halo-vest' traction. A halo fixed to the skull – attached to bars mounted on the chest.

> **REFLECTION 12.6**
>
> **First Aid for Accident Victims: The Effect on Outcome**
>
> Two 18-year-old men were brought into the emergency department on the same night. They had both sustained multiple injuries to the head and body in similar RTCs – the first (Dan) had been moved from his overturned vehicle by well-meaning people at the scene of the accident whilst waiting for the ambulance to arrive, whereas the second (Jamie) was supported in the position in which he was found until the ambulance team arrived. The paramedics applied a neck collar and maintained skeletal alignment whilst transferring him to the ambulance and at all times subsequently. Spinal X-rays showed that the men had identical injuries to the cervical spine.
>
> Two months later, Jamie walked out of the SIU; many months later, Dan was wheeled out of the same unit with quadriplegia.
>
> **Activity**
>
> • Think about the two scenarios and discuss with your practice supervisor/assessor the main reasons for such different outcomes of the two accident victims.

bladder, and urinary catheterisation and manual evacuation of faeces will be undertaken by suitably qualified practitioners.

Psychological Care

Spinal cord injury is a life-changing event, not only for the patient but also for the family. Two most important interventions for nurses are to always be truthful, ensuring all staff are providing the same information, and to reduce the effects of sensory deprivation through the use of therapeutic touch and aids such as mirrors (Rodger 2022). Long-term support and adaptation will be necessary and organisations such as the Spinal Injuries Association are vital in this.

⊕ See Evolve website Critical thinking question 12.1

Osteoporosis

Osteoporosis is a chronic, systemic skeletal disorder characterised by low bone mass and microarchitectural deterioration of bone tissue, with a consequent increase in bone fragility and susceptibility to fracture (van Oostwaard 2018). It is estimated that 1 in 3 women and 1 in 12 men in the UK will develop clinically significant osteoporosis.

Pathophysiology

An overall reduction in BMD is caused by both uncontrollable and modifiable factors. Eighty per cent of BMD is determined by genetically derived risk factors such as race, gender and stature. The remaining 20% is influenced by nongenetic factors which can be modified to enhance BMD (van Oostwaard 2018). Patients become susceptible to fragility fractures, with the wrist (e.g. Colles' fracture), vertebrae and hip being the most common sites.

Management

Prevention is aimed at ensuring patients have as high a BMD as possible. Modifications to diet such as increased calcium and ensuring sufficient weight-bearing exercise are key to this. Peak BMD is reached by a person's early 30s, so such modifications should ideally be made before this, although there are benefits in all age groups.

Early identification is also key. Any low-impact or fragility fracture (one sustained by falling from standing height or less, especially a distal radial fracture) is suggestive of osteoporosis and merits further investigation and patient education. All patients over 50 with a fragility fracture should have their bone density measured (by dual-energy X-ray absorptiometry [DEXA] scan) and appropriate treatment initiated by their GP or local osteoporosis unit.

When osteoporosis is diagnosed, medication therapy is prescribed to inhibit bone resorption by osteoclasts to slow down the rate of bone loss. A group of drugs known as bisphosphonates are widely prescribed and are designed to bind calcium to bone; in the UK, alendronate, etidronate and risedronate are commonly prescribed. Vitamin D and calcium supplements are also prescribed, as vitamin D is required for the absorption of calcium, and calcium supplementation is vital in the prevention and treatment of postmenopausal osteoporosis (van Oostwaard 2018). There are known racial differences in the prevalence of osteoporosis with BMD and access to osteoporosis treatment services being lower in some ethnic minority groups (Noel et al. 2021) requiring health services to ensure such individuals are supported in accessing osteoporosis prevention and management.

● See Evolve website Critical thinking question 12.2

Hormone replacement therapy (HRT) is often used to control hormonal symptoms but has also been shown to prevent osteoporosis. However, questions about the long-term safety of HRT remain, especially regarding increased risk of breast, ovarian and endometrial cancer, coronary heart disease, VTE and stroke.

❖ Nursing Management and Health Promotion: Osteoporosis

Prevention

Nurses play a key role in educating the population about the importance of diet and exercise in the prevention of bone fragility later in life. Community nurses, school nurses and health visitors can make a significant contribution, but all nurses can use time spent with patients as a health promotion opportunity.

Early Detection and Treatment

Many hospitals have now developed 'Fracture Liaison Service' schemes through which patients identified as at risk of osteoporosis, especially patients who have had an 'index' fracture (e.g. Colles' or vertebral fracture), are screened for osteoporosis, diagnosed and treated appropriately so that further fragility fractures can be prevented. Many of these schemes are nurse led (Santy-Tomlinson et al. 2018).

Bone Tumours – Osteosarcoma

Primary bone tumours (osteosarcoma) can be benign or malignant, although some benign tumours may become malignant. Sarcoma is a primary cancer which originates from one of the cells of connective tissue – including bone tissue. It is a rare form of cancer which affects all age groups and all parts of the body. Annually, there are around 160 new diagnoses of osteosarcoma in the UK (Bone Cancer Research Trust (BCRT) 2016). Sarcomas are usually classified according to the cell type from which they originate. Malignant bone tumours (osteosarcoma) are more common in children and young adults (under 30 years), while soft tissue sarcomas are more common in later life (Stradling 2023). Their treatment requires multidisciplinary care and nursing plays a key role in coordinating care and supporting the patient through their journey.

Metastatic bone disease is treated very differently to sarcoma. This is malignant bone disease due to secondary deposits in bone tissue from a primary cancer elsewhere, such as those in the breast or the lung (see Chapter 31, Nursing the Patient With Cancer). The focus here is on primary sarcoma – particularly osteosarcoma.

Pathophysiology

Cancer is a collection of disorders that share a common feature of uncontrolled cell proliferation leading to the formation of a mass of cells known as a tumour which can invade adjacent tissues. Osteosarcoma can originate from a specific cell type within the bone tissue but may then involve a variety of bone cells.

Medical/Surgical Management

Diagnosis and Assessment

The first symptom of osteosarcoma is local pain. As a bone sarcoma grows, eruption into the surrounding tissues can occur, possibly becoming a warm swelling of the affected area. Pain at night and pain not relieved by rest are common indications of osteosarcoma. There may also be swelling, reduction in movement of the affected limb and reduced sensation. Patients are, however, rarely unwell in the early stages and a painful limb may have many causes. Because of the relative rarity of sarcoma, general practitioners may not immediately consider it as a potential diagnosis. All practitioners need to be more aware of this condition and its presenting symptoms so that sarcoma can be considered as a condition to be ruled out early in the diagnostic process. (For further information see Sarcoma UK, www.sarcoma.org.uk.) The later diagnosis has been made, the more likely the disease is to have spread. Osteosarcoma becomes life-threatening once metastatic disease is present (Stradling 2023).

Investigations

X-rays do not always show osteosarcoma, especially early in the disease. Any patient with suspected osteosarcoma should be referred to a specialist centre where a biopsy can be taken, and histological diagnosis made to inform the most effective treatment.

Management

This will depend on the type of bone tumour but should be led by an oncology team in a specialist centre.

Benign Bone Tumours

Osteochondroma, the most common type of benign bone tumour, is managed by wide excision. Osteoclastoma, common in the

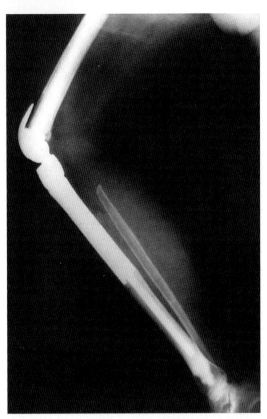

Figure 12.13 Endoprosthetic replacement of the proximal tibia (lateral view) with distal femoral component and excision of head of fibula.

femur and tibia, may require excision and insertion of an endoprosthesis (Fig. 12.13). Prostheses are now extendable, allowing for growth in skeletally immature patients.

Osteosarcoma

The treatment of osteosarcoma will depend on the histological diagnosis. Once a diagnosis has been made, the patient will have staging scans and scans (computed tomography (CT) or positron emission tomography (PET)) of the chest. Low-grade tumours may be treated with surgical excision alone. Higher-grade tumours will be treated with a combination of chemotherapy and surgery with or without endoprosthesis, or amputation.

❖ Nursing Management and Health Promotion: Osteosarcoma

Once the patient has seen their GP, immediate referral to a specialist centre will be needed. The care of a patient undergoing cancer diagnosis, chemotherapy and/or radiotherapy is described in Chapter 31.

The care of a patient who has a custom-built prosthetic implant will be specific to the implant, but the principles of postoperative care are similar to care joint arthroplasty.

Psychological care is vital for patients with osteosarcoma, as treatment can last for several months and is likely to be very debilitating, for example chemotherapy alongside major orthopaedic surgery. Concerns about self-concept and body image are likely and there will be many fears, including fear of death, the unknown and of dependence.

Amputation of a Limb

With the development of new treatments, amputation is becoming less common, but it can still be necessary in some instances. The most common reasons are osteosarcoma, crushing injury, peripheral vascular disease, congenital anomaly, severe osteomyelitis with systemic complications and intractable pain following limb trauma.

❖ Nursing Management and Health Promotion: Amputation of a Limb

Coping With Loss

Loss of a limb through amputation is like any other major loss. As most amputations are carried out as elective procedures, the team can make physiological, psychological and social assessments of the patient, and plan care to assist in the adjustment and adaptation process for the patient (Schober and Abrahamsen 2022) This may include arranging for the patient to visit the local prosthetic department or to meet a patient who has had an amputation and is coping successfully.

Sometimes amputation is an emergency procedure following a severe crushing injury. In this case, the psychological preparation of the patient and family is very limited and extra support and understanding during the postoperative period will be needed.

Wound Care

A crepe 'stump' bandage is used for the first few days and is then replaced with a compression sock, which is lighter and has better elastic properties. This maintains uniform compression on the wound, thus reducing oedema, promoting wound healing and beginning to shape the stump, to help with fitting of a prosthetic limb.

Phantom Sensation (Phantom Limb)

Painful sensations are experienced by some patients following limb amputation (see Chapter 19, Pain Management). If this becomes chronic, the patient will be referred to a chronic pain service for treatment in the form of transcutaneous electrical nerve stimulation (TENS), ultrasound, local nerve blocks, relaxation therapy or medication, such as the adjuvant analgesic carbamazepine, which may be effective (Richardson and Kulkarni 2017).

Pneumatic Postamputation Mobility Aid

Some centres use a prosthesis known as a pneumatic postamputation mobility (PPAM) aid to help the patient regain balance, reduce oedema of the stump and encourage early walking after amputation (Scott et al. 2017). The aid consists of an inflatable plastic tube which is placed around the patient's stump. The tube is encased in a metal frame with a rocker foot. The use of the PPAM aid can help with adjustment to the change in body image as the time without an artificial limb is reduced.

Bone Infections

Antibiotic resistance, the re-emergence of tuberculosis (TB) even in higher income countries and the increased use of implants in orthopaedic surgery mean that the potential for orthopaedic infections is ever present. This section will outline the three most common types: osteomyelitis, septic arthritis and TB.

Osteomyelitis

Osteomyelitis is a local or generalised infection affecting bone tissue and bone marrow.

Pathophysiology

Osteomyelitis can be acute or chronic and is a major complication of trauma and orthopaedic surgery as it can be associated with biofilms attached to implanted devices or haematogenous seeding (spread of bacteria from the bloodstream to implant sites). Like all infections, identifying osteomyelitis early makes it more likely to respond well to antibiotics. If the condition is untreated, or treatment fails, it usually becomes chronic. Infection prevents bone from healing, leading to long-term pain and disability and possible amputation of the affected limb. Preventing infections that may lead to osteomyelitis is vital in the care of all orthopaedic patients. Microorganisms usually gain entry during surgery or trauma but can also spread from existing infection or via the bloodstream. In the early stages the patient develops pyrexia and severe pain, and the affected area is hot and swollen. If untreated, the infection spreads through the bone marrow and erodes the cortex and periosteum. An abscess forms, which will eventually discharge through the skin. By this stage the condition is chronic osteomyelitis. If the infection is close to a joint, it may track into the joint, causing septic arthritis; this most commonly occurs at the hip, knee, shoulder, elbow and wrist joints (Maffulli et al. 2016)

Management

Assessment

Patients may have had recent trauma affecting the bone or an infection elsewhere in the body. Local signs of infection may be pain, heat and redness, and systemic symptoms of pyrexia, nausea, sweating and/or malaise.

Blood cultures, wound swabs or needle biopsy samples are taken to identify the causative organism and ensure the appropriate antibiotics are prescribed. Blood tests will show raised inflammatory markers: WBC count, erythrocyte sedimentation rate (ESR) and C-reactive protein (CRP). A plain X-ray will exclude any other causes for the symptoms, and a CT scan will highlight bony abscesses or sinus wounds. An MRI scan may also be carried out to detect any soft tissue or bone marrow involvement.

Treatment

Antibiotic therapy is not always successful and surgical intervention may be necessary to remove infected tissue and/or implants followed by bone grafting and/or external fixation. In severe cases, amputation may be necessary.

Nursing Management and Health Promotion: Osteomyelitis

Patients and nurses need to be alert to the condition so that early referral and treatment can be instituted to prevent progression.

Elevation of the affected part will reduce pain and may involve the use of traction, splints or casts to rest the affected area.

Rest, gentle handling, use of bed cradles to relieve pressure, prompt administration of analgesics and antipyretics, reassurance and distracting activity will all help to relieve pain.

Antibiotics will initially be administered intravenously and may continue for several weeks. Increasingly, this is being carried out in the community by appropriately skilled nurses.

Managing Chronic Osteomyelitis

Patients with chronic infection may have many hospital admissions and procedures and be anxious about the long-term prognosis.

Nurses should ensure that patients are kept fully informed of their condition and its management by referring them for appropriate social and therapy support.

Joint Infection – Septic Arthritis

Septic arthritis is an acute bacterial infection of a joint.

Pathophysiology

Septic arthritis can be caused by a nearby infection from a penetrating wound such as an insect bite or bacteraemia from a distant site of infection.

Management

Assessment

Septic arthritis usually presents as a hot, swollen, red and painful joint which the patient is reluctant to move. Blood cultures, blood tests and aspiration of the joint will confirm the presence of infection and identify the causative organism. Imaging, such as X-rays, CT and MRI, will help to identify the extent of the problem.

Treatment

The joint is drained by needle aspiration, arthroscopic washout or open surgery. Antibiotic therapy is commenced, usually intravenously at first. If treatment is unsuccessful, patients may suffer long-term arthritic changes and associated disability.

Nursing Management and Health Promotion: Septic Arthritis

The priorities are similar to those for patients with osteomyelitis with a focus on pain management and supporting activities of daily living.

Tuberculosis and Bone Infection

Rates of TB have increased recently for several reasons, including movement of unvaccinated people between countries and susceptibility to infection of immunosuppressed patients such as those with HIV (see Chapter 3, Nursing Patients With Respiratory Disorders, Chapter 7, Nursing Patients With Disorders of the Lymphatic and Immune Systems). The emergence of strains of multidrug-resistant TB (MDR-TB) and extensively drug-resistant TB (XDR-TB) limits treatment options and is a significant concern.

Pathophysiology

TB usually occurs in the lungs and may spread to the skeletal system, especially the vertebral (spinal) column, where half of all cases of skeletal infections occur (Jester et al. 2021). The course of the disease is like osteomyelitis, but at a slower pace. It weakens bone and so can lead to vertebral fractures and, in some cases, paraplegia. Surgical treatment may be needed once the active disease has been controlled (vertebral fusion to prevent further collapse of vertebrae, or joint replacement).

Management

Assessment

Symptoms usually develop slowly with little redness or heat initially. Localised tenderness sometimes occurs. Blood tests, sputum/urine tests, X-rays and MRI are all used to aid diagnosis.

Treatment

A combination of antitubercular drugs, for example rifampicin, will be administered for a long period (sometimes several years) and the symptoms of the disease are managed.

❖ Nursing Management and Health Promotion: Tuberculosis and Bone Infection

Nursing management involves implementation of the principles of infection prevention and control (see Chapter 18, Infection Prevention and Control), health promotion and pain and comfort measures to manage symptoms. It may take up to 2 years to successfully treat skeletal TB and patients require support that includes regular supervision and monitoring of their medication regimen for side-effects to ensure concordance with and completion of treatment. In some areas specialist TB teams take this responsibility.

DISORDERS OF JOINTS

This section outlines the management of disorders of the lumbar spine, OA and RA.

Disorders of the Lumbar Spine – Back Pain

Lumbar spine disorders or 'back pain' account for more lost working hours than any other medical condition and a significant proportion of GP attendances and referrals to orthopaedic clinics (NICE 2016). The focus, here, is on management of acute back pain, recurrent back pain and prolapsed intervertebral disc (PID).

● *Pathophysiology*

Damage or trauma to the vertebrae, ligaments or intervertebral discs can result in instability and potential impingement on the spinal cord and nerves. Fig. 12.14 illustrates the major causes of low back pain (LBP). In the lumbar spine, mechanical causes are the most common but they do not usually have serious consequences.

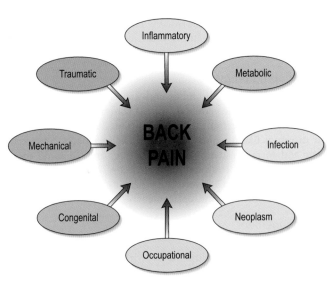

Figure 12.14 Causes of back pain.

Acute Back Pain

Acute back strain can be caused by a sudden sharp movement or an attempt to lift a heavy object in an extended body position, or when people with sedentary occupations indulge in bursts of exercise to which they are unaccustomed. This manifests as sudden severe pain in the lower back, due to acute muscle or ligament strain in the lumbar spine. When assessing patients with LBP, it is important that serious causes such as cancer and infection are ruled out. Acute LBP usually resolves within a few weeks or months, if management is led by up-to-date evidence-based advice.

● *Management*

Management includes (NICE 2016):

- rest for 24 hours maximum in the most comfortable position and then resumption of normal activity
- support in self-management symptoms
- analgesics, nonsteroidal antiinflammatory drugs (NSAIDs) which may be combined with paracetamol
- return to work or study as soon as possible
- engagement in group exercise programmes.

❖ Nursing Management and Health Promotion: Acute Back Pain

Nurses have many opportunities in the workplace, community and hospital to educate people about how to avoid acute back pain. This includes consideration of ergonomic living and working environments, manual handling techniques and appropriate exercise and activity. Many excellent materials to support education and health promotion activity are now available online to assist in this. Nurses are, themselves, at high risk of back injury and they have a responsibility to maintain their well-being by following recommendations for manual handling and appropriate personal health actions. Both employer and employee responsibilities are set out and there are specific guidelines for assessment and planning of patient care (Reflection 12.7).

Chronic Back Pain

Episodes of LBP can recur and up to one-third of sufferers of acute back pain complain of continued pain 1 year after onset (NICE 2016).

● *Medical Management*

Physiotherapy, exercise, medication and strategies for dealing with chronic pain are the mainstays of treatment. Pharmacological pain management will be prescribed according to the pain ladder (see Chapter 20, Pain Management). Patients may be referred to a chronic pain service where an interprofessional team aims both to relieve pain and to enable patients to live with their pain (Maher et al. 2017). This is achieved by helping patients to understand the reason for their pain, and by teaching behavioural techniques that can help to reduce it, such as pacing activities over time and learning to use relaxation techniques (Kamper et al. 2015).

❖ Nursing Management and Health Promotion: Chronic Low Back Pain

Within the multidisciplinary team, the nursing role within a chronic back pain management programme can encompass patient assessment, case management, pain monitoring and education.

REFLECTION 12.7

Moving and Handling of Patients

Assessment and Planning

Particularly heavy patients, or helpless immobile patients with no, or limited, ability to assist nurses, need to be individually assessed by a competent patient handling team to enable a patient handling plan to be put in place for the team. Student nurses and support workers should not be expected to undertake these assessments without competent supervision.

The care plan or profile should include the following information:

- The current weight of the patient.
- The nature of any manual handling tasks that might be needed, based on the patient's needs.
- The extent of the patient's ability to assist and weight-bear, and any other relevant information.
- The technique to be employed to handle that particular patient which should be consistent with the activity undertaken. This should be based upon:
  - the task
  - the individual
  - the load
  - the environment.

The Manual Handling Operations Regulations 1992 (Health and Safety Executive 2016) do not contain any weight limits or state that there is any threshold below which handling may be regarded as safe. All patient handling should be assessed by looking at all risk factors, not just the weight of the patient.

Mechanical handling devices or equipment should be used for moving totally dependent patients who cannot move for themselves in situations, for example, where they need to move from bed to chair, trolley, toilet, etc. Sliding equipment should be used for moving totally immobile patients in bed.

Activities

- Find out which moving and handling aids are available in the clinical area to which you are currently attached. How often are they used?
- Reflect on the different techniques for moving and handling patients you have seen or used. Discuss the safety, suitability and effectiveness of each technique with your mentor or practice supervisor/assessor.

Prolapsed Intervertebral Disc

A PID is the protrusion of the disc nucleus through a tear in the disc annulus fibrosus into the spinal canal.

Pathophysiology

The intervertebral discs act as shock absorbers between each of the vertebrae and consist of a gelatinous nucleus pulposus surrounded by fibrocartilage and fibrous tissue, the annulus fibrosus. Age-related loss of water content and an increase in collagen content lead to the discs drying out and being less elastic, so more prone to injury. The disc space becomes narrowed and distorted, leading to increased stress on the spine and intervertebral discs. Eventually, the disc may rupture and the pulposus will prolapse, potentially compressing nerve roots and/or fibres. Most lumbar disc protrusions involve L4–5 or L5–S1 (Fig. 12.15).

Management

Assessment

Patients usually present with acute lumbar pain radiating down the thigh and lower leg – sciatica. Muscle spasm and an intense focal area of pain may be evident. Straight leg raising will indicate painful restriction of hip flexion well below 90 degrees and there may be neurological signs such as numbness, tingling or

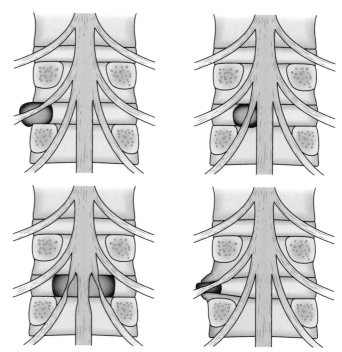

Figure 12.15 Disc prolapse and root compression in the lumbar spine. A laterally placed prolapse may compress the L4 root, a more central prolapse will compress L5 and a central prolapse will compress the cauda equina. Osteophytes in the lateral canal will also produce root compression.

diminished motor function of the leg/s. An MRI scan may be performed to confirm the diagnosis.

Treatment

A patient who presents with a central disc prolapse is an emergency as the prolapsed disc causes pressure directly on the spinal cord and prompt surgical decompression is required. For other prolapses conservative treatment for acute back pain as outlined above should be tried first.

The indication for disc excision is usually when there is proven disc protrusion with accompanying neurological signs and no improvement after 6 weeks of conservative treatment, or if any neurological deficit worsens. Surgical discectomy, microdiscectomy, open discectomy and minimally invasive discectomy are the most common procedures and the differences in patient outcomes between these are small (Rasouli et al. 2014). Removal of a portion or all of the disc means there will reduction in its shock-absorbing function with the result that some may suffer chronic stiffness and back pain.

Nursing Management and Health Promotion: Prolapsed Intervertebral Disc

Conservative Management

As most conservative treatment can be carried out at home, it is the primary care nurse who will have responsibility for advising and supporting the patient and family.

See Evolve website Critical thinking question 12.3

Surgical Management

As well as the general principles for perioperative care and for musculoskeletal care, the following advice is specific to postoperative management of patients having disc excision.

Pain. The use of patient-controlled analgesia (PCA) or of epidural analgesia following spinal surgery will help to ensure that pain is well controlled.

Positioning and Mobilising. Spinal alignment should be maintained after surgery. Normal movements can be gradually resumed as soon as the patient's general condition permits. A supportive brace may be needed before commencing mobilisation. Minimal flexion of the knees, using a knee rest or a pillow for support while in the supine position, allows spinal muscles to relax. A pillow between the knees provides comfortable alignment when in the lateral position.

Early mobilisation and a physiotherapist-led rehabilitation programme are usually recommended. The bed should be lowered, and the patient taught to roll to the edge, swing the legs to the floor and stand up in one smooth movement.

Degenerative and Inflammatory Joint Disorders

There are over 200 conditions that can affect synovial joints and tissues. This section focuses on two common joint diseases: OA and RA (Fig. 12.16).

Osteoarthritis

OA is the most prevalent joint disorder worldwide and is a leading cause of pain and disability (NICE 2022).

Figure 12.16 Some differences between rheumatoid arthritis and osteoarthritis. Rheumatoid arthritis affects small joints, is symmetrical and is more common in young women. Osteoarthritis mainly affects the weight-bearing joints and is more common in older people.

⬤ Pathophysiology

OA is characterised by a slow deterioration of the articular cartilage that covers the bone ends in synovial joints, particularly the hips, knees and joints of the hands and feet. It is a complex degenerative disease of synovial joints involving inflammatory processes, metabolism and other individual factors that appear to prevent the renewal and remodelling of articular cartilage (Mobasheri and Batt 2016). Much more than a disease of wear and tear of the articular cartilage, OA is now known to involve the whole joint, with changes in the local bone and surrounding soft tissues (Parsons and Roberts 2020).

OA may be classified as primary or secondary, the former being a progressive condition of unknown origin, more common in the older person, especially females. Secondary OA can affect people of any age or gender and is usually associated with a previous injury/condition of the joint, such as a fracture or childhood hip conditions such as Perthes' disease. It can also develop following repeated high-impact joint movements in sport or occupation, for example professional footballers are particularly prone to hip and knee OA.

⬤ Medical/Surgical Management

Assessment

Pain on movement, stiffness at rest and reduced joint function are the most common symptoms. The joint will have a reduced range of movement on examination, and this may be accompanied by pain.

There are no specific diagnostic tests for OA, and diagnosis is usually made on history and examination. X-ray of an osteoarthritic joint will show loss of joint space and bony outgrowths, known as osteophytes. However, the degree of destruction of the joint space does not always correlate to the degree of pain and disability a patient is experiencing (Parsons and Roberts 2020), so X-ray is usually reserved for patients where joint replacement is being considered or to rule out other disease such as a tumour or more aggressive type of arthritis. Blood tests are not necessary unless infection or inflammatory disease is suspected.

Treatment

The NICE has reviewed the evidence for effectiveness of treatments and provided good practice guidelines (NICE 2022; Evidence-Based Practice 12.2).

Surgery is considered when conservative methods are no longer effective in relieving the pain of OA and the disease is impacting on the person's quality of life. For hip and knee OA in younger people, consideration may be given to osteotomy, the realignment of the forces passing through the joint by cutting a wedge of bone out of the distal or proximal bone. The surgical treatment of choice for hip and knee OA is joint replacement (arthroplasty), the removal of the damaged ends of the bones and their replacement with a combination of metal (cobalt chromium or titanium) and plastic (polyethylene) components (Fig. 12.17). Total hip replacement/arthroplasty (THR) and total knee replacement/arthroplasty (TKR) prostheses are expected to still function well at 10–15 years following surgery (Jester et al. 2022). For OA of the hand, arthrodesis (fusing of the joint) or joint replacement may be considered if all other treatments have been ineffective.

Access to Services for Marginalised Groups

There is limited evidence about inequalities in access to services for management of chronic musculoskeletal conditions for marginalised communities. It is known that there is a higher prevalence of musculoskeletal conditions among some ethnic minority groups, reflecting social, cultural and psychological differences. Cultural perspectives relating to pain and chronic health problems

Figure 12.17 Examples of a total knee replacement (A) and a total hip replacement (B).

and factors affecting the experience and outcomes of services are important considerations for practitioners (Jeraj and Butt 2020). One marginalised group who frequently use orthopaedic services but often receive care that is not sensitive to their needs is people with a learning disability (Drozd et al. 2021).

❖ Nursing Management and Health Promotion: Conservative Treatments for Osteoarthritis

The key to early OA treatment is patient self-management and nurses can play a leading role in helping patients to develop the necessary skills and knowledge to do this. Nurses can provide education and support themselves or refer patients to a self-management programme. In the UK, there are several online programmes that aim to help patients to manage their disease. Some of these programmes are generic and some disease specific. Such programmes can increase patient self-efficacy, their belief in the ability to change behaviour and manage their disease, and this can lead to better symptom management and enhanced quality of life (McHugh et al. 2018).

❖ Nursing Management and Health Promotion: Joint Replacement

Preoperative Care

Preparation should begin as soon as a patient's name is added to the waiting list, with provision of written information and the opportunity to attend an assessment and information session. These are usually multidisciplinary but coordinated and led by orthopaedic nurse practitioners. Many elective orthopaedic surgery units base patient care following THR and TKR surgery on the principles of enhanced recovery pathways which aim to optimise patient safety and outcomes through preoperative evaluation and patient education and perioperative optimisation of recovery based on evidence based care. Such pathways focus on optimising preoperative assessment, fasting, bowel preparation, anaesthesia, prophylactic VTE prevention, postoperative nausea and vomiting, nutrition and fluid management (Kaye et al. 2019).

Postoperative Care

Postoperative care will follow the basic principles (see Chapter 25, Nursing the patient Undergoing Surgery) and the general principles of care for musculoskeletal disorders outlined earlier. A focus on VTE prevention is vital as hip and knee replacement surgery can have the highest reported rate of DVT if prophylaxis is not used.

Mobility and Rehabilitation

The patient may begin to mobilise as soon as their postoperative condition permits, which is usually on the first day postoperatively. This will be supervised by the nursing and physiotherapy teams nurse. After a hip replacement, there is a risk of dislocation of the prosthesis and it is important that the knee is not raised higher than the hip; a raised bed, chair and toilet seat are usually necessary. A walking frame may be used at first and the physiotherapist will re-educate the patient to use a normal walking gait. Depending on progress, the patient should practice using crutches or walking sticks and may practice on steps before discharge.

Aids to Living

The occupational therapist will provide aids for dressing, such as a stocking applicator, and any other aids needed after an assessment of the home environment and the patient's capabilities.

Discharge Planning

Discharge planning should begin preoperatively, and, in some centres, patients will be identified as suitable for an early supported discharge scheme where a 'hospital at home' environment is provided. Where such services do not exist, the community nurse will provide care, such as wound suture removal, and will liaise with the hospital team as necessary (Reflection 12.8).

REFLECTION 12.8

A Patient's Reflection on Having a Total Hip Replacement

Two months after an operation for hip replacement, I am trying to record my experiences, but one thought predominates to such an extent that everything else fades into insignificance. I can think of nothing other than the fact that I have no pain: no pain walking, no pain sitting, no pain lying in bed, no pain at all. Two ideas arise from this: one, that it does not seem at all healthy to be so conscious of the absence of pain. The hope must be that, sooner or later, being pain-free will become the normal unobserved fact of life. The other is a retrospective awareness of the debilitating effect of continuous chronic pain, the insidious way in which everything developed. People now keep exclaiming that I look so well, that my colour has improved so much. They never in the past told me that I looked old and grey. This must have been as unremarkable to others as the experience of continuous pain was to me.

There were many kinds of pain. The worst in intensity was probably the pain on weight-bearing, but somehow it did not bother me so very much. I felt I could anticipate it, control it by leaning on a stick or furniture, or by refraining from walking altogether. There were sudden and very acute bouts of pain, sharp like toothache, on sudden movements or jolts, but these passed and did not matter much. There was the impossibility of ever sitting or lying in comfort – much less severe pain, but the most difficult to bear. It was when that particular pain suddenly got much worse that I first told the GP how I felt. When, despite antiinflammatory painkillers, even the weight of the sheet became intolerable and lack of sleep became difficult to cope with, an appointment was made with the orthopaedic specialist services. I saw an orthopaedic nurse practitioner in the outpatient clinic and she asked me about my symptoms, examined me and talked through the X-ray with me. My hip joint was almost completely worn out and we agreed that it was time for a total hip replacement.

I was very apprehensive as I did not know a great deal about the operation. However, I was given a comprehensive information booklet and invited to the 'Hip Clinic'. At this session I met other people waiting for their operation and we had the opportunity to talk with two people who had already had theirs; it was very reassuring to hear about their experiences. The orthopaedic nurse practitioner answered any questions we had and showed us a hip replacement. There was also an occupational therapist there who explained what adaptations we would need to our home, such as a raised toilet seat, and a physiotherapist taught us the exercises we would have to do after our operation so that we could practice them before we came into hospital. At the end of this, I felt I knew what was going to happen, though I was still a little apprehensive.

Now, after the operation, I have joined the ranks of those who extol its virtue, but even the most enthusiastic supporters had not prepared me for the speed with which it would be possible to lead a normal life: walking within 24 hours, discharged from hospital within 5 days, fully independent by the time of the follow-up outpatient appointment 6 weeks after operation. Here, in summary, are the events which I now believe made the whole experience entirely positive: on first appointment at the orthopaedic outpatient clinic the thorough examination, the fact that the nurse practitioner appeared to

understand how much pain I had – perhaps even better than I did – and did not belittle what I was saying. The fact that I attended the Hip Clinic and that I was only on the waiting list for 12 weeks. Two weeks before the operation, there was a day of tests and examinations in the ward to which I was to be admitted, giving a good opportunity to allay anxiety.

On admission, I was immediately aware of the cordiality and friendliness of the nursing staff and of the community spirit of the patients who made me feel welcome and who augmented the very adequate information given to me by the staff, both in print and in discussion.

Preoperative relief of anxiety and postoperative pain control were superb; after the initial intravenous analgesic cover, painkillers were offered every 4 hours, but not really needed, except before physiotherapy, after the first few days. It was interesting to observe that all patients who had hip operations went through the same progression of skill acquisition and setbacks, learning how to get in and out of bed, how to turn in bed, how to walk, first with a Zimmer frame, then with two sticks, and later one stick, how to pick things up off the floor, to put on stockings and shoes, to shower independently, to dress and undress, to climb stairs and to get in and out of a car. It was evident that all the nurses knew exactly what each patient was capable of doing. All were willing to help but clearly expected and encouraged independence. The nurses' awareness of patients' progress and the supervision of the activities of less highly qualified staff were always in evidence. It was reassuring to notice that there was vigilance in case deep vein thrombosis arose. With the emphasis throughout on what one can do by oneself and encouragement to get moving, it was a boost to self-confidence to know that nurses were vigilant for complications and setbacks. I found it helpful to have been shown the X-ray of the new hip as it makes it possible to visualise what the joint is doing during various activities, and to understand why one is advised never to cross the legs, to get on all fours or to pick things up off the floor from the sitting position. A pillow between the legs during sleep helps prevent crossing the legs accidentally.

There were 12 women in the ward, most of them in for hip or knee operations. The impression gained on admission of a friendly, supportive group spirit was reinforced throughout. What a wealth of experience, what a reservoir of knowledge, what abundance of empathy, goodwill and helpfulness. There was also a tremendous amount of fun and humour, perhaps enhanced by the experience all had of being pain-free all of a sudden. On discharge, I was part of a supported discharge scheme, which meant that a physiotherapist and nurses visited me during my first few weeks at home to check that I was continuing to make progress. It was reassuring to have this support when I got home.

Activity

Using information from the chapter and this patient's reflection, write a concise discharge plan for a patient who has undergone an uncomplicated total hip replacement. Discuss the plan with your practice supervisor/assessor.

Rheumatoid Arthritis

RA is common autoimmune inflammatory disease that involves the synovium that lines joints, affecting around 1 million people in the UK. It is a chronic progressive condition that results in significant pain and disability and its causes are largely unknown (Jester et al. 2021).

🔵 Pathophysiology

RA is an autoimmune disease (the body's immune system attacks its own tissues and becomes self-destructive – see Chapter 7, Nursing Patients With Disorders of the Lymphatic and Immune Systems) that causes joint inflammation. The cause of this is not

fully known and research continues. The joints are initially acutely inflamed due to inflammatory changes in the synovial membrane leading to pain, stiffness and loss of function. The synovium becomes thicker, very vascular and a site of increased cell infiltration, causing joint swelling. The proliferative tissue spreads as a 'pannus' over the articular cartilage, slowly eroding it (Primdahl and Esbensen 2020).

Systemic inflammatory changes can affect many of the body's organs and lead to pericarditis, pleuritis and bowel vasculitis, as well as general malaise and anaemia. RA can be a very debilitating chronic disease with life expectancy potentially reduced due to associated infections, renal or respiratory disease, and RA itself. There is no one path of RA progression and some patients have permanent remission while others have severe relentless deterioration in symptoms; each patient must therefore be assessed individually.

Medical/Surgical Management

Assessment

The disease most commonly starts when a person is in their 30s or 40s with a gradual onset of pain and stiffness, particularly in the morning, affecting the small joints of the hands and feet. They may also present to their GP complaining of loss of appetite and weight, mild pyrexia and characteristics of anaemia. As the RA progresses, other joints may become involved, with inflammation, swelling and progressive loss of function. The wrists, elbows, shoulders, cervical spine, temporomandibular joints, knees and ankles are commonly affected.

For some patients the onset of RA is acute, with multiple joint involvement from the outset, with rapid progress to loss of function.

The affected joints appear swollen and warm to the touch. The patient will complain of pain when the normal range of movement is attempted.

X-rays of both hands and feet will usually confirm joint erosion. A blood sample will be taken for assessment of the presence of rheumatoid factor although this is not present in every patient with RA.

Diagnosis

NICE (2018) guidelines for the management of RA in adults recommend that patients should be referred for a rheumatologist opinion if they have any of the following criteria:

- the small joints of the hands or feet are affected by the symptoms of RA (see earlier)
- more than one joint is affected
- there has been a delay between onset of symptoms and seeking medical advice.

Management

There is no known cure for RA, and therefore intervention is directed towards relieving pain, modifying the level of disease activity and maintaining optimal functional ability for each individual (NICE 2018).

The aims of medical treatment are to:

- Reduce the patient's pain with the lowest effective dose of analgesics such as NSAIDs and COX II selective inhibitors.
- Reduce joint destruction with the use of disease-modifying antirheumatic drugs (DMARDs) such as oral methotrexate, leflunomide or sulfasalazine and/or early short-term use of local or systemic corticosteroid therapy. In newer treatments, biological agents that aim to alter the normal immune response by blocking the normal inflammatory process are under evaluation.
- Prevent or minimise deformity of a joint by splinting damaged or painful joints.
- Assist the patient to adapt their lifestyle.
- Correct anaemia.

The main surgical treatments are:

- synovectomy (removal of excess synovial membrane from within the joint capsule)
- osteotomy
- joint replacement or arthrodesis (most commonly of the ankle).

Nursing Management and Health Promotion: Rheumatoid Arthritis

The aim of care is to relieve symptoms and to maintain and, if possible, improve quality of life. A multidisciplinary approach is essential, but coordination of care and therapeutic interventions such as joint injections often fall within the remit of rheumatology nurse specialists.

Patient Involvement/Empowerment

As with OA, the current emphasis for RA management is on patient involvement and self-management through Expert Patient programmes.

Controlling Pain

A range of analgesics may need to be considered, from paracetamol/aspirin to compound analgesics, such as co-codamol, to NSAIDs. Corticosteroids are usually used in the short term in acute episodes of pain/inflammation. When they are used for long-term therapy, abrupt withdrawal must be avoided as the body may not have sufficient glucocorticoids to deal with stress (see Chapter 5, Nursing Patients With Endocrine Disorders). Various alternative therapies are tried by many patients but there is often little evidence for their effectiveness (NICE 2018) and some herbal medication can interact with prescribed drugs. Some patients do appear to gain at least short-term benefit from alternative and complementary therapies and nurses play an important role in ensuring that patients are aware of any potential side-effects.

Local pain control can be achieved in some joints by other methods, such as splints for the hand and wrist joints.

Maintaining Independence and Fostering Well-being

Exercise and Mobility. The principles of joint protection should be explained to the patient, such as respecting pain and not being fearful or ignoring it, balancing work and rest, using the larger or stronger joints rather than small ones and reducing the effort to a joint (Gay et al. 2016).

Adaptation of Living Space. The muscle power of the patient with RA is reduced, so the use of aids such as a variable-height bed, raised or ejector chair and raised toilet seat can be helpful.

Walking aids, such as a stick or elbow crutches, can help to retain the patient's level of mobility by reducing the weight load placed on specific joints. The handle sections of the aids may need to be adapted to accommodate the finger and wrist deformities that are common features of RA.

Diet. The patient with RA may require assistance in maintaining nutritional status due to anorexia and/or difficulty in using eating and drinking utensils. Frequent, light, appetising meals should be served. The occupational therapist can supply a variety of utensils, such as large-handled cutlery and a tilting kettle stand, which will help the patient to retain independence. A patient with RA is likely to develop anaemia due to the chronic inflammatory process of the disease and/or from gastrointestinal bleeding caused by non-steroidal anti-inflammatory medication therapy, and iron supplements may be prescribed.

Sexual Activity. Counselling regarding sexual activity may be needed. The Arthritis Research Campaign has produced booklets containing useful information for RA patients and their partners (see Useful Websites).

SOFT TISSUE INJURIES

This section of the chapter outlines a range of soft tissue injuries, including those affecting ligaments, muscles and tendons and peripheral nerves.

Ligament Injuries

Injuries to ligaments may involve a partial or complete rupture of the ligament.

Pathophysiology

Ligament injuries are often called 'sprains' and are usually caused by excessive extension, flexion and/or rotation of a joint which stretches a ligament, or group of ligaments, beyond the boundaries of their elasticity, damaging or tearing their fibres, or the entire ligament (Jester et al. 2021). 'Whiplash injury' is the term used to describe a ligamentous injury to the cervical spine area often occurring after an RTC. This injury is due to excessive flexion and extension movements to the neck. The knee and ankle are both heavily dependent on ligaments for stability and they are susceptible to injury. Injured ligaments have poor blood supply so rarely heal well enough to regain their former strength and the scar tissue that forms at the site is never as strong as the original tissue.

Medical Management

History and Examination

People who suffer ligament injuries are often young and will complain of severe pain around the injured area after feeling or hearing something snap or tear. Limitation of normal joint movement may be found with swelling of the injured part and joint instability may be noted during the physical examination.

Investigations

Plain radiographs are taken to rule out a bony injury to the area. An MRI scan or examination of the joint under general anaesthesia may be performed.

Treatment

The injured area will often be supported, for example using a cervical collar for a whiplash injury (Fig. 12.18) or a POP cylinder/knee brace for a knee injury. Short-term rest, elevation and ice packs can be helpful in managing swelling and pain can usually be

Figure 12.18 Cervical collar.

managed with simple analgesia such as paracetamol. Physiotherapy may be prescribed to build up muscle groups that surround the joint which the injured ligament normally supports. Surgical intervention is usually needed only when the injury affects the knee joint or where there is damage to more than one ligament and/or gross instability of the joint.

Nursing Management and Health Promotion: Ligament Injuries

If no other injury has been sustained, the patient may be treated and discharged from the ED to attend as an outpatient.

Pain Relief. Pain will be the major patient problem on presentation at hospital. Such pain should be assessed (see Chapter 20, Pain Management) and appropriate analgesic prescribed. Ligament injuries can be sustained following significant trauma to the body part, so the surrounding soft tissues will also be involved, causing further bleeding and haematoma/bruising which will increase swelling and irritate the surrounding tissues, thus increasing pain. NSAIDs can be useful to reduce the inflammatory response.

Muscle Spasm. This is a common sign of soft tissue irritation and, if severe, the patient may need to be prescribed a mild antispasmodic as well as an analgesic.

Support/Immobilisation. There is no evidence that tubular elastic bandages help with ligament injuries, so these are no longer used in EDs and clinics. Refer to priorities and management of patients in casts. When a cervical collar is worn, it can usually be removed to allow daily skin care. Following anterior cruciate ligament repair, a patient may wear a knee brace for the first 6–8 weeks, which prevents flexion greater than 90 degrees, and nurses should ensure that the patient can correctly apply the device.

Psychosocial Care. Ligament injury can take up to a year to heal completely, and work and financial status, as well as social interaction, can be affected (Craig et al. 2023b).

Muscle and Tendon Injuries

Pathophysiology

Ligament injuries are most often caused by a sudden sharp movement of the joint that places the joint under stress, most commonly during sports and leisure activities. The large tendons and muscles of the lower limbs, such as the Achilles tendon that inserts the gastrocnemius and soleus muscles into the heel bone, are the most common sites of injury.

Medical Management

History and Examination

The patient will experience a distressing tearing sensation or a 'snap' at the site of the injury and often an inability to put the foot down. Swelling and tenderness will develop quickly following the injury. Bruising will appear later and may be extensive and alarming for the patient. On examination, a gap between the ends of the muscle or tendon may be felt in superficial muscle injuries. MRI or ultrasound may be used to determine the extent of the injury.

Treatment

For muscle injuries the principles of RICE – rest, ice, compression and elevation – should be followed to control haemorrhage and limit haematoma formation. Early mobilisation within pain limits is important, as muscle healing occurs through aerobic metabolic pathways and therefore needs adequate circulation. Surgery may be necessary if there is a large intramuscular haematoma or if there is a large muscle tear affecting movement.

Tendon injuries are usually treated conservatively, with a cast or splint holding the ends together until healed. Surgery may be required for a complete tendon rupture, particularly of the Achilles tendon. Surgical versus conservative treatment of Achilles tendon injury is a matter of continued debate. While surgery can reduce the risk of rerupture, it significantly increases the risk of other complications such as infection.

❖❖ Nursing Management and Health Promotion: Muscle and Tendon Injuries

Comfort. The nurse has a key role in helping the patient to institute and maintain RICE.

Mobility. Once activity is commenced, the physiotherapist will teach the patient to use the most appropriate walking aid, usually a pair of crutches, and nurses should ensure that the patients use these correctly.

Assessment of the patient's home circumstances with regard to mobility will be required and referral to an occupational therapist may be necessary.

Following surgery, routine postoperative care will be needed (see Chapter 25, Nursing Patients Undergoing Surgery). The use of a cast or brace will require education of the patient in its care and management.

Peripheral Nerve Injuries

Nerves can be damaged due to underlying disease or following trauma. In this section, the focus will be on nerve injuries following trauma.

🔴 Pathophysiology

A single nerve or group of nerves may be damaged depending on the site of injury. Nerve injuries can be due to either direct or indirect force and can be divided into three types (Craig et al. 2023b):

- neuropraxia – intact nerves with temporary damage usually due to compression
- axonotmesis – divided axons with maintenance of the endoneural tubes, usually due to severe blow or traction, a pulling injury; prognosis is good
- neurotmesis – the whole nerve is divided, usually from a penetrating wound such as a stabbing; no recovery is possible without surgical repair.

🔴 Medical Management

History and Examination
Following trauma, a patient may become aware of tingling (paraesthesia), numbness and/or loss of movement of the affected part. Examination of the distribution of the loss of sensation and movement will aid diagnosis of the extent of the injury.

Investigations
Plain radiographs can assess bony injury and the presence of foreign material, such as glass fragments, which may have caused the injury.

Diagnosis
Diagnosis is confirmed by the absence or alteration of neurological function and sensation of the affected part. Nerve conduction studies, which involve stimulating a nerve with a wave pulse to evaluate the sensory and motor responses along the course of the peripheral nerve, may be carried out. Electromyography (EMG), which records motor activity at rest and on attempted muscle contraction, may also be used (Craig et al. 2023b).

Treatment
Nonoperative management involves immobilisation of the affected part in the anatomical position, using a lightweight cast or splint. Peripheral nerves are capable of regenerating at a rate of 1–2 mm/day (Jester et al. 2021). It is possible to calculate roughly the length of time to recovery although there is no guarantee that each nerve cell will heal. Primary surgical repair is indicated only when a nerve has been cleanly divided. Secondary repair may include suturing and grafting of nerve tissue from a less important nerve within the patient's body.

❖❖ Nursing Management and Health Promotion: Peripheral Nerve Injuries

Complete recovery may occur but can take a few weeks, months or years. However, the patient may need to adapt to permanent and severely disabling physical, psychological and social changes (Craig et al. 2023b).

In the short term, as the patient will have been involved in some form of trauma, nursing care as outlined in Chapter 26, Nursing the Patient Who Experiences Trauma, will apply. Should the patient require surgery, general perioperative care will be needed (see Chapter 25, Nursing the Patient Undergoing Surgery).

Health Promotion – Preventing Further Injury
The patient will have partial or complete loss of the protective mechanisms of touch and pain, and care must be taken to prevent further injury to the affected part. Movement of the injured limb must be through the normal range of passive joint movements, otherwise joints, muscles, tendons, ligaments and other nerves could be damaged further. To prevent the development of joint contracture and deformity, the patient may be fitted with a lightweight splint which holds the joints in their anatomical position. This may be needed for a long period. Exposure to extremes of temperature should be avoided, to prevent a skin burn.

Other Considerations
Pain. Sharp, shooting pain and a constant tingling sensation can be very troublesome, and the patient may need prolonged use of analgesics. Antidepressant medication, such as amitriptyline, and adjuvant analgesics are known to be beneficial as a supplementary medication in the relief of neuropathic pain (see Chapter 20, Pain Management).

Washing and Dressing. Advice and information can assist the patient in their usual mode of personal cleansing and dressing. For example, a patient with a median nerve injury due to a laceration of the wrist of the dominant hand may have difficulty in brushing their teeth or combing their hair. The occupational therapist can provide advice and appropriate aids.

Splints. If a splint is used, the patient will need information and advice about the correct method of application and removal.

Support. As recovery from a peripheral nerve injury may be prolonged, the patient will require support and understanding from family, friends and members of the healthcare team to relieve boredom and prevent the development of depression. Group sessions for patients with similar injuries who are receiving physiotherapy, occupational therapy and/or diversional therapy can be an excellent psychological support mechanism. The social worker can assist with social and/or financial problems which may develop due to possible lengthy absence from employment.

Permanent Disability. If the nerve injury prevents return to the previous occupation, it will be necessary to ensure that the patient has access to specialist advice about retraining and new employment opportunities. In some instances, alteration to body image could have a severe psychological effect. Nurses should be aware of this and provide support and counselling as needed by the patient.

Summary: Key Nursing Issues

- The overall aims of nursing care of patients with musculoskeletal injury or disorder are to prevent further injury, reduce the risk of complications, promote healing, maximise independence and promote optimal rehabilitation.
- Three key potential complications which must be considered with musculoskeletal injury or the treatment of musculoskeletal disorders are CS, VTE and fat embolus. Nurses play a key role in reducing the risk of these complications and their early identification.
- Fracture treatment consists of reducing the fracture, maintaining its position whilst it heals, and restoring function. Nurses caring for patients with fractures need an understanding of the various methods used to achieve fracture healing, including casts, traction and internal or external fixation.

Many fractures are fragility fractures occurring in older people with osteoporosis. It is vital to treat the osteoporosis so that future fractures are less likely to occur.

- The management of joint disorders such as OA and RA requires patients to play a central role in the management of their condition. Nurses can help to ensure that patients have the necessary knowledge and self-management skills to achieve this.
- Patients with musculoskeletal injury or disorder will be cared for in a wide variety of settings and not just an orthopaedic ward. All nurses need some understanding of the common conditions such as osteoporosis and OA and their attendant treatments such as medication and joint replacement.

Reflection and Learning – What Next?

- **Test** your knowledge by visiting the Evolve website 🌐 and answering the multiple-choice questions and critical thinking questions.
- **Consolidate** your learning by looking at some of the further reading suggestions, references, and specialist websites.
- **Revisit** some of the additional material on the Evolve website.

- **Consider** what you have learnt and how this will help your professional development.
- **Reflect** on how you can apply this knowledge to the care of your patients.
- **Discuss** your learning with your practice supervisor/assessor/supervisor, lecturer and colleagues.

References

BCRT (Bone Cancer Research Trust) (2016). Osteosarcoma. https://www.bcrt.org.uk/information/information-by-type/osteosarcoma/?gclid=EAIaIQobChMI7aDw5cnH_QIVT-vtCh35HA5mEAAYASAAEgJ7h_D_BwE.

Cone J, Inaba K. Lower extremity compartment syndrome. *Trauma Surg Acute Care Open*. 2017;2(1):e000094. doi: 10.1136/tsaco-2017-000094.

Craig J, Clarke S, Moore P. Principles of fracture management. In: Clarke S, Drozd M, eds. *Orthopaedic and Trauma Nursing: An Evidence-Based Approach to Musculoskeletal Care*. 2nd ed. Oxford: Wiley–Blackwell; 2023a:240–255.

Craig J, Gray Linnecor B, Neil M. Soft tissue, peripheral nerve and brachial plexus injury. In: Clarke S, Drozd M, eds. *Orthopaedic and Trauma Nursing: An Evidence-Based Approach to Musculoskeletal Care*. 2nd ed. Oxford: Wiley–Blackwell; 2023b:304–315.

Drozd M, Chadwick D, Jester R. A cross-case comparison of the trauma and orthopaedic hospital experiences of adults with intellectual disabilities using interpretative phenomenological analysis. *Nurs Open*. 2021;8(2):858–869.

Duperouzel W, Gray B, Santy-Tomlinson J. The principles of traction and the application of lower limb skin traction. *Int J Orthop Trauma Nurs*. 2018;29:54–57.

Falaschi P, Marsh D, eds. *Orthogeriatrics. The management of older patients with fragility fractures*. 2nd ed. Cham, Switzerland: Springer; 2021. Open access ebook.. https://link.springer.com/book/10.1007/978-3-030-48126-1.

Gay C, Chabaud A, Guilley E, Coudeyre E. Educating patients about the benefits of physical activity and activity for their hip and knee osteoarthritis: systematic literature review. *Ann Phys Rehabil Med*. 2016;59(3):174–183.

Gray B, Santy-Tomlinson J. The Thomas' splint: application and patient care. *Int J Orthop Trauma Nurs*. 2018;30:20–22.

Health and Safety Executive (HSE). *Manual Handling: Manual Handling Operations Regulations 1992 – Guidance on Regulations*. London: Health and Safety Executive; 2016.

Hertz K, Santy-Tomlinson J. Fragility Hip Fracture In: Clarke, S. Drozd, M, eds. *Orthopaedic and Trauma Nursing: An evidence-based approach to musculoskeletal care*. 2nd ed. Wiley-Blackwell. Oxford; 2023:268–287.

Jeraj S, Butt J. Musculoskeletal conditions and Black, Asian and minority ethnic people: addressing health inequalities. *Race Equality Foundation*. 2020. https://raceequalityfoundation.org.uk/wp-content/uploads/2022/10/MSK-Report-Addressing-Health-Inequalities.pdf.

Jester R, Flynn S, Drozd M. Elective orthopaedic surgery. In: Clarke S, Drozd M, eds. *Orthopaedic and Trauma Nursing: An Evidence-Based Approach to Musculoskeletal Care*. 2nd ed. Oxford: Wiley–Blackwell; 2022:180–200.

Jester R, Santy-Tomlinson J, Rogers J. *Oxford Handbook of Orthopaedic and Trauma Nursing*. 2nd ed. Oxford: Oxford University Press; 2021.

Kamper S, Apeldoorn A, Chiarotte A, et al. Multidisciplinary biopsychosocial rehabilitation for chronic low back pain. *BMJ*. 2015;350:h444.

Kaye AD, Urman RD, Cornett EM, et al. Enhanced recovery pathways in orthopedic surgery. *J Anaesthesiol Clin Pharmacol*. 2019;35(Suppl 1):S35–S39. doi:10.4103/joacp.JOACP_.

Large P. A 'new focus' in casting – an introduction to the concepts of focus rigidity casting. *Orthop Nurs*. 2001;5:176–179.

Maffulli N, Papalia R, Zampogna B, et al. The management of osteomyelitis in the adult. *Surgeon*. 2016;14:345–360.

Maher C, Underwood M, Buchbinder R. Non-specific low back pain. *Lancet.* 2017;389(10070):736–747.

Marsh D et al. The Multidisciplinary Approach to Fragility Fractures Around the World: An Overview. In: Falaschi, P., Marsh, D, eds. *Orthogeriatrics. Practical Issues in Geriatrics.* Springer, Cham. 2021. https://doi.org/10.1007/978-3-030-48126-1_1.

MASCIP (Multidisciplinary Association for Spinal Cord Injury Professionals); 2009. Moving and Handling Patients With Actual or Suspected Spinal Cords Injuries. www.mascip.co.uk, https://www.mascip.co.uk/wp-content/uploads/2015/02/MASCIP-SIA-Guidelines-for-MH-Trainers.pdf.

McHugh G, Conaghan P, McConville M, et al. Promoting self-management in older people with arthritis: preliminary findings of the Northern Ireland Staying Connected Programme. *Musculoskeletal Care.* 2018;16(4):489–493.

Mobasheri A, Batt M. An update on the pathophysiology of osteoarthritis. *Ann Phys Rehabil Med.* 2016;59:333–339.

Murphy C, Mullen E, Hogan K, O'Toole R, Teeling S. Streamlining an existing hip fracture patient pathway in an acute tertiary adult Irish hospital to improve patient experience and outcomes. *Int J Qual Health Care.* 2019;31(Suppl 1):45–51.

Myhre Jensen C, Hertz K, Mauthner O. Orthogeriatric nursing in the emergency and perioperative in-patient setting. In: Hertz K, Santy-Tomlinson J, eds. *Fragility Fracture Nursing. Holistic Care and Management of the Orthogeriatric Patient.* Cham, Switzerland: Springer; 2018:53–66.

Newton-Triggs L, Rogers J, Timms A. Key musculoskeletal interventions. In: Clarke S, Drozd M, eds. *Orthopaedic and Trauma Nursing: An Evidence-Based Approach to Musculoskeletal Care.* 2nd ed. Oxford: Wiley–Blackwell; 2022:86–100.

NHFD (National Hip Fracture Database). Annual Report 2022. 2022. https://www.nhfd.co.uk/2022report.

National Institute for Health and Care Excellence (NICE) 2016. Low back pain and sciatica in over 16s: assessment and management. NICE guideline [NG59]. https://www.nice.org.uk/guidance/ng59.

National Institute for Health and Care Excellence (NICE) 2018. Rheumatoid arthritis in adults: management. NICE guideline [NG100]. https://www.nice.org.uk/guidance/ng100.

National Institute for Health and Care Excellence (NICE) 2022. Osteoarthritis in over 16s: diagnosis and management. Clinical guideline [CG226]. https://www.nice.org.uk/guidance/ng226.

Noel SE, Santos MP, Wright NC. Racial and ethnic disparities in bone health and outcomes in the United States. *J Bone Miner Res.* 2021 Oct;36(10):1881–1905. doi:10.1002/jbmr.4417.

Parsons G, Roberts D. *Osteoarthritis. In: Ryan, S. Nursing Older People with Arthritis and Other Rheumatological Conditions.* Cham: Springer; 2020:3–16.

Primdahl J, Esbensen BA. Rheumatoid arthritis. In: Ryan S, ed. *Nursing Older People with Arthritis and other Rheumatological Conditions.* Cham: Springer; 2020:17–30.

Rasouli M, Rahimi-Movaghar V, Shokraneh F, et al. Surgery for leg and back pain caused by damage to spinal discs. *Cochrane Database Syst Rev.* 2014(9) Art. No. CD010328.

Richardson C, Kulkarni J. A review of the management of phantom limb pain: challenges and solutions. *J Pain Res.* 2017;10:1861–1870.

Rodger, S. Spinal cord injury. In: Clarke S, Drozd, M , eds. Orthopaedic and Trauma Nursing: An Evidence-Based Approach to Musculoskeletal Care. 2nd ed. Oxford: Wiley-Blackwell; 2022:288-303.

Santy-Tomlinson J, Clarke S, Davis P. The complications of musculoskeletal conditions and trauma: preventing harm. In: Clarke S, Drozd M, eds. *Orthopaedic and Trauma Nursing: An Evidence-Based Approach to Musculoskeletal Care.* 2nd ed. Oxford: Wiley-Blackwell; 2022:101–116.

Santy-Tomlinson J, Hertz K. Fragility Fractures. In: Clarke, S. Drozd, M, eds. *Orthopaedic and Trauma Nursing: An evidence-based approach to musculoskeletal care.* 2nd Ed. Wiley-Blackwell. Oxford; 2023:256–267.

Santy-Tomlinson J, Speerin R, Hertz K, et al. Falls and secondary fracture prevention. In: Hertz K, Santy-Tomlinson J, eds. *Fragility Fracture Nursing: Holistic Care and Management of the Orthogeriatric Patient.* Cham, Switzerland: Springer; 2018:27–40.

Santy-Tomlinson J, Vincent M, Glossop N, et al. Calm, irritated or infected? The experience of the inflammatory states and symptoms of pin site infection during eternal fixation: a grounded theory study. *J Clin Nurs.* 2011;20(21–22):3163–3173.

Schober T-L, Abrahamsen C. Patient perspectives on major lower limb amputation – a qualitative systematic review. *Int J Orthop Trauma Nurs.* 2022;46:100958.

Scott H, Hebenton J, Seenan C, Colvin J. Early PPAM aid use post unilateral transtibial amputation is associated with reduced time to prosthetic fitting and finishing rehabilitation. *Physiotherapy.* 2017;103:e1255.

Smith M. Care of patients with acute spinal cord injuries. In: Kneale J, Davis P, eds. *Orthopaedic and Trauma Nursing.* 2nd ed. Edinburgh: Churchill Livingstone; 2004:390–410.

Stradling H. Musculoskeletal oncology over the lifespan. In: Clarke S, Drozd M, eds. *Orthopaedic and Trauma Nursing: An Evidence-Based Approach to Musculoskeletal Care.* 2nd ed. Oxford: Wiley–Blackwell; 2023:201–213.

Tarling M, Aitken E, Lahoti O, et al. Closing the audit loop: the role of a pilot in the development of a fractured neck of femur integrated care pathway. *J Orthop Nurs.* 2002;6(3):130–134.

Timms A, Pugh H. Pin site care: guidance and key recommendations. *Nurs Stand.* 2012;27(1):50–55.

van Oostwaard M. Osteoporosis and the nature of fragility fracture. In: Hertz K, Santy-Tomlinson J, eds. *Fragility Fracture Nursing. Holistic Care and Management of the Orthogeriatric Patient.* Cham, Switzerland: Springer; 2018:1–13.

Further Reading

Clarke S, Drozd M, eds. *Orthopaedic and Trauma Nursing: An Evidence-Based Approach to Musculoskeletal Care.* 2nd ed. Oxford: Wiley Blackwell; 2022.

Jester R, Santy-Tomlinson J, Rogers J. *Oxford Handbook of Orthopaedic and Trauma Nursing.* 2nd ed Oxford: Oxford University Press; 2021.

Marieb EN, Hoehn K. *Human Anatomy and Physiology.* 11th ed. Cambridge: Pearson; 2019.

NICE (National Institute for Health and Care Excellence). Venous thromboembolic diseases: diagnosis, management and thrombophilia testing. NICE guideline [NG158]. 2020. Available at: https://www.nice.org.uk/guidance/ng158.

Useful Websites

Fragility Fracture Network, www.fragilityfracturenetwork.org
MASCIP (Multidisciplinary Association for Spinal Cord Injury Professionals) Guidelines, www.mascip.co.uk
National Osteoporosis Society (NOS), www.nos.org.uk
Sarcoma UK, www.sarcoma.org.uk
Spinal Injuries Association, www.spinal.co.uk
Versus Arthritis, https://versusarthritis.org/

13

Nursing Patients With Blood Disorders

CLARE BUTLER, VICKY MACARTHUR

CHAPTER OUTLINE

Introduction

Disorders of the blood are diverse and the nursing care of a patient with a blood disorder will depend on the type and nature of the condition. They can be acute or chronic and can affect all age groups. Some blood disorders, such as haemophilia, are sex-linked. Others, such as the hereditary haemoglobinopathies, sickle cell disease and thalassaemia, are more prevalent among certain ethnic groups whereas others, such as iron-deficiency anaemia, occur generally. Some blood disorders, such as acute leukaemia, are life-threatening and require urgent treatment. Nursing patients with a blood disorder is challenging and requires expert knowledge and skills in order to ensure individualised, holistic care. This chapter provides a brief overview of the anatomy and physiology of blood and haematopoiesis (blood cell production) (see Further Reading, e.g. Tortora and Derrickson 2023).

Disorders of blood, investigations and treatments are also described with a focus on nursing management and health promotion.

Anatomy and Physiology

The haematological system comprises the blood, bone marrow and lymphoid tissue. The three primary functions of blood include:
- Transportation of oxygen, carbon dioxide, essential nutrients, enzymes and hormones. Blood also carries waste products to the excretory organs.
- Regulation of water, electrolyte and acid–base balance and body temperature.
- Protection against infection. As blood contains coagulation factors, it also protects the body from excessive blood loss.

All blood cells originate from pluripotent haematopoietic stem cells. Stem cells are capable of self-renewal, proliferation and differentiation into separate cell lineages, which give rise to distinct blood cell populations. This multistep process, known as haematopoiesis, is stimulated and regulated by a range of cytokines, hormones and growth factors including erythropoietin, thrombopoietin, colony-stimulating factors (CSFs) and interleukins (Hoffbrand et al. 2019).

Blood cells have a limited lifespan and an estimated 100 billion new blood cells are required daily in order to maintain a healthy, steady state (Huether and McCance 2019). Consequently, haematopoiesis is a continual process which takes place in different anatomical sites throughout the lifespan. These include the embryonic yolk sac, the fetal liver and spleen, and all bone marrow during infancy. From childhood onwards, red bone marrow is progressively replaced with fat. In adults haematopoiesis occurs primarily in the medullary cavity of flat bones. Sites include the:
- ends of the humerus and femur
- pelvis
- vertebrae
- ribs
- sternum
- skull.

Additional sites may be recruited when there is an increased demand for blood cells, such as in the case of illness.

Blood constantly circulates around the body and the normal total blood volume depends on the size of the individual, for example, 5–6 L in an average adult male. Blood is composed of both cellular and fluid elements.

Cellular Components of Blood

The three main cellular components of blood are:
- erythrocytes (red blood cells)
- leucocytes (white blood cells)
- thrombocytes (platelets).

Erythrocytes (Red Blood Cells)

Erythrocytes, the most numerous of all blood cell types in the blood, constitute approximately 40% of total blood volume. Biconcave in shape, erythrocytes are responsible for the transportation of oxygen to the tissues and some carbon dioxide to the lungs. Haemoglobin, the oxygen-carrying molecule contained within the cell, contributes to a third of its weight and gives blood its characteristic red colour. Iron is an essential component of haemoglobin. Erythrocytes are soft and pliable, allowing them to travel easily through capillaries, and their thin cellular membrane facilitates gaseous exchange between the cell and surrounding tissues.

The total number of circulating erythrocytes remains fairly stable at $3.8–6.5 \times 10^{12}$ cells/L, with women having fewer than men. Erythropoietin has a vital role in the regulation of red cell production (erythropoiesis) and is produced mainly by the kidneys in response to tissue hypoxia. During maturation, the erythrocyte synthesises haemoglobin and extrudes its nucleus, thereby rendering the mature cell incapable of reproduction, repair, growth or haemoglobin production (Fig. 13.1). The average lifespan of a red blood cell (RBC) is 120 days, after which it is sequestered in the spleen where it is destroyed by the phagocytic cells of the reticuloendothelial system (also known as mononuclear–phagocytic system).

Leucocytes (White Blood Cells)

Leucocytes or white blood cells (WBCs), of which there are several distinct types, make up approximately 1% of blood volume and are instrumental in defending the body against infection. The total number of WBCs is between 4.0 and 11.0×10^9 cells/L. Leucocyte maturation is regulated by specific haematopoietic growth factors such as granulocyte colony-stimulating factor (GCSF), and their lifespan will vary according to type (Fig. 13.2). For example, neutrophils circulate for about 7–8 hours in the blood before migrating into the tissues, where they die after a few days. Lymphocytes may live from 100 days to several years, whereas macrophages can survive for many years.

Leucocytes are classified according to their structure as either granulocytes or nongranulocytes or in relation to their function (phagocytes or immunocytes).

Granulocytes. These cells contain enzyme-rich granules within their cytoplasm, which assist with phagocytosis (the process of engulfing and destroying harmful substances) and inflammatory and immune functions. Subtypes of granulocytes include neutrophils, eosinophils and basophils (the polymorphonuclear cells). (See Appendix for the normal numbers of each type.)

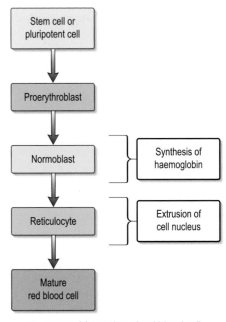

Figure 13.1 Maturation of red blood cells.

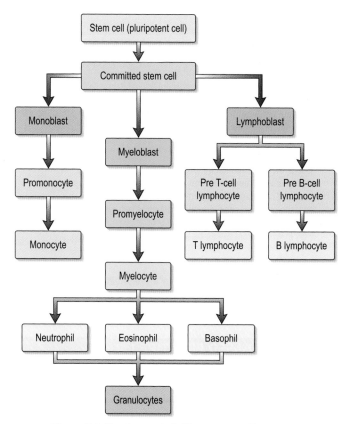

Figure 13.2 Development of different types of leucocyte.

Neutrophils are the largest component of the WBC population, and the primary phagocytes of infection control. These cells spend 8–10 hours in circulation before migrating to the tissues where they are responsible for nonspecific defence against bacterial and fungal infections.

Eosinophils circulate in the peripheral blood for approximately 5 hours. Phagocytic eosinophils exit to the tissues where they are responsible for defence against infestation by parasites. Eosinophils also have a role in allergic responses (see Chapter 7).

Basophils comprise the smallest number of WBCs. Basophils and mast cells contain heparin and histamine and are involved in anaphylactic, hypersensitivity and inflammatory responses (see Chapter 7, Nursing Patients With Disorders of the Lymphatic and Immune Systems).

Agranulocytes. These WBCs have a large nucleus and, as their name suggests, do not contain granules in their cytoplasm. They include monocytes and lymphocytes, both of which perform a range of protective functions. (See Appendix for the normal numbers of each type).

Monocytes. The largest of the WBCs, monocytes start as immature macrophages which are present in the blood for 20–40 hours before travelling to tissue sites where they mature into powerful phagocytes. Tissue macrophages also process and present antigens to lymphoid cells and play a role in the production of cytokines and growth factors important for haematopoiesis, inflammation and cellular responses (Mehta and Hoffbrand 2014).

Lymphocytes are the chief cells of the immune response and make up approximately 36% of total leucocyte count. Lymphocytes mature in either bone marrow (B lymphocytes or B cells) or the thymus gland (T lymphocytes or T cells). B lymphocytes

are responsible for antibody-mediated (humoral) immunity while T lymphocytes play an integral role in specific cell-mediated (cellular) immunity (see Chapter 7). Natural killer (NK) cells are a subset of lymphocytes which share many features of cytotoxic T cells, a type of T lymphocytes.

Thrombocytes (Platelets)
Platelets are very small, non-nucleated cell fragments that play a vital role in haemostasis (arrest of bleeding). The normal platelet count is $140–400 \times 10^9$/L.

Originating from the pluripotent stem cell, these cells differentiate and mature into megakaryocytes, which then fragment to form platelets. Platelets are involved in the first three phases of haemostasis, but not the final phase:
- vasoconstriction of the injured vessel
- formation of a platelet plug
- coagulation – formation of a fibrin clot
- fibrinolysis – dissolution of the fibrin clot.

Information about blood coagulation factors and haemostasis is available on the companion website.

About one-third of platelets are stored in the spleen, from which they are released in response to cellular damage or injury. Platelets survive for about 10 days before being destroyed by macrophages.

Plasma
Plasma comprises 50%–55% of total blood volume and is a straw-coloured aqueous solution containing plasma proteins, i.e. albumin, globulins and fibrinogen. It also contains inorganic ions that regulate cell function, blood pH and osmotic pressure. These ions include sodium, potassium, chloride, phosphate, magnesium and calcium. Small amounts of nutrients, waste products, drugs, hormones and gases are also present in plasma.

Blood Groups
ABO Blood Groups
RBCs have specific inherited antigens (also known as agglutinogens) on their membrane. These are important in terms of defining the ABO blood group classification system and a person can possess the A or B antigen, neither, or both. As such there are four main blood groups: A, B, AB and O.

A person with the antigen A (blood group A) has anti-B antibodies (also called agglutinins) in the plasma whereas a person with antigen B (blood group B) has the anti-A antibodies. A person with both antigens A and B (blood group AB) has no antibodies in the plasma, whilst a person with neither A nor B antigens (blood group O) has both anti-A and anti-B antibodies in the plasma (Table 13.1).

TABLE 13.1 Antigens and Antibodies Present in ABO Blood Groups

ABO Blood Group	Antigen on Red Blood Cell Membrane	Antibodies Present in the Plasma
A	A	Anti-B
B	B	Anti-A
AB	A and B	None
O	None	Anti-A and anti-B

The importance of the A and B antigens is evident when one person receives blood from another. If a person receives a transfusion of ABO-incompatible blood, the transfused red cells will clump together (agglutinate) and break down (haemolyse), which may be fatal. Thus if the recipient's plasma contains anti-B antibody, they must only receive blood from a group A or O donor.

WBCs and platelets also possess ABO antigens. Therefore if a patient is to receive a transfusion of other cellular components, the correct blood group must also be used.

The recipients and donor ABO group are also taken into consideration when transfusing plasma and where possible matched.

The RhD Factor
In the UK, 85% of the population have a second important class of antigen present on their red cells: the Rh (previously referred to as Rhesus) D factor. Thus a person may be either RhD-positive or RhD-negative.

The antibody, anti-D, does not occur naturally in the plasma of RhD-negative blood, but stimulation to produce it can occur if a RhD-negative person receives a RhD-positive blood transfusion or if, during pregnancy or childbirth, RBCs from a RhD-positive fetus cross the placental barrier into the circulation of a RhD-negative woman. In these circumstances later exposure to RhD-positive RBCs will result in agglutination and haemolysis. Blood products to be transfused must therefore be carefully cross-matched for the RhD factor as well as ABO groups.

Other Blood Groups
In addition to the ABO and RhD factor blood groupings there are several further blood classification systems, for example, Duffy, Kell and other Rh antigens. These do not usually cause agglutination unless multiple blood transfusions are required, in which case it would be essential to check that donor blood is compatible with the recipient's blood serum antibodies.

(See Further Reading, e.g. Daniels and Bromilow 2013.)

Blood Transfusion

Blood transfusion, the administration of whole blood or blood products donated by one person to another, makes it possible to save lives. Transfusion does, however, expose patients to the risk of potentially fatal complications, for example, TACO (transfusion-associated circulatory overload), infection, haemolytic reactions or receiving an incompatible unit of blood (Reflection 13.1). Evidence-Based Practice 13.1 provides an opportunity for you to consider how nurses can improve safety during transfusion.

🌐 **See Evolve website Critical thinking question 13.1**

Many people who require blood transfusions fear being infected with a transmittable disease, such as HIV, hepatitis or variant Creutzfeldt–Jakob disease (vCJD). It is therefore necessary that the screening procedures undertaken on all blood donors and the testing and processing of donated blood are explained. For instance, in the UK, white cells are routinely removed from donated blood to minimise the risk of transmitting vCJD. Some religious groups such as Jehovah's Witnesses may refuse blood transfusions while others may wish to consult family and religious leaders before giving consent. In this case, where the need for a blood transfusion is required to treat anaemia, erythropoietin can be given (NICE 2015). The blood transfusion products readily available are listed in Table 13.2.

Before a patient receives a transfusion of a blood product their blood is grouped. The donated blood is then tested for compatibility with that of the recipient. The donor's blood should be of the same ABO blood group and a RhD-negative recipient should receive RhD-negative blood products. Details of the cross-matching are recorded along with the blood unit number on the documentation sent with the unit of blood. After the transfusion, this documentation is retained in case of a transfusion reaction. Patients may be able to donate their own red cells prior to elective surgery. This is known as an autologous transfusion and avoids the risks associated with allogeneic blood transfusions.

(See Further Reading, e.g. Brown and Cutler 2012.)

TABLE 13.2	Blood Transfusion Products Available	
Product	Indications for Use	Special Points
Whole blood (infrequently given)	Acute, severe bleeding requiring replacement of red blood cells and plasma and coagulation factors	Stored at 4°C for up to 35 days Platelets and coagulation factors have much reduced viability
Fresh whole blood (infrequently given)	As above	Blood <24 h old, therefore more likely to contain viable coagulation factors
Red cell concentrate	Replacement of red blood cells only. Therefore used when haemoglobin level is low	Up to 200 mL plasma removed per 500 mL blood
Washed red cells	As for red cell concentrate Specially prepared to remove antigens	Prevents anaphylactic transfusion reactions
Frozen red cells	As for red cell concentrate	Storage lifespan lengthened, therefore useful for rare blood groups
Platelet concentrate	Patients with platelet count $<20 \times 10^9$ cells/L but not actively bleeding	Platelet units from blood banks contain platelets from many units of blood, therefore there are frequent reactions. Patients may require i.v. hydrocortisone plus i.v. chlorphenamine prior to transfusion. Stored at 20°C. Viability of platelet concentrate only 24 h. Never place in fridge
Other Blood Components		
Fresh frozen plasma	Hereditary or acquired bleeding disorder Volume replacement Liver disease Disseminated intravascular coagulation (DIC)	Frozen within 6 h of cell separation and viable for 1 year. Once thawed, use within 30 min
Cryoprecipitate (factor VIII, fibrinogen)	Haemophilia	From fresh frozen plasma Last part to thaw is cryoprecipitate
Factor VIII	Haemophilia A	From fresh frozen powder (half-life 12 h)
Factor IX	Haemophilia B (Christmas disease)	
Human immunoglobulin	Passive immunity, especially immunosuppressed patients	
Albumin solution	Hypoproteinaemic oedema, ascites, acute volume replacement	

DISORDERS OF THE BLOOD

The following sections address a range of blood disorders affecting RBCs, WBCs and platelets. Although the specific responsibilities of nurses caring for patients with blood disorders will depend on their particular role and workplace setting, key elements will include:
- detecting and monitoring signs of illness and response to treatment
- assisting with medical investigations
- administering treatment and supportive therapies
- providing information and patient education
- health promotion regarding nutrition, lifestyle and the prevention of complications
- assessment and management of pain
- implementing strategies aimed at infection prevention and control
- providing emotional support and reassurance
- liaising with and making referrals to multidisciplinary health team members.

Investigations Used in the Diagnosis of Blood Disorders

A range of investigations are used for the diagnosis of blood disorders. Specific tests will depend on the nature of the suspected disorder but may include:

Blood Tests

- Full blood count (FBC) – to establish the total number of red cells, white cells and platelets.
- Haemoglobin concentration – a level 10% below normal is considered indicative of anaemia.
- Packed cell volume (PCV) or haematocrit – the volume of RBCs expressed as a percentage of the total volume of blood.
- Reticulocyte (immature RBCs) count – a small percentage are normally present in the blood, but a larger percentage may indicate increased bone marrow activity if the red cell count is low.
- Mean cell volume (MCV) – measures the average red cell volume.
- Mean cell haemoglobin (MCH) – measures the average haemoglobin concentration.
- Erythrocyte sedimentation rate (ESR) – measures the rate of fall of red cells in plasma left standing for an hour.
- Ferritin (an iron storage protein) – measures the amount of iron stores.
- Vitamin B_{12} and folate.

Blood Film

This is the examination of blood cells under a microscope to examine cell morphology in order to detect abnormalities in their size, structure or shape.

Bone Marrow Aspiration and Trephine Biopsy

This involves the removal of a small amount of bone marrow from the posterior iliac crest or sternum. This is mounted on slides and stained for microscopic examination. This test is not done routinely but is indicated if there is evidence of severe anaemia or of another blood disorder such as aplastic anaemia or leukaemia (Information 13.1).

Other Investigative Techniques

These include cytogenetic studies, immunophenotyping and molecular studies which assist in the detection of chromosomal and genetic abnormalities and are important prognostic indicators for many haematological malignancies.

Disorders of Red Blood Cells – Anaemias (General Aspects)

Anaemias are a complex group of blood disorders found in all age groups resulting from a reduction in the number of RBCs and/or haemoglobin concentration in the blood (Fig. 13.3). Defined by the World Health Organisation (WHO 2011) as haemoglobin level less than 130 g/L in males over 15 years of age, less than 120 g/L in nonpregnant females over 15 years and children aged 12–14 years, and less than 101 g/L in pregnancy, anaemia may be caused by:

- decreased red cell production
- excessive destruction of red cells
- chronic or acute blood loss.

Anaemia may be the primary presenting illness or may occur secondary to another condition such as cancer, chronic renal failure or an inherited disorder of haemoglobin synthesis. Anaemia may also be acquired due to environmental, iatrogenic or nutritional factors.

INFORMATION 13.1
Bone Marrow Aspiration

Purposes

- Diagnosis – to examine cell populations and thus determine the type of anaemia, leukaemia or lymphoma.
- Monitoring – to assess the progress of disease and response to treatment.

Sites

Red bone marrow is found in the cavities of the flat bones of the adult, for example skull, clavicle, scapula and iliac crest. The site usually chosen (for ease of access to minimise trauma to nearby structures) is the iliac crest – left and right, anterior and posterior.

The Nurse's Role

The patient may be anxious about this investigation, especially if there is awareness that the results may show a malignant condition. This anxiety may be heightened if the patient has been talking with others who have undergone the procedure.

Providing the patient with information on all aspects of the test – the use of premedication and local anaesthetic, the site to be used, the degree of discomfort to be expected, the time that it will take and when the results will be reported – will help to reduce anxiety.

It is the policy of some doctors, especially where repeated aspiration will be required, to give a sedative such as lorazepam or a light general anaesthetic. The individual may undergo the procedure as an outpatient, inpatient or as a day case. Whatever the setting, the nurse's role will include:

- Assessing the patient's understanding of the test and providing more information if necessary.
- Ensuring that the patient's platelet count has been checked prior to the procedure and that the results are available.
- Preparing the equipment.
- Ensuring that the patient is comfortable and is positioned correctly.
- Observing the patient throughout the procedure and drawing attention to any change in condition.
- Assisting the doctor.
- Applying a pressure dressing and making the patient comfortable after the procedure.
- Inspecting the aspiration site frequently for signs of haemorrhage or haematoma formation.
- Documenting the patient's response to the procedure.
- Preparing the patient for discharge by explaining care of puncture site, what discomfort may be expected, who to contact if ill-effects arise, when results will be available and timing of the next appointment.

Possible Complications

- Haemorrhage – the patient's platelet count should be checked before aspiration.
- Infection.

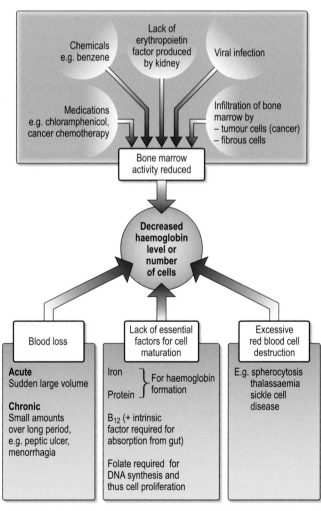

Figure 13.3 Main types of anaemia.

Interestingly, many people are diagnosed with anaemia by chance when they seek medical advice for an unrelated symptom or during a routine medical examination.

Pathophysiology

Anaemia arises when the oxygen-carrying capacity of the RBCs is reduced. Symptoms stem from a lack of oxygen in the tissues and are primarily due to compensatory mechanisms that occur in response to hypoxia (reduced levels of oxygen in the tissues). The severity of symptoms will depend on the haemoglobin concentration of the RBC and the ability of the person to adapt to a lower oxygen concentration.

Clinical Presentation

The clinical presentation of anaemia is diverse and each type of anaemia has specific attributes. However, features common to all types include:

- tiredness and lethargy
- pallor
- breathlessness
- palpitations
- tachycardia
- dizziness, fainting and dimness of vision
- headache and lack of concentration
- angina and/or intermittent claudication.

Medical Management

History and Examination

A diagnosis of anaemia requires a thorough patient assessment. A detailed history, looking at the patient's past and present health and lifestyle, should be undertaken. It is important to identify the use of medications such as aspirin or phenytoin as these may contribute to anaemia. Assessing the person's social circumstances and nutritional intake is also important.

Physical examination may reveal:

- pallor of the skin and mucous membranes
- signs of complications of anaemia such as jaundice, dyspnoea and cardiac failure
- bleeding
- changes to hair and skin texture or pigmentation
- signs of underlying disease or conditions such as cancer or pregnancy.

Investigations

An FBC will be taken for, haemoglobin level, MCV, MCH, and PCV. If this indicates anaemia iron studies will then be done including serum iron and a blood film. Bone marrow aspiration is not undertaken routinely but is indicated if the anaemia is severe.

Treatment

Treatment will depend on the cause, type and severity of anaemia. Some patients may need to be hospitalised but most can be treated in the community with medication, dietary and lifestyle changes and health education. The underlying cause of the anaemia must also be treated. Blood transfusions may be needed either initially or repeatedly over a period of time. Follow-up care for all anaemic patients is important to encourage and monitor compliance with medication and to prevent recurrence and long-term adverse effects.

❖ Nursing Management and Health Promotion: Anaemia

Patients may experience some general problems common to most anaemias in addition to those specific to their type of anaemia.

This section outlines the nursing management of general problems. The specific problems and nursing management are discussed in subsequent sections. It is vital that the patient is treated as an individual and that care is holistic. A nursing assessment of the patient's background, lifestyle, illness, needs and goals should be undertaken, after which a care plan will be agreed.

General Problems Associated With Anaemia

Tiredness

Patients may tire easily because of hypoxia. It is important that their daily routine in hospital or at home includes periods of rest. If cardiac failure is evident, the patient may need to be nursed in bed or in a chair. The nurse should be aware of the potential problems of immobility, paying particular attention to pressure areas and the prevention of venous thromboembolism (VTE). Assistance with personal hygiene and dressing may also be needed. Patients should be reassured that their tiredness is not imaginary but is part of the anaemia and that it will lessen as treatment progresses.

Breathlessness

Breathlessness may be mild, occurring only on exertion, or it may be a major problem causing considerable distress and debility. Nursing priorities will focus on ensuring maximum perfusion of oxygen to the tissues and reducing the patient's distress. These can be achieved by nursing the patient in an upright position, administering oxygen as prescribed, explaining to the patient the reason for the breathlessness and giving reassurance that it will lessen as the anaemia improves.

Nutrition

The anaemic patient will require a high-protein diet which includes all the nutrients necessary for red cell production (see Erythrocytes [red blood cells]). Breathlessness, a lack of energy to shop and prepare food, a sore mouth and dysphagia may all contribute to anorexia. A sore mouth can be especially distressing and the nurse will need to carry out an oral assessment using an appropriate assessment tool. Care should include not only that which will improve and heal the mouth but also relevant health education about oral hygiene including teeth cleaning and/or care of dentures, mouthwashes and lip care.

Patients who have a poor understanding of nutrition may need referral to a dietitian or specialist nutritional nurse for specific guidance about nutrition and diet.

Safety

Faintness, light-headedness and sensitivity to cold make the anaemic patient prone to injury. As the body responds to poor oxygenation by preserving the blood supply to the essential organs, anaemic patients will have poor peripheral circulation and, consequently, fragile skin. The reduced attention span typical of anaemic patients will also make them vulnerable to falls, minor injuries and hypothermia. Anaemic patients should be warned against changing position suddenly, especially from lying to standing, and should be given instruction on first aid for minor injuries and on the prevention of hypothermia.

Skin Integrity

The anaemic patient's reduced oxygen and nutrient supply to the skin increases the risk of pressure ulcers. Hypoxic skin will not necessarily break down quickly, but if damaged it will take longer than usual to heal. An initial and continuing assessment of all pressure areas should be undertaken using appropriate risk assessment tools.

Once the patient's level of risk of developing pressure ulcers has been determined, it is important to instigate appropriate interventions. These will include ensuring that the patient's position is changed regularly, the use of appropriate pressure-relieving devices and instructing the patient about the importance of moving regularly (European Pressure Ulcer Advisory Panel, National Pressure Injury Advisory Panel and Pan Pacific Pressure Injury Alliance [EPUAP/NPIAP/PPPIA] 2019).

Anxiety and Communication

Prior to diagnosis, the anaemic patient may fear the presence of a life-threatening illness, particularly if frightening symptoms such as breathlessness, palpitations and chronic headaches have been experienced. The disorientation and confusion arising from cerebral hypoxia can be distressing. Explanation of the causes of these symptoms and reassurance that they should improve as the anaemia responds to treatment may help to reduce the anxiety suffered by both the patient and the family.

Specific Anaemias

The section outlines some specific anaemias: iron deficiency, megaloblastic, aplastic, haemolytic, including inherited haemoglobinopathies (sickle cell disease and thalassaemia), and anaemia caused by blood loss.

Iron-Deficiency Anaemia

In 2019 there were 1.8 billion cases of anaemia globally (of a global population of 7.7 billion) with iron deficiency being one of the largest causes (Global Health Metrics 2019).

Pathophysiology

Iron is a constituent of haemoglobin and is essential for cellular function and erythropoiesis. Iron-deficiency anaemia arises when the absorption of iron from food does not meet the daily requirements. This may be due to chronic blood loss (discussed more fully on Section: Anaemia Resulting from Chronic Blood Loss) or malabsorption, although the most common cause is inadequate dietary intake (Mehta and Hoffbrand 2014).

Clinical Presentation

As the onset of iron-deficiency anaemia is usually very gradual, the patient may not seek medical attention until sometime after symptoms appear. The most common presenting features are tiredness and pallor, although any of the other general symptoms of anaemia (see Disorders of Red Blood Cells – Anaemia [general aspects], sub section, Clinical Presentation) may be apparent. Signs and symptoms specific to iron-deficiency anaemia include:
- glossitis – a smooth, sore tongue
- hair brittleness and thinning
- angular cheilosis – maceration at the angles of the mouth
- koilonychia – spoon-shaped (concave) and brittle nails
- pica – a strong desire to eat unusual substances such as ice or coal.

Medical Management

History and Examination

The patient may give a history suggestive of inadequate iron intake or chronic blood loss, for example, menorrhagia or bleeding from the gastrointestinal tract. Examination may reveal general signs of anaemia.

Investigations

Blood samples will be taken for tests, such as FBC, haemoglobin level, MCV, MCH, blood film, serum iron and total iron-binding capacity (TIBC). Estimates of ferritin (an iron storage protein) measure iron stores and a subnormal level is caused by iron deficiency (Watson et al. 2022). Other investigations such as faecal occult blood (FOB) testing, endoscopy or barium studies may be undertaken to establish the cause of the deficiency. Adults over 60 or those under 50 with rectal bleeding should be referred using a suspected cancer pathway for an appointment within 2 weeks.

Treatment

If dietary changes are insufficient to correct the anaemia, oral iron (ferrous salts) supplements, usually ferrous sulphate, will be prescribed. Medication is typically continued for 3 months after the haemoglobin level has returned to normal to replenish iron stores. Side-effects, which include constipation, nausea, abdominal pain and diarrhoea, often lead to poor compliance with medication and these should be explained to the patient. Intramuscular iron injections are usually given only where there is proven malabsorption syndrome or poor compliance. If the anaemia is very severe (less than 7 g/dL) blood transfusions may be required.

❖ Nursing Management and Health Promotion: Iron-Deficiency Anaemia

Many of the nursing considerations for the general care of anaemic patients (see Section: Nursing Management and Health Promotion: Anaemia) are relevant for iron-deficiency anaemia. Other nursing management strategies will focus on patient education and discharge planning with an emphasis on health promotion.

Patient Education and Health Promotion

Helping the patient to understand the disorder will assist in promoting compliance with treatment. Information about foods that are rich in available iron should be given and advice on selecting and budgeting for a well-balanced diet may also be needed (Reflection 13.2). Assessing the patient's perception of the problem, level of knowledge and sociocultural background can help to ensure that the advice offered is relevant and comprehensible. Referral to a social worker may also be appropriate.

Clear instructions should be given to reinforce the prescriber's directions regarding medication. Patients should also be made aware that ferrous salts of iron cause blackened stools and discolouration of the urine.

If inpatient treatment has been required the following should be discussed with the patient and family/carers before discharge:
- conditions at home and the availability of support services if family or friends are unable to help
- the importance of follow-up appointments with health professionals
- the importance of taking prescribed medication.

In older people, there is often a link between recent bereavement and the onset of iron-deficiency anaemia, as loneliness, grief and depression may lead to self-neglect. Such patients should have the necessary follow-up and support from the health visitor, social worker or bereavement support counsellor.

Nutrition and the Prevention of Iron-Deficiency Anaemia

Tom is 45 years old and has been diagnosed with iron-deficiency anaemia. He tells you that he works as a long-distance lorry driver and is often away from home for long periods of time. Subsequently he does not eat regular meals and most of his diet comprises chips, sweets and take-away meals.

You have been asked to provide Tom with advice about his diet and improving his intake of iron-rich foods.

Activity

- Access the *Food Fact Sheet – Iron* on the British Dietetics Association website (see below) and consider the following issues:
  - foods rich in iron
  - absorption of iron
  - the role of vitamin C in iron absorption
  - foods and beverages that inhibit iron absorption
  - suggestions for meals and snacks.
- Consider the advice that you would give to Tom about his diet. Plan some iron-rich meals and snacks that fit into Tom's work pattern.

Resource

https://www.bda.uk.com/resource/iron-rich-foods-iron-deficiency.html

Anaemia Resulting From Chronic Blood Loss

Iron-deficiency anaemia may result from blood loss. This may either be:

- acute – the loss of a large volume of blood over a short period of time, as in haemorrhage (Chapters 19, The Deteriorating Patient, Recognising and Managing Shock, and Chapter 26, Nursing the Patient Who Experiences Trauma), or
- chronic – the loss of small amounts of blood over an extended period of time.

Chronic blood loss, which will be addressed in this section, is not uncommon and may present secondary to a number of other disorders. Frequently, it is only when a diagnosis of iron-deficiency anaemia has been established that the underlying cause is suspected. The most common causes of chronic blood loss are listed in Information 13.2.

Pathophysiology

It is unlikely that the ill-effects of chronic blood loss will be noticed until it has caused depletion of the body's iron stores. The pathophysiology is similar to that of iron-deficiency anaemia caused by poor dietary intake of iron (see Specific Anaemias, subsection: Iron Deficiency Anaemia).

Clinical Presentation

In addition to those of iron deficiency anaemia, clinical features of anaemia occurring as a result of blood loss occur in accordance with the underlying disorder. Examples include indigestion, abdominal pain, menorrhagia, weight loss, blood in stools or haematuria.

Medical Management

History and Examination

These are similar to those used for the diagnosis of iron-deficiency anaemia (see Iron Deficiency Anaemia, subsection: Medical Management – History and Examination).

Common Causes of Chronic Blood Loss

Gastrointestinal blood loss is the most common cause in men and postmenopausal women (Liu and Kaffes 2012).

Gastrointestinal Bleeding (see Chapter 4)

- Gastritis – excessive alcohol intake, drugs such as NSAIDs and aspirin
- Peptic ulceration – infection with the bacterium *Helicobacter pylori*, corticosteroid therapy
- Oesophageal varices (blood loss may be acute)
- Inflammatory bowel disease
- Diverticulitis
- Gastric or colorectal cancer
- Intestinal parasites such as hookworm infestations are important causes worldwide

Genitourinary Bleeding (see Chapters 9 and 10)

- Menorrhagia (heavy regular menstrual flow) – a common cause
- Haematuria – bladder cancer

Respiratory Bleeding (see Chapter 3)

- Chronic haemoptysis – lung cancer, tuberculosis, bronchiectasis, pulmonary infarction.

Reference

Liu K, Kaffes AJ. Iron deficiency anaemia: a review of diagnosis, investigation and management. *Eur J Gastroenterol Hepatol*. 2012;24(2):109–116.

Investigations

These are as for the diagnosis of iron-deficiency anaemia (see Iron Deficiency Anaemia, subsection, Medical Management – Investigations).

Treatment

Treatment will depend on the specific cause of the blood loss; however, treatment options include oral iron preparations to replenish iron stores and possibly blood transfusion.

Nursing Management and Health Promotion: Anaemia Due to Chronic Blood Loss

The patient may be feeling apprehensive and frightened, and providing clear information about investigations, especially invasive procedures such as endoscopy (see Chapter 4, Nursing Patients With Gastrointestinal, Liver and Biliary Disorders), may help to alleviate anxiety. Information should address any pre-investigative preparation such as fasting, approximate durations of tests and what they will involve. It is also important to discuss whether the patient will be fit to return home unaccompanied after investigative procedures and when the results can be expected.

When planning care, the nurse must prioritise the patient's needs and be sensitive to their individual values and perceptions. Comprehensive assessment will help to establish the cause of bleeding and this will incorporate sensitive questioning, observation, monitoring of vital signs and discussion with the patient's family and friends as appropriate.

Megaloblastic Anaemias

Megaloblastic anaemias are characterised by large, immature and dysfunctional RBCs (megaloblasts) in the bone marrow.

Pathophysiology

Megaloblastic anaemias are due to defective DNA synthesis, commonly caused by a deficiency of either:
- vitamin B_{12} (cobalamins), or
- folates (group of B vitamins).

Although in these conditions the haemoglobin content of the cells is typically normal, the defective cells have a considerably reduced lifespan, which decreases their numbers in the bloodstream resulting in anaemia.

Vitamin B_{12} Deficiency

As vitamin B_{12} is found predominantly in meat, eggs and dairy products, vegans are at particular risk; however, the most common cause of vitamin B_{12} deficiency is malabsorption due to pernicious anaemia. This condition, caused by autoimmune gastritis, occurs when the gastric mucosa atrophies, resulting in a failure to produce intrinsic factors required for vitamin B_{12} absorption. Whilst predominantly a disease associated with older age, deficiency in younger people is increasing due to the popularity of vegan diets and the recreational use of nitrous oxide which inactivates vitamin B_{12}. Table 13.3 outlines other causes.

Folate Deficiency

Folates are found in green leafy vegetables, potatoes, fruits, fortified breakfast cereals and bread, liver, milk and dairy products and yeast extract. Deficiency is commonly due to an inadequate dietary intake of folic acid. (See Table 13.3 for other causes.) This may occur either alone or in conjunction with a condition such as pregnancy, in which folate utilisation is increased. Fetal abnormalities, for example, neural tube defects (NTDs), are associated with inadequate folate intake around the time of conception and during the first few weeks of pregnancy.

Clinical Presentation

As vitamin B_{12} and folic acid are essential for all dividing cells, a deficiency of these not only affects RBCs but also the gastrointestinal epithelium, leading to glossitis, anorexia, diarrhoea and malabsorption. In addition to these and other general signs of anaemia, megaloblastic anaemia may cause mild jaundice and skin pigmentation.

Pernicious anaemia develops gradually so the condition may be very advanced when treatment is sought. Because vitamin B_{12} is important for myelin production, up to 40% of people with this deficiency may develop spinal cord damage or peripheral nerve problems causing:
- paraesthesia
- coldness or numbness in limbs
- ataxia
- atrophy of optic nerve
- dementia.

Medical Management

History and Examination

History and examination are similar to that for anaemia (see Disorders of Red Blood Cells – Anaemias [general aspects] subsection: Medical Management – History and Examination). However, if megaloblastic anaemia is suspected the doctor will

TABLE 13.3	Causes of the Megaloblastic Anaemias
Type	**Causes**
Folate deficiency	Inadequate dietary intake Malabsorption • disease of small bowel, e.g. coeliac disease, extensive surgical resection of small bowel • alcohol misuse Increased demands • very active cell proliferation, e.g. in haemolytic anaemia or leukaemia • pregnancy Excessive loss • heart failure • long-term dialysis Drugs • the cytotoxic drug methotrexate • antiepileptic medications, e.g. phenytoin • oral contraceptive
Vitamin B_{12} deficiency	Inadequate vitamin B_{12} in diet (especially vegans) Malabsorption • reduced gastric acid (hypochlorhydria) • gastric surgery • pernicious anaemia caused by autoimmune gastritis that leads to gastric atrophy and intrinsic factor deficiency • pancreatic insufficiency • inflammatory disease of terminal ileum where vitamin B_{12} is absorbed, e.g. Crohn's disease • small bowel resection involving the ileum Drugs • recreational use of nitrous oxide inactivates vitamin B_{12} • metformin affects intestinal mobility • proton pump inhibitors and histamine 2 receptor antagonists (H2RA) affect release of vitamin B_{12} from proteins within ingested food • alcohol impairs absorption from the intestine

be alert to a history of gastrointestinal surgery, alcohol misuse or epilepsy and to the specific features identified in Clinical Presentation.

Investigations

Blood tests will be similar to those for the diagnosis of iron-deficiency anaemia. Additional specific diagnostic blood tests for megaloblastic anaemia include serum B_{12} levels and folate assays. Other investigations may include:
- gastric parietal cell antibodies
- Schilling test (to determine cobalamin absorption)
- endoscopy
- bone marrow aspiration (see Information 13.1)
- neurological examination (see Chapter 11, Nursing Patients With Disorders of the Nervous System).

Treatment

Vitamin B_{12} deficiency is usually treated with injections of hydroxycobalamin until blood count improves. Maintenance doses of hydroxycobalamin are usually required every 3 months for life.

Folate deficiency is conventionally treated with oral folic acid, for 4 months. This is usually continued as a weekly maintenance dose if the underlying cause cannot be rectified.

❖ Nursing Management and Health Promotion: Megaloblastic Anaemias

Patients with vitamin B_{12} and intrinsic factor deficiency may need to be admitted to hospital for diagnosis and treatment in the initial stages, but most will be diagnosed by their GP. If the anaemia is not yet advanced, treatment can be started immediately by a community or practice nurse, who will administer prescribed vitamin B_{12} injections. Assistance with personal care and other activities of living may be needed if the patient is experiencing breathlessness or fatigue.

The patient and family should be encouraged to participate in their management, possibly by learning how to administer the hydroxycobalamin injections themselves.

Advanced stages of pernicious anaemia are rarely seen today; however, if cardiac failure and severe neurological problems develop, specific nursing and medical interventions will be required (see Chapter 2, Nursing Patients With Cardiovascular Disorders, and Chapter 11, Nursing Patients With Disorders of the Nervous System).

Health promotion and education regarding a healthy diet, abstinence from alcohol or recreational nitrous oxide use where appropriate, and compliance with medication are nursing priorities when managing patients with folate deficiency anaemia. Patients will need to know which foods contain folic acid, how to shop and budget for these and how to avoid destroying folic acid during food preparation and cooking (see Useful Websites, e.g. British Dietetics Association). An understanding of how to take folic acid supplements correctly is also essential. The importance of follow-up checks should also be emphasised.

Aplastic Anaemia

Aplastic anaemia is a rare and life-threatening condition. It manifests when haematopoietic stem cells in the bone marrow fail to mature and proliferate and are replaced by fat cells. This results in pancytopenia – lack of RBCs (anaemia), WBCs (leucopenia) and platelets (thrombocytopenia).

● Pathophysiology

Aplastic anaemia may be due to an inherited condition such as the rare Fanconi anaemia. However, it may also be acquired, and in 20%–50% of all cases onset is thought to be associated with exposure to one of the following:
- chemicals, especially benzene, coal tar derivatives and petroleum products
- drugs, including chloramphenicol, certain cytotoxic chemotherapeutic agents, phenothiazines and anticonvulsants
- ionising radiation (see Chapter 31, Nursing the Patient With Cancer)
- viral infection, notably hepatitis viruses and Epstein–Barr virus (EBV).

The remaining 50%–80% of cases have no detectable cause. The incidence of aplastic anaemia varies worldwide and is estimated to be between 1.5–2.3 per million in Western countries and 2–3 times higher in Asia possibly related to genetic or environmental factors (Norasetthada et al. 2021).

Clinical Presentation

The onset of aplastic anaemia is usually insidious and months may elapse between exposure to the causal agent and the development of symptoms. It can occur at any age and the presenting symptoms will vary relative to the extent of the pancytopenia. These may include:
- general symptoms of anaemia
- infections
- bleeding – especially from the nose, gums or gastrointestinal tract.

● Medical Management

History and Examination

Initial examination may detect no abnormality other than the presenting symptoms. However, further assessment may reveal exposure to chemicals or the use of over-the-counter medication and a thorough drug history is essential.

Investigations

These are those undertaken to provide a definitive diagnosis and assess the severity according to the Camitta criteria (1988) include among others:
- FBC including a reticulocyte count
- blood film
- bone marrow aspiration and trephine biopsy.

Treatment

Immediate admission to hospital may be required once a diagnosis of aplastic anaemia is made, particularly if the condition is advanced. Supportive therapy with blood and platelet transfusion will be given based on clinical need. Broad-spectrum antibiotic therapy and antifungal drugs may be needed prophylactically and to treat any infections. Other medications that may be prescribed include antithymocyte globulin, ciclosporin and haematopoietic growth factors (Killick et al. 2015).

Allogeneic haematopoietic stem cell transplantation (HSCT) has become the treatment of choice for younger patients with severe or very severe aplastic anaemia when an appropriate donor is available (Killick et al. 2015). Immunosuppressive therapy (IST) is recommended for patients with nonsevere aplastic anaemia who are transfusion-dependent, patients with severe or very severe disease who are over 40 years old and for younger patients with severe or very severe disease who do not have an appropriate donor (Killick et al. 2015).

❖ Nursing Management and Health Promotion: Aplastic Anaemia

Nursing management of patients with aplastic anaemia requires expert skills and knowledge to prevent the development of serious life-threatening complications. Nursing care will include the:
- prevention and early detection of infections (Chapter 18, Infection Prevention and Control, and Chapter 31, Nursing the Patient With Cancer)
- initiation of immediate treatment for septic patients
- prevention and early treatment of haemorrhage.

The nurse will play an important role in the coordination of the numerous tests necessary for diagnosis and will be instrumental in the care of the patient if HSCT is undertaken. Further details regarding transplantation and the care of profoundly pancytopenia patients are included in the subsequent section on leukaemia.

Communication and Psychological Support

Supporting the patient and their family psychologically is an important aspect of care and sensitivity is required as the patient comes to terms with their diagnosis, prognosis and effects of treatment.

Education

Patients and their families need information about how to prevent fatigue, infection and haemorrhage and to identify signs of these should they occur. The nurse should also assess the patient's understanding of the need for medication, what action to take if medication is inadvertently missed and how to obtain new supplies. It is important that the patient is advised to inform their doctor or dentist about prescribed corticosteroids and always to carry information with details of their medication.

Rehabilitation and Health Promotion

Patient rehabilitation will involve the multidisciplinary team and it is important that this is planned before discharge in response to the patient's specific needs and potential for recovery. Realistic goals should be set in partnership with the patient, as it may be necessary to make lifestyle or career changes. Before discharge, it is important to discuss with the patient, family and carers any fears or apprehensions and to clarify details of whom to contact if there are any further episodes of illness. Information about support outside the hospital including support groups should also be provided.

Haemolytic Anaemias

Haemolytic anaemias are rare and result from the premature destruction of RBCs in response to an inherited or acquired defect. The most common inherited anaemias are the haemoglobinopathies – sickle cell disease and thalassaemia. These are outlined in this section. The most common acquired forms result from direct cell injury following infection or medical treatment (Information 13.3).

INFORMATION 13.3

Causes of Haemolytic Anaemia

Inherited

- RBC membrane fragility
  - spherocytosis (RBCs round in shape)
  - elliptocytosis (RBCs elliptical in shape)
- Haemoglobinopathies (haemoglobin defects: structure or synthesis)
  - sickle cell disease
  - thalassaemia
- RBC enzyme defects
  - glucose-6-phosphate dehydrogenase (G6PD) deficiency
  - pyruvate kinase deficiency

Acquired

- Antibody attack, e.g. mismatched blood transfusion
- Autoimmune haemolytic anaemia (warm or cold antibodies)
- Nonimmune haemolytic anaemia
  - traumatic (disruption of RBCs), e.g. prosthetic heart valve, burns injury, intense exercise
  - chemical- or drug-induced, e.g. sodium chlorate, dapsone, sulfasalazine, nitrites
  - infection, e.g. malaria (*Plasmodium falciparum*), etc.

Pathophysiology

Haemolytic anaemia is characterised by a reduced lifespan of the RBCs, due to fragility and excessive breakdown (haemolysis). This results in a reduced oxygen-carrying capacity and tissue hypoxia. The production of erythropoietin, a growth factor that stimulates erythropoiesis, is increased; however, if the RBC lifespan is greatly reduced (<15 days) the bone marrow will not be able to compensate adequately and the person will experience symptoms of anaemia. Because the products of RBC breakdown are retained in the body, signs of increased bilirubin and urobilinogen may be evident.

Thalassaemia

The thalassaemias are a group of inherited autosomal recessive disorders that cause an impaired rate of synthesis of one of the two globin chains (alpha, α or beta, β) of adult haemoglobin (Huether and McCance 2019). The resultant imbalance leads to ineffective erythropoiesis and a reduced RBC lifespan. Thalassaemias are among the most common genetic disorders in the world. Cases occur sporadically in the general population; however, they are more common in people who originate from around the Mediterranean, the Middle East, South and East Asia. In the UK the condition occurs most often among people of Cypriot, Italian, Greek, Indian, Pakistani, Bangladeshi and Chinese descent. This is because the mutations that cause thalassaemia originally occurred in countries in which *falciparum* malaria was common (Hoffbrand et al. 2019).

Pathophysiology

A haemoglobin molecule comprises four ferrous iron-containing haem groups and four matching globin (protein) chains. To function effectively haemoglobin requires two α globin chains and two β globin chains. There are two forms of thalassaemia – α thalassaemia and β thalassaemia. Both types have major or minor subtypes, depending on how many genes are defective and whether the defects are inherited homozygously (thalassaemia major) or heterozygously (thalassaemia minor).

Clinical Presentation

There are a number of clinical syndromes associated with thalassaemia and clinical presentation will depend on the mode of inheritance. β thalassaemias occur more frequently than α thalassaemias.

Medical Management

Treatment

Blood transfusion is the mainstay treatment for thalassaemia and a patient typically requires three units of blood every 3–4 weeks. This carries an increased risk of transfusion-related reactions due to the development of antibodies against donor blood. Excessive accumulation of iron can also be problematic, particularly if it affects the heart, liver and endocrine organs. This risk can be minimised by the regular administration of an iron-chelating drug, e.g. desferrioxamine, which is usually administered overnight via subcutaneous infusion (Hoffbrand et al. 2019).

Nursing Management and Health Promotion: Thalassaemia

Thalassaemia and its treatment can have a disruptive impact on the individual's life and requires expert, supportive nursing care.

In many areas this will be provided by specialist nurses and will involve:

- The safe administration of blood and vigilant monitoring for transfusion reactions in accordance with national and local policy.
- Sensitivity to the patient's fears or concerns regarding the transmission of infections during blood transfusions.
- Educating the patient and their family/carers how to administer drugs safely and the provision of support to encourage compliance.
- Referral to relevant support groups (see Useful Websites).
- Health promotion and advice regarding nutrition, lifestyle and compliance with medication and treatments.

Sickle Cell Disorders

Sickle cell disorders (SCDs) comprise a group of disorders caused by an inherited structural abnormality in the haemoglobin molecule. The abnormal haemoglobin (HbS) causes a characteristic sickle shape of the RBC when it is deoxygenated (Fig. 13.4).

It is inherited as a recessive, autosomal disorder of which there are two types. In the heterozygous variant, the person inherits the abnormal haemoglobin gene (HbS) from one parent and the normal (HbA) gene from the other parent. This person has sickle cell trait (HbSA) and usually is unaware of the abnormality unless tested for the trait or if they develop symptoms when exposed to hypoxic conditions, such as during an anaesthetic. In the homozygous type, the abnormal gene is inherited from both parents and the person will have sickle cell anaemia.

A crucial factor in diagnosing this haemoglobinopathy is knowledge of the family's genetic history. SCD occurs more commonly among people of African, Caribbean, Eastern Mediterranean, Middle Eastern, Indian and Pakistani origin. In the UK, it affects 1 in 2000 live births and there are currently estimated to be about 15,000 people living with sickle cell disease in England, making it one of the most common genetic disorders (Sickle Cell Society 2018).

🕮 Pathophysiology

The amino acid sequence in the beta globin chains of haemoglobin is altered in HbS by a substitution of one amino acid for

INFORMATION 13.4

Trigger Factors in Sickle Cell Anaemia

- Reduced oxygen, e.g. during strenuous exercise
- Anaesthesia
- Dehydration
- Infection
- Fever
- Pregnancy
- Sudden change in temperature
- Alcohol – possibly because of dehydration
- Emotional stress
- Extreme fatigue

another. HbS has certain properties which distinguish it from normal HbA haemoglobin. When it becomes deoxygenated, crystals are formed within the RBC making it more rigid and distorting it into a sickle shape (Hoffbrand et al. 2019). Affected RBCs are destroyed prematurely and have a lifespan of between 5 and 30 days (normally 120 days).

Clinical Presentation

Sickle cell disease normally presents in childhood. It is characterised by chronic haemolytic anaemia in which mild jaundice and splenomegaly may be evident and intermittent painful crises in response to a triggering factor (Information 13.4). People with sickle cell anaemia have an increased risk of infection, tissue necrosis and renal insufficiency.

During a sickle cell crisis large numbers of RBCs become sickle-shaped, causing subsequent blood vessel occlusion and tissue ischaemia. Pain is caused by the obstruction of small blood vessels in the tissues and is typically characterised by the acuteness of its onset and unresponsiveness to mild analgesics. The location of the pain depends on the location of the obstruction.

Acute chest syndrome (ACS), a common form of acute lung injury that may lead to acute respiratory distress syndrome (ARDS), is a leading cause of death in people with sickle cell disease (Information 13.5). Central to its effective management is an awareness of its clinical presentation, anticipation of its development and prompt intervention. Nurses and medical teams should be educated to recognise and manage ACS, and patients and their carers should be taught about it and to seek urgent medical attention should symptoms arise.

🕮 Medical Management

Investigations

Investigations for diagnosis include FBC, blood film and reticulocyte count. The presence of HbS can be demonstrated when the RBCs are mixed with a solution of sodium metabisulphite. The screening test for sickle cell anaemia and sickle cell trait uses electrophoretic analysis to measure the rates of movement of the different haemoglobins in an electrical field.

Treatment

Management is based on alleviation of symptoms, the prevention of complications and the promotion of a lifestyle that minimises crisis events. This includes:

- avoiding situations that may trigger a crisis (see Information 13.4)
- prompt treatment of any infections, even minor ones
- prophylactic penicillin and pneumococcal vaccination

Figure 13.4 Blood film showing a sickle cell. (Reproduced with permission from Watson HG, Craigg JIO, Manson LM. Blood disease. In: Walker BR, Colledge NR, Ralston SH, Penman ID, eds. *Davidson's Principles and Practice of Medicine.* Edinburgh: Churchill Livingstone; 2014:989–1056.)

INFORMATION 13.5

Acute Chest Syndrome (ACS) in Sickle Cell Disease

The characteristic presentation includes:
- tachypnoea
- chest pain
- cough
- dyspnoea
- fever
- hypoxia.

Early recognition is vital and all patients admitted to hospital should be assessed for these signs and symptoms and a chest X-ray performed if chest pain, respiratory symptoms or reduced oxygen saturations are found. All patients should be monitored for the development of ACS using regular pulse oximetry and observation of pulse and respiratory rates throughout admission, especially if they are having opiate analgesia.

Protocols should be in place for the management of ACS and will include:
- analgesia
- measurement of arterial blood gases (ABGs)
- nursing observations (respiratory rate and effort, colour, temperature, pulse, blood pressure, oxygen saturation, level of reported pain, fluid balance, etc.)
- fluid management
- oxygen and respiratory support (see Chapters 3 and 28)
- incentive spirometry
- bronchodilator therapy for patients with evidence of wheeze, reversible airway disease or a history of asthma, antibiotics and indications for blood transfusion.

See Further Reading suggestions, e.g. Sickle cell society 2018.

- education on general health and nutrition. Prophylactic folic acid may be recommended for those whose diet does not contain adequate folic acid or with a proven folate deficiency.
- recognising complications of sickle cell disease including: bone and joint pains, leg ulcers, priapism (prolonged penile erection without sexual stimulation), gallstones, blurred vision, kidney disease in patients over 50 years of age, and peptic ulceration
- frequent follow-up in special clinics to monitor disease
- genetic counselling and vigilant antenatal care
- alerting other relevant health professionals to the condition
- obtaining support from sickle cell centres and support groups.

Patients experiencing a severe sickle cell crisis will need hospitalisation and management with adequate analgesics, antibiotics, oxygen therapy, rehydration and close observation. An exchange blood transfusion may be needed if the crisis does not resolve or if there is continued hypoxia. Some patients are prescribed hydroxycarbamide in an attempt to reduce the frequency and severity of crises. Allogeneic HSCT is the only available therapy that can cure sickle cell disease. It is currently offered in the UK to children and adults with severe sickle cell disease who have a related fully matched donor.

❖ Nursing Management and Health promotion: Sickle Cell Disease

A patient or the parents of a child newly diagnosed with sickle cell disease will require comprehensive education about the disorder, addressing ways to minimise complications and necessary lifestyle changes.

All family members should be offered screening if this has not been done previously and genetic counselling should be available.

REFLECTION 13.3

Minimising the Risk of a Sickle Cell Crisis

Josh, a 16-year-old male with sickle cell disease, is studying for school exams which start next month. He is worried that he might experience a sickle cell crisis in the lead-up to his exams.

Activity
- Reflect on the trigger factors for sickle cell crisis (see Information 13.4). What advice can you give Josh?

Some areas with a high incidence of sickle cell disease employ specialist nurses and nurse counsellors to carry out these roles. The emphasis for care is on promoting health and minimising ill health.

Sickle cell crisis is an emergency and must be treated as such. Accordingly, nurses need to act promptly to manage symptoms and initiate treatment in order to prevent complications. This will involve:
- Vigilant observation and monitoring.
- Assessing the severity of the pain and likely need for opiates, and administering these regularly as prescribed. Vitally, appropriate pain relief should be administered to individuals experiencing an acute episode within 30 minutes of presenting at an emergency department (Sickle Cell Society 2018).
- Commencing an intravenous infusion to rehydrate the patient to aid the reduction of blood viscosity.
- Administering antibiotics and other prescribed medications.
- Administering oxygen therapy to alleviate hypoxia.

Patients experiencing a sickle cell crisis are often frightened and require considerable emotional support. Some patients may have had several previous episodes and may know the best way that they should be treated when in a crisis and nurses should be mindful of this.

Males may be admitted with priapism due to thrombosis in the corpora cavernosa (two lateral columns of spongy erectile tissue in the penis). This requires both the administration of analgesics and intravenous hydration as well as possibly exchange blood transfusion to reduce the percentage of sickle cells. Chronic priapism can occur and the man's sexual function may be impaired.

Before discharge, patients should be made aware of the importance of recognising and avoiding situations that may trigger a sickle cell crisis and of the need to seek medical advice at the onset of further painful episodes (Reflection 13.3).

🌐 **See Evolve website Critical thinking question 13.2**

See Sickle Cell Society Standards for the Clinical Care of Adults with Sickle Cell Disease in the UK (2018) for information about the care of patients with sickle cell disease. This can be downloaded from the Sickle Cell Society website.

Disorders of Red Blood Cells – Overproduction

Excessive RBC production is referred to as polycythaemia or erythrocytosis. Relative polycythaemia occurs when there is an increased concentration of blood cells due to dehydration. Absolute polycythaemia occurs as a physiological response to hypoxia such as in people living at high altitudes, those with congenital heart disease or those with chronic pulmonary disease, and is referred to as secondary polycythaemia. It may also be caused by inappropriate production of erythropoietin or similar substances in certain conditions such as cancer. The overproduction of erythrocytes with no erythropoietin stimulus is called polycythaemia vera (PV) (or primary proliferative polycythaemia).

Polycythaemia Vera

This is a myeloproliferative disorder (a condition characterised by the overproduction of one or more of the cellular components of the bone marrow) which originates from a neoplastic haematopoietic stem cell due to a mutation of the JAK2 gene. This disease is distinguished by hypercellularity of the bone marrow and an overproduction of erythrocytes. Increased WBC (leucocytosis) and platelet counts (thrombocythaemia) are not uncommon and the spleen is often enlarged as a result of the increased number of blood cells (splenomegaly). The condition occurs most frequently in White males aged between 55 and 80 years (Huether and McCance 2019).

Pathophysiology

The raised RBC, WBC, platelet count and haemoglobin level have a number of implications. These include hyperviscosity of the blood, thrombosis and hypertension, all of which could precipitate cardiac failure or peripheral vascular disease.

Clinical Presentation

Often characterised by a ruddy appearance and suffused conjunctiva, hyperviscosity of the blood can also give rise to symptoms associated with sluggish circulation and arterial and venous thrombosis. The patient may therefore present with symptoms of:
- cerebral vascular disease, e.g. headaches, dizziness, blackouts, visual disturbances
- peripheral vascular disease, e.g. intermittent claudication
- hypertension, e.g. headaches, epistaxis, dyspnoea
- angina and cardiac failure.

Gout may also arise due to increased cell turnover and raised uric acid levels. Excess histamine production released from basophils can cause gastric ulceration and pruritus, especially on exposure to temperature extremes.

Medical Management

History and Examination

The patient may be found to have hypertension during a routine check-up. A ruddy complexion may be evident and the palms of the hands and the oral mucosal membrane may be deep red. Splenomegaly may also be detected.

Investigations

Diagnostic criteria for PV require that the Hb or haematocrit is above normal, the bone marrow shows hypercellularity and either the presence of JAK2 mutation in blood cells or subnormal erythropoietin levels (Tefferi and Barbui 2023).

Treatment

Treatment is aimed at preventing thrombosis and reducing symptoms. Venesection is the simplest form of treatment and involves the drainage of 300–500 mL of whole blood, usually via a needle in the arm. This procedure is normally carried out in the outpatient setting and will typically be repeated regularly until the PCV drops sufficiently and there is an alleviation of symptoms. Thereafter, less frequent but regular venesection will maintain this level. Low-dose aspirin is recommended for all patients without contraindications and is prescribed to reduce platelet activity and prevent clot formation (Tefferi and Barbui 2023).

Once the diagnosis is established, the underlying myeloproliferation may be managed in some patients with a high risk of thrombotic events with treatments such as interferon, hydroxycarbamide, ruxolitinib or alkylating agents to suppress bone marrow function (Tefferi and Barbui 2023).

All patients will require frequent monitoring to minimise the effects of the disorder.

Nursing Management and Health Promotion: Polycythaemia Vera

Psychological support may be needed as the patient and their family come to terms with the diagnosis of a chronic disorder that may impact lifestyle and longevity. Clear information regarding investigations, treatment and monitoring should be provided to the patient and their family. It is important to teach the patient how to monitor for signs and symptoms of thrombosis, such as pain or swelling. If medication has been prescribed detailed instructions about taking this should be provided. The necessity of continued monitoring, via blood tests and outpatient appointments, should also be emphasised.

While undergoing venesection, the patient must be monitored closely for signs and symptoms of shock (see Chapter 19, The Deteriorating Patient, Recognising and Managing Shock). If admission to hospital is required, the need for isolation to protect other patients, visitors and staff must be tactfully explained to the patient.

Disorders of White Blood Cells and Lymphoid Tissue

Disorders of the WBCs and lymphoid tissue are highly diverse and specific nursing management will vary as discussed in subsequent sections. However, nurses have an essential role throughout the disease trajectory and are central to providing the continuity and coordination essential for efficient patient care. The prevention and management of specific disease- and treatment-related complications are also of utmost importance.

This section of the chapter provides an outline of:
- leukaemia
- lymphoma
- multiple myeloma
- myelodysplastic syndrome.

Leukaemia

The leukaemias are a group of blood disorders in which there is an abnormal and excessive proliferation of malignant WBCs. Leukaemia is typically divided into acute and chronic types. These are then further subdivided into myeloid or lymphoid classifications depending on the type of WBC affected. Leukaemia is uncommon, representing less than 3% of cancers in the UK but it occurs in all ages, in both sexes and in all races. Leukaemia accounted for 4830 deaths in 2017–2019 (Cancer Research UK nd (a)).

Aetiology

The aetiology of leukaemia is not fully understood but, like other cancers, appears to be a multistep process involving accumulated genetic mutations that disrupt normal cellular functions controlling proliferation and differentiation (Howard and Hamilton 2013). Exposure to factors such as ionising radiation, viruses, petroleum-based chemicals and some cytotoxic medications has been associated with increased incidence. Congenital factors or genetic disorders such as Down's syndrome are also implicated in the development of leukaemia although this is very rare.

Acute Leukaemia

Acute leukaemia is subdivided into acute myeloid (myelogenous) leukaemia (AML), originating in the myeloid stem cell, and acute lymphoblastic leukaemia (ALL), arising from the lymphoid stem cell. In adults, AML is more common than ALL with around 3089 people diagnosed with AML in the UK each year in 2016–2018 (Cancer Research UK n.d. [b]) while in children ALL accounts for most cases (Howard and Hamilton 2013). The internationally recognised 2016 WHO classification system categorises acute leukaemia into subgroups according to morphological, cytogenetic and molecular characteristics, which have gained recognition as significant prognostic factors (Emadi and Law 2022).

Pathophysiology

Acute leukaemia is characterised by uncontrolled malignant proliferation occurring at the blast level of cell maturity and is defined as the presence of over 20% of blast (immature) cells in the blood or bone marrow (Hoffbrand et al. 2019). It is thought to arise from a genetic alteration in a stem cell which proliferates to produce a clone of identical cells. As these abnormal cells proliferate, they gradually crowd out the bone marrow, affecting the production of normal blood cells. This leads to anaemia, thrombocytopenia and neutropenia (reduction in the number of neutrophils).

Clinical Features

There is little uniformity in the presentation of acute leukaemia; however, clinical features, which derive from the effects of the disease on the bone marrow, include:
- acute infection, associated with fever
- bleeding of the gums, epistaxis or bruising
- anaemia – pallor, breathlessness and lethargy.

Other signs and symptoms may occur if leukaemic cells infiltrate tissues and organs leading to:
- bone pain
- hepatosplenomegaly (enlargement of liver and spleen) causing abdominal pain
- hypertrophy or swelling of the gums
- skin lesions.

Medical Management

History and Examination

During a detailed medical assessment, the patient may describe either:
- an acute onset of symptoms occurring over the previous 72 hours with pallor, pyrexia and tachycardia and exhibiting other signs and symptoms of acute infection, or
- a 2–3-month history of minor recurrent infections.

Physical examination may reveal pallor, lymphadenopathy (enlargement of the lymph nodes), splenomegaly, gum bleeding, petechiae, purpura and bruising.

Investigations

Typically, a diagnosis of leukaemia will be established through a series of investigations, including blood count, biochemistry and microscopic examination of a blood film.

This diagnosis will be confirmed by examination of a bone marrow aspirate and biopsy (see Information 13.1).

See Evolve website Critical thinking question 13.3

Further laboratory testing of the marrow using cytochemistry, immunophenotyping, cytogenetic analysis and molecular studies will lead to a precise diagnosis of a particular subtype of acute leukaemia.

Further aspirations of bone marrow are taken and examined during and after treatment to assess the response of the disease and help to indicate the prognosis.

If the patient has ALL, further diagnostic investigations will be carried out. These include:
- lumbar puncture, as there is a high risk of central nervous system (CNS) involvement, especially in the cerebrospinal fluid
- examination of the testes, as this is a region to which leukaemia may spread.

Treatment

Acute leukaemia is a serious life-threatening condition and such a diagnosis requires urgent treatment. The aim is elimination of the disease and involves hospitalisation, intensive chemotherapy and, in some cases, HSCT (Information 13.6 and see Table 13.4). Research into the use of novel therapies, such as monoclonal antibodies, is currently ongoing.

Cytotoxic chemotherapy is the mainstay treatment in the management of acute leukaemia. Chemotherapeutic agents act on the cell cycle disrupting cell growth and replication. As many chemotherapy agents are nonselective, normal cells undergoing cell division are also damaged, giving rise to potentially life-threatening complications. These include infection and haemorrhage caused by bone marrow suppression and side-effects such as nausea and vomiting, mucositis, alopecia and infertility (see Chapter 31, Nursing the Patient With Cancer).

Before treatment commences, several issues need to be considered including:
- A detailed, holistic assessment to determine the patient's general state of health and organ function.
- The insertion of a long-term central venous access device (CVAD) such as a Hickman catheter.
- Referral for a wig fitting due to the likelihood of alopecia.
- Fertility issues must be discussed with patients of child-bearing age; male patients should be offered sperm banking facilities and female patients the opportunity to review the strategies available to them to maintain the possibility of future fertility (Freeman and Postma 2018).

The chemotherapy regimens used to treat acute leukaemia are based on national protocols of treatment devised by the Medical Research Council (MRC) and change over time in light of ongoing research and drug development. At the time of diagnosis, most patients will be entered into a clinical trial. Typically, several cycles of treatment, each lasting several days, are required using a combination of agents that induce cell death by different means.

Initial treatment for AML, known as the induction phase, is aimed at achieving disease remission. The International working group (IWG) response criteria that indicated complete remission (CR) was updated in 2003 (Cheson et al. 2003) and still applies.

INFORMATION 13.6

Haematopoietic Stem Cell Transplant

In some cases, HSCT may be considered the sole chance of a cure for a number of haematological conditions, including acute leukaemia. It involves the transplantation of healthy haematopoietic progenitor cells to re-establish healthy bone marrow function in someone whose bone marrow has been destroyed or depleted as a result of a disease or its treatment. Prior to receiving the stem cells, a preparatory regimen, known as conditioning, is administered. This typically consists of high-dose chemotherapy and/or total body irradiation. Consequently, myeloid and lymphoid blood cells are destroyed leaving the patient extremely vulnerable to infection. Administered in a similar way to blood transfusion, the stem cells are then given with the goal of repopulating the patient's marrow to restore normal haemopoietic function.

The type of transplant is defined according to the donor and source of stem cells. Stem cells may be donated from a related or unrelated HLA (human leucocyte antigen)-compatible donor (allogeneic) or they may be obtained from the patient (autologous). Haematopoietic stem cells can be harvested from the peripheral blood following mobilisation using growth factor injections. They can also be obtained from the bone marrow or umbilical cord blood.

There are many potential life-threatening complications associated with stem cell transplantation which are largely due to the myeloablative (describes the therapy used intentionally to destroy the patient's bone marrow) effects of conventional conditioning regimens. As such, guidelines identify which patients are most likely to benefit from this procedure. Although these are constantly being refined, they typically exclude older patients and those with comorbidities. Reduced intensity conditioning, also known as 'mini transplants', which use less toxic doses of chemotherapy and radiation than standard full intensity transplants, has emerged as a treatment strategy. This approach has extended the chance of cure to patients with acute leukaemia and other blood disorders who are ineligible for transplant due to age or comorbidity. Reduced intensity transplants attempt to utilise an immunological 'graft versus leukaemia' effect to eradicate the malignant cell clone and have resulted in a reduction in transplant-related mortality (Watson et al. 2022).

For different types of transplant see Table 13.4.

See Further Reading, e.g. Brown and Cutler 2012.

Reference

Watson HG, Culligan DJ, Manson LM. Haematology and transfusion medicine. In: Penman ID, Ralston SH, Strachan MWJ, Hobson RP, eds. *Davidson's Principles and Practice of Medicine*. 24th ed. London: Elsevier; 2022: 921-989.

TABLE 13.4	Transplantation for Malignant Haematological Disease
Type of Transplant	**Explanation**
Bone marrow transplantation	A term to describe the transplantation of bone marrow, which contains haematopoietic progenitor cells, to re-establish haematopoiesis in someone whose bone marrow has been destroyed or damaged by high-dose therapy. Donor marrow is usually harvested from the posterior iliac crests in the pelvis under general anaesthetic and infused intravenously to the recipient
Haematopoietic stem cell transplantation	The transplantation of haematopoietic stem cells to re-establish haematopoiesis in someone whose bone marrow function has been destroyed or damaged by high-dose therapy. Stem cells may be obtained from peripheral blood or the umbilical cord and are infused intravenously
Syngeneic transplant	Transplantation of bone marrow or haematopoietic stem cells between identical twins
Allogeneic sibling transplant	The use of bone marrow or haematopoietic stem cells from a matched sibling donor obtained from a bone marrow harvest or peripheral blood stem cell collection
Matched unrelated donor transplant (MUD)	Where a matched related donor is not available, a volunteer donor of bone marrow or stem cells may be found from national or international donor registries
Autologous transplant (rescue)	The use of a patient's own bone marrow or blood stem cells following high-dose therapy to reduce the period of pancytopenia. The cells are usually harvested during a period of remission, preserved and returned at a later date

CR is defined as fewer than 5% blast cells in the bone marrow, absence of circulating blasts and extramedullary leukaemia (tumours outside of the bone marrow), and recovery of neutrophil and platelet counts. This is followed by further chemotherapy (the consolidation phase) which aims to eliminate any remaining leukaemic cells. However, some patients may undergo HSCT once induction is complete. Examples of chemotherapies used in the treatment of AML include daunorubicin, idarubicin, cytarabine, thioguanine, amsacrine and etoposide. Newer chemotherapies and biological therapies are currently being investigated in clinical trials in the UK in relation to their role in the treatment of AML and may be prescribed for some patients (Cancer Research UK 2020).

Treatment regimens for ALL are principally the same as for AML but may include an intensification phase, after the induction phase. This is then followed by consolidation therapy. Drug regimens will vary but may conventionally include vincristine, asparaginase and doxorubicin during induction with the addition of methotrexate and etoposide during consolidation therapy. Maintenance therapy is administered to patients with ALL for a further 1–2 years after the completion of consolidation chemotherapy (Cancer Research UK 2021). Additionally, regular doses of chemotherapy via the intrathecal (within the subarachnoid space) route are given prophylactically with the aim of treating or preventing the spread of leukaemia to the CNS. Cranial irradiation may also be used.

Tumour Lysis Syndrome

Tumour lysis syndrome (TLS) is the most common oncologic emergency and can be life-threatening. It occurs as a result of the release of intracellular material such as potassium, phosphate and uric acids from tumour cells disintegrating (lysis) due to chemotherapy. Signs and symptoms of TLS result from electrolyte imbalances and include cardiac arrhythmias, muscle cramps, seizures, reduced urine output, nausea and vomiting. Regular monitoring of urea and electrolyte levels, renal function and vital signs should be done after initiation of cancer treatment. Treatment of TLS consists of electrolyte management but may include haemodialysis and delaying cytotoxic therapy temporarily. Patients at high risk of TLS may be given allopurinol prior to treatment to reduce uric acid levels (Rivera-Gamma and Davis 2023).

Supportive Therapy

Leukaemic disease and aggressive treatment result in the suppression of normal blood cell production and, as outlined earlier, the patient will be predisposed to bleeding caused by thrombocytopenia, anaemia and infection. Supportive interventions will be required as detailed below.

Bleeding Caused by Thrombocytopenia. Platelet transfusion will be required if the platelet count falls below 10×10^9 cells/L (BSH 2016). Platelets will also be required with higher counts in other specific instances, such as bleeding gums or epistaxis.

Anaemia Caused by Reduced Numbers of RBCs. RBC transfusions are used to minimise the effects of anaemia by maintaining the haemoglobin level above 7 g/dL (NICE 2015). As for platelet transfusions, some patients may require cytomegalovirus (CMV)-negative and/or irradiated blood products.

Infection Caused by Neutropenia. To reduce the incidence of infection, prophylactic antibiotics are often administered from the start of chemotherapy and for some time after the completion of treatment. Prophylactic antifungal and antiviral agents are also typically prescribed.

Neutropenic patients are extremely vulnerable to infection and once an infection develops, the lack of normal defence mechanisms means that the patient's condition can rapidly deteriorate, leading to septic shock. A temperature of >38°C or any symptoms and/or signs of sepsis may indicate neutropenic sepsis and requires urgent intervention. Treatment protocols for the management of neutropenic sepsis are specific to individual haematology units; however, these typically involve implementation of the UK Sepsis Trust 'Sepsis Six' bundle within the first hour (UK Sepsis Trust 2022). To reduce the period of neutropenia for select patients, GCSF may be administered by subcutaneous injection.

❖ Nursing Management and Health Promotion: Acute Leukaemia

Nursing care for patients with acute leukaemia must meet their individual physical and psychological needs throughout the disease trajectory. Treatment is intensive and has potentially life-threatening side-effects, thereby requiring expert care. Nurses are instrumental in administering treatments and supportive therapies, monitoring condition and providing appropriate information, emotional support and reassurance to the patient and their family.

Prevention of Infection

An essential aspect of nursing patients undergoing treatment for acute leukaemia is to minimise the risk of infection. Some patients may require protective isolation in a single room to reduce contact with environmental microorganisms, while others will be nursed in general areas away from infectious patients. Other interventions to reduce the risk of infection include:

- Meticulous hand hygiene and decontamination using bactericidal solutions prior to patient contact and between tasks performed for the same patient.
- Use of protective clothing such as disposable plastic aprons and gloves during close contact with the patient or when blood and body fluid are present.
- Use of sterile gloves and aseptic technique for invasive procedures.
- Restricting visitor numbers.
- Encouraging compliance with food safety advice recommended for neutropenic patients ($<1.5 \times 10^9$/L); this includes, for example, unpasteurised dairy products, probiotics and soft

---

REFLECTION 13.4

Dietary Restrictions for Patients With Neutropenia

Dietary restrictions are required for neutropenic patients as part of the measures put in place to minimise the risk of infection.

Activities

- Access the British Dietary Association's (2020) policy statement on safer eating with neutropenia and consider the foods that are excluded.
- Reflect on having to exclude so many food items from the diet – how would you feel and what would you most miss?

Resource

BDA Policy Statement: Safer Eating With Neutropenia, 2020. https://www.bda.uk.com/uploads/assets/9f7e021a-2edf-4d62-9bd5fba841d7472c/52d14410-d3b7-45cb-a3a0e09e15eeda2b/Neutropenic-Diets-Guidance-Jan-2020.pdf.

---

cheeses, raw or partially cooked eggs, damaged or bruised fruit, smoked fish or sushi, raw or undercooked meat, unpackaged loose brought products e.g. spices, cereals, nuts (British Dietary Association 2020) (Reflection 13.4).
- Removal of flowers and pot plants which may harbour fungal spores and infection.

As the patient's own microflora will also pose a threat to the immunosuppressed patient, the risk of infection can be reduced by:

- regular and vigilant observation of the patient, e.g. 4-hourly recordings of temperature, pulse, respirations and blood pressure
- management of CVADs according to local protocol
- encouraging attention to personal hygiene including daily showers and regular handwashing
- regular assessment and care of the oral cavity using appropriate solutions

Prevention of Haemorrhage

The patient should be closely monitored for bleeding and any indication of this must be acted on promptly. Such actions will include:

- immediately reporting signs and symptoms of bleeding to medical staff
- administering prescribed platelet transfusions promptly in accordance with national and local policy
- monitoring pulse and blood pressure readings at least 4-hourly
- undertaking daily urinalysis for blood
- testing stools for occult blood
- observing for changes in levels of consciousness or development of headaches which may indicate cerebral haemorrhage
- inspecting sputum and vomit for blood
- assessing the skin daily for purpura and bruising
- monitoring pain, especially in the abdomen, as this may be an indication of haemorrhage
- avoiding intramuscular injections and the use of aspirin-based medications
- advising the patient against the use of wet razors or harsh toothbrushes.

Communication and Psychological Support

The nature of acute leukaemia means that chemotherapy is often started before the patient has had time to fully assimilate their diagnosis and its associated implications. Treatment typically lasts several months and the impact of this on the patient and their family can be devastating and should never be underestimated. Treatment usually involves repeated admission to hospital and patients may find this difficult to cope with. Periods of social isolation and lengthy disruptions to normal life may promote anxiety and this may be coupled with feelings of uncertainty about the future or a fear of death. Helping the patient to understand their illness and its treatment may help them to retain a sense of control, even when very ill. This can be achieved through effective communication and the provision of support and reassurance. Providing patients and their families with information relevant to their needs in relation to investigations, treatment strategies and expected side-effects is also essential.

Minimising the Side-effects of Chemotherapy

General side-effects of chemotherapy are discussed in Chapter 31, Nursing the Patient With Cancer. Common short-term side-effects experienced by patients receiving chemotherapy for leukaemia are outlined here.

Nausea and Vomiting. If left untreated, nausea and vomiting may lead to fluid and electrolyte imbalance (see Chapter 21, Maintaining Fluid, Electrolyte and Acid–Base Balance), malnutrition (see Chapter 22, Nutrition and Health) and a possible reluctance by the patient to accept further treatment. However, control is possible through the use of antiemetic medications given prior to, during and after the administration of treatment. A wide range of antiemetics are currently available and alternatives can be used if first-line medications are ineffective. The use of relaxation techniques or distraction therapies may also help.

Compromised Nutritional Intake. Loss of appetite is common during and after chemotherapy and may be influenced by factors such as nausea and vomiting, stomatitis and anxiety. Advice should be sought from the dietitian about appropriate food and drinks and nutritional supplements. Occasionally it may be necessary for the patient to receive enteral or parenteral nutrition for a short period of time (see Chapter 22, Nutrition and Health). In such circumstances, the patient will require careful assessment and monitoring to ensure fluid and electrolyte balance. Daily or weekly weight monitoring may also be indicated.

Mucositis/Stomatitis. Chemotherapy inhibits cell replication of the mucosa lining the oral cavity and may lead to inflammation known as stomatitis. The production of saliva is also reduced leading to changes in the normal microflora of the mouth, thus increasing the possibility of infection. Ulcers, which often develop within the oral cavity, increase the risk of microorganisms entering the circulation. Mouth ulcers may also compromise nutrition and cause considerable pain which is sometimes severe enough to merit the administration of opioid analgesia. Baseline and daily oral assessment using a specialist tool will help to ensure that changes are detected promptly and that appropriate management strategies are implemented. Patients may be required to use a bactericidal mouthwash several times a day, often in conjunction with an antifungal agent.

Patient Education

Providing clear, accurate information about treatment, procedures and expected side-effects is essential. The active involvement of the family should be encouraged as the patient is given guidance in the following areas:

- monitoring body temperature
- recognising and responding to the symptoms of infection and haemorrhage
- maintaining a high standard of personal hygiene and oral care
- recognising and responding to complications associated with a CVAD
- adhering to the oral medication regimen.

Discharge Planning

On discharge, patients should receive a date for an outpatient appointment. The patient's GP and community nurse will be informed of discharge and arrangements made regarding continuing care. It is also important that patients receive information about whom to contact in the event of an emergency.

Chronic Leukaemia

Unlike acute leukaemia, the onset of chronic leukaemia is insidious and the disease may be present for some time before medical attention is sought. Diagnosis may result from incidental blood testing for other conditions. Chronic leukaemia is subdivided into chronic myeloid leukaemia (CML), and chronic lymphocytic leukaemia (CLL).

Pathophysiology

CML is a disease of the pluripotent stem cells leading to an overproduction of granulocytes and their precursors in the peripheral blood. CML is a rare disease, accounting for less than 1% of new cancers in 2016–2018 (Cancer Research UK n.d. [c]). Since the 1980s the incidence rates for CML in the UK have been decreasing considerably. The incidence is highest in people aged 85–89 years, and it is reported that there were 829 new cases of CML diagnosed in 2016–2018 (Cancer Research UK n.d. [c]).

In CML, over 95% of the leukaemic cells have an abnormal chromosome known as the Philadelphia (Ph) chromosome (a shortened chromosome 22) (Mehta and Hoffbrand 2014). The disease is characterised by three stages. After a chronic phase, which may last 2–3 years, the disease enters an accelerated stage and finally transforms into acute leukaemia, which is often the main cause of death. Life expectancy has significantly improved over the past decade, with advancements in targeted therapies and improved management of the disease (Hochhaus et al 2020). With appropriate management and regular medical care, many people with CML can lead relatively normal lives and achieve long-term remission.

CLL is a malignant disorder of the mature B lymphocytes which proliferate and accumulate in the blood, bone marrow, lymph nodes and spleen. Since 2005, the incidence rates for CLL in the UK have been slowly increasing. The incidence is strongly related to age, and most new cases occur in adults aged over 75 years. CLL is the most common type of leukaemia in Western countries, with an incidence higher in White ethnic group than in other racial groups. Approximately 3800 new cases of CLL were reported yearly in the UK in 2016–2018 (Cancer Research UK n.d. [d]).

In CLL the abnormal B cells have a prolonged lifespan, and as CLL progresses, the accumulating abnormal B cells crowd out healthy blood cells, leading to a decrease in the production of normal WBCs, RBCs, and platelets. The aetiology of CLL is unknown but it is believed to result from a combination of genetic and environmental factors. CLL is typically slow-progressing leukaemia, and many people may not require immediate treatment and can have a good quality of life.

Clinical Presentation

Presentation of chronic leukaemia is extremely variable. Presentation may be similar to that of acute leukaemia and include:
- fatigue
- anaemia
- weight loss
- infection, sweats and fevers
- painless lymphadenopathy (in CLL)
- abdominal discomfort due to splenomegaly.

Medical Management

History and Examination
During a detailed medical assessment the patient may describe:
- easily bruising and bleeding
- fatigue
- frequent infections.

Physical examination may reveal pallor, lymphadenopathy (in the neck, axilla, groin), splenomegaly and hepatomegaly.

Investigations
A diagnosis of chronic leukaemia will be confirmed by further investigations, including peripheral blood count, reticulocyte count, examination of bone marrow aspirate and trephine biopsy, biochemical tests, computed tomography (CT) scans and chest radiography. Lymph node biopsy may also be needed in some cases. Staging is important in CLL as it assists with prognostic information and treatment decisions (Howard and Hamilton 2013).

Treatment of Chronic Myeloid Leukaemia
Targeted therapies using tyrosine kinase inhibitors (TKIs), such as imatinib, are now the most commonly used first-line treatment for CML. Other biological therapies such as nilotinib and dasatinib are recommended by National Institute for Health and Care Excellence (NICE) for some patients who cannot have imatinib or if their disease is resistant to it. Newer TKIs such as ponatinib and bosutinib may also be prescribed as an alternative for some patients (NICE 2016a). For patients in the accelerated phase, treatment is highly problematic. Patients in blast crisis may be treated with chemotherapy suitable for treating acute leukaemia, however, the response is usually short-lived.

Allogeneic HSCT is a potentially curative option and may be used for younger patients who have a matched sibling donor. The best results have been seen when a transplant has been performed during the early chronic phase within 1 year of diagnosis (NICE 2016a). For those who do not have a sibling donor, matched unrelated donor HSCT may offer the possibility of a cure.

Treatment of Chronic Lymphocytic Leukaemia
Although there is no curative treatment for CLL, evidence suggests that there is no advantage to early treatment of asymptomatic patients. Hence, current practice follows a 'wait and watch' or 'active monitoring' approach during which the patient is monitored regularly for signs of disease progression.

Chemoimmunotherapy, a combination of chemotherapy and monoclonal antibodies, is now recommended as first-line treatment for patients who need treatment for CLL and is started when the patient develops an advancing disease (BSH 2018). This is typically manifested by progressive bone marrow failure, enlarged spleen and lymph nodes, increasing lymphocyte counts and systemic symptoms such as weight loss, fatigue, fever and night sweats (Leukaemia Care UK 2019). Splenectomy, leucopheresis and supportive care may be used alongside chemotherapy. The administration of intravenous immunoglobulins and antibiotics for patients experiencing recurrent infections, allopurinol to control hyperuricaemia and radiotherapy to relieve local obstruction may also be required.

❖ Nursing Management and Health Promotion: Chronic Leukaemia

A diagnosis of chronic leukaemia is a significant, life-changing event. Unless intensive treatment is required many patients remain at home but they require regular monitoring. Hospital-based nurses may be involved in assisting with diagnostic procedures and the administration of supportive therapies. However, if more intensive treatment or transplantation is pursued the nursing responsibilities will include:
- providing information about tests, diagnosis and treatment options
- administering treatment such as chemotherapy and immunotherapy
- providing psychological support to help the patient come to terms with a chronic and potentially life-threatening illness
- educating the patient about medication, including the importance of continuing with intermittent courses of chemotherapy
- assisting with activities of living
- giving advice about the level of work and activity that can realistically be attempted
- reinforcing the importance of follow-up in outpatient clinics.

Lymphoma

The lymphomas are a group of malignant disorders characterised by a proliferation of lymphoid cells originating in the lymph nodes or lymphoid tissue. Most often the disease is of B-cell origin. Traditionally, lymphomas are divided into two groups:
- Hodgkin lymphoma (HL)
- non-Hodgkin lymphoma (NHL).

HL is uncommon and accounted for fewer than 1% of all cancers in the UK in 2016–2018. The annual incidence of HL in the UK is around 2100 cases (Cancer Research UK n.d. [e]). It is more common among men than women and among people aged between 20 and 30 years, peaking again after 75 years of age.

NHL is the sixth most common cancer in the UK, representing 4% of all cancers in 2016–2018. Incidence increases with age with in excess of a third of people diagnosed with NHL aged 75 years and older and, as with HL, it seems to be more common in males than in females (Cancer Research UK n.d. [f]).

Pathophysiology
Lymphomas arise from the uncontrolled growth of lymphocytes and in both HL and NHL, cells in the affected lymph tissue (usually lymph nodes) reveal a disruption of normal structure, can infiltrate other sites and interfere with the normal functioning of the immune system. HL is characterised by the presence of large, malignant, multinucleated cells of B-cell origin known as Reed–Sternberg cells within the lymphoma tumour mass (Fig. 13.5). HL has two main types:
- classic HL, of which there are four subtypes
- nodular lymphocyte-predominant lymphoma.

NHL is more difficult to classify as it encompasses a wide range of diseases, encompassing a diverse group of lymphomas with different subtypes. The WHO (Alaggio et al. 2022) group lymphomas by cell type:

Figure 13.5 Hodgkin lymphoma showing a typical Reed–Sternberg cell. (Reproduced with permission from Watson HG, Craigg JIO, Manson LM. Blood disease. In: Walker BR, Colledge NR, Ralston SH, Penman ID, eds. *Davidson's Principles and Practice of Medicine.* Edinburgh: Churchill Livingstone; 2014:989-1056.)

- B cells, such as diffuse large B-cell lymphoma (DLBCL), mantle cell lymphoma (MCL), Burkitt lymphoma (BL), mucosa-associated lymphoid tissue (MALT) lymphoma and follicular lymphoma (FL)
- T cells NK cells, such as peripheral T-cell lymphoma (PTCL), angioimmunoblastic T-cell lymphoma (AITL) and cutaneous T-cell lymphoma (CTCL)

NHL can be further classified by according to how quickly they grow and spread. Low-grade (indolent, slow-growing) or high-grade (aggressive, fast-growing).

Clinical Presentation

Hodgkin Lymphoma. For 80%–90% of patients with HL, the most common manifestation is a painless enlarged lymph node, often described as 'rubbery'. Such nodes are found in the neck and supraclavicular fossae, axillae or inguinal regions. These may grow slowly or rapidly and compromise other organs by compression or obstruction. Other symptoms include pruritus and pain in the diseased lymph nodes on consuming alcohol. The reasons for this are unclear (Hoffbrand et al. 2019), but are thought to be related to vasodilatation within the lymph node.

Some patients also present with systemic symptoms, which are medically known as B symptoms. These may include one or more of the following:

- persistent unexplained fever, often at night
- drenching night sweats requiring the patient to change bed linen and night clothes
- weight loss >10% of body weight.

These symptoms are important when staging the disease and give some indication of prognosis.

Non-Hodgkin Lymphoma. Patients with NHL may present similarly to those with HL with painless lymphadenopathy. However, NHL is often widely disseminated at presentation and a wider range of symptoms can occur and will depend on the extent and site of the diseased nodes. Examples include:

- breathlessness due to enlarged mediastinal lymph nodes or obstruction of the superior vena cava
- lymphoedema in the arms or legs due to obstructed lymph drainage in the axillary or inguinal node

- anaemia or pancytopenia due to bone marrow involvement
- infection caused by defective humoral and/or cell-mediated immunity (see Chapter 7, Nursing Patients With Disorders of the Lymphatic and Immune Systems).

Like with HL, some patients also present with B symptoms.

🔵 *Medical Management*

Investigations

Diagnosis of lymphoma is generally made by means of:
- lymph node biopsy
- blood tests including FBC, ESR, renal function, liver function, bone profile tests, HIV, Hepatitis B and C
- bone marrow aspiration (see Investigations Used in the Diagnosis of Blood Disorders, subsection: Other Investigative Techniques)
- chest X-ray
- CT scan of chest, abdomen and pelvis
- positron emission tomography (PET) scan.

After clinical examination and once results of the investigations are known, the disease is staged. For both NHL and HL this is typically based on the Lugano classification (Information 13.7). This important prognostic indicator determines the extent of the disease by examining the number of involved lymph nodes, if located on one or both sides of the diaphragm, or extra lymphatic involvement and takes into account the presence or absence of B symptoms.

An international prognostic index (IPI) based on age, stage, bulk of disease, performance status and the serum lactate dehydrogenase (LDH) level is used as a predictor of adverse outcomes in NHL (Kahl and Mehta-Shah 2021).

Fertility preservation and counselling should be considered if appropriate.

Treatment

Hodgkin Lymphoma. Treatment depends on the stage of the disease. For early-stage disease, a short course (two to four cycles) of combination chemotherapy is typically given and is normally followed by involved-field radiotherapy (IFRT). Doxorubicin, bleomycin, vinblastine and dacarbazine (ABVD) and escalated bleomycin, etoposide, doxorubicin, cyclophosphamide, vincristine, procarbazine and prednisolone (eBEACOPP) are now considered standard treatments. An interim PET scan is now used to identify patients who may not need radiotherapy, due to concerns over radiotherapy effects (Follows et al. 2022).

Advanced-stage disease is typically treated with six to eight cycles of combination chemotherapy, either ABVD or eBEACOPP, the choice is dependent on the individual risk profile. An interim PET scan then determines further chemotherapy cycles and radiotherapy. Patients with 'bulky' (i.e. large diseased lymph nodes) mediastinal disease historically were managed as 'advanced stage disease' but newer trials confirm good outcomes when treated with early-stage protocols (Follows et al. 2022).

Patients who develop progressive disease are considered for intensive management and transplantation.

Non-Hodgkin Lymphoma. Specific chemotherapy regimens are prescribed according to the type of lymphoma and the stage of the disease. Regimens are continually being refined as clinical understanding improves.

'Low-Grade' NHL (FL, MCL, CTCL). Patients who are asymptomatic with 'low-grade' NHL are generally monitored closely without treatment until symptoms indicate the need. Local disease may be treated with radiotherapy. When required, chemotherapy (e.g. cyclophosphamide, vincristine and prednisolone) and/or immunotherapy (e.g. rituximab) can be used to manage low-grade NHL (NICE 2016b). Relapsed patients may respond to the same treatment that induced remission.

'High Grade' NHL (DLBCL, BL, PTCL). Most patients with high-grade NHL are treated as if they have advanced disease. The exact management depends on the type of NHL, but many are treated with a combination of CHOP (cyclophosphamide, doxorubicin hydrochloride, vincristine and prednisolone), with targeted immunotherapy, rituximab. This protocol is known as R-CHOP (NICE 2016a).

❖ Nursing Management and Health Promotion: Lymphoma

As lymphoma comprises such a diverse group of disorders and treatment is so varied, nursing care cannot be prescriptive. Some patients will be treated as outpatients, whereas others will be hospitalised throughout the course of treatment. Regardless of the setting in which the patient is treated, nursing interventions will include:

- explanation of diagnostic and staging investigations
- information about the disease
- administering specific treatment and managing side-effects with care and skill
- offering psychological support to patients and their families who may be shocked by the possibility of serious illness.

After the course of treatment patients should be given detailed information about postradiotherapy/chemotherapy care (see Chapter 31, Nursing Patients With Cancer). This should include:

- a contact number for help or advice
- the signs of infection or bleeding and whom to contact should either of these occur
- medication and details about how and when to take it, and potential side-effects
- dietary advice
- advice regarding skin care
- recommended level of activity and when to return to employment
- the importance of attendance at follow-up clinics
- appropriate self-help and support groups
- sex and fertility counselling as appropriate
- referral to community nurse, social worker and GP.

Whatever the outcome of treatment, patients with HL or NHL require high-quality physical and psychological care from nursing staff who are able to recognise and meet their individual needs and concerns.

Myeloma

Myeloma, sometimes also referred to as multiple myeloma, is an uncommon malignant disorder characterised by an abnormal and unregulated proliferation of plasma cells which develop from mature B lymphocytes. Myeloma accounted for 2% of all new cancer cases diagnosed in the UK in 2016–2018, with 6000 new cases each year (Cancer Research UK n.d. (g)). The disease is rare in young people and primarily occurs over the age of 40. In the UK incidence rates are highest in people aged 85–89 years, and most common in Black racial groups compared with White and Asian groups.

🔵 *Pathophysiology*

Normal plasma cells develop from B lymphocytes following antigen stimulation. Each plasma cell produces a specific immunoglobulin, which contains a variety of heavy and light chains. In myeloma, there is a malignant proliferation of one clone of plasma cells, which produce a single heavy or light chain known as a paraprotein. Depending on the type secreted, the abnormal paraprotein may be detected in the serum. It may also be present in the urine where it is referred to as Bence Jones protein. Measurement of paraprotein is commonly used to monitor the course of the disease.

The majority of malignant plasma cells exist in the bone marrow. Here they produce cytokines which stimulate osteoclasts, which are responsible for bone resorption in balance with bone formation by osteoblasts. Myeloma cells disrupt this balance by promoting osteoclast activity. This results in increased bone resorption and a reduction in bone formation. Multiple lytic bone lesions, hence the term 'multiple myeloma', also occur due to the secretion of bone-damaging cytokines by the myeloma cells.

Although the cause of myeloma is unknown there appears to be some connection with occupational exposure to certain products such as pesticides, radiation and benzene.

Clinical Presentation

The onset of myeloma is often insidious and it is not uncommon for the disease to be advanced at the time of presentation. Some patients may experience a sudden onset of bone pain caused by pathological fractures or severe bone tenderness throughout the body. Others present with pneumonia due to neutropenia and lowered immunoglobulin levels, and yet others may present with clinical features of renal failure and/or hypercalcaemia.

The most common presenting signs and symptoms associated with multiple myeloma are:

- bone pain, especially in the lower back region, and pathological fractures
- spinal cord compression (SCC) due to vertebral collapse
- anaemia, mediated by cytokines rather than by marrow replacement
- acute kidney injury
- hypercalcaemia
- infection
- amyloidosis (deposition of the abnormal protein, amyloid, in organ systems) affecting the kidney and leading to proteinuria and nephrotic syndrome.

🔵 *Medical Management*

Investigations

Investigations undertaken to diagnose myeloma include:

- whole-body MRI or CT-PET (X-ray skeletal survey, CT if MRI is unsuitable)

- bone marrow aspiration and trephine biopsy with plasma cell phenotyping
- blood tests – FBC, urea and creatinine, calcium, albumin, immunoglobulins, serum electrophoresis, serum free light chains

To confirm the diagnosis of myeloma and determine its stage, the following is required (Sive et al. 2021):
- clonal bone marrow plasma cells ≥10% or biopsy-proven plasmacytoma
- one or more myeloma-defining events (≥60% plasma cells in marrow; involved/uninvolved light chain ratio ≥100; two or more focal lesions on MRI; hypercalcaemia; renal insufficiency; anaemia; one or more lytic bone lesion)

Treatment

Myeloma is currently incurable. Patients with minimal symptoms may not require intervention. In more advanced disease, management is aimed at controlling symptoms of the disease, particularly pain. High fluid intake of 3–4 L of fluid a day is recommended to prevent and treat renal impairment and hypercalcaemia, and in some cases, intravenous fluids may be needed.

Chemotherapy. Recommended first-line treatment for newly diagnosed myeloma is dexamethasone, either used alone or in combination with the chemotherapy agents bortezomib and/or thalidomide (NICE 2018).

Lenalidomide, in combination with dexamethasone, may be considered for people with myeloma who have received two or more prior therapies (NICE 2018).

Haematopoietic stem cell harvesting and more intensive treatment using high-dose melphalan and autologous stem cell rescue may then follow. Allogeneic transplantation may cure some patients and should be considered for patients with suitable performance status and fitness (NICE 2018).

To manage relapsed myeloma, Bortezomib is recommended by NICE (2018) as a possible treatment for people who have had a bone marrow transplant, or if transplant is not suitable for them.

Bisphosphonates have been shown to substantially reduce bone destruction by inhibiting osteoclast activity and are recommended for all patients requiring treatment (NICE 2018). VTE prophylaxis should also be considered for people with myeloma who are receiving chemotherapy to prevent thrombosis (NICE 2019).

Surgery. Internal fixation of fractured bones or areas of lytic lesions that are liable to fracture may be necessary to stabilise bones that are diseased (see Chapter 12, Nursing Patients With Musculoskeletal Disorders).

Plasmapheresis. may be used to reduce a high blood viscosity, as the removal of the patient's plasma will also reduce the paraprotein level. This is done only as a temporary measure whilst other treatment is given.

❖ Nursing Management and Health Promotion: Myeloma

Myeloma is a very complex disorder with multisystem effects, some of which are potentially life-threatening. In order to plan and implement care, it is important that the nurse has a thorough knowledge of the disease and its effects on the patient.

Pain Management

Often the most distressing and debilitating symptom for the patient is pain. Assessment should take into account the multidimensional effects of pain and that the pain may have been present for some time. Pain management strategies will depend on the cause and severity of the pain but may include the use of analgesia including opioids and nonsteroidal anti-inflammatory drugs (NSAIDs), and nonpharmaceutical methods such as relaxation, massage and the application of hot or cold packs. Palliative chemotherapy and/or radiotherapy may be used to reduce pain.

Maintaining Mobility Whilst Preventing Fractures

Whilst prolonged periods of bed rest should be avoided to decrease the risk of hypercalcaemia and pulmonary embolism, so too should activity which increases the risk of fracturing weak bones. Management strategies include:
- ensuring pain is controlled prior to exercise and being aware that increased activity may increase the level of pain and the need for analgesics
- working with the physiotherapist and occupational therapist to help the patient attain an optimal level of activity
- provision of lightweight braces which provide support for the spine for patients with multiple lytic lesions
- maintaining a safe environment
- ensuring that a home assessment has been carried out prior to discharge to identify any modifications that may be needed within the patient's home.

Prevention of Infection

Preventative strategies include:
- monitoring the patient for signs and symptoms of infection and treating these promptly with prescribed antibiotics if required
- offering the seasonal influenza vaccination and considering the pneumococcal vaccination ensuring maintenance of adequate hydration
- avoiding urinary catheterisation to prevent the possibility of infection
- maintaining a diet high in calories and essential nutrients to support the immune system.

Fatigue Due to Anaemia

Anaemia causing fatigue will be corrected by regular blood transfusion. Patients may need reassurance about
the frequency of transfusion and to be assisted in establishing strategies to maximise their energy by ensuring a balance between rest and activity.

Prevention of Spinal Cord Compression

SCC is an oncological emergency which can occur in patients who have myeloma. Nurses need to know the presentation of SCC, which includes spinal pain, impaired sensation, limb weakness, or bladder or bowel dysfunction, and must recognise the importance of urgent reporting to medical staff and immediate interventions.

Communication and Psychological Support

In addition to coping with distressing and debilitating symptoms, the patient faces a diagnosis of a malignant disease which is probably incurable. Nursing management strategies include listening to the patient's anxieties and answering questions honestly, in a way that is appropriate for the patient.

Patient Education

Acquiring knowledge about the disease and its management may help the patient to feel more in control. The patient should receive information about:

- side-effects of treatment and self-monitoring
- preventing or minimising complications, e.g. sufficient oral fluids
- safe techniques for moving and handling
- reducing muscle weakness
- the importance of follow-up with the GP and hospital outpatient clinics and relevant support groups (see Useful Websites).

Discharge Planning

This will depend on the patient's physical and psychological state, the type of treatment received and the availability of carers at home or in the community. Planning needs to address the following:

- the patient's level of dependency
- the availability of home carers – the type and degree of support needed
- the skills needed by carers, e.g. safe moving and handling of the patient.

Myelodysplastic Syndromes

Myelodysplastic syndromes (MDSs) are a group of disorders derived from an abnormal stem cell which retains the capacity to differentiate into end-stage cells. However, this differentiation is disordered and ineffective and leads to peripheral blood cytopenias of RBCs, WBCs and platelets (Hoffbrand et al. 2019). Morphological abnormalities and impaired maturation of RBCs, WBCs and platelets are common and these form the basis for diagnosis. Disease progression is extremely variable but during the course of MDS the abnormal clone is prone to lose its ability to differentiate, with some cases transforming into acute leukaemia.

MDS is a very rare condition, with an incidence in the UK of only 3.72 cases per 100,000 population per year. It is more common in men than women, and although it can affect all ages tends to be a disease affecting older people (Roman et al. 2016).

It occurs most often as a primary condition with an unknown cause, but may also develop secondary to exposure to cytotoxic medications (e.g. alkylating agents), chemicals (e.g. benzene) and radiation.

Pathophysiology

MDS occurs as a result of DNA damage to a pluripotent stem cell leading to more rapid cell division in the abnormal clone of cells when compared to normal cells. The disease is classified into subgroups by the WHO based on the combination of bone marrow and peripheral blood morphology (Hoffbrand et al. 2019). This newer classification, compared to the French–American–British classification (FAB), lowers the threshold for AML diagnosis, with an improved prognostic value.

Clinical Presentation

The clinical presentation of MDS is highly variable. Some patients may have symptoms of bone marrow failure such as fatigue caused by anaemia, infection caused by neutropenia, or bruising due to thrombocytopenia. Others may be diagnosed through unrelated routine blood tests. In some cases, hepatosplenomegaly may be present and occasionally gum hypertrophy, pleural and pericardial effusion, and painful, swollen joints.

The course and prognosis of MDS are variable and unpredictable. Some patients remain stable for many years, whilst others experience rapid progression to AML.

Medical Management

Investigations

After a thorough history, diagnosis is made on findings from the following investigations:

- bone marrow aspiration and trephine biopsy
- FBC and film
- cytogenetic analysis.

Vitamin B_{12} and folate levels are usually checked to eliminate any deficiency that would affect the blood results.

Treatment

Treatment of MDS depends on the patient's health status, comorbidities and severity of the myelodysplasia. The Revised International Prognostic Scoring System (IPSS-R) is used to categorise patients into low, intermediate or high risk disease groups according to percentage of blasts in the bone marrow, the number and severity of cytopenias present and abnormal karyotypes (Hoffbrand et al. 2019) and this will be used to guide treatment strategies. Treatment is most often aimed at supportive care in order to prolong survival and delay transformation to acute leukaemia (Killick et al. 2021). Interventions include:

- regular blood transfusion, to improve symptomatic anaemia
- platelet transfusion administered when spontaneous bleeding occurs (no longer recommended for prophylaxis)
- infection prevention strategies and swift treatment in the event of detection
- immunosuppression with antithymocyte globulin
- erythropoiesis-stimulating agents, for symptomatic anaemia
- thrombopoietin receptor agonists to reduce bleeding events in thrombocytopenic patients
- low-dose or intensive chemotherapy
- ongoing supportive care and emotional health needs assessment

Other potential treatments include lenalidomide, luspatercept, iron chelation and hypomethylating agents.

Allogeneic stem cell transplantation is the only curative treatment and may be considered for patients with a suitable donor.

Nursing Management and Health Promotion: Myelodysplastic Syndrome

Nursing a patient with MDS requires specific skills and expert knowledge in relation to the disease process, treatment options and side-effects. Due to the unpredictability of the disease and the seriousness of its effects, MDS may have significant psychological and social implications and the effect of these on the patient and their family should not be underestimated. Strategies aimed at promoting health and minimising the risk of complications should be provided to the patient with an emphasis on maintaining quality of life. As such, nursing priorities will include:

- monitoring the patient for signs of anaemia, infection and bleeding and acting promptly if these are detected
- educating the patient and their family about the disease, treatment and associated risks and what to do if complications arise
- administering prescribed treatment and supportive therapies such as blood transfusion in line with national and local policy guidance
- demonstrating flexibility when planning hospital appointments and treatment in order to minimise disruption to daily life

- referral to a social worker or counsellor for psychological support and assistance with financial issues if required.

Disorders of Coagulation

Disorders of coagulation can be subdivided into three types:
- disorders due to lack of coagulation (clotting) factors, such as haemophilia or von Willebrand disease
- platelet disorders, such as thrombocytopenia
- disorders due to other causes such as lack of vitamin K or liver disease (see Chapter 4, Nursing Patients With Gastrointestinal, Liver and Biliary Disorders).

These disorders may be inherited or acquired and all age groups are affected. Some problems with coagulation are caused by genetic disorders, for example, haemophilia A. Coagulation factor disorders involve a deficiency in one or more of the blood factors required for haemostasis. Inherited coagulation disorders result from the lack of specific coagulation factors. The acquired disorders involve the failure of certain coagulation factors to be activated, usually as a result of vitamin K deficiency or liver disease.

This section provides an outline of haemophilia and thrombocytopenia (deficiency of platelets).

Haemophilia

The haemophilias are a group of inherited disorders in which an essential coagulation factor is either partly or completely missing. This causes a person with haemophilia to bleed for longer than normal. A rare acquired autoimmune haemophilia can also occur, where there is no bleeding history, and is most commonly seen in older people (NORD 2022). Haemophilia is evident worldwide and occurs in all racial groups, and is most common in males.

🔴 Pathophysiology

Haemophilia is a recessive X-linked condition (sex-linked inheritance) which nearly always affects males, while females carry the defective gene (Reflection 13.5). Notably, it is possible for a female to have haemophilia or a tendency to bleed (Haemophilia Society 2023). There are two types of haemophilia, the most common being haemophilia A (classic haemophilia), in which factor VIII is lacking. This type affects approximately 1/5000 of the male population (Haemophilia Society 2023). In haemophilia B, also known as Christmas disease, factor IX is lacking, this is rarer affecting 1/30,000 of the male population. Both types of the disorder share similar symptoms.

Clinical Presentation

Despite haemophilia being an inherited disorder, it is unusual for excessive bleeding to occur before 6 months of age, when superficial bleeding or bruising may occur (Carcao et al. 2018). A FBC and coagulation assays will be required for diagnosis and a family history must be taken to ascertain whether the condition is inherited.

Haemophilia is classified as mild, moderate or severe and clinical presentation will vary accordingly. In mild cases, superficial bruising and excessive bleeding after minor injuries or procedures may be evident, while if haemophilia is severe, spontaneous recurrent bleeding in major joints and muscles is common. Serious long-term effects of this include pain, arthritic changes and mobility problems.

🔴 Medical Management

There is no cure for haemophilia. Treatment involves replacing the deficient coagulation factors and is dependent on the degree of factor deficiency and severity of the bleeding. People with mild haemophilia A may be prescribed desmopressin (DDAVP), a synthetic hormone which stimulates factor XIII release and may be given in combination with tranexamic acid. More severe cases will require regular intravenous infusions of factor VIII or IX concentrate. These are in recombinant form, not from blood, which is considerably safer in terms of reducing viral contamination. A serious consequence of regular factor VIII replacement therapy is the development of antibodies to factors which may render treatment ineffective. In such cases higher doses may be required or an alternative treatment. Immune tolerance therapy (ITT) or Emicizumab may be required (Haemophilia Society 2023).

Thrombocytopenia

Any disturbance in the number or function of circulating platelets will affect the normal coagulation process. Thrombocytopenia implies a reduction in the number of platelets and may be inherited or acquired.

🔴 Pathophysiology

Inherited thrombocytopenia is fortunately rare. Acquired thrombocytopenia may occur as a result of factors that either decrease normal platelet production or increase platelet consumption/destruction (Information 13.8).

Decreased production is usually caused by drugs or some other agent whereby the bone marrow is suppressed. The most common cause of increased platelet consumption/destruction is immune (idiopathic) thrombocytopenic purpura (ITP). This commonly affects individuals in their teens or early 20s and is thought to be autoimmune in origin. Whatever the cause, ITP will result in a prolonged bleeding time, giving rise to bruising, purpura or petechiae and, more seriously, gastrointestinal, retinal or intracranial bleeding.

Clinical Presentation

Patients may present with a history of bleeding gums, epistaxis, melaena and haematuria. In contrast to haemophilia, if pressure is applied to the bleeding point, the bleeding will stop and not recur unless further trauma occurs.

REFLECTION 13.5

Haemophilia and Health Promotion

Belinda and Marvin are expecting their first baby. One of Belinda's brothers has haemophilia A, as do several other male relatives. She has been tested and knows that she is a genetic carrier of the disorder. Belinda and Marvin are worried that their baby will be affected and that, if this is the case, he or she will not be able to have a fulfilling life.

Activity

- Access *Understanding Haemophilia* (Haemophilia Society 2023) and find out (a) how likely it is that their baby will be affected, (b) information about the management of haemophilia and lifestyle if they have a son who has haemophilia.
- Reflect on Belinda and Marvin's situation. Are their concerns valid and what information and advice should they be given?

Causes of Acquired Thrombocytopenia

Decreased or Abnormal Platelet Production

- Malignancy
- Myelofibrosis
- Sarcoidosis
- Nutritional deficiency
- Congenital disorders.

Increased Platelet Destruction

- Immune thrombocytopenic purpura (ITP)
- Disseminated intravascular coagulation (DIC)
- Thrombotic thrombocytopenic purpura (TTP)
- Autoimmune thrombocytopenia
- Drug induced – for example quinidine, quinine, nonsteroidal anti-inflammatory drugs (NSAIDs), penicillin and anticonvulsants.

Increased Platelet Sequestration

- Splenomegaly, due to portal hypertension
- Hepatic vein thrombosis or vena cava thrombosis
- Cirrhosis
  Thrombocytopenia can also be dilutional (caused by blood transfusion, or pregnancy), or cancer-related (caused by myelosuppression due to bone marrow infiltration or myelodysplasia) (NICE 2021).

Reference

National Institute for Health and Care Excellence (NICE) What are the causes of thrombocytopenia? 2021. https://cks.nice.org.uk/topics/platelets-abnormal-counts-cancer/background-information/causes-of-thrombocytopenia/

Medical Management
History and Examination

A thorough clinical history is required to identify any recent minor illness or drug therapy, including over-the-counter medicines. Clinical examination is carried out to detect any signs of bruising, petechiae, purpura or any underlying disorder.

Investigations
These will include:
- FBC and blood film
- bone marrow aspiration
- coagulation screen
- biochemical screen.

Treatment
Some cases of ITP resolve spontaneously; however, it usually becomes a chronic condition. In cases where an exacerbating factor such as a medication is withdrawn, spontaneous remission may also occur.

Corticosteroids improve platelet survival and a short course may be given until resolution occurs. However, thrombocytopenia may recur when the corticosteroids are withdrawn. Second-line therapies include a thrombopoietin receptor agonist, or monoclonal antibody rituximab (Neunert et al. 2019). Splenectomy may also be required in some cases, as the spleen is a major site of platelet destruction. Platelet transfusions are given if bleeding is severe.

❖ Nursing Management and Health Promotion: Thrombocytopenia

Nursing priorities for the hospitalised patient with platelet disorders include:
- controlling any superficial bleeding by the application of external pressure
- ensuring that the patient is protected from injury by advising on environmental safety and that feeling faint may indicate anaemia or low blood pressure
- providing explanations and support during tests and treatment
- observing the patient for evidence of bleeding by:
  - regular monitoring of patient's pulse (note: caution should be used if blood pressure measurement is required as this may cause bruising and petechiae)
  - inspection of the skin for petechiae, purpura and bruises, and of the mouth for bleeding and infection
  - regular testing of urine, stools and vomit for blood
  - being alert to complaints of headaches and drowsiness, as these may indicate intracranial bleeding.

Health promotion is of utmost importance and the importance of monitoring all episodes of bleeding must be stressed, along with the need for regular follow-up.

Specific points that the patient should be advised about include:
- taking medicines as prescribed
- avoiding aspirin preparations
- avoiding intramuscular injections
- carrying identification such as a MedicAlert card/bracelet
- minimising potential for soft tissue injury
- avoiding contact sports.

The family should be included in the education programme to ensure that all members understand the necessity of certain restrictions on lifestyle. However, it should also be stressed that it is important for the patient to maintain a balance between being overcautious and taking unnecessary risks.

Summary: Key Nursing Issues

- Haematology is a challenging and constantly developing area of practice in which ongoing research continues to improve patient outcomes.
- Nurses are instrumental in the planning, delivery and evaluation of care of people with blood disorders and require a range of skills underpinned by a sound knowledge of blood and haematopoiesis as well as an understanding of disorders, treatment and potential complications.

- Anaemia is a common blood disorder. It is associated with various factors including diet and disease and can impact on physical and psychological well-being.
- An understanding of infection prevention and control by nurses is vital when caring for patients with WBC disorders. Signs of infection require prompt action.
- The nature of acute leukaemia means that chemotherapy is often started before the patient has had time to fully assimilate

the diagnosis and its implications. Nurses can assist by providing accurate information and ongoing psychosocial support in response to the needs of the patient and their family.
- HSCT or bone marrow transplantation may be the only curative treatment for a number of blood conditions. It typically involves preparatory regimens which render the patient extremely vulnerable to infection and other complications.

- Some blood disorders are inherited and this may have implications for the family members.
- Many blood disorders are incurable and in such cases, effective symptom control and maintaining quality of life should be a priority.

Reflection and Learning – What Next?

- **Test** your knowledge by visiting the Evolve website 🌐 and answering the multiple choice questions and critical thinking questions.
- **Consolidate** your learning by looking at some of the Further Reading suggestions, references and specialist websites.
- **Revisit** some of the additional material on the Evolve website.

- **Consider** what you have learnt and how this will help your professional development.
- **Reflect** on how you can apply this knowledge to the care of your patients.
- **Discuss** your learning with your assessor/supervisor, lecturer and colleagues.

References

Alaggio R, Amador C, Anagnostopoulos I, et al. The 5th edition of the World Health Organisation Classification of Haematolymphoid Tumours: Lymphoid Neoplasms. *Leukemia*. 2022;36(7):1720–1748.

British Dietary Association. Policy Statement: Safer eating with neutropenia; 2020. https://www.bda.uk.com/uploads/assets/9f7e021a-2edf-4d62-9bd5fba841d7472c/52d14410-d3b7-45cb-a3a0e09e15eeda2b/Neutropenic-Diets-Guidance-Jan-2020.pdf

British Society for Haematology (BSH). Guidelines for use of platelet transfusion. *Br J Haematol*. 2016;176:365–394.

British Society for Haematology (BSH). Guidelines for diagnosis and management of chronic lymphocytic leukaemia. *Br J Haematol*. 2018;182:344–359.

Camitta BM Criteria for severe aplastic anaemia. *Lancet*. 1988 Feb 6;1(8580):303–304.

Cancer Research UK. Leukaemia (all sub-types combined) statistics; n.d. (a). https://www.cancerresearchuk.org/health-professional/cancer-statistics/statistics-by-cancer-type/leukaemia.

Cancer Research UK. Acute myeloid leukaemia (AML) statistics; n.d. (b). https://www.cancerresearchuk.org/health-professional/cancer-statistics/statistics-by-cancer-type/leukaemia-aml.

Cancer Research UK. Chronic myeloid leukaemia (CML) statistics; n.d. (c). https://www.cancerresearchuk.org/health-professional/cancer-statistics/statistics-by-cancer-type/leukaemia-cml/incidence

Cancer Research UK. Chronic lymphocytic leukaemia (CLL) statistics; n.d. (d). https://www.cancerresearchuk.org/health-professional/cancer-statistics/statistics-by-cancer-type/leukaemia-cll#heading-Zero

Cancer Research UK. Hodgkin lymphoma statistics; n.d. (e). https://www.cancerresearchuk.org/health-professional/cancer-statistics/statistics-by-cancer-type/hodgkin-lymphoma.

Cancer Research UK. Non-Hodgkin lymphoma statistics; n.d. (f). https://www.cancerresearchuk.org/health-professional/cancer-statistics/statistics-by-cancer-type/non-hodgkin-lymphoma.

Cancer Research UK. Myeloma statistics; n.d. (g). https://www.cancerresearchuk.org/health-professional/cancer-statistics/statistics-by-cancer-type/myeloma.

Cancer Research UK. Research into AML; 2020. https://www.cancerresearchuk.org/about-cancer/acute-myeloid-leukaemia-aml/research-clinical-trials/research-aml.

Cancer Research UK. Chemotherapy for acute lymphoblastic leukaemia (ALL). 2021. https://www.cancerresearchuk.org/about-cancer/acute-lymphoblastic-leukaemia-all/treatment/chemotherapy-acute-lymphoblastic-leukaemia-ALL.

Carcao M, Moorehead P, Lillicrap D, Hemophilia A and B. In: Hoffman R, et al, eds. *Hematology: Basic Principles and Practice*. 7th ed. Philadelphia: Elsevier; 2018:2001–2022.

Cheson BD, Bennett JM, Kopecky KJ, et al. International Working Group for Diagnosis, Standardization of Response Criteria, Treatment Outcomes, and Reporting Standards for Therapeutic Trials in Acute Myeloid Leukemia. Revised recommendations of the International Working Group for Diagnosis, Standardization of Response Criteria, Treatment Outcomes, and Reporting Standards for Therapeutic Trials in Acute Myeloid Leukemia. *J Clin Oncol*. 2003 Dec 15;21(24):4642–4649.

Emadi A, Law JY. Overview of Leukemia; 2022. www.msdmanuals.com/en-gb/professional/hematology-and-oncology/leukemias/overview-of-leukemia

Haesler Emily, ed. *European Pressure Ulcer Advisory Panel, National Pressure Injury Advisory Panel and Pan Pacific Pressure Injury Alliance. Prevention and Treatment of Pressure Ulcers/Injuries: Quick Reference Guide*. EPUAP/NPIAP/PPPIA; 2019. https://internationalguideline.com/2019.

Follows GA, Barrington SF, Bhuller KS, et al. Guideline for the first-line management of Classical Hodgkin Lymphoma - A British Society for Haematology guideline. *Br J Haematol*. 2022;197(5):558–572.

Freeman L, Postma B. Talk about fertility options. *Cancer Nurs Pract*. 2018;17(3):12.

Global Health Metrics. Anaemia–Level 1 impairment. 2019;393. https://www.healthdata.org/results/gbd_summaries/2019/anemia-level-1-impairment.

Haemophilia Society. Understanding Haemophilia; 2023. https://haemophilia.org.uk/wp-content/uploads/2023/07/THS_A5_understanding_JCv1_interactive.pdf.

Hill B, Derbyshire J. Blood transfusions in adults: ensuring patient safety. *Br J Nurs*. 2021;30(9):520–524.

Hochhaus A, Baccarani M, Silver RT, et al. European LeukemiaNet 2020 recommendations for treating chronic myeloid leukemia. *Leukemia*. 2020;34:966–984.

Hoffbrand AV, Moss PAH, Pettit JE. *Essential Haematology*. 8th ed. Oxford. Wiley Blackwell; 2019.

Howard MR, Hamilton PJ. *Haematology: An Illustrated Colour Text*. 4th ed. Edinburgh: Churchill Livingstone; 2013.

Huether SE, McCance KL. *Understanding Pathophysiology*. 7th ed. St. Louis: Elsevier; 2019.

Kahl BMehta-Shah N 'Non-Hodgkin Lymphoma' in Govindan R, Morgensztern D, Ghobadi A. *The Washington Manual of Oncology: Therapeutic Principles in Practice*. Wolters Kluwer Health; 2021.

Killick SB, Brown N, Cavenagh J, et al. 2015, Guidelines for the diagnosis and management of adult aplastic anaemia. 172(2):187–207.

Killick S, Ingram W, Culligan D, et al. British Society for Haematology guidelines for the management of adult myelodysplastic syndromes. *Br J Haematol*. 2021.

Leukaemia Care UK. Chronic lymphocytic leukaemia (CLL); 2019. https://www.leukaemiacare.org.uk/support-and-information/information-about-blood-cancer/blood-cancer-information/leukaemia/chronic-lymphocytic-leukaemia/.

Mehta A, Hoffbrand V. *Haematology at a Glance.* 4th ed. Chichester: Wiley; 2014.

Neunert C, Terrell DR, Arnold DM, et al. American Society of Hematology 2019 guidelines for immune thrombocytopenia. *Blood Adv.* 2019;3(23):3829–3866.

National Institute for Health and Care Excellence (NICE). *Blood Transfusion* 2015. https://www.nice.org.uk/guidance/ng24.

National Institute for Health and Care Excellence (NICE). Guidance on the use of imatinib for chronic myeloid leukaemia; 2016a. https://www.nice.org.uk/guidance/ta70/resources/guidance-on-the-use-of-imatinib-for-chronic-myeloid-leukaemia-pdf-2294751800005.

National Institute for Health and Care Excellence (NICE). Non-Hodgkin's lymphoma: diagnosis and management 2016b. https://www.nice.org.uk/guidance/ng52/chapter/Recommendations

National Institute for Health and Care Excellence (NICE). Myeloma: diagnosis and management 2018. https://www.nice.org.uk/guidance/ng35

National Institute for Health and Care Excellence (NICE). Venous thromboembolism in over 16s: reducing the risk of hospital-acquired deep vein thrombosis or pulmonary embolism 2019. https://www.nice.org.uk/guidance/ng89/chapter/Recommendations

National Organisation for Rare Disorders (NORD). Acquired hemophilia 2022. https://rarediseases.org/rare-diseases/acquired-hemophilia/.

Norasetthada L, Wongkhantee S, Chaipokam J, Charoenpraset K, Chuncharunee S, Rojnuckarin P, et al. Adult aplastic anaemia in Thailand:incidence and treatment outceom from a prospective nationwide population-based study. *Ann Heamatol.* 2021;100(10):2443–2452.

Rivera-Gamma S, Davis ME. CE: Tumor Lysis Syndrome: An Oncologic Emergency. *Am J Nurs.* March 2023;123(3):30–35.

Roman E, Smith A, Appleton S, Crouch S, Kelly R, Kinsey S, et al. Myeloid malignancies in the real-world: Occurrence, progression and survival in the UK's population-based Haematological Malignancy Research Network 2004–15. *Cancer Epidemiol.* 2016;42:186–198.

SHOT (Serious Hazards of Transfusion). Annual report 2022; 2022. https://www.shotuk.org/shot-reports/

Sickle Cell Society. *Standards for the Clinical Care of Adults with Sickle Cell Disease in the UK.* 2nd ed.; 2018. https://www.sicklecellsociety.org/sicklecellstandards/.

Sive J, Cuthill K, Hunter H, Kazmi M, Pratt G, Smith D. Guidelines on the diagnosis, investigation and initial treatment of myeloma: a British Society for Haematology/UK Myeloma Forum Guideline. *Br J Haematol.* 2021.

Tefferi A, Barbui T. Polycythemia vera:2024 update on diagnosis, risk stratification, and management. *Am J Hematol.* 2023;98:1465–1487.

UK Sepsis Trust. https://sepsistrust.org/

World Health Organisation. *Haemoglobin concentrations for the diagnosis of anaemia and assessment of severity. Vitamin and Mineral Nutrition Information System.* Geneva: World Health Organisation; 2011. http://www.who.int/vmnis/indicators/haemoglobin/en/index.html.

Further Reading

Brown M, Cutler T, eds. *Haematology Nursing.* Chichester: Wiley; 2012.

49 Cancer Research UK. Cancer statistics for the UK. n.d. https://www.cancerresearchuk.org/health-professional/cancer-statistics-for-the-uk.

Daniels G, Bromilow I. *Essential Guide to Blood Groups.* 3rd ed. Chichester: Wiley; 2013.

Guinan EC. Diagnosis and Management of Aplastic Anemia. *Hematology Am Soc Hematol Educ Program.* 2011(1):76–81.

Haemophilia Society. Understanding haemophilia; 2023. https://haemophilia.org.uk/wp-content/uploads/2023/07/THS_A5_understanding_JCv1_interactive.pdf.

Leukaemia Foundation. Acute lymphoblastic leukaemia; 2023. https://www.leukaemia.org.au/disease-information/leukaemias/acute-lymphoblastic-leukaemia/.

Leukaemia Foundation. Acute myeloid leukaemia; 2023. https://www.leukaemia.org.au/disease-information/leukaemias/acute-myeloid-leukaemia/.

Leukaemia Foundation. Chronic lymphocytic leukaemia; 2023. https://www.leukaemia.org.au/blood-cancer/leukaemia/chronic-lymphocytic-leukaemia/.

Leukaemia Foundation. Chronic myeloid leukaemia; 2023. https://www.leukaemia.org.au/disease-information/leukaemias/chronic-myeloid-leukaemia/.

Sickle Cell Society. Standards for the Clinical Care of Adults with Sickle Cell Disease in the UK; 2018. https://www.sicklecellsociety.org/resource/standards-clinical-care-adults-sickle-cell-disease-uk/standards-for-the-clinical-care-of-adults-with-sickle-cell-disease-in-the-uk/.

Tortora GJ, Derrickson B. *Principles of Anatomy and Physiology. 16th ed. International Adaptation.* Hoboken, NJ: Wiley; 2023.

Useful Websites

Bloodwise, https://bloodwise.org.uk/
British Dietetics Association, https://www.bda.uk.com
British Nutrition Foundation (BNF), www.nutrition.org.uk/
Cancer Research UK, www.cancerresearchuk.org
Haemophilia Society, www.haemophilia.org.uk
Leukaemia Foundation, www.leukaemia.org.au/
Lymphoma Association (UK), www.lymphomas.org.uk
Myeloma UK, www.myeloma.org.uk
NHS Blood and Transplant, www.nhsbt.nhs.uk
NICE (National Institute for Health and Care Excellence), www.nice.org.uk
SHOT (Serious Hazards of Transfusion), www.shotuk.org
Sickle Cell Society, www.sicklecellsociety.org
United Kingdom Thalassaemia Society, www.ukts.org
World Health Organisation, www.who.int/

14

Nursing Patients With Skin Disorders

JILL PETERS

CHAPTER OUTLINE

Introduction

This chapter introduces dermatology nursing and the most common conditions encountered. Skin disorders range from minor conditions, resolved with over-the-counter (OTC) preparations, to potentially life-threatening skin conditions requiring intensive care and treatment (skin failure). Many conditions are of a cyclical, long-term nature with patients requiring care in different settings: inpatient, outpatient, community and self-care. Dermatology is a visual specialty and readers can access colour images in Further Reading, for example *ABC Dermatology*, from the companion website and Useful Websites. Dermatology nursing is a still developing into exciting specialist roles that have clinical descriptions to support their development regardless of clinical setting (British Association of Dermatologists [BAD] 2020).

Skin disorders are encountered in all fields of nursing. A good knowledge base helps the nurse to dispel myths about the contagious nature of skin disorders, and the psychosocial implications of skin disease should not be dismissed lightly. Success, power and achievement are often dependent on 'image'. The media support images of the soft-skinned baby, blemish-free teenager and smooth sophisticated adult, and such images are reflected in money spent by all genders who aspire to cosmetic perfection.

Various research-based tools, for example, Dermatology Life Quality Index (DLQI) (Chernyshov 2019), are used to investigate the quality of life (QoL) of patients with skin disorders and how skin disease impacts on their life. The Patient Health Questionnaire (PHQ) 9 is used to measure mental well-being when on systemic biologic and nonbiologic medications, for example retinoids and biologics; both groups can give remission from physical disease but not always psychological fear of relapse.

The experience of skin disease may restrict social, professional and personal activities and impact on careers and relationships. Problems with sexuality and relationships can be linked to low self-esteem and the self-concept of an altered body image associated with having a skin condition. The psychological morbidity of skin disease is often underestimated by health professionals (Green 2010) despite patients reporting their experiences of ostracism, stigmatisation and isolation – the 'unclean leper' status of having a skin disorder (Reflection 14.1).

Epidemiology of Skin Diseases

Skin disease is common. One in four people (13.2 million) see their general practitioner (GP) for a dermatological condition in England and Wales each year, with 3.5 million attending dermatology outpatients and minor surgery each year (GIRFH 2021). The type, incidence and prevalence of skin disorders depend on social, economic, geographical, racial and cultural factors (Gawkrodger and Ardern-Jones 2020). The economic implications of skin disease can be considerable for individuals, families and employers. Skin diseases are the most common group of occupational health problems leading to absence from work (Lachapelle et al. 2017). Age is an important factor in diagnosing disorders, some conditions being exclusive to a particular age group, and others persisting throughout life. Atopic eczema, for example, is most common in infancy but can be cyclical in nature throughout life, while acne develops in adolescence and normally wanes by the late 40s. Older people show expected degenerative skin changes, with 27% having malignant skin lesions.

For malignant melanoma, the deadliest form of skin cancer, 46 new cases are diagnosed every day (2016–2018), 16,700 cases in the UK every year (Melanoma UK 2022), equalling 4% of all new cancers. It is largely preventable and may be curable if found, diagnosed and treated early, with one-stop clinics for skin lesions being very effective in reducing missed appointments as lesions are examined and surgically removed if needed in one visit (Elective Care

Transformation Team, Operations & Information NHS England 2019). Over the last decade, nonmelanoma skin cancer incidence rates have increased by around three-fifths (61%) in the UK (Cancer Research UK 2018). UK online campaigns aim to change behaviour in relation to sunlight exposure and sunbed use by educating people that a suntan is a sign of damaged skin rather than a desirable fashion statement.

Genetic or hereditary factors can be relevant to the diagnosis, and a family history should be part of the assessment. Psychological stress (e.g. exams and financial concerns) is common as a trigger, but most skin disorders are stressful conditions in their own right. Certain skin disorders are recognised as being entirely of psychogenic origin, for example trichotillomania (breaking of hair).

Social factors impact on skin disorders, and improvements in standards of living, personal hygiene and nutrition have reduced the rate of certain skin disorders (Gawkrodger and Ardern-Jones 2020). The current rise in the number of patients with asthma and eczema appears to be associated with environment changes of the home, for example central heating, decrease in humidity, carpeting and so forth. Unemployment and low wages restrict job mobility and people with industrial skin diseases may have difficulty in changing jobs to alleviate the condition. Homelessness and poor housing and loneliness create problems in maintaining skin care, the former often resulting in limited access to healthcare.

The Nurse's Role

Patients with skin disorders and support groups have asserted their right to access specialist staff and be nursed in specialist areas (Department of Health (DH) 2018), but dermatology training is not compulsory within registered nurse education and it is difficult to attain courses to support development even with the development of independent nurse prescribing. If nurses can spend time talking with the patient, educating and demonstrating skin care techniques, it increases their confidence, and potentially the patient becomes the 'expert' and the burden of skin care can be alleviated by supported self-management, a strategy that fits with government position on long-term conditions (DH and Social Care 2015).

Cure is not a word widely used in dermatology given the cyclical nature of many conditions, So nurses involved often forge long-term relationships with patients. Nurses with experience of chronic skin disease can help patients who require empathy and guidance from specialist practitioners who have the time, knowledge and willingness to share clinical skills with this motivated client group who may achieve remission with the use of systemic biologic and nonbiologic immunosuppressive drugs. Woollenberg et al. (2018) reported inpatient management as improving QoL for dermatology patients.

It is important to share this specialist knowledge with primary care nurses as 'care moves closer to the patient' within dermatology, including the uptake of nonmedical prescribing over the last 20 years. Self-medication, OTC therapies and nonmedical prescribing mean that, for many, pharmacists and community teams are the first contact for most patients. Patients from Black, Asian and minority ethnic populations or the homeless may not easily access healthcare as there might be cultural, language or religious barriers, which might hamper history taking and physical examination. Females are often brought by male chaperons with limited understanding of English, their children by their fathers. Access to interpreter services is essential, as well as sufficient time to enable questions and answers to occur through interpreter services, plus demonstrations of how to carry out treatments or discussing how these treatments could be carried out by those who are homeless or have no access to bathing facilities (see also https://qni.org.uk/nursing-in-the-community/transition-community-nursing/homeless-health/).

The dermatology nurse specialist/practitioner/liaison uses educational input to support the primary care team in providing information and therapies that are valid, accurate and up-to-date, acts in an advisory and consultative capacity and helps sustain continuity of care. Dermatology nurse practitioner/specialists play a vital role of direct specialist care by introducing initiatives in many areas of practice such as nurse-led clinics for chronic disease management (eczema, psoriasis and acne), utilising nonmedical prescribing, managing patients with skin cancer, undertaking surgery and supporting those with melanoma in joint roles like Macmillan nurses. One-stop clinics for skin lesions can be effective, especially if the patient has the lesion removed the same visit, thus reducing the number of unattended appointments (Elective Care Transformation Team, Operations & Information NHS England 2019).

Anatomy and Physiology

A brief outline of the structure and functions of the skin is provided. For further information, readers should consult their own anatomy and physiology textbook.

Structure of the Skin

The skin is composed of two layers: epidermis and dermis. Beneath these layers, a layer of subcutaneous fat protects and insulates the underlying structures.

Epidermis

The epidermis is composed of stratified epithelium and varies in thickness between different parts of the body; skin on the palms and soles is thicker than that on the face or back. The epidermis is avascular, the cells being nourished by means of diffusion of materials. Structures passing through the epidermis include hair follicles and sebaceous and sweat glands (Fig. 14.1A).

The epidermis has several layers, its health depending on three factors:
- regular division and migration of epidermal cells to the skin surface
- gradual keratinisation of these cells
- desquamation or rubbing away of these cells.

The layers of the epidermis are (Fig. 14.1.B):

Basal Layer (Stratum Basale). The cells lying nearest the dermis form the germinative layer where cell division occurs. Cells migrate upwards from this layer, becoming keratinised over a period of 21–28 days before being shed.

Prickle Cell Layer (Stratum Spinosum). Cells in this layer have intercellular connections that protect against shearing forces or trauma to the skin.

Granular Layer (Stratum Granulosum). This layer contains keratohyalin, a precursor of keratin, which gradually replaces the cytoplasm of the cells.

Clear Cell Layer (Stratum Lucidum). Present only where the skin is thickened, for example the soles of feet. The cells exhibit nuclear degeneration and contain large amounts of keratin. Skin injury or friction increases cell production, resulting in a callus or corn.

Cornified, Horny Layer (Stratum Corneum). Comprises thin, flat, nonnucleated cells, the cytoplasm of which has been totally replaced by keratin.

The epidermal/dermal junction is convoluted into dips and ridges which help to prevent damage to the skin from shearing forces. The configuration of these ridges is visible at the epidermal surface as corresponding characteristic, individualised patterns, for example at the fingertips.

Dermis

The dermis is composed of fibrous connective tissue providing a supportive meshwork for the structures and organs within. The

Figure 14.1 (A) The structure of the skin. (B) The layers of the epidermis.

papillary layer has many capillaries and lies next to the basal layer of the epidermis. The reticular layer, lying above the subcutaneous fat layer, has fewer blood vessels and is less reactive.

The ground substance of the dermis is a jelly-like material acting as a support and a transport medium. Tissue mast cells are often found near hair follicles and blood vessels, producing heparin and histamine when damaged. Tissue macrophages engulf foreign particles within the dermis.

Fibroblasts generate collagen fibres, a process requiring vitamin C. These strong fibres bind with water molecules to give skin its tight, 'plump' appearance. Elastin fibres are also formed by fibroblasts. They are bound loosely around bundles of collagen and, in combination with the ground substance and collagen, help the dermis to maintain its characteristic properties.

Lymph vessels drain excess tissue fluid and plasma proteins from the dermis, thereby maintaining correct volume and composition of tissue fluids.

Specialised nerve endings (sensory receptors) present in the dermis and basal layer of the epidermis detect mechanical and thermal changes.

Glands

Sweat Glands are coiled tubes of epithelial tissue opening as pores onto the skin surface. They have individual nerve and blood supplies and secrete a slightly acid fluid containing excess excretory products (water, salts). Sweat glands are of two types: eccrine and apocrine. Eccrine glands are controlled by the sympathetic nervous system, producing secretions in response to temperature elevation or fear. Apocrine glands in the pubic and axillary areas are not functional until puberty. They are thought to secrete pheromones, chemical signals released into the external environment.

Sebaceous Glands are lined with epidermal tissue, secreting sebum, a greasy, slightly acid substance which helps to form a waterproof covering over the skin and, like sweat, to keep the keratin supple. The acid sebum has antibacterial and antifungal properties. Most sebaceous glands open into hair follicles (collectively a pilosebaceous unit). Sebum production is influenced by sex hormone levels.

Functions of the Skin

Intact skin is vital to health and well-being. As the largest organ in the body, weighing approximately 4 kg or 16% of body weight and having a surface area of 2 m², the skin has many vital functions.

- Protection
- Sensation
- Vitamin D synthesis
- Temperature regulation
- Insulation and protection of internal organs
- A barrier to harmful external factors

Protection

The horny layer forms a waterproof seal against undue entry or loss of water. The skin surface protects against microorganisms (through its acidity) and acts as a barrier to chemicals, gases and gamma and beta radiation. Internal structures are shielded by the skin from minor mechanical trauma, and repeated pressure or friction stimulates an increase in cell division, producing thickened areas of skin, for example corns and calluses. Melanin produced in the basal layer of the epidermis screens the dermis from ultraviolet light (UVL).

Sensation

Nerve endings continually monitor the environment and are most highly concentrated in areas such as the fingertips and lips.

Innervated hair follicles help the individual to avoid injury by stimulating reflex action in response to touch.

Vitamin D Synthesis

Epidermal cells produce 7-dehydrocholesterol, which is slowly converted to vitamin D when skin is exposed to UVL (see Chapter 12, Nursing Patients With Musculoskeletal Disorders and Chapter 22, Nutrition and Health).

Temperature Regulation

The skin is vital in temperature regulation. In cold conditions, heat is conserved by vasoconstriction and generated by the involuntary muscular action of shivering. Body hair becomes erect to trap warm air on the skin. During overheating, sweating is induced and vasodilatation occurs. As sweat evaporates from the skin, latent heat is lost from the skin surface, causing it to cool. Vasodilatation allows large quantities of blood to circulate in the uppermost layers of the dermis. Heat is then lost through convection, radiation and conduction. Blood flow is controlled to direct blood either to the capillary bed closer to the skin surface (maximum heat loss) or to the deeper tissues of the skin (minimising heat loss).

Other Functions

During starvation, subcutaneous fat is utilised both as an energy source and as a water reserve. The dermis functions as a water reservoir which may also be utilised by the body in an emergency, for example haemorrhage. The skin is able to absorb various substances, a property utilised for the administration of various drugs. The skin also has an excretory function, with urea and salts being excreted in small amounts through sweat.

Skin Assessment

In completing a comprehensive skin assessment, it is important to obtain a full history, which should include:

- onset, initial site and duration of the condition
- associated symptoms, e.g. itch, redness
- actions that worsen the condition, e.g. sunlight exposure
- family history, e.g. genetic predisposition, allergies
- associated systemic disorders, e.g. asthma, hay fever
- current medication – oral and topical therapies, prescribed, OTC or illegal
- social history – occupation, hobbies, housing, alcohol/drug intake
- impact of the disorder on daily life – personal coping strategies, self-esteem and self-image
- allergies.

History Taking

The history should reveal the person's description and understanding of the disorder as well as their perception of living with it. It can often be a symptom of systemic disease or a condition in its own right; for example pruritus may indicate liver disease/low ferritin or dry skin. An effective assessment should determine the impact of the skin disorder on those around the patient. Skin disease, with all its social implications, has a major cultural impact that varies within a multicultural society. Cultural beliefs need to be identified if treatment programmes are to be adapted to acknowledge such issues. It is important to ask patients what they have already used to treat their skin disorder.

Many OTC preparations or treatments, borrowed from well-meaning friends, can exacerbate an existing skin condition. When examining skin, the nurse must have knowledge of 'normal' skin to be able to identify the abnormal at any age. Patients often now record their condition on their mobile phones and use them in the consultation to illustrate how bad the skin has been which is helpful if they are in remission or have difficulty with language.

Physical Examination

The entire skin surface is examined to determine the extent of the disorder. Touch is very important – lightly run the tips of the fingers over the skin surface. Palpation of skin lesions will determine changes in skin texture with associated crusting or scaling. In skin disorders, the term 'lesion' describes a small area of disease, while an 'eruption' or 'rash' describes widespread skin involvement.

Skin assessment includes routine examination of the hair and nails as changes can aid diagnosis, for example nail changes in psoriasis or fungal infection. The distribution of lesions can vary. Psoriasis tends to localise on the outer aspects of elbows and knees, while eczema is most common in the skin flexures.

During assessment, the nurse should recognise that skin changes can be a manifestation of systemic disorders, for example pruritus = liver disease. It is important to remind ourselves to recognise the wide diversity of skin colour and pigmentation in society. The pathophysiology of the disorder will be unchanged, but skin pigmentation can influence skin changes during illness. Clinical presentation can also be altered by skin colour or can look less florid, and thus, the severity of the presentation can be underestimated. A useful tool for exposure to skin presentations in skin of colour is found on a website for those new to skin diseases in any care setting: https://blackandbrownskin.co.uk/mindthegap.

Communication with patients is important for accurate assessment, as a patient's description of symptoms is relevant to diagnosis and management (they often say blister when in fact it is a pustule). Initial nursing management involves alleviation of distressing symptoms while awaiting diagnosis.

The nurse should also recognise that the effect of the physical appearance of a skin disorder on QoL is often viewed by the patient as being of greater importance than the discomfort of having abnormal skin as viewed by the patient.

Investigations

Investigations assist with the process of elimination or act as supporting evidence to develop a working diagnosis. Interpretation of the result is important, while identifying the relevance to the current clinical picture and the patient.

Common investigations include:
- skin swabs (bacterial or viral)
- skin scraping/nail clippings/hair debris (mycology)
- skin biopsy (histopathology)
- blood tests, e.g. full blood count, immunoglobulin E (IgE)
- patch testing
- prick testing (done by allergists).

🌐 See Evolve website Figs. 14.1–14.5

Principles of Therapy in Skin Disorders

This section outlines the range of treatments used to treat skin disorders. They are often used in combinations of topical and systemic treatments.

Topical Therapies

Topical therapies are usually known as first-line treatments and are applied directly on the skin which is the target organ and readily accessible. Various classes of topical preparations are used (Information 14.1).

Ongoing commitment is needed to maintain treatment as topical therapies can be messy, time-consuming and malodorous (Reflection 14.2). Treatment programmes often have to be customised because therapeutic responses can differ with each patient.

INFORMATION 14.1

Classification of Topical Preparations

- Creams – have a light effect due to high water content. They rub in easily and cool the skin.
- Lotions – used if skin is 'weeping'. Good for scalp treatment as they are not greasy to apply.
- Ointments – greasy preparations used as a base for the drug being applied. They last for 6–8 hours on the skin, encouraging absorption by a barrier effect.
- Pastes – ointments applied to medicated bandages for occlusive use or used in combination as a stiffer paste to apply treatment directly to lesions. This permits a slower, more effective absorption on the target sites.
- Gel – oil and water held together with a carbomer gelling agent – cool evaporation.
- Foam – liquid and cream with tiny bubbles
- Spray – liquid and cream in a mist

REFLECTION 14.2

Advantages and Disadvantages of Topical Therapy

Advantages
- Drug delivered directly to the target area
- Reduces systemic absorption
- Patient can view improvement
- Side-effects easily identified

Disadvantages
- Time-consuming
- Messy and potential to stain clothing
- Preparations smell or stain the skin
- Patient can see deterioration or lack of improvement
- Inability to apply to oneself due to lack of dexterity

Activities
- Reflect on the advantages that would motivate you to persevere with topical therapy, and the disadvantages most likely to stop you using the treatment.
- Discuss with your mentor how you would deal with the disadvantages while teaching a patient how to use their medication.

Regular nursing assessment will identify improvements or deterioration and allow treatment to be amended appropriately. A maintenance programme is needed as well as the treatment response for a flare. The patient needs to have the therapies at home so they can also use them immediately a flare occurs – step-up step-down. In order to achieve the desired outcome, the skilled practitioner needs a sound knowledge of dermatology therapies balanced with abilities to educate, support and motivate the patient to complete lengthy treatment programmes.

A fire hazard associated with the use of paraffin-based skin products (containing over 50%) was initially highlighted in 2007. Nurses must alert patients and assess fire risk if they are a smoker or have lighted flames in the home (Peters 2018), are aged over 60 and have reduced mobility (Medicines and Healthcare Products Regulatory Agency [MHRA] 2020). Fire can spread through paraffin-soaked clothes and bedding and there have been 15 deaths caused by this (London Fire Brigade 2017). However, liquid paraffin has a low potential for allergy, is absorbed into the epidermal barrier and is used in the majority of skin preparations. The fire warning has been extended to all emollient products (National Fire Chiefs Council 2020).

Emollients

Agents that moisturise and lubricate the skin are the mainstay of dermatological treatment. They are used in different forms such as soap substitute/bath additives or leave-on preparations. They can be used in skin maintenance programmes and are vital in preparing the skin for the specific therapies available for different disorders, for example tar and corticosteroids. The choice of emollient depends on the disorder:

- Dry, hyperkeratotic skin – use oily occlusive ointments or those with humectants.
- Flaky, rough, excoriated skin – use grease-based preparations.
- Erythematous, inflamed skin – benefits from the cooling effect of water-soluble creams.

Patients may use a combination of emollients for different areas of the body. Taking time to demonstrate application technique and trial different moisturisers so the patient is involved in choice is key for compliance. In terms of overall satisfaction with formulation, it was highest with lotions (67%), gels (46%) and lowest in cream (34%) in both adults and children (Tucker 2022). Demonstrating to patients in the clinic on how to apply their topical leave-on emollients is now supported by web-based tools (Guy's and St Thomas's NHS Foundation Trust 2017).

Since 2010 at least 56 UK recorded fire deaths have been linked to emollient use, with corners' reports linked to contamination of clothing and bedding. Many of those involved were found to be elderly smokers (over 60; MHRA 2020) with reduced mobility (National Fire Chiefs Council [NFCC] 2020). All emollients can act as an accelerant; the MHRA toolkit and campaign were launched in 2020

WHAT YOU NEED TO KNOW

- Advise patients to continue using emollients but to be aware of burn risks, avoid naked flames, and stop smoking.
- Emollients are not flammable themselves but, when impregnated into fabric, can act as an accelerant.
- People most at risk are those with reduced ability to react quickly when emollient impregnated fabric is exposed to naked flames.

From Ridd MJ, Hall S, Lane ME, Roberts A, Williams HC. Burns with emollients. BMJ 2022:376:e066102.

---

and it is worth it for all health professionals to look at this resource and see what their local fire and rescue service is doing to communicate these messages to the local population (Housam 2022).

Topical Corticosteroids

Topical corticosteroids should be applied after the topical emollient or bathing with a bath oil or soap substitute to the affected areas only. Advice given about the use of topical corticosteroids should be balanced: they are safe to use but often patients are anxious because there is emphasis on thinning of the skin, which relates more systemic corticosteroids.

The potential side-effects, such as skin thinning, bruising/purpura, hirsutism, systemic effects and others, depend on the age of the patient, site and frequency of the product used. A review (Bewley 2008) stated that 'the intermittent use of topical corticosteroids is highly effective, bears little risk, and is relatively inexpensive'.

A concern with children is that they are more prone to the development of systemic reactions based on their higher ratio of total body surface area to body weight. Epidermal thinning does occur within 1–3 weeks of treatment with potent or very potent topical steroids on normal skin but reverses within 4 weeks of stopping. It is recognised that emollient therapy is potentially steroid-sparing and this potentially corrects the defect in the skin barrier, so using emollient therapy for washing, bathing and as a leave-on preparation is key to the day-to-day management with intermittent use of topical corticosteroids (Herbert and Galindo 2022).

Other Topical Therapies

Other topical therapies used include:
- vitamin D analogues or dithranol for psoriasis
- cleansers, vitamin A analogues or antibiotics for acne
- fluorouracil, diclofenac sodium, imiquimod for sun-damaged skin or basal cell carcinoma (BCC).

Each therapy has to be applied in a different manner and the nurses advising/prescribing the patient must know the difference and the potential effect it has on the skin in order to advise the patient (see Useful Websites, www.bdng.org).

Systemic Therapies and Biological Therapies

A range of oral medication, from antibiotics to immunosuppressants (e.g. ciclosporin, methotrexate, azathioprine) to biological drugs (medical products produced by living cells e.g. dupilumab and baricitinib), is used to treat long-term inflammatory conditions as well as acute inflammatory or bullous conditions. Monitoring of patients on oral medication is often undertaken by dermatology nurses who work as nonmedical prescribers: they interpret blood results and alter doses or initiate alternative therapies used in conjunction with topical therapies. Nurses must know the potential side-effects of topical and systemic therapies in order to provide safe care and when necessary be able to adjust therapy accordingly.

Phototherapy (Ultraviolet Light B)

Certain skin disorders, most commonly psoriasis and eczema, can be treated with ultraviolet light B (UVB) in measured doses. UVB is the wavelength in natural sunlight responsible for sunburn. Treatment requires outpatient attendance two to three times weekly over a period of weeks. Phototherapy is given in a cabinet with fluorescent lamps emitting UVB or with panels so that targeted areas only are treated (hands/feet/shins).

● See Evolve website Fig. 14.6

A test dose administered to the patient's back determines a safe starting dose. This dose is gradually increased over the treatment period.

Photochemotherapy (Psoralen and Ultraviolet Light A)

The treatment combination of psoralen and ultraviolet light A (PUVA) requires the patient to take oral psoralen (a natural plant extract) 2 hours before exposure to UVA. Photochemotherapy is given in a cabinet with fluorescent lamps emitting UVA.

● See Evolve website Fig. 14.7

Bath PUVA (methoxypsoralen lotion) is a treatment in which a measured amount of psoralen is added to 150 L of bath water. Patients soak for a specific time, pat the skin dry and then treatment is given in a UVA light cabinet. Again, psoriasis and eczema can both be treated with PUVA. A test dose is administered to determine a safe starting dose and treatment is given in twice-weekly sessions.

Patients having light therapy wear protective goggles during UVB/PUVA exposure. After PUVA, they must also wear dark glasses for 24 hours to protect the eye if oral psoralen is taken. UVB/PUVA is administered in specialist units to ensure accurate recording of the amount of light therapy given, as guidelines exist that restrict the amount a patient may receive.

Complementary Therapies

The increasing interest in complementary therapies to treat skin disorders reflects a rise in public awareness of nontraditional approaches to treatment, perhaps stimulated by the failure of orthodox medicine to provide 'cures'. The nurse is ideally placed to discuss both the orthodox and complementary options. Discussion should focus on the safe use of complementary therapies initiated by a practitioner who has undergone accredited training and is a licensed practitioner with insurance. It is very easy to order products over the internet being influenced by the visuals used. Complementary therapy should be considered as an adjunct and not as an alternative to routine therapies.

DISORDERS OF THE SKIN

Psoriasis

Psoriasis is a chronic, relapsing, inflammatory, noninfectious T-cell autoimmune skin disease (Dilworth et al. 2015), characterised by well-demarcated erythematous plaques with adherent silver scales. The epidermal cell proliferation rate increases greatly, while epidermal turnover time is reduced. Psoriasis is prevalent in 2% of the UK population, yet the cause remains unknown. It can occur in any age group and is characterised by exacerbations and remissions. Genetic influences predispose to the condition, with 35% of patients showing a family history.

Precipitating/aggravating factors include:
- infection – streptococcal throat infection
- medications – can exacerbate or trigger psoriasis, e.g. beta-blockers
- sunlight – in some patients, psoriasis improves during the summer and relapses during the winter; however, others report that sunlight aggravates the condition

- hormonal change – psoriasis can get better or worse during pregnancy or during the climacteric
- alcohol – can exacerbate the condition
- smoking is associated with a 70% increased risk of developing psoriasis (Keyworth et al. 2014)
- psychological stress – can exacerbate psoriasis, but the condition itself is recognised as stressful
- trauma – creates the 'Köebner effect' where psoriasis is triggered in damaged skin, e.g. the site of an injury or surgical scar.

Psoriasis varies from mild forms, with plaques localised to the knees and elbows, to severe forms which are potentially life threatening. Classification of psoriasis is made on clinical presentation (Psoriasis Area Surface Index, PASI) or location such as nails (National Institute for Health and Clinical Excellence (NICE) 2012).

Guttate presents as drop-like symmetrical lesions on the trunk and limbs. It is most common in adolescents and young adults and is often triggered by a streptococcal throat infection.

Plaque presents as well-demarcated, erythematous plaques covered in dry, white waxy scale often localised to the knees and elbows (Fig. 14.2) Plaques vary in size and extend to cover the trunk and scalp. Plaque psoriasis tends to be chronic, with exacerbations and periods of remission.

Flexural affects the axillae, submammary and anogenital areas. Plaques are sharply defined but the skin has a thin glistening redness, often with painful fissures in the skin folds.

Pustular is a localised form affecting the hands and feet. It is characterised by yellow/brown pustules which dry into brown scaly macules (Fig. 14.3). It is a painful condition, difficult to treat and linked to smoking and very debilitating.

Generalised pustular is a rare yet serious form of the disease. Sheets of sterile pustules develop, merging on an erythematous background. These areas of skin shear and the patient will present with pyrexia and malaise and require hospital admission. It is often triggered when attempts are made to withdraw oral or topical corticosteroids, or may just reflect the instability of the condition.

Figure 14.2 Plaque psoriasis – erythema with silvery scale and a well-demarcated edge.

Scalp can often be the sole manifestation of the disorder. Thick scale adheres to the scalp and can extend to the scalp margin and behind the ears.

Nail Changes. Psoriasis can involve pitting of nails and onycholysis, where the distal edge of the nail separates from the nail bed. There is no effective topical treatment for psoriatic nail changes.

Erythrodermic is a rare but severe form of skin failure that can be life-threatening and warrants hospital admission. The skin becomes uniformly red due to high blood flow volume. The patient feels unwell and maintaining body temperature is difficult. It can be triggered by the irritant effects of therapies, or by withdrawal of oral/systemic corticosteroids or by a medication reaction. The condition can progress to a generalised pustular psoriasis.

Psoriatic Arthropathy. Within approximately 10 years of developing psoriasis, an estimated 20%–30% of individuals develop psoriatic arthritis. Joint changes occur in hands, feet, spine and sacroiliac joints. This arthropathy mimics rheumatoid disease but notably the rheumatoid factor test is negative (see Chapter 12, Nursing Patients With Musculoskeletal Disorders). Psoriatic arthropathy

Figure 14.3 Pustular psoriasis – sterile pustules along the demarcated edge.

is difficult to treat, meriting the combined expertise of a rheumatologist and a dermatologist.

Pathophysiology

The epidermis thickens, with an associated increased blood flow to the skin, and becomes raised to accommodate skin changes (parakeratosis) (Fig. 14.4). Epidermal cell proliferation rate increases and infiltration of T cells which produce inflammatory cytokines such as tumour necrosis factor-alpha (TNF-α). The transit time of epidermal cells maturing through normal skin is approximately 21–28 days, whereas in psoriasis, it is 4 days. The increased cell production and transit time mean that cells do not keratinise completely and so cannot be shed, causing the build-up of a white, waxy silver scale as immature skin cells remain adherent to the skin. Psoriasis results from an increase in activity of dividing cells associated with an increase in their rate of reproduction. Interleukin (IL)-17A can upregulate keratin 17 expressions on keratinocytes along with other T-cell subsets. Th1, Th17, Treg and Th22 interplay and contribute to the disease development (Cai et al. 2012). Further work is ongoing into TNF-α biological agents in the treatment of psoriasis to target the pathway of development.

Common Presenting Signs/Symptoms

These may include:

- *Pain.* Fissures form, particularly on hands and feet, because of loss of flexibility in the thickened epidermis.
- *Erythema.* Generalised redness and heat loss.
- *Scaling.* A build-up of cells creates the silver-scale appearance diagnostic of psoriasis.
- *Pustules.* In inflammatory conditions, an infiltration of white blood cells is normal. Increased infiltration in pustular psoriasis accumulates as microabscesses in the outer layer of the skin.
- *Pruritus (itch).* Patients often report itch to be troublesome.
- *Sore throat.* In guttate psoriasis.

Medical Management

With the introduction of biological/new antiinflammatory medications, the treatment options have expanded and the majority of psoriasis patients are managed on an outpatient basis, but the severity of activity in erythrodermic/pustular psoriasis may result in hospital admission to prevent potential life-threatening complications of an unstable psoriatic state and to move the patient into remission with nonbiological systemic therapies as per NICE guidelines (NICE 2012). There are now 11 licensed biological therapies NICE approved for use in psoriasis (Smith et al. 2020) which has changed life outcomes.

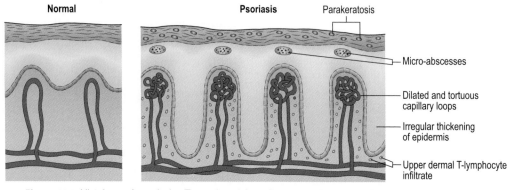

Figure 14.4 Histology of psoriasis. (Reproduced from Boon NA, Colledge NR, Walker BR. *Davidson's Principles and Practice of Medicine.* 20th ed. Edinburgh: Churchill Livingstone; 2006, with permission.)

Investigations

Diagnosis can be made from the clinical picture and relevant history:

- skin biopsy
- throat swab
- Auspitz sign – gentle removal of the silvery scale from a plaque reveals pinpoint bleeding from the dilated superficial capillaries
- blood tests – if considering systemic therapy.

Treatment

This may involve topical and systemic medication and phototherapy. PUVA and UVB are effective therapies for psoriasis. The combination of prescribed therapies chosen depends on the diagnosis and severity of the disorder, with corticosteroids, in combination with vitamin D in foams/gels therapies, being the mainstay of psoriasis treatment (see Nursing Management and Health Promotion section).

Medications. Combined systemic and topical medication is useful in the management of psoriasis. Systemic medications used include:

- antihistamines – alleviate itch and promote sleep and rest
- analgesics – reduce the pain and discomfort of inflamed skin
- antibiotics – for streptococcal throat infections
- nonbiological methotrexate, ciclosporin, retinoids (e.g. acitretin)
- biological (e.g. adalimumab) (BAD Guidelines, Smith et al. 2020).

The majority of patients with psoriasis respond to topical therapies, but the more extensive forms of psoriasis may require a systemic approach. When commencing patients on systemic medication, it is important to raise patients' awareness of links to obesity. This can hamper the effectiveness of anti-TNF agents (Juan and Jiabi 2019) and has an increased tumour potential from immunosuppressant medications (that patients will have previously been on, e.g. methotrexate and ciclosporin). It is important to highlight shared care with the GP for monitoring the patient's general health, with an annual screen to monitor body mass index (BMI) and review of cardiac risk.

❖ Nursing Management and Health Promotion: Psoriasis

The goals of nursing management will vary depending on the type and severity of the person's psoriasis. If the epidermal barrier is breached, as in severe erythroderma leading to acute skin failure, measures are needed to support the epidermal barrier (see Skin Failure). Generalised pustular psoriasis and erythrodermic psoriasis can be life-threatening conditions requiring skilled nursing. Dermatology nurse specialists run nurse-led systemic monitoring clinics for nonbiologic and biological therapies in conjunction with the consultant dermatologists.

🌐 **See Evolve website Critical thinking question 14.1**

Intensive nursing care is essential for comfort, preventing infection and monitoring and acting on the early signs or noting change in general health status.

However, the majority of people manage their condition at home by themselves or with the help of family members. Applying topical therapies can be time consuming and messy with the need to carry out additional washing and vacuuming to remove shed skin scale. The role of the nurse is to:

- support self-care, exchanging explanations on techniques of application of the different therapies
- discuss life activities/style to reduce potential causes of exacerbations while promoting confidence and reducing stress
- work in collaboration with the patient/family to achieve the maximum benefit for the minimal risk of the therapy (topical or systemic)
- work in collaboration with the patient/family to raise awareness of comorbidities, e.g. diabetes, hypertension, obesity and cardiac disease and what steps to undertake to avoid them.

Many patients who have a long-term skin disorder such as psoriasis may wish to use a complementary treatment and should only do this via a qualified and insured practitioner.

Psychological Support

People react to events differently and so it is important to ask the patient about how the psoriasis affects their everyday life. This sometimes can be obvious in that they are too self-conscious to expose their skin to go to the gym or swimming. This can also impact on their physical health with unhealthy options that can lead to cardiac disease and obesity. Use of excessive clothing hides their skin from public view or even from their partners through embarrassment. A referral to a clinical psychologist may be needed to work with the patient on areas of body image, sexuality, QoL and personal coping strategies. These are all management considerations, and effective counselling can enhance the therapeutic effect. Just because systemic and biological therapies can now clear the skin, these does not always result in a healthier and happier lifestyle.

Management of Topical Therapies

A range of topical therapies are used for outpatient management of psoriasis. By talking together, the patient and nurse can choose the therapies that fit into the patient's lifestyle and if necessary ensure that there is someone at home to assist. It is important to review the patient once therapies are commenced and to adjust accordingly. Of course, all therapies take some weeks to cause improvement so a realistic timeframe is essential. The nurse should also explain the different preparations used, giving advice on correct application/location of use on the body and potential side-effects. By providing clear information and ongoing psychological support, the nurse can help to ensure the patient perseveres with treatment. Specific considerations in using topical preparations are as follows.

Emollients. Bland emollients (e.g. emulsifying ointment) moisturise and lubricate the skin, helping to ease scaling and promote comfort. Regular applications seal the stratum cornum, thus reducing transdermal heat and fluid loss, which is particularly relevant in erythrodermic psoriasis. Erythrodermic or generalised pustular psoriasis is often treated with emollients initially to allow fiery skin to 'settle' before other treatments. Emollient bath additives, for example Oilatum, and soap substitutes, such as Epimax cream, are available over the counter.

Coal Tar Ointments. are usually blended with white soft paraffin and have an antipruritic, antiinflammatory and keratolytic effect. Low concentrations are used initially and can be messy and smelly and can stain so they tend to be used for day-care/inpatient treatment. Proprietary blends of cleaner tar creams are available for home use and sensitive areas of skin.

Patients must be advised that if ointment irritates or burns the skin, it should be removed immediately in an emollient bath and advice sought.

Dithranol suppresses cell proliferation. It is available in many forms, but patients must be informed that it can stain skin and clothes; staining can last for 10–14 days after treatment has finished. If the patient is attending a day unit daily, then dithranol is applied by spatula to the affected skin and powdered or covered with stockinette gauze to prevent the ointment from spreading to surrounding skin. It then stays on for between 1 and 12 hours before being cleaned off. This procedure is time-consuming and messy but effective. For outpatient therapy, short-contact treatment is available. Cream/ointment is applied to the plaque and removed 30–60 minutes later.

Vitamin D Analogues such as calcipotriol are applied as an ointment directly to plaques. They are nonmessy, nonstaining and well tolerated. Calcipotriol inhibits cell proliferation and stimulates epidermal cell differentiation, correcting the increased cell turnover time associated with psoriasis. Due to potential systemic absorption, there is a restriction on the quantities (100 g) to be applied over 1 week. This restriction will relate to the extent and severity of the psoriasis and it is important that patients are aware of the prescriptive guidelines. It can be combined with corticosteroids as a gel with an applicator or a foam so that it can be applied to scalp and body plaques.

Corticosteroids. Immunosuppressants can be useful to reduce itch on the body or scalp. Newer combinations of corticosteroids and vitamin D analogues in gel or foam can be useful in chronic plaque psoriasis but should be pulsed, for example 4 weeks daily then take a break, or if psoriasis is still present, switch to plain vitamin D analogues.

PUVA/UVB. The treatment programme varies for each individual depending on identification of skin type and tolerance of sunlight. Koek et al. (2009) found that UVB phototherapy administered at home is as safe and effective as that given in outpatient departments. Moreover, using the treatment at home reduced the burden of treatment and increased patient satisfaction found mainly in very rural areas of the UK. Retinoids can be given with PUVA to stimulate more rapid skin clearance at lower total doses of UVL.

Goeckerman Regimen. An effective combination treatment comprising a tar bath prior to exposure to UVL

Ingram Regimen. A combination therapy involving tar baths, UVL and dithranol applications.

Cocois Ointment. A blend of tar, emulsifying ointment and salicylic acid used to treat scalp psoriasis. It is gently massaged into the scalp, occluded from 1 hour to overnight with a showercap and removed with shampoo of the patient's choice to remove scale.

Eczema

Eczema describes a range of inflammatory skin disorders. The aetiology of eczema is unknown. Most classifications of eczematous skin disorders use the term 'eczema' synonymously with 'dermatitis', as both terms apply to the inflammatory skin changes provoked by either internal (endogenous) or external (exogenous) factors or a combination of both (Table 14.1) (Gawkrodger and Ardern-Jones 2020).

The priorities of medical and nursing management are similar for all classifications of eczema. In common with other skin conditions, some types of eczema can lead to life-threatening skin failure.

Endogenous Eczema

Atopic Eczema

Atopic eczema is a common inflammatory skin disorder affecting 20% of infants/children in the UK and 5%–10% adults (Cork

TABLE 14.1	External and Internal Factors Causing Skin Disease	
External	**Internal**
Ultraviolet light (UVL)/sunshine	Psychological factors/stress
Extremes of temperature – heat and cold	Genetic factors
Allergens	Systemic disease
Chemicals	Prescribed medications
Irritants	Herbal or over-the-counter products
Infections	Infections
Skin trauma/friction	Behavioural – scratching/picking

Figure 14.5 Atopic (subacute) eczema on the fronts of the ankle in a teenager. These are sites of predilection, along with the cubital and popliteal fossae, in atopic eczema. (Reproduced from Boon NA, Colledge NR, Walker BR. *Davidson's Principles and Practice of Medicine.* 20th ed. Edinburgh: Churchill Livingstone; 2006, with permission.)

et al. 2020); there are associated genetic and environmental factors, and in some babies, food allergens. The patient may have inherited a skin barrier gene mutation so may be affected for life. Atopy covers the classification of related disorders, for example asthma, eczema and hay fever. Atopic eczema can be a chronic itchy distressing disorder with learnt behaviour response to itch. Strict diagnostic criteria are followed (NICE 2023). Infantile eczema can resolve spontaneously but sometimes progresses to a chronic pattern of episodic exacerbations in adulthood (reoccurs at time of stress, e.g. exams, university, house moving.) The pattern of distribution can alter into adulthood and late onset can be very distressing to the older person (Fig. 14.5).

Pompholyx Eczema

This is a 'blistering' eczema localised to palms and soles. It develops rapidly, causes acute discomfort and can become secondarily infected. The cause is unknown and outbreaks can be linked to heat/humidity or reaction of contact dermatitis or fungal infections. It can be very debilitating and distressing causing problems in the work and social settings.

Discoid Eczema

Characteristic symmetrical coin-shaped lesions that can be wet or very crusty affect mainly the limbs and can be intensely itchy.

Asteatotic Eczema

This mainly affects older people, commonly on the lower legs. It appears to be associated with a deficiency of sebaceous secreting glands, resulting in excessive dryness and scaling of the skin. Central heating, diuretic therapy and over-frequent washing are also implicated as possible causes

Varicose Eczema

Chronic patchy eczema of the legs occurs, with or without the presence of a venous ulcer (see Chapter 23, Tissue Viability and Managing Chronic Wounds). It is associated with chronic venous stasis, and there may be varicose veins, oedema and pigmentation of the skin (due to haemosiderin from the blood leaking through capillary walls) (Gawkrodger and Ardern-Jones 2020). The area involved may become itchy and hot to touch and a secondary response may produce associated eczematous areas on other parts of the body and it may not resolve fully.

Exogenous Eczema

Irritant Contact Dermatitis. This is very common, especially in industrial/work settings. It usually erupts at the maximum point of contact, but presentation varies according to the nature of the irritant contact. The epidermis may be damaged by water or abrasion, and the effect of the irritant, for example cement, is exacerbated by rubbing against clothing. Epidermal necrosis may occur within hours of contact with strong chemicals, while eczema triggered by milder substances, for example detergents, may take longer to evolve. Many patients with atopic eczema appear prone to irritant contact dermatitis and should be advised to avoid work where exposure to irritants could occur.

Allergic Contact Dermatitis

In this condition the skin develops a specific immunological hypersensitivity. The most common allergy is to nickel (found in inexpensive jewellery/body piercing). Continued exposure to the allergen results in an eczematous response, ranging from mild to severe. Allergy patch testing may identify the allergen; in many cases a change of job or avoidance of the allergen may be necessary. The most difficult cases to treat are those in which allergic contact dermatitis is suspected but no definitive triggering factor is found.

🔵 *Pathophysiology*

The skin generally becomes drier to the touch and then erythema and swelling caused by vasodilatation and oedema occur. The erythema may be generalised or limited to localised areas. It can be exacerbated by scratching, extending to an exudative, scaling and crusting phase. Blistering can occur as part of the inflammatory process. Caused by the genetically altered filaggrin gene, discovered in 2006, this deficiency leads to a lifelong faulty epidermal barrier.

In chronic conditions involving recurrent exacerbations, the skin is scaly, excoriated, thickened and pigmented. The eczematous areas will be localised to more defined parts of the body and lichenification will be apparent (Fig. 14.6). Lichenification is the skin's response to mechanical damage (rubbing/scratching) in which the affected areas become thickened, toughened and show a marked exaggeration of normal skin markings. Painful fissuring of the skin occurs as normal elasticity is lost. For clinical scoring, the Eczema Area and Severity Index (EASI) is used along with DLQI as part of the assessment process of patients with severe eczema who have failed on systemic therapy and are prepared for dupilumab (a biologic) (NICE 2018a).

Common Presenting Symptoms

- *Itch (pruritus)* accompanies most eczematous conditions and can be acute and distressing. The itch–scratch–itch cycle quickly becomes established as a learnt behaviour. The skin is well supplied with sensory nerves that respond quickly to the mechanical stimulation of scratching or any external stimulation.
- *Redness.* Inflammatory skin diseases cause vasodilatation of blood vessels feeding the skin, leading to generalised total body redness (erythroderma). In atopic eczema, white dermographism can be evoked – firm strokes of the skin normally produce a 'wheal and flare' response, a pink raised wheal lasting about 30 minutes, but in atopic patients, a simple white line arises, with no erythema.
- *Fissures/lichenification.* In the chronic stages, there is also a generalised thickening of some layers of the skin over flexures or any area traumatised by scratching. Open fissures are painful and slow to heal.

Figure 14.6 The histology of acute (A) and chronic (B) dermatitis.

- *Infections.* Primary or secondary bacterial infections (e.g. *Staphylococcus* or *Streptococcus*) can exacerbate eczema. Patients with atopic eczema tend to be more susceptible to viral infections, e.g. eczema herpeticum. The skin of 90% of patients with atopic eczema is colonised by *Staphylococcus aureus* bacteria (Alexander et al. 2020), which thrives on dry skin, and functions as a superantigen.

🔴 Medical Management

Diagnosis is made from the presentation and the patient's history. Many of the exogenous conditions are managed in an outpatient setting; however, severe exacerbations warrant hospital admission.

Investigations

Laboratory investigations may include:

- Skin swabs – excoriated lesions may result in secondary infection
- Skin scrapings – to exclude fungal infection
- Skin biopsy – for immunohistological examination when the diagnosis is in doubt
- Blood test – to ascertain the level of IgE or the presence of specific antibodies to external factors, e.g. house dust mite, pollen, cat/dog or food proteins
- Prick tests – to ascertain type 1 reaction to specific allergens, e.g. grass

Patch Testing may be carried out to confirm allergic contact dermatitis. A range of patch tests is available in which suspected allergens, for example nickel, fragrance, hairdressing products, plant material and rubber, are made up in a concentration which would normally produce no reaction unless the patient was sensitive to them.

Treatment

This is topical, phototherapy, systemic, biological or combination.

Topical Therapies. (See later Nursing Management and Health Promotion section

- First-line treatment for dry skin is emollient therapy and the avoidance of products that contain sodium lauryl sulphate (SLS), e.g. soap, which remove the skin's natural moisturising factor (NMF). 'Emollients that contain urea, glycerol and colloidal oatmeal are more effective than placebo comparators' (Tucker 2018).
- Soap substitutes or bath additives cleanse the skin without removing the NMF. 'Leave-on' skin preparations help restore the epidermal barrier.
- Second-line treatment is the use of corticosteroids/immunosuppressants to suppress the inflammation and reduce itch. Sometimes combined with an antibiotic for local infection.
- Bandaging.

Systemic Medication Therapy.

- Antihistamines – to reduce itch; the side-effect of drowsiness may aid sleep and rest.
- Antibiotics – to treat bacterial infection, specifically *S. aureus*, for generalised infection.
- Analgesics – to ease heat, tenderness and localised pain.

❖ Nursing Management and Health Promotion: Eczema

The immediate priority is to alleviate discomfort. A tired, hot, itchy patient is not in an ideal state to absorb information and learn self-care techniques, and therefore an immediate and sympathetic approach to care is important. Ongoing support and reassurance are fundamental to achieving long-term goals. Informing the patient about eczema, triggers, treatments and techniques of applications creates greater understanding of the condition and its outlook as well as getting access to medication.

Substantial time and effort can be required to motivate, educate and empower the patient to share condition management. Patients and families should be informed of relevant support groups (see Useful Websites, e.g. National Eczema Society).

Nursing Considerations in Topical Therapy
Emollients

Emollients are used to rehydrate and smooth the epidermal barrier; take the form of bath oils, creams, gels, foams, sprays and ointments; and are the mainstay of treatment. Itch, heat and dryness all respond promptly to lubrication. Many emollients create a barrier for inflamed skin, preventing further fluid/heat loss. Eczema is a condition in which the skin is chronically dry, so long-term use of emollients is essential from birth to reduce the potential for atopic eczema (Simpson and Chalmers et al. 2014). Patients should be advised to avoid perfumed products and use bath additives and soap substitutes that are SLS-free. When bathing, water temperature should not be excessive as this causes the skin to become drier through evaporation causing water loss (Penzer 2012), length of immersion can also affect the skin barrier so 20 minutes is recommended. Very greasy preparations are used when the skin is very dry, for example paraffin or emulsifying wax base, or lighter/less greasy preparations, for example oil/water based, when less dry or over the summer months.

Emollient preparations should be applied lightly, with smooth downward strokes in the direction of hair growth to prevent follicle blockage and infection. Rubbing creates heat in the skin causing itch, and if emollient is applied thickly, it traps body heat causing itching. Frequent applications are needed throughout the day even if humectant emollients are used to reduce transepidermal water loss (NICE 2023).

Immunosuppressants

Corticosteroids. Topical corticosteroid therapy will have a major impact on the eczematous skin, therefore it is important that the patient understands the correct methods of application. Absorption of topical corticosteroid and the volume of cream used will be greater if the skin is dry and excoriated was established in 1998, thus the skin must be regularly moisturised with emollient during corticosteroid therapy. Corticosteroids should be applied to freshly bathed skin (if using emollient) or at least 60 minutes after the application of a leave-on emollient. Using the 'fingertip unit of approximately 0.5 g', measured amounts of cream are gently massaged into the affected areas for maximum effect but not rubbed in to irritate and cause itch or heat.

The best treatment advice is to be proactive and use the correct potency to match the location and extent of inflammation; however, many eczematous conditions require a potent corticosteroid to inhibit the inflammatory process. Treatment programmes start with a potent corticosteroid (moderate potent to face) applied twice daily, gradually reducing the strength as the condition improves. The 'step-up step-down' approach is recommended by NICE (2023). Many patients are aware of the side-effects of topical corticosteroids, for example systemic absorption and skin thinning. The nurse must emphasise that it is prolonged use of potent corticosteroids with or without inadequate use of emollients that potentially produces side-effects. This long-term use can cause red skin, burning sensation and itchiness with a different appearance to normal eczema (MHRA 2021). In eczema, secondary bacterial infection may be present and treatment may include a combined corticosteroid and antibiotic cream.

Topical Immunomodulators. These are nonsteroidal preparations that are applied topically. They reduce inflammation by suppressing the T-lymphocyte response. An option for treatment in individuals at risk of or with irreversible skin atrophy (NICE 2004).

Bandaging
A variety of occlusive, medicated bandages is available. Applied overnight, occlusive bandaging creates a moist environment which aids the absorption of medication. Bandaging is a mechanical barrier, preventing skin damage from scratching but must be applied correctly.

Other Considerations
Cardiovascular Risk in Severe Eczema on Systemic Therapies
A recent study also demonstrated such an association between severe atopic eczema in adulthood and all forms of nonfatal cardiovascular disease (Silverwood et al. 2018). Individuals with severe atopic eczema who have received systemic immunosuppressant medication or phototherapy are defined as being at risk, and they should be referred to secondary care, for assessment of the indicators of disease severity as well as the risk of stroke, unstable angina, atrial fibrillation, myocardial infarction and heart failure and death from cardiovascular disease.

Rest
Rest is imperative for recovery in more severe eczematous conditions. This involves taking a sick leave to allow the skin to heal by having time to concentrate on skin care. Patient and family may be distraught by itch and inadequate sleep which will affect concentration and behaviour. The nurse must give clear information about the safe use of antihistamine medication in children/adults but the judicious use of antihistamines will provide rest for the eczema sufferer and the family.

Diet
Diet is implicated in some forms of infantile eczema when the history strongly suggests the infant is allergic or intolerant to milk or milk products but may outgrow these as they age. Exclusion diets to identify food allergy are difficult and should be attempted only under the supervision of a dietitian (Wedgeworth et al. 2012).

Complementary Therapies
When conventional medicine cannot offer a cure, parents or adults with atopic eczema may turn to alternative therapies, for example homeopathy, herbal medicine and aromatherapy. Care needs to be taken as some products will contain corticosteroids despite being labelled as natural and sold in markets and on the internet. Researchers reported finding super potent topical steroids in 7 of 11 samples of such 'miracle creams'.

Behaviour modification for eczema is based on habit reversal (scratching/picking), creating awareness of the attitudes and circumstances that lead to scratching and intervention to change and allow the skin to heal.

The Contribution of the Nurse
In 2006, the DH recommend the provision of more care closer to home, places the primary care team at the forefront of skin care, and therefore their clinical skills and educational abilities must address the identified need by commissioners to ensure quality of service provision in terms of safety, effectiveness and patient experience.

School nurses can support and motivate the child to maintain skin care at school while educating teachers about the physical and psychosocial impact of eczema. There are information packs developed by the National Eczema Society for both parents and teachers (National Eczema Society 2016). Occupational health nurses advise on changes in work practice to reduce risk factors and the incidence of industrial-acquired skin disorders. In every setting, the nurse should utilise all available resources and refer patients appropriately to the relevant agencies and support groups (Nicol and Ersser 2010).

Skin Infections and Infestations
Many skin infections and infestations cause anxiety among sufferers because of their real or perceived social implications.

Fungal Skin Infections
These are a group of infections caused by fungi that include dermatophytes (*Trichophyton* (ringworm)), nondermatophyte moulds (*Aspergillus, Scopulariopsis*) and yeasts (*Candida albicans Pityrosporum (Malassezia)*).

Dermatophyte Infections
Dermatophytes are fungi responsible for superficial fungal infection occurring in keratin (i.e. stratum corneum, hair and nails). Some dermatophyte infections are confined to humans, while others principally affect animals and can transfer from animal to human, causing severe inflammatory skin reactions. 'Tinea' is the generic description given to these fungal infections. Fungal infections are usually unilateral. A dermatophyte can be identified by scaly erythema-defined edge plaques with central clearing, excessive scaling in the skin creases or, if by stretching the skin between two fingers (5 cm apart), fine scaling is seen.

Tinea pedis or athlete's foot. The patient complains of itchy, scaling skin between the toe webs.

Tinea capitis affecting the scalp, can result in loss of hair and scarring and emotional distress.

Tinea cruris, presenting as scaly erythematous lesions on the inner thighs and spreading to the perineum and buttocks, affects young males. The source of infection is usually athlete's foot and the fungus is transferred to the groins on fingers or towels.

Tinea unguium is a fungal dystrophy of the toenails in which the nail thickens, discolours and becomes very friable.

Cattle ringworm (tinea corporis) is common amongst farm workers or visitors to farms. The fungus is picked up from gates or fences where cattle have left keratin debris containing the organism.

Medical Management
Topical treatments (e.g. clotrimazole, miconazole creams) are usually first line for all, but for multiple nails or hair infection, then systemic therapy is effective with confirmation of mycology results, especially if considering treatment in children.

Investigations
Skin scarping/nail clippings/hair debris are sent for mycology to confirm dermatophyte infection.

🌐 **See Evolve website Fig. 14.2**

Blood monitoring is required for 'azole' drugs for liver and renal function tests for adverse effects.

❖ Nursing Management and Health Promotion: Dermatophyte Infection

Nursing management focuses on containment of infection and promotion of basic hygiene. Avoidance of shared face cloths/towels prevents further spread. The nurse can advise on prescribed and OTC therapies and their correct method of application. Treatment programmes may involve combined oral and topical therapies, and patients should be advised to persevere where therapies take time to resolve the condition. Conditions can recur, so educating the patient in management of the condition is beneficial in preventing this.

Candida Infection

Candidiasis (thrush) is a yeast infection of the skin and mucous membranes caused by *C. albicans*. The microorganism is a normal commensal of the human digestive system, only becoming pathogenic if the opportunity presents itself. Immunosuppressed patients, people with diabetes, and patients having broad-spectrum antibiotics or topical and systemic corticosteroid therapies are all at risk from this opportunistic infection. Yeast infections are often moist with pustules along the periphery and on nearby healthy skin or macerated in between skin webs. Yeast infections can be intensely itchy – scratching can cause secondary bacterial infection and spread.

Buccal Mucosal Candidiasis. Oral thrush presents as milky curd-like spots on the tongue and inner cheeks. It often affects babies, older people and patients having broad-spectrum antibiotics.

Candida Vulvovaginitis. Presents with a creamy vaginal discharge and itchy erythema of the vulva. It tends to be associated with pregnancy, use of oral contraceptives, antibiotics and diabetes.

Candida Balanitis is a thrush infection of the foreskin and glans. It tends to be more common in uncircumcised males and may be associated with poor hygiene or diabetes. It can recur if a sexual partner also has candidiasis.

Candida Paronychia is a candidal infection of the nail plate which is common in people whose occupation involves repeated immersion of the hands in water, for example hairdressers, nurses and bartenders. The nails become distorted and the nail base is painful, red and swollen.

Intertrigo. Candidal infection is common where two skin folds are in contact and there is increased heat and humidity, such as the groins (nappy rash), axillae and beneath the breasts or pendulous abdomen. Obesity and poor hygiene exacerbate the problem. The skin displays erythematous, well-demarcated erosive lesions and is tender, moist and painful in these areas.

Angular Chelitis is a common condition of older people where the deep grooves at the side of the mouth tend to be moist with saliva; a *Candida* infection exacerbates the problem. It can also be a feature of vitamin B_2 deficiency.

🌑 Medical Management

The diagnosis is confirmed from the clinical picture and skin swab results. The use of topical preparations can be effective.

Investigations
- Skin swabs. 🌐 **See Evolve website Fig. 14.1**
- Urinalysis and fasting blood sugar to exclude diabetes.

- A full blood count must be carried out in older people including vitamin B_2.

Treatment

Treatment is specific to the affected area. Antifungals in the form of creams, ointments and pessaries are very effective. A combined moderate corticosteroid/antifungal, for example Trimovate, is appropriate to treat intertrigo, reducing both inflammation and infection. Combination packs of vaginal pessary and cream are available for vaginal thrush, for example clotrimazole, and these are usually single applications, depending on the dose/strength of the preparation. Newer OTC preparations include a single dose of the antifungal drug fluconazole.

❖ Nursing Management and Health Promotion: Candidiasis

The nurse must be able to identify those at risk of opportunistic infection, for example older people, babies and patients on immunosuppressants. The nurse's role as counsellor is vital in the treatment of genital candidiasis and confidential information should be respected when sexual partners are treated concurrently to prevent reinfection.

Bacterial Skin Infections

Cellulitis

Cellulitis is an acute, spreading and potentially serious infection of dermal and subcutaneous tissue, characterised by red, oedematous, tender skin that is hot and painful. Patients feel unwell with rigors and fever and local lymph nodes may be enlarged. Microorganisms implicated in cellulitis include *S. aureus* and *Streptococcus pyogenes* (group A β-haemolytic streptococcus). In adults, the most common presentation is cellulitis affecting the lower limbs. Cellulitis is common in older people who have lower limb oedema. Infection enters the skin in a variety of ways, including surgical wounds, stasis eczema or leg ulcers, insect bites, minor abrasions between the toes and intravenous drug injection sites. A superficial streptococcal infection of the skin is called erysipelas.

🌑 Medical Management

Management involves the prompt administration of appropriate oral or intravenous antibiotic therapy (sometimes involving several different antibiotics). Analgesics reduce the pain of inflammation.

Investigations
Where appropriate:
- Blood culture – bacterial growth
- Doppler – to rule out deep vein thrombosis

❖ Nursing Management and Health Promotion: Cellulitis

Initial care includes bed rest, monitoring of temperature and dealing with rigors. Pain assessment and administration of regular analgesics will ease discomfort. Early intervention teams often initiate intravenous antibiotics in the patient's own home to prevent admission into hospital. A limb affected by cellulitis requires elevation to reduce oedema. Exercising (passive exercises) reduces the complications of bed rest but mobilisation should occur as soon as possible. Once the condition resolves, general advice on basic skin care and avoidance of predisposing factors is helpful.

Patients can have recurrent cellulitis and may be prescribed prophylactic antibiotic therapy to prevent future episodes.

Other Staphylococcal Skin Infections

Impetigo is a superficial skin infection caused by *S. aureus*, sometimes with *S. pyogenes*. The head and neck are the most common sites. The condition starts as a small but gradually enlarging pustule that ruptures to leave a raw exuding surface. The exudate dries and forms the yellow golden crust typical of impetigo. It can also occur as a secondary infection, for example associated with eczema and scabies.

Folliculitis. Infection of superficial hair follicles by *S. aureus* presents as a small pustule on an erythematous base centred around the follicle. Folliculitis may be exacerbated by the use of greasy ointments that may have been rubbed into the skin; this is why technique of application is important, that is application in the direction of hair growth.

Medical Management

Treatment involves the use of topical and/or oral antibiotics depending on whether the bacterial infection is localised or generalised. Careful selection of antibiotics (see local policies) reduces antibiotic resistance and healthcare-associated infection (HCAI).

Viral Skin Infections

Warts

Infection by the human papillomavirus (HPV) affects the DNA in epidermal cells, creating warts. Warts are benign, highly contagious and can be unsightly or catch on clothing.

See Evolve website Fig. 14.8

Some are self-limiting and are nonscarring. Transmission occurs during direct contact, for example in gyms, swimming baths or schools. The classification of warts is outlined in Information 14.2.

Medical Management

Diagnosis is based on history and clinical appearance. Treatment may involve topical application of ointments or premedicated plasters containing salicylic acid to soften and remove the wart, or liquid nitrogen (cryotherapy).

❖ Nursing Management and Health Promotion: Warts

The nurse should explain virus transmission and encourage the meticulous continuation of treatment. Many patients become disheartened by the slow resolution of the problem and discontinue treatment. Regular assessment by the practice nurse may encourage adherence to treatment. If warts occur on hands, especially of people in the catering trade, then the use of liquid nitrogen is viable but can cause scarring and is available OTC. The economic cost to the NHS and primary care is greater for cryotherapy compared to salicylic acid but less tolerable to children and it not nationally available so recent study recommends the use of salicylic acid as first line treatment (Dillon 2020).

See Evolve website Figs. 14.9 and 14.10

Molluscum Contagiosum

A pox virus produces solid, skin-coloured or pearly-white papules on the skin. It affects adults but is more common in children, arising over a period of 2–3 months. The lesions may be single or multiple, occurring on the neck and trunk more resistant in those with atopic eczema.

Medical Management

Initial diagnosis is based on history and clinical appearance. The condition should resolve spontaneously and patients or parents can be reassured that it tends to be self-limiting. Normal basic hygiene rules prevent further spread. It can be treated with potassium hydroxide OTC.

Herpes Simplex Virus (HSV)

There are two types of HSV – HSV-1, oral labial herpes (cold sores) and HSV-2, genital herpes – but either can cause genital herpes. Initial contact with the herpes simplex virus is usually in childhood and often goes unnoticed. However, development of primary cutaneous herpes simplex can occur and, in a patient with atopic eczema, it can be a severe life-threatening condition. Following primary infection, HSV-1 can establish itself in sensory ganglia (trigeminal) and be reactivated by, for example, sunlight, stress and colds. Reactivation of the virus is preceded by a tingling sensation before a cluster of small vesicles develops. The vesicles burst and lesions then crust, usually resolving in 10–14 days. Genital herpes is a sexually transmitted infection affecting the penis, vulva, perianal area and rectum.

Medical Management

Recurrent herpes simplex is treated with topical aciclovir which is now available OTC. It must be used immediately on awareness of the tingling sensation, and applied five times daily for 5 days to inhibit vesicle eruption. Patients with genital herpes should be referred to a sexual health clinic for investigations, management and expert counselling.

❖ Nursing Management and Health Promotion: Herpes Simplex

The nurse can advise patients at risk of recurrent episodes of herpes simplex on the use of topical aciclovir and should recommend completing the course. The patient should be reminded of basic hygiene standards to avoid further transmission of the virus during the active phase. Patients with genital herpes should be encouraged to access specialist support and counselling at the sexual health clinic. A pregnant woman with genital herpes requires effective liaison between herself, the midwife and obstetrician, to acknowledge the condition and its potential complications and

---

INFORMATION 14.2

Classification of Warts

- Common warts – hyperkeratotic nodules occurring on the hands and feet of children. These often resolve spontaneously.
- Plane warts – smooth flat-topped warts appearing on the face and hands.
- Plantar warts (verrucae) – the HPV is pressured into the dermis, creating a callus. The most common site is the feet.
- Genital warts – a mass of warts with a cauliflower-like appearance present on the perianal and genital areas.

to initiate appropriate action to minimise virus transfer during delivery (Gawkrodger and Ardern-Jones 2020).

Eczema Herpeticum

Eczema herpeticum is a widespread cutaneous HSV infection occurring in patients with atopic eczema. In children, it can be life-threatening, and any patient can be systemically unwell and febrile. Vesicles erupt rapidly over the face and neck and can extend over the rest of the body. The skin is taut, red and painful. As vesicles erupt and rupture, the patient becomes susceptible to secondary bacterial infection.

⬤ Medical Management

Treatment depends on the severity of illness and is a combination of antiviral drugs and antibiotics. The patient who is pyrexial and systemically unwell should be hospitalised. A side room with effective standard (universal) precautions is required (see Chapter 7, Nursing Patients With Disorders of the Lymphatic and Immune Systems). Oral aciclovir is adequate in minor cases, but if the patient is unwell, aciclovir is given by the intravenous route. Prompt referral to an ophthalmologist is vital for the patient with any eye involvement (see Chapter 15, Nursing Patients With Disorders of the Eye and Sight Impairment). Patients with eczema discontinue topical corticosteroids until the virus resolves. Secondary bacterial infection should be treated with topical antibiotic cream and/or oral antibiotics. Appropriate analgesics may be required.

❖ Nursing Management and Health Promotion: Eczema Herpeticum

The nurse's role is to maintain effective infection prevention and control procedures in order to reduce the transmission of infection. The patient who is systemically unwell requires regular observations of temperature, fluid intake and rest until infection resolves. The nurse should assist in cleansing the skin, removing crusty skin and applying topical applications of prescribed creams as the patient feels too unwell or too distressed by pain to manage this independently. Once the infection resolves, the nurse can advise the patient on restarting topical corticosteroids for the eczema. Patients who have had HSV previously and are at risk of cold sores should keep aciclovir in reserve to use promptly if a cold sore develops and avoid contact with people who have them. Aciclovir is available OTC so effective treatment is easier to achieve. Delay in seeing the GP can be detrimental as this condition erupts quickly.

Herpes Zoster (Shingles)

Herpes zoster is caused by the varicella-zoster virus (VZV). After an attack of childhood chickenpox, the virus remains dormant in the dorsal root ganglia of the spinal cord but can be reactivated later in life to cause shingles. The trigger factor is unknown, but the condition occurs in immunosuppressed people, stress and serious illness, and commonly affects middle-aged and older people.

Once reactivated, VZV multiplies within host cells. The cells lyse and virus particles are released to invade other cells. The virus particles migrate along the sensory nerve fibres causing nerve damage and pain. Fluid-filled vesicles erupt along a thoracic and/or cranial dermatome with a characteristic unilateral band-like distribution of the sensory nerve. Pain and tenderness often precede the vesicular erosions, and patients may have fever and feel unwell. As the vesicles crust over, the infective risk resolves over a period of 2–3 weeks.

⬤ Medical Management

Early treatment with antivirals such as topical aciclovir, ideally 72 hours before the development of the vesicles, can reduce the intensity. Diagnosis is confirmed by clinical history and viral culture. Oral or intravenous aciclovir is essential management in immunosuppressed patients. The potential complications of herpes zoster are:
- herpes zoster ophthalmicus (causing corneal vesicles, ulceration and scarring)
- postherpetic neuralgia (requiring input from the specialist pain team).

❖ Nursing Management and Health Promotion: Herpes Zoster (Shingles)

In an acute attack of shingles, the patient may require hospitalisation. Standard (universal) precautions and isolation are required until the infectious stage resolves. The patient should be nursed by staff who have had chickenpox, as nonimmune people can develop chickenpox following contact with a patient with shingles. Nurses should encourage people to seek early treatment before the vesicles erupt (see earlier) and vaccinations are now available.

Certain groups of people are particularly susceptible to the transmission of herpes zoster, for example patients having radiotherapy and/or chemotherapy, and immunocompromised patients on oral or topical corticosteroids. Community nurses should be aware of the long-term problems associated with shingles. A small proportion of patients report persistent pain (postherpetic neuralgia) continuing for many years. Chronic pain has a major impact on daily living and requires full assessment (see Chapter 20, Pain Management). Treatment options available for postherpetic neuralgia include transcutaneous electrical nerve stimulation (TENS), topical capsaicin, ultrasound, antidepressants and/or anticonvulsant therapy. Referral to a pain control clinic is advisable for intractable pain.

Infestations

Scabies

Scabies is a skin infestation caused by the itch mite *Sarcoptes scabiei* and acquired by prolonged close physical contact with the mite. The female scabies mite burrows into the stratum corneum, and after fertilisation begins to lay eggs along the burrow. For the first 4–6 weeks after infestation, there may be no itching, but thereafter pruritus is intense, especially at night. This is thought to be due to a hypersensitive response to the mite. Skin examination usually reveals burrows, principally on the hands and feet, the sides of fingers/toes, between finger and toe webs, the wrists and the insteps. Burrows/papules can also present on the male genitalia. A scabies 'rash' may be present in the axillae, umbilicus and thighs. Excoriation can cause burrows to become eczematised and infected, which can often confuse diagnosis.

⬤ See Evolve website Fig. 14.11

Crusty scabies is the form of scabies presenting in patients who have sensory deficits where the sensation of itch is absent, for example in spinal injuries, or in patients who are immunosuppressed either because of disease or treatment, for example HIV disease, lymphoma, systemic corticosteroids or transplantation. Absence of scratching leads to large numbers of mites remaining on the skin in crusted lesions.

During skin shedding, mites are shed into the environment, and therefore any person in contact is at considerable risk of developing scabies from the patient.

Medical Management

Diagnosis can be confirmed by using a needle to remove a mite from a burrow and examining it microscopically, or a burrow can be visualised with a dermatoscope. Current topical therapies are permethrin and malathion. In resistant cases, oral ivermectin is prescribed. Once the infestation is treated, further therapy with a combined corticosteroid/antibiotic cream may be necessary to reduce itch and treat excoriated lesions until the skin is healed. Antihistamine tablets are appropriate if itch disturbs sleep. Soothing topical preparations, for example Eurax or Dermacool cream, can be useful until residual itch disappears.

❖ Nursing Management and Health Promotion: Scabies

The priority is to treat the patient and identify close contacts requiring treatment (especially in nursing homes). The nurse combines practical advice with psychological support, recognising the social embarrassment associated with scabies. The nurse must identify current treatments and their correct method of application (Reflection 14.3). As recurrent scabies is often due to poorly applied treatments, both patient and nurse should read carefully the advice leaflets provided with topical scabicides, always remembering to leave some preparation to reapply to the hands if they are washed after initial application. Treatments are usually repeated after 7 days. Transient contact with the patient is unlikely to cause transmission. However, the patient with crusty scabies is highly contagious and should avoid contact with others while treatment is ongoing. Normal washing of linen and clothes is adequate.

Head Lice (Pediculosis Capitis)

Head lice are transmitted by close contact. The adult female louse lays eggs which are cemented to the hair approximately 0.5 cm from the root. Scalp irritation and itch are due to the saliva produced as the louse bites the scalp. The 'nit' is the empty case left once the larva has hatched – the case becomes white and is more easily detected.

🌐 See Evolve website Fig. 14.12

Head lice are an emotive topic, as infestation continues to be endemic amongst school children.

❖ Nursing Management and Health Promotion: Head Lice

The priority is to treat the patient and appropriate contacts. Treatment usually consists of an insecticide lotion applied to the scalp, for example malathion or pyrethroid (phenothrin), which is left on for a number of hours and then shampooed out. Treatment is repeated after 7 days to destroy newly hatched lice. Combing with a fine-tooth comb assists in the final removal of nits. The practice of rotating products to prevent the development of resistance is no longer advocated: current advice is that if an insecticide does not destroy the lice, a different one should be used for the next course (British National Formulary [BNF] 2020-21). Education of parents regarding the guidelines for each product is essential as the burden of treatment falls on them. Some will opt to use nightly wet combing after conditioning, rather than use chemicals.

BULLOUS DISORDERS

Bullous disorders are characterised by large watery blisters (bullae) arising within or immediately under the epidermis (Weller et al. 2015). The aetiology of autoimmune bullous diseases remains unknown; genetic factors may have a role – and histological location influences the classification of the disorder. Early detection and treatment are essential, as many of the bullous conditions are severe and potentially life threatening. Blistering may be caused by insect bites, burns, oedema, cellulitis, erythema multiforme and contact dermatitis.

Pemphigus (Intraepidermal Bullae)

Pathophysiology

This autoimmune disease occurs in adults. It is characterised by the development of autoantibodies against epidermal cell surface molecules creating superficial erosions and blisters on epidermal and mucosal surfaces.

Common Presenting Symptoms

Superficial fluid-filled blisters are present within the epidermis. These blisters are flaccid and thin roofed and offer little resistance; consequently, they shear, leaving raw, denuded skin. Pain from the exposed sites is a major factor. Oral lesions are common affecting nutrition and hydration. Diagnosis is confirmed by a positive Nikolsky's sign – when lateral pressure is applied to the skin surface with a thumb, the epidermis shears and appears to slide over the dermis.

Pemphigoid (Subepidermal Bullae)

Pathophysiology

This is more common in older people: 80% of patients are aged 60 and over, and like pemphigus, pemphigoid is an autoimmune disease and can be triggered by certain drugs (Weller et al. 2015). Antibodies bind to the junction between dermis and epidermis, and blisters are formed in response to enzymes released from inflammatory cells

Figure 14.7 Bullous pemphigoid. Large tense and unilocular blisters clustered in and around the axilla. (Reproduced from Boon NA, Colledge NR, Walker BR. *Davidson's Principles and Practice of Medicine*. 20th ed. Edinburgh: Churchill Livingstone; 2006, with permission.)

(Fig. 14.7). Diagnosis can be confirmed by biopsy with immunofluorescence studies and blood test for pemphigoid antibodies.

Common Presenting Symptoms
Symptoms may include generalised intense itch, followed by erythematous plaques on the skin (pre-pemphigoid stage), followed by the development of tense intact blisters affecting any area of the body. Nikolsky's sign is negative.

Toxic Epidermal/Epidermolytic Necrolysis (TEN) (Subepidermal)

Pathophysiology
TEN presents as a dermatological emergency and is often precipitated by drug hypersensitivity (severe form of Stevens–Johnson syndrome). The skin split is subepidermal and the entire epidermis shears off in layers, leaving raw, denuded areas. A review of the patient's medication and removal of the causative factor(s) are essential.

Common Presenting Symptoms
The skin is erythrodermic and painful, with the skin shearing off in sheets.

See Evolve website Fig. 14.14

Nikolsky's sign is positive. There is pain and erosions may be present in the mouth, oesophagus and bronchus.

Medical Management of Bullous Disorders
Early diagnosis and treatment either in the home or hospitalisation due to the life-threatening potential of bullous disorders are essential.

Investigations
Investigations include:
- skin biopsy – to identify the type of skin split
- blood tests – full blood count, urea and electrolytes to monitor fluid loss from eroded skin; presence of antibodies in pemphigus
- skin swab – to diagnosis secondary infection.

Treatment
Treatment might involve the following
- Antibodies – for secondary infection.
- Corticosteroids – in pemphigus and pemphigoid, high-dose oral corticosteroids, e.g. prednisolone, are the first line of management and are maintained until blistering stops. The dose is gradually reduced, aiming for low-dose maintenance therapy.
- Doxcycline 200 mg daily for 6 weeks (in elderly/diabetics). Given as an antiinflammatory long-term.
- Analgesics – to control pain from eroded skin lesions.
- Antihistamines – to reduce itch and aid rest.
- Immunosuppressants, e.g. cyclophosphamide, azathioprine, are used in combination with oral corticosteroids to control the disease process of pemphigus and pemphigoid.
- Plasmapheresis to remove antibodies is considered in severe cases; it also allows monitoring of circulating pemphigus antibodies.

❖ Nursing Management and Health Promotion: Bullous Disorders

The general nursing care of bullous disorders is outlined. Although rare, they are more commonly seen in dermatology units. In severe cases the nursing priorities are similar to those needed by patients with severe burn injuries (see Chapter 29, Nursing the Patient With Burn Injury) and are often care for in burn units.

Major Nursing Considerations

Analgesia
Analgesia must be effective and consistent. Pemphigus and TEN are distressing, painful conditions when shearing of the skin is active. Pain assessment tools (see Chapter 20, Pain Management) permit the nurse and patient to determine pain control needs, ensure accurate delivery of analgesics, and evaluate their efficacy, which is particularly relevant prior to dressing changes.

Bed Rest, Special Beds/Pressure-Relieving Equipment
Facilitating rest and comfort is a primary aim to avoid further trauma to the skin. The use of low-pressure, air-fluidised beds enhances comfort and reduces the need for positional changes which contribute to shearing forces on the skin. The temperature regulator in these beds maintains an appropriately warm environment, helping the patient to maintain body temperature. This warm environment also increases the amount of insensible fluid loss, so the patient's fluid intake must be increased to compensate. Dressings remain moist with the use of these beds, and are usually easily removed.

Hygiene
The maintenance of good personal hygiene and the prevention of infection are extremely important. Gentle washing or the application of soaks, i.e. potassium permanganate, for their mild antiseptic/antipruritic effect can be soothing and help to minimise further trauma.

Infection Prevention and Control (see Chapter 18)
Isolation may be necessary due to skin loss. The patient will be susceptible to infection and the use of immunosuppressants will increase this susceptibility. Patients with TEN are often cared for in burns units.

Diet

Approximately 20% of an adult's dietary protein is used for skin repair and growth in normal health. Therefore, an increased intake of protein is advisable in bullous conditions. Referral to a dietitian will ensure the prescription of any necessary supplements. Constipation induced by fluid loss, or as a side-effect of analgesics, is an associated problem. Mild laxatives may be indicated to prevent discomfort.

Monitoring Vital Signs

Regular measurement of body temperature is required, as fluctuations may occur due to fluid and heat loss from the skin. Variations in environmental temperature can be reduced by nursing the patient in a side room.

Blood pressure is checked regularly if there is associated fluid loss, corticosteroid-induced hypertension or hydration by intravenous fluids.

Monitoring Electrolyte and Fluid Balance

This is imperative in any condition associated with skin loss. Rehydration may initially be achievable by increasing the patient's oral intake and monitoring output. An intravenous infusion may be necessary in severe cases. If skin loss presents problems in siting a peripheral infusion, a central line may be required, with monitoring of central venous pressure providing an accurate assessment of fluid requirements.

Urine should be tested for glycosuria in order to detect a potential diabetic state induced by oral corticosteroid therapy.

Dressings and Topical Therapy

A dressing procedure provides the best opportunity to complete a skin assessment and evaluate disease activity. In pemphigus and TEN, raw areas are recorded and dressed. The tense bullae of pemphigoid are identified and left intact to permit reabsorption of blister fluid, thereby minimising trauma and infection risk. Daily reassessment is based on blister count. Blisters restricting movement are uncomfortable for the patient and can be aspirated using a sterile syringe and needle, leaving the blister roof intact (Ro et al. 2018). Administration of analgesics prior to the application of topical therapy is important to reduce the patient's apprehension about dressing changes. Individual needs and disease severity determine dressing requirements, but the aims are to:
- keep dressing changes to a minimum
- maximise comfort
- ensure dressings are removable without traumatising the skin, so NO tape.

Meeting these aims ensures that further trauma is minimised and healing is promoted. Simple applications of soothing emollients or a nonadherent/silicone dressing secured by gauze stockinette will possibly be all that is tolerated. Dressing choices (see Chapter 23, Tissue Viability and Managing Chronic Wounds) should be guided by the patient's comments and nurses will adjust dressings appropriately to prevent constriction and pain.

Care in the Community

Although these conditions are rare, as numbers of older people increase, the incidence will rise. The community nurse has a dual role: firstly, in identifying disorders and coordinating referral for specialist help; and secondly, the nurse may support the family in providing care in the home or after discharge from hospital, in ensuring the patient understands the rationale behind long-term maintenance medication, encouraging adherence to and monitoring side-effects of systemic therapies.

ACUTE SKIN FAILURE

This life-threatening condition is associated with a number of serious skin disorders, for example erythrodermic psoriasis, eczema, bullous diseases and others.

❖ Nursing Management and Health Promotion: Acute Skin Failure

The nursing goals will vary depending on the type and severity of the presenting condition. If the epidermal barrier is breached, as it is in severe erythroderma associated with types of psoriasis and eczema or autoimmune blistering conditions, the nursing interventions need to support the epidermal barrier:
- loss of body temperature control – bed rest, use of warmth, management of rigors
- loss of water through the skin surface – increase oral fluid
- loss of protein – high-protein diet
- discomfort and pain – analgesia, emollient therapy hourly and antihistamines if itchy.

Intensive nursing care is essential for the safety and comfort of the patient, including infection prevention and monitoring and acting on early signs of deterioration in the patient's condition (Information 14.3).

INFORMATION 14.3

Monitoring Patients With Acute Skin Disorders/Failure

The type and frequency of observations and investigations depend on the severity of the person's condition.
- Level of consciousness
- Temperature and shivering
- Heart rate
- Respiratory rate
- Blood pressure
- Gastric emptying
- Fluid balance
- Urinary volume may be measured hourly
- Urinary osmolality
- Extent of skin lesions
- Body weight
- Calculation of fluid loss
- Arterial blood gases
- Chest X-ray
- Blood tests
  - full blood count
  - urea and electrolytes
  - glucose
  - serum proteins
  - liver enzymes
- Urine tested for glucose (glycosuria).

ACNE

Acne is a disorder of the pilosebaceous units. It is a common condition, usually developing during adolescence, with an average age range 14–30 years, and can persist for many years (Tomlinson 2021). It reaches a peak between 17 and 21 years, gradually improving and disappearing. However, 6% of adults between 25 and 40 years still experience persistent acne.

The psychosocial impact of acne should not be underestimated, as its onset during the years when visual appearance is important to developing new relationships can have a devastating effect on the young adult. Acne can also impact on an individual's personal identity and affect psychological well-being, causing distress, depression and anxiety, so early intervention in primary care for those with mild disease might reduce this impact.

🔷 Pathophysiology

During puberty, circulating androgen hormones stimulate sebum production. Hyperkeratosis occurs at the mouth of the hair follicle and the dilated chamber fills with sebum. The organism *Propionibacterium acnes* grows in large numbers, creating the comedone. *P. acnes* acts on sebum to produce inflammatory chemicals which leak into the surrounding dermis or out through a rupture in the follicle wall (Gawkrodger and Ardern-Jones 2020) (Fig. 14.8).

Common Presenting Symptoms

Acne affects the face, neck, upper back and front of the chest. In more severe cases, these lesions may spread further. Lesions can include comedones, papules, pustules, nodules, cysts and residual scars.

🌐 See Evolve website Figs 14.14–14.16

🔷 Medical Management

Mild acne is managed with topical therapies, antiseptic washes and antibiotic preparations, whereas moderate/severe acne requires both topical (combination therapies) and systemic therapies.

Antibiotics. Oral tetracyclines given over a 6-month period reduce the inflammatory process. Side-effects of and contraindications to tetracycline should be noted (see BNF 2020-21).

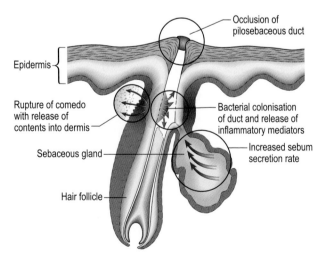

Figure 14.8 The pathogenesis of acne. (Reproduced from Boon NA, Colledge NR, Walker BR. *Davidson's Principles and Practice of Medicine*. 20th ed. Edinburgh: Churchill Livingstone; 2006, with permission.)

If patients are intolerant of tetracycline, erythromycin can be prescribed.

Isotretinoin (a Retinoid) reduces sebum production. Its side-effects necessitate regular monitoring of liver function and blood lipid levels. The medication is teratogenic: pregnancy must be ruled out before starting treatment and female patients must use reliable contraception (see BNF 2020-21). Isotretinoin clears acne in most patients with no reoccurrence but you can have more than one course if there is a relapse.

❖ Nursing Management and Health Promotion: Acne

Nurses are key to educating patients and dispelling misinformation about acne. The patient should be reassured that acne is not linked to poor diet, an excess of sweets or chocolate (per se) or poor hygiene. Indeed, most acne sufferers are overzealous in personal hygiene. The nurse should encourage continuation of therapies for the full treatment course. Nurses prescribing must ensure that females starting a course of isotretinoin understand that they must not become pregnant and that they are enrolled into the pregnancy prevention programme (PPP) prior to commencing treatment. The nurse must respond empathetically to the acne sufferer. The degree of distress may not always equate with the severity of disease, and care must address the psychosocial impact of acne. Emotional distress due to skin disease has provoked suicide, and the nurse working with acne patients should recognise that individuals can become so disturbed that they are pushed to this extreme but it does not mean they should be denied isotretinoin (Paljarvi et al. 2022). Part of the monitoring of isotretinoin is around the emotional impact that the drug has in magnifying moods and could lead to sadness and potential self-harm so the use of PHQ-9 is used to help with the monitoring as well as involving GPs or mental health services with the patient's care.

PHOTODERMATOSES

Photodermatoses are skin disorders induced or aggravated by sunlight. They are relatively common and can impose severe limitations on daily life. Nursing management focuses on assisting the patient to maintain independent living within the limitations imposed by photosensitivity.

Sunlight

Sunlight is composed of different wavelengths of UVL, divided into UVA, UVB and visible light. UVA in larger doses can produce erythema, passes through window glass and is less variable in intensity. UVB causes sunburn. Visible light easily penetrates the epidermis, usually with minimal significance. Some conditions, however, demonstrate an abnormal sensitivity to visible light. Factors affecting the intensity of sunlight include:
- time of day – strongest between 1100 and 1500
- geography – weaker in northern latitudes
- season – UVB less intensive in winter months
- reflective effect of snow, water and sand.

Note that clouds do not protect against sunburn as UVB penetrates cloud cover.

Types of Photodermatosis

Polymorphic Light Eruption (PLE) is very common, with women being affected twice as frequently as men. It affects patients in early spring, disappearing in autumn. Several hours after exposure to sunlight, the patient develops an itchy papular rash, which persists for 7–10 days. The rash is provoked by UVB or UVA wavelengths, and it should be remembered that UVA also penetrates window glass and thin clothing.

Photo-Aggravated Dermatoses. Some preexisting skin conditions, for example atopic eczema, psoriasis and herpes simplex, can be exacerbated by sunlight.

Photo-Contact Dermatitis. In these disorders, direct contact of the skin with a substance, for example tars and sunscreens, followed by exposure to UVL provokes dermatitis. Certain genetic disorders, for example xeroderma pigmentosum, also produce a photosensitive reaction.

Chronic Actinic Dermatitis usually affects men over 50 years of age but can also occur in women. Patients are sensitive to sunlight (all components) and artificial light and have allergies to substances in direct contact with their skin, for example plants, wood, perfumes, sunscreens and rubber. Sparing of the shaded skin can be present, for example behind the ears and under a watch strap. The condition presents with marked erythema, eczema and thickening of the skin of the face, neck and hands. Skin changes may be less evident in areas covered by clothing.

Medical Management

A full history is required and assessment of related factors, such as skin type, sites involved, drugs, hobbies, occupation, and so on.

Signs and Symptoms include eczema, erythema, heat, itch, oedema, pain and urticaria.

Investigations.
- *Phototesting* – available in specialist photobiology/dermatology units. Phototesting involves the use of a monochromator to identify if abnormal light sensitivity is present and establish which wavelengths are responsible, i.e. UVA, UVB or visible light. Varying doses at different wavelengths are irradiated to small areas on the back and delayed erythema is noted at 7 and 24 hours. Responses are compared with those of a control group, to determine the degree of photosensitivity and wavelengths responsible.
- *Patch testing.*

Treatment involves:
- systemic and topical therapy and/or phototherapy
- antihistamines, immunosuppressants and oral and/or topical corticosteroids
- sunscreens – offer a sun protection factor (SPF) either chemically (absorbing/filtering UVL) or physically (reflecting/scattering UVL) to protect the skin. A combination sunscreen creates a more effective sun block.

Some light-sensitive conditions, for example PLE, can be treated with a course of phototherapy desensitisation and patients should be encouraged to continue exposure to maintain their new tolerance level. Unfortunately, this is lost during winter and repeat phototherapy is needed the following spring.

❖ Nursing Management and Health Promotion: Photodermatoses

Many patients are relieved that investigations have produced a diagnosis rather than a dismissal of symptoms as merely 'a bit of sunburn'. Information from nursing staff is vital if the patient is to cope with lifestyle changes imposed by the diagnosis. Advice includes:
- regular use of emollients
- meticulous, regular (every 2 hours) application of prescribed sunscreens to exposed sites

- treatment with topical corticosteroid if the condition flares
- sun avoidance between 1100 and 1500
- wear closely woven clothing as an effective barrier; a wide-brimmed hat, scarf and gloves may prove helpful
- apply clear museum film (blocks UVL) to windows (home, workplace and car).

Psychological Support

Social isolation is a major problem for individuals with severe photosensitive disorders. Many patients, distressed by their diagnosis and the restrictions it entails, reject management regimens which would lead to a life indoors or only leaving home after sundown. Others accept the limitations and persevere with the use of sunscreens to permit them some freedom, albeit restricted daily living.

The nurse must display an empathic understanding of the psychological impact of the diagnosis and restrictions. Nursing support should aim for the patient to control skin management in an informed way, with easy access to professional help as needed.

URTICARIA

Urticaria is a common condition. Lesions are described as 'hives' or nettle rash. The skin feels irritable with white raised wheals that turn pink with a bordered edge.

🌐 See Evolve website Figs 14.17 and 14.18

There are many causes, and it often resolves spontaneously. Severe cases may lead to swelling around the eyes, mouth and throat known as angioedema (see Chapter 7, Nursing Patients With Disorders of the Lymphatic and Immune Systems). In severe attacks, the airway is compromised, so immediate emergency treatment is needed. Urticaria may also be associated with anaphylaxis (see Chapter 7).

Pathophysiology

In response to the initial trigger factor, the dermis becomes oedematous, blood vessels dilate and mast cells release histamine. The wheal of urticaria is oedema of the dermis and can extend rapidly into the subcutaneous tissues causing angioedema.

Classification of Urticaria (Information 14.4)

Acute contact urticaria is related to contact factors, for example animal fur, plants and insect stings. Extensive urticaria associated with angioedema is usually idiopathic but can be related to the

---

INFORMATION 14.4

Classification of Urticaria

- Chronic – idiopathic
- Acute – IgE mediated, e.g. food allergy, drug reaction (see Chapter 5, Nursing Patients With Endocrine and Metabolic Disorders)
- Physical – dermographism, cholinergic, cold, solar, heat, delayed pressure
- Contact – immune (e.g. animal saliva) or nonimmune (e.g. nettle sting)
- Pharmacological – aspirin, penicillin, food additives
- Systemic cause – lymphoma, hyperthyroidism, infection, infestation
- Inherited – hereditary angioedema
- Other – vasculitis, insect bites, pregnancy

ingestion of food or drugs (strawberries, nuts, penicillin). Cold, heat, sun, pressure and water can all induce physical urticaria. Sweating after physical exercise or eating spicy food may also induce urticaria with isolated facial swelling.

🌑 Medical Management

History and skin examination assist in determining the provoking factors. Antihistamines are essential; they suppress histamine release and some, for example desloratadine, are nonsedating. In acute attacks, the patient requires oral antihistamines until the condition resolves, usually in a few days. In chronic (more than 6 weeks) urticaria, maintenance antihistamines (up to 4 times the normal dose) may be needed for several months. Severe urticaria may also require second-line treatments with methotrexate or ciclosporin for longer-term treatment and even biologic therapy in accordance with NICE guidance for urticaria (NICE 2018b). The management of anaphylaxis and administration of adrenaline are outlined in Chapter 7.

❖ Nursing Management and Health Promotion: Urticaria

The nurse in every setting will encounter the patient with allergies. Angioedema and anaphylaxis can prove fatal, so professionals must recognise the urgency of the situation and be trained and competent in emergency procedures. On a day-to-day basis the nursing role is to provide factual information and manage the condition.

Dietitians provide dietary advice about avoiding foods that trigger urticaria. Dietary exclusion is difficult, as food labelling is not always helpful. Public pressure has persuaded food companies and supermarkets to provide accurate food labelling, for example to protect those with nut allergy. Nut allergy and sensitisation can lead to anaphylaxis and death. In cases of severe allergic reactions the patient/parents should be trained to use adrenaline pens. The nurse can help the patient and family in relation to all aspects of the allergy, in particular to recognise warning symptoms and to use the adrenaline promptly whilst seeking medical assistance (see Chapter 7).

SKIN TUMOURS

The skin can develop a wide diversity of tumours, both benign and malignant, within the epidermis and dermis (e.g. seborrheic warts, actinic keratoses, BCC, squamous cell carcinoma (SCC), malignant melanoma and others.). Skin biopsy for histology is necessary in the diagnosis, prognosis and management of skin tumours (NICE 2011) involving multidisciplinary teams and skin cancer nurse specialists.

🌐 **See Evolve website Figs 14.9–14.23**

Malignant Melanoma

Malignant melanoma is the most serious of the skin tumours and its incidence is rising. Melanoma is responsible for most skin cancer deaths – over 2400 per annum in the UK (2014–2016) (Cancer Research UK 2018). UK survival figures for 2013–2017 indicate that 87% of patients with melanoma are alive 10 years following diagnosis (Cancer Research UK 2022). Melanoma commonly arises in a naevus (mole) (Fig. 14.9), involves the pigment-producing melanocytes and can metastasise rapidly via the blood and lymph (unlike other skin tumours). Early detection and excision of thin tumours (less than 1 mm thick) carry an excellent

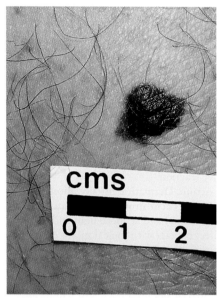

Figure 14.9 Malignant melanoma. A changing mole which fails the ABCDE test (**A**symmetry, **B**order irregular, **C**olour irregular, **D**iameter often greater than 0.5 cm and **E**levation irregular). (Reproduced from Boon NA, Colledge NR, Walker BR. *Davidson's Principles and Practice of Medicine*. 20th ed. Edinburgh: Churchill Livingstone; 2006, with permission.)

Figure 14.10 Superficial spreading melanoma. Note the irregular, asymmetrical shape and different hues, including depigmented areas signifying spontaneous regression. (Reproduced from Boon NA, Colledge NR, Walker BR. *Davidson's Principles and Practice of Medicine*. 20th ed. Edinburgh: Churchill Livingstone; 2006, with permission.)

prognosis and potential cure. Late-stage untreated melanoma with metastases has a poorer outcome and treatment is often palliative, for example radiotherapy (Fig. 14.10).

Health Promotion

Research (Green et al. 2011) suggests that excessive childhood sun exposure is an important factor in the aetiology of melanoma. Current campaigns such as #OwnYourTone (Cancer Research UK 2018) encourage people to protect themselves and their children from the sun's harmful rays and so reduce their risk of skin

DERMATOLOGY LIFE QUALITY INDEX (DLQI)

Hospital No.
Date: ....
Name: ....
Score: ....
Address: ....
....
Diagnosis: ....

The aim of this questionnaire is to measure how much your skin problem has affected your life OVER THE LAST WEEK.

Please tick (✓) one box for each question.

1. Over the last week, how itchy, sore, painful or stinging has your skin been?
   Very much
   A lot
   A little
   Not at all

2. Over the last week, how embarrassed or self-conscious have you been because of your skin?
   Very much
   A lot
   A little
   Not at all

3. Over the last week, how much has your skin interfered with you going shopping or looking after your home or garden?
   Very much
   A lot
   A little
   Not at all
   Not relevant

4. Over the last week, how much has your skin influenced the clothes you wear?
   Very much
   A lot
   A little
   Not at all
   Not relevant

5. Over the last week, how much has your skin affected any social or leisure activities?
   Very much
   A lot
   A little
   Not at all
   Not relevant

6. Over the last week, how much has your skin made it difficult for you to do any sport?
   Very much
   A lot
   A little
   Not at all
   Not relevant

7. Over the last week, has your skin prevented you from working or studying?
   If 'No', over the last week how much has your skin been a problem at work or studying?
   If Yes
   A lot
   A little
   Not at all
   Not relevant

8. Over the last week, how much has your skin created problems with your partner or any of your close friends or relatives?
   Very much
   A lot
   A little
   Not at all
   Not relevant

9. Over the last week, how much has your skin caused any sexual difficulties?
   Very much
   A lot
   A little
   Not at all
   Not relevant

10. Over the last week, how much of a problem has the treatment for your skin been, for example by making your home messy, or by taking up time?
    Very much
    A lot
    A little
    Not at all
    Not relevant

Please check you have answered EVERY question. Thank you.

DERMATOLOGY LIFE QUALITY INDEX (DLQI)

Instructions for Use
The Dermatology Life Quality Index questionnaire is designed for use in adults, i.e. patients over the age of 16. It is self-explanatory and can be simply handed to the patient who is asked to fill it in without the need for detailed explanation. It is usually completed in 1 or 2 minutes.

Scoring
The scoring of each question is as follows:
Very much – scored 3
A lot – scored 2
A little – scored 1
Not at all – scored 0
Not relevant – scored 0
Question 7, 'prevented work or studying' – scored 3

The DLQI is calculated by summing the score of each question resulting in a maximum of 30 and a minimum of 0. The higher the score, the more quality of life is impaired.

How to Interpret the Meaning of DLQI Scores
0–1: no effect at all on patient's life
2–5: small effect on patient's life
6–10: moderate effect on patient's life
11–20: very large effect on patient's life
21–30 extremely large effect on patient's life

References
Basra MK, Fenech R, Gatt RM, Salek MS, Finlay AY. The Dermatology Life Quality Index 1994–2007: a comprehensive review of validation data and clinical results. *Br J Dermatol.* 2008;159:997-1035.
Finlay AY, Khan GK. Dermatology Life Quality Index (DLQI): a simple practical measure for routine clinical use. *Clin Exp Dermatol.* 1994;19:210-216.

cancer. However, it is important to recognise the importance of safe exposure to UVL and adequate vitamin D in older people at risk of osteoporosis and falls (see Chapter 12, Nursing Patients With Musculoskeletal Disorders, and Chapter 32, Nursing Older Patients). Campaigns stress the importance of the individual being aware of the appearance of their own moles, emphasising the fact that all moles change slowly over the years (See Figs 14.9 and 14.10) and promote 'safe sun' and encourage behavioural and social changes that might prevent or reduce the incidence of melanoma.

Advice includes:

- avoidance of direct sun between 1100 and 1700
- use of high SPF sun creams
- use of T-shirts/sun hats.

Nurses can encourage regular checking of moles as a preventive strategy, which could have a profound impact on the early detection, incidence and mortality rates of malignant melanoma. Nurses also should raise awareness of other skin cancers that can occur without a mole present and advise patients to seek medical advice if they develop a nonhealing lesion or lesions that are red and get very scaly rather than ignoring them. There are new tools on the internet that enable monitoring, for example Skin Test.

⊕ **See Evolve website Critical thinking question 14.2**

Summary: Key Nursing Issues

- This chapter focuses on some of the more common skin disorders.
- Dermatology is a major specialty and all nurses will encounter people with skin conditions.
- When assessing and managing skin conditions, it is important to consider the psychosocial and economic impact on patients and families.
- A sound knowledge and skills in dermatology are important for all nurses, particularly so for nurses who are nonmedical prescribers.

- Publication of competency frameworks to underpin clinical development (Further Reading, for example RCN Competencies: An Integrated Career and Competency Framework for Dermatology Nursing 2005 and BAD Clinical Dermatology Nursing Roles Descriptors: Guidance on Scope of Practice 2020) aims to open up this specialty, so increasing access for patients.

Reflection and Learning – What Next?

- **Test** your knowledge by visiting the Evolve website ⊕ and answering the multiple-choice questions and critical thinking questions.
- **Consolidate** your learning by looking at some of the further reading suggestions, references and specialist websites.
- **Revisit** some of the additional material on the website.

- **Consider** what you have learnt and how this will help your professional development.
- **Reflect** on how you can apply this knowledge to the care of your patients.
- **Discuss** your learning with your mentor/supervisor, lecturer and colleagues.

References

Alexander H, Paller AS, Traidl-Hoffman C, et al. The role of bacterial skin infection in atopic eczema: expert statement and review from the International Eczema Council for Skin Infection Group. *Br J Dermatol*. 2020 June;182(6):1331–1342.

Bewley A. Expert consensus: time for a change in the way we advise our patients to use topical corticosteroids. *Br J Dermatol*. 2008;158:917–920.

British Association of Dermatologists (BAD). https://cdn.bad.org.uk/uploads/2021/12/29200130/BAD-BDNG-RCN-NURSING-WORK-STREAM-A4-LANDSCAPE-FINAL.pdf.

Clinical dermatology nursing role descriptors: guidance on scope of practice (2020).

British National Formulary (BNF). 2020-21. https://bnf.nice.org.uk/drugs.

Cai Y, Fleming C, Yan J. New insights of T cells in the pathogenesis of psoriasis. *Cell Mol Immunol*. 2012;9(4):302–309.

Cancer Research UK. Sun, UV and cancer: #Own Your Tone. 2018. https://www.cancerresearchuk.org/about-cancer/causes-of-cancer/sun-uv-and-cancer/own-your-tone/.

Cancer Research UK. Melanoma skin cancer statistics. 2022. https://www.cancerresearchuk.org/health-professional/cancer-statistics/statistics-by-cancer-type/melanoma-skin-cancer#heading-Two.

Chernyshov PV. The Evolution of quality of life assessment and use in dermatology. *Dermatology*. 2019;235:167–174. https://doi.org/10.1159/000496923.

Cork MJ, Danby SG, Ogg GS. Atopic eczema epidemiology and unmet need in the United Kingdom. *J Dermatolog Treat*. 2020;31(8):801–809.

Department of Health. The NHS Improvement Plan. Putting people at the heart of public services (Section 2); 2018. https://www.dh.gov/uk/en/Publications/PublicationsPolicyAndGuidance/Browsable/DH4097241.

Department of Health and Social Care. 2010 to 2015 government policy: long term health conditions; 2015. https://www.gov.uk/government/publications/2010-to-2015-government-policy-long-term-health-conditions.

Dillon MJ. Salicylic acid versus cryotherapy for common and plantar wart treatment: Which should we recommend? A meta-analysis. *Dermatol Nurs*. 2020;19(4):38–44.

Dilworth D, Caruana D, Borg J, et al. Psoriasis guidelines: can they improve the delivery of better holistic care? *Dermatol Nurs*. 2015;14(3):32–36.

Elective Care Transformation Team, Operations & Information NHS England. Transforming Elective Care Services Dermatology. 2019. England. https://nhs.uk/wp-content/uploads/2019/01/dermatology-elective-care-handbook-v1.pdf.

Green L. The effect of skin conditions on patients' quality of life. *Nursing Standard*. Nov 3-9 2010;25(9):48–55.

Green AC, Wallingford SC, McBride P. Childhood exposure to ultraviolet radiation and harmful skin effects: epidemiological evidence. *Prog Biophys Mol Biol*. 2011;107(3):349–355.

GIRFH. Dermatology. GRIFH Programme National Speciality Report. 2021. https://www.gettingitrightfirsttime.co.uk/wp-content/uploads/2021/09/DermatologyReport-Sept21o.pdf.

Guy's and St Thomas' NHS Foundation Trust. Emollients and how to use them. 2017. https://www.guysandstthomas.nhs.uk/resources/patient-information/der,atology/emollients.pdf.

Gawkrodger D, Arden-Jones MR. Dermatology. ABC Elsevier 7th Edition. 2020.

Herbert AA, Galindo EG. Eczema. *BMJ*. 2022. https://bestpractice.bmj.com/topics/en-gb/87.

Housam N, Housam M, Housam H. Emollients and flammability: answering the burning question. *Dermatol Nur*. 2022;21(3):42–47.

Juan S, Jiabi Z. Impact of obesity on the efficacy of different biologic agents in inflammatory diseases: a systemic review and meta-analysis. *Joint Bone Spine*. 2019;86:173–183. doi:10.1016/j.jbspin.2018.03.007 pii: S1297-319x(18)30050-2.

Keyworth C, Nelson P, Chisholm A, et al. Providing lifestyle behaviour change support for patients with psoriasis: an assessment of the existing training competencies across medical and nursing health professional. *Br J Dermatol*. 2014;171(3):602–608.

Koek MB, Buskens E, van Weelden H, Steegmans PHA, Bruijnzeel-Kooean CAFM, Sigurdsson V. Home versus outpatient ultraviolet B phototherapy for mild to severe psoriasis: pragmatic multicentre randomised non-inferiority trial (PLUTO) study. *BMJ.* 2009;338:b1542.

Lachapelle JM, Gimenez-Arnau A, Metz M, et al. Best practices, new perspectives and the perfect emollient: optimizing the management of contact dermatitis. *J Dermatolog Treat.* 2017;29(3):241–251.

London Fire Brigade. Skin creams and fire deaths; 2017. https://www.tinyurl.com/yaposr4y.

Medicines and Healthcare Products Regulatory Agency. Skin creams dried on fabric can lead to fire deaths. Press release 29 July 2020. https://www.gov.uk/government/news/skin-creams-dried-on-fabric-can-lead-to-fire-deaths.

Medicines and Healthcare Products Regulatory Agency. Topical steroid withdrawal reactions – a review of evidence. September 2021. https://www.gov.uk/government/publications/topical-steroid-withdrawal-reactions-a-review-of-the-evidence.

Melanoma UK. Statistics. 2022. https://www.melanomauk.org.uk/statistics.

Nicol NH, Ersser SS. The role of the nurse educator in managing atopic dermatitis. *Immunol Allergy Clin N Am.* 2010;30(3):369–393.

National Eczema Society. *All about eczema: information pack for schools.* London: National Eczema Society; 2016. https://www.eczema.org/eczema-at-school.

National Fire Chiefs Council. UK NFCC warns of fire risk when using emollients. 2020. https://www.nationalfirechiefs.org.uk/News/nfcc-warns-of-fire-risk-when-using-emollients.

National Institute for Health and Clinical Excellence (NICE). Atopic dermatitis (eczema): pimecrolimus and tacrolimus. Technology appraisal guidance [TA82]. 2004. https://www.nice.org.uk/guidance/index.jsp?action=download8ro=3290.

National Institute for Health and Clinical Excellence (NICE). Improving outcomes for people with skin cancer including melanomas: Evidence Update 2011. https://www.nice.org.uk/guidance/csg8/evidence/evidence-update-october-2011-pdf-2188923229.

National Institute for Health and Clinical Excellence (NICE). Psoriasis: assessment and management. Clinical guideline [CG153]. 2012. https://www.nice.org.uk/CG153.

National Institute for Health and Clinical Excellence (NICE). Dupilumab for treating moderate to severe atopic dermatitis. Technology appraisal guidance [TA534]; 2018a. https://www.nice.org.uk/guidanceta534.

National Institute for Health and Clinical Excellence (NICE). CKS. Urticaria. 2018b. https://cks.nice.org.uk/topics/urticaria.

National Institute for Health and Clinical Excellence (NICE). Atopic eczema in the under 12s: diagnosis and management. 2023. https://www.nice.org.uk/guidance/CG57.

Paljarvi T, McPherson T, Luciano S, Herttva K, Fazel S. Isotretinoin and adverse neuropsychiatric outcomes: retrospective cohort study using routine data. *Br J Dermatol.* 2022;187(1):64–72.

Peters J. Eczema and the influence of environmental factors. *General Practice Nursing.* 2018;4(2):40–45.

Ro H-S, Shin JYS, Sabbagh MD, Roh S-G, Chang SC, Lee N-H. Effectiveness of aspiration or deroofing for blister management in patients with burns. *Medicine.* April 2018;97(17):pe0563. doi:10.1097/MD.0000000000010563.

Simpson EL, Chalmers JR, Hanifin JM, et al. Emollient enhancement of the skin barrier from birth offers effective atopic dermatitis prevention. *J Allergy Clin Immunol.* 2014;134:818–823.

Smith CH, Yiu ZZ, Bale T, et al. British Association of Dermatologists guidelines for biologic therapy for psoriasis 2020: a rapid update. *Br J Dermatol.* 2020;177(3):628–636. doi:10.1111/bjd.19034 183(4).

Tomlinson J. Acne vulgaris: isotretinoin and nurse monitoring. *Dermatol Nurs.* 2021;20(4):17–20.

Tucker R. What's the best emollient for eczema? *Dermatol Nurs.* 2018;17(1):40–41.

Tucker R. Which is the most clinically effective emollient formulation? *Dermatol Nurs.* 2022;21(3):55–56.

Wedgeworth EK, Sharp H, Powell AM, Flohr C. What's new in eczema? Part 1: epidemiology and pathophysiology. *Dermatol Nurs.* 2012;11(4):9–15.

Woollenberg A, Barbarot S, Bieber T, et al. Consensus-based European guidelines for treatment of atopic eczema (atopic dermatitis) in adults and children part II. *J Eur Acad Dermatol Venerol.* 2018;32(6):856–878.

Further Reading

Chouliara Z, Stephen K, Buchanan P. The importance of psychological assessment in dermatology: opening of Pandora's box. *Dermatol Nurs.* 2017;16(4):30–34.

May RJ, Franklin A. Fundamentals of skin immunology in psoriasis: part 1. *Dermatol Nurs.* 2018;17(2):40–47.

Morris-Jones R, ed. *ABC Dermatology.* ed 6. London: British Medical Journal; 2014.

NHS Education for Scotland. *Caring for People with Dermatological Conditions: A Core Curriculum.* Edinburgh: NHS Education for Scotland; 2003.

Penzer R. *Best Practice in Emollient Therapy. A Statement for Health Professionals.* London: Dermatological Nursing; 2012. https://www.researchgate.netpublication/291043200/Best-practice-in-emollient-therapy.

Penzer R, Ersser S. *Principles of Skin Care: A Guide for Nurses and Health Care Practitioners.* Oxford: Wiley–Blackwell; 2010.

Ridd MJ, Santer M, MacNeill SJ, et al. Effectiveness and safety of lotion, cream, gel and ointment emollients for childhood eczema: a pragmatic, randomized phase 4, superiority trial. *Lancet Child Adolesc Health.* 2022;6(8):522–532.

Royal College of Nursing (RCN). *Caring for Children and Young People With Atopic Eczema: Guidance for Nurses.* London: RCN; 2008.

Silverwood RJ, Forbes HJ, Abuabara K, et al. Severe and predominantly active atopic eczema in adulthood and long term risk of cardiovascular disease: population based cohort study. *BMJ.* 2018;361:k1786. https://doi.org/10.1136/bmjk1786.

Weller RPJB, Hunter HJA, Mann MW, Hunter JAA. Clinical/Dermatology 5th Edition. 2015. Oxford:Wiley-Blackwell.

Useful Websites

APPGS Mental Health and Skin Disease report, https://eczema.org/blog/appgs-mental-health-and-skin-disease-report/

Skin for Health, https://www.skinhealthinfo.org.uk/

Dr C Bridgett, Behaviour modification/habit reversal, www.atopics-kindisease.com

British Association of Dermatologists (BAD), www.bad.org.uk

British Dermatological Nursing Group, www.bdng.org.uk

EASI online calculator, https://www.easiderm.com/

National Eczema Society, https://www.eczema.org

New Zealand Dermatological Society Inc., www.dermnetnz.org

Nottingham University Hospitals, www.nottingham.ac.uk/dermatology

Psoriasis Association, www.psoriasis-association.org.uk

Skin Care Campaign, www.skincarecampaign.org

Wessex Cancer service sponsoring MARC's Line, www.wessexcancer.org

Dermatology videos, Guy's and St Thomas' NHS Trust via hospital website, http://www.gstt.nhs.uk/dermatologyvideos

Emollient video via YouTube link, https://www.youtube.com/watch?v=nj4JSWGL5KQ

Scalp psoriasis video via YouTube link, https://www.youtube.com/watch?v=hMUPuqt-khY

Topical steroids video via YouTube link, https://www.skinhealthinfo.org.uk/support-resources/video-guides

15

Nursing Patients With Disorders of the Eye and Sight Impairment

ALLYSON SANDERSON, PENELOPE STANFORD

CHAPTER OUTLINE

Introduction

Understanding vision, visual impairment and its impact on a person's life is essential for patient care across all healthcare environments. Eyesight is essential to aid walking, learning, working and many essential aspects of life (World Health Organisation (WHO) 2019). Visual impairment occurs when ophthalmic conditions alter the visual system and subsequently its function (WHO 2019).

Although the majority (80%) of eye conditions are considered to be preventable (WHO 2018), ophthalmic disorders causing permanent or temporary visual impairment continue to impact on population eye health.

The COVID-19 pandemic had negative impacts on eye health across the world and the extent in the UK reported in the State of the Nation's Eye Health in 2021. COVID-19 lockdown delayed access to assessment and treatment and directly caused 2986 people in the UK to lose their eyesight. The report also estimates the numbers of people living with eye conditions such as cataract (713,000), chronic glaucoma (708,000), diabetic retinopathy (1.33 million), age-related macular degeneration (2.95 million). As people age, so does their susceptibility to age related eye conditions and subsequent vision impairment (Office for National Statistics 2020, Royal National Institute of the Blind 2021b)). People of Black and Asian minority ethnic (BAME) groups are more susceptible to systemic eye diseases and sight loss. Organizations such as BravoVictor (https://www.bravovictor.org/) are working with Moorfield's Eye Hospital Trust to research and support this community. Also the Royal National Institute for Blind people (RNIB) are supporting sightline directory, a service aimed at helping people from BAME communities with sight impairments (https://www.sightlinedirectory.org.uk/Listings/Details/5962/bame-vision).

People with eye conditions and those with a visual impairment are cared for in all healthcare settings. Healthcare professionals should aim to develop knowledge and understanding about ophthalmic nursing care to provide holistic patient care. This chapter sets out to inform the reader about essential ocular anatomy, physiology, related conditions, and nursing care.

This chapter aims to inform the reader with the specialised knowledge to support and care for any person and their carers living with an ophthalmic problem, to raise awareness of sight impairment (SI) and how SI affects all aspects of living, and to consider the implications for practice relating to the Equality Act 2010. The term 'sight impaired' will be used throughout this chapter as an alternative term for people who do not wish to be labelled as 'blind' or 'partially sighted', as they can feel these terms are deemed negative and misleading (RNIB 2021).

It is estimated globally that 253 million people live with sight impairment; of those, 36 million are severely sight impaired (SSI) and 217 million are sight impaired (SI). Within the UK, 250 people start to lose their sight every day (State of the Nation Eye Health 2017) and estimated sight loss in England alone is 1.7 million (Office of National Statistics [ONS] 2020). The World Health Organisation (WHO) (2020) states that 80% of all sight loss is preventable or curable, with the main causes of sight loss being refractive error (39%), age-related macular degeneration (AMD) (23%), cataracts (19%), glaucoma (7%), diabetic retinopathy (5%) and other eye diseases (7%) (The State of the Nation Eye Health 2017). These ocular diseases are discussed in detail in this chapter.

As life expectancy increases in the UK, there is a higher incidence of eye diseases and, therefore it is increasingly important for early recognition of adverse ocular signs and symptoms by all healthcare professionals, and to encourage prompt referral for specialised assessment and care. In addition, lifestyle is recognised as contributing to sight loss, with cardiovascular diseases, smoking and obesity being known risk factors for chronic eye diseases, especially AMD (Yip et al. 2015). Yip et al. (2015) continue to suggest that poor vision is strongly associated with social deprivation, with the incidence of glaucoma being higher in this social group due to late presentation of symptoms, limited knowledge and limited services available. As the incidence of dementia continues to increase, with 900,000 people currently living with dementia (Alzheimer's Society 2023), many will have associated sight loss and visual symptoms.

It is recognised that the recruitment of nurses, especially specialised ophthalmic nurses, is a challenge for the National Health Service (NHS) and at a time when a large percentage of the population will be over 60 years of age and by association there will be a higher incidence of eye disease. In order to continue to provide quality healthcare services, the global driver to develop workforce is linked to service improvement, with evolution of tradition roles by orthoptists; optometrists, ophthalmic technicians and ophthalmic nurses (Kunjumen et al. 2022). For example, optometrists now lead with glaucoma clinical services, ophthalmic nurses lead on Lucentis clinical services for people with treatable macular disease and ophthalmic assistants will assess visual acuities, visual fields and intraocular pressures. These roles are evolving in response to the influence of technological, statutory and organisational change.

The World Health Organization remains at the forefront of Vision 2020 – The Right to Sight: A Global Initiative for the Elimination of Avoidable Blindness. The aim is to eliminate avoidable blindness as a public health problem by the year 2020 (IAPB 2018). With this date drawing nearer, the State of the Nation Eye Health Report (2017) highlights the ongoing financial cost of direct healthcare at £3 billion per annum, as well as the realities of sight loss still being that only one in four people with SI or SSI of working age has employment, and only 17% are offered emotional support in regard to their sight loss (RNIB 2021). So, we, as healthcare professionals, have to work collaboratively and provide a person-centred approach to the care needs for people living with sight loss, ensuring duty of care to be up to date in practice, to facilitate health promotion, screening, primary and secondary care (Health and Care Professions Council [HCPC] 2016, Nursing and Midwifery Council [NMC] 2018).

Anatomy and Physiology

The structures of the eyeball do not themselves produce sight but act as a gateway for visual impulses, which are processed via the optic nerves and tracts, the visual cortex, the occipital lobe of the brain. Accessory structures such as eyelids and extraocular muscles play a vital role in our visual function.

The Eye

The Eyeball

The eyeball is generally spherical in shape and approximately 24 mm in length. It is protected within the bony structures of the orbit and behind the eyelids. It receives light stimuli through the clear anterior structures of the cornea and lens, which refract or bend the light to direct the light stimuli through the clear posterior structure of the vitreous. The light is focused on to the

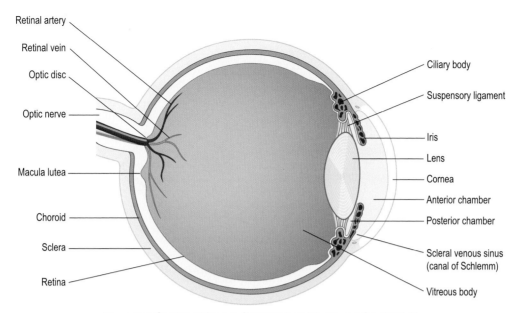

Figure 15.1 Section of the eye. (Adapted from Waugh and Grant 2014.)

photoreceptor cells of the retina and especially the macula, which is responsible for detailed, colour vision.

The eyeball or globe is a structure composed of three main layers of tissue (Fig. 15.1):

1. The outer layer of the globe consists of the fibrous white sclera posteriorly and the transparent cornea anteriorly. The junction of the two is called the limbus. The cornea is transparent due to its avascularity and is supplied with nerve endings from the trigeminal nerve, cranial nerve V, ophthalmic branch. Attached at the equator/mid-point, are the six extraocular muscles which allow for movement of the eyes. They work in pairs, and include the superior and inferior recti, medial recti and lateral recti, plus superior and inferior oblique muscles.

Extraocular Muscle	Direction of Gaze	Cranial Nerve Innervation
Superior rectus	Upwards	CN III (oculomotor)
Inferior rectus	Downwards	CN III (oculomotor)
Medical rectus	Inwards/convergence	CN III (oculomotor)
Lateral rectus	Outwards/divergence	CN VI (abducens)
Superior oblique	Downwards and outwards	CN IV (trochlear)
Inferior oblique	Upwards and inwards	CN III (oculomotor)

2. The middle vascular layer, known as the uveal tract, consists of the choroid, the ciliary body and the iris. The choroid lines the sclera in the posterior compartment of the eye and continues into the muscular ciliary body, into which are inserted the suspensory ligaments. These ligaments, known as the zonules, extend to the lens and hold it in position. The contraction or relaxation of the ciliary body changes the shape of the lens controlling its refractive and focusing power. The iris is the pigmented anterior portion of the uveal tract. It contains circular and radial muscle fibres, which control the size of the pupil.

3. The inner layer of the eyeball is the retina. It contains several million photoreceptive cells that are responsible for converting light into electrical impulses. The retina arises just behind the equator of the eyeball: the ora serrata. This leaves a small

anterior section of the choroid – the pars plana – exposed, which allows surgical access without retinal damage. The two retinal layers are the pigmented outer layer, which lines the choroid, and the innermost neural layer, which is in contact with the vitreous humour. Rod cells in the periphery function best in dim light. Cone cells near the macula are adapted for bright light and colour vision. These photoreceptor cells are linked through a series of synapses to ganglion cells whose axons run together to form the optic nerve. For further anatomy and physiology see (Peate and Evans 2020).

The Two Segments of the Eye

Inside the globe the lens acts to divide the eye into two main segments:

- The anterior segment, which is divided into two chambers: the anterior chamber in front of the iris and the posterior chamber behind the iris.
- The posterior segment behind the lens, which contains the clear jelly-like substance vitreous humour. In conjunction with the aqueous this exerts sufficient pressure to maintain the shape of the eye.

Internal Environment and Intraocular Pressure (IOP)

The anterior chamber (AC) is full of clear aqueous fluid (humour) produced by the ciliary body and provides nutrients to the lens and cornea. Aqueous flows from the posterior chamber through the pupil to the AC. This drains away through the sieve like fibrous trabecular meshwork located in the angle between the iris and cornea around the circumference of the eye. This then drains into the vascular canal of Schlemm and into the systemic venous circulation. The production and drainage of aqueous must be constant to maintain a normal IOP within the range of 10–20 mmHg (Peate and Evans 2020).

The functioning of the drainage system depends on the depth of the AC and the angle between the cornea and iris. The larger, elongated eye of the myope (short-sighted person) has a naturally deeper AC with an open angle, whilst the small eye of the hypermetrope (long-sighted person) has a shallow AC with a narrow angle (Information 15.1). Any interference with normal drainage

INFORMATION 15.1

Terms Associated With Visual Acuity and Refractive Errors

- Emmetropia – normal sight; light rays focus on the retina
- Ametropia – defective sight due to refractive error
- Myopia – short-sightedness; light rays focus in front of the retina
- Hypermetropia – long-sightedness; light rays focus behind the retina
- Presbyopia – loss of focused reading/near-sight capacity, resulting from loss of lens elasticity due to ageing
- Astigmatism – irregular curvature of the cornea which prevents light rays from focusing at a single point

of the aqueous humour raises the IOP, leading to the decreased blood supply, pain and impaired vision associated with conditions such as glaucoma.

The Visual Pathways and Interpretative Centres

The optic nerve runs from the posterior of the globe, entering the cranial cavity via the optic foramen. The medial nerve fibres cross over to the opposite side at the optic chiasma (Fig. 15.2) to join with the lateral fibres and form the optic tract before synapsing in the lateral geniculate body of the thalamus. The fibres then run in the optic radiations to the occipital cerebral cortex of the brain. The main blood supply to the eye is via the ophthalmic artery, a branch of the internal carotid artery.

Accessory Structures

The eyeball is protected by the eyebrow, eyelids and eyelashes. The conjunctiva, a mucous membrane, lines the eyelids (palpebral conjunctiva) and reflects back on itself (bulbar conjunctiva) to cover the sclera. This fold forms the conjunctival sac or fornix and is an ideal site for the instillation of topical drugs. At the limbus, the conjunctiva is modified to form the epithelial layer of the cornea. The conjunctiva allows movement of the eyelids over the globe.

The exposed surface of the eye is covered by a three-layered film of tear fluid. Mucous secretion from conjunctival goblet cells forms the first layer of the tear film and ensures an even spread of tears over the cornea. The middle layer is the watery fluid secreted by the lacrimal glands (situated under the upper orbital rim) and by the accessory glands in the conjunctiva. The outer lipid layer of tear film is secreted by the meibomian glands of the lids. This is thought to reduce the evaporation rate of tears and to prevent the lids sticking together during sleep. The main functions of tear fluid are to lubricate the eye, to facilitate O_2 and CO_2 exchange, to provide an optically smooth corneal surface and to cleanse the eye with a bacteriostatic enzyme called lysozyme. Excess tears are drained from the eye via the lacrimal punctum and apparatus at the inner canthus (nasal end of the lid margins) into the lacrimal sac and thence into the nose through the nasolacrimal duct (Fig. 15.3). Posteriorly and laterally the globe is protected by the bony orbit and orbital fat.

The Physiology of Vision

Light rays are bent (refracted) as they pass through the clear media of the cornea, aqueous, lens and vitreous to focus on the retina. The cornea is relatively constant in shape and is responsible for about two-thirds of the refractive power of the eye. The zonules extend from the ciliary body into the lens through 360 degrees

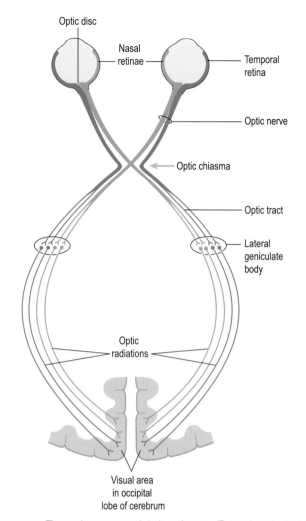

Figure 15.2 The optic nerves and their pathways. (Reproduced with kind permission from Waugh and Grant 2014.)

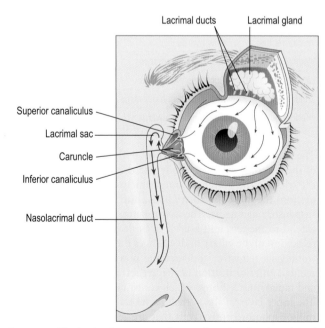

Figure 15.3 The lacrimal apparatus. *Arrows* show the direction of the flow of tears. (Reproduced with kind permission of Waugh and Grant 2014.)

so that any contraction or relaxation of the body will change the shape of the lens and affect focusing (refractive) power. The normal eye in its relaxed state brings rays of light from distant objects into sharp focus. However, for clear focusing on near objects, an autonomic reflex known as the synkinetic near reflex comes into play. This reflex involves accommodation, miosis and convergence, as follows:

- Accommodation – the ciliary body contracts and changes shape, thus releasing tension on the zonular fibres and allowing the lens to thicken and increase its refractive power. This allows objects at different distances to be visualised with equal clarity.
- Miosis, or constriction of the pupil, accompanies accommodation and ensures that light rays are concentrated to pass through the centre of the lens, focusing on the macula.
- Convergence, or in-turning of the eyes, seeks out the object to be focused on.
- Failure to focus may be described as ametropia, or refractive error (see Information 15.1).

Once the rays of light are focused on the retina, their energy is converted into neuroelectrical energy by the photoreceptor cells. These nerve impulses are transmitted via the visual pathway to the visual cortex. Here, they are interpreted as sensations of light, form and colour and are processed into images of objects that are given meaning by other cerebral areas (see Chapter 11, Nursing Patients With Disorders of the Nervous System).

⊕ **See Evolve website for multiple choice questions**

Assessing the Eye and Visual Function

Examination of Structure

It is necessary to know what a normal eye looks like, as well as the normal ocular recovery from surgery or disease. The eye should be examined in a systematic way, using a good light source and be methodical with all ocular structures from outermost to innermost. This will aid in recognition of abnormalities. The clinical features and possible implications from an eye examination are listed in Table 15.1.

Testing Visual Function
Visual Acuity
Obtaining an accurate visual acuity (VA) assessment is vital, as a baseline of the patient's ability and forms the basis of the clinical decision-making process for treatment options. VA is the mathematical estimation of visual function for different distances.

Distance Vision. This is tested using Snellen test-type charts, which display letters or pictures arranged in rows of precise and diminishing size (Fig. 15.4A). Each eye should be tested separately, with the benefit, if worn, of any spectacles or contact lenses, to ensure that 'best corrected vision' is being checked. The eye not being tested must be completely occluded. In normal testing, patients are positioned 6 m away from the chart and asked to read each line aloud, until they can no longer make out the letters. The result is recorded as a fraction of the distance from the chart in metres over the normal reading distance of the last complete line read, plus the number of extra letters read from the line below or minus the number of letters read incorrectly, e.g. 6/9 – 2 (see Fig. 15.4A). If glasses or contact lenses are worn this is also recorded.

Normal distance acuity is accepted as 6/6. If the patient sees less than 6/12 or 6/9 (there may be variations from one eye unit to another), they should be asked to read the chart again, looking

TABLE 15.1	Significance of Clinical Features Found on Eye Examination	
Structure	Clinical Features	Possible Significance
Lids	Bruising (ecchymosis) Swelling Drooping Increased lacrimation Discharge	Surgical handling Trauma Neurological deficit Infection
Conjunctiva	Redness (injection) Swelling (chemosis)	Surgical handling Trauma Allergy Infection
Cornea	Cloudy Crinkled Fluorescein staining Suture line not intact Penetrating injury	Increased IOP Infection Loss of AC Ulceration Chemical injury
Anterior chamber (AC)	Hyphaema (blood in AC) Hypopyon (pus in AC) Shallow AC	Hyphaema due to surgery should gradually resolve Increasing IOP = bleeding/inflammation Hypopyon = infection Shallow = possible aqueous loss or ACAG
Iris	Muddy/lack of detail	Inflammation
Pupil	Irregular shape	Iris prolapse Pharmacology Adhesions Trauma

ACAG, Acute closed-angle glaucoma; IOP, intraocular pressure.

through a pinhole. A pure refractive error should improve with this simple method of sharpening focus by cutting out peripheral light stimulation, but a posterior segment problem, such as AMD will not improve using pinhole.

If the patient cannot read the top letter (6/60) then ability to count fingers (CF) at 1 m, detect hand movements (HM) or perceive light (PL) is tested. If the patient does not read or understand English or has learning difficulties, poor concentration or expressive dysphasia, then VA testing can be done by using a Sheridan–Gardiner singles booklet in which single letters or pictures of varying size are presented one at a time and the patient is asked match them on a card with a limited choice of symbols. The Log-MAR system is used as frequently as the Snellen chart in many eye clinics, at a distance of 4 m (see Fig. 15.4B). It is conducted in a similar fashion to the Snellen test, but the scoring system for every letter missed is more rigorous.

Near Vision is tested in good illumination and the patient is asked to read text in various sizes of standard print that are prefixed with the letter N. N5 is accepted as normal reading acuity.

Binocular Vision involves simultaneous perception of an image by both eyes and fusion of the two images in the visual cortex to form a single image. Binocular vision is important for stereopsis (depth perception). Having two eyes with good sight also widens the field of vision and omits deficits caused by natural blind spots. (Try the activity in Reflection 15.1.)

The visual field (perimeter) refers to what the eye can see with respect to angle of view (rather than distance). Normally

Figure 15.4 Eye testing charts. (A) Snellen test-type chart; the standard method for testing visual acuity in the UK. (B) The logMar vision testing chart.

---

this is about 60 degrees nasally, 90 degrees temporally, 50 degrees superiorly and 70 degrees inferiorly. Assessment of the visual field is essential in the management of glaucoma, intermittent loss of vision, transient ischaemic attack (TIA), cerebral vascular accident (CVA), diagnosis of neurological disease and retinal detachment. In the ophthalmic setting, it is performed by means of perimetry, a field analyser to gain accurate measurements of visual field defects known as scotomas (Chen and Gedde 2023). In the primary care environment, during the confrontation test, the examiner sits directly in front and approximately 1 m from the patient and compares the patient's field of vision with their own.

Colour Blindness

Colour vision depends on the normal functioning of the retinal cones. A colour-blind person is unable to distinguish between some colours – usually red and green. While approximately 8% of the male population is born with defective colour vision, this problem is estimated at only 1% in females. Colour blindness can be congenital or acquired through certain conditions such as optic neuritis or drug dependency. For further information on colour vision deficiency, see http://www.color-blindness.com/color-blindness-tests/.

The most common method of testing is by means of a series of Ishihara colour-dotted plates, but with emerging technology there are apps and electronic assessment tools used in screening for colour blindness. A person with defective colour vision would be unable to distinguish the numbers from the surrounding background. Some occupations, such as pilots and electricians, require normal colour vision, usually for reasons of safety but there are no restrictions on driving, as traffic lights have a fixed sequence and can be recognised by position rather than colour. (For more on driving and vision see the DVLA website, listed in Useful Websites.)

Bedside Vision Test

The bedside vision test is a simplified visual assessment published by the Royal College of Physicians (2017) in collaboration with professional organisations including the Royal College of Nursing. This eyesight test assesses a patient's risk of falling due to poor eyesight and guides the healthcare professional to ask open questions about eyesight, vision assessment and plan appropriate interventions.

VA is an objective measurement, but a person's real-world vision is also important. A conversation with the person about how their vision affects their activities of daily living activities, is their vision worse in bright/dim light, for example.

It is estimated that visual impairment could have been prevented in half of the visually impaired global population (WHO 2019). This emphasises the importance of eye health awareness is essential for healthcare professionals and the people they care for. Healthcare environments can foster health promotion, health prevention and diagnosis of eye disease and strategies for rehabilitation underpin eye health promotion (Burton et al. 2019).

Patients should be encouraged to have a regular eye test at the opticians. Eye tests are more than a test to see if the person needs glasses; it is an overall assessment of eye health.

The correct glasses prescription and wearing glasses as prescribed by an optometrist can enhance a person's general well being, as they will have the optimum vision to live their life. An eye test can detect eye conditions such as glaucoma, cataracts, age-related macular degeneration.

Eye health can be promoted by creating awareness of potential risk factors of eye disease. These may include damage of sunlight, smoking, poor nutrition, and risk of trauma to eyes from gardening, DIY and employment.

The next parts of this chapter explain some of the most common eye disorders and the promotion of eye health.

Eye Changes With Ageing

Loss of sight is associated with age (Kandel et al. 2022) and it is recognised that after the age of 50 people will need some form of refractive correction. Focusing is affected as the cornea flattens, causing astigmatism (see Information 15.1). Retinal cells become less efficient due to deposits laid down by ageing pigment epithelial cells. Tear film is reduced in volume and altered in structure, with the result that tears evaporate more quickly, leading to dryness and irritation of the eye. As age progresses, people may complain of watering eyes due to muscle laxity and malposition of eyelids (see Entropion and Ectropion sections), but it is important to note that systemic changes such as the menopause can cause dry eyes. With a high incidence of dementia within society, RNIB (2022c) highlight how these impact on sight changes, including sight loss, colour defects, visuospatial awareness and visual hallucinations, especially in Lewy body dementia (DLB).

❖ Nursing Management and Health Promotion: Preservation of Vision

Healthcare professionals can do a great deal through health education and active intervention to help people preserve their sight by initially taking a full history of the person and observing individual behaviour and general appearance; noting missed appointments, unkempt clothes and a reluctance to go out, which may suggest ocular problems. There are strong links between low psychological mood and social isolation associated with people living with sight loss (Senra et al. 2022) (Reflection 15.2).

Should any changes be noted, prompt action and referral to an optician to ensure early screening and accurate diagnosis are vital. The following will contribute to health education and promotion.

- Annual eye examinations, especially in people over 40 years of age and individuals in high-risk groups such as those with diabetes or hypertension. In the UK, free sight testing is available for those over 60 years as well as for those in high-risk groups, lower income groups and people over 40 years old who have a family history of glaucoma.
- Smoking causes hypoxia and increased inflammatory cytokines within the orbit (Dave et al. 2022), therefore is linked to eye diseases such as glaucoma and age-related macular degeneration

(AMD), with risk of sight loss caused by this lifestyle choice. Encouraging smoking cessation can be beneficial to preserve sight.
- Encourage a well-balanced nutritional intake, sensible alcohol consumption (see DrinkAware website, listed in Useful Websites), and regular exercise in minimising the risk of cardiovascular disease and high cholesterol which are linked to age-related sight loss.
- Provide advice and ensure the correct use, storage and cleaning of glasses and contact lenses. It is vital that contact lenses are properly maintained and used according to optometrists' and manufacturers' guidance. If guidance is not followed, there is a risk of long-term, possibly permanent, damage to the cornea, due to infection, ulceration or abrasion (Kates and Tuli 2021).
- Encourage the prompt self-referral, assessment, and treatment of eye problems to prevent long-term ocular damage.
- Both work- and leisure-related eye injuries can be prevented by wearing eye protection. The wearing of eye protection is mandatory in certain work environments, e.g. chemical laboratories and any area where grinding of metal occurs (Health and Safety at Work Act 1974 and Personal Protective Equipment Work Regulations 2002). The healthcare professional must be aware that education is vital to help to reduce the number of eye injuries, as lack of eye protection remains a problem (Public Health England 2018). The reporting of any incidents to comply with the Environment and Safety Information Act 1988 and Reporting of Injuries, Diseases and Dangerous Occurrences Regulations (RIDDOR) 2013 is essential.
- Advocate the correct and safe labelling of chemical products, and ensure first aid (e.g. eye irrigation) is available for emergency use. Individuals in the workplace and at home should be urged to read any labels on chemical products to indicate if harmful to the eyes and make a careful note of first aid instructions in case of accidental splashing (see Information 15.3 for eye irrigation). By law, it is essential to comply to the Control of Substances Hazardous to Health (COSHH) Regulations (2002) as defined in the Health and Safety Executive (2018).
- Ensure that display screen equipment (DSE) is used in accordance with the Health and Safety Executive (2013) recommendations for short, frequent rest periods to prevent eye fatigue. Employers must provide an annual sight test for all VDU users.
- Promote the wearing of sunglasses, as exposure to sunlight can contribute to long-term ocular changes, such as cataracts and macular degeneration (RNIB 2019).
- Some people with sight loss can experience visual hallucinations, known as Charles Bonnet Syndrome (CBS). The condition was initially recognised by philosopher Charles Bonnet in the 18th century. It is thought that the hallucinations are the brain reacts to loss of vision. Hallucinations may seem very real and often are scary. CBS is not widely known meaning that

---

REFLECTION 15.2

Sight Impairment and Cognitive Impairment Recognition

Consider the changes in behaviour or appearance that may be indicative of both visual and cognitive abilities.

INFORMATION 15.2

Eversion of an Eyelid

This should be done if a foreign body (FB) is suspected or a gritty sensation reported under the upper eyelid. With the patient's eyes open and looking down, the upper lid lashes are grasped. At the same time, the upper edge of the tarsal plate (at the crease of the eyelid) is depressed, using a cotton bud, with one end dampened with saline. This allows the lid to be turned over to expose the subtarsal conjunctiva and allows for inspection, irrigation and FB removal (RCO 2022).

people who experience the hallucinations may not tell anyone resulting in low mood and isolation (Jones 2021).

The Sight-Impaired Person (SIP)

Living with good sight can be taken for granted. Unless we have a SI or refractive error, it can be difficult to understand the physical, social, and psychological impact of sight loss.

Certification of Sight Impairment

Most SIP have some residual sight. Only a small percentage of SIPs will have a VA of no perception of light (NPL). An ophthalmologist is required to certify the degree of impairment, using standards to decide whether the patient is either severely sight impaired (SSI, previously known as blind) or sight impaired (SI, previously known as partially sighted). In England and Wales, a 'certificate of vision impairment' form is used and in Northern Ireland and Scotland it is a BP1 form. For information regarding definitions of SSI and SI, see the RNIB website, listed in Useful Websites.

Registration is completely voluntary, entitling the individual to many local and national benefits; however, rehabilitation support can be obtained without registration. The Equality Act 2010, makes it unlawful to treat disabled individuals in a discriminatory way, stating that all health and social care employers and service providers must make reasonable adjustments to their services, ensuring for example equal access for disabled persons. The RNIB (2021) support this stance adding that a reasonable adjustment is an adaptation to facilitate a person living with any disability to do their job safely and effectively.

People with impaired sight should be referred to a low-vision clinic and seen by an optometrist, specialist nurse or an Eye Clinic Liaison Officer (ECLO) to assess for low visual aids (LVAs) (RNIB 2021a). These can vary depending upon the person's individual requirements, but can include a monocular telescope, to aid distance vision, or a magnifying glass for near-sight tasks such as reading. Closed circuit television (CCTV) allows the SIP a magnified image of material such as photographs or objects with added clarity helping individuals to make best use of their residual sight. These professionals may also provide information and advice on adaptation or retraining for employment. Employers should be advised by various agencies, including the Royal National Institute of Blind People, about technology available for SI employees. Within a community setting, the multidisciplinary team may include the social worker, occupational therapist, ECLO and Rehabilitation Officers visiting individuals in their homes, helping to arrange the appropriate support related to their holistic needs, which may include mobility and communication, incorporating technology including 'Alexa', so they can move about safely in their own environment. If appropriate training in the use of special canes or guide dogs will be offered. The focus of these services is to offer a person-centred approach, enabling the SIP to function as independently as possible. Sight loss does not always equate with lack of ability to live a full life.

Considering the Needs of the Sight-Impaired Person

Fully assessing the needs of the SIP and their family is essential. By using frameworks such as the Biopsychosocial Model (Makivić and Klemenc-Ketiš 2022) in conjunction with the Activities of Living (AL), this can facilitate a realistic account of their needs, supporting the concepts of empowerment and promoting independence.

🌐 See Evolve website Critical thinking question 15.1

Some general principles of care for the SIP are outlined below:

- *Communication.* Approximately 80% of sensory information is obtained visually, perception through focused use of other senses, especially hearing and touch, will therefore be heightened. Ensure the person has choices and access to radio, talking books/newspapers, information in large print, Braille, audiotape, or other technologies as required.
- When approaching the individual, address them by name and identify yourself, gaining consent to interact and help if needed. By describing what you are doing, this prompts respectful and dignified care. Please inform the SIP when you are leaving, as otherwise they may not be aware of this.
- *Orientation to place.* If the person is at home the environment is familiar and it is important to keep things in their usual place. Assistance should be given to help SIPs move around the community and workplace until they are confident to do so independently. Safety is always the priority. Appropriate visual aids such as magnifiers should be used. If the person is admitted to hospital, it is the duty of the healthcare professional to orientate them (NMC 2018). Increased support and reassurance may be needed for anyone living with a learning disability, mental health challenge or cognitive changes, as they may become confused and agitated. (NICE 2022a).
- *Mobility.* Safe mobility should be encouraged in the home and hospital with appropriate assistance given (Lindsay et al, 2022). SIPs are at increased risk of falls, so use the falls risk assessment tool (NICE 2017) and ensure effective assessment of their ability. (Waterman et al. 2016). The preferred method of guiding a person with visual impairment is illustrated in Fig. 15.5.
- *Maintaining a safe environment.* It is essential to be aware of any hazards in the environment. Doors should be fully open or closed. Fires should have guards. Trip hazards such loose flooring must be secured.
- *Eating and drinking.* Bearing in mind the person's functioning visual field, the content and position of food on the plate should be described using a clock-face analogy. Plate guards, nonslip mats and using crockery that contrasts with the food colour can be helpful for those with SSI. Many safety devices are available for use in the home to help with cooking. (For more information, visit the RNIB website, listed in Useful websites).

With effective rehabilitation and family support, the SIP should be able to get around in their environment safely and effectively. It will take confidence, time and patience to achieve this level of ability, with the SIP requiring understanding and ongoing support. A key philosophy is to always ask what the SIP needs help with, do not assume they are not able.

❖ Nursing Management and Health Promotion: Ophthalmic Care

The following principles should be followed when performing ophthalmic nursing care procedures. These apply in any clinical setting. The reader is encouraged to read specialist ophthalmic nursing texts listed in the references section.

General Principles for Ophthalmic Care

This chapter focuses on cataract, retinal detachment, glaucoma, and corneal transplant. Please note the term 'intraocular surgery' describes procedures that are performed inside the globe of the eye involving structures in the anterior and/or posterior segments. All patients should be assessed prior to any medical, surgical, or

Figure 15.5 Guiding a sight-impaired person (SIP). Before you set off, offer your arm to the SIP. Ask which side they prefer. They should hold your arm just above the elbow. Check that the SIP is ready to go. Always walk one pace in front and at the same pace as the person. Describe the environment and warn the SIP of any obstacles or changes in the journey, i.e. stairs – up or down, doors, kerbs. In this way, the SIP can sense any turning of the guide's body and can walk more confidently. The long cane or guide dog is in the SIP's 'free' hand. (Reproduced with permission from the Medical Photography Department, St John's Hospital.)

Figure 15.6 Instilling eye drops into the lower central fornix.

emergency procedure. The assessment process should incorporate key aspects of holistic assessment, development of discharge plan, education and awareness of support services available and follow-up review (Centre for perioperative care 2021). These general priorities for ophthalmic nursing management are outlined below, but specific priorities relating to each condition are within this chapter.

Alleviating Stress and Giving Information

Anxiety levels for ophthalmic patients attending or admitted to hospital may be exacerbated by fear of sight loss and loss of independence. The patient and their family should be offered the opportunity to discuss concerns and provided with honest and realistic information that does not raise false expectations. In addition, reassurance and information about available support and resources should be discussed.

Often surgery is under topical or local anaesthesia. The person may naturally be concerned about their ability to lie still and cooperate. This should always be discussed as part of the assessment process. To aid effective communication, hand holding is routine practice during surgery, so the patient can squeeze the healthcare professionals' hand if they need anything. See Chapter 25, Nursing the Patient Undergoing Surgery, for further discussion of the principles of perioperative nursing, anxiety, informed consent and information giving.

Asepsis and Infection Control Issues

Aseptic and infection prevention measures must be maintained to reduce the risk of infections. Education regarding self-care on discharge, safe eye drop instillation and good asepsis should be tailored to each individual and their family.

Each eye should be treated separately, for example, eye bathing, a sterile, moist, dental roll or gauze is used to wipe from inner to outer canthus along the eyelash line then discarded after a single use. Cotton wool balls can be used only if they have been thoroughly soaked and squeezed out to ensure that no dry fibres are protruding. These precautions and simple handwashing measures (see Chapter 18, Infection Prevention and Control) will reduce the risk of ocular infections.

Instilling Eye Drops and Ointments

If the patient wants to and is able to instil eye drops, then teaching for postoperative self-care should commence at assessment. Eye drops and ointments are inserted into the middle of the lower conjunctival sac. The patient needs to tilt the head back and look up while the lower lid is gently pulled down (Fig. 15.6). Avoid dropping the eye medication onto the sensitive cornea as this causes discomfort and triggers a reflexive response, squeezing the eye shut. After drop instillation the patient is asked to close their eyes gently for 30 seconds to maximise absorption. To reduce the risk of systemic absorption, punctal occlusion can be applied (Davis et al. 2018). Contact of the tip of the tube or bottle with the eye should be avoided. Drops and ointments should only be used in the eye for which they are prescribed. In hospital, topical medication should be dated upon opening and discarded after 1 week (after 4 weeks in the community).

It is essential that all eye medication regimes are completed, even if symptoms have settled. For information about topical and systemic drugs and other ophthalmic preparations consult the British National Formulary (see Useful Websites).

Eye Dressings

Asserting pressure on the eyeball must be avoided. The principle is to keep eyelids closed for comfort when photophobia or lacrimation (tear production) is excessive.

The term 'double padding' means that two pads are applied to the treated eye. Avoid padding both eyes at the same time, as it is unsafe, disorientating and distressing. Eye pads are applied after bathing, examined and treatment instilled, for certain conditions such as large corneal abrasion. Ensure that the eye is closed underneath the pad, to prevent corneal damage, as the cornea is sensitive, particularly after the instillation of local anaesthetic drops. The eye pad is held in position with tape applied by attaching one end to the forehead, then stretching diagonally across the eye pad towards the lateral aspect of the cheek, where it is secured. The downward movement aids lid closure and the diagonal position of the tape permits facial muscle movement. To aid removal a tab should be made by turning under the top of the tape. The skin on the forehead and cheek are supported during removal of the tape to reduce any dragging movement on the eyeball. When an eye pad is removed, both eye and pad must be inspected for signs of infection or haemorrhage. Patients should avoid rubbing their eyes.

When the eye cannot be closed voluntarily, for example in sedated patient, this impairs the blink reflex and tear production increasing risk of exposure keratopathy (Kousha et al. 2018). Interventions such as keeping the cornea moist by the instillation of eye lubricants, and lid closure using moist gauze can reduce this risk. Plaszewska et al. (2021) suggest that for a sedated patient, after 4 days, risk of corneal and ocular problems increases significantly.

Alternatively, a plastic 'cartella' shield can be used depending upon the ocular condition and procedure. Dark glasses are useful to reduce the discomfort of glare; and patients should be taught to put the glasses on over their forehead to avoid accidentally pushing the earpieces into the eye.

Irrigation

This procedure is urgently required when acidic or alkaline substances have entered the eye. In this instance, do not assess VA first, as it is vital to irrigate as soon as possible. Please see Information 15.3 and Ocular Burns section.

Patient Positioning and Activity

Any activity that increases venous pressure in the head should be avoided in patients postophthalmic procedures. Usually, an upright head position is recommended. Except in cases of retinal detachment, macular hole surgery and following vitrectomy (removal of some of the gel-like substance in the posterior segment of the eye) when the surgeon's instructions for face-down positioning must be followed precisely to aid a positive outcome (Shimada et al. 2017). For patients with COVID-19 who need nursing in the supine position, this increases chemosis and corneal oedema (Sansome and Lin 2020) so ocular review is vital.

Nausea and Vomiting

This can be associated with raised IOP, in acute glaucoma, postintraocular surgery, and trauma, so prompt assessment and appropriate referral is required. The head-down position can raise intraocular pressure (IOP), resulting in damage to ocular structures. Management with antiemetics is required (see BNF for details) and reassurance. Effective discharge and an explanation of any restrictions on activity must be clear and concise.

Assessing Sight

It is important to assess the patient's sight, as a baseline for diagnosis and care planning. VA for distance should be assessed using Snellen or Log Mar charts, as discussed earlier. It may also be appropriate to assess near or colour vision, depending upon the presenting history. Any significant change in acuity must be reported.

INFORMATION 15.3

Irrigation of an Eye

Copiously irrigate the affected eye(s), preferably with 1 L of sodium chloride 0.9% via an IV giving set or ideally a Morgan lens (http://www.morganlens.com). Ensure the patient is comfortable, reclining with their head and neck supported. Clothing should be protected by a waterproof cape and towels. Check pH for levels in both eyes, even when one eye is affected as the unaffected fellow eye will show the normal pH measure for the affected eye. It should read 7.5 or below (Dua et al. 2020). Ask the patient to hold the receiver dish and to turn their head slightly to the affected side. Instil topical anaesthetic drops, e.g. proxymetacaine one to two drops. Pull down the lower eyelid and irrigate with a steady flow of fluid, while asking the patient to move their eye around and to evert the upper lid to ensure thorough irrigation. Continue irrigation for at least 15 minutes, re-instilling local anaesthetic drops as required. Remove particles or foreign bodies with moistened cotton bud or forceps. Wait 5 minutes prior to checking pH levels again. Continue irrigation until neutral pH is indicated when reading the colour reaction of a strip of universal pH paper when it touches the tear film in the lower fornix of the eye.

Examining the Eye

Using a pen torch this should be systematic and allow the healthcare professional to check external ocular structures. If there is no underlying pathology it is helpful to use the unaffected eye as a baseline to compare the operated or injured eye. The unaffected eye may react in sympathy with the affected eye (sympathetic ophthalmitis), so looking at both eyes is essential. The patient should be asked to describe how each eye feels; providing a pain score is useful using an appropriate pain assessment tool. As eye complications can develop rapidly, early recognition and reporting of abnormalities including increasing pain, or blurred vision are vital in reducing the risk of potential permanent loss of sight. Look at Table 15.1 for clinical features and diagnostic significance.

The eye should be examined from outer to inner, so from looking at face, eyelids, moving to conjunctiva, cornea, AC, pupils and checking for a red reflex with an ophthalmoscopy. Key ocular features to consider are bruising or swelling of the eyelids, subconjunctival haemorrhage, particularly in patients post cataract surgery under local anaesthetic. If a hyphaema (bleeding into the AC) is present this should be recorded with a digital image or diagram showing size relative to the AC, then documented. Conjunctival redness (injection) and oedema (chemosis) can be signs of allergy, infection or postoperative antibiotic injection site. The cornea and AC should be clear. A fine suture line may be evident, although cataract wound size is so small, that sutures are not usually required. Glaucoma surgery wounds are concealed under the top lid and examined by asking the patient look downwards, gently retracting the upper lid. The depth and shape of the AC should be noted, with the eclipse test, as a shallow AC (one in which there appears to be a decreased space between the cornea and the iris) may indicate that aqueous from the AC is leaking from the site of the wound. Photophobia (sensitivity to light) is to be expected postoperatively and following trauma.

Conditions Requiring Surgical Intervention

Cataract

Cataracts are an opacity of the lens, which can develop as part of the ageing process. NICE (2017) (Salmon 2019) acknowledge many risk factors including diabetes mellitus, trauma, long-term eye conditions such as iritis, steroidal medications, smoking, poor diet, excessive alcohol intake and lifelong overexposure to sunlight. The lens of the eye is normally transparent due to the regular arrangement of its crystalline fibres and the nature of the proteins inside them. These fibres, which originate in the epithelium of the lens capsule, continue to develop throughout life. This results in thickening and a loss of elasticity, linked to ageing.

Clinical Features

Cataracts are seen as a dull red reflection when examining the eye using ophthalmoscopy, as the lens's nucleus and cells become opaque.

Common Presenting Symptoms

Symptoms of age-related cataract are as follows:
- Gradually decreasing acuity affecting distance sight more than near sight
- General dimming of sight because of the reduction of light reaching the retina
- More frequent refractive errors because of reduced lens elasticity
- Increased glare in bright light and appearance of haloes around lights at night
- Monocular diplopia (double vision or a 'ghosting' effect in one eye)
- Difficulty recognising faces, colour and depth perception (Nizami and Gulani 2022)

Surgical Management

During the developmental stages of cataract, changing spectacles may provide a degree of improvement in sight but, as it is impossible to reverse the opacification process, surgical removal of the cataract is the only effective treatment (RNIB 2022b). Wood (2022) highlights the impact of COVID-19 on waiting times for cataract surgery and recognises this increases the detrimental impact on daily life, including loneliness and social isolation.

Local anaesthetic day care is most prevalent, although within the older age group cognitive changes, hearing loss and lack of cooperation must be considered and in rare cases general anaesthetic could be a safer option. The most recent UK guidelines on cataract surgery by NICE (2022b) have been adopted by the Royal College of Ophthalmologists.

Cataract removal and lens implantation are performed when the cataract affects the person's AL. Surgery will still be considered in the presence of coexisting ocular pathology such as age-related maculopathy or glaucoma, even though the visual outcome may be poor (guarded prognosis). Nizami and Gulami (2022) advise that with this group improved general health status, increased safety, and improved visual function are of benefit.

Before the operation, the pupil is dilated to improve access to the lens and to reduce the risk of damage to the iris. An incision is then made into the globe at the limbus in the 12 o'clock section of the eye. The main method of lens removal is *phacoemulsification*, when ultrasonic fragmentation breaks up the nucleus and aspirates the soft lens material, leaving the posterior capsule intact.

On rare occasions, a technique of *extracapsular extraction* is used for mature cataracts. This is the removal of the entire nucleus and cortex through a large incision, leaving the posterior capsule intact.

Intraocular Lens Implantation

The best visual correction is achieved by the insertion of an intraocular lens (IOL) positioned in front of the posterior capsule at the time of cataract removal. The IOL is calculated for each patient based on a combination of biometry (measurement of the axial length of the eye along the visual axis), keratometry (measurement of the corneal curvature) and their previous optical history, using a biometer. Occasional surgical complications, such as posterior capsular rupture with the vitreous moving into the AC, are one reason why IOL cannot be inserted. The healthcare professional must have a sound knowledge and understanding of the tests, as accuracy is vital in obtaining the best postoperative sight for both eyes (Chang et al. 2023)

An IOL may be inserted as a secondary procedure. In the rare situation when no IOL is inserted, a contact lens or corrective spectacle may be used.

❖ Nursing Management and Health Promotion: Cataract Extraction and Implantation of Intraocular Lens

Day case cataract surgery is routine and ophthalmic units have developed care standards based on national clinical guidelines NICE (2022b). The principles of care relating to intraocular surgery are detailed in the Nursing Care Plan on the website.

The following points are specific to cataract extraction and IOL implantation.

Intraocular Lens Management

The nurse must also be aware if surgery has deviated from the routine course, by carefully reading notes and receiving detailed handover. If the IOL has not been implanted, the postoperative eye drop regimen will be different from the normal care plan.

Problems that may arise following IOL implantation include:
- A secondary rise in intraocular pressure, usually accompanied by severe one-sided headache above the brow of the operated eye.
- Cystoid macular oedema, which results in the patient noting reduction and distortion of sight.
- Infection with the rare, but sight-threatening, possibility of endophthalmitis (severe infection inside the eye).

Patients and relatives need to know who to contact promptly should any of these signs and symptoms occur for advice and to prevent complications (NICE 2022b). It should be explained that during the healing process there is a period of adaptation as the brain adjusts to changes in visual perception. Although there are generally no restrictions on mobility the patient should take care and avoid bending during this period, especially if they have any pre-existing conditions that affect their balance.

Postoperative Medication

The inflammatory response during the healing process is managed by a combination of topical steroids and antibiotics. As a day case, procedure is normally a 2–3-hour visit, with no fasting requirements if under local anaesthetic and a gown is worn over the patient's clothing. This can be misinterpreted as a simple and low risk operation. There is a risk that the postoperative eye drop administration is not followed, therefore part of the nurse's role to ensure that patients and their carers understand the importance of completing the prescribed medications, as well as the need to follow postoperative short-term restrictions.

Refractive Laser Treatments

People who have myopia, hypermetropia or have an astigmatism (see Information 15.1) have options other than glasses or contact lens to correct refractive errors. Laser surgery is now common practice, with techniques developing through research. Laser energy is used to reshape the cornea, for photorefractive keratectomy (PRK), which alters corneal curvature by ablating surface corneal tissue and results in a reduction of refractive power. Laser in situ keratomileusis (LASIK) consists of cutting a hinged flap of cornea under very precise conditions, performing the laser ablation in the corneal bed and then replacing the flap (Royal College of Ophthalmologists 2022). Other treatments include Epi-LASIK (epithelial laser in situ keratomileusis), SMILE (Small Incision Lenticule Extraction) and FLEx (Femtosecond lenticule extraction) (Sharma et al. 2020). These treatments have risks associated with them, especially dry eye disease (Sharma et al. 2020), so patients need psychological preparation to be fully informed for the outcomes and medicolegal requirements (Lake 2018). Any corrective surgery is deemed as cosmetic, so is regulated by clinical standards from the General Medical Council (GMC) (2016) and the Royal College of Ophthalmologists (RCO) (2022).

Glaucoma

Glaucoma is an overarching term for a number of conditions caused by impaired flow of aqueous through the trabecular meshwork (Batterbury and Murphy 2018). Impaired aqueous drainage causes a buildup of intraocular pressure causing damage to the neural tissue of the retina optic nerve. The most common glaucoma is chronic and is responsible for the cause of visual impairment in 7 million people, worldwide (WHO 2022)

Glaucoma is a term applied to a group of conditions which may be acquired or genetic in origin. Glaucoma may be acquired or genetic in origin, and include ocular hypertension (OHT), chronic open-angle glaucoma (COAG), primary closed-angle glaucoma (PCAG – both acute and chronic) and glaucoma secondary to pathological processes (secondary glaucoma). Early detection and adherence to treatment in some cases can help prevent further deterioration of vision. There are a number of different types of glaucoma; some of the most common are discussed in the following sections.

Chronic Open-Angle Glaucoma

Defined symptoms include raised IOP, optic disc cupping and gradual irreversible loss of peripheral vision (Batterbury and Murphy 2018). The normal range of IOP is 12–20 mmHg and this varies throughout the 24-hour period. In COAG, the pressure is generally elevated and the diurnal variation may show considerable fluctuation (Marsden 2017). Loss of vision is slow and deteriorates from the periphery. Patients therefore do not notice the permanent visual impairment that ensues. Raised IOP decreases the blood flow in the optic disc capillaries damaging nerve fibres passing through it (cupping).

Signs and Symptoms

The outward appearance of the patient's eye is normal. On examination, if there is cupping of the optic disc, peripheral visual field loss, raised IOP, a diagnosis of chronic glaucoma may be made (NICE 2022c).

There is usually a gradual and painless loss of peripheral sight; the patient may not notice until there is irreversible damage. Regular eye tests by an optometrist (and subsequent annual eye tests) are essential to detect the disease and refer the patient onto the appropriate local eye care pathway for support, nursing care and management.

Current Nursing Care and Management

Patients and their family should always be fully aware of their treatment options and involved in decision making about their treatment. The main aim of treatment is to reduce IOP to allow better capillary perfusion at the optic nerve head and although this will not repair the damaged vision, it can prevent further loss.

Tests and Investigations

Several patient assessments can confirm a diagnosis of COAG (NICE 2022c)

- Tonometry – measurement of IOP with instruments that allow for corneal contact
- Visual field analysis (perimetry)
- Ophthalmoscopy to examine the optic nerve head at the back of the patient's eye and estimate the degree of cupping
- Optical coherence tomography (OCT), which can predict disease outcomes through detailed analysis of neural tissues and blood flow
- Central corneal thickness (pachymetry) is measured as this is important in IOP control
- Gonioscopy – examination of the state and depth of the angle of the AC (NICE 2022c)
- Genetic risk on families after 40 years of age
- Ethnicity
- Age (after age of 40)

Treatment

NICE (2022c) recommend Selective Laser Trabeculoplasty (SLT) as the first line of treatment for patients with an IOP of 24 mmHg and above who are at 'risk of visual impairment within their lifetime' and can delay the need for eye drops. However, if a patient is not suitable for or chooses not to have SLT then prescription eye drops are essential as part of a patient-centred plan of treatment.

Eye drops such as Prostaglandin Analogue (PGA) may be prescribed to enhance the drainage of aqueous and reduce the IOP. Additional or alternate eye drops such as the beta-blocker called timolol and systemic carbonic anhydrase inhibitors (such as acetazolamide) may be required to reduce aqueous production. Eye drops are prescription drugs and should be treated as such. For example, eye drops such as those to treat glaucoma should only be instilled (in care settings) by registered professionals with awareness of the actions, side-effects, contraindications, and infection control aspects of eye drops.

Patient education underpins the effectiveness of eye drops and supports adherence to the prescribed drop regime. Patients and their family/carers should be taught about their eye drops, the importance of safe and timely instillation (Waterman et al. 2013)

Some patients may prefer to continue to self-administer their eye drops and should be supported to do so as prescribed.

Laser Treatments. Involves applying short bursts of a laser beam through a special lens, targeting selected areas of the trabecular meshwork; argon laser trabeculoplasty has been found to be effective in selected cases in reducing IOP. The scarring caused by the laser appears to stretch the tissues between the burns, opening up spaces in the trabecular meshwork and aiding drainage of aqueous. Cyclodiode laser is when a probe is applied to the ciliary body and destroys the tissues, resulting in significant reduction in aqueous production.

❖ Nursing Care, Management and Health Promotion: Chronic Open-Angle Glaucoma (COAG)

There are three major nursing considerations for patients with COAG: eye health, adherence to eye drop therapy, and postoperative education.

Patient Adherence to Eye Drop Therapy

Adherence to glaucoma eye drop therapy is associated with preferential patient outcomes in reduction of IOP and consequent progression of visual loss (Waterman et al. 2013). Education and support can prevent further visual deterioration and promote eye health (Newman-Casey et al. 2020). Glaucoma eye drops are essential. It is the healthcare professional's responsibility to assess the patient's understanding of their condition, treatment and their ability to instil the eye drops, with educational aspects, including occlusion of lid puncta after beta-blocker eye drops are instilled to reduce the risk of the drug being absorbed into the body (systemic absorption). Self-administration of eye drops requires arm and neck flexibility and hand dexterity to successfully manage the bottle. Using devices such as auto droppers can help, as well as encouragement of patients and carers with low confidence.

Postoperative Observation and Monitoring

A surgical intervention such as trabeculectomy may be indicated for some patients in order to control their IOP

Postoperative care includes a holistic patient assessment with a detailed eye assessment performed by a registered eye care professional, including:

- The depth of the AC. The operated eye should be compared to the unoperated eye and variations must be reported. It is possible for over-drainage of the bleb to result in a shallow AC or for under-drainage to result in a deeper AC. Using the eclipse test, a pen torch is shone laterally across the AC. If the iris is fully illuminated then the AC is deemed safe.
- IOP. Raised IOP, which can present as severe postoperative pain, accompanied by a cloudy cornea and flat AC, is abnormal and must be investigated.
- Signs of postoperative infection such as discharge, pain.

Retinal Detachment

Retinal detachment (RD) can be described as the separation between the neurosensory retina and the retinal pigmented epithelium (RPE) layers of the retina.

The light-sensitive cells in the neurosensory layer are detached from the RPE layer as fluid effusion between the layers gradually causes more separation. RDs are most frequently associated with holes or tears in the retina, due to lattice degeneration, as the retina thins. Predisposing factors include myopia, when the eyeball is elongated. Other causes of RD can be posterior vitreous detachment (PVD); trauma; acute ocular inflammation; postoperative after eye surgeries; vitreous traction or retinal/choroidal tumour.

If one eye is affected, the other may also be at risk. RD is an eye emergency and with an annual incidence of around 10–15 cases per 100,000 people is cited as one of the most common ocular emergencies in the UK (NICE 2019).

The patient may present with any of the following, particularly new onset (NICE 2019):

- painless and sudden and often developing visual loss
- reduced vision, distorted vision, blurred vision
- floaters, which are flakes of pigment in the vitreous
- flashing lights, caused by using at the retina by the vitreous
- loss of sight either central or field, often described as a curtain sensation.

The external appearance of the eye is unchanged, unless recent traumatic injury or surgery has occurred. A specialist ophthalmic retinal team should assess patients with symptoms of a retinal detachment within 24 hours of experiencing symptoms (NICE 2019). A full ophthalmic assessment including the patient's VA, visual fields and slit-lamp examination with IOP check. Identification of Relative Afferent Pupillary Defect (RAPD) (a swinging light source) will determine a difference between the pupils, that is constricted/fixed or fixed pupils. This may suggest an extensive RD; a fundoscopy, with the patient's pupil dilated will facilitate an assessment of and diagnosis of the type of RD and determine the best care and management for the patient (NICE 2019).

Surgical Procedures

The type of surgical intervention is indicated by the nature of the RD and the macular attachment or nonattachment (Salmon 2023). The aim of surgery is to produce a controlled inflammatory response to seal the detachment, release the subretinal fluid and reattach the retinal layers, and reduce virtual traction (Idrees et al. 2020). Surgical intervention is essential and should be undertaken at the earliest opportunity to give the best possible visual outcome, especially in those situations where the macula is still attached. If the macula is off, visual prognosis can be limited. The surgery is often performed under local anaesthesia (LA) as a day case procedure. Depending upon assessment there are various options available.

Current treatments for retinal tears as recommended by NICE cause a reaction on the tissue between the retina and retinal epithelial layers producing scar tissue, which acts as an adhesive causing the layers to come together.

- Laser photocoagulation, when contiguous laser burns are applied around the hole/tear. This may be is performed under local anaesthetic for smaller tears/holes.
- External cryotherapy in the form of a CO_2 freezing probe is applied to the sclera behind the detached retina again to induce adhesion of the detached neurosensory and pigment epithelium layers.

Retinal surgery aims to repair holes and tears, reduce traction of the vitreous, and reattach the retina.

- Scleral buckling surgery when a silicone band is sutured externally over the area of detachment.
- A vitrectomy (removal of some of the vitreous humour) to reduce traction from the vitreous humour to the retina.
- Pneumatic retinopexy, a small gas bubble is injected into the vitreous humour. The bubble expands and altering posture, for example a head-down position, causes the it to rise, pressing against and closing the retinal break.

❖ Nursing Management and Health Promotion: Retinal Detachment

There are four major nursing considerations for patients with RD: positioning, education and counselling, pain management and observation of the eye.

Patient Positioning

Following a vitrectomy with gas inserted, a patient will require an individualised care plan and this includes head positioning. The surgeon determines the position according to location of the RD.

Adherence to positioning can improve the success of surgery. The head-down positioning may be necessary for 2–6 weeks postoperatively, with 50 minutes out of every hour in this posture.

Patients must be well educated about the reasons for adhering to positioning as essential to the success of the reattachment. Appropriate education and posturing aids support patients to establish and maintain the required position. Posturing itself may be uncomfortable and regular assessment for discomfort and skin integrity is an essential aspect of patient care.

Patient Education and Support

Control of the postoperative inflammatory response is achieved by dilating (mydriatics) and steroid eye drops, so patients and their carers must be fully aware of the regimen. Patients may have concerns about sutures being left in place, but they should be advised that non-absorbable sutures are used and left in place in order to sustain their compressive effect over time. Patients should be advised that the sight may be temporarily poorer than before surgery and will gradually improve, due to the manipulation of the eye, the postoperative mydriatic drops and the alterations to the focusing power of the eye resulting from any scleral buckling.

Postoperative Pain

Postoperative pain is an individual experience and the patient's pain should be assessed at regular intervals using an appropriate pain assessment tool. Prescribed analgesia should be administered regularly and effectiveness monitored. Severe pain, accompanied by nausea and vomiting may indicate acute rise in IOP. Patients, their families, carers, and the healthcare team should be aware of this potential postoperative complication and know to report it as a matter urgency.

Patients may be anxious about the results of their surgery and should expect that their vision may not reach its full potential for several weeks. Postoperative eye coverings and/or reduced vision initiates an assessment of a patient's activities of daily living and consideration of nursing interventions such as help with personal hygiene and falls prevention.

Patients may be prescribed postoperative eye drops to prevent infection and inflammation. As part of a holistic nursing care plan, patients, family and carers are taught how to instil eye drops safely and effectively along with appropriate infection control.

Postoperative Appearance of the Patient's Eye

The external appearance of the patient's eye postretinal surgery may show chemosis (conjunctival swelling) with bruising and swelling of the eyelids. The patient's eye should be assessed regularly for signs of infection and inflammation. Education about signs and symptoms of postoperative infection will support patients to identify signs of infection and inflammation and where to seek advice.

Corneal Transplant (Keratoplasty)

Indications for corneal transplant include corneal injury or disease, some cases of keratoconus (conical cornea) and corneal opacity. The corneal has six layers, so transplants can vary depending on patient's condition, for example an endothelial keratoplasty (EK) replaces the inner most layer, a deep anterior lamellar keratoplasty (DALK) replaces the front layers and a penetrating keratoplasty (PK) is full thickness (Liu et al. 2022). All require donor tissue, which has to be harvested within 24 hours of death, then processed at Bristol or Manchester Eye banks, ensuring robust screening and suitability for donation (Armitage et al. 2019). Keratoplasty is dependent upon the availability of suitable donor material. Current UK law is an opt-out system for organ and tissue donation, also known as Max and Keira's law (see Useful Websites for more information). Expectations now are that everyone aged 18 plus must register their choice about organ and tissue donation online (https://www.organdonation.nhs.uk/register-your-decision/donate/confirmation/?v=715). It is straight forward and so important to have made this decision, as well as informing your loved ones, as per the *Leave them certain public health campaign* (NHS Blood and Transplant, 2021). English et al. (2019), acknowledge that a lack of organ and tissue availability is a NHS challenge, especially for corneal transplantation. They suggest the new opt out system will not make a positive difference. Corneal cross linking (CXL) can be used for people with keratoconus (Bradford et al. 2020). This procedure uses topical vitamin eye drops and ultraviolet light to alter corneal cell structure and reshape, so removes the need for corneal transplant in some individuals.

❖ Nursing Management and Health Promotion: Corneal Transplant

The perioperative period is managed as for other intraocular surgery but there are some important considerations following keratoplasty, including informed consent to discuss risks of rejection and healing times (Liu et al. 2022).

The Use of Donated Tissue

The use of donor corneas can be an emotive issue, and recipients may ask questions. Healthcare professionals must be ready to give reassurance, whilst remembering the Data protection act (2018), and the Human Tissue Authority, code F, part two (2020). The website https://www.organdonation.nhs.uk/ offers a good resource for patients or potential donors who want more information.

Postoperative Examination

Following the procedure, any conjunctival redness (injection) should gradually lessen. There are risks of transplant rejection, cataract and glaucoma associated with keratoplasties (Liu et al. 2022), so close monitoring of the wound to ensure the suture line remains intact and the corneal disc (transplant) has stayed in position, is required. Disruption of either may affect the optical (visual) power of the transplant, and subsequent quality of sight.

Patient Involvement

Patients and their carers should be educated that any corneal transplant requires a lengthy follow-up period, taking up to 12 months to fully recover (Salmon 2019). The cornea is an avascular structure, and healing will be slow. The corneal sutures will remain in situ for several months or, if a good visual result has been obtained, it may be decided to leave the sutures in indefinitely rather than risk disturbing the transplant.

It is vital to continue any topical medication prescribed to avoid rejection of the transplant, usually corticosteroids (Bradford et al. 2020), and to prevent infection with effective handwashing standards. Initially sight may seem worse than before transplant, so reassurance is vital for the patient and their carers. They need to attend review appointments, full contact details must be provided for early self-referral if any symptoms of transplant rejection occur, which include:
- increased redness of the conjunctiva
- cloudiness of the cornea
- reduction of visual function
- discomfort in the operated eye.

Red Eye

This section focuses on the acute aspects of eye care, and the most common presentation is the 'red eye'. There are numerous diagnoses for the red eye, but a general principle is that a painful red eye is often more serious than a nonpainful eye (NICE 2021a). It should be noted that the more injection and redness does not necessarily equate to a more serious eye condition. For example, a subconjunctival haemorrhage can present as a completely red sclera, but this is not usually urgent. Yet redness around the limbal, corneal area can be acute glaucoma which is sight threatening. It is essential to work within your competency and seek advice from experts if unsure (Shirodkar 2019).

Triage. The Manchester triage system is an effective tool to aid clinical decision making (Please see Useful Websites for more information) to ensure prompt assessment and intervention of required care. In some ophthalmic emergency departments, an electronic self-triage is used to manage waiting times and prioritise care (Dickson et al. 2022). A detailed patient holistic and clinical history, as well as the ophthalmic vital signs of VA, pupillary check and IOP are required to aid safe clinical decision making.

Anxiety. Suffering eye injuries can cause high levels of anxiety, so the role of the healthcare professional is to provide reassurance and emotional support. This should be done by explaining the procedures, answering questions, ensuring adequate pain control and contacting the patient's family. It is essential to acknowledge that the patient may experience pain and fear at the potential loss of sight (State of the Nation Eye Health 2017). It is important that equal consideration is made for physical and mental health needs; 'parity of esteem' (RCN 2022).

Education and Safe Environment. Some conditions will require the patient to have their eye padded and have dilated pupils, the latter of which causes photophobia (sensitivity to light) and glare especially when driving. It is a medicolegal requirement in the UK to avoid driving and operating heavy machinery during this treatment regimen (Gov.UK 2022) so ensure the patient and carer are well informed and document your advice (NMC 2018).

Prevention of cross-infection and hospital-acquired infection (HAI) is a priority. Standards for hand hygiene, using antibacterial gels, wearing gloves, correct storage and instillation of eye drops and correct aseptic technique should be maintained. Please refer to Chapter 18, Infection Prevention and Control, for further information.

The patient and their carers must be fully informed about any prescribed treatment and understand the need to attend follow-up outpatient appointments.

In cases of sight loss, ensure that the patient and carers are fully supported and are offered appropriate advice.

Acute Closed-Angle Glaucoma (ACAG)

This is an ophthalmic emergency requiring immediate referral to ophthalmology to prevent permanent ocular damage. This presents as an acute episode of severe raised IOP, usually unilateral. Prophylactic treatment is also given for the unaffected eye.

Raised IOP develops as a result of disruption of the circulation of aqueous humour in the AC, which can be associated with hypermetropia. Pupil dilatation is accompanied by forward displacement of the iris, which blocks the trabecular meshwork, reducing or stopping the flow of aqueous to the canal of Schlemm.

The pupillary margin of the iris touches the lens, causing the pupil to become semidilated and fixed, further blocking the flow of aqueous and increasing forward displacement of the iris. Aqueous buildup results in corneal oedema and disturbance of sensory nerve fibres.

According to NICE guidelines (2022c) the typical symptoms and signs include:

- Eye pain, often severe, and associated with headache, nausea, and vomiting caused by the pain.
- A red eye, especially around the limbal area.
- Impaired VA and lights are seen surrounded by haloes – caused by a hazy oedematous cornea.
- Photophobia.
- Semidilated and fixed pupil. Classically, the pupil becomes fixed in a vertically oval shape.
- A tender, hard eye (palpate very gently). When measured by an optometrist or ophthalmologist, the IOP is typically very high.

Management

Tests and investigations include the following:

- A full history (Table 15.2) including medications as benzodiazepines can be linked to ACAG (Park et al. 2019).
- Cannula must be in place as intravenous (IV) access will be needed.
- Systematic ocular examination using a slit lamp, which is a binocular microscope that illuminates and magnifies the ocular structures with a narrow band of light, facilitating examination for accurate diagnosis.
- Measurement of IOP.
- Gonioscopy (examination of the angle of the eye).
- A full set of observations including Blood pressure and temperature.
- Blood tests for inflammatory markers and infection.
  Acute signs and symptoms should be managed as follows:
- Intensive topical miotic therapy, pilocarpine 2% or 4% is commenced to constrict the pupil so the outflow of aqueous humour is increased by freeing the iris angle. Prophylactic therapy is prescribed for the other eye to prevent an acute attack (https://bnf.nice.org.uk/).
- Reduction in production of aqueous by administration of carbonic anhydrase inhibitors such as acetazolamide (Diamox) either orally or intravenously (https://bnf.nice.org.uk/) (NICE 2022c).
- Pain assessment and management with analgesics, including IV opioids.
- Control of nausea and vomiting with IV antiemetics.

Surgical Intervention

When the patient is stable, and acute signs and symptoms have been managed, then decisions about further procedures and tests, for example, if visual fields or surgery, should be made. The surgical decision depends on clinical presentation and may incorporate the following:

- laser iridotomy – small holes are created in the peripheral iris of the affected eye
- surgical procedures, including trabeculectomy (see Glaucoma), to improve aqueous circulation
- post laser iridotomy, topical steroid treatment and possible long-term antiglaucoma therapy (Royal College of Ophthalmologists (RCO) 2022) to reduce inflammation and stabilise the IOP.

TABLE 15.2	Systematic Approach to History Taking	
Assessment	**Question**	**Rationale**
Presenting complaint	How did the accident/change occur? When did the accident/change occur? Where did the accident/change occur? Which eye or associated structures are affected? Is the injury unilateral/bilateral? Were safety goggles worn? Do you have any pain? (use appropriate pain tool) Is your vision altered? How? Is it central, peripheral or colour?	To aid diagnosis For medicolegal reasons
Ophthalmic history	Are glasses or contact lenses worn? Why? What is refractive error? Has a similar problem occurred before? Has patient had a previous eye injury or operation?	To ascertain if preventive lessons are learnt To aid clinical examination and diagnosis, as some conditions are recurrent. If myopic, wears glasses for distance and they have floaters, flashing lights or visual field defect, this can be a PVD or RD. If hypermetropic, can be at increased risk of acute glaucoma, due to angle of the eye.
Medical and surgical history	Does patient have any general health problems? Has patient had previous surgery, including eye operations?	Some systemic disorders may affect the eye, e.g. diabetes mellitus, hypertension, altered thyroid activity Patient may require surgery and may have had a reaction to an anaesthetic previously. May be using eyedrops which alter normal pathophysiology.
Medications	Is patient taking medication at present? Prescribed, over the counter, self-administer, illegal, eye drops/ointments.	Some medications may affect the eye, e.g. opioids and pupil reactions Patient may have an allergy to a medication To ensure medicine optimisation and avoidance of any contraindications to use
Allergies	Is patient allergic to any substance, e.g. medications, Sellotape, Elastoplast?	A substance may inadvertently be given to which the patient is allergic, causing potential patient harm
Family history	Has anyone in patient's family got a diagnosed eye condition? Had a similar problem recently?	Some conditions are hereditary such as squints, glaucoma and refractive errors. If the person has conjunctivitis, the may have contracted from another family member, so health promotion is needed.
Recent foreign travel	Has patient travelled abroad recently? If so where?	To ensure accurate information about location of travel, and public health risks associated with these areas. For example, contact lens wearers can contract acanthamoeba keratitis, if not following contact lens care instructions.
Systemic enquiry	Ask about all the body systems	To promote a holistic approach and consideration of systemic causes for eye problem

PVD, Posterior vitreous detachment; *RD,* retinal detachment.

Uveitis

Uveitis is inflammation of the uveal tract, includes the iris and/or the ciliary body (anterior uveitis or iritis) or the choroid (posterior uveitis). It is an acute condition, often affecting one eye, which should be seen urgently, as it accounts for up to 10% of global sight loss (NICE 2021b). The aetiology is most commonly idiopathic or autoimmune, for example rheumatoid conditions, irritable bowel syndrome (IBS), and in approximately 8% of cases, the presence of HLA-B27 histocompatibility antigen; used to detect gene/antigen compatibility and autoimmune disease (College of Optometrists 2021).

Recurrent episodes are expected however, through effective patient education, prompt self-referral and treatment offer a good prognosis. Secondary uveitis may accompany other eye infections or trauma, so both are treated in these clinical cases.

Clinical features are as follows:
- pain (dull ache) due to ciliary body spasm
- sluggish pupil reaction on affected side
- photophobia
- limbal injection/redness
- decreased vision
- lacrimation.

The above are visible using a pen torch however, the following symptoms require a slit lamp providing a magnified view.
- Cloudy and shallow AC due to the increased inflammation of iris, aqueous protein content and presence of white blood cells (the debris floating in the aqueous is known as 'flare and cells').
- Cellular exudates (keratic precipitates or KPs) may be present on the posterior endothelial surface of the cornea.
- Inflammation of the iris may cause it to adhere to the anterior surface of the lens (synechiae formation); this will interfere with aqueous flow leading to possible raised IOP which, if untreated, may progress to secondary glaucoma.

🔴 Management

This will vary depending on the severity and potential cause of inflammation (Gamalero et al. 2019), but can include:
- Blood tests are used to determine the cause of new onset and recurrent uveitis: the most commonly used tests are HLA-B27 and erythrocyte sedimentation rate (ESR) or C-reactive protein (CRP) (NICE 2021a).
- Ocular examination, VA, fundoscopy with dilated pupils to exclude posterior uveitis and if IOP is raised this must be treated (see ACAG).

- Pharmacological treatment is with topical (eyedrops) and systemic corticosteroids (to reduce inflammation) and mydriates or cycloplegics (to dilate the pupils, prevent synechia and relax the ciliary body) (Gamalero et al. 2019) in severe cases, these may be given via subconjunctival injection.

Research trials advise immunosuppressants such as methotrexate, and TNF-α (tumour necrosis factor alpha) inhibitors for long-term prevention and management (Gamalero et al. 2019).
- Outpatient review is required, to manage condition.

Patients and their families must be educated to recognise the symptoms, and promptly self-refer, as this condition is recurrent especially when linked to a systemic health condition.

Please refer to the clinical management guidelines from the NICE, for Uveitis, May 2021 for further information.

Keratitis

Keratitis refers to inflammatory conditions of the cornea, associated with infections (bacterial, viral, fungal), trauma, external eye disease (blepharitis, entropion), dry eye and extensive contact lens wear (Jackson 2020). The cornea has six layers, severity of conditions varies, for example if the superficial layer (epithelium) alone is affected, there is minimal damage with little sight loss, but if the middle portion (stroma) is involved, loss of transparency and altered corneal curvature may lead to significant loss of sight. Severe inflammation can result in cells being deposited into the AC (hypopyon).

Clinical features are as follows and the severity of signs and symptoms will vary depending upon actual cause:
- red, injected and painful eye
- photophobia with spasm of the eyelid (blepharospasm)
- lacrimation/profuse tearing in most cases, although there are some instances of dry eye presentation
- cloudy cornea
- blurred vision.

Bacterial Keratitis

This is more prevalent with common causative agents being staphylococci, *Streptococcus* and *Pseudomonas*. They invade the cornea, resulting in an inflammatory reaction. This can recur, especially in contact lens use or with a history of corneal abrasion, injury or disease. The severity can vary from superficial to severe, which can result in corneal thinning and, in rare cases, perforation (Tuft et al. 2021).

Viral Keratitis

The most common form is dendritic (herpetic) ulcer, which is caused by the herpes simplex virus. Its distinguishing feature is the branching, tree-like pattern it forms on the cornea, which is visible on corneal staining with fluorescein (NICE 2021c).

Fungal Keratitis

The usual causes of fungal infections of the eye are *Candida*, *Aspergillus* and *Nocardia*. These are linked to people who are immunocompromised, have had minor trauma from vegetation or use contact lens. They cause severe corneal damage, and complications can develop rapidly. Urgent referral for clinical management and specific antifungal treatment agents is required. The distinguishing feature of this kind of ulceration is that it appears as fluffy, feathery extensions over the cornea.

Acanthamoeba

This free-living organism is found in soil, air, dust, sea water and drinking water, although rare, it is serious and sight threatening.

There are links to contact lens use, especially soft, disposable lenses, poor hygiene levels and excessive contact lens wear which breaches the manufacturer's guidance (Szentmary et al. 2019). Clinical features include ring abscess formation and corneal thinning resulting from inflammation, infection or degeneration, as well as typical signs and symptoms of keratitis listed above. Treatment is medical with an intensive antiseptic eye drop regimen (Moorfields 2021). If the treatment regime is not effective, then severe SI can occur, with the possibility of corneal graft.

Management

Patients should be managed, wherever possible, by an ophthalmic consultant.

Diagnosis must be sought by the following:
- Obtaining a thorough patient history, including contact lens care
- Taking of conjunctival, corneal swabs and corneal scrapings
- Slit-lamp examination, with fluorescein staining; this fixes to damaged corneal tissue and turns the affected area a bright fluorescent green, indicating the extent of the damage
- Sending away contact lens for culture and sensitivity

The most appropriate topical antibiotic, antiviral, antifungal or antiseptic therapy is commenced immediately to avoid rapid development of complications. As clinical signs can be similar and if there are any uncertainties in actual diagnosis, then a referral to an ophthalmic department is advised (NICE 2021c).

Possible secondary ocular complications of raised IOP or uveitis must be treated as necessary. It is important to note that steroids are contraindicated, as they suppress the response to infection (Jackson 2020).

❖ Nursing Management and Health Promotion: Keratitis

Patients are generally managed as an outpatient, unless they require intensive topical treatment day and night – this can be as frequent as eyedrops every quarter of an hour. The care and education for patients with keratitis should be as follows:
- Careful hygiene is essential to prevent cross-infection. Tears should be wiped from the cheek only, with a clean disposable tissue on each occasion. Principles of isolation and infection control will be observed in the hospital situation (see Chapter 18, Infection Prevention and Control) with correct handwashing techniques.
- The patient should be taught not to touch or rub the eye as this may extend the ulceration.
- Dendritic ulcers can occur due to an outbreak of cold sores (herpes simplex). Patients should be advised to guard against touching the sores and then rubbing their eyes. Any healthcare professionals with active sores should not have contact with ophthalmic patients.
- Education regarding contact lens wear is essential and the long-term use may be contraindicated for some patients. Contact lens education and care must be as per manufacturers guidance, incorporate the following (Specsavers 2022):
  - maintaining strict hygienic practice
  - not exceeding the recommended wearing time
  - cleaning with sterile water or lens cleaning products, not with saliva or tap water
  - removing lenses if the eyes become inflamed or sore, and not reinserting until advised by a specialist
  - removing soft lenses before administering drops containing preservatives.

Conjunctivitis

This is inflammation of the conjunctiva due to allergic or immunological reactions, infection (viral, bacterial, *Chlamydia or* parasitic), mechanical irritation or contact with toxic substances (NICE 2022d). These cause dilatation of the small conjunctival vessels, resulting in redness and oedema (chemosis) causing discharge.

Clinical features include:
- red eye
- pruritus (itching)
- gritty sensation, due to follicle formation
- discharge may be watery (viral) or mucopurulent (bacterial/chlamydial), with eyelids sticking together at night
- varying degrees of pain
- preauricular lymphadenopathy, usual in acute or chlamydial causes Photophobia, but the VA is not necessarily affected.

❖ Nursing Management and Health Promotion: Conjunctivitis

This includes diagnosis through history taking, VA assessment, lid eversion (Information 15.3) to reveal follicle formation and slit-lamp examination. If recurrent, a history longer than 2 weeks or nonresponsive to usual treatment, then conjunctival swabs may be considered. Also, enquire into sexual history, as chlamydial and bacterial have similar presentations, but require different treatments.

As a broad diagnostic guide, viral infections have watery discharge, and no treatment is required. Possible fungal infections need referral to ophthalmology specialist. Chlamydial and bacterial infections can be referred to primary care services, please note that both have a purulent ocular discharge. The Royal College of Optometrists have a useful referral guide (https://www.college-optometrists.org/clinical-guidance/guidance/guidance-annexes/annex-4-urgency-of-referrals-table).

The patient should be advised as follows:
- Bathe their eyes frequently using cooled boiled water.
- Complete the prescribed regimen of eye drops.
- Over-the-counter artificial tears can soothe the eye
- Wear sunglasses if photophobic.
- Prevent transmission of infection by strict handwashing and the use of individual towels and face cloths, as conjunctivitis is highly infectious (NICE 2022d).
- Return for review if the condition is not improving after 7 days. Acute cases usually settle under 4 weeks, however chronic cases can take longer, and a differential diagnosis needs to be considered.

As well as educating the patient in eye hygiene and self-medication, the healthcare professional must monitor for complications and refer.

Subconjunctival Haemorrhage (SCH)

This red eye condition presents suddenly, is unilateral, painless and does not change sight. As it looks dramatic, patients can be concerned that it is serious, however it is a minor eye condition resulting from a bleed between the conjunctiva and the sclera (NICE 2021a).

A history of poorly managed hypertension NICE (2023), excessive coughing, sneezing or vomiting, taking anticoagulant medications and in some cases mild trauma can be the causes.

The patient's VA should be checked, if unaltered then there is no topical ocular treatment. However, a referral to primary care should be made for blood pressure monitoring, medication review and blood tests to assess clotting factors. Importantly, the healthcare professional's role is reassurance and advising that reabsorption of the SCH can take several weeks, depending on severity.

Herpes Zoster Ophthalmicus (Ophthalmic Shingles)

This is an acute unilateral viral infection of the trigeminal ganglion, which extends from the scalp to the nose and includes the eye. It is caused by the chickenpox virus and its predisposing factors can be compromised immune systems and increased age. The lifetime risk of the population developing this is 20%–30% (NICE 2022e).

Common presenting symptoms and signs are:
- regional adenopathy and general malaise of the patient
- pain and tingling sensation
- skin rash of the forehead and around the eye
- swollen eyelids
- characteristic vesicular eruptions over the course of the nerve
- there may be serious ocular complications, resulting in SI, if the globe/eyeball is affected, including uveitis, keratitis and conjunctivitis.

🔵 Management

- Treatment with oral antiviral treatment (aciclovir, valaciclovir, or famciclovir) should begin immediately (Patil et al. 2022).
- Treatment with topical antiviral agents, usually commenced by the ophthalmologist.
- Analgesia for postherpetic pain, as this may persist for many weeks.
- Possibly ocular lubricants to relieve ocular discomfort.
- Regular eye bathing if there is ocular discharge.
- Encourage the patient to rest.
- Sunglasses can be worn if photophobia is a symptom.
- Determine any contributory factors and address these, such as stress or immune disorder.

Allergy to Topical Medication

This presents as chemosis (swelling of the conjunctiva) and inflammation of the eyelids extending to the cheeks. Common causative agents are neomycin, atropine and preservatives, (benzalkonium chloride) in eye drops (Goldstein et al. 2022).

Clinical signs include:
- red and oedematous eyelids
- chemosis
- epiphora (excessive watering) and intense itching in the acute stage.

🔵 Management

- Stop ocular medication and review medication regime, if clinically indicated.
- Substitute an alternative ocular treatment including a topical antihistamine.
- Systemic antihistamines to relieve itching.
- Cortisone lotion may be prescribed for the affected skin area to relieve itching and oedema.
- Cool eye bathing may be used as a therapeutic measure.
- Contact lenses should not be worn, until fully resolved.

External Eye Conditions

These are common and easily treated, once accurately diagnosed (Moorfields 2021). Nurse specialists in many ophthalmic units and optometrists within the community setting manage patients with such diseases.

Blepharitis

This is a chronic inflammatory condition of the rim of the eyelids, resulting in redness, itchiness and crusting of the eyelashes. This condition can lead to the patient having styes or chalazions (see below) and may recur especially with causes linked to acne rosacea, psoriasis or eczema (Moorfields 2021).

Long-term management is required and includes:
- lid hygiene and application of warm flannel compresses to remove crusting and excess oily secretions from the eyelids
- topical antibiotics such as chloramphenicol
- ocular lubricants, if associated with dry eye (refer to age-related conditions)
- systemic antibiotics.

It is important to refer to ophthalmology services if reoccurring (NICE 2021a).

Stye

This is an infection of an eyelash follicle. This should be treated with warm compresses and if needed, topical antibiotics.

Chalazion or Meibomian Cyst

This is a blocked duct from the meibomian glands. Treatment is as for blepharitis initially but may require 'incision and curettage' if the cyst remains. This procedure is performed under a local anaesthetic in the outpatient department. These are more prevalent in people who are pregnant, have rosacea, seborrheic dermatitis and diabetes mellitus (NICE 2020). As with any lesion or cyst, a careful history of the duration, any changes, systemic patient health are essential, and referral to an ophthalmic consultant for pathology is advised if malignancies are suspected.

Diplopia (Double Vision)

A patient may report seeing two images instead of one either vertically, obliquely, or horizontally in one or both eyes and this is described as diplopia (Batterbury and Murphy (2018). Acute onset diplopia may be a symptom of neurological, ischaemic disease requiring immediate referral to the appropriate specialist service (Margolin 2020) exclude serious systemic disease.

❖ Nursing Management and Health Promotion: Diplopia

The exact cause of diplopia requires investigation and diagnosis prior to any intervention or long-term treatment to alleviate symptoms. The orthoptist has a vital role in assessing and diagnosis of diplopia. Information about the role of the orthoptist is available on the British and Irish Association of Orthoptists website. Orthoptists advise interventions such as occlusion therapy and eye muscle exercises to assist patients with diplopia to maximise their visual potential.

Signs and Symptoms of Diplopia
- Ptosis (drooping eyelid)
- Inability to focus on fixed object (nystagmus)

- The patient may be dizzy, disorientated and at risk of falls, due to associated problems so preserving their safety is paramount

● Nursing Care and Management

After diagnosis which includes full eye assessment, blood tests and scans, the treatment is long term. The patient, family and their carers should have the diagnosis and management explained to them. These may include:
- Occlusion of one eye after assessment by an orthoptist and ophthalmologist.
- Use of prisms on the patient's glasses.
- Injection of botulinum toxin into overactive muscle. This results in temporary paralysis (approximately 3 months) and encourages increased function of the underactive muscle. The botulinum blocks the transmission of the nerve impulses at the neuromuscular junction by interfering with release of the neurotransmitter acetylcholine (see Chapter 11, Nursing Patients With Disorders of the Nervous System).
- Surgical intervention to correct squint (strabismus). This is either 'recession' or 'resection', the weakening or strengthening of extraocular muscles, by moving their attachment to the sclera backwards or forwards.

Eye Injuries

It is vital to record an accurate history (see Table 15.2) to rule out any nonvisible injury such as intraocular foreign body (IOFB). The VA must be measured, and a systematic eye examination made to establish a diagnosis and for medicolegal reasons. The Manchester triage system is used in clinical practice to prioritise care, based on presenting history to support the healthcare professional's judgement, in order to facilitate the preservation of sight (Reflection 15.3). Some of the more prevalent eye injuries are described below.

Hyphaema

This is an accumulation of blood cells in the AC of the eye (Chen and Fasiuddin 2021). Usually due to blunt trauma, but can be spontaneous, following penetrating injury or post intraocular surgery (Gragg et al. 2022) causing rupture of the small iris and ciliary body blood vessels. The severity of bleed will vary from microscopic, visible only with the aid of a slit lamp, or severe with a level of blood seen in the anterior chamber of the eye, sometimes completely filling the AC (Gragg et al. 2022). The severity of the bleed will determine pain levels, this is due to ciliary spasm and raised IOP (as the angle of eye is blocked, so aqueous cannot drain away) and VA.

REFLECTION 15.3

Triage Exercise

Using the Manchester triage system (Marsden 2017) list the following ophthalmic conditions in order of priority for emergency treatment: conjunctivitis, uveitis, retinal detachment, entropion, perforating eye injury, chemical injury.

Answers

Red = chemical injury; orange = perforating eye injury; yellow = retinal detachment, uveitis; green = conjunctivitis, entropion.

🌑 Management

This depends upon the severity. A detailed patient holistic and clinical history, associated with hypertension and cardiovascular problems, as well as the ophthalmic vital signs of VA, pupillary check and IOP, are required to aid the clinical decision-making process.

- A patient with microscopic or moderate hyphaema will be advised to rest at home for several days, to encourage reabsorption.
- A patient with a severe hyphaema may be admitted for observation, as there could be an associated rise in IOP or further bleeding.
- Investigations will include B-scan (an ultrasound technique in which a probe is used to detect vitreal or retinal haemorrhages), fundal examination, blood tests to estimate clotting time and international normalised ratio (INR) (NICE 2021a), and possibly CT scan to determine cause.
- Topical drops will be prescribed, including cycloplegics to dilate the pupil and alleviate pain and steroids to reduce ocular inflammation (Chen and Fasiuddin 2021).

A review appointment is required for all patients with any hyphaema.

❖ Nursing Management and Health Promotion: Hyphaema

It is important for the patient or their carer to monitor the level of the hyphaema and to assess visual function in the injured eye daily. Regular analgesia is required, as this condition can be painful. If the patient has nausea or vomiting, antiemetics are advised (Gragg et al. 2022). Education and advice should be provided about possible complications including RD or raised IOP. Gentle activity should be encouraged, as well as advice to bend at the knees to reach things from below waist height rather than bend over, lift or strain. On discharge, the patient will be advised to avoid active or contact sports until the first follow-up appointment and that protective eyewear will be necessary in the future, for example, whilst playing squash or working, if appropriate.

Penetrating Injuries

Depending on history taking, nature of injury and examination, a penetrating injury must always be treated as an emergency. Investigations including X-rays and ultrasound scanning to confirm the presence, location and type of any IOFB or cerebral involvement. It is essential to keep the patient nil by mouth (NBM), until reviewed by ophthalmology, and naturally offer reassurance and honest communication.

🌑 Management

Treatment is dependent on the cause and extent of the injury. It may include the administration of mydriatic (dilating), steroid or antibiotic eye drops, and possibly systemic antibiotics to reduce the risk of complications from inflammation and infection (Field et al. 2015).

Perforating Injuries

The patient will be admitted to hospital for surgical repair of the wound and possible excision of iris prolapse. If the lens is damaged; a traumatic cataract, this may be extracted at the same time. If facial or other injuries are present, then referral for review will be made to the appropriate specialists. In recent years, tattooing of the eyeball has become a lifestyle choice, this is risky and can result in ocular perforation (Ng et al. 2019).

Small Puncture Wounds

These may seal themselves, but review is required to ensure wound closure and intraocular infection do not develop. If the wound is not completely sealed, acrylic glue may be instilled onto the affected cornea and a 'bandage' contact lens (CL) placed over this site to seal the wound and hold the CL in place until the wound has healed. The glue gradually dissolves to allow for removal of the CL (Marsden 2017).

Intraocular Foreign Body (IOFB)

Admission is essential for surgical removal of the FB, as it could be embedded in the iris, vitreous humour or lens. If embedded in the lens, a cataract extraction is carried out. A vitrectomy may be necessary if the IOFB is posterior in the vitreous humour or has caused a haemorrhage.

Complications Following Penetrating Injury

The most common complications are corneal scarring, raised IOP, cataract formation, haemorrhage, hyphaema, hypopyon, iris prolapse and retinal detachments (see relevant sections for further detail).

Severe intraocular infections (endophthalmitis) can occur following any injury, making intensive treatment with antibiotic eye drops and systemic antibiotics necessary.

It is always essential to examine the uninjured eye for signs of 'sympathetic ophthalmitis', a rare complication that presents as a low-grade uveitis. The cause of the sympathetic inflammatory process is an immune response to damaged uveal tissue. The use of topical steroids can reduce the occurrence of this potentially sight-threatening condition, previously managed by enucleating the injured eye (Jackson 2020).

A severely damaged eye with prognosis of SI may become very painful and unresponsive to analgesics, in which case it may be necessary to enucleate the eye to give relief to the patient.

Following repair of large penetrating injuries (or severe infections), the eye may collapse entirely and shrink within (phthisis bulbi) the orbit. This can be distressing for the patient and enucleation for cosmetic reasons may be needed.

❖ Nursing Management and Health Promotion: Penetrating Injuries

The main considerations are the degree of SI, altered body image (see Changing Faces in Useful Websites), pain and potential impact on ALs and their everyday life. Effective, honest communication and answering any concerns are vital to prevent any misunderstandings, or to give any false hope related to their prognosis. A process of grieving and depression can be normal with any permanent sight loss (Rosie et al. 2022).

The primary healthcare team should be advised of the immediate practical measures regarding dressings, pharmacology regimes, wound care and how to refer the patient, if psychological support is required. The ECLO is a good resource for psychological support if the patient is struggling to accept their altered appearance or if they have queries about cosmetic results.

Ocular Burns

Chemical burns can vary from minor irritation to sight devastating, depending on the structures affected, but should all be treated as emergencies. If chemicals (acids, alkalis, solvents or detergents) are splashed into the eye, irrigation (see Information 15.3) must be started immediately (Dua et al. 2020). Then an urgent referral to an emergency department. Parker et al. (2018) reinforce that ocular chemical injuries can be preventable for sight loss and days adjusted life years (DALYS).

Ocular burns can be caused by either acid or alkali. Both damage, with acids causing superficial burns because coagulation of the tissues prevents further penetration. However, alkalis penetrate the conjunctivae, cornea, sclera and eyelids more deeply and can cause severe damage within 15 seconds (Kwok and Chew 2019). Other substances that cause burns include antifreeze, car battery acid, household cleaning agents, cement and superglue. Many chemical substances have antidotes, so the chemical label or details on the container, if available, should be taken to the emergency department along with the patient (see Toxbase in Useful Websites).

Clinical Signs and Symptoms
- Severe, burning pain due to the exposure of the pain receptors of the trigeminal nerve.
- Extreme watering of the eyes due to reflex action.
- Reduced VA due to disruption of cell membranes in the cornea.
- Lids will be very swollen and red.
- Burns to the surrounding skin may also be evident.

Absence of pain or a white eye, 'blanching', does not mean the burn is mild: it may be so severe that it has compromised conjunctival circulation and destroyed the nerve endings.

Management
The eye must be irrigated immediately (NICE 2021a) (see Information 15.2). This is the one time when VA is not assessed before treatment (Marsden 2017). Once the nurse is sure that all traces of the chemical have been removed, a full history can be taken and VA assessed. Post irrigation, ocular examination will be done using a slit lamp to assess the extent of the injury, with lid eversion recommended. Chemical injuries can be successfully treated without causing any long-term damage, especially when irrigation is prompt. Ocular burns can be graded I–IV using the Roper Hall classification depending upon structures involved (Baradaran-Rafil et al. 2017) and treatment will vary. Kwok and Chew (2019) recognise that chemical injuries take a long time to resolve and can cause permanent ocular damage. In some cases, the person will need limbal cell autograft or corneal graft.

Treatment for Minor Burns
An antibiotic ointment is prescribed and possibly guttae cycloplegics to relieve iris spasm, prior to an eye pad being applied. The topical treatment is prescribed for several days and the patient should be given a follow-up appointment.

Treatment for Severe Burns
Admission to hospital for intensive treatment, pain management and observation may be necessary. An antibiotic ointment is instilled at least four times daily to lubricate the inner eyelids and reduce the risk of secondary infection. In addition, guttae mydriatic are instilled to relieve iris spasm, which causes ocular pain. Topical steroids are often administered in addition to vitamin C eye drops, which are thought to aid collagen remodelling and speed healing time to promote better visual outcome in severe burns. A bandaged CL can be used for therapeutic reasons and to aid epithelisation (Baradaran-Rafil et al. 2017). Monitoring of IOP using a slit lamp by the specialised healthcare professional is required to detect complications such as uveitis, which can lead to secondary glaucoma.

Radiation Injuries
Irradiation from ultraviolet, infrared or laser light can cause eye damage. Natural UV rays can cause cataract and localised cancers, but can take years to develop (WHO (2019) and UVC rays protect our eyes to some extent. Turbert (2020) recommends use of sunglasses and eye protection if using sunbeds. Sunbeds emit both UVA and UVB rays, which according to the WHO (2017) can damage the DNA of the cells, causing irreversible retinal damage.

In any work environment where employees are exposed to hot material such as molten glass or metal, employers must comply with the Health and Safety at Work Act 1974 and local policies. Ultraviolet radiation causes corneal epithelial damage (arc eye, welder's flash) and most commonly occurs when approved eye goggles with protective sides are not worn during welding. Usually, the signs and symptoms do not appear until several hours after exposure, when the patient presents with photophobia, pain and excessive lacrimation. Fluorescein drops show dot-like staining of the cornea. Treatment is with topical antibiotics, oral analgesia and the use of eye pads or dark glasses. The corneal healing is variable but there should be no long-term effects.

Central Retinal Artery Occlusion (CRAO)
This condition is an ophthalmic emergency. The patient will experience sudden, complete and painless loss of sight in one eye, due to an obstruction of the central retinal artery. It is predominantly associated with embolus and thrombosis. Predisposing factors include diabetes mellitus, hypertension, GCA and lupus (Farris and Waymack 2022). Damage to the retinal artery, some of its branches and retinal cells may be irreversible.

Management
Naturally the patient and family will need reassurance yet honest dialogue. Farris and Waymack (2022) refer to CRAO as a CVA of the retina, so referral for treatment by an ophthalmic healthcare specialist must be urgent, with prompt interventions for any degree of sight to be restored. The aim is to reduce IOP rapidly by digital ocular massage, guttae timolol (beta-blocker), oral acetazolamide (Diamox), administration of osmotic medication of intravenous mannitol. These interventions aid osmosis to release aqueous from the AC, as with acute glaucoma. This should reduce the IOP, allowing dilation of the retinal artery, so any clots may be flushed along to a peripheral branch. Supplementary oxygen is advised, as well as effective management of pain, nausea and vomiting (Farris and Waymack 2022).

Nursing Care Assessment and Management
Patients may present with a sudden loss of vision, a distressing event and therefore they should receive psychological support at all stages of their treatment.

Emergency treatment in the initial 4–6 hours of onset is essential, in the first instance to prevent visual loss and for urgent referral to an acute stroke specialist unit (Batterbury and Murphy (2018)).

Batterbury and Murphy (2018) detail the emergency treatment led by the ophthalmologist aimed at dissolving the thrombosis and reducing the patient's IOP:
- External Ocular massage
- Paracentesis of the AC
- Topical apraclonidine and timolol eye drops

- Rebreathing into a paper bag. This can dilate the retinal blood vessels by increasing carbon dioxide
- YAG laser – if the embolus is visible

Once the emergency stage has passed the patient needs a systemic and ocular examination. Any underlying medical condition such as hypertension should be referred to, and treated in, primary care. In addition, blood tests for inflammatory markers erythrocyte sedation rate/c-reactive protein (ESR/CRP), INR, full blood count (FBC) and glucose should be checked.

Minor Eye Injuries

Corneal Foreign Body

There is usually a history of something entering the eye from DIY, gardening, or high velocity (RCOpto 2022). Signs and symptoms are typical unilateral including red eye, FB sensation on blinking, lacrimation, and blurred sight. Initial care is to gently remove FB with wet cotton bud, irrigation can help also. If the FB is well embedded, then anaesthetise the eye with topical drops, use a 10 G needle to remove FB or rust ring. This must be done by an experienced practitioner, using an appropriate magnification aid, ideally a slit lamp. It is necessary to check for possible corneal abrasion using fluorescein drops and Seidel test for diagnosis of possible perforation. Treatment is with guttae chloramphenicol and guttae cyclopentolate (BNF/NICE 2023). See Royal College of Optometrists (RCOpto) link for more detail.

Subtarsal Foreign Body

The presence of a FB should be considered when, despite the patient's complaint of something entering the eye, nothing can be seen on normal systematic inspection. There will be discomfort, especially on blinking. The upper lid should be everted and the FB removed (see Information 15.2). It is necessary to check for possible corneal abrasion, as per corneal FB.

Corneal Abrasion

This can be due to subtarsal FB, ingrown eyelashes, fingernail, CL damage or trauma (RCOpto 2022). It is extremely painful with excessive lacrimation and photophobia. Fluorescein eye drops should be instilled in order to determine the extent of the abrasion, this should be measured/documented. Antibiotic ointment may be prescribed to prevent infection, as well as mydriatics (NICE 2021a) if pain from ciliary spasm is severe. A follow-up appointment should be given depending on the severity of the abrasion.

An eye pad is not always required after treatment for abrasion or FB removal (Marsden 2017). The need depends upon the severity and location, for example if the abrasion is central and large.

Surgical Removal of an Eye

There are numerous reasons why an eye or the surrounding structures may need removal, including severe facial chemical burns, trauma, and malignancies and, so the type of operation is dependent upon the diagnosis (Sadiq et al. 2020). The three methods of removing an eye are:

- *Enucleation* is the surgical removal of the whole eyeball.
- *Evisceration* is the removal of the contents of the globe, leaving the scleral shell and extraocular muscles in situ, then an implant is inserted.
- *Exenteration* is a more extensive operation involving removal of the eye and surrounding tissues/bone.

A badly injured eye may be enucleated, whilst a blind infected eye may require to be eviscerated. Exenteration would be required when a malignant tumour extends beyond the globe. The need for good cosmetic appearance to facilitate positive psychological health and wellbeing is essential. Both the range of socket and orbital implants, and counselling/support services will aid this, as any of these operations are life-changing (NAES). Sadiq et al. (2020) highlight that restoration of the person's normal appearance is not always possible, for example in cases of facial burns. A person's psychological status should be monitored using an appropriate tool such as the Hospital and Anxiety Disorder Scale (HADS), as Senra et al. (2022) recognise the impact that sight loss has on mental health.

The management is as for extensive penetrating injuries. The nurse may find that if patients have suffered severe pain in the eye, the relief from pain after surgical removal should promote positive outcomes (Sadiq et al. 2020).

Ocular Prosthetic Care

Expert support is available from the National Artificial Eye Service (NAES) in Blackpool in the UK (see Useful Websites).

Ocular prosthesis are individually designed to fit the socket, and the type again depends on the actual operation. The acrylic prosthesis is painted by an ocular artist to match the patient's other eye, so gives an excellent cosmetic result. The prosthesis is shell-like in shape and form. If an orbital implant has been inserted, the prosthesis will move with the natural eye because the extraocular muscles have been preserved and attached to the scleral implant.

It can take up to 18 months for the eye socket to fully heal and inflammation to resolve, so long-term care and follow-up are required. In addition, the ocular prosthesis may need changing if socket size shrinks. See NAES in Useful Websites for further information.

Contact through support groups and counselling may help to support the patient through their grief and loss, affirming that adaptation to the changes are possible (see Changing Faces in Useful Websites). Education, support and follow-up services are also provided by technicians in local ocular prosthetic departments with the aim of reducing anxiety, ensuring independence and offering reassurance.

Principles of Ocular Prosthetic Care

Healthcare professionals should be prepared to assist in or advise on the care of an ocular prosthesis. Principles of daily management are as follows.

Moorfield's NHS Trust website 'Removal of an eye' and NAES have useful information.

Removal of an Ocular Prosthesis

A special extractor is provided by the ocular prosthesis department. The eyelids are opened with the thumb and forefinger, and the lower edge of the ocular prosthesis is gently levered out with the aid of the extractor. If an extractor is not available, then a finger will suffice (see Fig. 15.7A).

Insertion of an Ocular Prosthesis

The eyelids are opened with the thumb and forefinger. The ocular prosthesis is inserted under the upper lid with the curve of the prosthesis towards the nose. The lower lid is depressed slightly. The prosthesis can then be slipped into position (see Fig. 15.7B).

Care of the Ocular Prosthesis/Shell

Patients are encouraged to wear the ocular prosthesis all the time, as it maintains the socket and lid volume, as after 24 hours they

Figure 15.7 (A) Removing an artificial eye. (B) Inserting an artificial eye. (Reproduced with kind permission of the National Artificial Eye Service (NAES) 2018.)

can contract down. When not in use for any short period of time, the prosthesis should be carefully stored in cotton wool or tissue to prevent scratching.

An ocular prosthesis can be cleaned frequently if the eye is sticky or can be left longer if it is worn all the time. Too much cleaning can irritate the socket. Use ordinary soap and warm water, rinsed afterwards using sterile water (https://www.naes.uk/eye-care/artificial-eye-care/). Chemical cleansers or disinfectants must not be used.

The ocular prosthesis can lose its high polish, due to buildup of proteins and salts from tears, so will require occasional polishing by a trained technician. Replacements can be obtained cost-free from the same department.

Care of the Socket

The socket needs to remain healthy, so regular review is required. Infection or irritation of the socket may result from scratches on the ocular prosthesis leading to ulceration and pain, so the patient can self-refer for support.

The socket can be irrigated with sterile normal saline to keep it clean and then dried thoroughly. Topical or oral antibiotics can be prescribed as required. The ocular prosthesis should not be inserted until any infection or irritation has cleared up.

Age-Related Conditions

Age-Related Macular Degeneration (AMD)

According to the WHO (2019), the ageing process presents the greatest risk to several eye conditions. Macular degeneration is one such age-related condition and is one of the leading causes of global vision impairment (WHO 2022) affecting over 700,000 people in the UK (Macular Society 2022). It is accountable for 50% of individuals on the SSI or SI register and the incidence is increasing due to the following factors (NICE 2018):

- Age – as life expectancy increases so does the incidence of ocular disease
- Presence of cardiovascular diseases such as hypertension

- Diabetes mellitus
- Smoking AMD
- Poor nutritional intake
- High alcohol consumption above government recommendations
- Lack of exercise
- Body mass index (BMI) 30 kg/m² or higher

Central and colour sight are affected, with the patient noticing difficulty with activities such as reading as well as problems in identifying faces.

In some cases, a new blood vessel membrane may develop and cause lifting of the central retina, which results in distorted and blurred central sight, but peripheral sight is maintained. AMD can occur in dry and wet form, as shown below, and in the presence of other eye conditions such as cataract and glaucoma, complicating the diagnosis, treatment and visual prognosis. The Macular Disease Society website is a patient information site that covers aspects of both clinical and psychosocial support through member discussion (see Useful Websites).

Dry AMD (Geographic Atrophy)

Dry AMD develops slowly and in most cases causes mild symptoms. However, advanced dry AMD can cause marked visual loss. If dry AMD is unilateral, there is an increased risk of developing it in the other. So referral to the ECLO service and long-term support is vital to empower the patient and their family (RNIB 2021a), as there is no current treatment for this type but research on stem cell and gene therapy may offer the possibility of viable treatment in the future.

Wet AMD (Neovascular)

Wet AMD is less common than dry AMD, but patients with this condition are most likely to develop severe visual impairment (Salmon 2023).

Retinal pigment epithelial cells (RPEs) degenerate with age and they deposit material on the underlying membrane, which accumulates to form yellowish white spots on the retina. Initially this process does not affect sight, but eventually the cell loss will result in atrophy of the RPE layer, as the cells are not replaced, which may then disperse pigment into the macula.

Nursing Care and Management

Assessment by the ophthalmic team determines the type of AMD and the necessary treatment. Full clinical history and nursing assessment including systemic health and lifestyle:

- Visual acuities for both near and distance
- Amsler grid – which is a grid pattern used to detect small changes in central sight
- Colour sight, as the majority of the cones (receptors for colour) are around the macula
- Clinical ocular examination using slit lamp and fundoscopy
- OCT for macula assessment (see Glaucoma)
- Fundal fluorescein angiogram (FFA) (see Diabetic retinopathy)

Clinical management guidelines for both dry and wet AMD are comprehensive yet complex and dependent on VA and ocular diagnosis, but an overview includes:

- NICE recommends options for treatment of wet AMD including ranibizumab, aflibercept and faricimab (NICE 2022f), which are classified as anti-vascular endothelial growth factor inhibitors or anti-VEGF therapy. These medications are given directly into the eye by intravitreal injection, every 8 weeks (NICE 2022f) and new injectable such as faricimab there is potential for longer gaps between treatments.
- *Photodynamic therapy (PDT)* – this treatment is the process of intravenous injection of verteporfin, a light-sensitive drug, circulated into the retinal vessels to allow photodynamic laser treatment of the degenerated tissue (Salmon 2019, Marsden 2017). However, PDT is not offered to patients who have late AMD and already receive in addition to anti-VEGF treatment.
- *High-dose vitamin and mineral supplements* – are believed to reduce the progression in advanced AMD and are recommended for use by those with intermediate AMD in one or both eyes, and those with advanced disease in one eye but not the other eye but not in early AMD (NICE 2018). Discussion with the ophthalmologist or specialist nurse is essential prior to starting treatment, as the AREDS-recommended vitamins have been linked with certain systemic side-effects (AREDS/AREDS2 2023). For example, high-dose beta carotene has been linked with an increased risk of lung cancer and is contraindicated in smokers.
- *LVA and referral to an ECLO* – to discuss registration as sight impaired, and to assess their individual needs and required support.
- Consider eccentric-viewing training, as this utilizes the peripheral retina, which still has functioning sight (NICE 2018).

Whilst SSI can now be prevented in a large number of people with wet AMD, a healthcare professional's supportive and educational role is key, especially at the point of diagnosis and possible registration, as grief, fear and depression are common (NICE 2018). Smoking cessation is recommended by NICE (2018) as deemed beneficial and linked to disease progression. Liaison with the ECLO and social services is essential to ensure that the SIP and their family are fully supported and empowered to live as independently as possible.

See Evolve website Critical thinking question 15.2

Malposition of the Eyelids

Entropion and ectropion are prevalent conditions in the older population, therefore early recognition is essential so an effective treatment plan and education can be implemented. Both conditions cause 'red eye', so it is important to consider differential diagnosis, to avoid misdiagnosis and management. The instillation of ocular lubricants or minor corrective lid surgery is often effective in treating the discomfort associated with the conditions.

Entropion

The eyelid, with the lid margin and lashes turned towards the globe, usually affects the lower lid and is caused by reduced elasticity of the connective tissue. Causes include the ageing process, trauma or a badly applied eye pad. The inturned eyelashes irritate the cornea, potentially causing discomfort, ulceration and keratitis (NICE 2021a).

Management

Discomfort can be relieved in the following ways (Bergstrom and Czyz 2022):

- Short-term intervention by the application of tape to the affected lid margin, to retract it in such a way that downward traction of the tape, when applied to the cheek, restores the normal position.
- Ocular lubricants, either ointment or drops to lubricate the eye.
- Topical antibiotics if the cornea is damaged by infection or abrasion.
- Botulinum toxin injection, as a short-term measure and alternative to taping.
- Repositioning of the lid by either a simple surgical procedure or eversion sutures.

Ectropion

This is the malposition of the eyelid when the lid margin is turned away from the globe, again mainly affecting the lower lid and associated with reduced elasticity of the connective tissue. Because the lid and punctum are malpositioned, tears overflow and run down the cheeks causing localised skin irritation. The individual constantly wipes their eyes, drawing the lid even further down and exacerbating the condition (McKelvie et al. 2018).

Management

The use of ocular lubricants may be required if the eye is infected or sore. Topical cream to the skin is soothing if excessive watering (epiphora) is causing excoriation. Cautery to the inner eyelid contracts the tarsal conjunctiva and inverts the lid. Minor oculoplastic surgery may be required to reposition the eyelid (Jackson 2020).

Dry Eye Syndrome (Keratitis Sicca)

This is a common and painful condition resulting from altered anatomical structure, function or disease (Craig et al. 2017). It is thought that 5%–50% of the global population affecting women more than men and prevalent in people with Asian heritage (Stapleton et al. 2017).

DED is commonly due to a tear film stability. Causes are the quantity of tear production, poor quality of tear film, or both, which results in symptoms of dry, burning and gritty eyes, occasionally with excessive epiphora, exacerbated by underlying systemic diseases, as well as environmental aspects of humidity, wind and smoke.

The diagnosis can be complex as the condition is associated with systemic disease such as rheumatoid arthritis and Sjögren's syndrome. Symptoms are dry eyes and mouth, as well as dryness of joints and major organs (Salmon 2023).

Nursing Assessments and Management

Dry eyes can impact on a person's activities of daily living and psychological well being.

Diagnosis includes the assessment of tear film, which should be performed by an appropriately trained health care professional.

The assessment involve a Schirmer's test, using filter paper to check tear production and quality. The tear break up time is tested by instilling fluorescein eye drops and then using a cobalt blue light to look at tear distribution across the cornea.

Nursing Care and Management

The patient's care is dependent upon the severity and actual cause of the condition, but consists of one or more of the following (not exhaustive) as advised by Salmon (2023):

Patient Education

Explanation of DED and the causes; adherence to prescribed treatment, regular breaks from screen use; workplace environmental support, advice on conserving tears, for example reducing room temperature.

Hypromellose eye drops and viscose type ointments can be used at night to lubricate eyes. In more severe cases, topical cyclosporine is used to reduce inflammation.

- Instillation of ocular lubricants four times a day or as required and at night. Often a preservative-free preparation is needed as some types of artificial tears contain preservatives such as benzalkonium hexachloride, and may cause a toxicity reaction within the cornea.
- Often topical steroids or antibiotics are required in cases of ocular inflammation or infection.
- Punctal occlusion, inserting collagen or silicone plugs into the upper and lower punctum, preventing drainage of tears. These can last 2–6 months.
- Punctal cautery to seal the puncta, in extreme cases of dry eye.
- Corrective surgery, e.g. tarsorrhaphy, which involves partial closure of the lids, thereby decreasing the surface area of the cornea from which the tear film evaporates.
- Long-term use of CL may be contraindicated, due to the quality of tear film. However, this should be assessed on an individual basis.
- Sunglasses to reduce glare can be beneficial.

Systemic Disease and Disorders of the Eye

The eye is a sensitive indicator of systemic disease, as sight changes or abnormal appearance of the retina or optic disc may be the first manifestation. In this section, ophthalmic conditions associated with some of the more common systemic diseases will be described. Other conditions are described in Table 15.3. The reader should refer to relevant chapters in the present text for further information on the underlying systemic disease.

Diabetes Mellitus

The incidence of diabetes, especially type 2, is increasing globally and nationally due to complex systemic diseases and lifestyle factors (see Chapter 6). It is recognised that poorly controlled diabetes can lead to diabetic retinopathy, early cataract development, vascularisation of the iris (rubeosis) and a high incidence of minor eye conditions such as chalazion.

Diabetic Retinopathy (DR)

Elevated blood sugar levels, associated with prolonged poor diabetic control and poorly managed systemic diseases such as hypertension and hyperlipidaemia, damage the blood vessel basement membrane. In the retina, this leads to leakage and the formation of fatty and haemorrhagic lesions. The patient will usually complain of gradual and painless loss of sight – unless there is bleeding into the vitreous, in which case sight loss is sudden. The diagnosis of DR can be confirmed by assessment of central and peripheral vision, fundal imagery and in some cases fluorescein angiography, whereby photos of the retinal blood vessels are taken immediately after intravenous injection of fluorescein dye (NICE 2022f). DR is the leading cause of preventable blindness in the working population in developed countries.

Background or Nonproliferative Diabetic Retinopathy (NPDR)

The small retinal vessels become fragile, microaneurysms form and leakage occurs, causing localised oedema and haemorrhages. If these changes are in the peripheral retina they may not cause vision loss. Moderate to severe NPDR can have ischaemic features that can cause changes to the fovea and macula.

Maculopathy

This is the commonest cause of blindness in type 2 diabetes. The leakage round the macula will result in the subsequent deposit of hard exudates within the macula, thereby reducing central visual function

Proliferative Retinopathy

This stage of DR can result in sight-threatening vision loss. In this phase, there is further deterioration as new blood vessels and fibrous bands form in response to breakdown and occlusion of the normal retinal circulation.

Advanced Diabetic Retinopathy

The main complications arising from the proliferative phase are bleeding into the vitreous and tractional RD which is a result of scar tissue formation from the bleeding. Eventually, proliferative vascularisation can affect the angle of the eye by blocking the trabecular meshwork and causing secondary glaucoma.

Nursing Care and Management

Early diagnosis is critical and patients are encouraged to attend their annual DR screening programme (Public Health England 2021). In relation to health status, NICE (2022g) advocate the following health promotion strategy must be monitored: blood pressure, dietary advice, exercise, control of cardiovascular/complex health needs, HbA1c measurements, self-monitoring of blood capillary glucose (BCG) and compliance with medication.

Severe vitreous haemorrhage with subsequent scar formation and tractional RD may be treated by removing the vitreous (vitrectomy), as previously discussed.

Nursing Management and Health Promotion: Diabetic Retinopathy

Patient Education

As diabetes can affect many body systems, patient education is a collaborative MDT approach. The resulting effects on the patient's vision from the retinopathy can be worrying but they must be aware of the predisposing factors. Patients, their families and

TABLE 15.3	Further Eye Problems Secondary to Systemic Diseases		
Disorder	**Main Ophthalmic Clinical Features**	**Cause**	**Treatment**
Thyroid function imbalance (Graves' disease)	Upper lid retraction Exposure keratitis Swelling of lids and conjunctiva Exophthalmos compression of optic nerve Diplopia	Sympathetic nerve innervation Exposure of eyeball Infiltration of lymphocytes in orbital tissue and associated oedema Infiltration of lymphocytes in muscle tissue leading to fibrosis	Lubricating drops during day and antibiotic ointment nightly As above Partial tarsorrhaphy Systemic steroids Surgical decompression Prism spectacles Botulinum A neurotoxin injection into the appropriate lid muscle Strabismus surgery
Nephritis	Blurred vision Papilloedema Retinal haemorrhage Retinal detachment	Hypertension	Reduce hypertension Laser treatment Vitrectomy Surgical repair of detachment
Multiple sclerosis	Uniocular Small unequal pupils: do not react to light but do with accommodation, unable to dilate with atropine Optic neuritis Rapid reduction of central sight Sudden onset of pain especially when looking upwards Central scotoma Diplopia	Localised demyelinating lesion to the cranial nerves III IV VI	Symptoms may recover spontaneously but will always recur Systemic painkillers Prism spectacles Botulinum A neurotoxin injection Strabismus surgery
Intracranial aneurysm	Uniocular/binocular – diplopia Blurred sight Ptosis Visual field defects	Pressure on visual pathway Pressure on cranial nerves III IV VI	Detection and clipping of aneurysm Botulinum A neurotoxin injection Strabismus surgery
Migraine	Headache with visual disturbances – Characteristic aura: multicoloured, jagged shape, firework-like	Idiopathic; possibly chemical changes in the brain caused by various triggers, e.g. stress, or dietary, e.g. eating oranges or chocolate	Feverfew herbal remedy Medication Rest

carers should be aware of the signs and symptoms of retinal bleeds and how to seek emergency advice. Annual attendance at a diabetic screening appointment is essential to assess and monitor diabetic eye health.

Laser is often the first line of treatment to limit the growth of new blood vessels. However, as Batterbury and Murphy (2018) point out, the success of DR screening programmes has been pivotal in improving sight outcomes and need for surgical interventions.

Cerebrovascular Accident (CVA) or Cerebrovascular Insult (CVI)

A CVA/CVI involves an interruption of the blood supply to a part of the brain and may be caused by blockage or rupture of a blood vessel, either ischaemic or haemorrhagic. If the damage has involved the visual pathways, then sight will be affected and the damage may be permanent. When a patient suffers a TIA, sight may be temporarily affected but will usually be restored when the attack subsides (see Chapter 2, Nursing Patients With Cardiovascular Disorders). Using the Face, Arm, Speech and Time (FAST) assessment tool can identify changes, which require urgent medical attention, such as ptosis and abnormal pupillary reactions (NICE 2022i).

❖ Nursing Management and Health Promotion: CVA/CVI

The extent of any sight deficit can vary from hemianopia, meaning a loss of half the visual field in both eyes, diplopia which is double vision due to cranial nerves III, IV and VI, and extraocular muscles being affected and visual processing, when an object can be seen but not interpreted due to an altered visual pathway to the occipital lobe. Individualised assessment of the patient's activities of daily living, including visual assessment is essential to holistic patient care. Patients with diplopia will have blurred vision; people with a hemianopia may ignore the affected side. The nursing care therefore must include psychological support and physical interventions for visual impairment and falls prevention strategies.

🌐 **See Evolve website Critical thinking question 15.3**

Hypertension and the Eye

Hypertensive retinopathy is a clinical diagnosis, resulting from visual assessment and fundoscopy, which reveals changes to the ophthalmic arteries, as choroidal and retinal blood supply is impaired. On fundoscopy, haemorrhages and exudates can be visible and widespread narrowing of the arteries.

This is linked to systemic health conditions of smoking, atherosclerosis, dyslipidaemia and hyperglycaemia, so a holistic management pathway is required.

Signs and symptoms can present as blurred altered sight, visual field defects, headaches and facial flushing, and in severe cases, sudden, painless and unilateral loss of sight which can be central retinal vein occlusion (CRVO) or central retinal artery occlusion (CRAO).

Hypertension can cause subconjunctival haemorrhages (SCH), when capillaries between the conjunctiva and sclera rupture. Also hypertension can cause cataracts, ocular hypertension and glaucoma. However, effective management of hypertension may prevent these ocular diseases and systemic complications (NICE 2016a).

Temporal Arteritis (Giant Cell Arteritis (GCA))

Salmon (2023) asserts that GCA is a progressive systemic disease affecting the over-50 age group in which the middle layer of medium-sized arteries arising from the aorta involving the ophthalmic artery, becomes inflamed. This leads to ischaemia causing optic neuropathy and permanent loss of vision. This sudden sight loss can be preceded by, or accompany, polymyalgia rheumatica (stiff aching muscles, especially around the shoulders) (Ameer et al. 2021).

Clinical Features

Patients often complain of general malaise, unintentional weight loss and lethargy, or a 'flu-like' illness which may last for a few days or weeks and which precedes a sustained sight disturbance. This is in contrast to the prodromal phase during which symptoms, which signal the impending onset of the condition, include:
- Episodes of blurred sight.
- Unilateral temporal or occipital headache (of varying severity).
- Absent temporal pulses.
- Scalp tenderness.
- Jaw claudication whereby pain is experienced on chewing due to insufficient blood supply to the muscles of the jaw.
- Blood tests to detect inflammation include ESR (erythrocyte sedation rate) and CRP (creatine reactive protein). The results will be raised (Ameer et al. (2021).

The loss of sight is sudden in onset, usually affecting one eye before the other. The length of time between both eyes being affected is extremely variable, ranging from several hours to several days (Ameer 2021; Salmon 2023).

Nursing Care and Management
- Pain assessment and management
- Visual assessment and support
- Psychological support
- Oral/IV corticosteroids and associated care of the IV, observation of medication side-effects

HIV

Ophthalmic complications affecting both the adnexa, anterior segment and posterior segment of the eye and the retina and can be the first sign of an immunity disorder, often before a HIV diagnosis (Batterbury and Murphy 2018). As treatments for HIV advance, it is thought that severe ophthalmic complications may be prevented.

HIV Retinopathy

Clinical signs are yellowish-grey, cotton wool-like spots, dot-like haemorrhages and microaneurysms over the retina. Sight remains normal unless the macula is involved. Some patients respond to antiviral agents.

Opportunistic Infections

HIV/AIDS patients are prone to all types of eye infections. The most common infections include severe herpes zoster ophthalmicus, herpes simplex, *Candida* retinitis, *Toxoplasma* chorioretinitis and cytomegalovirus (CMV) retinitis.

AIDS-Related Neoplasms

Kaposi's sarcoma may involve any of the ocular structures. Treatment may include combined antiretroviral therapy (cART), a combination of medications that block and delay the development of the condition.

Nursing Management and Health Promotion: HIV-Related Eye Diseases

The general principles of nursing a patient with HIV, together with the principles of nursing a patient with eye infections, apply in all of the above. Holistic and individualised care should be available for the patients and their family/partners/carers. Patients may need psychological and practical support regarding temporary or permanent sight loss arising from the HIV/AIDS-related ophthalmic conditions.

Summary: Key Nursing Issues

- The impact of sight loss on activities in everyday life should not be underestimated. SI patients will need additional support with regard to the practical and communication issues that arise from sensory deficit. As this chapter has demonstrated, sight loss is associated with systemic and often complex health conditions, therefore making it every healthcare professional's responsibility to promptly recognise any changes in signs and symptoms (State of the Nation Eye Health 2021); then refer to the appropriate specialist service, as delay can result in irreparable damage and permanent loss of sight.
- The specialism of ophthalmology has been shown to be a leader in role development, with ophthalmologists, opticians, optometrists, orthoptists, ophthalmic nurses and ophthalmic technicians, working to provide high-level clinical services, which are evidence-based, holistic and person-centred, aiming to facilitate seamless care.

Reflection and Learning – What Next?

- **Reflect** upon what you have learnt and how this will support your professional development, it could be used for revalidation purposes.
- **Test** your knowledge by visiting the **Evolve** website 🌐, to see the additional materials, answer the multiple choice questions and critical thinking questions.
- **Apply and share** this knowledge in the management of patient care with professional colleagues and patients/carers.
- **Consolidate** your learning by looking at some of the references and specialist websites.

References

Age-related eye disease studies (AREDS/AREDS2) (2023). https://www.nei.nih.gov/research/clinical-trials/age-related-eye-disease-studies-aredsareds2.

Alzheimer's society (2023) About Dementia. https://www.alzheimers.org.uk/about-dementia/types-dementia/what-is-dementia.

Ameer MA, Peterfy RJ, Bansal P, et al. Temporal Arteritis. *StatPearls*. Treasure Island (FL): StatPearls Publishing; 2021:2022 PMID: 29083688.

Armitage J, Winton HL, Jones M, et al. Corneal transplant follow-up study II (CTFS II): a prospective clinical trial to determine the influence of HLA class II matching on corneal transplant rejection: baseline donor and recipient characteristics. *Br J Ophthalmol.* 2019;103(1):132–136.

Baradaran-Rafil A, Eslani M, Haq Z, et al. Current and upcoming therapies for ocular surface chemical injuries. *Ocul Surf.* 2017;15(1): 48–64.

Batterbury M, Murphy C. *Ophthalmology: An illustrated text.* 4th ed. Elsevier; 2018.

Bergstrom R, Czyz CN. *Entropion.* StatPearls Publishers; 2022. https://www.ncbi.nlm.nih.gov/books/NBK470352/.

Bradford S, Mikula E, Juhasz T, et al. Nonlinear optical crosslinking (NLO CXL) for correcting refractive errors. *Exp Eye Res.* 2020;199 Elsevier.

British National Formulary (BNF)/NICE (2023) Chloramphenicol. https://bnf.nice.org.uk/drugs/chloramphenicol/.

Burton MJ, Faal HB, Ramke J, Ravilla T, Holland P, Wang N, West SK, Bourne RR, Congdon NG, Foster A. Announcing the Lancet global health Commission on global eye health. *Lancet Glob Health.* 2019;7(12):e1612–e1613.

Centre for perioperative care (CPOC) (2021) Pre-operative assessment and optimization of adult surgery. https://www.cpoc.org.uk/preoperative-assessment-and-optimisation-adult-surgery.

Chang P, Qian S, Wang Y, et al. Accuracy of new-generation intraocular lens calculation formulas in eyes with variations in predicted refraction. *Graefes Arch Clin Exp Ophthalmol.* 2023;261:127–135. doi:10.1007/s00417-022-05748-w.

Chen EJ, Fasiuddin A. Management of traumatic Hyphaema and prevention of its complications. *Cureus.* 2021;13(6):e15771.

Chen RI, Gedde SJ. Assessment of visual field progression in glaucoma. *Curr Opin Ophthalmol.* March 2023;34(2):103–108.

College of Optometrists (2021). Clinical management guidelines. Uveitis (anterior, acute and recurrent). https://www.college-optometrists.org.

Control of Substances Hazardous to Health (COSHH) Regulations. 2002. https://www.hse.gov.uk.

Craig J, Kelly K, Esen K, et al. (2017) DEWS II Definition and Classification Report The Ocular Surface 15 (2017) 276e283.

Data Protection Act (2018) https://www.legislation.gov.uk/ukpga/2018/12/contents/enacted.

Dave S, Binns A, Vinuela-Navarro V, et al. What advice is currently given to patients with age-related macular degeneration (AMD) by eyecare practitioners, and how effective is it at bringing about a change in lifestyle? A systematic review. *Nutrients, [online].* 2022;14(21):4652. doi:10.3390/nu14214652.

Davis SA, Sleath B, Carpenter DM, et al. Drop instillation and glaucoma. *Current Opinion Ophthalmol.* 2018;29(2):171–177.

Dickson SJ, Dewar C, Richardson A, et al. Agreement and validity of electronic patient self-triage (eTriage) with nurse triage in two UK emergency departments: a retrospective study. *Eur J Emerg Med.* 2022. doi:10.1097/MEJ.0000000000000863.

Dua HS, Ting DSJ, Saadi AA, et al. Chemical eye injury: pathophysiology, assessment and management. *Eye.* 2020;34(11):2001–2019.

English V, Johnson E, Blair LS, et al. Is an opt-out system likely to increase organ donation? *BMJ.* 2019;364:1967.

Environment and Safety Information Act 1988. https://www.legislation.gov.uk/ukpga/1988/30/contents.

Equality Act 2010. www.gov.uk/guidance/equality act 2010.

Farris W, Waymack JR. Central Retinal Artery Occlusion. *StatPearls [Internet].* Treasure Island (FL): StatPearls Publishing; 2022. 2022 Jan-. https://www.ncbi.nlm.nih.gov/books/NBK470354/.

Field D, Tillotson J, Whittingham E. *Eye Emergencies: The practitioner's guide.* Keswick: M&K publishing; 2015.

Gamalero L, et al. Evidence-based treatment for uveitis. *IMAJ.* 2019;21 July.

General Medical Council (GMC) (2016) Guidance for doctors who offer cosmetic interventions. www.gmc.uk.org/Guidance_for_doctors_who_offer_cosmetic_interventions_210316.pdf_65254111.pdf.

Goldstein MH, et al. Ocular benzalkonium chloride exposure: problems and solutions. *Eye.* 2022;36:361–368. doi:10.1038/s41433-021-01668-x.

Gov.UK (2022) Eye conditions and driving. https://www.gov.uk/eye-conditions-and-driving.

Gragg J, Blair K, Baker MB. *Hyphaema. StatPearls [Internet].* Treasure Island (FL): StatPearls Publishing; 2022. https://www.ncbi.nlm.nih.gov/books/NBK507802/.

Health and Care Professions Council (HCPC). Standards of Conduct, Performance and Ethics; 2016. http://www.hcpc-uk.org/aboutregistration/standards/standardsofconductperformanceandethics/.

Health and Safety at Work Act (1974). https://www.legislation.gov.uk/ukpga/1974/37.

Health and Safety Executive. Working with Display Screen Equipment (DSE); 2013. www.hse.gov.uk/pubns/indg36.pdf.

Health and Safety Executive. COSHH assessment: Identifying hazard and assessing risk; 2018. http://www.hse.gov.uk/coshh/basics/assessment.htm.

Human Tissue Authority (2020) Code F, part two. https://www.hta.gov.uk/guidance-professionals/codes-practice-standards-and-legislation/codes-practice. Accessed 1/11/22.

IAPB (International Agency for the Prevention of Blindness). What is Vision 2020? 2018 accessed. https://www.iapb.org/global-initiatives/vision-2020/what-is-vision-2020/.

Idress S, Kuriyan A, Schwartz S, et al. Recent developments in vitero-retinal surgery. In: Grzybowski A, ed. *Current Concepts in Ophthalmology.* Cham: Springer; 2020.

Jackson TL. *Moorfields Manual of Ophthalmology.* 3rd ed. India: Jaypee Brothers Medical Publishers; 2020.

Jones L, Ditzel-Finn L, Enoch J, et al. An overview of psychological and social factors in Charles Bonnet syndrome. *Ther Adv Ophthalmol.* 2021;13. doi:10.1177/25158414211034715.

Kandel H, Nguyen V, Piermarocchi S, et al. Quality of life impact of eye diseases: a Save Sight Registries study. *Clin Experiment Ophthalmol.* 2022;50(4):386–397.

Kates MM, Tuli S. Complications of Contact Lenses. *JAMA.* 2021; 325(18):1912.

Kousha O, Kousha Z, Paddle J. Exposure keratopathy: Incidence, risk factors and impact of protocolised care on exposure keratopathy in critically ill adults. *J Crit Care.* 2018;44:413–418.

Kunjumen T, Okech M, Diallo K, et al. Global experiences in health workforce policy, planning and management using the Workload Indicators of Staffing Need (WISN) method, and way forward. *Hum Resour Health.* 2022;19(Suppl 1):152.

Kwok JM, Chew HF. Chemical injuries of the eye. *CMAJ.* 2019; 191(37):E1028.

Lake D. Medico-legal aspects of corneal refractive laser eye surgery. *J Patient Saf Risk Manag.* 2018;23(2):66–70.

Lindsay RK, Allen PM, Koyanagi A, Smith L. Feasibility of physical activity promotion in eyecare and sight loss services to improve the health of adults with sight loss: a survey. *Disabil Rehabil.* 2022. doi:10.1080/09638288.2022.2104939.

Liu S, Ling Y Wong, Walkden A. Current Perspectives on Corneal Transplantation, *Clinical Ophthalmology.* 2022;16:631-646.

Macular society (2022) Incidence of macular degeneration. https://www.macularsociety.org/macular-disease/macular-conditions/.

Makivić I, Klemenc-Ketiš Z. Development and validation of the scale for measuring biopsychosocial approach of family physicians to their patients. *Fam Med Community Health.* 2022;10(2):e001407.

Margolin E. Approach to patient with diplopia. *J Neurol Sci.* 2020;417.

Manchester Triage System (MTS). https://www.triagenet.net/classroom/mod/page/view.php?id=1884.

Marsden J. *Ophthalmic care.* 2nd ed. Keswick: M&K publishing; 2017.

McKelvie J, Papchenko T, Carroll S, et al. (2018) Cicatricial ectropion surgery: a prospective study of long-term symptom control, patient satisfaction and anatomical success.

Moorfields Eye Hospital (2021) Guidelines for blepharitis. https://www.moorfields.nhs.uk/condition/blepharitis-0.

Newman-Casey P, Niziol M, Lee P, et al. The impact of the support, educate, empower personalized glaucoma coaching pilot study on glaucoma medication adherence. *Presented at: American Glaucoma Society Annual Meeting, February 2020, Washington, DC*; 2020.

Ng JY, Ting DSJ, Vaideanu-Collins D, et al. (2019) Self-tattooing of eyeball with inadvertent corneoscleral perforation: the implication of social media Published online: 5 June 2019 The Royal College of Ophthalmologists 2019.

National Institute for Health and Care Excellence (NICE). Hypertension in adults: diagnosis and management. Guidance NG136. 2023. https://www.nice.org.uk/guidance/ng136.

National Institute for Health and Care Excellence (NICE) (2017) Falls in older people, QS86. https://cks.nice.org.uk/topics/falls-risk-assessment/.

NHS Blood and Transplant. https://www.organdonation.nhs.uk/get-involved/news/new-nhs-campaign-urges-people-to-talk-to-family-and-leave-them-certain-about-organ-donation/.

National Institute for Health and Care Excellence (NICE). Stroke and transient ischaemic attack in over 16s: diagnosis and initial management. NG128. April 2022i. https://www.nice.org.uk/guidance/ng128.

National Institute for Health and Care Excellence (NICE). Age related macular degeneration. NICE guideline [NG82]; 2018. https://www.nice.org.uk/guidance/ng82/chapter/Recommendations.

National Institute for Health and Care Excellence (NICE). Retinal detachment NICE guideline, 2019. https://cks.nice.org.uk/topics/retinal-detachment/.

National Institute for Health and Care Excellence (NICE) (2020) Chalazions. https://cks.nice.org.uk/topics/meibomian-cyst-chalazion/.

National Institute for Health and Care Excellence (NICE) (2021a) Management of red eye. https://cks.nice.org.uk/topics/red-eye/management/management-of-red-eye/2021.

National Institute for Health and Care Excellence (NICE) (2021b), Uveitis. https://cks.nice.org.uk/topics/uveitis/.

National Institute for Health and Care Excellence (NICE) (2021c). https://cks.nice.org.uk/topics/herpes-simplex-ocular/management/management/on 12/10/22.

National Institute for Health and Care Excellence (NICE) (2022a) Social work with adults experiencing complex needs. NG216. https://cks.nice.org.uk/topics/learning-disabilities/.

National Institute for Health and Care Excellence (NICE). Cataracts; 2022b. https://cks.nice.org.uk/topics/cataracts/.

National Institute for Health and Care Excellence (NICE) (2022c) Glaucoma: diagnosis and management NICE guideline [NG81] https://www.nice.org.uk/guidance/ng81/.

National Institute for Health and Care Excellence (NICE) (2022d) Conjunctivitis. https://cks.nice.org.uk/topics/conjunctivitis-infective/.

National Institute for Health and Care Excellence (NICE) (2022e) Shingles. https://cks.nice.org.uk/topics/shingles/management/management/#antiviral-treatment.

National Institute for Health and Care Excellence (NICE) (2022f) Faricimab for treating wet age-related macular degeneration Technology appraisal guidance [TA800]. https://www.nice.org.uk/guidance/ta800/resources.

National Institute for Health and Care Excellence (NICE) (2022g) Type 2 Diabetes in Adults, management. NICE [NG28]. https://www.nice.org.uk/guidance/ng28.

Nizami, A, and Gulani AC. (2022) Cataract. https://www.ncbi.nlm.nih.gov/books/NBK539699/.

Nursing and Midwifery Council (NMC) (2018). *The Code: Professional Standards of Practice and Behaviour for Nurses, Midwives and Nursing Associates.* https://www.nmc.org.uk/globalassets/sitedocuments/nmc-publications/nmc-code.pdf.

Office for National Statistics (2020) Population estimates for the UK, England and Wales, Scotland and Northern Ireland: mid 2020.

Park MY, Kim WJ, Lee E, et al. Association between use of benzodiazepines and occurrence of acute angle closure glaucoma in the elderly: A population-based study. *J Psychosom Res.* 2019;122(2019):1–5 Elsevier.

Parker RT, McCall DP, Samarawickrama C. Eye injury from toxic chemical mistaken for eye drops. *Med J Aust.* 2018;208:369.

Patil A, Goldust M, Wollina U. Herpes zoster: A Review of Clinical Manifestations and Management. *Viruses.* 2022;14(12):192.

Peate I, Evans S. *Fundamentals of Anatomy and Physiology: For Nursing and Healthcare students.* 3rd ed. Wiley Blackwell; 2020.

Personal Protective Equipment Work Regulations 2002. http://www.legislation.gov.uk/uksi/2002/1144/contents/made.

Płaszewska-Żywko L, Sega A, Bukowa A, Wojnar-Gruszka K, Podstawa M, Kózka M. Risk factors of eye complications in patients treated in the intensive care unit. *Int J Environ Res Public Health. [online].* 2021;18(21):11178.

Public Health England. Chemical hazards; 2018. https://www.gov.uk/topic/health-protection/chemical-hazards.

Public Health England (2021) NHS Diabetic Eye Screening Programme https://www.gov.uk/guidance/diabetic-eye-screening-programme-overview.

Reporting of Injuries, Disease and Dangerous Occurrences Regulations (RIDDOR) 2013. www.hse.gov.uk/riddor/.

Royal College of Nursing (RCN) (2022) Pariety of Esteem. https://www.rcn.org.uk/clinical-topics/Mental-Health/Parity-of-esteem.

Royal College of Ophthalmologists (2022) Professional standards for refractive surgery. https://www.rcophth.ac.uk/resources-listing/professional-standards-for-refractive-surgery/.

Royal National Institute of Blind People (RNIB). Protect your eyes from the sun; 2019. https://www.rnib.org.uk/eye-health/looking-after-your-eyes/protect-your-eyes-sun.

Royal National Institute of Blind People (RNIB) (2021a) Fact sheet for Reasonable adjustments/compliance with equality act. https://www.rnib.org.uk/professionals/health-social-care-education-professionals/equality-act-compliance/.

Royal National Institute of Blind People (RNIB) (2021a) Eye Clinic Liaison Officer (ECLO) service UK evaluation report. https://media.rnib.org.uk/documents/APDF-UK_ECLO_Evaluation_Report201920_March_2021_FINAL.pdf.

Royal National Institute of Blind People (RNIB) Sight Loss Data. (2021b) version 4.3. https://www.rnib.org.uk/datatool.

Royal National Institute of Blind People (RNIB) (2022) https://www.rnib.org.uk/your-eyes/how-to-keep-your-eyes-healthy/protect-your-eyes-from-the-sun/.

Royal National Institute of Blind People (RNIB) (2022a) Corneal transplant. https://www.rnib.org.uk/your-eyes/eye-conditions-az/corneal-transplant/#when-is-a-corneal-transplant-needed.

Royal National Institute of Blind People (RNIB) (2022b) Cataracts. https://www.rnib.org.uk/your-eyes/eye-conditions-az/cataracts/.

Royal National Institute of Blind People (RNIB) (2022c) Dementia and sight loss information. https://www.rnib.org.uk/your-eyes/navigating-sight-loss/dementia-and-sight-loss/.

Royal College of Optometrists (RCOpto). (2022). Ocular foreign bodies. https://www.college-optometrists.org/clinical-guidance/clinical-management_guidelines/corneal_orothersuperficialocular_foreignbody.

Royal College of Physicians. (2017) Bedside vision check for falls prevention: assessment tool https://www.rcplondon.ac.uk/projects/outputs/bedside-vision-check-falls-prevention-assessment-tool.

Sadiq SA, Pattinson R, Poole HM, et al. Psychological distress and coping following eye removal surgery. *Orbit.* 2020;39(3):175–182.

Salmon J. *Kanski's clinical Ophthalmology: A systematic approach.* 9th ed. Elsevier; 2019.

Salmon J. *Kanski's Synopsis of Clinical Ophthalmology*. 4th ed. Elsevier; 2023.

Sansome SG, Lin P-F. Eye care in the intensive care unit during COVID-19 pandemic. *Br J Hosp Med*. 2020;81(6). doi:10.12968/hmed.2020.0228.

Senra, H, HernandezMoreno, L, Moreno, N, Filipe Macedo, A., (2022) Anxiety levels moderate the association between visual acuity and healthrelated quality of life in chronic eye disease patients (2022). https://doi.org/10.1038/s41598-022-06252-1.

Sharma B, Soni D, Saxena H, et al. Impact of corneal refractive surgery on the precorneal tear film. *Indian J Ophthalmol*. 2020;68:2804–2812.

Shimada Y, Seno Y, Miizuguchi T, et al. Patient adherence to the face-down positioning after macular hole surgery. *Clin Ophthalmol*. 2017; 11:1099–1104.

Shirodkar A. The Red Eye: Basic Algorithm on How to Differentiate Main Conditions from Each Other. In: Shirodkar A, Williams G, eds. *Practical Emergency Ophthalmology Handbook An Algorithm Based Approach to Ophthalmic Emergencies*. Boco Raton: CRC Press; 2019.

Specsavers (2022) Contact lens care. https://www.specsavers.co.uk/contact-lenses/care/wearing-contact-lenses.

Stapleton F, Alves M, Bunya VY, et al. TFOS DEWS II Epidemiology Report. *Ocul Surf*. 2017;15(3):334–365. doi:10.1016/j.jtos.2017.05.003. 2017 Jul, Epub 2017 Jul 20. PMID: 28736337.

State of the Nation Eye Health (2017). A year in review. RNIB and Specsavers. https://www.rnib.org.uk/.

State of the Nation Eye Health (2021). https://www.specsavers.co.uk/eye-health/state-of-the-uks-eye-health-2021.

Szentmary N, et al. Acanthamoeba keratitis – Clinical signs, Differential diagnosis and treatment. *J Curr Ophthalmol*. 2019;31:16–33. www.sciencedirect.com.

Tuft S, Somerville TF, Li O, et al. Bacterial keratitis: identifying the areas of clinical uncertainty. *Prog Retin Eye Res*. 2021;89:101031.

Turbert (2020) The Sun, UV Light and Your Eyes. https://www.aao.org/eye-health/tips-prevention/sun. 8/11/22.

Waterman H, Evans JR, Gray TA, et al. Interventions for improving adherence to ocular hypotensive therapy. *Cochrane Database Syst Rev*. 2013;30(4).

Waterman H, Ballinger C, Brundle C, et al. A feasibility study to prevent falls in older people who are sight impaired: the VIP2UK randomised controlled trial. *Trials*. 2016;17(1):464.

Wood R. Modelling the impact of COVID-19 on elective waiting times. *J Simulation*. 2022;16(1):101–109.

World Health Organisation (WHO). More can be done to restrict sunbeds to prevent increasing rates of skin cancer; 2017. https://www.who.int/phe/news/sunbeds-skin-cancer/en/.

World Health Organisation (WHO). Blindness and vision impairment: key facts; 2018. https://www.who.int/news-room/fact-sheets/detail/blindness-and-visual-impairment.

World Health Organisation (WHO) (2019) World Report on Vision. Geneva: World Health Organisation; 2019. Licence: CC BY-NC-SA 3.0 IGO.

World Health Organisation (WHO; 2022). Blindness and vision impairment: key facts; 2022. https://www.who.int/news-room/fact-sheets/detail/blindness-and-visual-impairment#.

Yip JLY, Khawaja AP, Chan MPY, et al. Cross sectional and longitudinal associations between cardiovascular risks factors and age-related macular degeneration in the EPIC-Norfolk Eye study. *PLoS One*. 2015;10(7). https://doaj.org/article/20b2868b7798458829f728406361d1415.

Useful Websites

Alzheimer's Society, www.alzheimers.org.uk

British National Formulary, https://bnf.nice.org.uk/

Changing Faces, https://www.changingfaces.org.uk/

College of Optometrists, https://www.college-optometrists.org/guidance/clinical-management-guidelines.html

Colour vision, www.colour-blindness

DrinkAware, www.drinkaware.co.uk

Driver and Vehicle Licensing Agency (DVLA), www.gov.uk/DVLA

Equality Act 2010, https://www.gov.uk/guidance/equality-act-2010-guidance

General Medical Council, https://gmc-uk.org

Guide Dogs, https://www.guidedogs.org.uk/

Health and Care Professions Council, https://www.hcpc-uk.org

Henshaws Knowledge Village, https://mft.nhs.uk/royal-eye/services/henshaws/

Macular Disease Society, https://www.macularsociety.org/age-related-macular-degeneration

Manchester Triage tool, https://www.triagenet.net/classroom/

Max and Keira's law. https://www.organdonation.nhs.uk/uk-laws/organ-donation-law-in-england/timeline-for-max-and-keiras-law/

Morgan lens for eye irrigation, http://www.morganlens.com

National Artificial Eye Service (NAES), https://www.naes.nhs.uk/

National Eye Institute, https://nei.nih.gov

NHS, www.nhs.uk/conditions/vision-loss/

National Institute for Health and Care Excellence (NICE), https://www.nice.org.uk/guidance

Organ and tissue donation, https://www.nhsbt.nhs.uk/

Patient UK, https://patient.info/

Royal College of Ophthalmologists, https://www.rcophth.ac.uk

Royal National Institute of Blind People (RNIB), https://www.rnib.org.uk

Toxbase: Toxicology database of the National Poisons Information Service, www.toxbase.org

World Health Organization, https://www.who.int/news-room/fact-sheets/detail/blindness-and-visual-impairment

16

Nursing Patients With Disorders of the Ear, Nose and Throat

HILARY HARKIN, LUCY VICTORIA JAMIESON

CHAPTER OUTLINE

Introduction

Problems of the ear, nose and throat (ENT) are very common; most people at some time in their lives suffer from nosebleeds, sore throats or earache. Many of these problems will be dealt with successfully at home, often with the advice of a pharmacist, practice nurse or general practitioner (GP). Other ENT problems, however, can be life-threatening, requiring an immediate visit to an emergency department (ED), surgery and, in some cases, a period of nursing care at home following discharge.

To nurse ENT patients effectively in a home or hospital setting, a basic knowledge of the anatomy and physiology of the relevant structures, along with a thorough understanding of the clinical features of common disorders, is essential. The health visitor, community nurse, school nurse or occupational health nurse is often in a position to detect problems before the medical practitioner or even the patient is aware of them. ENT symptoms are being commonly seen in patients with long COVID. Ten per cent of patients still have issues with taste and smell after being infected with the COVID virus (Tan et al. 2022).

This chapter will outline the basic structure and function of the ENT, describing the most commonly encountered disorders of each, and outlining appropriate medical and nursing interventions. As in every area of nursing care, one of the most important contributions that nurses can make is in the area of communication and education. They provide support and reassurance to the patient and family and convey information about the causes of the patient's condition, its treatment and measures to reduce the chance of recurrence. Understanding ENT is vital to be able to help and encourage patients to take part in decisions about their care which is a very important part of our Nursing and Midwifery Code of Practice (Nursing and Midwifery Council [NMC] 2018).

THE EAR

Anatomy and Physiology of the Ear

The ear is divided into three connecting sections: the external ear, the middle ear and the inner ear. The external and middle ears are primarily involved with the transmission of sound. The inner ear contains the organ of hearing as well as structures concerned with body balance (Fig. 16.1).

The ear can start to develop from the sixth week of pregnancy. The external ear comprises the pinna and the external auditory canal/meatus (EAC) which is lined with skin and is on average 2.4 cm long. In continuation with the pinna the outer third of the EAC is composed of cartilage while the inner two-thirds is housed within the temporal bone of the skull. The skin lining the cartilage has hair follicles and wax-producing glands but these are absent in the inner two-thirds of the bony area of the EAC. The purpose of the pinna and canal is to capture sound waves and funnel them to the tympanic membrane, which is located at the end of the ear canal and divides the external from the middle ear. Unlike the external ear which is lined with skin, the middle ear is lined with mucosa in continuation with the upper respiratory tract.

The middle ear is ventilated by the eustachian tube, which communicates with the nasopharynx. Three small bones, called the auditory ossicles, pass on sound vibrations received by the tympanic membrane to the inner ear. The first of these, the malleus, is attached to the tympanic membrane and articulates with the incus, which in turn articulates with the stapes. The 'footplate'

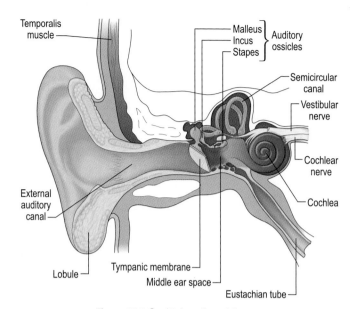

Figure 16.1 Sagittal section of the ear.

of the stapes lies against the membranous oval window of the inner ear.

The inner ear houses the cochlea, which is shaped like a snail shell and is the organ of hearing. The cochlea contains the organ of Corti, which consists of cells with hair-like projections on a membranous layer and connects with the terminal ends of the auditory nerve. The canals of the cochlea and the organ of Corti are bathed in endolymph. Perilymph is the fluid contained within the bony (osseous) cavities of the inner ear, whereas endolymph is the fluid within membranous cavities. As sound waves are transmitted by the ossicles, they travel along this fluid and disturb the hair cells. This disturbance changes to impulses, which travel along the auditory nerve to the brain stem and cortex, where they are interpreted as meaningful sound.

The posterior part of the inner ear is formed by three semicircular canals and by the vestibular apparatus. It is responsible for the balance of the body and is essential for coordinating the position of the head and the movement of the eyes. The vestibular apparatus consists of the utricle and saccule and is sensitive to linear acceleration. The semicircular canals are sensitive to rotatory acceleration. Balance is also maintained by the adjustment of muscles, joints, tendons and ligaments in response to information gathered by the vestibular apparatus and the canals as well as that received by the eyes. For further information, see Harkin (2021).

Disorders of the External Ear

Otitis Externa

Otitis externa is inflammation of the external ear commonly caused by infection and allergy. Infection may be caused by excess wax trapping water in the EAC or scratching the ear with contaminated fingernails, cotton buds or other sharp objects. Itching is an early symptom of allergy and is more common in dry skin and dermatological conditions. In otitis externa, multiple bacteriological flora are usually present. The condition most commonly occurs in hot, humid climates, where it tends to be recurrent and may be severe. Patients usually present with a sensation of a blocked ear and a history of localised pain and itching with a burning sensation followed by a discharge, which initially may be watery and then becomes thicker. If the EAC is very swollen or a large amount of debris is present, the patient may suffer from conductive hearing loss.

❖ Nursing Management and Health Promotion: Otitis Externa

The first priority of the nursing staff is to clean the EAC so that an examination can be carried out and any prescribed treatment administered effectively. This procedure is called aural toilet and should only be carried out by an appropriately qualified nurse. Cotton wool can be tightly applied to an instrument specifically designed for aural toilet such as the ProScoop (Fig. 16.2). This looks similar to a cotton bud; however, the area of cotton is designed to be narrower to ensure the ear canal is not occluded once the cotton-tipped instrument is inserted into the canal. Care must be taken not to damage the skin. Gentle pulling of the pinna will straighten the canal and allow easier access (as demonstrated in Fig. 16.3). A good light source should be used or an operating microscope. Gentle irrigation with water can clean the EAC but large amounts of discharge and debris are best removed by an appropriately qualified nurse using a microscope or magnifying glasses (called loupes) and suction via a fine-bore tube.

It may be necessary to administer an oral analgesic before the EAC can be properly examined, as often any movement of the pinna is painful (see Reflection 16.1).

Figure 16.2 Aural toilet using cotton wool.

Figure 16.3 Straightening the ear canal.

REFLECTION 16.1

History of a Patient With Otitis Externa

At the end of August, Mr Bakshi had just returned from a short break in Cornwall. He had been swimming in the sea in the warm weather. His right ear felt blocked as if he had some water left in it, so he tried to dry his ear with a cotton bud. The ear continued to feel blocked and also became very itchy. On the Monday night, Mr Bakshi woke up in the early hours of the morning with severe earache and a ringing noise on the same side of his head. He was finding it painful to talk as jaw movement hurt his ear and paracetamol had not relieved the discomfort. There was a small amount of dried liquid on the outside of the ear and it was uncomfortable to touch the ear itself. He was worried that there was something dreadfully wrong as he had never had any problems with his ear before.

Mr Bakshi attended the minor injuries department and the triage nurse examined his ear. The nurse said that there was debris present and the ear canal was mildly swollen. She explained it would be necessary to clean the ear canal to optimise the chance of clearing the infection. The nurse gently irrigated Mr Bakshi's ear with water to remove the debris. Mr Bakshi found this quite relieving and the ear felt better once the nurse dried the canal with a cotton-tipped carrier. He was diagnosed with otitis externa and the nurse prescribed an ear spray with combined steroid and antibiotic. The nurse advised Mr Bakshi to be careful not to allow water to enter the ear and to stop using the cotton buds. The nurse warned that he was to follow this advice forever or the ear infection might reoccur. The pain in the ear subsided very quickly and within 3 days Mr Bakshi's ear was better; however, he continued to use the spray for the full 10 days of the prescription.

Activities

Look at the website (irrigation guidelines and ear care advice) before attempting to answer the following questions and think about what questions the nurse will have asked Mr Bakshi about his ear prior to carrying out irrigation with water.
- How would you have advised Mr Bakshi to keep his ears dry from any entry of water?
- Is there any further advice you would give Mr Bakshi about taking care of his ears?

Since the vast majority of patients are seen in the community or outpatient department, the nurse's involvement will range from the total management of ear conditions in a nurse-led clinic to demonstrating how to administer topical preparations effectively. The nurse should also teach the patient to keep the ear dry from water entry and not to insert implements into the ear and stress the importance of frequent, thorough cleansing of any appliances, including hearing aids, that are put in the ear.

Cerumen Excess

Cerumen, or wax as it is more commonly called, is a normal secretion from the ceruminous and sebaceous glands located in the outer third of the EAC. It is produced to protect the EAC from bacteria and fungi (Sjovall et al. 2021), and along with shed skin and hair, the wax normally migrates naturally out of the EAC. This process can be hindered by coarse hair, narrow or abnormally shaped ear canals, hearing aids or misguided attempts to clean the ears with cotton wool buds or other instruments. Nurses should provide patients with health education information regarding the normal cleansing mechanism of the EAC and avoiding fiddling with the ears. It is estimated that 1 in 10 children, 1 in 20 adults and more than one-third of older adult and developmentally delayed people suffer problems with wax (Schwartz et al. 2017). Symptoms of a build-up of wax can cause patient distress as research has found that the wax build-up can cause vertigo (disturbance of balance), tinnitus, discharge, pain, hearing loss and otitis externa (Krouse et al. 2017). Persistent hard wax has also caused erosion in the EAC and patients who have had radiotherapy to the area of the head and neck would be more vulnerable to this occurring.

● Medical Management

If there is an excessive amount of wax, or the patient needs to have a hearing test or hearing aid review, the community nurse or outpatient nurse will need to clear the EAC. The wax can be removed manually with instruments, by irrigation with water using an electronic irrigator or by magnification and suction (microsuction). If the wax is too hard and compacted for this to be carried out, water can be inserted into the EAC for 15 minutes to soften the wax (Harkin 2019). To improve patient comfort, advice can be given at the time of booking recommending they use olive oil for two nights before and on the morning of the procedure. Spray dispensers have been found to have better distribution of the liquid in the ear and improved patient compliance so an olive oil spray can be recommended to be purchased over the counter. An advice sheet regarding ear care and how to insert ear drops is available on the website.

❖ Nursing Management and Health Promotion: Wax Build-up

Individuals with wax build-up are usually seen in general practice or, more rarely, in the outpatient department, for removal of the impacted wax. Ear syringing with a metal syringe is now obsolete and impacted wax is removed by instrumentation, ear irrigation with water or microsuction.

The clinician who performs the irrigation with water should first take a full history to ensure there are no contraindications to the procedure. The nurse should obtain valid consent and be seated at the same level as the patient with a disposable cape/apron placed over the patient's shoulders to keep them dry. The contraindications to irrigation with water and full guidelines for the procedure are available on the website.

Patients should also be advised that, following effective wax removal, they should prevent water entry to the EAC for approximately 5 days to reduce the chance of an ear infection and they may be hypersensitive to even quite normal sounds for a short time.

Foreign Bodies in the Ear

Small objects may become lodged in the ear by some mishap or, as frequently occurs among children, by accident during play. Such objects may lie undetected for years unless they have caused discomfort or the child has informed an adult. Sometimes gentle irrigation with water or microsuction will remove the foreign body, but if the child is uncooperative or it has become impacted, it may be necessary for the patient to be admitted to hospital as a day case and for the object to be removed under general anaesthetic (GA). A foreign body such as a small battery (as found in small toys or hearing aids) needs to be removed as an emergency. The battery fluid is corrosive so the battery requires urgent removal before it starts to leak and cause potentially fatal damage. Only objects that will not expand when in contact with water should be irrigated. Hydroscopic matter such as peas and lentils will absorb the

water and become enlarged and often impacted in the canal; as a result, removal from the EAC will be through microsuction and/or instrumentation.

Deafness and Hearing Loss

Although total deafness is comparatively rare, many people suffer hearing loss to varying degrees. Deafness can affect both adults and children. There are 840 babies born each year in the UK with profound hearing loss. Many children who are deaf continue to be so for all of their lives, but some can be helped to maximise auditory function. This section will concentrate on hearing problems among adults.

There are estimated to be over 11 million deaf and hard-of-hearing adults in the UK. This figure is rising as the number of those over 60 increases and 5% of the world's population will have a disabling hearing loss (Calvino et al. 2022). A high proportion of severely or profoundly deaf people have other disabilities as well and research has demonstrated the link between hearing loss and mental health. People with hearing loss are more likely to experience emotional distress, loneliness and depression and they are twice as likely to develop dementia (Amieva and Ouvrard 2020).

● Pathophysiology and Medical Management

Deafness is usually classified into conductive and sensorineural disorders. Conductive hearing loss can often be helped by removing any obstruction (cerumen or a foreign body, see earlier) or by amplifying sounds by means of a hearing aid. Because the external and middle ear are fairly accessible, surgical intervention may also be an option. Hearing loss generally develops gradually and people often do not notice the deterioration to their hearing but their families and friends may notice that they are struggling to hear or the television has been turned up loudly. People with conductive hearing loss can find benefit from their local audiology department. Conductive hearing loss can find interventions such as hearing aids of benefit so it is vital that they attend their local audiology department for a hearing test and this is available as an adult on the National Health Service (NHS).

By contrast, in sensorineural deafness, where the damage is to the organ of Corti or the cochlear portion of the VIIIth cranial nerve, the patient would need to be referred to a specialised hearing implant clinic to assess if surgery would be of benefit. There are medical advances all the time for hearing loss. If the patient is struggling with wearing their hearing aids due to ear infections or inadequacy, a referral to an implant centre for hearing assessment can be worthwhile. A patient who was previously assessed for a hearing implant can still benefit from a new referral. National Institute for Health and Care Excellence (NICE) guidelines (NICE 2018) have changed the criteria for hearing loss for a cochlear implant for patients that only hear sounds at 80 db at two or more frequencies (pre-2019, the criteria was 90 db). Patients may not have previously been eligible for the implant but now fall into the criteria.

Diagnosis of the type of hearing loss will be by examination and audiometry.

Hearing Tests

Voice tests are a simple method of establishing if the patient has a degree of hearing impairment. The charity Royal National Institute for the Deaf (RNID) offers free simple hearing checks on their website for people to complete while they are online; local libraries can assist people with accessing this hearing test.

Tuning Fork Tests. These tests are a simple means of determining a patient's basic auditory status. They may be performed in a clinical or home environment. Audiologists, nurses and doctors can perform these tests however, an audiometric assessment of hearing is generally carried out by the audiologist.

Rinne Test. Air conduction is tested by holding a vibrating 512-Hz tuning fork first to the front of the ear and then by placing the base of the tuning fork against the mastoid bone, which is located behind the ear. Patients should hear sound louder to the front of the ear. A Rinne positive result indicates normal hearing.

Weber Test. Bone conduction is tested by placing the base of a vibrating 512-Hz tuning fork to the middle of the forehead. This sound should be heard centrally within the head. A conductive hearing loss is indicated if the sound is lateralised to the ear that has reduced hearing. If sensorineural hearing loss is present, sound will typically be localised to the better hearing ear.

Audiometry

Audiometric tests measure hearing acuity. These tests, which include delivering tones of variable frequency and intensity, the spoken word and measuring middle ear pressures, are amongst the methods used to determine the type and source of any hearing loss. Electric response audiometry measures the patient's response to an acoustic stimulus by way of an electroencephalogram and can provide reliable and exact information on the site of a disorder, for example the cochlea, auditory nerve tract or brain stem. Detailed descriptions of these tests can be found in Sami (2017).

Conductive Hearing Loss

This results from a reduced ability of the sound waves to reach the fluid in the cochlea. The sound is quieter but not distorted. This can be due to:
- congenital abnormality
- otitis externa
- foreign bodies
- excessive cerumen
- otitis media (secretory and suppurative)
- damage to the tympanic membrane, incus, malleus or stapes.

Sensorineural Hearing Loss

This is a term used to describe a problem with the processing of sound. It is caused by a defect of the cochlea or its connecting nerves. It is a loss of the ability to convert sound into electrical impulses that the brain can understand or a loss of the brain's ability to transmit and process the electrical impulses. The sound heard is quieter and is also distorted. This is a result of the loss of the high frequencies, which register consonant sounds. In severe cases, patients may not be able to hear the sound of their own voice. This can be due to:
- ageing
- medication
- trauma, including head injury and noise
- infection
- Ménière's disease
- congenital malformation.

Presbycusis. The most common type of sensorineural deafness, this develops as a consequence of ageing and is becoming increasingly prevalent in Western society. In the UK, hearing loss affects 12 million people, with 1.1% of people over 70 and 41.7% of people over the age of 50 years having some kind of hearing loss. Audiometry initially shows loss of ability to hear high tones, but there is gradual deterioration of lower tone hearing as well. Degeneration of the nervous tissue leads to loss of intelligibility in the sounds that are heard. Hearing loss in this disorder is symmetrical; that is, it affects both ears. A hearing aid may be of slight advantage, but distortion and poor discrimination may cancel out any benefit from amplification. When communicating with these patients, it is important to speak a little slower and more distinctly and to try to eliminate any background noise. Because the high tones are affected first, the individual may have trouble hearing consonants, as these are usually of higher tone than vowels. Szeto et al. (2021) advise of a link between low levels of vitamin D and hearing loss in the elderly. Martinez-Vega et al. (2015) have found that taking a daily folic acid supplement (800 µg) may be helpful in slowing down the progression of presbycusis.

Medication. It has been recognised for some time that salicylates and quinine can cause deafness, but this can be reversed by discontinuing these medications. Other drugs, such as antibiotics of the aminoglycoside group (for example gentamicin), some diuretics, such as intravenous frusemide, and cytotoxic agents of the nitrogen mustard group, are ototoxic and can cause irreparable damage.

Trauma. Noise-induced hearing loss is well documented and has become recognised as an industrial disease. Socioacusis, the term used to describe the hearing loss caused by sources of noise outside work (loud music, traffic), can be as great a risk as loud noise in the workplace. A single exposure to a loud noise such as an explosion or gunshot can cause permanent deafness, or the injury may be temporary. Tinnitus usually accompanies this injury and often takes longer to resolve than any deafness. Exposure to loud noise over a period of time leads to destruction of the hair cells in the organ of Corti. The Control of Noise at Work Regulations (2005) laid down strict standards of noise control and protection for employers in the UK, who are liable to be prosecuted if they do not comply (see Useful Websites for more information). Occupational health nurses have a role to play in monitoring noise levels and encouraging auditory health through education. On audiometry, early changes in hearing caused by exposure to noise are seen as a dip that gradually deepens and involves adjacent frequencies.

Head Injuries or other trauma resulting in deafness usually involve fractures or penetrating injuries of the temporal bone. Occasionally, concussion (see Chapter 26, Nursing the Patient Who Experiences Trauma) can cause deafness due to haemorrhage into the middle ear or cochlea. These injuries are often accompanied by severe vertigo, nausea and vomiting.

Infection. Deafness caused by infection is usually viral in origin. The typical causative viruses are those associated with mumps, measles, meningitis, chickenpox and rubella.

Sudden-Onset Sensorineural Hearing Loss. This hearing loss can affect one or both ears and develops over seconds or hours. Sudden-onset hearing loss in one or both ears is a serious ENT emergency and the patient will need urgent intervention in an emergency ENT service. The patient will require audiometry to assess the degree of hearing loss and also to measure the response to treatment. There is ongoing national research regarding this type of hearing loss and currently intratympanic steroid injections weekly for 3 weeks with hearing tests is the recommended course of treatment. In 88% of cases, no obvious cause is found (Tysome and Kanegaonkar 2018) but a careful history and assessment should be taken. Patients may be treated with steroids (oral and/or intratympanic), betahistine, antivirals or inhaled carbogen (oxygen mixed with 5% carbon dioxide). When both ears are affected, patients tend to be admitted for investigation (blood tests and magnetic resonance imaging [MRI] scanning).

The NICE (2018a) hearing loss guidelines suggest that adults with sudden onset or hearing loss in one or both ears should be referred urgently to an ENT ED.

Ménière's Disease. Discussed later.

❖ Nursing Management and Health Promotion: Deafness and Hearing Loss

In the case of conductive deafness, the nurse's role may be to prepare the patient for surgery and facilitate postoperative recovery (see Chapter 25, Nursing the Patient Undergoing Surgery). Some of the surgical procedures that may benefit patients are myringoplasty (repair of the tympanic membrane), ossiculoplasty (repair to the ossicular chain in the middle ear) and stapedectomy (a prosthetic stapes is inserted to replace the damaged bone). A patient for whom surgery is not feasible may be fitted with a hearing aid and educated in its use by members of the audiology department, including the hearing therapist. In this case the nurse, as a member of the multiprofessional team, should also explain how to obtain the greatest benefit from the aid (see guide to looking after hearing aids on the website).

Most patients in this situation also benefit from learning how to lip-read. Lip-reading sessions are usually available as a day or evening class at audiology departments or a local college. It can take many months to become proficient at lip-reading, so the earlier the patient starts the better. Slow progress, combined with deteriorating hearing, can be very demotivating.

Communicating effectively with a hearing-impaired patient is a very important nursing priority (Information 16.1). In the assessment, the nurse should obtain and record information about the patient's preferred method of communicating, for example lip-reading, finger-spelling or sign language. It may be necessary, if the nurse is wearing a face mask, to remove this if infection control policies allow. A study by the charity (Abou-Abdallah and Lamyman 2021) suggested that deaf adults who used sign language were dissatisfied with and disadvantaged in their communication with healthcare staff, including nurses. Bigelow et al. (2020) has researched that hearing loss increases psychological distress and utilisation of mental health services.

The BSL Act (2022) is a vital step towards inclusion and equality for deaf people in society. British sign language (BSL) is now a recognised language in England, Wales and Scotland.

Deafness can have a profound psychological impact and hearing-impaired individuals may require support to help resolve problems. Many deaf people would prefer to have counselling from a counsellor who is deaf, and attempts should be made to find such a professional if preferred (via the British Association for Counselling and Psychotherapy [BACP] if necessary, see Useful Websites). Older adults and their carers have complained of symptoms such as depression, anxiety, decreased social activity and emotional turmoil (Niazi et al. 2020). NICE (2018a) recommends that patients with cognitive impairment or a diagnosis of dementia should have a hearing assessment every 2 years if they have are not already receiving care for hearing loss.

Community nurses can provide tremendous help and support for patients and their relatives when sensorineural deafness is a problem. They should be able to assist their patients to obtain many of the aids available, including a hearing dog for deaf

---

INFORMATION 16.1

Talking With Someone Who Has a Hearing Deficit

- Do not speak until you have the person's attention and they can see your full face.
- Ensure they are wearing their glasses and the lenses are clean.
- Never turn your back on the person when you are speaking or cover your mouth.
- Ask the person if they can lip-read.
- Do not exaggerate your lip movements.
- Direct your voice to one ear if it has better hearing than the other.
- Speak slowly, enunciate clearly and do not shout.
- Remember that vowels are heard more easily than consonants.
- Check that the person has understood what you have said.
- If the person has difficulty in understanding, try rephrasing the sentence.
- Do not laugh at misinterpretations.
- Have patience. Give the person time to adjust their hearing aid if necessary.
- Encourage the person to participate in group conversations when the occasion arises.
- If verbal communication is impossible, explore alternative means, e.g. sign language.
- Check with the patient that they have all the help that they need and they have a flashing fire alarm at home.

---

individuals, which can help to overcome communication difficulties in everyday life. There are many associations, both voluntary and professional, which can provide support and help. The nurse working in the community should be a resource person for patients and guide them to the support that is available. There are assistive listening devices such as personal loops, telephone devices, fire alarm and doorbell sensors with phone apps and streamers that can benefit people who are hard of hearing (see Useful Websites and Evidence-Based Practice 16.1).

Hearing Aids

About 2 million people in the UK have hearing aids, but only 1.4 million use them regularly. There are at least another 4 million people who do not have hearing aids but experience significant hearing difficulties in everyday life. They would be likely to benefit from hearing aids. Hearing aids have a microphone, which picks up the sound; the sound is processed electronically by digital circuits to make it more audible. This is then delivered to the receiver, converted back to sound and reaches the ear via an ear piece. Current NHS hearing aids have features that can help hear in background noise, such as directional microphones and noise reduction settings. For further information on hearing aids, see the website.

Disorders of the Middle Ear

Otitis Media With Effusion (Glue Ear)

Glue ear is the most common cause of hearing impairment and the most common reason for elective surgery in children. About 50% of children will have had at least one ear infection by the time they reach their second birthday (Paul and Moreno 2020). Fluid that becomes trapped within the middle ear space is commonly known as glue ear because it is characterised by a thick,

EVIDENCE-BASED PRACTICE 16.1

Are We Being Heard?

RNID. *A Simple Cure. A National Report Into Deaf and Hard of Hearing People's Experiences of the National Health Service.* RNID: London; 2004.

- The RNID decided to commission this report because of the frequency with which it received examples of poor communication experienced by deaf and hard-of-hearing people when attempting to use the NHS. The study took place within the context of the Disability Discrimination Act 1995, which came into force in 2004 and places a legal obligation on the NHS to meet the needs of disabled people. The NHS in England, Wales and Scotland has acknowledged defects in services that affect disabled people, including difficulties in communication with staff and in finding their way around premises. There are thought to be approximately 9 million deaf and hard-of-hearing people in the UK. As one in every seven people in the UK has some level of hearing loss, and it is known that the average GP will have up to four patients with hearing loss in their surgery daily, it is important that healthcare professionals in all care settings are aware of the particular needs for effective communication of those who have reduced hearing.
- The RNID and the UK Council on Deafness conducted this research in collaboration with 21 UK-based deaf and hard-of-hearing groups and charities; a total of 866 participants completed the survey.
- The main findings reported by deaf and hard-of-hearing people when using GP services were that 35% had experienced difficulty communicating with their GP or practice nurse and 15% avoided going to see their GP because of communication problems. Making and keeping appointments were another problematic area, with 28% reporting that they found their hearing loss made it difficult for them to make an appointment: of 24% who stated they had missed an appointment, 19% had missed more than five. Of those who did see their GP or nurse, 35% reported being unclear about their condition because of communication problems. Of those who used British Sign Language (BSL), 33% were either unsure about medication instructions or had taken inaccurate doses.
- The situation in NHS hospitals is equally disturbing, as 42% of the deaf and hard-of-hearing patients who had visited a hospital for nonemergency treatment found it difficult to communicate with staff.

- BSL users experienced even more difficulties, with 77% of this group reporting communication problems for emergency and nonemergency overnight stays and 70% of those admitted to EDs were not provided with a BSL/English interpreter to facilitate effective communication.
- Overall, the picture is one of poor communication, resulting in people having inadequate access to healthcare and insufficient information about their health condition and treatment, thus limiting their ability to make informed choices, and being placed in higher risk situations than their hearing counterparts. It is also unacceptable that family, including young children, and friends have to act as interpreters and on occasion convey critical health information. The financial cost to the NHS of missed appointments is put at approximately £15 million a year. The financial and nonfinancial costs to the patient, family and friends will never be known.
- The report notes that NHS staff do wish to deliver a better and more equitable service to deaf and hard-of-hearing patients but that, often, the necessary resources and infrastructure are not available. Solutions recommended include increasing the number of BSL/English interpreters, using video phones, providing improved written information, installing loop systems to allow better use of hearing aids in noisy environments, providing visual displays in appointment areas and clear lighting and providing deaf awareness education, including communication skills, for all healthcare staff, whether working in hospital or community settings. Deaf awareness seminars should be provided for appropriate hospital departments and GP surgery staff, so that these areas have at least one formally trained 'front line' staff member.
- Action on Hearing Loss (formerly RNID) researched the effect the Accessible Information Standard (2015) had on patients attending their GP. The Standard states that health and social care services should make a dramatic improvement in meeting the communication and information needs of people with disabilities and sensory loss including deaf and hearing loss. Overall, the results of their survey remain unchanged. There are still dramatic changes to be made to improve access to health and social care for people who are deaf or have hearing loss.

---

tenacious fluid that collects in the middle ear. Normally, the middle ear pressures are maintained by opening of the eustachian tube on swallowing (see Fig. 16.1). It is not certain whether the abnormal accumulation of this fluid is caused by the viscosity of the fluid, congestion of the eustachian tubes, low-grade viral or bacterial infection or obstruction caused by enlarged adenoids or, in rare cases, a tumour.

Common Presenting Symptoms

Pain is rarely associated with this condition. The adult patient usually complains of hearing loss. A child might never complain, and their condition might be discovered only upon investigation into poor speech, developmental delay or during routine screening of hearing at school. It is more common in children with cleft palate (underdeveloped facial skeleton leading to impaired eustachian tube function), Trisomy 21 (Down syndrome – more horizontally-lying eustachian tube and increased susceptibility to infection), primary ciliary dyskinesia (impaired ciliary function to the upper respiratory tract) and allergic rhinitis.

Medical Management

Examination of the tympanic membrane by otoscope usually confirms the diagnosis, as in this disorder the membrane has a

characteristic dull grey or orange appearance. It will also lose its normal translucence and become retracted.

Conservative Treatment. The fluid in the middle ear tends to last for at least 3 months (Vanneste and Page 2019).

The glue ear tends to settle spontaneously and there is no evidence to recommend prescribing antibiotics, antihistamines, mucolytics, decongestants or corticosteroids (Vanneste and Page 2019). Children will be referred to ENT if they have the associated medical problems listed previously and if they have a persistent hearing loss and/or a concern regarding developmental delay.

Hearing aids are often worn by children with persistent glue ear while they are being observed to see if the glue ear resolves spontaneously or if there is a reason not to perform surgery. Auto-inflation has been beneficial in children over 3 years of age who are cooperative and able to successfully blow their nose. A balloon device such as Otovent is inflated by blowing through the nose to improve the function of the middle ear. Although auto-inflation is often recommended, Cooper et al. (2022) refute this advice and have found that there is no evidence of improved outcomes for patients. Further information can be found in NICE (2016).

Surgical Intervention involves performing a myringotomy (incising the tympanic membrane) and suctioning of the glue. If a grommet

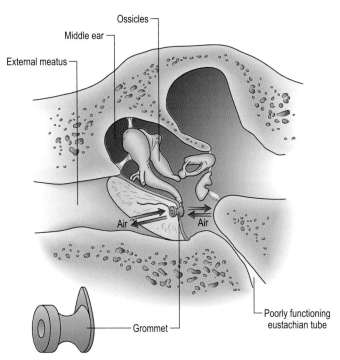

Ossicles

Middle ear

External meatus

Air Air

Grommet

Poorly functioning eustachian tube

Figure 16.4 Grommet and grommet in situ.

is not inserted, the delicate tympanic membrane heals within a few days. The fluid can accumulate again. A grommet allows aeration of the middle ear, thus restoring middle ear air pressure (Fig. 16.4). If a grommet is usually extruded from the tympanic membrane at 9–12 months, patients sometimes find it on their pillow when they wake one morning. Adenoidectomy will also be performed at the same time if the child has had sleep studies demonstrating disturbed sleep with/without apnoea and a persistent/frequent nasal obstruction/discharge. There is usually a marked improvement in hearing after this procedure, which is maintained in about 75% of patients. One-third to one-half of patients who have had grommets inserted will require a second set to be inserted within 5 years (NICE 2016). Parents should be advised of the risk factors of glue ear such as passive smoking, nursery attendance, bottle feeding, winter months, sibling history of glue ear, frequent upper respiratory tract infections and after an episode of acute otitis media (AOM).

❖ Nursing Management and Health Promotion: Otitis Media With Effusion (Glue Ear)

Only care specific to ENT patients is outlined in this chapter. The reader is referred to Chapter 25, Nursing Patients Undergoing Surgery, for details of routine perioperative care.

Preoperative Care

Most of this surgery is carried out on a day-case basis, and the nurse must ensure that the patient and family are adequately informed about what the surgical procedure will entail whilst providing support and reassurance. This may involve the use of diagrams and it may be helpful to show them a grommet if one is to be inserted. When communicating with the patient preoperatively, the nurse should make allowances for hearing loss (see Information 16.1). Patients should have their hearing aids removed when they are anaesthetised and replaced in the recovery room.

Postoperative Care

The anaesthetic for this operation is very light. Measures to prevent the spread of infection, for example washing the hands before and after touching the affected ear, how to change and dispose of cotton wool plugs in the EAC, and specific instructions about whether and when it is safe to allow water to enter the ear, must be discussed with the patient. When a grommet is in place, most surgeons allow swimming, as long as the patient does not dive or swim underwater. Usually, a cotton wool plug moistened with petroleum jelly is inserted in the external canal when the hair is being washed or when taking a shower. The nurse must ensure that the patient and family understand this advice and are given information booklets or advice sheets. ENT UK has produced superb evidence-based leaflets for patients (see Useful Websites). Patients should be told to see their GP if they experience any pain or if there is a bloodstained discharge from the ear. Most of these precautions apply to all patients who have undergone aural surgery. The patient may be asked to see their GP for regular checks of the position of the grommet rather than requiring them to attend the outpatient department.

Otosclerosis

Otosclerosis is a condition in which the ossicles in the middle ear, along with the temporal bone (see Fig. 16.1), begin to soften. This spongy bone gradually becomes a dense sclerotic mass; the ossicles may become fixed and less effective in passing on auditory vibrations. The individual with this condition will complain of increasing hearing loss. While this loss is conductive in origin, if the damage extends to the cochlea, sensorineural loss of hearing will also occur. Mild tinnitus may also be experienced, in which case some people find that they can actually hear better in a noisy environment where their tinnitus is masked.

This disorder commonly begins in adolescence and its cause is as yet unknown. Heredity, vitamin deficiency and otitis media have all been cited as significant factors.

🕭 Medical Management and Nursing Priorities

Although no cure for otosclerosis is known, surgery can often dramatically improve hearing. The surgery of choice, stapedectomy, involves freeing the stapes and replacing it with a prosthesis. This restores the vibration necessary to permit the transmission of sound waves. Surgery may be performed under local anaesthetic, and hospital admission may be no more than 24 hours.

Great care must be taken in the early postoperative period, as the patient may take a little while to regain their sense of balance. This short-term vertigo, if discussed and explained in the preoperative period, should cause minimal distress to the patient. Nursing staff will be able to support patients during the recovery period. Prior to discharge, advice should be given on the prevention of aural infection (keep the ears dry from water entry, do not insert implements into the ear) and the need to guard against blowing the nose until the operative site is completely healed. Violent nose blowing can force air up the eustachian tube, increasing middle ear pressure, which can affect the operated area and prosthesis. Patients should be advised to keep their mouth open when sneezing to reduce middle ear pressure, and also to avoid flight and Eurotunnel travel until they have discussed this at their outpatient follow-up appointment.

Acute Otitis Media (AOM)

This is an acute bacterial (62% of cases) or viral (5%) infection of the middle ear which mainly affects children. One in two children has had three episodes by the age of three (Venekamp et al. 2020). AOM tends to follow an upper respiratory tract infection. Young children are more prone to this as they have an underdeveloped eustachian tube. One quarter of all children will attend general practice with common ENT-related minor infections.

Common Presenting Symptoms

The patient usually presents with acute ear pain. Younger children are often seen pulling or rubbing the ear with irritability, a runny nose and fever. On examination, the eardrum is red and bulging due to the collection of pus in the middle ear. The tympanic membrane may perforate, releasing the discharge and dramatically and instantaneously relieving the pain.

Medical Management and Treatment

The NICE (2022) guideline has recommended a prescribing strategy for AOM and information for parents and carers. Reassuring parents that symptoms will settle in 50% of children at day 3 and 90% by days 7/8 in the absence of antibiotics is helpful. Regular painkillers are essential and complications such as mastoiditis are rare. Children under 5 years of age with fever should be assessed and managed using the NICE (2021) guideline on fever in under 5s.

NICE (2022) recommends the use of three antibiotic strategies (no prescribing, back-up prescribing or immediate prescribing). For initial presentation of AOM in children who are generally fit and well, prescribing will not be necessary. Advice should be given regarding the management of common coughs, colds and runny noses with or without ear infections. If time is spent explaining to the parents on a first occasion how to manage these common infections in their child, then care of siblings is more likely to be managed at home. Children under 2 years old with bilateral AOM should be considered for immediate antibiotics as should children with other health concerns and who are systemically unwell. A back-up prescription is commonly used in general practice. Patients can be advised that if the symptoms do not settle in 72 hours, they can have the prescription dispensed and start oral antibiotics. Advice should always be given to seek medical advice if the symptoms do not improve or the condition deteriorates.

Bulging Eardrum

If the infection has reached this stage, a myringotomy may be performed if the patient has other symptoms such as a facial nerve weakness. This involves applying a local anaesthetic before making an incision in the tympanic membrane to allow the pus to escape. If a myringotomy is performed in preference to allowing the eardrum to rupture, the membrane will heal with less scarring and hearing should not be impaired. The patient with a facial weakness will have been admitted and antibiotic ear drops prescribed with oral steroids.

Discharging Ear

By this stage the tympanic membrane will already have ruptured. A swab of the discharge will only be taken if the ear has not responded to the broad-spectrum antibiotics and continues to discharge. The ear is carefully mopped out of the discharge and the patient encouraged not to allow water into the ear and not to fiddle with the ear. Petroleum jelly or a medicated honey barrier cream can be advised to place around the entrance of the ear to protect the skin becoming excoriated from the discharge. The patient will have to visit the GP regularly so that healing of the membrane can be monitored. If the perforation does not heal, the patient may suffer with intermittent discharge from the ear which

would be unpleasant. If water enters the ear, this discharge will increase, making bathing and swimming difficult. If the perforation has not healed after 1 year, a myringoplasty (repair of the eardrum) will be performed.

❖❖ Nursing Management and Health Promotion: Acute Otitis Media (AOM)

Nurses who frequently treat children should be familiar with NICE guidelines so they can educate parents on management of common coughs, colds, sore throats and ear infections.

If the AOM has caused discharge from the ear, the nurse's role will include mopping out the external ear as often as required and carrying out microsuction clearance of the debris. Microsuction is performed using the same equipment and suction pressure as for tracheal suctioning. Looking down the microscope, the specialist nurse uses disposable thin suckers to remove any debris or wax from the ear canal. The benefit of the microscope is that it offers magnification and binocular vision and depth of field. If appropriate treatment is given early enough, AOM should resolve and hearing return to normal. Occasionally, complications do occur, including chronic suppurative otitis media (CSOM) and acute mastoiditis; descriptions of which follow.

Chronic Suppurative Otitis Media (CSOM)

This condition follows unresolved AOM.

Pathophysiology

The patient will present with a perforated tympanic membrane, a discharging ear and some degree of conductive deafness. Pain is not usually a complaint. The discharge may be intermittent and is mucoid, becoming purulent in the presence of secondary infection.

Medical Management

The recommended treatment is to keep the ear dry by the use of topical medication before correcting the hearing loss by performing a tympanoplasty.

Tympanoplasty

Following removal of diseased tissue, an attempt may be made to reestablish the sound transmission mechanism in the middle ear by reconstructing the tympanic membrane (myringoplasty) using a connective tissue graft taken from the fascia covering the temporal bone and reconstructing the ossicular chain (ossiculoplasty). This combined reconstruction is known as a tympanoplasty. For further information on middle ear surgery, see Tysome and Kanegaonkar (2018).

❖❖ Nursing Management and Health Promotion: Tympanoplasty

Preoperative Care

The patient is usually admitted on the day of surgery. In view of their obvious hearing deficit, the establishment of effective communication is very important. To help avoid complications, the ear must be dry and free from infection. Hearing tests will be carried out to confirm the degree of hearing loss. To help alleviate anxiety, the nurse should give the patient information about the procedure and warn about sensations that may be experienced afterwards, such as dizziness and tinnitus. It is also important to describe the very bulky bandage that will be present around the head and affected ear so that this does not alarm the patient and family. Hearing aids should be worn to the operating theatre. The theatre staff should remove the hearing aid as the patient is anaesthetised and place it in the patient's notes. Often, the ward nurse will take the hearing aid back to the ward and place it in the patient's locked bedside drawer if this is the patient's preference. If the hearing aid was worn in the ear that was not operated on, it should be reinserted by the recovery staff before the patient is extubated.

Postoperative Care

General postoperative care is as described in Chapter 25. The majority of patients undergoing ear surgery are given a hypotensive anaesthetic in order to reduce bleeding and thereby allow the surgeon a clearer view of the tiny operative field. This involves the intravenous administration of a hypotensive agent. Frequent blood pressure readings are therefore required until the preoperative baseline levels are regained.

Following the operation, the patient should be encouraged to lie with the affected area uppermost and should be observed for nausea, vomiting and vertigo, all of which might be present due to possible interference with the semicircular canals during surgery. The aim of the pressure dressing and bandage is to prevent bleeding and haematoma formation, but the nurse should always observe the patient's bandages and pillows for bloodstains.

Because of its location, the VIIth cranial (facial) nerve is at risk of damage during surgery to the middle or inner ear. Following this type of surgery, patients should be asked to smile, wrinkle their nose and shut their eyes tightly. The ability to perform these movements indicates that there has been no damage to the facial nerve. A record of the time of checking and level of function of the nerve should always be documented for medical and legal reasons and local policy and procedure must be adhered to.

Most patients are able to be up on the evening of surgery and return home the next day. The surgeon usually requests the nurse to remove the head bandage the morning after surgery. The patient should be advised that they may experience dizziness during the following 2 or 3 weeks and should avoid sudden movements such as quickly turning the head. Sutures are generally dissolvable but if the surgeon has inserted packing in the external auditory canal (EAC), it tends to be removed between 2 and 3 weeks following surgery. The patient will be shown how to change the piece of cotton wool at the entrance to the EAC as required, without disturbing the packing. The packing is removed by the surgeon in the outpatient department and the patient should be recommended to take a mild analgesic such as paracetamol before their appointment as this will be slightly uncomfortable. Surgeons often insert absorbable gel foam instead of ribbon gauze packing to support the tympanic membrane so they will not need to be reviewed postoperatively until 6 weeks.

CSOM With Cholesteatoma

This potentially dangerous condition is sometimes called atticoantral disease, because it is often found in the attic (upper) area of the middle ear. Cholesteatoma is an ingrowth of keratinising squamous epithelium from the external ear into the middle ear, usually from the site of a previous perforation. It may be possible to see this on examination. The squamous epithelium growing within the middle ear produces keratin, which has the ability to erode the bony ossicles and may even spread into the inner ear.

Common Presenting Symptoms

The patient will complain of a foul-smelling discharge from the ear and of hearing loss.

⊛ Medical Management

The treatment of choice is mastoidectomy (see later).

Acute Mastoiditis

This rare condition arises from AOM and is caused by the infection spreading to the bony walls of the cells of the mastoid process. The patient can present with serious complications such as meningitis, facial nerve palsy and severe vertigo.

⊛ Medical Management

Conservative management is by administration of antibiotics; surgical management is a mastoidectomy.

Mastoidectomy

There are three types: a combined approach tympanoplasty (CAT), which is also referred to as a canal wall-up mastoidectomy, an atticotomy or small cavity mastoidectomy and a modified radical mastoidectomy. Surgery involves incision, drainage and removal of unhealthy mucosa and bone cells from the mastoid process of the temporal bone, leaving the middle ear structures intact. A CAT tends to be performed if the disease is confined to the upper area of the mastoid and the patient has good hearing. This is currently the most common surgical procedure for middle ear infection.

Nursing care is for patients undergoing tympanoplasty.

Disorders of the Inner Ear

Tinnitus

Tinnitus is a little understood but most distressing feature of some ear diseases and disorders. It may also occur spontaneously or as a postoperative complication. Possibly because it is so puzzling, has no known cause and is not a visible symptom, sufferers often feel that they receive little empathy and understanding.

Tinnitus is a subjective sensation of sound in the ear. It is a relatively common complaint that may arise in association with a wide range of conditions, including inner and middle ear disease, overuse of medications such as aspirin and quinine, abnormalities of the auditory nerve, renal problems, cardiac problems and anaemia. It is often accompanied by vertigo and/or deafness. The Tinnitus Association helps sufferers and produces an excellent range of factsheets and a free newsletter for interested professionals (see Useful Websites).

Common Presenting Symptoms

Tinnitus can vary in severity from an intermittent mild ringing sensation in the ear to an incessant noise, loud enough to make life unbearable. The perceived sound varies in volume and character from one individual to another. Some patients are aware of the sound only during their waking hours, while others are aware of it mainly at night or when they are somewhere very quiet. Tinnitus may cause difficulty in sleeping, with irritability, tiredness and lack of concentration following restless nights. The persistent symptoms cause many tinnitus sufferers to feel anxious and depressed (Reflection 16.2). The feelings are exacerbated in some by fears that the tinnitus is an indication of a more serious underlying disease or that it will cause an increase in hearing loss. In the worst

An Experience of Tinnitus

I shall never forget the first time I experienced tinnitus. It was in the dead of night when I heard a high-pitched whine in my left ear. I was so taken aback that I got up out of bed and went in search of the source of the noise. Before long, however, I realised that the noise was being carried with me.

The tinnitus had been preceded about a month beforehand by nausea and severe vertigo which I had accepted as transitory. To find that I was left with this noise made me feel very anxious indeed. I had difficulty in coming to terms with the fact that it might always be present. My reaction was 'It can't be! There must be something to combat it and make the noise go away!'

When it became clear to me that I was now a 'tinnitus sufferer', I experienced a phase of reactive depression and felt that life was not worthwhile. Naturally, I searched for a cure and eventually joined the local branch of the British Tinnitus Association. This was a move which I made by myself, but the Association proved to be an invaluable source of emotional and practical support and information. A hearing therapist and a clinic psychologist have now joined the team at my audiology clinic and they are giving tinnitus sufferers like me a great deal of help in many ways.

Activities

- Reflect on the support you would offer the patient with tinnitus.
- How would you explain what tinnitus is to the patient's relatives?
- If the patient does not have a computer at home, how would you recommend they gain access to the internet?

cases, individuals with tinnitus may suffer total deafness because the noise in their ear eliminates all other sounds.

Medical Management

To aid diagnosis, a careful history must be taken, including information about all other symptoms and any medications. A hearing test and careful examination of the ear (including radiography) may help determine the cause. One-sided, pulsatile tinnitus is 30% more likely to have an identifiable cause (Sethi et al. 2017); however, in many instances, no treatable cause will be found.

❖ Nursing Management and Health Promotion: Tinnitus

Very few tinnitus sufferers will be patients in hospital, unless their condition has arisen as an early postoperative complication. The majority will attend their GP's surgery or the local ENT outpatient department. When nursing staff encounter these patients, high priority should be given to allowing them to express their fears and to recognising and relieving their anxiety and possible depression. Once an ENT specialist has carried out all the tests required to determine a diagnosis, any prescribed treatment and training can be commenced. Where there is no medical treatment, a planned programme of care, including counselling, tinnitus retraining therapy, hearing aids, cognitive behaviour therapy, explanations and information giving, such as details of support groups, will be necessary to help the patient adapt and to relieve any worries. There are more than 100 tinnitus support groups in the UK (see Useful Websites), and they can be of enormous help to sufferers by providing ongoing emotional support (see Reflection 16.2).

Vertigo

Vertigo is a disturbance of equilibrium, in the absence of an external cause, which creates a sensation of rotating motion of oneself or one's surroundings. It is usually caused by irritation of the vestibular apparatus and is most frequently associated with disorders of the bony labyrinth and with Ménière's disease. Cardiac, neurological or viral infections and therapeutic medications such as streptomycin can also cause vertigo. One-third of people will be affected by vertigo and dizziness before the age of 65 years and nearly two-thirds of women and one-third of men at 80 years (Tysome and Kanegaonkar 2018)

Common Presenting Symptoms

Vertigo is a disabling and often frightening sensation that may be transient or recurring. It is not the same as dizziness and may be relatively mild or quite severe. The motion perceived is often described as a whirling sensation, but rocking and swaying sensations are also reported. Sufferers may complain of a feeling that their body continues to move after they have stopped. Severe attacks of vertigo may be sudden and dramatic, accompanied by pallor, nausea and vomiting.

Medical Management

A careful history is required from the patient and must include any precipitating factors such as head and neck movements. Any other symptoms such as tinnitus or deafness should be ascertained. It is also helpful to know how long the periods of vertigo last. Details of medication and any recent trauma can also aid diagnosis. A neurological and cardiovascular examination and perhaps radiography, hearing tests and blood tests may be advisable.

There are a range of inner ear disorders that can cause vertigo and a common one is benign paroxysmal positional vertigo (BPPV). This is a condition where the calcium carbonate crystals located in the semicircular canals of the inner ear are dislodged and become free floating, causing vertigo on changes in head position. A specific range of head movements are performed by the GP or in the ENT outpatient department to try to encourage the crystals back into position. This series of head movements is called the Epley manoeuvre and the patient may be encouraged to do Cooksey Cawthorne head and neck exercises to help settle the fleeting episodes of vertigo. Occasionally, surgery will be required to treat the particular disorder of which vertigo is a symptom, but treatment is more commonly pharmacological. Research currently advocates an injection of steroid through the tympanic membrane into the middle ear space for debilitating vertigo. Vertigo sufferers can take as prescribed betahistine 3 mg buccal tablets at the acute stages of an attack.

❖ Nursing Management and Health Promotion: Vertigo

As is the case with tinnitus sufferers, the majority of individuals who suffer from vertigo will be distressed and incapacitated by their condition. They will usually be seen in their homes, as they are likely to feel unsafe venturing out. The first nursing priority for these patients is safety. The attacks of vertigo may be unpredictable, or may be associated with a particular head movement. For example, for one individual, a precipitating circumstance might be standing on a stepladder with their head back and to one side in order to change a light bulb; for another, it may be simply a quick movement to bend down and pick up a baby from its cot. The nurse should discuss with the patient and family how to avoid the particular head and/or other movements in order to eliminate attacks, if this is possible. An occupational therapy assessment of home safety may also be beneficial.

Ménière's Disease

In Ménière's disease, the membranous labyrinth is distended by an increase in the endolymph, at the expense of the perilymph, and the organ of Corti degenerates. The most widely held theory of its cause is that it arises as a result of local ischaemia, although it has been suggested that it may be due to viral infection, biochemical disturbance, vitamin deficiency or local physiological faults (Sethi et al. 2017). It is associated with fluctuating levels of hearing and vestibular function. It may arise at any age but is most common among individuals aged 30–50.

Common Presenting Symptoms

Ménière's disease is characterised by four disabling features:
- vertigo
- tinnitus
- sensorineural hearing loss
- nausea and vomiting.

As it runs its course over a period of many years, deafness increases. Although this hearing loss may initially affect only one ear, it will, in 10% of patients, eventually affect the other as well. Many patients have a warning that an attack is imminent (often described as an aura), for example there is a feeling of fullness in the ear or the character of the tinnitus changes. This can happen in vestibular migraines and patients can be referred to specialist audiological services or balance clinics for vestibular rehabilitation.

During an attack the patient will have vertigo, nausea and vomiting and will want to lie down and remain as still as possible, in order to relieve these distressing symptoms. Nystagmus (involuntary, rhythmic eyeball rolling) may be present and sweating, bradycardia and diarrhoea may occur.

🌑 Medical Management

It may be difficult to arrive at a conclusive diagnosis of Ménière's disease, as many other disorders, for example labyrinthitis, intracranial disease and acoustic neuroma, display similar symptoms. Given that, between attacks, clinical examination may prove negative, diagnosis will rely heavily on careful history taking and audiological investigations.

Treatment

The most common treatment for the symptoms of Ménière's disease is the prescription of medication, for example a labyrinthine sedative (medication to dampen the sensation of unsteadiness) such as cinnarizine, betahistine and diuretics. A vasodilator such as nicotinic acid or moxisylyte may be prescribed to alleviate local ischaemia. The majority of patients respond well to medication therapy and may have long periods of respite from severe symptoms. It had been thought that adherence to a low-salt diet would reduce the volume of endolymph but research is inconclusive.

Surgery may occasionally help to relieve symptoms. This may take the form of decompression of the endolymphatic sac, the creation of a fistula between the endolymph and perilymph reservoirs or a vestibular neurectomy.

❖ Nursing Management and Health Promotion: Ménière's Disease

The main nursing priority in case of an attack of Ménière's disease is to ensure the patient's safety. Attacks are often so severe that the patient needs to lie as still as possible, and, if in hospital, may gain a sense of security if the side rails on the bed are raised. Vomiting can be so severe as to cause dehydration. If the patient cannot take fluids orally, intravenous fluids and antiemetic drugs will be necessary until oral medication and feeding can be tolerated. It is necessary for the nurse caring for the patient to escalate their concerns to medical staff and ensure the appropriate medication and/or fluids are prescribed in a timely manner when necessary to minimise symptoms.

Patients suffering from Ménière's disease often have to make lifestyle changes in order to cope with some of the symptoms of the disorder. The nurse should be prepared to offer advice on lifestyle adaptations and provide useful websites or leaflets to give to the patient. As an individual faced with the problems associated with Ménière's disease is likely to feel anxiety, it is vital that the nurse provides clear information and explanations, particularly with regard to prognosis.

THE NOSE

Anatomy and Physiology of the Nose

The principal function of the nose is to provide a passageway for air entering and leaving the respiratory tract (Fig. 16.5). In so doing, it acts as an 'air conditioner', ensuring that inspired air is humidified, sufficiently warm, filtered and free from particulate matter.

The terminal fibres of the olfactory nerve are located in the roof of the nasal cavity. The lower two-thirds of the nose are supported by cartilage and the upper third is enclosed by bone. The cavity is divided in half by the septum which consists of cartilage anteriorly and bone posteriorly. The entrance is lined with stratified squamous epithelium and coarse hairs (termed vibrissae) and the passages are lined with a mucous membrane of ciliated columnar epithelium. These passages are highly vascularised. A branch of the maxillary artery supplies the lower posterior section of the cavity, and the anterior and posterior ethmoidal arteries supply the mucous membrane. All these vessels join at Little's area on each side of the septum (see Fig. 16.6). Unlike the smooth lining of the septum, the lateral wall of the nose has three bony projections called the inferior, middle and superior turbinates. Between these turbinates are the openings from the paranasal sinuses. The nasolacrimal duct drains below the inferior turbinate, the maxillary antrum between the inferior and middle turbinate and posterior to the middle turbinate the sphenoethmoidal opening.

Disorders of the Nose

Epistaxis

Epistaxis is bleeding from the nose. It is not a disease in itself but a symptom of some other disorder, which may be of a local or general nature. Local causative disorders include idiopathic, trauma caused by nose-picking, foreign bodies, a blow to the nose or surgery. More generalised disorders that sometimes give rise to nosebleeds can be:
- vascular, e.g. hypertension and cardiac failure
- congenital, e.g. haemophilia and hereditary haemorrhagic telangiectasia
- neoplastic, e.g. leukaemia, sino-nasal tumours
- endocrine, e.g. during pregnancy
- medication induced, e.g. a side-effect of anticoagulant therapy and chemotherapy
- infections, e.g. influenza, rhinitis, sinusitis and the common cold.

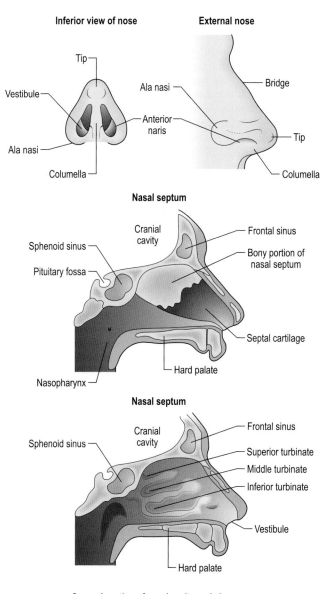

Inferior view of nose

External nose

Nasal septum

Nasal septum

Coronal section of nasal cavity and sinuses

Figure 16.5 The nose and paranasal sinuses.

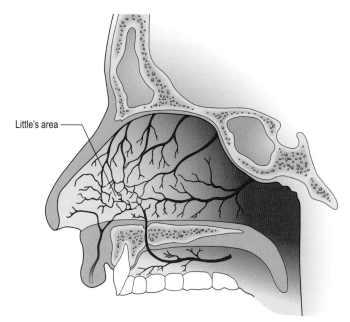

Figure 16.6 Blood supply to the nose (sagittal section).

Common Presenting Symptoms

Epistaxis can affect males and females equally and can occur at any age but is most common in childhood and early adolescence, when it usually occurs in Little's area (Fig. 16.6) and is often the result of trauma or infection. In middle-aged or older individuals, the bleeding often occurs in the posterior part of the nose and may be associated with hypertension. This form of epistaxis may be very frightening and can be life-threatening if it proves difficult to control. Epistaxis in elderly patients can prove fatal so it is essential to control the bleeding as soon as possible and monitor

for signs of shock (see Chapter 19, The Deteriorating Patient, Recognising and Managing Shock).

See Information 16.2 for the management of epistaxis.

Patients often present at clinics with a history of recurrent epistaxis, but are rarely actually bleeding at that time. On examination, dilated blood vessels may be apparent. The best treatment to prevent the bleeding recurring is cautery by the use of a chemical, such as silver nitrate, electrocautery or diathermy. Cautery will only be performed to one nostril to reduce the risk of a septal perforation.

Medical Management

The management of epistaxis can be divided into resuscitation of the patient, arrest of the haemorrhage and diagnosis and treatment of any underlying cause (Tysome and Kanegaonkar 2018). A patient with severe active epistaxis is usually admitted to hospital as an emergency. Vital signs are recorded to monitor for shock, as bleeding may be severe enough to necessitate blood transfusion. Treatment is by insertion of a nasal pack, commonly used brands include 'Rapid Rhinos' which work by ensuring even compression at the source of the bleed. Nasal packs are usually left in place for 24–72 hours. Prophylactic antibiotics are given if the packs are in longer than 48 hours, to prevent any risk of infection developing and spreading to the middle ear. Occasionally, when these measures fail to control the bleeding, arterial ligation is necessary. If the bleed is the result of some underlying medical condition, this will need to be investigated and treated at the same time.

Nursing Management and Health Promotion: Epistaxis

Nursing intervention will vary depending on the site, severity and cause of the epistaxis, and the patient's age. Most patients with anterior nosebleeds (bleeding from the front of the nose) are children or adolescents and will be treated as outpatients in their GP's surgery or at the hospital.

The first priority of nursing intervention is to stop the bleeding, whilst providing psychological support. The patient should

INFORMATION 16.2

Management of a Patient With Epistaxis

- Provide reassurance to the patient. Guide them to a bed and recommend they sit down, leaning slightly forwards so the blood drains out of the nose rather than into the back of the throat. Swallowing the blood will make the patient feel nauseous and they may vomit. Encourage the patient to breathe through their mouth and spit out the blood so the amount of blood loss can be monitored.
- Pinch all the soft parts of the nose (located below the nasal bones) between your thumb and forefinger (as if they were holding their nose to jump into a swimming pool). If the bleeding continues, apply ice to the forehead and back of the neck to constrict the blood supply to the nose. Monitor the patient's vital signs, ensuring they remain cardiovascularly stable. Speak gently with the patient, question them as to what the cause of the bleeding may be, what medication they take and if there is a history of nose bleeds or other medical issues.

Bleeding from nose → apply pressure to soft area towards the front of the nose for 10 minutes

Bleeding stops: vital signs normal, patient can go home with antibiotic nasal ointment and the following advice:
- Rest, and do not fiddle with, or pick your nose.
- Do not blow your nose. If you have to sneeze, open your mouth to reduce the pressure of air in your nose.
- Have cool showers or baths.
- Do not strain or bend down to lift anything heavy.
- No hot liquids for 72 hours.
- Do not strain during bowel movements; use a stool softener if necessary.
- If you take blood-thinning medication, ensure you have weekly blood monitoring until your blood levels have stabilised.
- If you are spending a lot of time in air-conditioned or heated environments, ensure your nose is well moistened or use a saline nasal spray.
 Bleeding continues despite compression of soft area of nose:
- Continue monitoring vital signs and take bloods.
- If the bleeding point is seen on examination of the nose, nasal cautery will be carried out.
- Bleeding stops; patient can go home if blood results are normal. Patient will require antibiotic nasal ointment and advice as above.
 Bleeding continues despite compression and no bleeding point is visible in the nose:
- Continue monitoring vital signs and take bloods.
- Nasal packing inserted into each nostril, apply bolster dressing under nose.
- Oral antibiotics and mild sedation prescribed.
- Encourage good oral hygiene and plenty of cold fluids.
- Packing removed after 24 hours. If no further bleeding the patient can go home with advice.
- Outpatient appointment to ensure underlying cause of epistaxis treated.
 Profuse bleeding from further back in nose:
- Continue monitoring vital signs and take bloods.
- Nasal packing and nasal catheter inserted with air used to inflate balloon, bolster dressing applied under nose.
- Encourage good oral hygiene and plenty of cold fluids.
- Oral antibiotics and mild sedation.
- Packing and catheter removed in 24–48 hours.
- If no further bleeding the patient can go home with advice as above and an outpatient's appointment.
 Profuse bleeding continues despite packing:
- Ensure patient's cardiovascular system remains stable.
- Prepare the patient for theatre to undergo ligation of nasal arteries (refer to Chapter 24 for details of routine perioperative care).
- Specific nasal postoperative care as above.

be helped to sit upright with the head slightly forward and asked to mouth breathe and spit out all blood. This helps to estimate the blood loss and prevents the blood from being swallowed and causing nausea and vomiting. Digital pressure with the thumb and forefinger should be applied to the soft part of the nose (as if they were holding their nose to jump into a swimming pool) which puts pressure on the bleeding blood vessels in Little's area (see Fig. 16.6). This area has many surface arterioles which may have weakened walls. Fifteen continuous minutes of this pressure is usually sufficient to control most nosebleeds. Ice wrapped in old material or something cold applied to the forehead or back of the nose will help constrict larger blood vessels. If these first aid measures fail, or if there are recurrent nosebleeds, the patient will probably be transferred to hospital for insertion of a nasal pack or cautery of the area.

Once the bleeding is under control, the nurse should explain to the patient and, where appropriate, to the parents how to prevent nosebleeds from recurring. Advice should be given about blowing the nose gently, avoiding picking the nose and trying to keep the nasal mucosa slightly moist by using soft petroleum jelly. An explanation of how to cope with and control a nosebleed should also be given (Information 16.2). The patient is often prescribed a simple antibiotic cream such as naseptin which contains both an antiseptic (chlorhexidine) and antibiotic (neomycin) with an emollient (arachis oil). The patient should gently insert the nozzle of the ointment into their nostril pointing it away from the septum to not traumatise the delicate lining. They should squeeze a small pea-sized amount into each nostril and pinch the soft bit of the nose after to distribute the ointment. The nurse can help the patient administer this the first time if necessary to reduce stress for patients when independently administering the ointment in the community. The patient should be questioned if they have a peanut allergy as peanut oil is contained in naseptin and bactraban could be used as an alternative.

Hospital Treatment

This will be necessary for severe epistaxis that cannot be controlled by the aforementioned measures. By providing clear and concise information, the nurse can help alleviate the patient's anxiety and aid recovery. Some patients admitted as emergencies with uncontrollable nosebleeds will be in hypovolaemic shock (see Chapter 19, The Deteriorating Patient, Recognising and Managing Shock).

A specialist nurse can pack the nasal cavity. When a nasal pack is in place, the patient will only be able to breathe through the mouth and may be afraid of suffocation. Frequent oral hygiene and plenty of cold oral fluids should be offered to prevent the oral mucosa becoming dry. These drinks must not be hot, as this can cause local dilatation of blood vessels and exacerbate the problem. Eye care may be necessary as the packing may obstruct the nasolacrimal duct, causing tears to overflow (see Chapter 15, Nursing Patients With Disorders of the Eye and Sight Impairment). Nasal packing can also cause hypoxia, leading to disorientation as well as alterations to vital signs. Oxygen therapy and blood gas monitoring with appropriate monitoring of O_2 saturation will be needed in this situation. Areas that have been cauterised may become encrusted. Naseptin or bactroban (if allergy to peanuts) should be applied to such areas twice a day for a few weeks until the mucosa has healed.

Although anxieties can be reduced by answering the patient's questions and giving information, sedatives may also be prescribed when necessary. Following epistaxis, patients are usually nursed propped up in bed to aid venous return from the area and to make it easier for them to spit out any blood. They should avoid swallowing blood as this can cause nausea and vomiting. Ice packs may be applied to the nose to help constrict the vessels and control bleeding. The nurse should explain to the patient how to breathe through the mouth and a vomit bowl or sputum carton as well as tissues and gauze should be on hand. Again, it is important to offer frequent oral hygiene such as mouthwash or mouth sponges, plenty of cool drinks and eye care as necessary. As these patients often have dysphagia because of the pressure of the nasal pack on the soft palate, eating and drinking must resume as tolerated but a nutritious soft or even liquid diet may be more appropriate. In severe cases, dietician input may be of benefit. Bed rest is usually advised, although patients should be allowed to gently mobilise to the toilet with support from a member of the nursing team when necessary. They should be advised not to strain and ask for stool softeners if they feel concerned.

Packing is usually removed in 2 or 3 days. If the bleeding has not been controlled, the patient will have the appropriate arteries ligated in theatre. This is performed using telescopes through the nostrils so the patient will not have to have incisions made in the skin. If a deviated nasal septum (see Fig. 16.5) has been a contributory cause, corrective surgery may be performed. If the patient continues to bleed, an interventional radiologist may be contacted to embolise the bleeding vessels using a guide wire to seal off bleeding points.

If hypertension, anticlotting medication (such as warfarin, clopidogrel or apixaban) or another medical disorder has caused the nosebleed, an appropriate specialist medical opinion is sought and treatment commenced. The nurse may, in the meantime, obtain appropriate patient education booklets or information sheets in relation to the relevant disorder from colleagues working in the ward(s) specialising in the care of such patients, so that the patient can be given appropriate advice (see Chapter 13, Nursing Patients With Blood Disorders).

Community Care

To prevent the recurrence of epistaxis, support should continue after the patient has returned home and resumed normal activities. If the patient is at home, the GP and practice nurse will be informed of their condition so that they can encourage the patient to implement the advice received in hospital and can monitor hypertension if present. Drinking a lot of alcohol can increase the risk of nosebleeds so the patient needs to be advised to reduce their alcohol intake. Refer to Reflection 16.3.

Disorders of the Paranasal Sinuses

The paranasal sinuses are a group of air spaces surrounding the nose which, it is said, make the skull lighter and add resonance to the voice. They consist of two frontal, two maxillary and two ethmoid sinuses and a single sphenoid sinus divided by a septum. These sinuses all drain into the nose (see Fig. 16.5).

Acute Sinusitis

Acute sinusitis is the inflammation of one or more of the paranasal sinuses. It usually develops as an infection secondary to an upper respiratory tract infection or dental disease. Because of the close anatomical connection of the sinuses with the nose, sinus infection is common. It may be acute or chronic.

Common Presenting Symptoms

Pain is a symptom, and it may be facial, supraorbital (above the eye) or intraocular (within the globe of the eye), depending on the sinus involved. Tenderness in the area of pain and nasal

---

REFLECTION 16.3

An Experience of Epistaxis

It first started on a Saturday morning. I bent down to pick up my bag from the floor and realised my nose was running. On wiping it, I saw fresh blood. Going into the bathroom, I could still feel it running and the tissue was getting soggy with blood. Remembering some first aid, I squeezed the soft front of my nose, sat down and leaned forward. At least it stopped the blood coming out of my nose, although I could taste some in my mouth now. After 10 minutes, I stopped squeezing and the bleeding stopped. I cleaned around the front of my nose, but spent the rest of the day not daring to blow my nose in case the bleeding started again.

All was well until Wednesday evening. I'd just had a bath and was watching TV, when I felt my nose running. Again, there was blood on the tissue and dripping from my nose. Like the previous time, I squeezed my nose, but after 10 minutes, when I released the pressure, the blood started dripping and I squeezed again. Again, on releasing the pressure, the blood continued to drip and I now had a pile of bloodstained tissues in the bin and patches of blood all over the bathroom floor as I tried stuffing tissues up my nose as well. By now an hour had passed and still the blood dripped. I didn't think it was ever going to stop and wasn't sure what to do.

My flatmate suggested ringing 111 for NHS advice. She phoned and we were advised to go to the ED of our local hospital. So my flatmate drove me to the hospital and I took the washing up bowl to catch the blood, as I didn't want to mess up the car!

On arriving at the ED, my flatmate booked me in and I was seen very quickly by a nurse. On releasing the squeeze on my nose, the blood still continued to drip out and the nurse said I would see an advanced nurse practitioner (ANP). The nurse then squeezed my nose for me. I was glad as my arms were aching from all the squeezing I had done. My blood pressure was taken and the doctor saw me.

Despite all the blood coming out of my nose, the ANP sprayed it with a local anaesthetic and had a look inside. They could see a blood vessel at the front of my nose that was bleeding, so they put a stick on it to cauterise the vessel and the bleeding stopped. It was a great relief and after an hour of no further bleeding I was allowed to go home with some nasal ointment and an outpatient's appointment for 4 weeks' time.

Activity

- Reflect on what advice you would give the patient with an active nosebleed if you had answered the telephone to them.

---

obstruction may also be features, and purulent nasal discharge is often present. The patient usually complains of general malaise and has a raised temperature.

Medical Management

A nasal swab may be taken for culture and sensitivity. Sinus radiography may also be performed to determine which sinuses are affected. Medical treatment usually consists of the prescription of mild analgesics, antibiotics and nasal decongestant drops.

Nursing Management and Health Promotion: Acute Sinusitis

The patient with acute sinusitis is usually nursed at home, and will be advised to rest in bed, to drink plenty of fluids, to take mild analgesics such as paracetamol and to self-administer any prescribed nasal drops/sprays. Oral hygiene is also important as the individual will probably be mouth breathing because of the nasal obstruction. Moist steam inhalations can also bring some relief and help to loosen crusting in the nasal cavities. Sinus rinses can also bring some relief and these can be purchased over the counter. Many sufferers find inhalations very soothing first thing in the morning and last thing at night. The patient can cover their head with a towel and leaning over a basin of hot water they should try to breathe the steam in through their nose and out through their mouth. They should blow their nose when necessary to release mucus rather than sniffing and swallowing. Patients need to take care that the hot water is placed on a stable surface to minimise the risk of burning themselves. Eucalyptus or olbas oil can be added to the water but there is no reliable research demonstrating that this is of benefit. After 2 or 3 days the person should have improved sufficiently to be fully active again.

Chronic Sinusitis

Chronic sinusitis is common and can be quite debilitating. It can develop for several reasons, including:
- inadequate treatment of an acute episode
- septal deviation or nasal polyps preventing adequate drainage of the sinuses
- pollution, e.g. cigarette smoke
- allergic nasal disease.

Common Presenting Symptoms

The main symptoms of chronic sinusitis are purulent nasal discharge, postnasal drip (mucus draining from the nose down to the back of the throat), facial pain, headache and recurrent throat infections.

Medical Management

Treatment is initially conservative, consisting of treating any infection with prescribed antibiotics and nasal decongestant sprays. Surgery may be necessary to remove all of the diseased mucosal lining and widen the opening to the nasal passage to allow more effective drainage. This is functional endoscopic sinus surgery (FESS). Computed tomography (CT) and/or MRI scans are vital for both diagnostic and intraoperative use. For further information, see Sethi et al. (2017).

❖ Nursing Management and Health Promotion: Chronic Sinusitis

Nursing priorities when caring for these patients are:
- To prepare the patient for surgery and to observe for any possible complications, including haemorrhage and infection.
- Removal of nasal packing (if competent) as per the surgeon's instructions.
- Administration of prescribed analgesics, education and assistance with nasal douching and antibiotics.

On discharge, the patient must be advised on the correct method for instillation of nasal drops/sprays and the importance of sinus rinses or steam inhalations. In addition, the patient should be provided with written information on sinusitis with self-help recommendations and advice to see the GP if they are concerned that the symptoms are returning.

Nasal Injury

Injuries to the nose are fairly common and usually occur in sporting activities, falls, accidents and assaults. A blow to one side of the nose may fracture and displace the bone, causing deviation on the other side. A direct blow to the front of the nose can splay out the nasal bones, resulting in a depressed bridge. Fractures of the nose account for 50% of facial fractures. An injury that is sufficiently severe to fracture the nasal bones will also cause soft tissue swelling and may cause epistaxis. It may take 3–5 days for the swelling to reduce so the bones can be assessed for fracture.

Medical Management

Investigations. Serious facial injuries will involve an X-ray however, it does not always reveal the nasal fracture or may simply reveal a previously undetected fracture. An examination of the nose using a nasal speculum will allow the practitioner to see if the airways are patent and if there is any damage to the septum. It is important to exclude a septal haematoma as this should be drained urgently. Palpation of the nasal bones must be carried out very gently, as they will be very tender and painful for up to 3 weeks following a fracture.

Treatment of a broken nose involves manipulating the fractured bones. Occasionally, this can be done at the time of the accident, but more commonly it is done a few days later, when the swelling has reduced. The fracture may not have caused a change to the shape of the nose but if it has, then movement of the nasal bones back into alignment can be successfully done in the outpatient setting under local anaesthetic. The manipulation must be performed within 14 days of injury to prevent calcification and fixation of the nasal bones. If the corrected fracture is unstable, a plaster of Paris cast is usually taped in position over the nose for about 10 days to allow the fracture to set correctly.

❖ Nursing Management and Health Promotion: Nasal Injury

First aid treatment of a fractured nose will involve measures to stop any epistaxis and to limit the oedema. This involves compressing the end of the nostrils gently between the thumb and forefinger, which unfortunately will be painful for the patient, and encouraging the patient to sit with the head slightly forwards and to spit out any blood. If ice is available, an ice pack applied to the bridge of the nose can help to control bleeding and swelling. Any epistaxis which results from a blow to the nose is usually short lived.

Disorders of the Nasal Septum

Deviation of the Nasal Septum

The nasal septum separates the nostrils. It is usually thin and quite straight. The posterior part is composed of bone and the anterior part of cartilage. Deviations of the nasal septum can range from a simple bulge to a marked S-shaped deformity. Most people have some degree of deviation; hence, when introducing a nasogastric tube, the patient should always be asked which nostril is easier to breathe through.

Developmental problems or trauma may result in a deviated nasal septum. Patients usually complain of nasal obstruction, infection of the sinuses or chronic otitis media due to the inability of the eustachian tubes to function properly. Any combination of these symptoms may be present, or there may be no symptoms; simply having a septal deviation is not a reason to operate on it.

Medical Management

An assessment by the specialist nurse of the symptoms, correlated with the degree of the deformity, should be carried out before a treatment plan is agreed. Inspection of the nose with a nasal speculum should reveal the extent of the deviation. If surgery is the chosen treatment, this is likely to be either a submucous resection or a septoplasty. For further details of these procedures, see Tysome and Kanegaonkar (2018).

❖ Nursing Management and Health Promotion: Deviation of the Nasal Septum

Septal surgery is often carried out as a day case and packs can be in place from 4 to 24 hours. Nursing care in hospital will be similar to that given for epistaxis. Patients are usually discharged 2–4 hours after the nasal tampon has been removed to ensure the patient can be monitored for post removal bleeding. It is the surgeon's preference as to whether packing or splints are used in the immediate postoperative period, but this will be documented in the patient's operation sheet. There will be a degree of nasal obstruction for 2 or 3 weeks after surgery, until the postsurgical swelling has subsided. Patients are usually advised to stay away from work or crowded places for 10–14 days after surgery to minimise the risk of infection. They are also advised to follow the surgeon's instructions with regard to steam inhalations, nasal douches (sniffing up a solution, usually water-based, into each nostril), sinus rinses or decongestant sprays.

Patients should rest when discharged home and take 10–14 days off work to recover. They should avoid hot showers and drinks and no strenuous exercise to reduce the chance of epistaxis for the first few weeks after the operation.

Septal Haematoma

This usually results from trauma or surgery, and is a collection of blood beneath the mucoperichondrium of the septum. The patient complains of nasal obstruction and pain. Examination usually reveals a bilateral swelling in the nasal cavities. Antibiotics are given to prevent infection and it is urgently necessary to incise and drain the haematoma.

Septal Perforation

Trauma, surgery or snorting illegal drugs is usually the cause of a hole in the septum. Although the patient is often symptom-free, excessive crusting or epistaxis may occur. Occasionally, the patient complains of whistling on inspiration. If symptoms are troublesome, surgical closure may be attempted.

Nasal Obstruction

Obstruction of the nasal cavities can result from a number of causes but patients usually present with similar symptoms, the most common being obstructed breathing and increased nasal discharge. Some of the most common causes are:

- infection
- allergy
- deviated nasal septum
- foreign bodies
- polyps
- neoplasms.

Infection and Allergy

Infection and allergy can cause an inflammatory reaction in the mucosa of the nose resulting in a sensation of blockage. This is one of the reasons that patients are often prescribed topical steroids and antihistamines in the form of intranasal sprays to reduce the swelling in the nose.

Foreign Bodies in the Nose

It is usually very young children, aged 2–4 years, or those with learning difficulties who insert foreign bodies into the nasal cavity. These objects may be organic or inorganic. Inorganic objects include buttons, beads and small plastic or metal objects which may lie undetected for a long time. Small button batteries such as found in small toys and hearing aids need to be removed as an emergency before the battery leaks its corrosive fluid. Organic bodies such as peas, wood, paper, cotton wool or sweets cause a local inflammatory reaction which will eventually lead to the formation of granulation tissue. The resulting nasal discharge will eventually become purulent, foul-smelling and bloodstained. Characteristically, the discharge is from only one nostril.

🔵 Medical Management

Following a thorough examination, the foreign body is usually removed in the outpatient department. Occasionally, it has been in place for such a long time that a GA is needed for smooth and safe removal.

❖ Nursing Management and Health Promotion: Foreign Body

Support and reassurance will be given to both the patient and the family as removal can be uncomfortable and the child will need to stay still. Epistaxis is a possible complication following removal, irrespective whether an anaesthetic was used.

Nasal Polyps

Nasal polyps come from the mucosal nasal lining and are projections of oedematous mucous membrane and may look like bunches of grapes. They tend to be triggered from prolonged infection or allergy and are usually bilateral and multiple. They occur more commonly in adult males than in females.

Common Presenting Symptoms

Nasal polyps are more commonly seen in patients who developed late-onset asthma, aspirin intolerance or cystic fibrosis. Patients usually complain of nasal obstruction and discharge. Occasionally, the size of the polyps may cause broadening of the external nose. The patient may complain of headaches if there is sinus involvement and there may be loss of smell and taste.

🔵 Medical Management

On examination, a characteristic glossy, greyish swelling will be visible. If probed, it will be found to be soft, insensitive and mobile. Medical management is the treatment of choice using intranasal steroid drops/sprays. If this fails to improve symptoms, then surgical removal may be appropriate. Recurrences are common and an attempt should be made to treat any underlying infection or allergy.

❖ Nursing Management and Health Promotion: Nasal Polyps

Nursing staff should be alert to epistaxis, which is the main postoperative complication of polyp removal. Given that polyps can be associated with allergies, many patients may also suffer from asthma and should be closely observed in this regard. It is dependent on the surgeon's preference if nasal packing is used in the immediate postoperative stage. As it is fairly common for polyps to recur, patients may be followed up in nurse-led telephone clinics. If the patient still complains of nasal obstruction, an appointment can then be made for the rhinology clinic.

Neoplasms

Nasal and sinus tumours are rare. When they occur, they are usually unilateral. Malignant tumours are often infected and ulcerated, in which case they usually produce epistaxis or a profuse purulent discharge. Headache may also be a feature if there is sinus involvement.

Treatment may consist of surgery, radiotherapy, chemotherapy or a combination of these. Patients receiving radiotherapy or chemotherapy are usually treated as outpatients and may be visited by community nurses, including Macmillan nurses, if they experience any side-effects of treatment requiring nursing intervention. For further information on nasal and sinus neoplasms and treatments, see Tysome and Kanegaonkar (2018).

Common Problems Caused by Nasal Surgery

- *Bleeding* – this occurs because the nasal mucosa has such a rich blood supply. It can be controlled by the use of ice packs. If the surgeon suspects that the bleeding might be severe, a nasal pack may be inserted.
- *Oedema* – oedema of the mucosa is likely to occur as a consequence of manipulation. Ice packs may help to minimise swelling.
- *Watery discharge* – the irritation of the mucosa, which results from surgery, will cause the production of an excessive amount of watery discharge known as rhinorrhoea. The nurse should provide an adequate supply of tissues or apply a nasal bolster made of gauze to absorb discharge. This helps to make the problem more manageable.
- *Pain* – as the nose is blocked after surgery, the patient may experience frontal headaches, which should be alleviated with prescribed analgesics, e.g. ibuprofen and paracetamol.

THE THROAT

Anatomy and Physiology of the Throat

The throat is usually considered to consist of the pharynx and the larynx. The pharynx may be divided into three parts. The nasopharynx extends from the nasal septum to the eustachian tubes and rests behind and above the soft palate. The oropharynx (middle part of the pharynx) extends from the soft palate to the hyoid bone; it contains the base of the tongue, the uvula and the tonsils and is surrounded by lymphoid tissue (Fig. 16.7). The lowest part of the pharynx is called the hypopharynx.

The larynx is the organ of voice production and airway protection. It is composed mainly of cartilage and muscle and is lined with a mucosa of stratified squamous epithelium (upper part) and ciliated pseudostratified columnar epithelium (lower part).

Disorders of the Throat

Benign Tumours

There is a wide breadth of pathology such as cysts, nodules, polyps and Reinke's oedema. Treatment options often include speech and language therapy (SALT), microlaryngoscopy surgery and vocal hygiene (reduce caffeine and low salt diet). These generally arise as a result of voice overuse and the patient usually presents with continued hoarseness. The tumours are usually attached to the vocal cords and vary greatly in size.

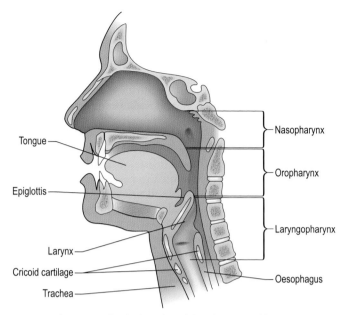

Figure 16.7 Sagittal section of the pharynx and larynx.

Resolution of small nodules may be achieved by voice rest and appropriate speech therapy. Larger nodules may require surgical removal. For further information on benign and malignant tumours, see Tysome and Kanegaonkar (2018).

Head and Neck Cancer

This refers to cancers that originate in the squamous cells that line the moist mucosal lining in the mouth, nose, sinuses and throat. Cancer of the salivary glands is included but these glands can have many different types of cancer (National Cancer Institute 2017). Risk factors include chewing betel quid (betel leaf and tobacco with a mixture of other leaves), poor dental hygiene, human papillomavirus (HPV), smoking and a high alcohol intake.

Laryngeal Cancer

Carcinoma of the larynx is classified according to its location and extent, that is supraglottic (above the vocal cords), glottic (confined to the vocal cords) or subglottic (below the vocal cords) (see Fig. 16.7). It accounts for 1% of all malignant disease and is more common in males than in females. The most common form of the disease is squamous cell carcinoma. About 10% of all patients with carcinoma of the larynx have a coexisting carcinoma of the bronchus.

Common Presenting Symptoms. Patients tend to present with a change in voice that has worsened over the last 2–3 months and they may also complain of earache, difficulty swallowing, a sensation of something in the throat when swallowing and possibly raised glands in the neck (Tysome and Kanegaonkar 2018). The majority of patients have a history of heavy smoking, although the disorder does occasionally occur in nonsmokers. ENT referral guidelines emphasise the importance of referring patients who present with change in voice, persistent sore throat (>3 weeks) and a lump in neck with an urgent 2-week wait suspected cancer referral. Otalgia (earache), dyspnoea (shortness of breath), dysphagia (difficulty swallowing), neck lumps and weight loss are all symptoms of advanced laryngeal carcinoma. The impact of the diagnosis and the community care needs of a patient newly diagnosed with cancer are discussed in chapter.

🌑 Medical Management

Carcinoma of the larynx has a high rate of cure if detected early. The form of treatment offered will depend on the site of the tumour and how early it has been detected. If the tumour is confined to the vocal cords, it is usually diagnosed as a result of the patient consulting their GP with a history of hoarseness. Patients who have suffered from hoarseness for more than 3 weeks should have a nasendoscopy (a flexible endoscope to examine the oropharynx and hypopharynx including the vocal cords) to investigate the possibility of carcinoma. Diagnosis is confirmed by an examination of the patient's larynx under sedation or general anaesthesia (direct laryngoscopy) and a histological examination of a biopsy of the tumour.

If the patient has a positive biopsy result, their case will be discussed within a multidisciplinary team and best management options considered and presented to the patient. Depending on the size and spread of the tumour, they may undergo CO_2 resection laser, radiotherapy, chemoradiation (chemotherapy given at certain points during a course of radiotherapy) or surgery with a total laryngectomy (see website). Laryngeal surgery may also have to be performed on patients who have a residual or recurrent tumour following radiotherapy. There is a wealth of information regarding tracheostomy and laryngectomy on the tracheostomy.org.uk website for all team members and patients and their families.

Office-Based Procedures in Laryngology

There has recently been a development of less invasive procedures for patients with benign and premalignant laryngological disease. There has been a shift of many procedures from the operating theatre to the outpatient setting as this has become a viable alternative with advances in technology and rising costs in inpatient procedures (Hamdan et al. 2021).

The term 'office-based setting' refers to a patient undergoing a procedure sitting in an upright position, receiving local anaesthesia and being able to communicate verbally throughout the intervention. These procedures tend to occur in the outpatients department. This has resulted in exciting developments for nurses in the ENT outpatient department as they assist with these procedures and monitor the patient's health and safety in the recovery period, providing support, reassurance and postprocedure care and advice.

Office-based laryngology procedures are performed under local anaesthetic and allow patients to be discharged straight after their procedure and avoid requiring an inpatient bed.

This transition has had a positive effect on laryngology departments within hospitals as theatre lists for cases requiring GA are reduced resulting in a more efficient system, shorter waiting times, significant cost reductions and happier patients.

Grewal et al. (2021) writes about the success of these office-based procedures and mentions the avoidance of GA as a key advantage to those with significant comorbidities and high GA risk, with nearly all patients discharged the same day and returning home straight away.

Very advanced tumours of the larynx may be considered inoperable, in which case the patient may be given palliative radiotherapy and/or chemotherapy to relieve some of the more distressing symptoms (see Chapter 31, Nursing the Patient With Cancer). Grier (2018) advises that 'although nurses can't eliminate the hardship that patients will face during treatment

for head and neck cancer, we can support them by providing compassionate and thorough care'. The most frequent symptoms and problems experienced by patients with head and neck cancer, in a palliative care situation, are pain, weight loss, feeding difficulties, altered body image, respiratory problems and communication difficulties. A tracheostomy is sometimes performed to relieve any respiratory obstruction and a percutaneous endoscopic gastrostomy (PEG) tube inserted to aid nutrition, hydration, administration of medications and patient comfort (see Chapter 21, Maintaining Fluid Electrolyte and Acid-Base Balance). For detailed information regarding the care of the patient with head and neck cancer and laryngectomy, please see the website.

Oropharyngeal Cancer

Carcinoma of the oropharynx is classified according to its location and extent, that is tonsil, soft palate, base of tongue or posterior pharyngeal wall. This disease is a squamous cell carcinoma. The incidence of oropharyngeal cancer is increasing and has done so over the past 15–20 years. Whilst smoking and alcohol are risk factors, the major drive for the increase in incidence has been from the increasing exposure of HPV through intimate contact. HPV is also associated with cervical, penile and anal cancers and certain subtypes are also associated with nonmalignant cutaneous warts. This disease is also a squamous cell carcinoma.

Common Presenting Symptoms. Patients may notice a neck lump associated with a lymph node metastasis from the primary tumour. Others may present with local symptoms such as a sore throat or earache. Occasionally, people just present by noticing in the mirror that there is something unusual in their throat. These HPV-driven cancers happen in a younger population group than a typical head and neck cancer patient.

🌑 Medical Management

HPV-driven carcinoma of the oropharynx has a better treatment success rate than other head and neck cancers, if localised and not spread further than the head and neck region. Treatments vary between hospital trusts but options include resection of the tumour (with a laser or robotic system) plus or minus radiotherapy versus radiotherapy plus or minus chemotherapy. Currently, trials are being run to decide on the best management options for patients.

Further metastatic disease may be managed in a palliative setting and a variety of treatments exist to manage the primary tumour but also the symptoms the patient may be incurring.

HPV vaccination has been introduced but is variable from country to country and it will reduce the incidence of HPV-driven disease but will take time for its effects to be seen. Ten years on from the vaccination of girls, boys are now included in the school vaccination programme in years 11 and 12. However, there is no catch up programme for older boys who have missed out on this vaccine opportunity.

Tracheostomy

The surgical procedure of tracheostomy involves making an opening through the skin and structures of the neck into the trachea. It is one of the earliest operations described; there is evidence that it was performed by the Egyptians in biblical times. A tracheostomy may be short- or long-term and may be planned as elective surgery or performed as an emergency procedure.

The pandemic resulted in a surge of patients requiring relatively prolonged intubation and ventilation, with around 10% of this patient group requiring a tracheostomy (McGrath et al. 2020). The highly infectious nature of the virus meant that usual considerations for tracheostomy and usual care for patients with a tracheostomy were adjusted.

There are recent publications regarding tracheostomy in patients infected with the COVID-19 virus. Research suggests that survival rates amongst ventilated patients with a tracheostomy were greater than in patients who did not have a tracheostomy performed (Molin et al. 2022).

See suggested reading.

Indications

The indications for a tracheostomy are as follows:

- *Airway obstruction* – this may be caused by the inhalation and impaction of a foreign body in the larynx. Severe inflammation may also cause obstruction, as might laryngeal cancer which is being treated by radiotherapy.
- *Bronchial toilet* – after head injury, drug overdose, cerebrovascular accident, coma or certain neurological disorders, the patient may require assistance with respiration and removal of bronchial secretions.
- *Need to improve respiratory efficiency* – when patients with impaired respiration are relying on their own efforts rather than assisted ventilation, the performance of a tracheostomy cuts down dead space and improves respiratory efficiency.
- *Artificial ventilation* – if artificial ventilation is required for more than 72 hours, a tracheostomy may be indicated, as it has been shown that endotracheal intubation for 72 hours or longer can cause laryngotracheal damage.
- *Major head and neck surgery* – a tracheostomy will maintain the airway and protect it from haemorrhage and obstruction due to oedema both during and after surgery (see also Chapter 25, Nursing the Patient Undergoing Surgery). Information 16.3 lists some indications for short- and long-term tracheostomy.

🔹 Medical Management

Prior to performing a tracheostomy, time must be spent with the patient and family explaining what is involved and the effect the procedure will have. In an emergency situation, such as when the patient presents with stridor or is unconscious, when there is minimal opportunity or time to prepare the patient preoperatively, a planned programme of support and explanation will be required afterwards. The National Tracheostomy Safety Project (NTSP) has excellent patient and family resources to help.

Tracheostomy is usually carried out with the patient under a GA, but in emergencies caused by severe airway obstruction, a local anaesthetic may be used. Tracheostomy involves making an incision into the trachea through the third and fourth tracheal rings. An appropriately sized tracheostomy tube is inserted. For the first 24–48 hours, a cuffed tracheostomy tube (Fig. 16.8) with cuff inflated is normally used to prevent blood and secretions from the wound being aspirated into the lungs and aspiration pneumonia developing (see Chapter 28, Nursing the Critically Ill Patient). Cuff inflation is often maintained for longer periods of time in patients with COVID-19 until viral shedding has subsided (David et al. 2020). A more permanent tract usually forms about 5 days postoperatively, at which time it is possible to change the tube. Tracheal dilators must always be to hand to keep the stoma open in case the tube is expelled accidentally. Most hospitals have

---

INFORMATION 16.3

Indications for Tracheostomy

Short-Term Tracheostomy

- Assisted ventilation
- Burns and scalds
- Foreign body lodged in trachea
- Major head and neck surgery
- Severe infection
- Trauma to larynx, face, mouth or oropharynx
- Vocal cord paralysis

Long-Term Tracheostomy

- Congenital abnormality
- Trauma causing permanent damage
- Untreatable tumours, causing airway obstruction
- Vocal cord paralysis
- Ventilatory support

Figure 16.8 Tracheostomy tubes in common use. (A) Noncuffed outer tube. (B) Cuffed outer tube. (C) Parts of tracheostomy tube set.

a policy regarding the first tube change, which is likely to be performed by medical staff or experienced nursing staff.

There are several types of tracheostomy tube available, and the most appropriate one will be chosen for each patient. As discussed earlier, a cuffed tube, preferably with a low-pressure cuff, may be inserted during the operation. Single-use disposable tubes are usually employed and may be cuffed or plain. All tubes have an introducer, which is removed immediately on insertion, and an inner tube, which can be removed for cleaning without necessitating removal of the whole tube. Most tubes are made of polyvinyl chloride (PVC) or silicone, although silver tubes are occasionally used (ensuring patient's do not have a metal allergy).

❖ Nursing Management and Health Promotion: Tracheostomy

Preoperative Priorities

Physical and psychological preparation of the individual for a tracheostomy is a priority of preoperative nursing care as the procedure can cause many difficulties. If the tracheostomy is short-term, these problems will be of limited duration, but if it is to be long-term, the patient and family will require additional information and education. They may need help in coming to terms not only with the problems presented by the stoma but also with a prognosis that might require additional care, for example cancer, which has necessitated surgical treatment. Patients who have been well prepared for a tracheostomy tend to cope better than those who have not. Unprepared patients may become insecure, withdrawn and depressed (Mills et al. 2021). Ideally, a patient undergoing tracheostomy should be assigned to one nurse who can gain the confidence of the patient and family. Many hospitals have tracheostomy clinical nurse specialists available to provide patient support. Every shift the patient's needs must be assessed and addressed both physically and psychologically. The main problems in the immediate postoperative period, for which the patient has to be prepared prior to surgery, are as follows.

Temporary Loss of Voice. Air will bypass the vocal cords following the tracheostomy, making speech impossible unless a tube with a speaking valve is inserted. Communication strategies whereby the patient can make themselves understood by staff and family members should be worked out beforehand (Freeman-Sanderson et al. 2018). This may be in the form of pen and paper or the use of technology, depending on patient preference.

Altered Body Image. Body image is concerned with the control and function as well as physical appearance of the body. The very thought of coughing out sputum, which most people usually go to great lengths to hide, but which in the case of the patient who has a tracheostomy must be done through an open hole and tube in their neck, as well as their need for suction, is not easy to understand and accept. High-quality information and education must be offered to help the patient and family adjust to the presence of a tube in the neck. A visit from a patient who has adjusted well to having a tracheostomy may help.

Increased Secretions. These are produced because of the irritation caused by the tube and air bypassing the nose. This should be explained to the patient along with the need for suction. It is helpful, if possible, to show the equipment required for this prior to surgery so that the patient is familiar with it.

Postoperative Priorities

Maintenance of the Airway. On return to the ward the patient should be nursed in a sitting position (usually at a 45-degree angle), with the neck well supported. The tracheostomy tapes are fixed to the flange of the tracheostomy tube and go around the neck and must be tied securely in position to avoid tube movement or displacement. The most critical incident regarding a tracheostomy is tube displacement when moving a patient (Lewith and Athanassoglou 2019), so the tube should always be checked to ensure it is in the correct position before, during and after moving the patient.

Tracheal suction should be carried out regularly to clear secretions from the tube. To prevent infection, it is necessary to perform this procedure with a sterile nontouch technique. The frequency of suction varies on each patient's clinical need. However, suction should be carried out at least once every shift to ensure the tracheostomy tube is patent. A sterile catheter should be used each time in open suction and should touch only the inside of the tracheostomy tube. Catheters are only reused when using the closed technique, which tends to be when caring for a ventilated patient. The catheter diameter should be no more than half that of the tube to allow adequate flow of gases around it. If it is too wide, it will draw air out of the lungs more quickly than it can be replaced, which can cause atelectasis. McGrath et al. (2018) gives a formula and chart to allow calculation of the correct catheter size. Tubes are now available with subglottic aspiration ports. Suction should be applied only as the catheter is being removed. Thumb-control catheters are ideal for this. Since the patient is unable to breathe during suction, it should be performed for no longer than 10–15 seconds; the patient should be allowed enough time to recover before it is repeated. The amount and type of secretions should be observed and recorded using bedside charts. Routine monitoring using capnography is now being used outside of the intensive care environment as immediate information is gained about adequate ventilation of the patient and assurance that the tracheostomy tube is in the correct position. Attentive nursing care is essential and the use of information over the patient's bed regarding their tracheostomy tube and a difficult airway plan should be routinely used. Bedhead information can be downloaded free of charge from the tracheostomy.org.uk website and the information has been produced for the National Tracheotomy Safety Project (2022).

The physiotherapist will teach the patient how to cough into a tissue; as the patient becomes competent at this, the need for suction will gradually be eliminated.

Continuous humidification at body temperature is given immediately postoperatively via a mechanical humidifier. When the patient begins to mobilise, a heat moisture exchange valve (HME) or protector over the stoma will humidify inhaled air, act as a filter and have a cosmetic effect by covering the tube.

Care of the Wound. The stoma (the surgically created opening into the trachea from the neck) into which the tube is inserted will require regular cleansing to prevent crusting and infection. A dressing beneath the tracheostomy tube can aid comfort and help to prevent sores caused by the tube and hard flanges as well as excoriation of the skin from tracheal secretions. However, there needs to be careful monitoring of the skin integrity as breakdown can occur quickly. Every shift, nurses should be checking the skin around the tracheostomy or stoma, and if exudate is seen a swab taken immediately for microbiological culture. Skin should be kept dry and can be protected with a barrier cream or film which should be applied regularly as part of the everyday stoma care. If sutures are present, these will be removed according to local policy (see Chapter 23, Tissue Viability and Managing Chronic Wounds). For further information on adult tracheostomy care, see McGrath (2020).

Complications

Blockage of Tracheostomy Tube. Tracheal dilators, a smaller size tracheotomy tube and a spare inner tube must always be kept to hand in case this problem arises. Sometimes, the blockage can be relieved by suction or by changing the inner tube. At other times, it will be necessary to change the whole tube.

Displacement of the Tube. The tube can become displaced into the pretracheal tissue or completely out of the stoma if the tapes holding it in place have not been secured adequately. The tracheostomy tube should be reinserted immediately and if necessary tracheal dilators can be used to keep the stoma open until the tube can be replaced. Details of the tracheostomy technique, tube size and airway management should be documented in the bed-head signs. Bedside equipment should always have spare tracheotomy tubes in event of displacement with one tube of the same size and one tube a size smaller in case there is difficulty reinserting the tracheostomy tube. There are further details available on the Tapes should be checked for correct fit at least twice daily. A 'good fit' is when you are able to fit two fingers underneath the tapes. Emergency algorithms have been produced by the NTSP (2022) to educate and familiarise staff on what to do in emergency situations when caring for a patient with a tracheostomy or laryngectomy.

Surgical Emphysema. Emphysema is the abnormal presence of air in the tissues. Surgical emphysema is iatrogenic in origin, being a result of faulty suturing, and can be corrected by releasing the sutures.

Haemorrhage. The insertion of a cuffed tracheostomy tube can help to control bleeding and prevent aspiration of blood. It is possible, however, for a major blood vessel to be eroded by a badly placed or poorly managed tube, causing a massive haemorrhage, and at that stage, treatment must follow the hospital major blood loss protocol.

Dysphagia, Nausea, Vomiting. If the tracheostomy tube is the wrong shape for the type of tracheostomy and the size of the patient, it may also tether the larynx and exert excess pressure on the posterior wall of the trachea and oesophagus, resulting in nausea, dysphagia and vomiting. These effects can be relieved by the insertion of a different type and/or size of tube.

Damage to the Tracheal Mucosa. This can result from poor suctioning technique, badly chosen or improperly inserted tubes or prolonged and/or over-inflation of the tube cuff. Ulceration of the anterior wall or a tracheo-oesophageal fistula may result and can lead to tracheal stenosis.

Infection. A wound or respiratory tract infection can result from poor technique when performing wound care to the stoma, changing the tube or applying suction or from inadequate management of respiratory problems. When a tracheostomy tube has a subglottic port, aspiration of secretions reduces the risk of hospital acquired infections.

Changing the Tracheostomy Tube
The first tube change should be performed by experienced medical or nursing staff, as it takes 5–7 days for a tract to form and there is a danger of the tube being misplaced or inserted into the pretracheal tissues. Two people should always be present for this procedure. One will carry out the tube change and feel for the position of the tract on removal in order for reinsertion to be less traumatic for the area as possible. The second nurse is present in case assistance is needed and to apply suction if necessary. The tapes are then securely tied.

Humidification
Humidification will prevent the tracheostomy patient breathing in cold dry air, which could cause the secretions of the trachea to become dry and difficult to remove and eventually lead to blockage and infection of the tube. A selection of HMEs and covers shaped like a small bib, which humidify and filter the air, are available and the patient should be introduced to these before discharge. A humidifying device can be worn under these covers.

Preparation for Discharge
It is important to include the patient in all aspects of caring for the tracheostomy to increase their independence and reduce reliance on nursing staff from the earliest possible stage after the insertion of the tracheostomy. Before discharge can take place, the patient and family must be well prepared for all foreseeable difficulties and should be proficient in total care of the tracheostomy tube. The teaching of self-care techniques can begin with the nurse demonstrating procedures while the patient watches in a mirror. Tracheostomy competencies for friends and family are commonly used in hospitals to ensure relatives are well prepared for the patient's discharge. Mosesso et al. (2014) published a book for the patient/family to help them with tracheostomy management and this can help them to use the book as a reference if they have any difficulty remembering all of the information. It is wise to teach not only the patient but also the family how to care for the tracheostomy in case the occasion arises when the patient is unable to do this themselves. However, some patients are managed by tracheostomy or head and neck specialist nurses. The psychological impact of having a tracheostomy cannot be underestimated and major head and neck surgery is very distressing for the patient and family. Education in self-care of the tube and planning for discharge has to be led by the patient's wishes with support and reassurance. For an outline of outpatient nursing care, see Russell et al. (2019).

The community nurse will be actively involved in the patient's discharge into the community. Ideally, they will visit the patient in hospital and arrange for suction apparatus and consumables to be installed in the home if necessary. After discharge, they should visit regularly to ensure that the patient is coping with the stoma and altered body image.

Decannulation or Removal of the Tube
The patient is gradually reintroduced to breathing through the nose and mouth prior to removal of the tube. A tube with a speaking valve allows the patient to breathe in through the tube and out through the larynx. Once the patient has become accustomed to this, the tube can be replaced by a cap so that the patient has to breathe in through the nose and mouth continuously. Once the patient is able to tolerate this continuously for 48 hours and oxygen saturation levels are satisfactory day and night, the tracheostomy tube can be removed.

After removal of the tube, an occlusive dressing must be applied to allow the tracheostomy site to heal. Initially, the dressing may need to be changed regularly due to the increased secretion load. This can be a very anxious time for patients, and support and encouragement are necessary. The stoma should shrink rapidly and close off in a short time. If a tract is still present after 14 days, the patient can be referred to the ENT surgeon for assessment for surgical closure of the tracheal fistula.

Tonsillitis
The tonsils are composed of lymphoid tissue and lie between the faucial pillars (Fig. 16.9). During early childhood, they enlarge in response to upper respiratory tract infections and in adulthood should become reduced in size. In old age, they normally atrophy. It is generally agreed that tonsils have a role to play in the body's defense system against infection.

Common Presenting Symptoms
Patients usually present with a sore throat. Tonsil pain increases with swallowing and is often referred to the ear because of the involvement of the trigeminal nerve, which supplies both sites. Patients may also present with pyrexia, inflamed tonsils with exudate, lethargy and the absence of a cough (NICE 2018b). Recurrent bouts

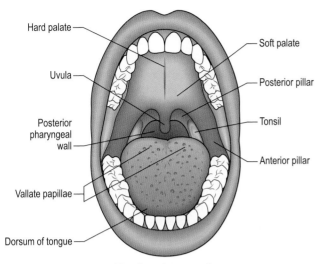

Figure 16.9 Tonsils and surrounding area.

Labels: Hard palate, Uvula, Posterior pharyngeal wall, Vallate papillae, Dorsum of tongue, Soft palate, Posterior pillar, Tonsil, Anterior pillar

of infection are the most common reason for the removal of tonsils. Infection may take the form of acute tonsillitis, AOM or a peritonsillar abscess. Streptococci, staphylococci and *Haemophilus influenzae* are the organisms most commonly present.

Patients with tonsillar tumours normally present with dysphagia. These patients usually also complain of weight loss and may have speech problems. They may also suffer from facial pain and deafness because of the involvement of cranial nerves.

🔴 Medical Management

There is some controversy among medical practitioners about when tonsil infections should be treated conservatively and when tonsillectomy, with or without adenoidectomy, should be performed. The size of the tonsils is not usually the main criterion, but rather the history of the effect of repeated infections on the general health of the patient. Consideration is also given to absence from school or work, loss of appetite, speech defects, nasal catarrh or colds, hearing loss, breathing problems and abdominal pain, the last a sign of mesenteric adenitis, which occurs because of transmission of infection through the lymphatic system (SIGN 2010). Generally, patients who suffer five or more episodes of tonsillitis per year are considered for tonsillectomy.

Tonsillectomy

Tonsillectomy is an elective operation and is not considered in the presence of respiratory tract infections, during the incubation period after contact with an infectious disease or if there is tonsillar inflammation. It is a common operation and there are a number of methods of surgical technique. The traditional method is where the tonsils are removed by dissection in comparison to a newer method called coblation where an electric instrument burns tissues at low temperatures (Bitar et al. 2022).

❖ Nursing Management and Health Promotion: Post Tonsillectomy

Airway. On returning from theatre, patients should be positioned in the posttonsillectomy position, that is semiprone, as this allows any blood or saliva to flow out of the mouth and helps keep the airway clear. When they are alert, they should be encouraged to sit upright and start drinking and eating.

Haemorrhage. Half-hourly recordings of pulse and blood pressure and observations of breathing, pallor, restlessness and frequent swallowing are carried out to ensure early diagnosis of haemorrhage. Frequent swallowing is one of the first signs of tonsil haemorrhage and can go unnoticed unless the patient is closely observed. Particular attention must be paid to the sleeping patient.

Chewing and Swallowing. Encouraging the patient to eat regularly and to swallow is important, as the exercising of the throat muscles seems to help keep the tonsil bed free from infection and to prevent the occurrence of secondary haemorrhage. It should be stressed to the patient and family to eat and drink normally as this reduces the likelihood of infection and bleeding (Tysome and Kanegaonkar 2018). Analgesia should be given regularly and then eating and drinking encouraged.

Infection. Pyrexia is not uncommon on the first postoperative day, as part of the general metabolic response to the trauma of surgery, but if it continues, antibiotics should be prescribed and the source of infection sought.

Analgesics. Prescribed analgesics should be administered and their effectiveness observed. They should be administered before meals, before going to sleep and first thing in the morning. Good pain management is vital in ensuring the patient has a comfortable and uncomplicated postoperative recovery.

Preparation for Discharge

Tonsillectomy is usually performed as a day-case procedure although patients with obstructive sleep apnoea will stay overnight for close monitoring. Patients are advised to avoid dirty, dusty atmospheres for approximately 2 weeks and to take a similar amount of time away from work or school/college. An advice sheet should be given on discharge with a contact number should any difficulties be experienced at home, including bleeding, pyrexia and otalgia (earache). Bleeding indicating a posttonsillectomy haemorrhage is a potentially life-threatening emergency and patients should be advised to immediately attend the ED where they will be assessed (see Chapter 19, The Deteriorating Patient, Recognising and Managing Shock). Patients should be advised that the pain will increase on leaving hospital and that is expected so to continue to take the painkillers and continue eating.

Peritonsillar Abscess (Quinsy)

This is a very painful condition and can be life-threatening. It usually occurs as a complication of acute tonsillitis. Pus forms in the space behind the capsule of the tonsil. The abscess is usually unilateral and affects males more than females.

The patient presents with a pyrexia high enough to cause a rigor. There is usually a history of an episode of acute tonsillitis that has subsided, only to return on one side. There is acute pain radiating to the ear on the affected side, trismus (spasm of the jaw muscles) is present and swallowing is so difficult that saliva dribbles out of the mouth. The voice becomes muffled because of the large swelling that affects the function of the palate. The neck glands on the affected side will be enlarged and tender.

🔴 Medical Management

Antibiotic cover must be prescribed and the abscess may need to be aspirated or incised and drained. Usually, it is necessary to administer intravenous fluids, and antibiotics are always given parenterally for the first 24 hours. Analgesics will be required when the pain is severe. Very rarely, the swelling will be so severe that it will obstruct the airway; it may then be necessary to perform a tracheostomy to enable the patient to breathe.

452 SECTION 1 Care of Patients With Common Disorders

❖ Nursing Management and Health Promotion: Peritonsillar Abscess

Nursing care of the patient with peritonsillar abscess will include:
- physical and psychological support of the patient
- administration of analgesics, antipyretics and antibiotics
- administration of prescribed intravenous fluids
- good oral hygiene
- observation and recording of the patient's airway, temperature, pulse, blood pressure, fluid intake and output
- care of the tracheostomy if this has been performed.

Patients who require admission to hospital will be very anxious, agitated and in pain. They will require explanations, reassurance and swift administration of analgesics. As many will be unable to swallow, observations must be made for signs of dehydration; if dehydration is present, it will be necessary to administer intravenous fluids as prescribed.

Good oral hygiene is important, especially once the abscess has been drained, as the patient will have had to spit out pus and will have a foul taste in the mouth. Once the pain has been relieved by analgesics and drainage of the abscess, the patient will be able to commence oral fluids and gradually begin taking a normal diet. Oral antibiotics will be substituted for intravenous administration.

The patient is usually discharged once apyrexial for 24 hours and able to eat and drink normally. If the abscess was severe enough to require a tracheostomy, this would be removed and the patient discharged only when the wound had healed. Patients are often sent home before they have finished their course of antibiotics; the importance of completing the course must therefore be clearly explained to them. Most patients who have a previous history of tonsillitis are readmitted in 6–8 weeks to have a tonsillectomy performed as peritonsillar abscesses have a habit of recurring.

Snoring/Obstructive Sleep Apnoea (OSA)

Over the last few years, the issue of snoring in association with OSA has been addressed as it has been recognised that these individuals may have a contributing anatomical defect. The patient may show signs of chronic sleep deprivation. The patient's partner and/or family may complain of loud snoring and periods of breath-holding when the patient is asleep. This may be as a result of the tissues of the soft palate and pharynx collapsing and causing a temporary obstruction of the oropharynx. When the patient breathes, this tissue, including the uvula and possibly large tonsils, may vibrate, resulting in loud snoring. Patients may hold their breath due to this obstructing tissue. This condition can be dangerous, due to the possible development of severe hypoxaemia and systemic and pulmonary hypertension.

🌑 Medical Management

Investigations

Untreated OSA increases the likelihood of the patient developing ischaemic heart disease, stroke and type 2 diabetes (Sethi et al. 2017). Treatment of choice for moderate or severe OSA is generally the use of CPAP (continuous positive airway pressure). Day-case sedation nasendoscopy may be necessary. By means of a nasendoscope, the oropharynx of the sleeping patient can be assessed and the activity and position of the tissues and structures observed. At this time, monitoring of oxygen saturation levels is also carried out.

Many centres now carry out sleep studies, which record the patient's breathing, snoring and pattern of electrical activity during overnight sleep. This is an excellent method of measuring the effect of obstruction on the patient.

Treatment

A variety of treatments is available. These include weight loss in overweight people, change of sleeping position, mandibular advancement splints and the use of nasal decongestants. CPAP may also be used (see next section).

If it is obvious that there is collapse of excess tissues in the oropharynx, then the surgical technique of uvulopalatopharyngoplasty, with or without tonsillectomy, may be performed at a later date. This involves tightening of the soft palate and pharyngeal tissue, removal of the uvula and possible tonsillectomy. Correction using a laser or punctate diathermy is an alternative procedure.

❖ Nursing Management and Health Promotion: Uvulopalatopharyngoplasty

The priorities and management are the same as for tonsillectomy. Patients may experience nasal regurgitation on swallowing. This will usually resolve over a short period of time.

Continuous Positive Airway Pressure (CPAP). This treatment avoids surgery and can be carried out by the patient at home each night. The patient requires a considerable amount of education and supervision during the initial stages and continuous ongoing support. This education and support are usually provided by a specialist nurse who plays a key role in coordinating and implementing continuity of care from the initial sleep investigation stage and throughout.

Nasal CPAP works as a pneumatic splint, as the continuous positive pressure stops the pharynx collapsing and vibrating. At night the patient wears a well-fitting nasal mask which is connected via tubing to a small machine which delivers the positive pressure airflow. The mouth is left uncovered. The nasal cavity needs to be free of obstruction.

Most patients tolerate CPAP well, despite occasional problems with nasal and face irritation. It is most commonly used for moderate to severe OSA.

Summary: Key Nursing Issues

- The specialty of ENT care is continually evolving and presents many challenges to the nurse, who will encounter patients of various ages and backgrounds, each with specific needs in regard to the intensity, duration and setting of treatment.
- The ENT nurse is likely to encounter a wide range of disorders, some of which will have profound implications for the patient's ability to function within family, work and social spheres and which will require thorough assessment and individualised care planning.

- The nurse's ability as communicator will do much to determine the effectiveness of interventions; the need for skill and inventiveness in communication is especially important.
- Underpinning all of the knowledge and practice in this chapter is The Code (NMC 2018).
- In order to successfully educate the patient about their ENT condition, a good knowledge of anatomy and physiology is required.
- The acoustics of the hospital and ward often make it difficult for older adults to hear. Turn off televisions and radios, shut

the door and, facing the patient with a positive attitude, repeat yourself as necessary. Ensure the patient is wearing their glasses and the lenses are clean.

- All older adults and children with a learning disability should have their ears examined on an annual basis. Patients who wear hearing aids or who have a history of wax build-up should have their ears checked on a more regular basis and wax or debris removed as necessary.
- Older adults with cognitive impairment or a diagnosis of dementia and children with a learning disability who have not been previously recognised hearing loss should have audiological assessments every 2 years.
- All hearing aid users and their families/carers should understand the basic care of the hearing aid and what to do if they encounter the common problems.
- Headphones are capable of producing the same volume of sound as a pneumatic drill, and thus present a serious risk of hearing impairment.
- Many ENT conditions are successfully managed within the primary setting. Health education and promotion are vital to maintain the patient's ability to function within the community.
- Most large ENT units also care for patients suffering from head and neck cancer. Guidance can be found on the NICE website

in regards to cancer pathways for suspected head and neck cancer patients. The guideline covers children, young people and adults with symptoms that could be caused by cancer. It outlines appropriate investigations that may be suitable for these patients and suggest a selection of people to refer for a specialist opinion (NICE 2022).

The guidance covers all kinds of cancer but focuses on specific head and neck cancers such as laryngeal cancer, oral cancer and thyroid cancer. In the UK, there is a 2-week-wait cancer pathway in place meaning anyone with suspected cancer should be seen by a specialist within 2 weeks of being seen in a primary care setting (Rapid Cancer Diagnostic and Assessment Pathways 2023).

- The NTSP website has excellent learning resources for healthcare workers, patients and their families.
- NICE has produced guidelines on a variety of ENT-related issues and recommends that practitioners take these into account alongside individual needs, preferences and values of their patients or service users.
- As the causes of certain ENT disorders become better understood, and as pharmacological and surgical treatments make further strides forward, ENT nursing will continue to offer challenges and rewards for nurses in a variety of care settings.

Reflection and Learning – What Next?

- **Test** your knowledge by visiting the Evolve website 🌐 and answering the multiple-choice questions.
- **Consolidate** your learning by looking at some of the further reading suggestions, references and specialist websites.
- **Revisit** some of the additional material on the website.
- **Consider** what you have learnt and how this will help your professional development.
- **Reflect** on how you can apply this knowledge to the care of your patients.
- **Discuss** your learning with your mentor/supervisor, lecturer and colleagues.

References

Abou-Abdallah M, Lamyman A. Exploring communication difficulties with deaf patients. *Clin Med* (Lond). 2021;21(4):e380–e383.

Amieva H, Ouvrard C. Does treating hearing loss in older adults improve cognitive outcomes? A review. *J Clin Med*. 2020;9(3):805. https://doi.org/10.3390/jcm9030805.

Bitar M, Nazir T, Abd-UI-Salam H. A retrospective observational cohort study evaluating the postoperative outcomes of intracapsular coblation tonsillectomy in children. *Sci Rep*. 2022;12:21134. doi:10.1038/s41598-022-25768-0.

Calvino M, Sanchez-Cuadrado I, Gavilan J, et al. Effect of cochlear implantation on cognitive decline and quality of life in younger and older adults with severe to profound hearing loss. *Eur Arch Otorhinolaryngol*. 2022;279:4745–4759.

Cooper H, Grifa I, Bryant C. Use of an autoinflation device does not lead to a clinically meaningful change in hearing in children with otitis media with effusion. *Clin Otolaryngol*. 2022;47(1):160–166. doi:10.1111/coa.13879.

David A, Russell M, El-Sayed I, Russell M. Tracheostomy guidelines developed at a large academic centre during the COVID-19 pandemic. *Head Neck*. 2020;42:1291–1296. doi:10.1002/hed.26191.

Freeman-Sanderson AL, Togher L, Elkins M, Kenny B. Quality of life improves for tracheostomy patients with return of voice. *Intensive Crit Care Nurs*. 2018;46:10–16.

Grewal R, Tantichirasakul N, Miller B, Watson N, Karagama Y. Office-based transnasal oesophagoscopy: evaluating the safety, efficacy and application in head and neck cancer patients. *Clin Otolaryngol*. 2021;47(1):218–223. https://doi.org/10.1111/coa.13868.

Grier M. Supportive care for patients with head and neck cancer. *Oncol Nurs News*. 8 May 2018. https://www.oncnursingnews.com/publications/oncology-nurse/2013/may-2013/supportive-care-for-patients-with-head-and-neck-cancer.

Hamdan AL, Jabbour C, Khalifee E, Ghanem A, El Hage A. Tolerance of patients using different approaches in laryngeal office-based procedures. *J Voice*. 2021. [Preprint]. https://doi.org/10.1016/j.jvoice.2020.12.009.

Harkin H. Earwax impaction: why it needs to be treated in primary care. *Nurs Times (online) Aug*. 2019;15(8):38–41.

Harkin H. The structure and function of the ear and its role in hearing and balance. *Nurs Times (online)*. 2021;117(4):56–59.

Krouse HJ, Magit AE, O'Connor S, et al. Plain language summary: earwax (cerumen impaction). *Otolaryngol Head Neck Surg*. 2017;156(1):30–37.

Lewith H, Athanassoglou V. Update on management of tracheostomy. *BJA Educ*. 2019.

Martinez-Vega R, Garrido F, Partearroyo T, et al. Folic acid deficiency induces premature hearing loss through mechanism involving cochlear oxidative stress and impairment of homocysteine metabolism. *FASEB J*. 2015;29(2):418–432.

McGrath BA. *Comprehensive Tracheostomy Care – National Tracheostomy Safety Project Manual (NTSP)*. Chichester: Wiley–Blackwell; 2018.

McGrath, et al. *Guidance for Tracheostomy Care*. Intensive Care Society London; 2020.

Mills CS, Michou E, King N, et al. Evidence for above cuff vocalization in patients with a tracheostomy: a systematic review. *Laryngoscope*. 2021. https://doi.org/10.1002/lary.29591.

Molin N, Myers K, Soliman AMS, Schmalbach CE. COVID-19 tracheostomy outcomes. *Otolaryngology and Head and Neck Surgery*. 2022;167(6):923–928.

Mosesso K, Von Euw E, O'Leary M, O'Wein R. *Tracheostomy Management Made Simple for the Head and Neck Cancer Patient.* Greenacres, WA: Provenir Publishing, USA; 2014.

National Cancer Institute. *Head and neck cancers*; 2017. www.cancer.gov.

NHS. (2023) Rapid cancer diagnostic and assessment pathways; 2023. England.nhs.uk.

Niazi Y, Ejaz B, Muazzam A. Impact of hearing impairment on psychological distress and subjective well-being in older adults. *Pak J Med Sci.* 2020;36(6):1210–1215. doi:10.12669/pjms.36.6.2457.

National Institute for Health and Clinical Excellence (NICE). *Tonsillectomy using laser.* Interventional procedures guidance [IPG186]; 2006a. https://www.nice.org.uk/guidance/IPG186.

National Institute for Health and Clinical Excellence (NICE). *Tonsillectomy using ultrasonic scalpel.* Interventional procedures guidance [IPG178]; 2006b. https://www.nice.org.uk/guidance/IPG178.

National Institute for Health and Care Excellence (NICE). *Otovent balloon for otitis media with effusion.* Medtech innovation briefing [MIB59]; 2016. https://www.nice.org.uk/advice/mib59.

National Institute for Health and Care Excellence (NICE). *Hearing loss in adults: assessment and management.* NICE guideline [NG98]; 2018a. https://www.nice.org.uk/guidance/ng98.

National Institute for Health and Care Excellence (NICE). *Sore throat (acute): antimicrobial prescribing.* Clinical guideline [NG84]; 2018b. https://www.nice.org.uk/guidance/ng84.

National Institute for Clinical Excellence. (NICE). Fever in under 5s: assessment and initial management. Clinical Guideline [NG143]; 2021. https://www.nice.org.uk/guidance/ng143.

National Institute for Health and Care Excellence (NICE). *Otitis media (acute): antimicrobial prescribing.* NICE guideline [NG91]; 2022. https://www.nice.org.uk/guidance/ng91.

Nursing and Midwifery Council (NMC). The Code: professional standards of practice and behaviour for nurses, midwives and nursing associates. 2018. https://www.nmc.org.uk/standards/code/.

Paul C, Moreno M. Acute otitis media. *JAMA Pediatrics.* 2020;174(3):308. doi:10.1001/jamapediatrics.2019.5664.

Russell C, MacGinley K, Meads C. Tracheostomy care in community settings Primary Health Care ; 2019. doi:10.7748/phc.2019.e1548.10.1111/jch.13487

Sami AS. *E.N.T. Made Easy.* Banbury: Scion Publishing Ltd; 2017.

Schwartz SR, Magit AE, Rosenfeld RM, et al. Clinical practice guideline (update): earwax (cerumen impaction). *Otolaryngol Head Neck Surg.* 2017;156(S1):S1–S29.

Sethi N, Pearson A, Bajaj Y. *Key Clinical Topics in Otolaryngology.* London: JP Medical; 2017.

SIGN (Scottish Intercollegiate Guidelines Network). *Management of Sore Throat and Indications for Tonsillectomy. Publication No. 117.* Edinburgh: SIGN; 2010.

Sjovall A, Aho V, Hyyrynen T, et al. Microbiome of the healthy external auditory canal. *Otol Neurotol.* 2021;42(5):609–614.

Szeto B, Valentini C, Lalwani AK. Low vitamin D status is associated with hearing loss in the elderly: a cross sectional study. *Am J Clin Nutr.* 2021;113(2):456–466.

Tan BKJ, Han R, Zhao JJ, et al. Prognosis and persistence of smell and taste dysfunction in patients with COVID-19: meta-analysis with parametric cure modelling of recovery curves. *BMJ;.* 2022;378:e069503.

The Control of Noise at Work Regulations. 2005. Available at: http://www.legislation.gov.uk/uksi/2005/1643/contents/made.

Tysome JR, Kanegaonkar R. *ENT: An Introduction and Practical Guide.* 2nd ed. London: Hodder and Stoughton; 2018.

Vanneste P, Page C. Otitis media with effusion in children: pathophysiology, diagnosis and treatment. A review. *J Otol. Jun.* 2019;14(2):33–39.

Venekamp R, Schilder A, Van den Heuvel M, Hay A. Acute middle ear infection in children. *Br Med J (Clin Res Ed).* 2020;371:m4238. doi:10.1136/bmj.m4238.

Further Reading

Bisogno A, Scarpa A, DiGirolamo S, Deluca P, et al. (2021) Hearing loss and cognitive impairment: epidemiology, common pathophysiological findings and treatment considerations. 11(10):1102. doi:10.3390/life11101102.

Corbridge R, Steventon N. *Oxford Handbook of ENT and Head and Neck Surgery.* Oxford: Oxford University Press; 2010.

Dobbins M, Gunson J, Bale S, et al. Improving patient care and quality of life after laryngectomy/glossectomy. *Br J Nurs.* 2005;14(12):634–640.

Harrison L, Sessions R, Kies MS. *Head and Neck Cancer: A Multidisciplinary Approach.* 4th ed. Philadelphia, PA: Lippincott Williams and Wilkins; 2014.

Kenney K, Gropman R. What immediate post-operative nursing care contributes to a better patient outcome after a child has had a daycase surgery tonsillectomy and adenoidectomy. *J Anesth Nurs.* 2013;28(3):e44.

Loveman E, Gospodarevskaya E, Clegg A, et al. Ear wax removal interventions. *Br J Gen Pract.* 2011;October:480–483.

Macmillan Cancer Support. *Rapid referral guidelines for suspected cancer.* Macmillan.org.uk; 2022.

Manchaiah V, Arthur J, Williams H. Does hearing aid use increase the likelihood of cerumen impaction? *J Audiol Otol.* 2015;19(3):168–171.

Miller BJ, Abdelhamid A, Karagama Y. Applications of office-based 445 nm Blue Laser Transnasal flexible laser surgery: a case series and review of practice. *Ear Nose Throat J.* 2020;100(1_suppl). https://doi.org/10.1177/0145561320960544.

Okonkwo I, Cochrane L, Fernandez E. Perioperative management of a child with a tracheostomy. *BJA Educ.* 2020;20(1):18–25. doi:10.1016/j.bjae.2019.09.007.

Ringash J. Survivorship and quality of life in head and neck cancer. *J Clin Oncol.* 2015;33(29):3322–3327.

Rodgers R. Does olive oil prevent earwax build-up? *Pract Nurs.* 2013;24(4):191–196.

Semple CJ, McGowan B. Need for appropriate written information for patients with particular reference to head and neck cancer. *J Clin Nurs.* 2002;11:585–593.

Useful Websites

Action on Hearing Loss (previously RNID), www.actiononhearingloss.org.uk

Association of Teachers of Lip Reading to Adults (ATLA), www.lipreading.org

British Association for Counselling and Psychotherapy (BACP), www.bacp.co.uk

British Association of Head and Neck Oncology Nurses, www.bahnon.org.uk

British Deaf Association, www.bda.org.uk

British Tinnitus Association, www.tinnitus.org.uk

ENT UK ENT UK, www.ENTUK.org

Hearing Concern, www.hearinglink.org

Hearing Dogs for Deaf People, www.hearingdogs.org.uk

Let's Face It (a national and international group for the facially disfigured, including cancer sufferers), www.lets-face-it.org.uk

National Association of Laryngectomy Clubs (NALC) (for laryngectomy patients, but tracheostomy and head and neck cancer patients are also welcome), www.layngectomy.org.uk

National Deaf Children's Society, www.ndcs.org.uk

Royal College of Nursing ENT/Maxillofacial Nursing Forum, www.rcn.org.uk/ent

Scottish Council on Deafness, www.scod.org.uk

The Global Tracheostomy Collaborative, http://globaltrach.org/

SECTION 2

Core Nursing Issues

17

Pharmacology and Medicines Management

RUTH PATERSON

CHAPTER OUTLINE

Introduction

In the UK, people across the lifespan have complex health needs and managing medicines safely and effectively is fundamental to all fields of practice. Nurses have a legal responsibility to know about the medications they administer to patients, to ensure patients are aware of why they are receiving treatment and to minimise risk when managing medicines. At all times the nurse must ensure that local policy and procedure are adhered to. This chapter will provide a broad overview of core principles associated with:

- What drugs are, how they work, effects and side-effects
- Evidence-based, person-centred medicines management including prescribing practice and drug administration
- Wider issues associated with medicines management

This chapter will look at each of these, aiming to provide a broad overview of key concepts. This is by no means a comprehensive resource but instead will provide key skills and knowledge that can be furthered by using other resources, such as the British National Formulary (BNF) and national clinical guidelines, for example Scottish Intercollegiate Guidelines Network (SIGN) and National Institute for Health and Care Excellence (NICE) guidance. Please refer to Further Reading at the end of this chapter for more information.

Drugs, Medicines and Pharmacology

A drug is a substance or combination of substances presented as having properties of preventing or treating a disease in human beings (Medicines and Healthcare products Regulatory Agency [MHRA] 2023). A medicine is a chemical preparation which contains one or more of a drug with the intention of producing a therapeutic effect. Medicines contain substances other than the drug, for example stabilisers, binding agents or agents to modify release of the drug, thus making them more convenient to use. Drug development is costly and highly regulated in the UK by the MHRA. Before a drug receives a licence for use it has to go through many phases of testing, and begins with laboratory research progressing to human testing only when proven safe to do so.

Drugs often have many brand names for the same drug, for example Zocor is a brand name for the generic drug simvastatin. As there are many different brand names for the same drug, using the generic name will help the nurse to understand different categories of drugs. See Table 17.1 for examples of drugs categorised by name endings, and Table 17.2 for drug classifications.

TABLE 17.1	Examples of Drug Categories by Generic Name Endings	
Generic Name Ending	**Type of Drug**	**Common Action**
'Prils' (e.g. lisinopril)	ACE inhibitors	Antihypertensive that relaxes arterial vessels
'Sartans' (e.g. losartan)	Angiotensin-receptor blockers	Antihypertensive that blocks action of vasoconstriction effects of angiotensin II
'Olols', 'alols' (e.g. atenolol, labetalol, metoprolol)	Beta blockers	Antihypertensives/antianginals that block beta adrenergic receptors in vascular smooth muscle
'Statins' (e.g. atorvastatin)	Antilipemics	Inhibit HMG-CoA reductase enzyme, reducing cholesterol synthesis

Continued

TABLE 17.1	Examples of Drug Categories by Generic Name Endings—cont'd	
Generic Name Ending	Type of Drug	Common Action
'Dipines' (e.g. amlodipine)	Peripheral vessel calcium channel blockers	Antihypertensives/antianginals that produce relaxation of coronary smooth muscle and vascular smooth muscle; dilate coronary arteries
'Afils' (e.g. sildenafil)	Erectile agents	Peripheral vasodilator that promotes a penile erection
'Floxacins' (e.g. ciprofloxacin)	Broad-spectrum anti-infectives	Inhibit bacteria by interfering with DNA
'Prazoles' (e.g. esomeprazole)	Proton pump inhibitors	Suppress gastric secretions, preventing gastric reflux and gastric and duodenal ulcers
'Tidines' (e.g. famotidine, ranitidine)	Block histamine-2 receptors	Inhibits histamine at H_2-receptor sites, decreasing gastric secretions
'Azoles' (e.g. fluconazole)	Antifungals	Cause direct damage to the fungal membrane
'Cyclovirs' (e.g. acyclovir)	Antiherpetic	Interferes with DNA synthesis, causing decreased viral replication

ACE, Angiotensin-converting enzyme; *HMG-CoA*, 3-hydroxy-3-methylglutaryl coenzyme A.
Adapted from a presentation by Barb Bancroft at the California Vocational Nurse Educators Conference in Burlingame, California, 17 April 2015.

TABLE 17.2	Selected Groups of Drugs Classified by Action	
Classification	Action	Examples
Cardiovascular System and Heart		
Anticoagulants	Inhibit clotting of blood	Sodium warfarin, heparin
Antianginals	Increase blood flow to the heart	Nitroglycerine, isosorbide dinitrate, diltiazem
Antiarrhythmics	Regulate the heart rate	Lidocaine, atropine, amiodarone
Antihypertensives	Control high blood pressure	Atenolol, enalapril maleate, captopril, clonidine
Antilipidemics	Lower abnormal blood lipid levels	Simvastatin, atorvastatin
Antiplatelets	Inhibit platelet aggregation	Clopidogrel bisulphate
Cardiotonics	Strengthen the contraction of the heart	Digoxin digitalis
Diuretics	Reduce oedema and increase urine output	Furosemide, chlorothiazide, bumetanide
Hemostatics	Promote clotting of blood	Vitamin K_5, absorbable gelatine sponge (Gelfoam)
Emotional and Mental States		
Hypnotics, sedatives	Relieve anxiety, reduce activity and promote sleep	Chloral hydrate, secobarbital, flurazepam, zolpidem tartrate
Stimulants	Increase mental alertness and function	Caffeine, methylphenidate, dextroamphetamine, modafinil
Tricyclic antidepressants	Relieve depression	Amitriptyline doxepin
SSRIs	Relieve depression	Paroxetine, fluoxetine, citalopram, sertraline
Anxiolytics	Relieve anxiety	Lorazepam, buspirone, diazepam
Antipsychotics	Relieve psychotic symptoms	Aripiprazole, haloperidol, olanzapine, ziprasidone
Muscular System and Integument		
Antihistamines	Reduce congestion and allergic reactions	Diphenhydramine chlorpheniramine
Muscle relaxants	Control muscle spasms and tension	Baclofen carisoprodol
Neurologic System		
Narcotics (opioids)	Relieve moderate to severe pain	Morphine, codeine, meperidine, hydromorphone, fentanyl, oxycodone
Nonnarcotics (nonopioids) NSAIDs	Relieve mild pain Reduce inflammation and pain	Aspirin, paracetamol Ibuprofen, naproxen, sulindac
Alzheimer disease drugs	Slow progression of disease	Donepezil rivastigmine
Antiepileptics	Control epileptic seizures and tremors	Phenytoin, paramethadione, phenobarbital
Respiratory System		
Antitussives	Relieve cough	Codeine, dextromethorphan, guaifenesin
Bronchodilators and expectorants	Relieve obstruction of air passages	Terbutaline, salbutamol, metaproterenol

Continued

TABLE 17.2	Selected Groups of Drugs Classified by Action—cont'd	
Classification	**Action**	**Examples**
Endocrine System		
Adrenal hormones	All hormones act to regulate body growth, function, and metabolism	Corticotropin, aldosterone, epinephrine, cortisone
Female hormones	–	Oestrogen, oestrone, progestin, ethinyl oestradiol
Male hormone	–	Testosterone
Pancreatic hormone	Reduces blood glucose	Regular insulin, isophane insulin, Humalog, Humulin (NPH), lente insulin
Hypoglycaemics	Reduce blood glucose	Gliclazide, metformin, chlorpropamide
Gastrointestinal System		
Antacids	Neutralise stomach acids	Aluminium hydroxide, aluminium carbonate
Antisecretories	Decrease gastric acid secretion	Rantidine, omeprazole, pantoprazole, lansoprazole
Anticholinergics	Reduce spasms and secretions of stomach	Propantheline
Antidiarrhoeals	Reduce bowel irritability and movements	Kaolin and pectin, loperamide, octreotide
Antiemetics	Relieve nausea and control vomiting	Promethazine, metoclopramide, ondansetron
Cathartics, laxatives	Promote bowel movements	Bisacodyl, magnesium hydroxide, senna
Stool softeners	Add water or bulk to stool and aid defecation	Docusate calcium, docusate sodium
Antibiotics	Inhibit the growth of or kill microorganisms	Erythromycin, cephalosporin, penicillin, vancomycin, ciprofloxacin, clarithromycin

NSAIDS, Nonsteroidal anti-inflammatory drugs; *SSRIs,* selective serotonin reuptake inhibitors.
Adapted from Williams P. *deWit's Fundamental Concepts and Skills for Nursing.* 5th ed. St Louis: Saunders Elsevier; 2018.

Pharmacology

Pharmacology is the study of a drug, or the way the body handles a drug and how that drug acts. 'Pharmaco' is derived from the Greek meaning biologically active substance, remedy or poison or more simply, drug. There are two main parts to pharmacology:
- Pharmacokinetics
- Pharmacodynamics

Pharmacokinetics is what the body does to the drug. Pharmacodynamics is what the drug does to the body or where and how that drug acts to produce the desired therapeutic effect. These concepts help us to understand why there is variation in how individuals respond to the same drug and why some side-effects occur. It provides an insight into why there may be variation in route of administration, dose and frequency due to prolonged drug use, or organ dysfunction. This section will address these points, providing examples using named drugs to illustrate key points.

Pharmacokinetics

This term refers to how the drug moves through the body. The rate and extent that drugs go through this process will determine optimum dose regime. There are four main phases of passage of drug through the body, namely:
1. Absorption
2. Distribution
3. Metabolism
4. Excretion

Pharmacokinetics is dependent on route of administration and there are two main categories of drug administration, enteral and parenteral. Enteral administration is any drug administered via the gastrointestinal (GI) tract and parenteral is using any other body system, for example intravenous, transdermal and topical. Rate of absorption will be dependent on route of administration;

TABLE 17.3	Differences in Absorption According to Route
Route	**Rate of Absorption**
Skin (transdermal)	Slow absorption
Mucous membranes	Quick absorption
Respiratory tract	Quick absorption
Oral	Slow absorption (liquids are faster than pills, tablets or capsules)
Intramuscular	Depends on the form of the drug: aqueous is quicker compared with oil, which slows absorption
Subcutaneous	Slow absorption
Intravenous	Most rapid absorption

intravenous has very rapid absorption as given directly into the bloodstream whereas transdermal is much slower. Table 17.3 illustrates differences in absorption rates according to the route given.

Most drugs are given enterally and pass through the GI tract to be absorbed in the intestine in preparation for distribution of the drug into the circulation. The drug will enter the portal venous system and pass through the liver where it goes through a process of first-pass metabolism. This process breaks some or all of the drug in preparation for excretion by the kidney or in faeces, sweat or breast milk. Any drug that has not been metabolised will be distributed into the systemic circulation to exert the desired response.

The amount of drug entering the systemic circulation is termed its 'bioavailability', or how much of the drug is available to exert a response. Drugs not given via the GI tract will avoid first-pass metabolism and enter the systemic circulation direct.

This cycle will continue until the drug is eliminated from the body. The time it takes for a drug to be eliminated may vary between individuals as it is dependent on the four phases mentioned previously, but also on the known drug action.

Drugs that remain in the body will be continually exposed to this pharmacokinetic cycle. In order to achieve a constant therapeutic effect or 'steady state', drug dosing must be balanced against excretion of the drug. This means that the concentration in the plasma is constant provided the drug is taken at the prescribed intervals. Drug dosing is dependent on drug half-life and those with a longer half-life may require a larger first dose or 'loading dose' to achieve the therapeutic plasma concentration. Half-life also can estimate how long it takes for the concentration of a drug to fall by half or 50%. Generally, it takes four or five half-lives for a drug to be eliminated from the body (Reflection 17.1).

Absorption

For a drug to survive enteral administration and pass through the body, the gut has to have good blood flow and movement (peristalsis); it has to be able tolerate gastric acid, avoid binding to certain foodstuffs and resist breakdown by gastric enzymes. If any of these are inhibited, absorption of the drug may be reduced. Most drugs are absorbed in the small intestine, but during critical illness or trauma (e.g. surgery), blood flow and peristalsis are reduced. Hence, if a drug is given orally during these times, there is a risk that the drug will not be absorbed and the desired therapeutic effect will not be achieved. Conversely drugs designed to increase gastric motility, for example stimulant laxatives and metoclopramide, may reduce absorption because there is insufficient time for the drug to be absorbed. Some drugs are broken down to their inactive form by gastric enzymes if given orally. One example of this is insulin, which if given enterally will be broken down by gastric enzymes rendering it ineffective. Finally, some drugs such as proton pump inhibitors (PPIs), omeprazole, are intended to increase gastric pH, reducing symptoms of gastro-oesophageal reflux disease (GORD) however, the alteration in gastric pH affects the absorption of antifungals, and when given together the efficacy of the antifungal may be reduced.

Distribution

Once drugs have been absorbed, they travel around the body and enter tissues and cells until the site of action is found and the drug exerts its effect. Many drugs are bound to plasma proteins (mainly albumin) and transported around the body until they are released, and distributed, into the bloodstream. When a drug is released, or 'freed', from the plasma protein, the 'free drug' is now ready to exert its effect on the target cell. The rate of distribution is dependent on molecule size and fat (lipid) solubility and this partly determines the frequency of dosing of drugs.

Drug distribution is dependent on albumin levels, which are altered in certain conditions. In severe liver disease, pregnancy, the elderly and in malnutrition, albumin levels are low which means there are less plasma proteins for the drug to bind to. As a result, more of the drug is circulating in the bloodstream to exert an effect, which may result in a greater effect of the drug on the patient and more risk of side-effects. In these situations, giving a lower dose of the drug may be required.

Drug distribution can also be affected by drugs given together. For example, when warfarin and ibuprofen are given together, ibuprofen binds more closely to plasma proteins, displacing warfarin and resulting in more free drug in the bloodstream. As warfarin is an anticoagulant, an increased amount of warfarin available may put the patient at risk of increased bleeding time.

Metabolism

We have touched briefly on metabolism in the Introduction, identifying that it mostly takes place in the liver. It is in two phases: phase I involves oxidisation using enzymes from the cytochrome P450 group and phase II involves conjugation with compounds, with both phases aiming to detoxify the drug, making them water-soluble (hydrophilic) in preparation for excretion. Occasionally, metabolites are toxic, for example paracetamol, or metabolism of a drug converts it to its active form (pro-drug), for example codeine phosphate.

Any drug that is not metabolised will remain fat-soluble and be reabsorbed into the systemic circulation to exert an effect. The amount of drug available after metabolism, that is, bioavailability, is calculated as a percentage or fraction of one.

Any drug given enterally will undergo some metabolism by the liver before entering the systemic circulation. For some drugs, for example glyceryl trinitrate, the liver will metabolise all of the drug and none will be available to exert its effect. This is the reason for this drug being administered sublingually, transdermally or intravenously as these routes avoid first-pass metabolism. Some drugs are not metabolised by the liver at all; in these cases, bioavailability is 1.0 or 100%. Intravenous drugs have no contact with the gut or liver and will enter the systemic circulation directly resulting in 100% of the drug available to exert a response on the target cell.

Excretion

Excretion of drugs is the removal of drugs and their metabolites from the body. This predominantly occurs in the kidneys, but some excretion is through bile, faeces or expired air. Some drugs that are excreted in the bile will be reabsorbed ready for recirculation. Faecal excretion may occur for those drugs that have not been absorbed by the small intestine or those excreted in bile.

The majority of drugs rely on excretion by the kidneys and the rate at which they are excreted is dependent on renal function and glomerular filtration rate (GFR). If a person has renal impairment and a reduced GFR, drugs may take longer to be eliminated from the body. The ageing process has an effect on drug excretion as renal function decreases with age. Acute illness or dehydration in the elderly can lead to reduction in excretion of drugs resulting in greater susceptibility to toxic side-effects.

Pharmacodynamics

The principle objective of giving a drug is to alleviate the diseased cells. Pharmacodynamics, or what the drug does to the body, describes the action that the drug has on the target cell in the body. This is achieved by targeting those molecules to either stimulate or block a response. There are four principle targets for drugs to

TABLE 17.4	Targets for Drug Action and Examples	
Target for Drug Action	Mechanism of Action	Example
Receptor	Large molecules which are found on the cell membrane which are stimulated or blocked by a naturally occurring chemical or drug which elicits a response (e.g. receptor antagonist or receptor agonist)	Antagonist drugs Agonist drugs
Antagonist	Drug that binds to a receptor molecule to block a response	B1 and/or B2 antagonists or beta blocker, e.g. atenolol, bisoprolol
Agonist	Drug that binds to a receptor molecule to stimulate a response	B2 receptor agonists, e.g. salbutamol
Ion channels	Drugs that alter the conduction of ions within the cells	Sodium channel blocker, e.g. lidocaine Calcium channel blocker, e.g. verapamil
Membrane transport systems	Drugs that have specialised proteins that carry, or inhibit ions or molecules to induce or block a response	Proton pump inhibitors, e.g. omeprazole Serotonin reuptake transporter, e.g. fluoxetine
Enzymes	Enzymes are chemicals that catalyse (or create) a chemical reaction. Drugs that interfere with an enzyme will stimulate or inhibit the catalytic reaction	Cox I and II inhibitors, e.g. ibuprofen Angiotension-converting enzyme (ACE) inhibitor, e.g. ramipril

act in body cells, namely receptors (antagonist and agonists), ion channels, membrane transport systems and enzymes (Table 17.4).

Side-Effects

When a drug is given, it will target a cell and initiate the desired effect. Even when given at normal doses, this may produce some unwanted side-effects. For example, salbutamol is a B2 agonist, and binds to B2 cells to stimulate a response and activation of the sympathetic nervous system. The desired response is dilatation of the structures inside the lungs, the bronchioles, which causes dilatation and relaxation. This reduces bronchospasm, alleviates wheeze and improves the work of breathing. However, B2 cells are located throughout the body and all B2 cells will be stimulated when salbutamol is given. One common undesired effect of the drug when given in large doses via a nebuliser is tachycardia as stimulation of B2 cells also increases the rate and force of heart contractions (Fig. 17.1). This side-effect is explained by the drug action and thus is a predictable effect of drug treatment (Reflection 17.2).

Adverse Drug Reactions

An adverse drug reaction (ADR) is an unwanted reaction following administration of a drug that is suspected to be related to the drug. ADRs can occur when too much of the drug is given (toxicity), when the right amount of the drug is given (side-effect) or when not enough of the drug is given. There are many factors that

affect a person's reaction to a drug including individual physiology, liver and renal function and age.

Some drugs are commonly associated with ADRs. For example, nonsteroidal anti-inflammatory drugs (NSAIDs) are responsible for ADR-related hospital admissions. ADRs most commonly occur in the elderly, those prescribed many medications (polypharmacy) and those with other medical conditions (comorbidities) (Al Hamid et al. 2014). Between 7% and 10% of hospital admissions are related to adverse drug events (Aljadhey et al. 2013).

ADRs can also be attributed to drug–drug interaction (pharmacodynamics) or variations in physiology (pharmacokinetics) (e.g. age, gender and weight). As drug testing has identified the specific action of a drug, pharmacodynamic drug interactions are predictable but pharmacokinetic interactions are generally less predictable. This is because it is difficult to predict an individual's physiological response to a drug. Common drug interactions are detailed in Table 17.5.

TABLE 17.5	Common Pharmacodynamic and Pharmacokinetic Drug Interactions	
Pharmacodynamic Drug Interactions	Example	Effect
Two drugs competing for the same receptor	Salbutamol and atenolol	Reduction of bronchodilator effect and increased wheeze
Direct effect on the same organs	Alcohol and benzodiazepines	Increased sedative effect
Pharmacokinetic Drug Interaction		
Inhibition of drug metabolism	Simvastatin and grapefruit juice	Increased risk of myopathy (side-effect of simvastatin)
	Warfarin and clarithromycin	Increased risk of bleeding (side-effect of warfarin)
Inhibition of drug absorption	Fluconazole and omeprazole	Reduced effect of antifungals due to altered gastric pH when taking omeprazole
Displacement of drug from plasma protein by another drug	Warfarin and NSAIDs	Increased risk of bleeding, resulting from increased amount of free drug to exert a response
Reduced excretion from kidneys	Lithium and diuretics	Increased risk of lithium toxicity

NSAIDS, Nonsteroidal anti-inflammatory drugs.
Adapted from Qureshi Z, Maxwell S. *The Unofficial Guide to Prescribing*. Edinburgh: Churchill Livingstone Elsevier; 2014.

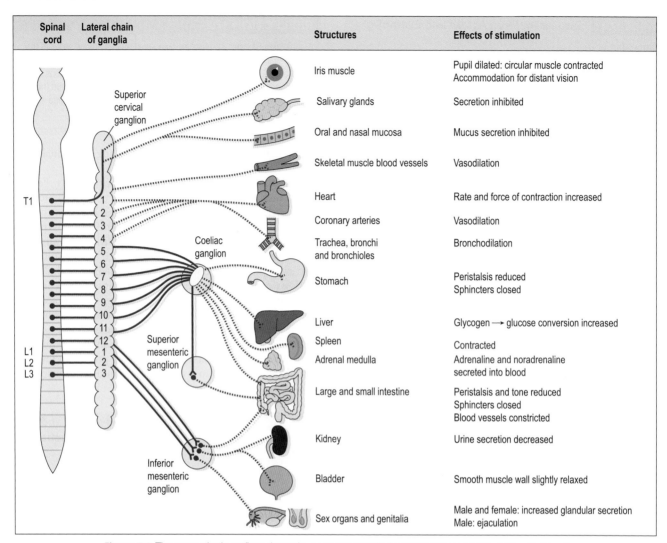

Spinal cord	Lateral chain of ganglia		Structures	Effects of stimulation
	Superior cervical ganglion		Iris muscle	Pupil dilated: circular muscle contracted Accommodation for distant vision
			Salivary glands	Secretion inhibited
			Oral and nasal mucosa	Mucus secretion inhibited
			Skeletal muscle blood vessels	Vasodilation
T1	1 2 3		Heart	Rate and force of contraction increased
	4		Coronary arteries	Vasodilation
	5	Coeliac ganglion	Trachea, bronchi and bronchioles	Bronchodilation
	6 7 8		Stomach	Peristalsis reduced Sphincters closed
	9 10 11		Liver	Glycogen $\longrightarrow$ glucose conversion increased
	12	Superior mesenteric ganglion	Spleen	Contracted
L1 L2 L3	1 2 3		Adrenal medulla	Adrenaline and noradrenaline secreted into blood
			Large and small intestine	Peristalsis and tone reduced Sphincters closed Blood vessels constricted
			Kidney	Urine secretion decreased
		Inferior mesenteric ganglion	Bladder	Smooth muscle wall slightly relaxed
			Sex organs and genitalia	Male and female: increased glandular secretion Male: ejaculation

Figure 17.1 The sympathetic outflow, the main structures supplied and the effects of stimulation. *Solid red lines* – preganglionic fibres; *broken lines* – postganglionic fibres. There are right and left lateral chains of ganglia. (Reproduced from Waugh A, Grant A. Ross and Wilson: Anatomy and Physiology in Health and Illness. 12th ed. Edinburgh: Churchill Livingstone Elsevier; 2014, with permission.)

Evidence-Based, Person-Centred Approaches to Medicines Management

Decision Support Tools for Safe, Effective Medicines Management

Medicines should only be given when necessary and when they will be of benefit to the patient. Knowledge of the evidence to support the prescribing of a particular drug is as important as knowledge of pharmacology and associated side-effects. National drug formularies will provide guidance on frequency and dose of the drug (see Reflection 17.3). Many of these are available as an 'app' and accessible from any smartphone device (e.g. BNF 2022).

National or local guidelines provide healthcare professionals with an appraisal of existing research to support the use of drug or drugs to help people to live with a condition. SIGN and NICE guidelines are recommendations for treatment underpinned by the best available research evidence that are also economically effective. Guidelines are often developed by an international consensus group and provide a structured, evidence-based and consistent approach to managing conditions wherever in the world they are treated. Examples of such guidelines are those developed

for management of diabetes, sepsis and acute coronary syndrome (NICE 2023, SIGN 2018).

Choice of treatment is often based on a confirmed diagnosis. However, treatments may be prescribed based on what is the most likely diagnosis (working diagnosis) from a number of different options (differential diagnoses). This may be because the prescriber has judged that the risk of waiting for a definitive diagnosis is outweighed by the benefit of starting treatment. For example, if the source of an infection is unknown at initial presentation, treatment with a broad-spectrum antibiotic may be the initial decision. Monitoring the patient's temperature, microbiological screening and cardiovascular response to treatment will establish whether the correct antibiotic has been selected, or whether an alternative should be considered. Once the source of the infection has been confirmed through microbiology, then antibiotics may be changed to provide more targeted treatment.

The role of the nurse is to have an appreciation of the evidence to support a particular treatment choice for a particular diagnosis and communicate this to the patient. If the evidence to support treatment is unclear, this should be explored further with the wider interprofessional team or referring to online clinical guidance prior to drug administration.

Aims of the Treatment

The aim of treatment will often be clear, particularly if the patient has presented with unpleasant symptoms. Abdominal discomfort due to constipation may be alleviated with laxative treatments and symptoms will resolve once treatment is given. Sometimes treatment is given to prevent progression of disease (e.g. angiotensin-converting enzyme (ACE) inhibitors for heart failure) or to destroy cancer cells or bacteria (e.g. chemotherapy or antibiotics). To ensure that the patient receives the right drug for them, it is important that the goals of treatment are agreed and the risks and benefits of taking treatment versus a different approach to managing their condition (e.g. high fibre diet and increased fluid intake) are discussed (see Reflection 17.4).

REFLECTION 17.4

Marion B, 26 years old, presents with a 3-day history with cold- or flu-like symptoms and thinks that she has tonsillitis. Her temperature and all other vital signs are within normal limits. She is reviewed by a nurse practitioner and following examination and history, the nurse discharges the patient with an information leaflet and advice to take plenty of fluid, 1 g of paracetamol 6–8 hourly (maximum 4 g in 24 hours) and ibuprofen 400 mg 3 times daily. She has been advised to return if her symptoms worsen, persist beyond 3 or 4 days, she develops a fever or has any difficulty breathing. She comes to you seeking to understand why this course of treatment has been made and why she has not been prescribed some antibiotics.

Activity

How would you explain this approach and what evidence is there to support the nurse practitioner's decision?

As a registrant, you will find patients often seek this reassurance. Fluid intake will assist in alleviating pain and reduce the risk of dehydration, and Marion may find cold drinks more palatable than hot. The analgesia will help with pain and swelling, and advising Marion to take the paracetamol 30 minutes before meals may make swallowing easier. Taking ibuprofen after food will minimise the risk of indigestion. The symptoms should resolve within 5–7 days, but having a safety net to advise that she return if symptoms persist or worsen is good advice.

A number of studies have investigated sore throat and its management in the community. Between 50% and 80% of sore throats are viral (Bird et al. 2014) and can be managed with the measures above. Sore throats are bacterial or viral in origin and with the symptoms that Marion B presents with, antibiotics may not be of benefit. A recent Cochrane review noted that although antibiotics may shorten the presence of symptoms by around 16 hours, a large number of patients require to be treated before a benefit was detected (Spurling et al. 2013). With the threat of antimicrobial resistance, vigilance when prescribing is important. Therefore antibiotics should only be prescribed if symptoms worsen or persist, or a fever or difficulty breathing develops (NICE 2018).

TABLE 17.6 Drug History Best Practice: Drugs Reconciliation

History From the Patient

Drug history	Prescribed drugs, type, dose, frequency and duration of treatment Herbal medication Over-the-counter medication How the drug is taken, e.g. orally, subcutaneously, inhaled
Medicines that are often forgotten ('pills, potions, lotions and sprays')	Inhalers Creams Contraception Vitamins
Recreational drug use	Alcohol Drugs Smoking history
Recent drug treatment discontinued	Check reasons for stopping
Adverse drug reactions	Type of reaction, allergies, side-effects
Adherence to treatment	Check that the patient takes treatment as prescribed

History From the General Practitioner or Pharmacist

List of medicines and adverse drug reactions	Check doctor's letter Repeat prescription

History From the Medical Record

Previous drugs and reasons for taking them	
Adverse drug reactions	

Inspection of Medicines

Check drug history with the patient's drug containers	The name of the medication on the container, dosage and who it was prescribed for When it was prescribed, how much of the medicine has been used and expiry date

Assessment of Drug History, Other Variables That Alter the Risks and Benefits to Treatment

Vigilance in medicines administration by carrying out a comprehensive drug and medical history is important. Allergies, intake of prescribed or over-the-counter medicines and recreational drug and alcohol use must be assessed prior to prescribing or administering medication. This is to ensure that ADRs are minimised. Medication history should also be verified with one other source so if the patient has provided a medication history this should be checked against the referring practitioner's letter, electronic patient record, family member or medications they have brought with them (Table 17.6). This process is known as medicines reconciliation and aims to create an accurate list of all possible medications the patient may be taking, assessing the appropriateness of these medications and ensuring that this list follows the patient through every transition point of care both in hospital and in the community (Care Quality Commission [CQC] 2023).

Often, there will be many drug choices based on the patient's diagnosis and local drug formularies. Healthcare professionals will also select drug, route and dose of administration based on patient preferences, medical history, previous ADRs and cost. Key considerations are:

- The ability of the patient to tolerate certain types of treatment. Age is a consideration when prescribing opioids as they may cause confusion in the elderly and are often avoided.
- How effective the drug is known to be: for people with GORD, PPIs (omeprazole) are often selected over H_2-receptor antagonists due to the greater efficacy of the former over the latter.
- Severity of disease: if a patient has a severe infection requiring hospitalisation, the preferred route of administration may be intravenous rather than oral.
- The weight of the patient: This is particularly important in the very young or underweight patient. Doses in children are mainly based on body weight (kg) and will be calculated on a unit (milligram, microgram) per kilogram basis.
- The presence of other conditions: liver and renal function will be taken into account when deciding on medications. If a person has asthma and requires treatment for hypertension, beta-blockers may be avoided as asthma symptoms may worsen.
- The willingness of the patient, or where relevant, the carer, to take their medication: frequency of dosing may be a factor to consider, a once-daily dose may be more realistic for a patient to manage than a three times daily dose.
- Cost: if there is a choice of two medications and they are equally effective, the cheaper of the two should be selected. This is to avoid unnecessary wastage of resources.

Shared Decision-Making and Medicines Adherence

It is important to discuss treatment options with the patient to ensure that the patient agrees to the proposed course of treatment. Shared decision-making and exploring with the patient their understanding, motivation and ability (cognitive and physical) are central to effective medicines management. Optimising medicines adherence is a key role for nurses as suboptimal adherence may result in overdose, progression of disease, unnecessary hospital admission, antimicrobial resistance, treatment failure and death (Holloway and Van Dijk 2011, Ryan et al. 2011). Medicines nonadherence is costly and reduces drug efficacy, resulting in increased mortality and morbidity in those who are nonadherent (Nieuwlaat et al. 2014).

'Medicines adherence' is the extent to which patients' actions match the prescribing recommendations from healthcare professionals. Optimum medicines adherence is when medicines are taken correctly 80%–95% of the time (Osterberg and Blaschke 2005). Worldwide, medicines adherence is poor and in the UK up to 30%–50% of medicines are not taken as prescribed (Jose and Bond 2021, NICE 2009).

There are a number of factors which are reported to influence medication adherence (or nonadherence) which include practical, psychological, cognitive and socioeconomic factors (WHO 2003).

Practical factors influencing adherence include the ability to open packs or bottles, the ability to swallow medication or whether or not a person has the time to adhere to a complex medication regimen. Psychological factors imply that a person's actions will be influenced by how they think, feel and behave (Bandura 1986). In the context of medicines adherence, this suggests that beliefs and attitude about illness and proposed treatment will influence how well a patient will adhere to their medication regimen. For example, if a person believes that the risk of side-effects outweighs the benefit of taking the medication, adherence to treatment will be reduced. With regard to cognitive factors, research has shown that patients with a poor understanding, or poor health literacy, of why they are taking their medicines are less adherent (Kim and Kang 2021,

Macleod et al. 2017, Paschal et al. 2016, Wu et al. 2016). Social factors such as cost, socioeconomic status, presence of family member and the relationship between the patient and healthcare professional will also influence how adherent a person is (Hung 2014).

A nurse caring for a person who is prescribed medication has an important role in optimising medication adherence. Spending some time exploring with the patient how easy they find the prescribed regimen, understanding of their condition and why treatment has been prescribed is an important aspect of nursing care.

There are some structured tools for monitoring adherence, for example the MMAS-8 (Morisky et al. 2008). This helps the healthcare professional understand the reasons why a person may be nonadherent, such as whether they forget to take their medication, whether they are unable to tolerate the side-effects or if they feel hassled when taking their medicine, and can often help to identify those who are at risk of nonadherence.

A nurse can optimise treatment by using strategies such as simplifying the drug regimen by reducing frequency of dosing, offering tips for reminders, for example alert systems on smart phones, or arranging for pharmacy to issue the patient with a dosette box or discussing alternatives to drug treatment. Education on self-management skills, counselling and enhanced follow-up after prescribing (Ryan et al. 2014) and screening for side-effects or effective communication with the patient about their understanding of the condition may also improve adherence (Reflection 17.5).

REFLECTION 17.5

Adolescent Case and Asthma Symptoms

Saskia is a 16-year-old girl who has attended her GP for an asthma review. Her triggers are known to be pet hairs and grass pollen and symptoms are worse when she has a cold or is tired. Current asthma management consists of a salbutamol inhaler (reliever) taken for relief of symptoms as well as a beclomethasone inhaler 50 micrograms (preventer) twice daily. She and her parents report an increase in night-time cough and less exercise tolerance in the last 2 months. This has been accompanied by an increased use of salbutamol and currently she is waking up and taking this in the middle of the night.

Questions

Q1. What questions would you ask Saskia?
Q2. What key steps would you take to help Saskia and her parents manage her medicines?

Answers

The following is an outline of areas to consider in answering Q1 and Q2 but it is not an exhaustive list.

Explore adherence to treatment: How well does Saskia manage to administer her own medications? At the age of 16 years, Saskia should be involved in recognising and managing her symptoms; this includes medicines administration. Adherence to asthma medication is particularly poor in this age group. If adherence to preventative treatment is poor or inconsistent, she will experience an increase in interval symptoms.

Exposures: Ask about exposure to known triggers and explore other related lifestyle and/or environmental factors, i.e. conditions in the home (damp), diet and exercise, family health, including any recent illness (viral or bacterial infections in particular) that may help explain the increase in symptoms.

Technique and understanding: Practitioners should explore how well the patient and family understand their condition, i.e. discuss signs and symptoms, how the patient and family recognise and respond to these, including treatment. Explore Saskia's technique and use of the inhalers to establish whether she understands the correct way of administration, as well as which medication is used for which purpose.

Adolescent Case and Asthma Symptoms—cont'd

Medication review: Where appropriate, practitioners should review the medications used to see if these suit the patient, and whether any alternatives could be offered and/or the dose is correct. It may be that Saskia requires an increased dose of her preventer inhaler (beclomethasone) to avoid recurrent asthma symptoms. This should only be considered if adherence is optimised and inhaler technique is good.

Written information: All patients and families should be provided with evidence-based written information related to their condition and medications. In relation to this case, practitioners would wish to review Saskia's written Asthma Plan and make sure that this is up to date in relation to her current management. This would include information related to each medication, when this should be given as well as escalation and de-escalation of treatment.

Practical Aspects of Medicines Administration: A Safe Prescription and Safe Drug Administration

A prescription is how the prescriber communicates to the dispenser (usually a pharmacist) and the person administering the drug (usually a registered nurse, carer or patient) how the drug treatment in intended to be given. It is a legal document and should be precise, clear, concise and written legibly in ink. If one or more of these are not satisfied, patient safety is at risk. Prescribing errors are the third most common cause of patient safety events and vigilance when administering drugs protects the patient from harm (Basey et al. 2014). Therefore the registrant has a responsibility to ensure that the prescription is accurate prior to drug administration.

Legislative authority to prescribe in the UK and globally is expanding and the UK has one of the most liberal approaches (Kroezen et al. 2011). A Cochrane Review suggested that there was no difference in service user outcomes (blood pressure, diabetes, medicines adherence and patient satisfaction) between medical prescribers and other professionals who had authority to prescribe (Weeks et al. 2016). Primary research and systematic reviews suggest that nurse prescribers are as effective as medical practitioners with regards to medication adherence, adverse events, overall satisfaction, quality of life and resource utilisation (Black et al. 2022, Duarte et al. 2017, Noblet et al. 2018). As pressures mount on existing healthcare resources, nonmedical prescribing is increasingly diversifying its range and scope with nonmedical prescribers increasing their contribution to prescribing practice in the community (Macvicar and Paterson, 2023).

From 2020, there has been greater emphasis on pharmacology and medicines optimisation in preregistration nursing programmes. In addition, all registered nurses can progress to a full prescribing qualification 1 year post registration, offering better access to medicines (Nursing and Midwifery Council [NMC] 2018). As a result, the nurse's role is evolving from one who only administered medication to one who may have the authority to prescribe or administer. Appreciating the key components of a 'safe prescription' is more important than ever.

A Safe Prescription

There are two types of prescription: those that are issued in hospital and those in the community.

Prescriptions can be issued in electronic or paper format but core information must be included (Table 17.7) and acceptable abbreviations must be used. Fig. 17.2 details the core information required. Further information on approved abbreviations is listed in the up-to-date BNF 'app'. Electronic prescribing is used more frequently in clinical

TABLE 17.7	Core Information Required for a Safe Prescription
Date	The date of issuing the prescription must be clear, and for community prescriptions the drug must be dispensed within 6 months of issue
Patient identifier	The name, date of birth and unique patient identification number are essential. Where possible the patient's address should also be detailed. The age of the person should be stated and is a legal requirement when drugs are prescribed for children under 12
The name of the drug	The generic name (e.g. ibuprofen) instead of the brand name (e.g. Nurofen) should be prescribed, clearly and legibly and, if handwritten, in block capitals
The formulation of the drug	Some drugs are prescribed in a particular way to have an effect over a longer period of time or reduce side-effects (e.g. a slow or modified release (MR), enteric coated (EC) or film coated (FC)). If this is the case the drug should be prescribed appropriately
The dose	Dose should be expressed avoiding the use of decimal points where possible, e.g. 5 mg not 5.0 mg Quantities less than a gram should be written in milligrams, e.g. 500 mg not 0.5 g Quantities less than a milligram should be written in micrograms, e.g. 500 micrograms not 0.5 mg The word microgram and nanogram should not be abbreviated When prescribing controlled drugs, the dose should be written in words and figures
The frequency	How often the drug should be taken should be in accordance with recommended intervals. If drug is given 'as required' the maximum dose in a 24-hour period is necessary
The route of administration	The route, oral, intravenous (IV), subcutaneous (SC), should be stated and abbreviations used should be only those listed in the BNF
The prescriber should be identifiable	Date, signature and printed name are a minimum requirement. Some prescriptions also require the prescriber's unique identifier (e.g. professional registration identifier)
Allergies	On a hospital prescription allergies and type of reaction should be detailed

BNF, British National Formulary.
Data from British National Formulary (BNF). BNF + BNFC app. 2018. https://www.bnf.org/products/bnfbnfcapp/, and NHS Lothian. Safe use of medicines and procedures. 2017. https://tinyurl.com/y75mytr6.

Figure 17.2 Sample prescriptions. (A) Front page of a Prescription and Administration Record. The correct identification of the patient is critical to reducing the risk of an administration error. This record also clearly identifies other prescription charts in use and previous adverse reactions to drugs in order to alert prescribers and reduce the risk of repeated exposure. Note also the codes employed by the nursing staff to indicate reasons why drugs may not have been administered. (B) 'Once-Only Therapy' box. This area is used for prescriptions for drugs that are unlikely to be repeated on a regular basis. Note that the prescriber has written the names of all drugs legibly in block capitals and signed and written their name clearly. The nurse who administered the prescription has signed to confirm that the dose has been administered. (C) 'Regular Therapy' box. This area is used for prescriptions for drugs that are going to be given regularly. Note the use of the notes box to communicate additional important information and the care with which the prescription for amlodipine has been cancelled with a clear explanation provided. (D) 'As Required Therapy' box. These prescriptions leave the administration of the drug to the discretion of the nursing staff. Note the clarity with which the indications for administration have been stated and, in the case of paracetamol, the importance of stating a maximum daily dose. (Reproduced from Qureshi Z, Maxwell S. The Unofficial Guide to Prescribing. Edinburgh: Churchill Livingstone Elsevier; 2014, with permission.)

PRESCRIPTION AND ADMINISTRATION RECORD
Standard Chart

(A)

Hospital/Ward: W26	Consultant: MAXWELL	Name of Patient: JOHN SMITH
Weight: 78kg	Height: 1.84 m	Hospital Number: WGH5522589
If re-written, date: 14.2.19		D.O.B.: 16.10.64
DISCHARGE PRESCRIPTION Date completed:-	Completed by:-	

OTHER MEDICINE CHARTS IN USE		PREVIOUS ADVERSE REACTIONS This section must be completed before any medicine is given		Completed by (sign & print)	Date
Date	Type of Chart	None known ☐			
		Medicine/Agent	Description of Reaction		
14.2.19	WARFARIN	PENICILLIN	SERIOUS REACTION (HOSPITALISED) AGE 15	SJ S Jones	14.2.19
		CEFALEXIN	RASH (DISCONTINUED)	SJ S Jones	14.2.19

(B)

ONCE ONLY

Date	Time	Medicine (Approved Name)	Dose	Route	Prescriber – Sign + Print	Time Given	Given By
14.2.19	16.00	MORPHINE	5 mg	IV	S JONES	16.20	ST
14.2.19	16.00	GLYCERYL TRINITRATE	2 mg	Buccal	S JONES	16.10	DK
14.2.19	16.00	METOCLOPRAMIDE	10 mg	IV	S JONES	16.20	ST

(C)

PRESCRIPTION		Date → Time ↓	14/2/19	15/2/19	16/2/19	17/2/19	18/2/19	19/2/19	20/2/19	21/2/19				
Medicine (Approved Name) **AMOXICILLIN**		6												
		(8)	X	DK	RB	RB	DK		X	X	X	X	X	X
Dose **500 mg**	Route **ORAL**	12												
Notes FOR 5 DAYS: STOP 20.2.19	Start Date 14.02.19	(14)	X	DK	RB	RB			X	X	X	X	X	X
		18												
Prescriber – sign + print S JONES		(22)	X	DK	RB	RB			X	X	X	X	X	X
Medicine (Approved Name) **AMLODIPINE**		6												
		(8)	X	DK	RB									
Dose **5 mg**	Route **ORAL**	12												
Notes	Start Date 14.02.19	14												
		18			DISCONTINUED DUE TO									
Prescriber – sign + print S JONES		22			PERSISTENT ANKLE OEDEMA SM S MAXWELL 16.02.19									
Medicine (Approved Name) **LISINOPRIL**		6												
		(8)	X	DK	RB	RB	DK							
Dose **20 mg**	Route **ORAL**	12												
Notes Review renal function on 16.2.19	Start Date 14.02.19	14												
		18												
Prescriber – sign + print S JONES		22												

(D)

AS REQUIRED THERAPY

Medicine (Approved Name) **PARACETAMOL**		Date	16.2.19	
		Time	11.15	
Dose **1g 4-HRLY**	Route **ORAL**	Dose	1 g	
Notes FOR PAIN MAXIMUM 4G/24HR	Start Date 16.02.19	Initials	DK	
Prescriber – sign + print S JONES		Date		
		Time		
Medicine (Approved Name) **GLYCERYL TRINITRATE**		Dose		
		Initials		
Dose **500 MICROGRAMS**	Route **SL**	Date		
Notes FOR CARDIAC ISCHAEMIA	Start Date 16.02.19	Time		
Prescriber – sign + print S JONES		Dose		
		Initials		

practice and appears to reduce the risk of adverse events although overall rates of prescribing errors may not be reduced (Slight et al. 2019).

Safety in Drug Administration

When a prescription is written the prescriber is responsible for prescribing the *right drug*, for the *right patient* at the *right time*, using the *right route*, with the *right dose* at the *right frequency*. These '6 rights' are essential during drug administration and are an additional safeguard to avoid adverse drug events (Table 17.8). All prescribers are required to adhere to the Royal Pharmaceutical Society (RPS) single competency framework (2021), which has the aim of a consistent approach to safe, effective evidence-based prescribing practice.

ADRs and prescribing errors can be minimised by the nurse practising safely during drug administration (see Fig. 17.3). This takes into account pharmacology, drug history, patient preferences and a safe legible prescription (see Reflection 17.6).

Preparation for drug administration is also important, ensuring that sufficient time is allocated and that interruptions are minimised. Checking that the correct dose has been prescribed by using the BNF and with a second person (registrant, patient or family member is important) is essential when administering drugs to the very young or when controlled drugs are prescribed (Reflection 17.7).

For some drugs, prior to administration, verification of vital signs or blood results is required to maintain patient safety, for example checking the heart before giving a beta-blocker or regular blood pressure checks for people receiving antihypertensives. For other drugs, prior to drug administration, specific blood tests are necessary. Chemotherapy for cancer treatments causes immunosuppression and an adequate white cell count is necessary to reduce the risk of infection or sepsis. As a result, the patient's serum full blood count will be measured prior to administration. Specific drug levels are measured for some treatments and are taken to prevent irreversible side-effects, monitor medication adherence or check drug sensitivity or tolerability. For example, gentamicin in toxic doses can cause deafness and, before each dose is given, serum gentamicin levels are measured to verify levels are sufficiently low to require a second dose of the drug. Fig. 17.4 provides an overview of what a nurse's role is for safe drug administration.

To optimise safety in drug administration, the person administering the drug should be different from the one prescribing. There are some circumstances where this may not be possible, for example in an emergency situation or when caring for people living in remote and rural areas, but the separation of these two provides an additional safety net when managing medicines.

Documenting accurately when the drug was given and by whom is important. If a drug is omitted for any reason, this should be clearly documented and reported in the patient's medical record. Hospital prescriptions will have a coding system that

TABLE 17.8	Principles Applied for Safe Drug Administration	
Domain	**Criteria**	
Right drug	The prescription, if handwritten, should be legible. If not, clarify the drug name or any other concerns with the prescriber	
	Make sure that the drug is appropriately labelled and the expiry date visible; if expired, do not administer and request replacement medication from pharmacy	
	Check that the patient does not have any allergies or sensitivities to the prescribed drug; this should be checked every time you give someone a drug	
	Ensure that there are no drug interactions between the drug that you are going to give and other drugs prescribed	
	Become aware of drugs with similar names and carefully check the original prescription and the reason why the patient is receiving the drug before administering it	
	If you are unsure what the drug is for, look it up or discuss with a more senior practitioner before administering	
	Never administer any medication if you any have doubts; refer back to the prescriber or a more senior healthcare professional	
Right patient	If the patient is able, ask them to state their full name and date of birth and check this against the name band. A red name band should be worn if the patient has a history of allergies. If the patient is cognitively impaired, sedated or unconscious, identification should be verified, using name band or with a relative or carer	
	Check the drug at the beside with the patient and against the medicine prescription chart	
	Only sign for the drug as being given one they have consumed the medication	
	Do not leave any drugs with the patient to take later	
Right time	Give the drug at the right time and, if a dose is missed, a double dose must not be given. If an additional dose is to be given as instructed by the prescriber, this should be prescribed as a one-off dose	
	Make sure the timing of the drug will optimise adherence, e.g. a drug may be more suitable to be taken at bedtime rather than midnight if the patient is usually asleep at midnight	
Right route	The route should to be used for administration as prescribed	
	If the patient has problems with swallowing, consider an alternative route of administration (intravenous (IV) as opposed to oral) or drug preparation (liquid as opposed tablet)	
Right dose	If dose unfamiliar, check dose in BNF or with a pharmacist	
	If a drug calculation is needed or a high-risk drug is prescribed, have a second person check the dose to be given independently	
	Ask the pharmacist or a second person if multiple tablets or vials are needed to give the prescribed dose it may be that the dose has been incorrectly prescribed	
Right frequency	The drug should be given regularly at the correct intervals. If drugs are given too infrequently, symptoms may recur by maintaining therapeutic drug levels	
	If drugs are given too frequently, the patient may experience side-effects	
	For patients who are self-administering, reducing the frequency of the drugs may optimise adherence, as the more complex the regimen the less likely the person will be fully adherent	

BNF, British National Formulary.

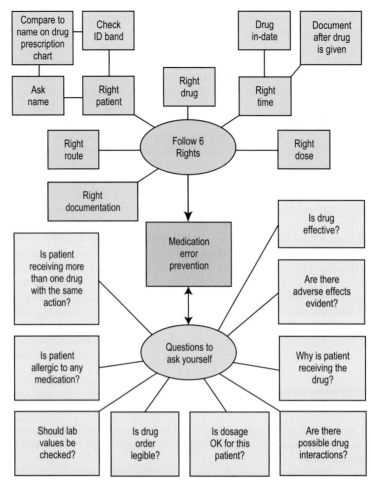

Figure 17.3 Factors to consider for safe drug administration. (Reproduced from Williams P. deWit's Fundamental Concepts and Skills for Nursing. 5th ed. St Louis: Saunders Elsevier; 2018, with permission.)

REFLECTION 17.6

You are working nightshift and Mr Smith has come into hospital with acute shortness of breath and heart failure. He has been prescribed furosemide 40 mg orally twice a day. A prescription has been issued and the dose is written as Furosemide 0.04 g orally. What would you do?

As a registrant, if you are unsure of the dose of a drug, this should be clarified with the prescriber and you should not administer a drug that is not in accordance with a safe prescription

Next stage: you go back to the prescriber and they cannot see the problem in this. How would you explain that this is not a safe prescription (see Table 17.7)?

What advice would you give to make the prescription safe to administer?

[Answer: This is an incorrect way to prescribe this drug. Decimal points should be avoided where possible and this should be prescribed as furosemide 40 mg or milligrams.]

REFLECTION 17.7

Work through the following drug calculations and write down the correct dose to be administered.

1. You are prescribing for an elderly patient and the BNF directs you to start treatment at 50% of the usual adult dose. The usual dose for Drug A is 750 mg daily. What daily dose of Drug A should be initiated for your elderly patient?

2. You wish to give antiviral Drug C to a 7-year-old child. The BNF suggests a dose of 6 mg/kg daily in three divided doses. The child weighs 21 kg. What exact dose of Drug C should be prescribed for each dose?

3. A patient is taking Drug E at a dose of 1.5 mg/kg/day. The patient weighs 120 kg. Calculate the correct daily dose.

4. A patient has been taking Drug H at a dose of 1000 mg twice a day. The patient has been getting toxic side-effects. The summary of product characteristics recommends that you decrease the dose by 60%. What is the new dose for this patient?

Your patient requires treatment of 7 days' duration and the recommended dose of Drug B is 500 mg three times daily. Drug B is only available as 250 mg tablets. How many tablets should you prescribe?

---

defines the reason for the omission, thus allowing accurate auditing of drug treatment. It is important that this is followed to allow for accurate reporting of reasons for treatment omissions.

Monitoring Drug Treatment and Reporting Adverse Drug Reactions

Monitoring the effect of drug treatment is required. As mentioned previously, this may be done by checking serum drug levels or taking specific investigations, for example cholesterol level for people prescribed cholesterol-lowering agents or haemoglobin A1C for people receiving antidiabetic treatment. Closer monitoring of drug effect and side-effects must be carried out for people with special requirements, for example renal or liver disease, the very young or old or those who are pregnant or breast feeding. Clinicians may

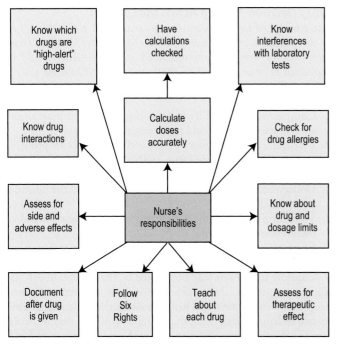

Figure 17.4 Nurse's responsibility in medication administration. (Reproduced from Williams P. deWit's Fundamental Concepts and Skills for Nursing. 5th ed. St Louis: Saunders Elsevier; 2018, with permission.)

recommend sick day rules for people with long-term conditions on certain drugs (Scottish Patient Safety Programme 2018) however, further research on the benefits of this is recommended (Martindale et al. 2017).

Patients and carers are also responsible for monitoring the effect the treatment has on their condition. It is important to inform the patient about how the medicine works, how long it will take to work and how the medicine should be taken to optimise efficacy. Precautions about when to report symptoms that may be an adverse drug event or interaction are all central to effective monitoring.

If an ADR is suspected, this should be reported in the UK through the Yellow Card system. This is an agency that monitors and reports all ADRs to a government body, the MHRA. The MHRA will review the product if necessary, and take action to minimise risk and maximise benefit to the patients. The MHRA is also able to investigate counterfeit or fake medicines or devices and if necessary take action to protect public health. Patients, carers or healthcare professionals can report any suspected ADRs electronically or on paper. The information is stored centrally and analysed to ensure continued drug safety, even after the product has been licensed. For the Yellow Card reporting suite, see Useful Websites.

Wider Issues of Medicines Management

Medicines management requires the practitioner to practise within professional codes of conduct, guidance and policy adopting an evidence-based patient-focused approach (NICE 2018, NMC 2018, RPS 2021). In this next section, we will explore the concepts of antimicrobial resistance, legalities and ethics, proxy decision-making, public health and clinical governance aspects of practice relating this to medicines management.

Antimicrobial Resistance

Globally, antimicrobial resistance is considered a significant public health concern. Previously treatable diseases, including major

surgery along with organ transplant, caesarean sections and hip replacements, cancer treatments and some chronic disease management, are all becoming high risk as a result. Recent international estimates report antimicrobial resistance-related deaths to be in the region of 700,000 per year (British Medical Association (BMA) 2017).

As a natural genetic process, antimicrobial resistance can be attributed to mutations that occur within microorganisms (i.e. bacteria, fungus, viruses or parasites); however, widely accepted accelerants include the extensive use of inappropriate antimicrobial agents (such as antibiotics, antifungals and antivirals) in both animal and human populations in addition to rising environmental pollution feeding a gene pool of resistance (Roca et al. 2015, World Health Organisation 2018).

International agencies and governments have recognised the need to tackle this through initiatives such as reducing the use of antimicrobial agents both in human and veterinary medicine, and investing in the monitoring and detection of resistant pathogens, sharing of information and endorsing research into newer antimicrobial agents.

In the UK, initiatives such as antimicrobial stewardship, medicines optimisation along with anticipatory guidance related to self-management and adherence to treatment are measures practitioners must harness to tackle this issue. Antimicrobial stewardship is the responsibility of all health and care practitioners. Indeed, NICE (2017) states it entails the following:

an organisational or healthcare system-wide approach to promoting and monitoring judicious use of antimicrobials to preserve their future effectiveness.

As a system-wide concept, it should be noted that antimicrobial stewardship should encompass a holistic approach to considering the patient, appropriate testing and recommending treatment based on robust evidence delivered over the shortest period as appropriate. Moreover, it is recognised that tackling health literacy is vital to empower patients and communities to better self-manage their conditions, understand their treatments whilst sharing decisions related to their medicines with the aim to reduce inappropriate use and harm and improve well-being (Public Health England 2015, Scottish Government 2017).

Vaccines

Vaccines are a way of protecting people from dangerous fungal, viral or bacterial microorganisms. The human body is continually exposed to the risk of these pathogens and the immune system recognises these organisms as 'foreign' and produces proteins called antigens. Lymphocytes respond to these antigens to defend the body against the infection and plasma cells make specific proteins against the antigen called antibodies and this contributes to the destruction of microorganisms. Vaccines are a form of active immunisation which promote the immune system to produce antibodies to a microorganism. Antibodies are produced by injecting the patient with killed or ineffective organisms in a controlled dose that will produce an immune response where antibodies are quickly produced protecting or minimising disease.

Vaccines lose their effectiveness quickly or become potentially dangerous if they become too hot or too cold at any time, especially during transport and storage. The 'cold chain' is a term used to describe the cold temperature conditions in which certain products need to be kept during storage and distribution. Maintaining the cold chain ensures that vaccines are transported and stored according to the manufacturer's recommended temperature range of +2°C to +8°C until the point of administration.

All vaccines must be refrigerated and protected from light. They must not be frozen. The efficacy of vaccines depends on their temperature being kept within the range +2°C to +8°C from manufacturer to patient. If storage recommendations are not followed, manufacturers will disclaim responsibility for any subsequent failure of the product. Use of a vaccine that has not been stored correctly is likely to be outside of the licensed use of the vaccine and therefore it cannot be used under a PGD.

Each site where vaccines are stored must have a trained and designated person responsible for receipt and safe storage of vaccines. This person should identify another trained person to deputise in times of absence. Public Health England (2018) provides a protocol that covers the minimum standards expected of professionals responsible for vaccination.

Legal and Ethical Aspects of Medicines Management

In the UK, a wide range of health and care practitioners may be involved in the delivery of care inclusive of medications. Medicines administration is one of the most common interventions between staff and patients of all ages. The need to prioritise people, practise effectively and preserve safety whilst promoting professionalism and trust forms the cornerstone of care delivery (NMC 2018).

The National Health Service (NHS) spend on medicines is growing significantly, The total cost of medicines and medical devices in England was £17.8bn in 2021/2022, up from £16.4bn in 2017/2018. (Robinson 2022). A variety of reasons are offered for this finding; these range from an increase in the product cost, supply and demand, prescriber behaviour, disease prevalence and changes in medical practices (Belloni et al. 2016). With this in mind, it is imperative that practitioners assist patients in getting the most out of their medicines for them and the health service. It is suggested that practitioners must understand the patient's experience, support choice based on evidence and promote safe use of medications (RPS 2021). Similarly, practitioners must align this practice to their professional standards which legally and ethically underpin their practice in this area (see Table 17.9).

All the standards convey the need to consider the four key ethical principles relating this to healthcare. These principles are:

- Autonomy – involves respecting the decision-making abilities of the person and facilitating informed choices.
- Beneficence – essentially, this reasons that all practitioners should ensure they act in a way that benefits the patient, balancing treatment against risks and associated costs.
- Nonmaleficence – this involves doing no harm; whilst all treatments may cause some degree of harm, this should proportionate to the benefits of treatment.
- Justice – this encompasses the fair distribution of benefits, risks and costs associated with treatment whereby the notion would be that patients in similar positions would be treated the same.

TABLE 17.9	UK Professional Standard Frameworks for Health and Care Practitioners
Nurses and midwives	Nursing and Midwifery Council (NMC) (2018). The Code: Professional Standards of Practice and Behaviour for Nurses, Midwives and Nursing Associates
Pharmacists	General Pharmaceutical Council (2017). Standards for Pharmacy Professionals
Allied health professionals	Health & Care Professions Council (HCPC) (2016). Standards of Conduct, Performance and Ethics

Proxy Decision-Making Across the Lifespan

The concept of informed consent is central and is closely aligned to the principle of 'autonomy' which necessitates that any treatment and/or intervention prescribed to the patient should be explained fully and agreed to. Beauchamp and Childress (2013) indicate five elements that should be considered when obtaining consent. These are:

1. Competence – the ability to grant consent, i.e. the practitioner should assess physical and psychological capacity.
2. Disclosure – all the effects, risks and benefits, both probable and possible, of a treatment and/or intervention should be explained by the practitioner to the patient.
3. Understanding – has the patient fully understood the information provided?
4. Voluntariness – does the patient agree to the treatment and/or intervention voluntarily?
5. Consent – considering the previous statements, does the patient then consent to this treatment and/or intervention?

Capacity to consent may be affected by the age and health status of your patient. Those vulnerable include children and young people, those with mental ill health, those with intellectual disability and older populations. In these circumstances, it may be necessary to refer to a proxy decision-maker. A proxy decision-maker is a person(s) who may make decisions on behalf of the patient when they are either deemed too young and/or no longer have capacity to do so (BMA 2019a). These persons may be a child's parent, a patient's wife or husband or someone legally responsible by legal agreement (BMA 2019b).

However, the law surrounding proxy decision-making varies considerably across Europe and internationally, and practitioners should familiarise themselves with the legalities related to practice wherever they are employed. Similarly, whilst patients may be too young and/or no longer have the capacity to make a decision related to their care, it is important that practitioners liaise closely with the proxy, that is, the parent(s), carer(s) and/or wider family, to appreciate the person's values, wishes and beliefs are adhered to (Weathers et al. 2016).

People with mental health issues are amongst the most vulnerable.

Public Health Aspects of Medicines Management

As discussed earlier in this chapter, medicines supply and demand incur a significant cost to the health service. Undoubtedly, substantial investment in the implementation of policies and guidance to try to tackle this has occurred, yet practitioners must fulfil a responsibility to educate, inform and guide patients in relation to their health. Indeed, it is vital patients and families understand their condition, risks, benefits and alternatives to drug therapy or treatment associated with their condition. The World Health Organisation (2018) defines health literacy as:

the cognitive and social skills which determine the motivation and ability of individuals to gain access to, understand and use information in ways which promote and maintain good health.

Interestingly, there is a strong correlation between low levels of health literacy and adverse health outcomes (National Voices 2017, Scottish Government 2017). Therefore practitioners must take steps to ensure patients and families are at the centre of planning for their care and an understanding related to treatment is assessed. Similarly, the concept of realistic medicine, which forms an integral component to public health and the management of medicines, focuses the need to shift from a didactic parental-led approach of care to one that harnesses an understanding of what matters to the patient to support care and treatment (Scottish Government 2017).

Two groups of society at particular risk of medicines related harm are people living with learning disabilities and people living with mental health conditions. With regards to people with learning disabilities, cognitive impairment, communication difficulties, multiple comorbidities, increased risk of depression and greater reliance on family or paid carers to optimise medicines taking, they are at risk of suboptimal medicines taking (Paterson et al. 2020). Nurses should be particularly aware of the risks of medication side-effects in this group, and supporting them to understand the importance of medicines taking by using communication aids such as easy-to-read materials, recorded conversations and talking mats is recommended.

In the context of mental health, psychiatric medications have significant physical side-effects and require close monitoring of cardiovascular health and weight control. The side-effects may have an impact on how adherent to treatment this population are and a recent systematic review of 14 qualitative studies reported patients stopped taking medicines to regain control of their life, citing breakdowns in the professional/service user relationship as a key factor linked to stopping medicines (Keogh 2022). They also cited the effects that psychotropic medication has on their

sense of self, describing 'blunting of emotions', loss of personality and significant side-effects. Shared decision-making and collaborative working with people with severe mental illness are vital for nursing practice to ensure medicines optimisation in this population.

Clinical Governance, Risk and Reporting of Drug Errors

Clinical governance involves the need for recognising and maintaining good practice whilst learning from and reporting mistakes to aid improvement (Scottish Government 2014). It is the responsibility of all individuals involved with care directly or indirectly. Practitioners must adhere to the best available evidence, assess the risk of any treatment and/or intervention and maintain a duty of candour (NMC 2018). Medicines errors and related adverse events pose a considerable challenge within the health service (Assiri et al. 2018), leading to a significant financial cost as well as physical and psychological harm for patients and families, ultimately resulting in inappropriate hospitalisation (Assiri et al. 2018). All practitioners have a duty to report errors factually, clearly and through the appropriate mechanisms. Electronic reporting mechanisms in hospital and community settings are used which allows the collation of incidents related to medication errors involving patient care. Again, vulnerable groups more at risk of adverse events related to medications include neonates, children and young people, as well as the elderly.

Summary: Key Nursing Issues

- In order to provide care that is safe and effective, the nurse needs to have solid understanding of the key issues associated with the management of medicines.
- Nurses are involved in the management of medicines in nearly every care setting; this includes acute, primary care, the general practice and in people's own homes.
- It is essential that nurses have knowledge of the regulatory, professional and legal and ethical frameworks that regulate and guide practice.
- The prescribing, storage, administration and safe disposal of medicines are laid down in law and the nurse must comply with these legal requirements.

- At all times the nurse must ensure that the patient is at the centre of all that is done and this is just as important when this concerns medicines administration.
- Effective medicines management is based on the nurse working in partnership with the patient as they assess, plan, implement and evaluate nursing interventions.
- Vulnerable groups such as people with learning disabilities or psychiatric conditions require specialist and focused support to optimise medicines.
- There is a need to work collaboratively with other members of the multidisciplinary team.
- Nursing students are required to achieve the knowledge and skills needed for effective medicines management during their pre-registration education.

Reflection and Learning – What Next?

- **Test** your knowledge by visiting the Evolve website 🌐 and answering the multiple-choice questions and critical thinking questions.
- **Consolidate** your learning by looking at some of the further reading suggestions, references and specialist websites.
- **Revisit** some of the additional material on the Evolve website.

- **Consider** what you have learnt and how this will help your professional development.
- **Reflect** on how you can apply this knowledge to the care of your patients.
- **Discuss** your learning with your mentor/supervisor, lecturer and colleagues

References

Al Hamid A, Ghaleb M, Aljadhey H, Aslanpour Z. A systematic review of hospitalization resulting from medicine-related problems in adult patients. *Br J Clin Pharmacol.* 2014;78(2):202–217.

Aljadhey H, Mahmoud MA, Mayet A, et al. Incidence of adverse drug events in an academic hospital: a prospective cohort study. *Int J Qual Health Care.* 2013;25(6):648–655.

Assiri G, Shebl N, Mahmoud M, et al. What is the epidemiology of medication errors, error-related adverse events and risk factors for errors in adults managed in community care contexts? A systematic review of the international literature. *BMJ Open.* 2018;8(5):e019101.

Bandura A. *Social Foundations of Thought and Action: A Social Cognitive Theory.* London: Prentice Hall; 1986.

Basey AJ, Krska J, Kennedy TD, et al. Prescribing errors on admission to hospital and their potential impact: a mixed-methods study. *BMJ Qual Saf.* 2014;23(1):17–25.

Beauchamp T, Childress J. *Principles of Biomedical Ethics.* 7th ed. New York: Oxford University Press; 2013.

Belloni A, Morgan D, Paris V. *Pharmaceutical expenditure and policies: past trends and future challenges. OECD Health Working Papers, no. 87.* Paris: Organisation for Economic Co-operation and Development; 2016. https://www.oecd-ilibrary.org/social-issues-migration-health/pharmaceutical-expenditure-and-policies_5jm0q1f4cdq7-en.

Bird J, Biggs T, King E. Controversies in the management of acute tonsillitis: an evidence based review. *Clin Otolaryngol.* 2014;39(6):368–374.

Black A, Gage H, Norton C, Franklin BD, Murrells T, Courtenay M. Patient satisfaction with medication consultations and medicines information provided by nurses working autonomously in sexual health services: a questionnaire study. *J Adv Nurs.* 2022;78(2):523–531. https://doi.org/10.1111/jan.15087.

British Medical Association (BMA). *Antimicrobial resistance.* London: BMA; 2017. https://www.bma.org.uk/collective-voice/policy-and-research/public-and-population-health/antimicrobial-resistance.

British Medical Association (BMA). *Best interest decisions of adults who lack capacity.* London: BMA; 2019. https://www.bma.org.uk/media/1850/bma-best-interests-toolkit-2019.pdf.

British Medical Association (BMA). *Children and young people ethics tool kit.* London: BMA; 2019. https://www.bma.org.uk/advice-and-support/ethics/children-and-young-people/children-and-young-people-ethics-toolkit.

British National Formulary (BNF). BNF + BNFC app. 2018. https://www.bnf.org/products/bnfbnfcapp/.

Care Quality Commission (2023). Medicines reconciliation. https://www.cqc.org.uk/guidance-providers/adult-social-care/medicines-reconciliation-how-check-you-have-right-medicine.

Duarte GS, Delgado RM, Costa J, Vaz-Carneiro A. Analysis of the Cochrane review: non-medical prescribing versus medical prescribing for acute and chronic disease management in primary and secondary care. *Cochrane Database Syst Rev.* 2016;11:CD011227 *Acta Medica Portuguesa, 30*(1), 7–11.

General Pharmaceutical Council. *Standards for pharmacy professionals.* London: GPC; 2017. http://www.pharmacyregulation.org.

Health & Care Professions Council. *Standards of conduct, performance and ethics.* London: HCPC; 2016. http://www.hcpc-uk.org/standards/.

Health England. National Minimum Standards and core curriculum for immunization training for Registered Healthcare Practitioners. 2018. https://assets.publishing.service.gov.uk/government/uploads/system/uploads/attachment_data/file/679824/Training_standards_and_core_curriculum_immunisation.pdf.

Holloway K, Van Dijk L. The world medicines situation 2011: the rational use of medicines. 2011. https://www.nivel.nl/en/publicatie/rational-use-medicines.

Hung C-I. Factors predicting adherence to antidepressant treatment. *Curr Opin Psychiatry [Internet].* 2014 Sep;27(5):344–349.

Jose J, Bond C. Medication adherence: still a problem. *Int J Pharm Pract.* April 2021;29(2):93–95. https://doi.org/10.1093/ijpp/riaa019.

Keogh B, Murphy E, Doyle L, Sheaf G, Watts M, Higgins A. Mental health service users experiences of medication discontinuation: a systematic review of qualitative studies. *J Ment Health.* 2022;31(2):227–238. doi:10.1080/09638237.2021.1922644.

Kim ES, Kang C. Improve medication adherence in older adults with chronic kidney disease by identifying and addressing underlying factors. *Drugs Ther Perspect [Internet].* 2021 Oct;37(10):460–464. https://search-ebscohost-com.napier.idm.oclc.org/login.aspx?direct=true&db=c8h&AN=152744952&site=ehost-live.

Kroezen M, van Dijk L, Groenewegen PP, Francke AL. Nurse prescribing of medicines in Western European and Anglo-Saxon countries: a systematic review of the literature. *BMC Health Serv Res.* 2011;11:127.

Macleod S, Musich S, Gulyas S, et al. The impact of inadequate health literacy on patient satisfaction, healthcare utilization, and expenditures among older adults. *Geriatr Nurs (Minneap).* 2017;38(4):334–341.

MacVicar S, Paterson RE. Characteristics of prescribing activity within primary care in Scotland 2013–2022 of general practitioners, nurse,

pharmacist and allied health prescribers: a retrospective cross-sectional study. *J Adv Nurs.* 2023;00:1–10. https://doi.org/10.1111/jan.15658.

Martindale A, Elvey R, Howard SJ, et al. Understanding the implementation of 'sick day guidance' to prevent acute kidney injury across a primary care setting in England: a qualitative evaluation. *BMJ Open.* 2017;7(11):e017241.

Morisky D, Ang A, Krousel-Wood M, Ward HJ. Predictive validity of a medication adherence measure in an outpatient setting. *J Clin Hypertens.* 2008;10(5):348–354.

Noblet T, Marriott J, Graham-Clarke E, Shirley D, Rushton A. Clinical and cost-effectiveness of non-medical prescribing: a systematic review of randomised controlled trials. *PLoS One.* 2018;13(3):e0193286. https://doi.org/10.1371/journal.pone.0193286.

National Voices. *Person-centred care in 2017: evidence from service users.* London: National Voices; 2017. http://www.nationalvoices.org.uk.

NHS Lothian. Safe use of medicines and procedures; 2017. https://tinyurl.com/y75mytr6.

National Institute of Health and Clinical Excellence (NICE). Medicines adherence: involving patients in decisions about prescribed medicines and supporting adherence. Clinical guideline [CG76]; 2009. http://www.nice.org.uk/CG76.

National Institute for Health and Care Excellence (NICE). Antimicrobial stewardship: changing risk-related behaviours in the general population, NICE guideline [NG63]; 2017. https://www.nice.org.uk/guidance/ng63/chapter/context.

National Institute for Health and Care Excellence (NICE). NICE guidance; 2018. https://www.nice.org.uk/guidance.

National Institute for Health and Care Excellence (NICE). 2023. https://www.nice.org.uk/.

Nieuwlaat R, Wilczynski N, Navarro T, et al. Interventions for enhancing medication adherence. *Cochrane Database Syst Rev.* 2014(11):CD000011.

Nursing and Midwifery Council (NMC). The Code: Professional Standards of Practice and Behaviour for Nurses, Midwives and Nursing Associates; 2018. https://www.nmc.org.uk/globalassets/sitedocuments/nmc-publications/nmc-code.pdf.

Osterberg L, Blaschke T. Adherence to medication. *N Engl J Med.* 2005;353(5):487–497.

Paschal AM, Mitchell QP, Wilroy JD, et al. Parent health literacy and adherence-related outcomes in children with epilepsy. *Epilepsy Behav.* 2016;56(C):73–82.

Paterson R, Taggart L, Hoyle L, Brown M. Characteristics of diabetes medication-taking in people with mild to moderate intellectual disability compared to those without: a mixed-methods study. *Diabet Med.* 2020;37:2035–2043. https://onlinelibrary.wiley.com/doi/10.1111/dme.14365.

Public Health England. Improving health literacy to reduce health inequalities; 2015. https://assets.publishing.service.gov.uk/government/uploads/system/uploads/attachment_data/file/460709/4a_Health_Literacy-Full.pdf.

Qureshi Z, Maxwell S. *The Unofficial Guide to Prescribing.* Edinburgh: Churchill Livingstone Elsevier; 2014.

Robinson, J. NHS Drug Costs see biggest rise for five years to almost £18bn. The Pharmaceutical Journal. 2022. https://pharmaceutical-journal.com/article/news/nhs-drug-costs-in-england-see-biggest-rise-for-five-years-to-almost-18bn.

Roca I, Akova M, Baquero F, et al. The global threat of antimicrobial resistance: science for intervention. *New Microbes New Infect.* 2015;6:22–29.

Royal Pharmaceutical Society (RPS). Prescribing Competency Framework; 2021. https://www.rpharms.com/resources/frameworks/prescriber-competency-framework.

Ryan R, Santesso N, Hill S, et al. Consumer-oriented interventions for evidence-based prescribing and medicines use: an overview of systematic reviews. *Cochrane Database Syst Rev.* 2011(5):CD007768.

Ryan R, Santesso N, Lowe D, et al. Interventions to improve safe and effective use of medicines by consumers, an overview of systematic reviews. *Cochrane Database Syst Rev.* 2014. https://pubmed.ncbi.nlm.nih.gov/24777444/.

Scottish Government. *Health and Social Care Integration: Public Bodies (Joint Working) Scotland Act 2014: Clinical and Care Governance Framework.* Edinburgh: ScotGov; 2014. https://www.gov.scot/Resource/0046/00465077.pdf.

Scottish Government. *Making It Easier: a Health Literacy Action Plan for Scotland.* Edinburgh: ScotGov; 2017. Available at: https://www.gov.scot/Resource/0052/00528139.pdf.

Scottish Intercollegiate Guidelines Network (SIGN). 2018. https://www.sign.ac.uk/.

Scottish Patient Safety Programme. Medicines Sick Day Rules Card. 2018. https://ihub.scot/improvement-programmes/scottish-patient-safety-programme-spsp/spsp-medicines/high-risk-situations-involving-medicines/medicines-sick-day-rules-card/.

Slight P, Tolley CL, Bates DW, Fraser R, Bigirumarame T, Kasim A. Medication errors and adverse drug events in a UK hospital during the optimisation of electronic prescriptions: a prospective observational study. *Lancet Digit Health.* 2019;1(8):e403–e412.

Spurling G, Del Mar C, Dooley L, et al. Delayed antibiotics for respiratory infections. *Cochrane Database Syst Rev.* 2013(4):CD004417.

Waugh A, Grant A. *Ross and Wilson: Anatomy and Physiology in Health and Illness.* 12th ed. Edinburgh: Churchill Livingstone Elsevier; 2014.

Weathers E, O'Caoimh R, Cornally N, et al. Advance care planning: a systematic review of randomised controlled trials conducted with older adults. *Maturitas.* 2016;91:101–109.

Weeks G, George J, Maclure K, Stewart D. Non-medical prescribing versus medical prescribing for acute and chronic disease management in primary and secondary care. *Cochrane Database Syst Rev.* 2016(11):CD011227.

Williams P. *deWit's Fundamental Concepts and Skills for Nursing.* 5th ed. St Louis: Saunders Elsevier; 2018.

World Health Organisation (WHO). *Health Literacy and Health Behaviour.* Geneva: WHO; 2018. http://www.who.int/healthpromotion/conferences/7gchp/track2/en/.

World Health Organization (WHO). 2003. Adherence to long-term therapies: evidence for action. World Health Organization. https://iris.who.int/handle/10665/42682.

Wu JK, Moser DA, DeWalt DK, et al. Health literacy mediates the relationship between age and health outcomes in patients with heart failure. *Circ Heart Fail.* 2016;9(1):E002250.

Further Reading

British National Formulary. Mobile application. British Medical Association and Royal Pharmaceutical Society. https://www.bnf.org/products/bnfbnfcapp/.

Lawson E, Hennefer DL. *Medicines Management in Adult Nursing.* London: Sage; 2012.

Pirmohamed M, James S, Meakin S, et al. Adverse drug reactions as cause of admission to hospital: prospective analysis of 18,820 patients. *BMJ.* 2004;329:15.

Qureshi Z, Maxwell S. *The Unofficial Guide to Prescribing.* Edinburgh: Churchill Livingstone: Elsevier; 2014.

Royal Pharmaceutical Society (RPS). *Medicines optimisation: helping patients to make the most of medicines.* London: RPS; 2013. https://tinyurl.com/y92w97t9.

Waugh A, Grant A. *Ross and Wilson: Anatomy and Physiology in Health and Illness.* 12th ed. Edinburgh: Churchill Livingstone Elsevier; 2014.

Williams P. *deWit's Fundamental Concepts and Skills for Nursing.* 5th ed. St Louis: Saunders Elsevier; 2018.

Useful Websites

BNF (British National Formulary), www.bnf.org/

Medicines and Healthcare products Regulatory Agency (MHRA), www.gov.uk/government/organisations/medicines-and-healthcare-products-regulatory-agency/services-information

NMC prescribing standards, www.nmc.org.uk/standards/standards-for-post-registration/standards-for-prescribers/

Royal Pharmaceutical Society, www.pharms.com/

Stockleys Drug Interactions, https://about.medicinescomplete.com/publication/stockleys-drug-interactions/

Yellow Card reporting suite, www.gov.uk/report-problem-medicine-medical-device

18

Infection Prevention and Control

EMMA BURNETT, PATRICIA KYDD

CHAPTER OUTLINE

Introduction

Infection prevention and control (IPC) measures are essential in everyday clinical practice to minimise the risk of infection to patients, their relatives/carers and healthcare staff. Any patient receiving healthcare, in hospital or community settings, could be at increased risk of infection due to many reasons such as their age, nutritional status, underlying illness or treatment needs. Additionally, patients being cared for in close proximity to other patients, for example in a hospital ward, are more likely to be exposed to infections harboured by others, particularly given the frequency of contact with healthcare staff, equipment and the environment. In all healthcare settings, to protect patients, themselves and others,

it is important for all healthcare professionals to understand the ways in which infection is spread and the precautions necessary to minimise the risk of spreading infection. Nurses, and all other members of the multidisciplinary healthcare team, are responsible for ensuring that IPC measures are implemented safely and correctly at all times. In this rapidly changing area of practice, it is also essential for health professionals to keep up to date with the latest evidence-based research and recommended best practice (Nursing and Midwifery Council (NMC) 2018). Throughout this chapter, reference is made to websites that provide current information, evidence-based guidance and other resources for use by healthcare professionals.

An Overview of the Challenges of Healthcare-Associated Infections

Healthcare-associated infection (HCAI) is the term used to refer to an infection acquired while receiving healthcare. There is ongoing concern and activity in the UK, and globally, in relation to HCAI and the prevention and control of all infectious diseases.

Microorganisms are capable of rapid spread within healthcare environments, cause major disruption on the provision of high-quality healthcare and compromise patient safety. Examples of such infections include methicillin-resistant *Staphylococcus aureus* (MRSA), *Clostridioides difficile*, *Escherichia coli*, *Klebsiella pneumoniae*, norovirus (known as winter vomiting disease) and respiratory syncytial virus (RSV, particularly in paediatric wards). HCAIs can also trigger sepsis, particularly among vulnerable people. Sepsis is a life-threatening medical emergency which can occur as a result of an infection anywhere in the body. It develops when the chemicals released by the immune system into the bloodstream to fight an infection cause inflammation throughout the body instead. If urgent treatment is not provided in a timely manner, the person will be at risk of death (Daniels and Nutbeam 2022).

Antimicrobial resistance (AMR) occurs when microorganisms continue to genetically mutate, developing resistance to antimicrobial agents in order to survive and continue to grow and spread in a changing environment. This means that the antibiotic will no longer be effective in treating that infection. It is important to note here that it is the antibiotic the microorganism becomes resistant to, not the human. The occurrence of antimicrobial-resistant microorganisms, such as Carbapenemase-producing Enterobacteriaceae (CPE), *E. coli*, MRSA and vancomycin-resistant enterococci (VRE) attributed in part to many years of use and misuse of antimicrobial agents, has also risen over recent years. These continue to cause significant patient safety concerns globally.

The most recent HCAI prevalence surveys in adult patients were conducted in 2006 in acute hospitals across England, Wales, Northern Ireland and the Republic of Ireland (Smyth et al. 2008) and in 2016 in both acute and nonacute hospitals in Scotland (Health Protection Scotland 2017). The results estimate the prevalence of HCAI to be between 2.7% and 8.2%, which means that at any one time, approximately one in eight patients could have an HCAI. Infections associated with invasive procedures and the use of medical devices such as catheter-associated urinary catheters and intravascular devices account for a high proportion of HCAIs. Prevalence and incidence results in the UK also reiterate that common microorganisms like those that have already been mentioned continue to cause significant problems.

It has been estimated that many HCAIs are preventable, and many can be eliminated by better IPC practices, such as standard infection control precautions (SICPs), transmission-based precautions (TBPs) and antimicrobial stewardship (AMS), thus saving thousands of lives (Haque et al. 2020). All healthcare professionals, in particular nurses, play a crucial role in achieving this, as described later in this chapter.

Infections such as pandemic H1N1 influenza, severe acute respiratory syndrome (SARS)-coronavirus and multidrug-resistant tuberculosis (MDR-TB) also continually pose challenges to public health as well as to healthcare settings. Specifically, in 2020, the WHO declared a Public Health Emergency of International Concern due to the rapid global spread of COVID-19. During the COVID-19 pandemic, the world then witnessed some of the most challenging years for IPC, with millions of confirmed cases and an estimated 14.83 million deaths (Msemburi et al. 2023). As a result, the pandemic caused a catastrophic impact on an already overburdened healthcare system and pushed healthcare professionals to emotional and physical exhaustion (Shreffler et al. 2020). Significant shortfalls in IPC practice during the pandemic were reported, such as inappropriate provision of personal protective equipment (PPE), inadequate training and inconsistent and lack of clear national guidance (Hoernke et al. 2021). The devastating impact of this pandemic continues (Prescott et al. 2021). This necessitates contingency planning both at population level and within all healthcare organisations. The ever-increasing world travel has added to concerns about the threat posed by infectious diseases, many of which have the ability to spread rapidly around the world affecting large numbers of people.

In the UK, the long-standing vaccine-preventable diseases including measles, mumps and rubella (MMR) affect only a small number of people in comparison to previous years. However, the uptake of MMR vaccine over recent years remains suboptimal and has resulted in lower 'herd immunity' (immunity across an entire population). Consequently, this has caused an increase in these diseases. Infections familiar mainly in older generations, for example smallpox, have also caused concern when there is heightened awareness of the risks from bioterrorism. Governments, both locally and globally, prepare for the possible reemergence of diseases that have previously been eradicated or controlled and the emergence of new infectious diseases.

Less common in the UK, but often with significant outcomes, are infections spread via the food-borne route. In the past, these have had a major impact on both hospital and community settings. It is estimated that there are around 2.4 million cases of foodborne illnesses each year in the UK, resulting in around 180 deaths caused by pathogens such as *Salmonella*, *Listeria monocytogenes*, *Clostridium perfringens* and *Campylobacter* (Holland et al. 2020). In healthcare facilities, guidance on proper food preparation, production and distribution is vital to prevent foodborne illnesses. An awareness of the food hygiene regulations is therefore essential for nurses and other healthcare professionals who handle food in healthcare settings (The Food Safety and Hygiene (England) Regulations 2013). Additionally, enteral feeding guidelines must be made available and followed at all times.

IPC measures aim to reduce the burden of HCAI and other infectious or communicable diseases, within all healthcare organisations (Loveday et al. 2014). Public Health England, Health Protection Scotland, Public Health Wales, Northern Ireland Public Health and Health Service Executive, Ireland coordinate many activities, such as national surveillance programmes to highlight and act upon the actual burden of HCAIs in specific settings (see Useful Websites). Nurses are well placed to contribute to the prevention, control and management of HCAIs within health and social care settings. Indeed, as nurses continue to occupy an ever-increasing diversity of roles, including those concerned with public health, they are in optimal positions to influence patient safety agendas.

For further information about the burden of HCAI in the UK and spread of other infectious diseases, see the recent national prevalence surveys (Health Protection Scotland 2017, Smyth et al. 2008), National Audit Office (2000, 2004, 2009) reports, the Care Quality Commission's work and the UK government department websites (see Useful Websites).

How Infection Spreads

The chain of infection is used to describe the circumstances that can lead to individuals developing a HCAI or any infectious disease. The rationale for applying IPC measures is based predominantly on this chain of events because it is crucial for healthcare professionals to understand how microorganisms spread and infection occurs. Only from this understanding can the right IPC measures be adopted. The chain of infection involves:

- The presence of *an infectious agent*, i.e. microorganisms that are capable of causing infection. These are often referred to as pathogenic microorganisms.
- *A reservoir or source* where microorganisms can be found. Within healthcare settings, this includes people such as patients, staff and visitors, and also the environment, such as dust, bedding, equipment, furniture, sinks, washbowls, commode chairs and surfaces.
- The potential for microorganisms to be transmitted from sources. This is often called a *'portal of exit'* and is the means by which microorganisms are expelled from the body, such as exhalation, aerosolisation (when liquid droplets are dispersed into the air, e.g. when coughing or sneezing), secretion and excretion.
- *A means or route of transmission* of microorganisms, categorised as contact, droplet, air-borne, blood-borne, food- and water-borne and vector-borne.
- The potential for microorganisms to enter the body through a susceptible site. This is often called a *'portal of entry'* and includes a breach in skin integrity such as a wound or open skin lesion, mucous membranes, ingestion and any breach in normal immune defences (Fig. 18.1), commonly through a variety of invasive devices, such as intravascular catheters, urinary catheters and respiratory devices.

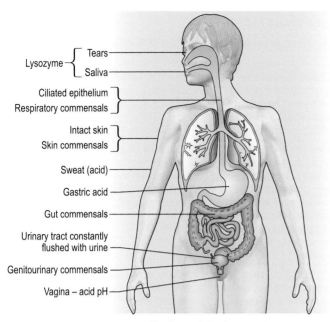

Lysozyme ⎱ Tears
⎰ Saliva
Ciliated epithelium ⎱
Respiratory commensals ⎰
Intact skin ⎱
Skin commensals ⎰
Sweat (acid)
Gastric acid
Gut commensals
Urinary tract constantly flushed with urine
Genitourinary commensals
Vagina – acid pH

Figure 18.1 Barriers to infection.

- *A susceptible host* refers to anyone who is at risk of infection by microorganisms, including those that would not normally cause them harm. Factors that affect the body's natural ability to fight infection include:
  - the presence of underlying disease, such as diabetes mellitus
  - being immunocompromised, for example if undergoing chemotherapy treatment
  - poor nutritional status
  - extremes of age, such as the very young and the very old.

The principles relating to all IPC measures are based on the interruption of this process. If these measures are not taken, the cycle will continue whereby individuals may be exposed to potentially pathogenic microorganisms that can cause harm, and the spread will continue.

Microbiology

Microbiology is the study of microorganisms and the interaction they have with humans, animals, plants and the environment. These include bacteria, viruses, fungi, protozoa, prions and helminths.

Bacteria

Bacteria are a large and diverse group of small single-celled organisms. They are commonly found living inside or outside the human body and in the environment, for example in soil and water. Bacteria capable of causing disease in humans are known as 'pathogens', with some being more pathogenic than others. Most bacteria are acquired though contact with other people or the environment (i.e. 'exogenous' sources). Table 18.1 gives some examples of pathogenic bacteria commonly encountered in healthcare settings. Microorganisms that are found on, and in, the human body which do not cause harm and can help prevent infection are called commensals which are considered 'normal flora'. Table 18.2 shows sites and commensal organisms. However, in certain situations, when these bacteria gain access to a different anatomical location outside or inside the human body, they can cause clinical infections. This is known as 'endogenous' infection.

Viruses

Viruses are a group of infectious agents so small that they are visible only through a microscope. They contain genetic material, either DNA or RNA, and must invade a host in order to multiply. Examples of viral infections include COVID-19, influenza, norovirus, rotavirus and RSV. Viruses have no independent metabolic activity and may replicate only within the cell of a living plant, animal or human. Viruses in humans therefore tend to spread due to close human contact, although some can also survive and be spread through environmental contamination.

Fungi

Fungi are simple plants that are parasitic on other plants, animals and humans. They can cause superficial skin infections such as ringworm or deep infection such as *Aspergillus*. Fungi can cause 'opportunistic' infection in people with increased susceptibility to infection (i.e. those with a weakened immune system). For example, in a postoperative patient, where antibiotic therapy may not only eradicate the infective organism but also protective normal flora, fungi such as *Candida albicans* can proliferate and cause infection.

Protozoa

Protozoa are single-cell microbes, which are the smallest organisms in the animal kingdom. Some species can cause human disease, particularly in hot climates, and can cause severe diarrhoea with the presence of blood. Most infections from parasitic infections affect people in developing countries, particularly in places where there are poor sanitary conditions. Gaining a travel history of people who are suspected to have an infection of this kind is vital. Protozoal infections do not pose a risk of person-to-person spread within healthcare settings, as depending on the type, they are spread via contaminated water or food, insect bites or sexual intercourse.

Prions

Prions are minute protein particles that cause transmissible spongiform encephalopathies (TSEs) in humans and animals. Creutzfeldt–Jakob disease (CJD) is a human TSE which is fatal. It causes the destruction of neural tissue, leading to progressive brain damage. Variant CJD (vCJD) has been associated with cases in young people. Healthcare professionals must follow the strict infection prevention measures in healthcare settings when caring for patients with known or suspected CJD.

Helminths

Helminths are worms, some of which can be a major cause of morbidity in humans, mainly in developing countries. In the Western world, many species of helminths can infest humans. These are most frequently spread within a household or shared living space and are not commonly encountered in the context of healthcare.

For further information on all microorganisms, see Gillespie and Bamford (2022) and VanMeter and Hubert (2021).

Epidemiology

Epidemiology is the study of disease in relation to populations, for example who is being affected by MRSA or influenza, and when and where they are being affected. Epidemiological data are crucial in targeting and implementing evidence-based IPC measures. Healthcare professionals should therefore support the collection of epidemiological data and understand feedback in order

TABLE 18.1	Examples of Common Bacteria Encountered in Healthcare Settings		
Organism	Main Sources	Main Mode of Spread and Means of Entry	Examples of Resulting Disease/Conditions
Staphylococcus aureus including MRSA	Found in people, in skin, wounds and at times in sputum and urine Environmental dust	Direct and indirect contact with persons carrying the organism or from the environment. Entry through susceptible sites, e.g. open wounds, invasive devices	Wound and skin infection, bacteraemia, endocarditis, osteomyelitis and septic arthritis
Clostridioides difficile	Found in people, in the lower bowel, therefore faeces and any faecally contaminated areas. Especially found in hospitalised patients who have received antibiotic therapy that has disturbed their normal bowel flora	Direct and indirect contact with persons carrying the organism or from the environment, especially as it forms spores that survive for long periods in the environment. Often also called faecal–oral spread if ingestion occurs resulting in further gastrointestinal (GI) upset/infection	GI infection, characterised by loose, foul-smelling green stools and abdominal pain. The most common diarrhoeal cause of healthcare-associated infection (HCAI). Can lead to pseudomembranous colitis
Streptococci	Found in people, at various sites, and in the environment	Direct and indirect contact with persons carrying the organism or from the environment. Through droplets from infected respiratory tract	Pharyngitis, wound infection, rarely necrotising fasciitis, septicaemia toxin-mediated disease, e.g. scarlet fever, toxic shock syndrome, pneumonia and associated bacteraemia
Escherichia coli	Found in humans, particularly the GI tract, and in the environment	Direct and indirect contact with persons carrying the organism or from the environment	Urinary tract infection, bacteraemia, GI infection (uncommon in the healthcare environment)
Enterococci, including glycopeptide-resistant enterococci (VRE)	Mainly environmental sources but also in the human GI tract. In the lower bowel of animals and humans, most commonly in hospitalised patients who have received antibiotic therapy Moist sites in the environment, but especially poorly draining shower areas and open fluid containers	Direct and indirect contact with persons carrying the organism or from the environment	Urinary tract infection Wound infection Endocarditis Eye and ear infections Wound infections, e.g. in burns Septicaemia Respiratory infections, especially in the immunocompromised, e.g. cystic fibrosis patients
Pseudomonas aeruginosa	Mainly environmental sources (soil and ground water). Contaminates moist/wet reservoirs in hospitals such as respiratory equipment and indwelling catheters	Direct and indirect contact with persons carrying the organism or from the environment	Urinary tract infection Wound infection Endocarditis Eye and ear infections Wound infections, e.g. in burns Septicaemia Respiratory infections, especially in the immunocompromised, e.g. cystic fibrosis patients
Mycobacterium tuberculosis (TB)	Found in humans, animals and in the environment	Through the air-borne route when respiratory infection is present. Through direct contact when other systems are infected	Respiratory or pulmonary tuberculosis (TB); can be termed as open TB. Closed TB, where another system or site of the body is infected. It can infect any organ in the body (see Chapter 3, Nursing Patients With Respiratory Disorders)

to enhance patient safety. A population considered at risk, for example from *C. difficile*, could be monitored using epidemiological methods to gather information that relates the disease to the population by studying both ill and healthy individuals.

In order to identify infectious diseases and HCAIs, robust approaches must be in place to gather appropriate information. There are various ways to monitor disease.

- *Incidence* is the number of new cases in a defined period within a specific population, e.g. incidence of wound infections postoperatively in all patients undergoing surgery in the next financial year.

- *Prevalence* is the number of cases that occur either at a particular time (point prevalence) or over a defined period of time (period prevalence), for example the number of patients with urinary tract infection (UTI) at any one time within a hospital.
- *Surveillance* is the ongoing systematic collection and analysis of data about an infectious disease that is essential to the planning, implementation and evaluation of public health practice and can lead to action being taken to control or prevent the disease.

Data collected over time will show the changing patterns of infectious diseases and HCAIs, providing information about newly

Site	Organism
Skin	*Staphylococcus epidermidis* Diphtheroids *Corynebacterium* spp.
Mouth and throat	Staphylococci Streptococci Anaerobes *Neisseria* spp.
Nose	Staphylococci Diphtheroids
Gut	*Escherichia coli* *Klebsiella* spp. *Proteus* spp. *Streptococcus faecalis* *Clostridium perfringens* Yeasts (*Candida*)
Kidneys and bladder	Normally sterile
Vagina	Lactobacilli Streptococci Staphylococci Anaerobes

TABLE 18.2 Normal Commensal Microorganisms

emerging diseases and identifying specific problem areas, such as outbreaks and seasonality of diseases. This informs the risk management process (discussed later in this chapter), which contributes to the prevention of the spread of infections and the control of outbreaks.

Mandatory surveillance systems are in place throughout the UK and globally, and comprehensive tools are provided to support the collection and collation of data. It is important that principles, including definitions, for epidemiological monitoring are followed to allow for reliable and comparable data to show improvement or deterioration over time.

Routes of Transmission

Clear understanding of the routes of transmission of microorganisms can ensure that appropriate IPC precautions are taken to minimise the risk of spread of the transmission of infection in all situations.

- *Contact* – contact transmission can be direct or indirect. This is the most common route of transmission related to HCAI. Direct contact is the transfer of microorganisms from one person to another through direct body contact without the involvement of an object or a third person. An example is direct contact between colonised skin of one individual and the mucous membranes of another. Colonised skin means that microorganisms have grown on the body but it has not caused an infection. Indirect contact means the transfer of microorganisms via objects in the environment (otherwise known as 'fomites'). Any inanimate object can carry pathogenic organisms, such as a contaminated commode chair or any patient-associated equipment, or from another person, such as the hands of healthcare workers.
- *Air-borne* – air-borne transmission is by small particles within the respirable size range (less than or equal to 5 μm). They can remain infectious in the air for long periods of time and can be widely dispersed by air currents and cause infection by entering the respiratory tract of susceptible individuals.
- *Droplet* – droplet transmission differs from air-borne transmission as the particles are larger (greater than 5 μm) and therefore do not remain suspended in the air and only travel short distances (less than 1 m). Transmission is therefore through close

contact with infected persons who may be sneezing, coughing, talking or undergoing airway procedures such as intubation or bronchoscopy. The droplets can also settle in the environment close to where they have originated, e.g. within 1 m of an infected coughing person.
- *Blood-borne* – through sexual transmission, injury or inoculation (penetration through the skin). The main concern within healthcare settings or for healthcare workers in the community is the transmission of hepatitis B, hepatitis C and HIV through sharps injuries or blood exposure.
- *Food- and water-borne* – food and water are common reservoirs for microorganisms, which includes medication, parenteral feeds and enteral feeds.
- *Vector-borne* – this spreads via insects such as mosquitoes and ticks, but cockroaches, ants and flies can also transmit infection. This mode of transmission is not common in the UK but should be considered in pest control policies.

Certain organisms can be transmitted through more than one of these routes and all modes of spread must be considered when carrying out risk assessments and providing safe care.

The Infection Prevention and Control Team

Healthcare professionals, patients, relatives and carers have a significant contribution to make in the prevention, control and management of the spread of infection. This includes nurses, doctors and dentists, allied health professionals, microbiology laboratory scientists, healthcare assistants, domestic and catering services, estates management, sterile services staff, administrative and management staff, education and training staff. This applies within all health and social care settings.

The role of the infection prevention and control team (IPCT) is vast, and priorities are driven by the need of the organisation, national policies and mandated requirements (Curran et al. 2020). IPCTs provide specialist advice, guidance and support, ensure that appropriate measures and action plans are in place and support sustained improvement through a change of culture throughout their healthcare organisation. The team has clear accountability for reporting IPC progress and issues through relevant committees and senior management structures. There are various roles within IPCTs which may vary depending on the needs of each organisation. These roles include IPC nurses, IPC Doctor, Microbiologist, Director of IPC, Deputy Director of IPC, Nurse Consultant, IPC Manager, IPC Matron, IPC Practitioner, Audit and Surveillance Staff, Health Protection Staff and IPC Support Staff. Each healthcare organisation will have their own local policy outlining their IPC team structure.

Many healthcare settings also have IPC link staff to enhance the effectiveness of the work of the team. The link person collaborates closely with the IPCT and receives additional education to improve the communication between IPC teams and the clinical setting and will assist with various IPC-related activities such as clinical audit and education (Dekker et al. 2022).

The Nurse's Role in Infection Prevention and Control

Nurses have a pivotal role in all aspects of IPC in clinical practice, both in hospital and community settings, acting as role models and influencing others:

- Maintaining and updating their knowledge based on the best evidence to ensure clinical practice is of the highest standard.

- Reporting and acting upon incidents when it has not been possible to implement best practice.
- Assessing infection risks to patients, staff and others and identifying and implementing appropriate actions required to minimise them.
- Promptly identifying signs and symptoms of infection and taking the appropriate actions (e.g. working with the multidisciplinary healthcare staff, collection of clinical specimens and interpretation of laboratory forms).
- Seeking specialist advice for support when required.
- Involvement in the promotion of best practice and monitoring of IPC standards.
- Communicating and educating patients, carers and other healthcare professionals about IPC.

As one of the largest group of healthcare professionals, nurses have a responsibility to deliver care based on the best available evidence or best practice (NMC 2018). They therefore have a duty of care to prevent and control infection. Effective IPC practice must be an integral part of everyday practice and be applied consistently by everyone. Nursing assessment is vital to IPC and patient safety, whether the healthcare setting is in a person's home, a hospital, a clinic or a care home, as it can reveal crucial information about patients, their surroundings and their behaviours. Nursing models and processes must incorporate approaches to the prevention, control and management of infection, for example within care plans and pathways.

The health of all healthcare professionals while at work is also important, as there are implications for IPC. They should therefore:

- Stay away from work if unwell, particularly if the illness could be transmitted to others, for example cough, flu-like symptoms, vomiting or diarrhoea.
- Be aware of their own immunity to infectious diseases such as rubella, chickenpox, measles, tetanus and hepatitis B. Nurses can obtain advice from their general practitioner (GP) or from their employer's occupational health department.
- Discuss other health concerns that may have an impact upon the ability to work, or upon others, with the Occupational Health Department, e.g. allergies that may be caused by products used during work and skin conditions that may harbour and spread microorganisms.

Specimen Collection

The collection of specimens for microbiological examination is an important element of a nurse's role. It enables identification of microorganisms to aid diagnosis and ensure appropriate treatment and specific IPC measures are commenced in a timely manner (Reflection 18.1). In the case of a bacterial infection, accurate diagnosis enables the use of narrow-spectrum rather than broad-spectrum antimicrobial agents, which optimises treatment and reduces problems associated with antimicrobial use, such as development of AMR. Samples may also be taken for screening purposes, for example to exclude previous known infections or as part of contact tracing. The UK countries currently have a range of policies on screening for antimicrobial-resistant organisms and, in particular, MRSA and CPE (see Useful Websites).

Samples may be taken from various sources according to the person's presenting symptoms or, in the case of screening, the most likely sites of colonisation. These include swabs from sites such as the ear, nose, throat, eye, vagina, skin or wound. A fluid specimen or, in some instances, a sample of tissue may be taken from the respiratory tract (e.g. nasopharyngeal aspirate, sputum),

---

REFLECTION 18.1

Mr Abadi's Journey

The following scenario concerns an infectious condition that is commonly encountered, both in community and hospital settings. From the information provided, consider (1) Mr Abadi's susceptibility to infection before admission to hospital; (2) how Mr Abadi's susceptibility to infection will be affected by his hospital admission and need for surgery; and (3) the ways in which infection risks can be minimised both to Mr Abadi and other patients on the ward.

Mr Abadi is due to be admitted to hospital for total hip replacement surgery. He is assessed in the outpatients' clinic 2 weeks before his operation is due. He is 62 years old with type 2 diabetes, treated by hypoglycaemics. On assessment, the significant factors noted are as follows: he is overweight and is a smoker, he states that he eats well and controls his diabetes and his skin is dry in places.

His wife is with him and is recovering from a hysterectomy, for which she was discharged from hospital 2 weeks ago. It later transpires that she is continuing to see the practice nurse for an ongoing postoperative wound problem.

Mr Abadi is found to have a foot ulcer. During examination of the foot ulcer, signs and symptoms of infection are present, that is erythema (redness), swelling and heat, with evidence of scanty serous exudate. Samples are taken and sent to the laboratory. Also, a nose swab is taken to screen for MRSA. The multidisciplinary team are eager to manage and treat the ulcer appropriately in order to progress with Mr Abadi's proposed hip surgery and are considering antibiotic therapy on results of the samples taken.

The results from Mr Abadi's MRSA screen and foot ulcer confirmed he has MRSA.

Activities

- What further information do you think the team needs to know to ascertain the epidemiology of the MRSA infection?
- Reflect on how you would manage discussions with Mrs Abadi and the rest of his family.

---

the gastrointestinal tract and biliary system (e.g. faeces), the genitourinary tract (e.g. urine) and the circulatory system (e.g. blood). Samples of vomit are not normally sent for testing as the results are of limited analytical value.

In order to ensure accurate laboratory results, it is important to ensure that there is no contamination from other microorganisms while obtaining samples. Additionally, an adequate amount of a sample should be taken and sent promptly to the laboratory or stored appropriately until it is sent. The storage requirement for different samples varies, so it is important to ensure the correct procedure is followed. For example, a sputum specimen must be sent to the laboratory immediately, as respiratory pathogens do not survive for long periods. Although urine ideally should be examined in the laboratory within 2 hours, it can be stored in a specimen fridge for up to 24 hours to prevent bacteria multiplying and giving misleading results. Likewise, a wound or MRSA screening swab can be stored overnight in a specimen fridge. Blood cultures differ, as they must be sent to the laboratory immediately or stored at room temperature but must not be refrigerated. All specimens must be placed in the appropriate container with the lid securely closed, and the transport pack should be sealed using the integral sealing strip. All specimens must be treated as a potential infection risk, therefore they should be collected using standard precautions.

If contamination occurs, for example, from intact skin surrounding a suspected infected wound, or not enough sample is sent to the laboratory, inaccurate results may be reported, and the patient may be commenced on the wrong treatment. This can then delay recovery, increase healthcare stay and contribute to AMR. Accurate completion of laboratory forms is also essential to provide laboratory staff with all the information needed to select appropriate diagnostic tests. Whilst demographic information about the patient is often computer generated in many healthcare settings, relevant information about the patient's condition, current medication or treatments (e.g. antibiotics), the source of the specimen and its purpose (e.g. screening or confirming the diagnosis of infection) is very important to include.

Underpinning much of the work undertaken in clinical practice are the policies and procedures that guide best practice related to IPC, such as surveillance, hand hygiene, isolation of infectious patients, aseptic technique and insertion and maintenance of medical devices, including urinary and intravascular catheters. These are informed by robust evidence and have specified timescales for review. Many nurses are involved in policy development and implementation. IPC policies must be communicated, learned, applied and closely monitored to aid continuous quality improvement for patient care (Reflection 18.2). It is part of being professionally accountable that each member of the multidisciplinary healthcare team adheres to policies and procedures.

Training and Education

In order for healthcare professionals to address the challenges of HCAIs and adhere to correct and safe IPC practice, they must be appropriately trained and educated. Additionally, healthcare professionals, including nurses, have a responsibility to train and educate others. This can take many different forms, including face-to-face lecture-style sessions and seminars, online programmes and shorter, interactive sessions within clinical settings. Not only is it important that nurses and other healthcare professionals are provided with IPC training and education, IPCTs must also be included (Tsioutis et al. 2020). To facilitate this, the Infection Prevention Society (IPS) developed a competency framework which reflects a broad range of competencies that IPCTs should possess (Infection Prevention Society 2020).

Quality Improvement

The correct and reliable implementation of evidence-based practice by all healthcare professionals is a cornerstone of high-quality patient care and safety. Quality improvement adopts a systematic and coordinated approach to identifying and addressing a problem using specific methods and tools so that improvements can be made (The Health Foundation 2021). Quality improvement strategies aim to change behaviour and create and sustain reliable systems of care. In order to be effective, such strategies must be aimed not only at individual level but also at group and institutional levels. This requires commitment from all healthcare professionals and senior management. There are many quality improvement models, one of which is the approach used by the Institute for Healthcare Improvement (IHI). The IHI Model for Improvement features key questions that must be asked in order to frame the overall improvement process, along with the use of rapid 'plan, do, study, act' (PDSA) cycles. Other strategies also ensure improvement, including the use of care bundles and checklists. Nurses are an important part of the multidisciplinary team in implementing and evaluating quality improvement strategies, in order to constantly improve patient care.

For further information on quality improvement approaches as applied to the prevention and control of infection, see the following websites:

> https://du.nhs.wales/patient-safety-wales/
> https://ihub.scot/improvement-programmes/
>   scottish-patient-safety-programme-spsp/
> https://www.ahrq.gov/hai/quality/tools/cauti-ltc/infection-prevention.html

Infection Prevention and Control Measures

In everyday clinical practice, specific IPC measures are routinely required to minimise the risk of infection to patients, their relatives/carers and healthcare professionals. This includes the use of SICPs, TBPs, AMS, aseptic technique, decontamination of reusable medical devices, outbreak recognition, investigation and management and use of evidence-based practice guidelines. All the following points must be considered in both hospital and community settings. There are also other specific targeted measures pertaining to key areas of concern related to HCAI incidence and prevalence, and their prevention.

Standard Infection Control Precautions (SICPs)

SICPs are the measures which must be always applied by all healthcare professionals in all care settings to minimise the risk of transmitting pathogenic organisms and prevent HCAIs to patients, healthcare professionals and others. They should be applied routinely in all situations, whether infection is known to be present or not, to ensure the safety of those receiving care, healthcare staff, visitors as well as the care environment (Reflection 18.3). There are 10 elements to SICPs. Some of these will now be covered in detail (see also Table 18.3).

Hand Hygiene

Hands play a major role in the transmission of infection within healthcare settings. It is universally acknowledged that they are the principal route in which microorganisms might be transported and cause infection to those who are susceptible. Therefore hand hygiene is considered to be the single most important intervention in preventing cross-infection and HCAI. Hand hygiene includes both handwashing with soap and water and the use of

TABLE 18.3	Standard Infection Prevention and Control Precautions (SICPs)	
Element	**Action**	**Rationale**
1. Patient placement/ assessment for infection risk	The infection risk for each patient must be assessed on arrival. Refer to your local policy for screening requirements. Choosing the most appropriate place to care for a patient is influenced using a risk management approach at all times. Consider the route of transmission of any known or suspected infections, how these might then spread to others, the potential outcomes of this spread, the availability of resources to site patients in the right place	To prevent exposure of both individuals and the environment to potentially infectious microorganisms and to protect the patient as far as possible from cross infection
2. Hand hygiene	In accordance with WHO '5 moments for hand hygiene', perform hand hygiene: (1) before touching a patient; (2) before clean/aseptic procedures. If alcohol-based hand rub (ABHR) cannot be used, then antimicrobial liquid soap should be used; (3) after body fluid exposure risk; (4) after touching a patient; and (5) after touching a patient's immediate surroundings	Frequently referred to as the single most important action to prevent, control and manage infection in healthcare settings
3. Respiratory and cough hygiene	When sneezing or coughing, the nose and mouth should be covered with a disposable tissue. If a disposable tissue is not available, use the elbow to cover the nose and mouth. Patients showing symptoms of respiratory illness should be encouraged to wear a surgical (TYPE II R FRSM) face mask as appropriate	Respiratory and cough hygiene is designed to minimise the risk of cross-transmission of respiratory illness (pathogens)
4. Personal protective equipment (PPE)	Prior to undertaking any care task or procedure, staff should assess any likely exposure to blood and/or body fluids and ensure PPE is worn that provides adequate protection against the risks associated with the procedure or task being undertaken	Remember that the use of gloves does not negate the need for hand decontamination and all PPE must be disposed of safely and properly immediately after being removed; often, this is into clinical waste
5. Safe management of care equipment	Ensure no reuse of single-use devices Prevent single-patient use devices being used on other patients Ensure that reusable devices are handled safely and decontaminated between use on the same patient and before use on others, following local policies Basic cleaning measures are a vital part of healthcare and should also be performed before any required disinfection processes	Care equipment is easily contaminated enabling the transfer of infectious agents from care equipment during care delivery. Therefore we need to ensure that items used during care are not a factor in the spread of potentially infectious microorganisms directly to patients or a factor in the contamination of patients' environment leading to indirect spread of infection
6. Safe management of the care environment	Cleanliness and maintenance of the environment must be kept at an optimum level to enable safe care to be delivered. Maintenance and audit schedules are required as per local policies, and must be applied routinely and in the case of outbreaks/incidents.	To ensure that the care setting, its fixtures and fittings and other items within it are adequately decontaminated and maintained to prevent cross-infection occurring through this route.
7. Safe management of linen	To ensure safe handling, transport and processing, linen should: • never be held against the body or shaken, even if protective clothing is worn • always be disposed of into appropriate receptacles immediately after being removed and never placed on the floor/other surfaces • removed from the bed one item at a time and not rolled/folded together	To prevent the risk of inappropriate, avoidable exposure to microorganisms when linen is being handled or reused, thus protecting healthcare workers and others and preventing contamination of the environment. Linen can be heavily contaminated with potentially pathogenic microorganisms; items such as urinary catheters, needles, etc., are often found in linen by laundry staff, putting them at unnecessary risk. Use of PPE when handling used linen is essential
8. Safe management of blood and body fluid spillages	Utilise cleaning products and disinfectants (often found in 'spillage kits') immediately after spillages occur, following local policies	Spillages must be safely decontaminated immediately to prevent the transmission of blood-borne viruses

Continued

TABLE 18.3	Standard Infection Prevention and Control Precautions (SICPs)—cont'd	
Element	Action	Rationale
9. Safe disposal of waste (including sharps)	Waste is categorised by regulations so that it will be segregated and subsequently destroyed safely and effectively: • clinical waste generated in the home and community is often dealt with differently from that generated in hospital settings; local policies reflecting current regulations must be followed • the area around the opening of clinical waste bags and sharps containers is often the most contaminated in healthcare settings and should never be touched; 'hands-free' waste sack holders, e.g. foot-operated, must always be in place Attaching waste bags to other pieces of furniture, e.g. trolleys, is not generally acceptable, nor is overfilling of bags	To prevent the risk of inappropriate, avoidable exposure to the microorganisms found contaminating clinical waste in particular, thus protecting all healthcare workers and others. The use of PPE when handling waste is essential
10. Occupational safety: prevention and exposure management (including sharps)	Avoid sharps injuries: • Never resheathe sharps such as needles • Utilise sharps receptacles close to the point of use • Never try to retrieve any items from sharps receptacles. • Use safety devices where possible	Sharps handling should be kept to a minimum and safety devices used where possible to eliminate the risk of transmission of a blood borne virus

alcohol-based hand rub (ABHR) containing at least 60% alcohol by volume. Undertaking hand hygiene is a simple but effective way to help prevent infections however, it is recognised that compliance of healthcare workers is suboptimal. The World Health Organisation (WHO) reports that appropriate hand hygiene prevents up to 50% of avoidable infections acquired during healthcare delivery and has produced guidelines on hand hygiene in healthcare. The First Global Patient Safety Challenge *Clean Care Is Safer Care* has identified '5 moments for hand hygiene' to highlight the most fundamental times when hands should be cleansed during care delivery and daily routines (WHO 2009). These moments are:

1. before touching a patient
2. before clean/aseptic procedures
3. after body fluid exposure/risk
4. after touching a patient
5. after touching patient surroundings.

For more information on the '5 moments for hand hygiene', the technique for performing adequate hand hygiene and hand hygiene campaigns going on throughout the UK, see the following websites:

https://www.washyourhandsofthem.com/home.aspx
https://www.who.int/health-topics infection-prevention-and-control#tab=tab_1

Two types of microorganisms colonise the hands: transient and resident. Transient microorganisms colonise the superficial layers of the skin and can be acquired from direct contact with people, equipment or the environment. These are the organisms most frequently associated with HCAIs (WHO 2009). They do not survive for long periods on the hands but can be effectively transferred if not removed. Resident microorganisms are found in the deeper layers of the skin, sweat glands and hair follicles. It is not necessary to remove these from the hands when providing routine clinical care. To remove transient microorganisms from the hands, you must perform hand hygiene using either soap and water or ABHR.

Within the healthcare setting, ABHRs are the preferred method for hand hygiene unless hands are visibly soiled or when there

is likely to be exposure to spore forming organisms such as *C. difficile* or diarrhoeal illness. In these situations, hands must be washed with soap and water as alcohol hand rubs are not effective. In most situations, plain (non-antimicrobial), liquid soap is the cleansing agent of choice to physically remove visible soiling and the 'transient' microorganisms from the skin. An effective hand hygiene technique is important in ensuring optimal removal of microorganisms, as detailed in Table 18.4. This technique ensures that all surfaces of the hands are covered and, if using soap and water, the hands are not recontaminated when closing taps and disposing of paper towels.

The UK Department of Health introduced 'bare below the elbows' in 2008 recommending that all staff providing care would have no jewellery or clothing below the elbow as they inhibit correct handwashing technique. This aimed to improve the effectiveness of hand hygiene performed by healthcare workers and thereby reduce the incidence of HCAIs. To facilitate effective hand hygiene, healthcare workers should not wear artificial fingernails or extensions. Nails should be kept short and natural to facilitate effective decontamination.

Personal Protective Equipment

PPE is defined as equipment that is intended to be worn or held by a person to protect them from risks to their health and safety while at work. Examples commonly used within healthcare include gloves, aprons and eye and face protection (Reflection 18.4). As well as protecting healthcare professionals, use of PPE also minimises microbial contamination of hands and clothing. Therefore it plays a key part in preventing the spread of microorganisms to patients and others.

The use of PPE is based on a risk assessment, depending on the task in hand and according to the likelihood of exposure to blood and/or body fluids or other infectious substances. Following this assessment is important to select the most appropriate PPE which provides the maximum protection for each procedure/situation. The incorrect use of PPE (including overuse) may increase the risk of infection to patients and cause contamination to both equipment and the environment. All PPE should be located close to the point of use to ensure it is not donned prematurely. It should always be changed immediately after each task for which it was

TABLE 18.4	Steps Involved in Performing Effective Hand Hygiene
Preparation for Hand Hygiene	**Healthcare Staff**
Procedure for handwashing with soap and water	Turn on tap(s) and adjust to a comfortable temperature (warm/tepid). Wet hands and wrists. Apply liquid soap Vigorously rub hands together, generating a good lather. Wash all surfaces of the hands (front and back) for 15 seconds: • Rub hands palm to palm • Rub the right palm over the back of the other hand with interlaced fingers and vice versa • Rub palm to palm with the fingers interlaced • Rub the backs of fingers to opposing palms with fingers interlocked • Use rotational rubbing of the left thumb clasped in the right palm and vice versa • Use rotational rubbing, backwards and forwards with clasped fingers of the right hand in the left palm and vice versa Rinse well under running water Turn off taps using a 'hands-free technique' (elbows or disposable paper towel) Dry thoroughly all parts of the hands and wrists, paying particular attention to interdigital surfaces of the fingers and thumbs Dispose of paper towel in a bin without re-contaminating hands
Procedure for hand hygiene with alcohol-based hand rub	Ensure hands are visibly clean Apply hand rub to all surfaces of the hands in the same way as described Allow to dry naturally (do not shake) Alcohol-based hand rubs are not reliable against spore-forming organisms (e.g. *Clostridioides difficile*) and viral causes of gastroenteritis (e.g. norovirus)
Application in community settings	Carry a supply of alcohol-based hand rub at all times In a patient's/client's home, whenever possible, request a freshly laundered hand towel and liquid soap for use during your visit Disposable paper hand towels can be carried if required

of infection posed by microorganisms, such as bacteria and viruses. It is vital to ensure that the environment and all equipment in it are clean to prevent the spread of microorganisms and ensure it is safe for practice. Environmental decontamination is the process by which the healthcare environment is made free from a harmful level of contamination that may result in the transfer of pathogens that can cause HCAIs.

The responsibilities for ensuring that the patient's environment is clean must be made clear to all. Assigning the specific responsibilities of healthcare organisation and cleanliness to domestic services staff and other clinical staff including nurses is important to avoid confusion about whose role it is to clean what. It is also important that healthcare staff are aware of the terminology and understand what is required for the particular situation:

Cleaning is the removal of 'dirt' from surfaces, which may include microbial (e.g. bacteria) and nonmicrobial (e.g. body fluids) contamination.

Disinfection is the killing of microbes on surfaces, via chemicals, heat, or another process.

Cleaning is usually conducted using a general-purpose detergent, warm water in a clean receptacle and clean or disposable cloths or mops. Disposable wipes impregnated with detergent offer a convenient alternative, although owing to the wide variety of wipes now available, care should be taken to select a suitable product for use.

Drying is also an important part of the cleaning process when using the detergent and water method, although large surfaces such as floors may have to be 'air-dried'. Stagnant moisture or fluid can be a focus for microorganisms and could potentially lead to HCAI (see example in Reflection 18.5). Disinfectants should be used routinely on sanitary equipment such as toilets, sinks, basins and baths. However, they need to be cleaned with detergent prior to disinfection. An alternative to this is to use a combined detergent and disinfectant. It is also important that equipment should be rinsed and dried after disinfection. In some situations, there may be specific areas which require routine cleaning with disinfection. Further guidance can be obtained from the IPCT and from local policies and procedures. The use of alcohol wipes is commonplace in healthcare environments. This is acceptable, in keeping with local policy, if the wipes are used for hard surface disinfection where the surface is physically clean, and wipes are moist throughout use.

If any visible contamination of the environment or equipment is observed, decontamination must take place immediately.

required and/or after each patient. To prevent contamination, it is just as important to remove PPE in the correct manner as it is to select the correct PPE in the first place. See the National Infection Prevention and Control manual for guidance:

https://www.nipcm.scot.nhs.uk/about-the-manual/

On removal of PPE, hand hygiene should always be performed. Remember that wearing gloves does not negate the need for hand hygiene.

Management of the Care Environment and Equipment

The cleanliness of the environment is important to support IPC, help reduce the incidence of HCAIs and ensure patient confidence. A clean environment reduces the cumulative risk of transmission

Particular attention must be given to frequently touched horizontal surfaces, such as bedrails, commodes, bedside cabinets, chair arms and tables, as well as other equipment at the point of care, such as infusion pumps. Other equipment within the healthcare setting may also become contaminated and will require regular cleaning such as computer keyboards and telephones. Cleaning and decontamination schedules must reflect specific risks, including the volume of activity, the patient's infectious condition and the procedures being undertaken. This applies to clinical areas as well as local or central storage areas for supplies such as PPE, waste and linen. Cleaning of soft furnishings such as curtains, chairs and carpets should include vacuuming and/or laundering as appropriate. Increasing the frequency of cleaning and reviewing methods of cleaning are essential during outbreaks or when there is increased risk of cross-infection, such as from incontinent patients or the presence of antimicrobial-resistant microorganisms. Schedules for the collection of linen and waste bags are also important and must be agreed, recorded and monitored.

Many disciplines are involved in environment control, and 'service level agreements' for example can ensure that all are aware of the standards to be achieved and tasks to be undertaken. Many reports, including findings of audits, have been published about the lack of cleanliness and hygiene in healthcare premises, particularly NHS hospitals, often focusing on the potential effects of the reduced numbers of dedicated cleaning staff. Roles such as the modern matron, director of IPC, nurse consultant in infection prevention and infection control manager, as well as the infection prevention team, should help to create a positive culture towards cleaning as one part of the broad range of IPC measures.

Standard Precautions for Control of Respiratory Infections – Respiratory and Cough Hygiene

The recent COVID-19 pandemic has brought respiratory precautions to the forefront of IPC. Precautions to prevent the spread of respiratory infections such as influenza are required and apply to every person with signs and symptoms of a respiratory tract infection (cough, congestion, runny nose, increased production or respiratory secretions), including patients, healthcare staff and visitors. Suggested preventative measures include:

- Covering the mouth and nose with a disposable tissue when coughing or sneezing. If not available, use the crook of the elbow to cover the nose and mouth.
- Encouraging patients showing symptoms of respiratory illness to wear surgical face mask where possible if tolerated (type IIR fluid-resistant surgical mask [FRSM]).
- Promptly disposing of tissues and facemasks into a bin.
- Avoid touching the face.

- Performing hand hygiene after any contact with respiratory secretions, used tissues and/or potentially contaminated surfaces.

The proximity of patients to one another in areas such as waiting rooms is also a consideration for the spread of respiratory infections. It is recommended that patients with respiratory symptoms who are confirmed or suspected to have a respiratory infection maintain a distance of at least 1 m from others (NHS England 2022). Key standard precautions points representing good practice in preventing infection are shown in Table 18.3.

Transmission-Based Precautions

TBPs are additional measures taken in addition to SICPs. They are grouped into categories which are focused on the mode of transmission of a particular microorganism:

- contact
- droplet
- air-borne.

Knowledge of the route of transmission will allow an understanding of the IPC measures to be taken without the need for more in-depth knowledge of the specific microorganism or infection. However, it is important to remember that some microorganisms are spread by more than one route and may therefore require a combination of precautions. For example, respiratory viruses spread via the air-borne or droplet route may also arrive at susceptible portals of entry (i.e. nasal mucosa, conjunctivae and the mouth) by the contact route, via hands that have become contaminated by the virus. Noroviruses are transmitted by contact, food- and water-borne routes, but may also be spread through aerosolisation of infectious particles from vomit or faecal material.

Full details of the IPC measures to be adopted in addition to standard precautions should be available within local IPC policies and from the IPCT. Although internationally accepted, recommendations are specific with regards to measures to prevent and control the spread of infection through identified routes of transmission; slight variations may occur due to local situations and facilities.

Contact precautions are the measures directed towards prevention of spread via the contact route of transmission. They are particularly important, as it has been found that 'contact', particularly via contaminated hands, is the most common route of spread in relation to HCAI (Wilson and Prieto 2021). If contact precautions are applied appropriately and correctly, infections such as MRSA and *C. difficile* can be prevented and controlled. Measures to control diarrhoea are extremely important due to the number of infections presenting that are spread through this route. Steps such as appropriate single room isolation as well as targeted hand hygiene, use of appropriate PPE, decontamination of equipment and the environment and prompt treatment for patients are crucial.

For further information, visit the NHS Scotland website to access the National Infection Prevention and Control Manual.

People being cared for under TBPs, whether in hospital or in the community, may be embarrassed or depressed because they feel that they are in some way 'dirty'. They may require additional psychological support, including more regular 'social' visits by nursing staff, particularly when cared for in single room isolation (see next section). Nurses are legally responsible for keeping patient information confidential and may divulge such information only if it is essential for the benefit of the patient or the safety of others. Nurses should explain this to patients to minimise embarrassment or unease. Avoiding unnecessary use of PPE, positioning the call bell within easy reach and involving visitors in helping find ways to relieve boredom may all help to minimise the adverse effects of single room isolation and should be part of the routine care of the isolated patient (Purssell et al. 2020). Patients in their own home may be concerned about friends and family visiting when they have an infection. Correct and appropriate advice and information can be obtained from the IPCT.

Nursing a Patient in a Single Isolation Room

The use of single isolation room for a patient who poses a risk of infection to others is an important element of TBPs. This is known as source isolation. There is also 'protective isolation' which aims to protect an immunocompromised patient at risk of acquiring microorganisms from the environment, other patients, staff or visitors. The Health and Social Care Act (2008) requires that all healthcare providers who deliver in-patient care can ensure that they can physically separate patients to minimise or prevent the spread of infection. Before isolation is implemented, there are several factors that must be considered. A risk assessment should be carried out by the IPCT.

However, implementing isolation can be challenging. It can have negative effects on the physical, social and psychological wellbeing of the patient. Patients have been reported to show signs of anxiety and even depression because of isolation and even reports of feeling that they are a threat to others because of their 'dirtiness' (Shaban et al. 2020). Patients can also feel that they do not receive the same level of care and attention as those not in isolation. The nurse's role in providing accurate information, support and reassurance is vital to ensure the patient experience is improved. It is important to explain to the patient and their visitors the rationale for the IPC procedures being used and offer enhanced support, both social and emotional, to minimise the negative effects that may be experienced. Nurses should ensure they maintain frequent contact with the patient to prevent feelings of social exclusion and receiving reduced nursing care. However, there are also positive effects, with some patients reporting they prefer the privacy of a single room (Cusack et al. 2019).

Isolation procedures can cause confusion amongst healthcare staff, especially in relation to the use of PPE, and this can prove challenging for the delivery of safe and effective care (Gammon and Hunt 2018). Other healthcare professionals and visitors to the patient in isolation often look towards nurses to guide them in the correct use of isolation procedures. It is therefore especially important for nurses to understand the rationale underpinning isolation procedures to promote their correct and consistent use. This will also likely reduce anxiety amongst colleagues, visitors and the patient, and minimise the risk of spread of infection. Ensuring that all staff have access to readily available information on the steps to be taken is important. Additionally, ensuring continued and regular communication with the IPCT will help them adhere to policies and guidance in place.

It must be acknowledged, however, that on some occasions, despite the requirement for isolation for IPC purposes, it may not be appropriate for a patient to be isolated, for example if isolation becomes detrimental to mental or physical health or will affect patient safety. In situations like this, advice should be sought from the IPCT where best to place the patient so not to put others at risk of infection.

Antimicrobial Stewardship

The last century saw the golden era of antibiotics. The WHO warns that without urgent action, we are heading for a postantibiotic era, in which common infections and minor injuries can once again kill. They define AMR as 'resistance of a microorganism to an antimicrobial drug that was originally effective for treatment of infections caused by it' (WHO 2015). AMR is accelerated by the overuse and misuse of antibiotics. Poor adherence to IPC practices

---

REFLECTION 18.6

Antimicrobial Use and Resistance

Antimicrobial therapy can work in different ways to treat infections. They can be bacteriostatic – stopping bacteria from multiplying – or they can be bactericidal – interfering with the cell wall of bacteria, thus killing them. It is important to remember that antimicrobial resistance **does not** mean the human body is resistant to antibiotics; it means the bacteria causing the infection are resistant to the antibiotic.

Bacteria mutate and change to protect their cell structure against antimicrobials, thus becoming resistant. Drug-resistant organisms can not only spread and cause further harm but can also transfer their resistance to other organisms. Even as new antimicrobials are introduced, it is anticipated that bacteria will continue to protect themselves by mutating and again become resistant.

Misuse and overuse of antimicrobials have contributed to the problem of resistance. Pressure from patients to be given antimicrobials, the contribution of topical antimicrobials to antimicrobial resistance and over-the-counter availability of antimicrobials in many countries outside the UK are all considerations. Some resistance, however, will be inevitable.

Policies should include guidance on the appropriate use of antimicrobials for treatment in all clinical eventualities, including the use of 'broad-spectrum' and 'narrow-spectrum' antimicrobials, and the length of time antimicrobials should be taken. Guidance on use of antimicrobials for prophylaxis is equally important, for example the use of antimicrobials before, during and after surgery to prevent rather than treat infection.

Nurse prescribing and its role in antimicrobial resistance are important at this time when nurse prescribing is being extended. Points for consideration include the difficulties associated with diagnosing infection accurately, awareness of allergies to and toxic effects of antimicrobials, the potential side-effects and the reduction in effectiveness of other medications when taking antimicrobials, for example the oral contraceptive pill. Patient education is also important; for example, there is often no point in taking antimicrobials for viral complaints such as a sore throat, and completing an entire course of antimicrobials as prescribed is essential.

---

also contributes (Courtenay et al. 2020). The key principles which underpin IPC are fundamental in preventing the developing or spread of infection because if infections can be prevented, this will avoid the use of antimicrobial agents. The NMC (2018) requires that nurses protect health through understanding and applying the principles of IPC and antimicrobial stewardship and resistance.

AMS is one of the key strategies to overcome resistance. It involves the care and responsible management of antimicrobial use (Nathwani 2018). The role of the nurse in AMS is often misunderstood (Gotterson et al. 2021). AMS encompasses all activities intended to improve patient outcomes from infection while minimising negative consequences such as HCAIs and limiting the development of bacterial resistance. Ultimately, the goals for AMS are to improve patient safety, improve patient outcomes, reduce resistance and reduce healthcare costs. Nurses have a vital role to play in AMS such as promoting good IPC practices; working with the multidisciplinary team to promote the effective use of antibiotics (right drug, right time, right dose, right duration); promoting appropriate and correct microbiological sampling; ensuring good nursing care such as nutrition, hydration and pressure area care; and ensuring good communication with patients and their carers (McEwen and Burnett 2018, Summer et al. 2018). (See Reflection 18.6.)

Aseptic Technique

Asepsis is defined as the absence of bacteria, viruses and other microorganisms. An aseptic technique is employed by healthcare professionals to undertake a procedure in a way that prevents the transfer of potentially pathogenic organisms which could cause infection. The application of an aseptic technique is pivotal in reducing the acquisition of HCAIs and reducing infections associated with invasive devices.

Aseptic nontouch technique (ANTT) is a critical skill which protects key-parts and key-sites from contamination. Key-parts are defined as the critical parts of the equipment used in the procedure and key-sites are open wounds and medical device access/insertion sites. ANTT must be employed when undertaking any procedure which bypasses the body's natural defences such as:

- urinary catheterisation and urine sampling via catheter port
- dressing wounds healing by primary intention, e.g. surgical wounds, burns, lacerations
- application of dressings to wounds healing by secondary intention, e.g. leg ulcers, pressure sores
- venepuncture and cannulation
- insertion/access vascular devices.

Before undertaking the procedure, healthcare staff should identify the key parts to prevent the risk of contamination.

The key principles of ANTT are:

Always ensure the hands are decontaminated effectively prior to the procedure.

Never contaminate key parts of sterile materials/equipment or the patient's susceptible key sites.

Touch non-key parts with confidence.

Take appropriate IPC precautions.

Whilst performing the procedure, it must be ensured that:

- all equipment and fluids used are sterile, in date, with packaging intact
- sterile packaging is opened in a manner which does not contaminate the contents
- key parts are identified and are always protected with caps, covers and never touched
- if a key part must be handled, sterile gloves should be worn (also if a key site requires to be touched)
- sterile items do not come into contact with nonsterile items
- PPE must be removed immediately after the procedure and hand hygiene performed
- the procedure is accurately documented in the patient's notes.

If sterile gloves are worn, they should be removed and renewed following hand hygiene if the sterility is compromised. Double gloves should never be worn (the only exception is within some surgical settings for Exposure Prone Procedures).

Decontamination of Reusable Care Equipment

The equipment used in providing care can become contaminated with organic material such as blood, bodily fluids, as well as dust, dirt and microorganisms. This can then present a risk of HCAI acquisition. Care equipment is classified in one of four ways:

- **Single-use** – equipment which is used once and then disposed of in the correct manner. It must never be reused, even on the same patient such as needles and syringes. The packaging carries the following symbol ②.
- **Single patient use** – equipment which can be reused on the same patient following the manufacturer's instructions for decontamination.
- **Reusable invasive equipment** – used once then decontaminated such as surgical instruments.
- **Reusable noninvasive equipment** (often referred to as communal equipment) – reused on more than one patient following

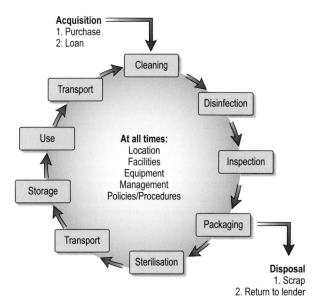

Figure 18.2 Decontamination cycle.

decontamination between each use for example, vital signs monitors and commodes.

Decontamination is defined as the process of removing contamination, from an item or surface, rendering it safe for reuse. Healthcare workers require specific guidance on the processes involved in the decontamination of care equipment. Decontamination encompasses cleaning, disinfection and sterilisation. The most frequent decontamination undertaken by nurses is that of reusable noninvasive equipment. All equipment should be decontaminated following manufacturer instructions, and generally, cleaning with neutral detergent is sufficient. However, it may be necessary to disinfect equipment on occasion when there is an increased risk of infection such as when the equipment has been in contact with mucous membranes; has been contaminated with blood or other body fluids; is contaminated with particularly virulent or readily transmissible organisms; or is to be used on or by immunocompromised patients. Cleaning should always precede disinfection to remove soiling and organic matter (Fig. 18.2).

The main areas to consider when undertaking decontamination include:

- The risk of HCAI from a reusable device and the most appropriate technique to protect patients from infection: cleaning, disinfection or sterilisation. General patient and staff safety to protect them from potentially infective microorganisms where devices are in use and to ensure that devices are safe to be handled and only used following decontamination.
- Recognition of the symbols that guide healthcare workers in relation to handling and reprocessing medical devices, such as the symbols for 'do not reuse', 'single use only' and 'sterile', which can be found on the packaging of all items.

Outbreak Detection, Investigation and Management

An outbreak is the occurrence of more cases of disease than would be expected within a specific place or group of people over a given period of time. The purpose of outbreak management is to protect public health by identifying the source and implementing control measures to prevent further spread or recurrence of the infection.

When an outbreak of infectious disease occurs, a prompt, well-coordinated, multidisciplinary response will help to minimise its impact. An outbreak may have minimal impact or major, widespread implications, including death or serious illness. Local IPC policies state the response that will be mounted when an outbreak is suspected or confirmed, including the definition of what is considered an outbreak, as this can vary between settings (Curran 2018).

An outbreak may be defined as an incident in which two or more people experiencing a similar illness are linked in time or place. However, the factors that constitute an outbreak depend upon a number of considerations, including the number of people involved, the pathogenicity of the organism and its potential for spread. Some infections should be automatically regarded as outbreaks, for example suspected food poisoning related to food supplied, such as salmonellosis, or serious communicable disease, such as viral haemorrhagic fever or polio. Other examples include organisms with a higher AMR profile (e.g. epidemic strains of MRSA) or an increase in infectious conditions that may be caused by different organisms (such as wound infections).

Policies on outbreak management should include details of the personnel involved and their roles during the incident, the communication processes and the actions to be taken, including risk assessments. Effective communication is crucial in these situations, as it is within all healthcare provision. Regular meetings are convened during an outbreak to facilitate the response and this will likely include extraordinary meetings of the IPCT. Involvement of staff from the local public health protection unit is especially important for outbreaks affecting primary care settings and the wider community. Similarly, outbreaks in the community often spread to healthcare settings, where patients may be more susceptible to infection, in an environment already conducive to the spread of infection.

As described earlier, the nurse's role in supporting IPC includes taking corrective action when outbreaks are suspected or proven. This entails alerting the IPCT to any concerns over increasing numbers of infections and following the specific direction given on the care and treatment of patients involved in an outbreak.

Infection Prevention and Control Measures in Community Settings

HCAI is not restricted to the hospital setting; pathogenic organisms can also be present in community settings. Nursing care is delivered in a wide variety of settings including the patient's home and other community settings such as long-term care facilities, including those for the elderly, individuals with mental health or learning disabilities. Also to be taken into consideration are prisons and places of detention. Within these settings, there is also a risk of the spread of infections and outbreaks. It is important that all staff working within these areas have adequate support and resources available to enable them to comply with SICPs. However, within the community setting, there are many factors which may inhibit the implementation of SICPs such as handwashing facilities, furnishings and of course pets (Wendt et al. 2022).

Care/Residential Homes
Within the care home setting, it is important to promptly assess an individual for infection risk on their arrival. It is imperative that local IPC policies and procedures are adhered to, the infection risk is documented and the appropriate action is taken. This assessment should also be reviewed throughout the individual's

stay. Individuals living within a residential or care home may be more susceptible to infection due to their age and the possibility of other underlying health conditions. Within a care setting such as this, pathogenic organisms may spread readily between residents causing an outbreak (Daker-White et al. 2021).

Ensuring patient safety is paramount, therefore it is important that good IPC practices are implemented to ensure the safety of those being cared for. As within the hospital setting, SICPs must be adopted to reduce the risk of infection regardless of healthcare setting. There may also be larger volumes of visitors and ancillary staff such as podiatrists and hairdressers.

IPC in the Patient's Home
Within the patient's home, it may not be possible to achieve some of the fundamental requirements for hand hygiene or environmental cleanliness; however, nurses can adopt innovative and inventive approaches to maintain the delivery of safe and effective care after completing a risk assessment. Education and support from the community nurse are essential to provide people at home with the information necessary to prevent the spread of infection while ensuring a clean and safe environment for those who are vulnerable. Diplomacy and tact should be always employed when making a suggestion or providing advice on how implementation of SICPs may be facilitated (see Reflection 18.7).

IPC in Prisons/Detention Centres
Prisons and other places of detention pose significant risks for both the transition and acquisition of infection due to the nature of both the environment and the population.

There are a number of factors which may contribute to the risk of infection within places of detention, including overcrowding, sharing cells and toilet areas, poor environmental decontamination and inadequate ventilation amongst others. There is also a greater prevalence of communicable disease as the individuals within these centres are often at a higher risk of certain infectious diseases such as blood-borne viruses and tuberculosis. It is important that SICPs are adopted within these areas to protect both staff and prisoners (Beaudry et al. 2020). Compliance with these greatly reduces the risk of transmission of infection. Hand hygiene is particularly important, and prisoners should also be provided with access to hand hygiene facilities. However, the use of ABHR for this group is not recommended and should only be available for staff. A risk assessment should be made for alternatives to soap and water which may include wipes or solutions which are alcohol free.

Use of Evidence-Based Practice Guidelines to Ensure Targeted Measures to Prevent HCAI

The evidence to support best practice in relation to HCAI prevention is well defined. Procedures associated with a high risk of infection are a focus for the production of a range of guidelines. These include the prevention of UTI, surgical site infection (SSI) and bloodstream infection (BSI). The IHI developed the concept of 'bundles' to assist healthcare providers to deliver the best care possible. The overarching aim is to improve the standard of care and patient outcomes by promoting the clear and consistent implementation of a set of effective interventions. A bundle generally consists of three to five evidence-based practices that when undertaken accurately have been proven to improve patient outcomes and minimise or eliminate the risk of HCAI acquisition. The use of care bundles that feature evidence-based criteria is one way in which to implement improvement and should reduce variation in how care is delivered (Shaw et al. 2020).

The prevention of UTIs, SSIs, skin and soft tissue infections, respiratory tract infections, particularly those associated with mechanical ventilation, and intravascular line infections is of concern, and clear plans of action are required to ensure these infections are minimised as far as possible.

- UTIs are one of the most common bacterial infections, affecting 150 million people each year worldwide. Many of these originate from indwelling urinary catheters. It is important to use a urinary catheter only when necessary and remove it as soon as it is no longer needed. Catheters should only be inserted once all other alternatives have been considered. Selection of the most suitable catheter for the patient is also essential. Both insertion and ongoing maintenance of the urinary catheter system must be conducted using aseptic technique (Atkins et al. 2020). A catheter passport should be used for patients with indwelling urinary catheters. This is a person-held record which contains a section for guiding the patient on how to look after their catheter and a section for healthcare professionals to document any catheter-related care that has been delivered.
- SSIs occur after an invasive surgical procedure. The impact of SSIs can range from liminal wound discharge to life-threatening complications. Surveillance data on SSI rates will allow healthcare organisations to monitor SSIs closely, which will then inform and influence the necessary actions required to minimise the risk of infection. There is much that nurses

can do to minimise infection risks before, during and after surgery. For further information, see NICE guideline NG15 (NICE 2020). Lower respiratory tract infections, including pneumonias, are also a leading cause of morbidity and mortality among patients. Ventilator-associated pneumonia accounts for a large proportion of healthcare-associated pneumonias. Nurses have a key role in minimising the risk of lower respiratory tract infection, such as encouraging all postoperative patients to take deep breaths, move about the bed and ambulate unless medically contraindicated. For mechanically ventilated patients, the nurse must ensure the patient is positioned correctly (elevating the head of bed to 30–45 degrees) and must adhere to standard precautions during care of the patient and their breathing apparatus, changing ventilator breathing circuits when soiled. The most common cause of ventilator-associated pneumonia is microaspiration of bacteria that colonise the oropharynx and upper airways in critically ill patients (Wu et al. 2019).

- BSI, also known as a bacteraemia, is associated with a higher mortality rate than most other HCAIs. A significant proportion of BSIs are related to the use of an intravascular device. As with urinary catheters, a peripheral or central intravascular device should be inserted only when necessary and removed as soon as no longer needed. Aseptic technique and thorough disinfection of the skin around the insertion site are essential. Care should be taken to avoid contamination of the dressing used to cover the device and of all other equipment (such as during attachment of the administration set and infusion fluid). Nurses have a vital role in regularly assessing the insertion site for signs of phlebitis and infection, recording the visual infusion phlebitis or 'VIP' score and taking the appropriate actions promptly when signs first appear. Routine replacement of an intravascular device should be conducted in accordance with agreed protocols, and clear documentation to support this, including documenting the date of insertion, is crucial. IPC practice continues to change and evolve, particularly in relation to new and emerging infections.

Summary: Key Nursing Issues

- The prevention and control of all infectious diseases and, in particular, HCAI are an essential part of safe, high-quality patient care.
- Standard precautions form a cornerstone of safe and effective IPC practice and are used in combination with risk management strategies to ensure the safety of patients, healthcare workers and visitors/family.
- Hand hygiene is part of SICPs and is widely regarded to be the most important step in preventing HCAI.
- Nurses, along with other members of the multiprofessional team, have a key role to play in ensuring that IPC measures are implemented consistently and reliably in whatever setting care is being delivered and that they are practicing

in accordance with the latest evidence and best practice recommendations.
- Nurses should feel confident to challenge their own practices and the behaviours of others to ensure recommended infection prevention measures are embedded into day-to-day routines. Education, training and communication are key to achieving this.
- By working closely with IPCTs and specialists, nurses can enhance their understanding of prevalent hazards and risks which must be considered and addressed in order to adapt to the ever-changing challenges and threats posed by infectious diseases and HCAI.

Reflection and Learning

- **Consolidate** your learning by looking at some of the further reading suggestions, references and specialist websites.
- **Revisit** some of the additional material on the website.
- **Consider** what you have learnt and how this will help your professional development.

- **Reflect** on how you can apply this knowledge to the care of your patients.
- **Discuss** your learning with your assessor/supervisor, educators and colleagues.

References

Atkins L, Sallis A, Chadborn T, et al. Reducing catheter-associated urinary tract infections: a systematic review of barriers and facilitators and strategic behavioural analysis of interventions. *Implement Sci.* 2020;15(44):1–22. doi:10.1186/s13012-020-01001-2.

Beaudry G, Zhong S, Whiting D, Javid B, Frater J, Fazel S. Managing outbreaks of highly contagious diseases in prisons: a systematic review. *BMJ Global Health.* 2020;5(11):e003201.

Courtenay M, Burnett E, Castro-Sanchez E, et al. Preparing nurses for COVID-19 response efforts through involvement in antimicrobial stewardship programmes. *J Hosp Infect.* 2020;106(1):176–178.

Curran E. Outbreak Column 22: how to manage an outbreak. *J Infect Prev.* 2018;19(5):244–251.

Curran E, Burnett E, Robinson J, Loveday H. A comparison of the nationally important infection prevention and control documents in NHS England and NHS Scotland. *J Infect Prev.* 2020;22(2);75–82. https://doi.org/10.1177/1757177420971849.

Cusack L, Wiechula R, Schultz T, Dollard J, Maben J. Anticipated advantages and disadvantages of a move to 100% single-room hospital in Australia: a case study. *J Nurs Manag.* 2019;27(5):963–970.

Daker-White G, Panagioti M, Giles S, et al. Beyond the control of the care home: A meta-ethnography of qualitative studies of infection prevention and control in residential and nursing homes for older people. *Health Expect.* 2021;25(5):2095–2106.

Daniels R, Nutbeam T. *The Sepsis Manual: Responsible Management of Sepsis, Severe Infection and Antimicrobial Stewardship.* 6th edition. United Kingdom Sepsis Trust; 2022. https://sepsistrust.org/wp-content/uploads/2022/06/Sepsis-Manual-Sixth-Edition.pdf.

Dekker M, van Mansfeld R, Vandenbroucke-Grauls CM, et al. Role perception of infection control link nurses; a multi-centre qualitative study. *J Infect Prev.* 2022;23(3);93–100. https://doi.org/10.1177/17571774211066786.

Gammon J, Hunt J. A review of isolation practices and procedures in healthcare settings. *Br J Nurs.* 2018;27(3):137–140.

Gillespie S, Bamford K. *Microbiology at a Glance.* 5th ed. Hoboken, NJ: Wiley–Blackwell; 2022.

Gotterson F, Buising K, Manias E. Nurse role and contribution to antimicrobial stewardship: an integrative review. *Int J Nurs Stud.* 2021;117:103787.

Haque M, McKimm J, Sartelli M, et al. Strategies to prevent healthcare-associated infections: a narrative overview. *Risk Manag Healthc Policy.* 2020;13:1765–1780.

Health and Safety at Work Act 1974 (Application outside Great Britain Order 2001). http://www.legislation.gov.uk/uksi/2001/2127/made.

Health and Social Care Act 2008. https://www.legislation.gov.uk/ukpga/2008/14/contents.

Health Protection Scotland. *National point prevalence survey of healthcare associated infection and antimicrobial prescribing 2016.* Glasgow: Health Protection Scotland; 2017. https://www.nss.nhs.scot/publications/national-point-prevalence-survey-of-healthcare-associated-infection-and-antimicrobial-prescribing-2016/.

Hoernke K, Djellouli N, Andrews L, et al. Frontline healthcare workers' experiences with personal protective equipment during the COVID-19 pandemic in the UK: a rapid qualitative appraisal. *BMJ Open.* 2021;11(1):e046199.

Holland D, Thomson L, Mahmoudzadeh N, et al. Estimating deaths from foodborne disease in the UK for 11 key pathogens. *BMJ Open Gastroenterol.* 2020;7(1):E000377.

Horner DL, Bellamy MC. Care bundles in intensive care. *BJA Educ.* 2012;12(4):199–202.

Infection Prevention Society. Competencies Framework for Infection Prevention & Control Practitioners. 2020. https://www.ips.uk.net/ips-competencies-framework.

Loveday HP, Wilson JA, Pratt RJ, et al. Epic3: national evidence-based guidelines for preventing healthcare associated infections in NHS hospitals in England. *J Hosp Infect.* 2014;86(Suppl):S1–S70.

McEwen J, Burnett E. Antimicrobial stewardship and pre-registration student nurses: evaluation of teaching. *J Infect Prev.* 2018;19(2):80–86.

Msemburi W, Karlinsky A, Knutson V, Aleshin-Guendel S, Chatterji S, Wakefield J. The WHO estimates of excess mortality associated with the COVID-19 pandemic. *Nature.* 2023;613:130–137.

Nathwani D, ed. *Antimicrobial Stewardship: From Principles to Practice.* Birmingham: BSAC; 2018.

National Audit Office. *Report by the Comptroller and Auditor General: The Management and Control of Hospital Acquired Infection in Acute NHS Trusts in England.* London: NAO; 2000.

National Audit Office. *Report by the Comptroller and Auditor General: Improving Patient Care by Reducing the Risk of Hospital Acquired Infection: A Progress Report.* London: NAO; 2004.

National Audit Office. *Report by the Controller and Auditor General: Reducing Healthcare Associated Infection in Hospitals in England.* London: NAO; 2009. https://www.nao.org.uk/reports/reducing-healthcare-associated-infections-in-hospitals-in-england/.

NHS England. National infection prevention and control manual (NIPCM) for England. 2022. https://www.england.nhs.uk/national-infection-prevention-and-control-manual-nipcm-for-england/chapter-2-transm.

National Institute for Health and Clinical Excellence (NICE). 2020. Surgical site infections: prevention and treatment. Clinical guideline [NG125]. https://www.nice.org.uk/guidance/ng125.

Nursing and Midwifery Council (NMC) (2018). The Code: Professional Standards of Practice and Behaviour for Nurses, Midwives and Nursing Associates. https://www.nmc.org.uk/standards/code/.

Prescott K, Gray J, Mahida N, et al. Lessons learned from the COVID-19 pandemic through the JHI and IPIP. *J Hosp Infect.* 2021;119:80–83.

Purssell E, Gould D, Chudleigh J. Impact on hospitalised patients who are infectious: a systematic review with meta-analysis. *BMJ Open.* 2020;10(2):e030371.

Shaban R, Nahidi S, Sotomayor-Castillo C, White E, Hackett K, Bag S. SARS-CoV-2 infection and COVID-19: the lived experience and perceptions of patients in isolation and care in an Australian healthcare setting. *AJIC.* 2020;48(12):1445–1450.

Shaw A, Morton K, King A, et al. Using and implementing care bundles for patients with acute admission for COPD: qualitative study of healthcare professionals' experience in four hospitals in England. *BMJ Open Resp Res.* 2020;7.

Shreffler J, Petrey J, Huecker M. The impact of COVID-19 on healthcare worker wellness: a scoping review. *West J Emerg Med.* 2020;21(5):1059–1066.

Smyth ETM, McIlvenny G, Enstone JE, et al. on behalf of the Hospital Infection Society Prevalence Survey Steering Group. Four country healthcare associated infection prevalence survey 2006: overview of the results. *J Hosp Infect.* 2008;69(3):230–248.

Summer S, Forsyth S, Collette-Merrill K, et al. Antibiotic stewardship: the role of clinical nurses and nurse educators. *Nurse Educ Today.* 2018;60:157–160.

The Food Safety and Hygiene (England) Regulations 2013. No. 2996. https://www.legislation.gov.uk/uksi/2013/2996/contents/made.

The Health Foundation. *Quality Improvement Made Simple: What Everyone Should Know About Health Care Quality Improvement.* The Health Foundation; 2021.

Tsioutis C, Birgand G, Bathoorn E, et al. Education and training programmes for infection prevention and control professionals: mapping the current opportunities and local needs in European countries. *Antimicrob Resist Infect Control.* 2020;9(183).

VanMeter K, Hubert R. *Microbiology for the Healthcare Professional.* ed 3. London: Elsevier; 2021.

Wendt B, Huisman-de Waal G, Bakker-Jacobs A, et al. Exploring infection prevention practices in home-based nursing care: A qualitative observational study. *Int J Nurs St.* 2022;125:104130.

Wilson J, Prieto J. Re-visiting contact precautions –25 years on. *J Infect Prev.* 2021;22(6). https://doi.org/10.1177/17571774211059988.

World Health Organisation (WHO). *Global Action Plan on Antimicrobial Resistance*. Geneva: WHO; 2015. https://www.who.int/publications/i/item/9789241509763.

World Health Organisation (WHO). *WHO Guidelines on Hand Hygiene in Health Care*. Geneva: WHO; 2009. https://www.who.int/publications/i/item/9789241597906.

Wu D, Wu C, Zhang S, Zhong Y. Risk factors of ventilator-associated pneumonia in critically ill patient. *Front Pharmacol*. 2019;10:482.

Useful Websites

Antimicrobial prescribing and stewardship competencies, https://www.gov.uk/government/publications/antimicrobial-prescribing-and-stewardship-competencies

Advisory Committee on Dangerous Pathogens, www.gov.uk/government/groups/advisory-committee-on-dangerous-pathogens

Association of Medical Microbiologists, www.rcpath.org/profession/committees/medical-microbiology.html

British Society of Antimicrobial Chemotherapy, www.bsac.org.uk

British Thoracic Society, www.brit-thoracic.org.uk/

Care Inspectorate, www.careinspectorate.com

Care Quality Commission, www.cqc.org.uk

Centers for Disease Control and Prevention (USA), www.cdc.gov

Department for Environment, Food and Rural Affairs, https://www.gov.uk/government/organisations/department-for-environment-food-rural-affairs

Department of Health, www.dh.gov.uk

Department of Health, Social Services and Public Safety in Northern Ireland, www.dhsspsni.gov.uk

Public Health Wales, https://phw.nhs.wales/services-and-teams/health-protection/health-protection-team/

The Green Book (for up-to-date information on immunisation against infectious disease), www.gov.uk/government/collections/immunisation-against-infectious-disease-the-green-book

Health Products Regulatory Authority, www.hpra.ie

Public Health Scotland, https://publichealthscotland.scot/

Health and Safety Executive (including Care of Substances Hazardous to Health Regulations), www.hse.gov.uk/coshh

Health in Wales, www.wales.nhs.uk/

Healthcare A–Z, www.nhs.uk/conditions/

Healthcare Infection Society, www.his.org.uk

Healthcare Improvement Scotland, www.healthcareimprovementscotland.org/

Infection Prevention Society, www.ips.uk.net

Institute for Healthcare Improvement, www.ihi.org

Medicines and Healthcare products Regulatory Agency (MHRA), www.gov.uk/government/organisations/medicines-and-healthcare-products-regulatory-agency

National Institute for Health and Care Excellence (NICE), www.nice.org.uk

National Resource for Infection Control, www.nric.org.uk

NHS Health Facilities Scotland, www.hfs.scot.nhs.uk

NHS Improving Quality, www.gov.uk/

NHS Scotland (Fit for Travel) travel advice for the public on infectious diseases around the world, www.fitfortravel.nhs.uk

NHS Supply Chain, https://www.supplychain.nhs.uk/

NHS National Services Scotland National Infection Prevention and Control Manual, www.nipcm.scot.nhs.uk

Public Health England, https://www.gov.uk/government/organisations/public-health-england

Public Health Ireland, www.hpsc.ie

Scottish Government Health and Social Care Directorates, www.sehd.scot.nhs.uk

World Health Organisation, www.who.int

19

The Deteriorating Patient, Recognising and Managing Shock

RACHAEL LEAR, SUZAN THOMPSON

CHAPTER OUTLINE

NMC FUTURE NURSE STANDARDS OF PROFICIENCY FOR REGISTERED NURSES

This chapter/section will address the following platforms and proficiencies

Platform 3: Assessing Needs and Planning Care

Registered nurses prioritise the needs of people when assessing and reviewing their mental, physical, cognitive, behavioural, social, and spiritual needs. They use information obtained during assessments to identify the priorities and requirements for person-centred and evidence-based nursing interventions and support. They work in partnership with people to develop person-centred care plans that take into account their circumstances, characteristics and preferences.

At the point of registration, the registered nurse will be able to:

3.2: demonstrate and apply knowledge of body systems and homeostasis, human anatomy and physiology, biology, genomics, pharmacology, and social and behavioural sciences when understanding full and accurate person-centred nursing assessments and developing appropriate care plans.

3.3: demonstrate and apply knowledge of all commonly encountered mental, physical, behavioural, and cognitive health conditions, medication usage and treatments when undertaking full and accurate assessments of nursing care needs and when. Developing and reviewing person-centred care plans.

3.9 recognise and assess people at risk of harm and the situations that may put them at risk, ensuring prompt action is taken to safeguard those who are vulnerable.

Platform 6: Improving Safety and Quality of Care

Registered nurses make a key contribution to the continuous monitoring and quality improvement of care and treatment in order to enhance health outcomes and people's experiences of nursing and related care. They assess risks to safety or experience and take appropriate action to manage those, putting the best interests, needs and preferences of people first.

At the point of registration, the registered nurse will be able to:

6.5: Demonstrate the ability to accurately undertake risk assessments in a range of care settings, using a range of contemporary assessment and improvement tools.

NMC FUTURE NURSE STANDARDS OF PROFICIENCY FOR NURSING ASSOCIATES (2018)

This chapter/section will address the following platforms and proficiencies.

Introduction

The aim of this chapter is to provide an overview of shock. By the end of this chapter, the reader should be able to:

1. Understand the evolving pathophysiology of shock
2. Identify the different types of shock and the differences between them
3. Identify the signs and symptoms of the patient developing shock and the features of the deteriorating patient
4. Understand the issues in providing nursing care to a patient in shock
5. Understand and meet the standards of Proficiency for Registered nurses (Nursing and Midwifery Council [NMC] 2018) as identified in the following.

As long ago as 1885, shock was described by John Collins Warren as being 'a momentary pause in the act of death'. Shock is not a primary diagnosis but is a physiological consequence of a range of pathophysiological events, therefore it is now most commonly defined as being a life-threatening state in which the circulation is unable to deliver sufficient oxygen to meet the demands of the tissues – resulting in cellular dysfunction (Cecconi et al. 2014, Stratton 2017). Inadequately treated or untreated shock can have devastating consequences. Prompt management starts with early recognition; this is often highly challenging and reliant on the nurse identifying the subtle signs of deterioration.

Research studies from the 1990s identified that nursing and medical staff's failure to recognise, report and manage patient deterioration appropriately resulted in deaths (avoidable). These claims were supported by the National Patient Safety Agency (NPSA) in 2007, who provided continuing evidence through investigation that the recognition and timely management or referral of acutely ill and at-risk patients were often delayed or missed completely. More recently, an investigation undertaken by the Health Service Investigation Branch (2019) found that the issues in recognising and responding to deteriorating patients continued to be a major source of severe harm and preventable deaths in hospitals.

Therefore it is important that nurses from all areas of clinical practice have and maintain the knowledge required to identify at-risk and deteriorating patients promptly and implement timely and appropriate interventions (National Institute for Health and Clinical Excellence [NICE] 2007, 2017b, NMC 2018).

It is essential when caring for acutely unwell patients or patients at risk of deterioration that practitioners adopt a recognised approach to patient assessment. The airway, breathing, circulation, disability and exposure (ABCDE) methodology provides a rapid and systematic method of clinical assessment that shares a common language and structure and is therefore understood by the wider multidisciplinary team (Resuscitation Council [UK] 2021). This uniform approach provides the practitioner with the structure to identify and treat life-threatening issues in order of priority and manage these before moving onto the next component of the assessment. However, an understanding of the normal and abnormal physiological parameters is essential if the information collected is to be appropriately interpreted and acted upon (Peate and Dutton 2021, p. 2).

Aggregated Early Warning Scores (Track and Trigger tools) have been developed and advocated to facilitate the early identification, escalation and continued monitoring of patients who are acutely unwell or are at risk of deterioration (NICE 2007, Royal College of Physicians [RCP] 2017). The National Early Warning Score (NEWS2) is based on an aggregate scoring system reflecting the patient's observations against six physiological parameters (RCP 2017):

1. respiratory rate
2. oxygen saturation
3. systolic blood pressure
4. pulse rate
5. level of consciousness:
   A: Alert
   C: New-onset confusion, disorientation and/or agitation
   V: Responds to voice
   P: Responds to painful stimuli
   U: Unresponsive
6. temperature.

As each parameter is measured, the practitioner documents the scores on a standardised observation chart – the NEWS2 chart. Scores reflect the degree of derangement from the normal range. After checking and documenting all parameters, scores are aggregated. An additional 2 points is added for patients requiring supplemental oxygen to maintain their recommended oxygen saturation. The NEWS2 chart has a specific oxygen saturation section (SpO_2 Scale 2) that should be used for patients with hypercapnic respiratory failure (generally due to chronic obstructive pulmonary disease (COPD)) whose target oxygen saturation is 88%–92%. The aggregated NEWS2 score guides the clinical response, including the frequency of clinical observations, the urgency of clinical review and the competency requirements of the clinical team reviewing the patient, and the most appropriate clinical setting for ongoing care of the patient. For example, an aggregate score of 5–6 meets the threshold for an urgent response. In line with local escalation policies, the practitioner should immediately inform the medical team and the patient should be reviewed by a clinician with competence in assessing and treating acutely ill patients who can recognise when escalation of care to a critical care team is required. The ability to escalate concerns and communicate information succinctly and accurately is essential. The SBAR (situation, background, assessment and recommendation) tool (Resuscitation Council [UK] 2021) enables the practitioner to structure and compose the information concisely, at the right level of detail whilst reducing repetition.

The Evolving Pathophysiology of Shock

In this section, the evolving pathophysiology and associated signs and symptoms of shock are outlined within four stages:

1. the initial stage
2. the compensatory stage
3. the progressive stage
4. the refractory stage.

It is important to note that although shock can be considered within these four stages, it is a complex and continuous process and patients may progress rapidly from one stage to the next.

The Initial Stage

In the initial stage of shock, the patient may be asymptomatic, or the changes to the haemodynamic values may so subtle that they may be overlooked unless a high index of suspicion is applied. The patient may demonstrate signs of mild anxiety and restlessness and there may be a slight increase in heart rate above the patient's baseline level. Blood pressure may be normal or slightly depressed and the skin may be cool. These signs usually arise from activation of compensatory mechanisms that cause mild vasoconstriction and the shift from aerobic to anaerobic metabolism at the cellular level. In general, a normally healthy individual can compensate for approximately 10% reduction in blood volume by means of these compensatory mechanisms.

The Compensatory Stage

In this stage of shock, physiological adaptions occur in an attempt to mitigate the adverse effects of shock and return the body to a state of homeostasis. These physiological adaptions include the spontaneous activation of neuronal, hormonal and biochemical mechanisms.

Firstly, the patient in shock will begin to hyperventilate in order optimise oxygen delivery to the alveoli, and to rid the body of carbon dioxide (CO_2), thereby raising the blood pH (lowering the acidity). In the context of tissue hypoperfusion, this helps to combat the lactic acidosis that results from anaerobic cellular metabolism. An arterial blood gas (ABG) taken at this stage may indicate hypocapnia (a partial pressure of carbon dioxide ($PaCO_2$) less than 4.7 kPa) due to hyperventilation.

A 10–15 mmHg reduction in mean arterial pressure (MAP) will be detected by the baroreceptors in the aortic arch and carotid sinuses. This information is relayed to the cardiovascular centre in the medulla oblongata of the brain, which forms part of the brain stem. Activation of the sympathetic nervous system leads to the release of epinephrine (adrenaline) and norepinephrine (noradrenaline). Noradrenaline will predominantly cause vasoconstriction and a mild increase in heart rate, whereas adrenaline causes an increase in heart rate, with a small effect on the vascular tone. The combined effect results in an increase in blood pressure. Therefore this compensatory stage strives to maintain cardiac output (CO) (which comprises of stroke volume (SV) and heart rate (HR); CO = SV × HR). The effects of vasoconstriction can be seen in the patient with pale, cool peripheries and a narrow pulse pressure (PP) (PP = the difference between the systolic and the diastolic pressures).

At this stage, the renal and biochemical compensating mechanisms are activated because early compensatory mechanisms are insufficient in isolation to maintain CO. Reduced renal perfusion stimulates the release of renin from the kidneys and antidiuretic hormone (ADH) from the hypothalamus, in order to conserve fluid via the kidneys. The release of these hormones ultimately results in sodium and water reabsorption in the renal tubules, which is reflected in reduced urine production.

The Progressive Stage

The progressive stage of shock can also be considered as late decompensated shock (Stratton 2022). In early compensated shock, the body's homeostatic mechanisms (e.g. tachycardia and peripheral vasoconstriction) are able to maintain blood pressure and

CO – thus preserving end-organ perfusion. However, as shock progresses, the body's compensatory mechanisms begin to fail – the blood pressure drops, resulting in inadequate perfusion of the body tissues and vital organs.

Inadequate perfusion of the brain leads to confusion and drowsiness. Prolonged hypoxia suppresses the sympathetic nervous system and the cardiovascular and respiratory centres in the medulla oblongata – leading to impaired conscious levels (Tait et al. 2022). Poor renal perfusion eventually leads to acute kidney injury, which is manifest through a fall in urine output (oliguria) and a rise in serum creatinine levels. At this stage, the patient's peripheries will also be cold and there may be evidence of peripheral cyanosis caused by prolonged and intense vasoconstriction (Tait et al. 2022).

In decompensated shock, tissue hypoperfusion results in a variety of additional adverse effects. In response to hypoxia, cells begin to metabolise anaerobically. Lactic acid is produced as a byproduct of anaerobic cellular metabolism, eventually leading to a state of metabolic acidosis, which further impairs the basic function of the cells (Tait et al. 2022). At this point, an ABG may indicate an acute lactic acidosis (lactate greater than 2 mmol/L and pH less than 7.35). The patient's respiratory effort will have noticeably increased in an attempt to blow off carbon dioxide and water in order to reduce circulating hydrogen ions. Initially, an ABG may demonstrate hypocapnia (a partial pressure of carbon dioxide ($PaCO$) less than 4.7 kPa). However, the adverse effects of decompensated shock eventually lead to type II respiratory failure (evidenced by a raised $PaCO_2$).

A massive inflammatory response is triggered by the damage to cells caused by lactic acidosis and tissue ischaemia. As a result, fluid and plasma proteins leak out of the capillaries into the alveoli, causing pulmonary oedema and acute lung injury. Gaseous exchange is impaired, and this is evident in reduced peripheral oxygen saturation (SpO_2). In the shocked patient, caution should be applied when interpreting pulse oximeter values as peripheral vasoconstriction can lead to inaccurate readings. Impaired gaseous exchange is reflected in a reduced partial pressure of oxygen (PaO_2) and a rise in $PaCO_2$ on ABG results.

At this stage, myocardial workload will be increased due to the compensatory tachycardia and the effort made to eject blood from the left ventricle against the high peripheral resistance caused by vasoconstriction. In the late stages of shock, the heart will eventually fail as coronary perfusion and oxygen supply become inadequate to meet the demands of the myocardium.

Eventually, the patient may also develop a paralytic ileus which is manifested in the absence of bowel sounds and the appearance of abdominal distension. Ischaemic damage to the intestinal mucosa can result in the release of bacteria and toxins from the gut into the circulation.

The extent of tissue damage and organ failure that occur in the late stages of shock is influenced by the severity of the cause of shock, and how quickly the patient is assessed and treated. If late shock is not recognised and treated promptly, there may be overwhelming damage to the body's cells leading to multiorgan failure (Stratton 2022).

The Refractory Stage

Refractory shock can develop if the multidisciplinary team treating the patient are unable to reestablish haemodynamic stability. In this scenario, tissue hypoperfusion and cellular damage will ultimately lead to irreversible failure of the organ systems (Tait 2016). In this stage of shock, pathophysiological processes are set in motion that cannot be arrested and the patient will no longer respond to treatment. If the refractory stage is reached, shock is irreversible and death will occur.

TYPES OF SHOCK

Shock is generally classified according to its cause. There are four major pathophysiological mechanisms that can result in a state of shock (Stratton 2022):
1. hypovolaemia (loss of intravascular volume from internal or external fluid loss)
2. cardiogenic factors ('pump failure')
3. obstruction (barriers to cardiac filling or circulatory flow)
4. distributive factors (due to failure of vasoregulation and loss of vascular tone).

The distinguishing feature of the first three types of shock is low CO, which leads to tissue hypoxaemia (Suh and Lee 2018). On the other hand, distributive shock is characterised by reduced systematic vascular resistance, which can occur in the presence of a normal or high CO. The type and cause of shock may be apparent from taking the patient's history and conducting a comprehensive assessment.

The following sections describe the key causes and distinguishing features of hypovolaemic shock, cardiogenic shock, obstructive shock and the different forms of distributive shock. Within each section, key priorities for the management of each type of shock are highlighted.

Hypovolaemic Shock

Hypovolaemic shock is characterised by loss of intravascular volume of 15% or more leading to inadequate perfusion of the tissues (Moruzzi and McLeod 2017). Reduced circulating blood volume leads to a decrease in venous return and subsequent reduction in CO – resulting in reduced tissue perfusion.

Loss of fluid from the circulation may be external or internal. When there is significant external fluid loss, the cause of shock may be immediately apparent – for example: traumatic haemorrhage, massive gastrointestinal bleed, extensive burns, severe vomiting and diarrhoea. Conducting a comprehensive assessment, including taking the patient's history and performing a thorough examination, can provide valuable information to indicate a loss of intravascular volume that may otherwise go unnoticed. For example, in the case of paralytic ileus, 1 L or more of fluid may shift from the intravascular space into the gastrointestinal tract leading to a relative hypovolaemia that is not immediately apparent. In trauma, there will be a higher suspicion of internal fluid loss: internal bleeding occurs in patients with haemothorax, long bone and pelvic fractures and arterial injuries. Internal blood loss may be sudden and catastrophic – for example, a ruptured aortic aneurysm will progress rapidly to circulatory collapse. The patient with a ruptured aortic aneurysm will require immediate transfer to an operating theatre if there is to be any chance of survival.

Signs and Symptoms of Hypovolaemic Shock

In early hypovolaemic shock, the compensatory mechanisms discussed earlier are triggered in response to falling blood pressure and reduced tissue perfusion. These compensatory mechanisms lead to:
- Tachycardia as the body tries to increase the CO in response to the reduced circulating volume.

- A weak, thready pulse, due to low blood flow and peripheral vasoconstriction. Vasoconstriction occurs in an effort to increase systemic vascular resistance and maintain blood pressure.
- Pale, cool and clammy skin as a result of peripheral vasoconstriction, poor peripheral perfusion and sympathetic activation of the sweat glands.
- Narrowing of the PP (i.e. a reduced difference between the systolic and diastolic pressures) due to a reduction in SV and an increase in peripheral vascular resistance.
- SA fall in urine output – initially a result of endocrine compensatory mechanisms (i.e. the renin–angiotensin–aldosterone system and secretion of ADH from the hypothalamus).
- Anxiety, restlessness and confusion, which may indicate decreased cerebral perfusion and oxygenation.

It is essential that the nurse is able to recognise these clinical features of early shock, so that urgent treatment can be initiated to prevent its progression. Without prompt treatment to halt the fluid loss and correct the hypovolaemia, the body's compensatory mechanisms eventually fail to maintain the MAP, resulting in inadequate end-organ perfusion, lactic acidosis and multiorgan failure. By this stage, oliguria may indicate acute kidney injury rather than a compensatory endocrine response to conserve body fluid. Blood tests, including urea and creatinine levels, will be required to assess the extent of organ damage due to hypoperfusion.

Management of Hypovolaemic Shock

As in all types of shock, the ABCDE approach should be used to re-assess and treat the patient, and the underlying cause should be identified and treated as early as possible (Stratton 2022).

Fluid Resuscitation

Fluid resuscitation should be commenced as early as possible to restore the circulating volume and improve CO. Crystalloid solutions are the fluid of choice (NICE 2017a, Stratton 2022) unless the patient is actively bleeding, in which case administration of blood products is the first-line treatment to restore the oxygen-carrying capacity of the blood and to prevent coagulopathies. Fluid therapy should be administered as fluid challenges initially – with close monitoring to identify response to, and the adverse effects of, treatment. To ascertain whether a patient is responding to treatment with fluid therapy, the nurse should look for an increase in systematic arterial pressure, a decrease in the heart rate and an increase in urine output. Fluid challenges can be repeated as needed while the patient is responding to treatment; smaller volumes (e.g. 250 mL) should be administered in patients with known cardiac failure (Stratton 2022). Pulmonary oedema may be suspected if the patient develops acute dyspnoea and worsening hypoxia, which may be secondary to fluid accumulation in the lungs that impairs gaseous exchange in the alveoli (Purvey and Allen 2017). A chest X-ray may be performed to confirm the pulmonary oedema diagnosis.

Vasoactive Agents

If the patient is not responding to fluid therapy or if hypotension persists despite adequate filling, the use of vasopressors is generally indicated (Stratton 2022). Vasopressors such as noradrenaline (norepinephrine) work by improving vascular tone, thereby increasing systematic vascular resistance and improving blood pressure. Patients receiving vasopressor support must be cared for within critical care settings, where they can undergo advanced haemodynamic monitoring (see later section).

Controlling Blood Loss

Uncontrolled bleeding is the leading cause of potentially avoidable death in patients suffering traumatic injury (Spahn et al. 2019). Interventions to slow down life-threatening bleeding include (NICE 2016, Spahn et al. 2019):

- the use of dressings to apply local compression
- the use of devices to control bleeding such as tourniquets and pelvic binders
- pharmacological interventions to promote clotting and reverse the effects of any anticoagulation medication that the patient may have been taking
- urgent escalation of the patient to a surgeon and subsequent transfer to the operating theatre or interventional radiology suite for interventions to restore haemostasis.

In some cases, aggressive fluid resuscitation should be delayed until the source of fluid loss has been corrected (NICE 2016, Kudo et al. 2017). In patients with ruptured aneurysms or with traumatic haemorrhage, aggressive fluid resuscitation may worsen bleeding by increasing the CO and the hydrostatic pressure within damaged vessels and impeding the formation of a haemostatic clot (Kudo et al. 2017). In these patients, the practice of 'permissive hypotension' is usually appropriate (Chaikof et al. 2018). This approach allows patients to maintain a blood pressure within a range that is lower than normal until definitive treatment to achieve haemostasis can be implemented. Although this approach aims to prevent exacerbation of bleeding by restricting the volume of fluid administration, it does carry the potential risk of tissue hypoperfusion (Kudo et al. 2017).

Cardiogenic Shock

Cardiogenic shock is a low CO state leading to life-threatening end-organ perfusion that is caused by disorders that impair the function of the heart (Van Diepen et al. 2017). Acute myocardial infarction (MI) is the underlying cause in 81% of patients with cardiogenic shock (Vahdatpour et al. 2019). Damage to the myocardium prevents the heart from pumping effectively, resulting in a fall in CO and blood pressure, and tissue hypoperfusion. Paradoxically, the compensatory mechanisms that would usually function to maintain end-organ perfusion are actually pathological in the case of cardiogenic shock. The release of catecholamines produces tachycardia, vasoconstriction and increased cardiac contractility. These compensatory responses increase myocardial oxygen demand and the workload of the left ventricle, potentially causing extension of the infarct and further compromising left ventricular function. Because there is an increase in afterload due to peripheral vasoconstriction and increased systemic vascular resistance, the left ventricle does not empty effectively. As a result, pressure rises in the left atrium, the pulmonary circulation and the right side of the heart. Pulmonary oedema ensues – gaseous exchange in the alveoli is impeded due to the presence of fluid in the lungs, and the problem of tissue hypoxia in the context of shock is exacerbated.

Signs and Symptoms of Cardiogenic Shock

The signs of cardiogenic shock include:

- systolic pressure <80 mmHg
- tachycardia and a weak, thready pulse
- dyspnoea
- old, clammy skin
- oliguria – urine output <0.5 mL/kg per hour

- confusion
- mottling of the extremities, particularly the legs
- raised jugular venous pressure.

Management of Cardiogenic Shock

The most important intervention in the management of cardiogenic shock associated with MI is early revascularisation – by percutaneous coronary intervention (PCI) or coronary artery bypass grafting (CABG) to restore blood flow to the myocardium (Jones et al. 2019, Vahdatpour et al. 2019). This usually necessitates the transfer of an unstable patient between departments, or even between hospitals – an inherently risky procedure in critically ill patients. The nurse must be able to prepare the patient and any equipment required for the transfer in a timely fashion. At times, the nurse may be required to accompany the doctor and the patient during transfer, and if this is the case, they must possess a sound working knowledge of the principles of safe transfer.

Numerous pharmacological interventions will also be required to treat the patient with cardiogenic shock. In the case of MI, these treatments will include antiplatelet and antithrombotic medication. Other pharmacological interventions include the basic initial treatments to support circulatory and respiratory function – including supplemental oxygen therapy, vasodilators (nitrates) and diuretic treatment (in acute heart failure) (McDonagh et al. 2021). Vasopressors, such as noradrenaline, and inotropic support may also be given to improve blood pressure and heart contractility, but invasive blood pressure monitoring in a cardiac care unit or high-dependency setting is required as they can rapidly induce hypotension (Vahdatpour et al. 2019).

Obstructive Shock

Obstructive shock is a form of shock associated with mechanical obstruction of blood flow to the heart (Kim 2018). Causes of obstructive shock include pulmonary embolism, pericardial tamponade and tension pneumothorax. Pulmonary embolism is usually the result of migration of thrombus from the venous system of the legs to the pulmonary arterial tree, where it impedes blood flow and leads to haemodynamic compromise. Pericardial tamponade is a condition, commonly caused by trauma to the chest, in which the pericardial sac fills with fluid or blood – this compresses the chambers of the heart and prevents it from filling effectively. With tension pneumothorax, air leaks into the pleural space and is unable to escape. As well as compressing the lung and causing it to deflate, the presence of air in the pleural space puts pressure on the blood vessels in the chest and reduces venous return to the heart. All these conditions can lead to shock due to impaired blood flow and resultant haemodynamic compromise leading to tissue hypoperfusion. Signs of obstructive shock are similar to hypovolaemic and cardiogenic shock: that is, rapid, thready pulse; pale, cool peripheries; oliguria; hypotension; and hypoxia. Rapid identification and immediate treatment to remove the obstructive lesion are vital. Management is dependent on the underlying cause (Kim 2018). Treatment of tension pneumothorax is the decompression of accumulated air in the pleural space using a needle inserted over the superior margin of the third rib in the midclavicular line. Anticoagulant therapy is the primary treatment for pulmonary embolism; thrombolysis may be administered in severe cases. If cardiac tamponade is suspected, pericardiocentesis is performed to treat the build-up of fluid in the pericardium.

Distributive Shock

Distributive shock can be divided into four different categories:
1. Septic shock
2. Neurogenic shock
3. Anaphylactic shock
4. Spinal shock

All of these are characterised overtly in patients by warm peripheries and a rapid bounding pulse. In contrast with other types of shock, these symptoms are caused by vasodilation. Normally, the circulating volume of blood in the body is approximately 5 L (70 mL × body weight = circulating blood volume). In distributive shock the vascular compartment has expanded due to vasodilation while the blood volume has remained the same. This decrease in systemic vascular resistance contributes to the hypotension seen in distributive shock. The physiological compensatory mechanisms (described previously) are activated however, these are usually insufficient to maintain end-organ perfusion without supportive treatment.

Septic Shock

Septic shock is a 'subset of sepsis where particularly profound circulatory, cellular and metabolic abnormalities substantially increase mortality' (Singer et al. 2016). Septic shock is the most common cause of shock, accounting for an estimated 48,000 deaths in the UK per annum (UK Sepsis Trust 2022b).

Sepsis is the collective term for a number of physiological responses to an invading pathogen (e.g. chest, wound or urinary tract infection), involving the immune system and the coagulation cascade. It is characterised by a process known as inflammation.

Inflammation in response to an infection is activated by receptors in the endothelium, which detect antigens on the cell membranes of invading pathogens. The response from the immune system is to trigger the production of histamine and proteolytic enzymes, leading to vasodilatation and increased capillary permeability. The result of this is redistribution of circulating fluid as it leaks out of the intravascular spaces into the interstitial spaces.

Vasodilatation is the first step in the inflammatory process in order to increase blood flow to the affected area. This is necessary to ensure that white blood cells, fibrin and platelets are transported to where they are needed. Overtly, the patient will appear flushed and will feel warm. However, this will also cause the patient to be hypotensive.

Increased Capillary Permeability (Capillary Leakage). In addition to vasodilation the capillaries become more permeable; this essential component of the inflammatory response ensures that leucocytes (white blood cells) are able to move into the tissues where they are required to combat infection. This movement of fluid into the tissues not only causes oedema (swelling) – it also further exacerbates the problem of hypotension.

Screening for Septic Shock

Screening for septic shock must be initiated when the NEWS2 (RCP 2017) has triggered and the patient is likely to have an infection. The additional factors that should prompt screening for sepsis include:
• Carer or relative concern
• Recent chemotherapy or known to be neutropenic
• Known (or risk of) immunosuppression

• There is evidence of organ dysfunction (e.g. lactate >2 mmol)
• Recent surgery or trauma
• Indwelling lines

The most contemporary screening tools are available from the UK Sepsis Trust and should be used in conjunction with the organisation's policy and procedures and clinical guidelines.

Red Flag Sepsis

The concept of 'red flag sepsis' was developed by the UK Sepsis Trust, who developed a number of screening tools, for use in a variety of clinical settings, to identify those patients who are at risk of developing sepsis and subsequent shock and organ dysfunction. The screening tools aid healthcare professionals in recognising patients with hallmark signs and symptoms of sepsis or septic shock; they do not provide a formal diagnosis.

In patients with a suspected infection, the presence of *one* or more red flags alerts the healthcare professional to commence immediate treatment for sepsis to prevent organ dysfunction. Other patients who may be at risk of sepsis, but in whom the vital signs are less acutely deranged, can also be identified in a second stage of screening – the presence of a single 'amber flag' alerts the health practitioner to assess the patient for signs of organ dysfunction. If the lactate is raised or the patient is displaying signs of acute kidney injury, immediate treatment for sepsis should be given.

Signs and Symptoms of Septic Shock

• Reduced or altered mental status
• Tachypnoea
• Dyspnoea
• Hypotension
• Tachycardia (bounding pulse)
• Prolonged capillary refill time
• Widened PP >50 mmHg
• Low MAP <70 mmHg
• Reduced urine output or oliguria
• Warm, flushed skin or as noted previously

Management of Septic Shock

Sepsis is a time-critical condition; for every hour that appropriate antibiotic administration is delayed in patients with septic shock, the risk of mortality has been shown to increase by 8% (UK Sepsis Trust 2022b). 'The Sepsis Six Pathway' (UK Sepsis Trust 2022a) is a bundle of six interventions known to improve outcomes in patients with sepsis if implemented as soon as sepsis is recognised. These interventions are outlined here:
1. Ensure a senior clinician attends.
2. Administer oxygen as required. Oxygen should be commenced if the saturations are less than 92%; the aim is for the oxygen saturations to be between 94% and 98% (if at risk of hypercarbia, aim for saturations of 88%–92%).
3. Send blood tests (blood glucose, lactate, full blood count (FBC), urea and electrolytes (U&Es), C-reactive protein (CRP) and clotting and other tests as required) including cultures.
4. Give intravenous (IV) antibiotics; think source control (within 1 hour) to control the underlying infection.
5. Give IV fluids – administer up to 20 mL/kg in divided boluses (administer more if indicated). Use lactate to help guide further fluid therapy.
6. Monitor – use NEWS2 (RCP 2017) to monitor and escalate response, measure urinary output (this may require a catheter), with strict fluid balance, repeat lactate at least hourly if the initial lactate is >2 mmol or clinical condition changes.

Anaphylactic Shock

Anaphylactic shock is a serious systemic hypersensitivity reaction that is usually rapid in onset and may cause death. Severe anaphylaxis is characterised by potentially life-threatening compromise in airway, breathing and/or circulation and may occur without typical skin features or circulatory shock being present. These severe allergic reaction symptoms are caused by an antigen–antibody reaction and are triggered by environmental, iatrogenic (including drugs, foods, blood transfusion of incorrectly cross-matched or administered blood) and hereditary (hereditary angioedema) causes. In some cases of anaphylactic shock, the cause is unknown.

The antigen–antibody complex causes tissue mast cells (found in the loose connective tissues, bronchi and gastrointestinal mucosa) and basophils to release large quantities of vasogenic substances including histamine, serotonin and bradykinin. These toxic substances cause an increase in capillary permeability, widespread and massive vasodilatation and a consequent drop in blood pressure (hypotension). The associated vascular permeability can result in mucosal and laryngeal oedema, which may threaten airway patency, and can cause bronchospasm and impaired myocardial contractility.

Signs and Symptoms of Anaphylactic Shock

The individual developing anaphylactic shock may present with some or all of the following symptoms:
Airway
- Hoarse voice
- Laryngeal stridor

Breathing
- Increased work of breathing
- Dyspnoea
- Cough
- Cyanosis (occasionally)
  - o Cyanosis refers to the blue or grey ('ashen') discolouration of the skin and mucous membranes due to high levels of deoxygenated haemoglobin. Note that it is particularly difficult to detect in dark skin (Mukwende et al. 2020). It is best to look for cyanosis in the lips or oral mucous membranes where the epidermis is thin and there is abundant vasculature.
- Wheeze
- Oxygen saturations (<94%)

Circulation
- Localised oedema (particularly around the face)
- A weak and rapid pulse
- Low blood pressure

Disability
- Fatigue
- Confusion
- Reduced level of consciousness

Exposure
- Skin eruptions, large weals (may be absent in 10%–20% of all reactions)

Management of Anaphylactic Shock

The treatment for anaphylactic shock is (refer to the UK Resuscitation Guidelines 2021) prompt recognition.
- Call for help.
- Remove the trigger (for example, stop the IV Infusion).
- Lie the patient flat.
- The administration of adrenaline (IM in the anterolateral thigh). Adrenaline causes an increase in blood pressure by producing vasoconstrictor effects and inhibiting the mediators released by the immune response. It also causes smooth muscles to relax, leading to bronchodilation of the airways.
- Establish a patent airway, administer high flow oxygen therapy and apply monitoring.
- If no improvement administer further IV adrenaline and IV fluids.

Spinal Shock

Spinal shock is defined as the sudden onset of complete loss of motor and sensory functions below the level of the lesion, as well as the complete loss of tone with absent tone with no deep and superficial reflexes (Ko 2018). Spinal shock usually lasts from 4 to 12 weeks but may last up to 6 to 12 months postinjury with a gradual return of reflex activity (Hills 2020).

The degree and type of force exerted on the spine at the time of injury will determine the nature and severity of the injury. The mechanism of injuries includes:
- Subluxation of the vertebra, which causes a 'pincer-like' damage to the cord, which can result in complete cord transection in extreme cases.
- Hyperextension – extreme extension which can cause compression of the cord.
- Axial loading – vertical compression caused by a direct force to the top of the head; this force is then transferred through the spine.
- Rotation – extreme lateral flexion.
- Penetrating injury, which can cause direct compression and vascular injury.

Signs and Symptoms of Spinal Shock

Somatic
- Flaccid paralysis
- Loss of sensory function
- Loss of deep tendon and cutaneous reflexes
  Autonomic – loss of sympathetic tone and unopposed parasympathetic function
- Hypotension
- Bradycardia
- Skin hyperaemia
- Altered genital and urinary symptoms

Management of Spinal Shock

The treatment for spinal shock revolves around treating the underlying spinal cord injury (SCI), and the prevention of any further injury exacerbation. Specific treatment will be dependent on the level of spinal injury but will include:
1. Management of airway, breathing and circulation as priorities – by adopting the ABCDE approach to assessing and treating the acutely ill patient.
2. Spinal precautions (logrolling, cervical collar) and protection from further injury.
3. Management of gastrointestinal function as a paralytic ileus may be present: patients should be nil by mouth until bowel sounds return and a nasogastric tube should be inserted (Bonner and Smith 2013).
4. Urinary management: patients in spinal shock are unlikely to have bladder-emptying reflexes therefore it is important that they are catheterised. Because of the lack of sympathetic

activity, oliguria may be present; practitioners need to be aware that this may not reflect poor circulatory volume and the administering intravenous fluids needs to be undertaken cautiously. Strict fluid balance is required.

5. Bowel management: bowel function is likely to be affected and will require careful and appropriate management. The accumulation of faeces in the rectum can result in overdistension of the stretch receptors in the bowel; however, the sensation and ability to defecate will be absent. Because the bowel will not respond to chemical stimulation, careful digital removal of faeces will be required (Hills 2020).

6. Monitoring for signs of DVT and administration of low-molecular-weight heparin (LWMH) as per local policy.

7. Pressure area care – Patients who have sustained a SCI are at high risk of developing pressure damage as a result of impaired circulation and muscular disuse. Therefore meticulous pressure area care and monitoring should be initiated from admission (Eckert and Martin 2017).

8. Psychological and emotional care.

Neurogenic Shock

Neurogenic shock refers to the immediate loss of sympathetic tone that occurs after a SCI most commonly at the level of T6 (Hills 2020). Neurogenic shock occurs because of the loss of sympathetic nerve activity from the brain's vasomotor centre due to disease, a drug or traumatic injury. The loss of sympathetic impulses causes massive vasodilatation of the arterioles and venules, as the vasoconstrictor tone has been interrupted. The result is a significant decrease in peripheral vascular resistance and a reduction in venous return. There will be a concurrent decrease in CO with hypotension.

There are a number of preconditions, which include:

- spinal anaesthesia
- cerebral trauma
- spinal cord trauma.

Signs and Symptoms of Neurogenic Shock

- Hypotension due the loss of blood vessel tone with resultant venous pooling
- Bradycardia due to reduced cardiac sympathetic input
- Warm dry skin

Management of Neurogenic Shock

The treatment for neurogenic shock will include treating the underlying SCI and preventing any further injury exacerbation. Specific treatment (in addition for those identified for spinal shock) will include

- Management of airway and breathing
- Management of circulation to include:
  - Fluid therapy (crystalloid) to manage the blood pressure, although this rarely results in an increase in the central venous pressure.
  - The use of vasoconstrictor inotropes to support circulation and will compensate for the loss of sympathetic nerve activity; this treatment should only be commenced under the direct supervision of an intensivist.
  - Management of bradycardia.
- Observing for signs of autonomic dysreflexia and initiating prompt treatment. Autonomic dysreflexia is a life-threatening syndrome that potential affects all patients with SCI at the level of the sixth thoracic vertebrae (T6) or above; it is caused by

spinal reflex mechanisms that remain intact despite the injury (Hills 2020). Noxious (painful) stimuli (e.g. blocked catheter, constipation) below the level of injury produce an afferent impulse causing vasoconstriction below the level of the injury (vasodilation above). Patients may present with:

- anxiety
- severe headache
- sweating above the level of the injury (pallor below)
- blurred vision
- palpitation.
- Management includes:
  - monitor blood pressure
  - loosen tight clothing
  - remove noxious stimulus
  - administer antihypertensive agents as prescribed.

To conclude this section on types of shock, now look at Reflection 19.1.

MONITORING THE PATIENT IN SHOCK

Close monitoring of the patient in shock will enable the nurse to monitor the patient's response to treatment and to identify signs and symptoms of further deterioration. It is important to monitor the following aspects of a patient's condition to assess the level of organ perfusion and the severity of shock:

- cardiac status
- respiratory status
- haemodynamic status
- level of consciousness
- renal function
- body temperature
- skin condition.

Strategies to monitor each of these aspects of the patient's condition are considered in more detail in following sections.

Monitoring Cardiac Status

Manual Pulse Check

The manual assessment of an arterial pulse, usually the radial artery, is the most fundamental and vital form of cardiac monitoring. It can demonstrate not only the rate but also the rhythm of the heart, together with an impression of blood pressure and whether this is 'bounding' (strong) or 'thready' (weak). A bounding pulse represents a raised blood pressure, whereas a 'thready' one denotes a low blood pressure.

Electrocardiography

An electrocardiogram (ECG) is a recording of the electrical activity of the myocardium and indicates the changes that occur as a result of contraction. The contraction of any heart muscle is associated with electrical changes called depolarisation and these can be detected by electrodes attached to the surface of the body (see Chapter 2, Nursing Patients With Cardiovascular Disorders). An ECG can be obtained quickly in an emergency department or with a portable electrocardiograph at the patient's bedside. It can provide further useful information about the rate and rhythm of the heart. Thus if arrhythmias arise, they can be detected and treated immediately. However, electrocardiographs should only be used by specialist staff who can interpret waveforms accurately. Thus ECG monitoring is usually only performed in coronary, high-dependency or intensive care units.

Monitoring Respiratory Status

Respiratory rate is an extremely sensitive indicator of deterioration and should *always* be monitored together with haemodynamic observations. Unfortunately, if automated devices are used respiratory rate is often omitted because it is not measured by the device (Palmer et al. 2022). The nurse should always be alert to hypo- or hyperventilation, and additional airway noises such as snoring, gurgling or stridor (Tait et al. 2022). Although hyperventilation may occur as a compensatory response to metabolic acidosis, it will eventually result in fatigue of the respiratory muscles. This may lead to shallow breathing and the risk of respiratory distress, necessitating mechanical ventilation. Hypoventilation may be a very late sign of shock, as the patient begins to tire and has insufficient reserve to maintain ventilation. Hypoventilation may also be associated with the administration of opiates, such as morphine, often administered in cardiogenic shock.

Monitoring Oxygen Saturation

The level of O_2 saturation in the patient's blood (SpO_2) will give some indication of respiratory status. Continuous monitoring will provide valuable information related to the individual's response to interventions and can provide early warning of hypoxaemia. However, poor oxygen delivery to the tissues may also occur in the presence of a normal SpO_2. It is, therefore, also important to know the patient's haemoglobin level in order to assess whether the oxygen-carrying capacity of the blood is adequate (Hb 9–10 g/dL).

Pulse Oximetry

Arterial O_2 saturation along with pulse rate can be monitored continuously by means of a noninvasive electronic device called a pulse oximeter. This functions by measuring the absorption of red and infrared light passed through living tissue, usually a finger, toe or ear lobe however, the accuracy of the reading can be affected by nail varnish, movement and artificial light. Results usually correspond closely to ABG values and this instrument reduces the need for blood samples. Vasoconstriction can impair SpO_2 readings, and if this is the case then ABGs should be taken. Readings can be distorted by high blood bilirubin levels, as in jaundice, and in cases of carbon monoxide poisoning and smoke inhalation. Results for very heavy smokers may also be difficult to interpret. Importantly, there is increasing evidence that the accuracy of pulse oximetry is impacted by skin colour and nurses should be aware that pulse oximetry may underestimate hypoxaemia in Black patients.

Monitoring Haemodynamic Status

The importance of monitoring the blood pressure has already been established through its use not only to recognise deterioration but also to evaluate the effectiveness of fluid resuscitation. MAP and PP are also very useful measures of haemodynamic status. The MAP is considered to be a better indicator of end-organ perfusion than the systolic blood pressure. It may be calculated using the following equation: MAP = ([diastolic blood pressure × 2] + systolic pressure) divided by 3. For example, in a patient with a BP of 110/80 mmHg, the MAP would be calculated as ([80 × 2] + 110) / 3 = 90 mmHg. A 'normal' MAP of 75–100 mmHg suggests that there is good end-organ perfusion. However, the patient's MAP should be considered within the context of their baseline blood pressure – for instance, patients with chronic hypertension may require a higher MAP to achieve good end-organ perfusion. The PP is the difference between the systolic and diastolic pressure. Thus if the BP is 110/80 mmHg, the PP will be 30 mmHg ('normal' is 30–50 mmHg). If this narrows, it indicates the activation of the sympathetic nervous system and vasoconstriction. If it widens, it can denote vasodilatation, indicating a reduction in circulating volume and the need for fluid resuscitation. The absolute values of the PP are of less significance than the trend. Therefore in documenting the blood pressure, it is important to establish the status of the PP. In addition to noninvasive BP monitoring, MAP and PP, invasive monitoring of CVP and blood pressure are also useful adjuncts in the monitoring and management of shock, these are outlined here.

Central Venous Pressure (CVP) and Invasive Blood Pressure Monitoring

CVP is the pressure within the right atrium and superior vena cava. Its measurement can provide valuable information about circulating blood volume. It can also give an indication of vascular tone and pulmonary vascular resistance, as well as the effectiveness of the right myocardium. However, it does not measure left ventricular function and it can be unreliable in the critically ill patient with chronic lung disease, right and left heart failure or valve disease. CVP monitoring reflects the rate of blood return to the right side of the heart and can be an accurate guide for fluid replacement. A CVP of approximately 2 cmH_2O in the presence of a low arterial blood pressure usually indicates hypovolaemia, whereas a CVP above 14 cmH_2O in the presence of a low arterial blood pressure indicates cardiogenic shock.

Technique. A large-bore catheter is inserted under strict aseptic conditions into the internal or external jugular, or subclavian vein, using ultrasound techniques to correctly site the catheter. In wards, the CVP can be measured as shown in Fig. 19.1. In critical care settings, a transducer can be attached to the central line in order to obtain a waveform and digital display of the CVP reading in mmHg (see Chapter 28, Nursing the Critically Ill Patient). Continuous monitoring will indicate the effectiveness of treatment.

Similarly, a thin catheter called an arterial line can be inserted into an artery (usually the radial or the femoral artery) and attached to a transducer to facilitate monitoring of blood pressure in real time and to obtain blood samples for blood gas analysis.

Arterial and central venous lines, although extremely important for a critically ill patient, present a danger of bacterial infection (see Chapter 18, Infection Prevention and Control). Nurses can make an important contribution to care by ensuring that aseptic techniques are adhered to when the line is inserted and that the insertion site is kept clean and dry. Once it is no longer needed,

Figure 19.1 Diagram of a central venous pressure (CVP) water manometer. (A) Before measuring CVP, the infusion flow is to the patient and the three-way stopcock is closed to the manometer. (B) To measure CVP, the stopcock is turned so that it is closed to the patient. This allows the manometer to be refilled with fluid. (C) The stopcock is turned so that it is closed to the infusion fluid. This allows a free flow of fluid from the manometer to the intravenous catheter. The fluid level will fall until the level corresponds with the pressure in the right atrium or superior vena cava. (Adapted from Jamieson EM, McCall JM, Blythe R, White LA. Guidelines for Clinical Nursing Practices. 4th ed. Edinburgh: Churchill Livingstone; 2004.)

the line should be removed as quickly as possible to reduce the risk of infection.

Monitoring Level of Consciousness

In the early stages of shock, the patient may still be quite alert and anxious. They may complain of pain and may be able to give a history, which will help the clinician to establish a diagnosis. However, if cerebral perfusion pressure falls, with resulting cerebral hypoxia, the patient will gradually become less coherent and may eventually become comatose. The nurse should observe the patient carefully to ensure changes in the state of consciousness are noted as they occur, and management escalated to the appropriate personnel (e.g. senior ward nurse, specialist registrar, critical care outreach team, anaesthetist). There is a danger that if a patient has been agitated, due to hypoxia, and then becomes quiet the nurse may consider the patient is responding to treatment, whereas the opposite may be the case. Once the conscious level drops, it is vital to ensure that the airway is maintained and a Guedel airway or intubation may be required. It may be advisable to place the patient in the left lateral position. The Glasgow Coma Scale is a useful tool with which to assess the patient's cerebral function (see Chapter 11, Nursing Patients With Disorders of the Nervous System, and Chapter 27, Nursing the Unconscious Patient). The mnemonic ACVPU is also now widely used because it is easier to calculate than the GCS (RCP 2017). ACVPU refers to an assessment of consciousness in which the patient is **A**lert, has new-onset **C**onfusion, disorientation and/or agitation, is alert to **V**oice only, is roused by **P**ain, is **U**nconscious.

Monitoring Renal Function

Renal function is a very good indicator of tissue perfusion and should therefore be monitored carefully in patients suffering from shock (see also Chapter 21, Maintaining Fluid, Electrolyte and Acid–Base Balance). A urinary catheter and accurate fluid balance chart are therefore vital to the patient's management. Since the kidneys are dependent on adequate tissue perfusion, a drop in urinary output indicates poor perfusion. The urinary output

should be 0.5–1.0 mL per kg per hour or not less than 200 mL in the last 6 hours. A lower figure may represent dehydration, as well as shock; however, both conditions require fluid resuscitation and dehydration may lead to hypovolaemic shock. Urinary catheterisation and hourly urine measurement greatly assist the early detection of decreasing renal perfusion.

Measurement of specific gravity (SG) reflects the concentration of the urine. The normal urinary SG is between 1.002 and 1.028. In the early stages of shock, when urine volume falls, the concentration of excreted waste products rises. This is reflected in a raised SG and osmolality. However, if the shocked state progresses and urine volumes remain low, the ability of the kidneys to concentrate the urine is fixed or low. Levels of creatinine and urea in the blood will also rise in the presence of decreased renal perfusion and function.

Monitoring Body Temperature

The importance of obtaining accurate body temperature measurements should not be underestimated, as many clinical interventions are based on these readings.

Observing Skin Condition

Direct observation of the skin colour, temperature and condition will reflect the stage of shock that the patient is in. Intense activation of the sympathetic nervous system will result in pale, clammy skin and a dry mouth. In dark skin, pallor may be easier to identify by observing the palms of the hands; there will be pale skin, and in particular, reduced darkness in the palmar creases (Mukwende et al. 2020). Capillary refill time is a common measure of peripheral perfusion. It is the rate at which blood refills the empty capillaries. It is measured by pressing on the fingernail bed until it turns white and noting the time it takes for the colour to return. Refill should occur within 2 seconds once the nail bed is released. Failure of capillary refill indicates sustained and prolonged vasoconstriction. If oxygen delivery is severely impaired, the skin will become cold, mottled and cyanosed. However, it should be noted that the clinical picture in septic, neurogenic and anaphylactic shock is different. In these types of shock, the skin is warm, dry and flushed due to vasodilatation.

Laboratory and Diagnostic Tests

ABG analysis provides a guide to oxygenation, tissue perfusion and aerobic or anaerobic respiration by the cells. In all types of shock, it is not uncommon to find a fall in the partial pressure of oxygen (PaO_2) and a rise in the partial pressure of carbon dioxide ($PaCO_2$) (although a fall in $PaCO_2$ may be seen in the early stages of shock as a result of hyperventilation). With an increase in anaerobic metabolism resulting in the production of lactic acid, metabolic acidosis is frequently seen in the severely shocked patient.

Summary: Key Nursing Issues

- Fundamental to the recognition and effective management of shock is the accurate recording and documentation of physiological parameters and fluid balance.
- In assessing the patient, continual review of the airway, breathing, circulation and disability (conscious level) is vital, together with the exposure of the patient to ascertain alteration in skin colour, or the presence of oedema, urticaria (rash) or inflammation.
- If shock is established, then treatment must be swift as this is a medical emergency and effective communication is imperative.
- Use of the SBAR system enables complex information to be escalated efficiently.
- Once management is instigated the nurse again plays a crucial role in monitoring the effectiveness of treatment. Successful resuscitation of the patient relies heavily on the vigilance of the nurse.

Reflection and Learning – What Next?

- **Test** your knowledge by visiting the Evolve website 🌐 and answering the multiple-choice questions and critical thinking questions.
- **Consolidate** your learning by looking at some of the further reading suggestions, references and specialist websites.
- **Revisit** some of the additional material on the Evolve website.
- **Consider** what you have learnt and how this will help your professional development.
- **Reflect** on how you can apply this knowledge to the care of your patients.
- **Discuss** your learning with your mentor/supervisor, lecturer and colleagues.

References

Bonner S, Smith C. Initial management of acute spinal cord injury. *Contin Educ Anaesth Crit Care Pain.* 2013;13(6):224–231.

Cecconi M, De Bracker D, Antonelli M, et al. Consensus of circulatory shock and haemodynamic monitoring. Task Force of the European Society of Intensive Care Medicine. *Intensive Care Med.* 2014;40(12): 1795–1815.

Chaikof EL, Dalman RL, Eskandari MK, et al. The Society for Vascular Surgery practice guidelines on the care of patients with an abdominal aortic aneurysm. *J Vasc Surg.* 2018;67(1):1–78.

Dutton H, Peate I. Acute Nursing Care Recognising and Responding to Medical Emergencies (2nd Edition). 2021. London: Routledge.

Eckert MJ, Martin MJ. Trauma: spinal cord injury. *Surg Clin North Am [online].* 2017;97(5):1031–1045. https://doi.org/10.1016/j.suc.2017. 06.008.

Health Service Investigation Branch (HSIB). Recognising and Responding to Critically Unwell Patients. Independent report by the Healthcare Safety Investigation Branch. 2019. https://hssib-ovd42x6f-media. s3.amazonaws.com/production-assets/documents/hsib_report_recognising_responding_critically_unwell_patients.pdf.

Hills TE. Caring for patients with a traumatic spinal cord injury. *Nursing (Lond).* 2020;50(12):30–40. doi:10.1097/01.NURSE.0000721724. 96678.5a PMID: 33497093.

Jamieson EM, McCall JM, Blythe R, White LA. *Guidelines for Clinical Nursing Practices.* 4th ed. Edinburgh: Churchill Livingstone; 2004.

Jones TL, Nakamura K, McCabe JM. Cardiogenic shock: evolving definitions and future directions in management. *Open Heart.* 2019;6:e000960.

Kim KS. Obstructive shock. In: Suh GJ, ed. *Essentials of Shock Management: A Scenario-Based Approach.* Singapore: Springer Nature; 2018;pp 45–54.

Ko H-Y. Revisit spinal shock: pattern of reflex evolution during spinal shock. *Korean J Neurotrauma [online].* 2018;14(2):47–54. https://doi. org/10.13004/kjnt.2018.14.2.47.

Kudo D, Yoshida Y, Kushimoto S. Permissive hypotension/hypotensive resuscitation and restricted/controlled resuscitation in patients with severe trauma. *J Int Care.* 2017;5(11):1–8.

McDonagh TA, Metra M, Adamo M, et al. 2021 ESC guidelines for the diagnosis and treatment of acute and chronic heart failure. *Eur Heart J.* 2021;42:3599–3726.

Moruzzi M, McLeod A. Hypovolaemic shock: assessment, pathophysiology and nursing care. *Br J Neurosci Nurs.* 2017;13(3):126–132.

Mukwende M, Tamony P, Turner M. Mind the Gap: a Handbook of Clinical Signs in Black and Brown Skin. 2020. https://figshare.com/articles/online_resource/Mind_the_Gap_A_handbook_of_clinical_signs_in_Black_and_Brown_skin/12769988.

National Institute for Health and Clinical Excellence (NICE). Acutely ill adults in hospital: recognizing and responding to deterioration. Clinical guideline [CG50]. 2007. https://www.nice.org.uk/guidance/cg50.

National Institute for Health and Care Excellence (NICE). Major trauma: assessment and initial management. NICE guideline [NG39]. 2016. https://www.nice.org.uk/guidance/ng39/resources/major-trauma-assessment-and-initial-management-pdf-1837400761285.

National Institute for Health and Care Excellence (NICE). Intravenous fluid therapy in adults in hospital. Clinical guideline [CG174]. 2017a. https://www.nice.org.uk/guidance/cg174.

National Institute for Health and Care Excellence (NICE). Sepsis: recognition, diagnosis and early management. NICE guideline [NG51]. 2017b. https://www.nice.org.uk/guidance/ng51.

Nursing and Midwifery Council (NMC). The Code: Professional Standards of Practice and Behaviour for Nurses, Midwives and Nursing Associates. 2018. https://www.nmc.org.uk/globalassets/sitedocuments/nmc-publications/nmc-code.pdf.

Palmer JH, James S, Wadsworth D, Gordon CJ, Craft J. How registered nurses are measuring respiratory rates in adult acute care health settings: an integrative review. *J Clin Nurs*. 2022. https://doi.org/10.1111/jocn.16522.

Purvey M, Allen G. Managing acute pulmonary oedema. *Aust Prescr*. 2017;40(2):59–63.

Royal College of Physicians (RCP). *National Early Warning Score (NEWS) 2: Standardising the Assessment of Acute-Illness Severity in the NHS*. London: RCP; 2017. Available at: https://www.rcplondon.ac.uk/projects/outputs/national-early-warning-score-news-2.

Singer M, Deutschman CS, Seymour CW, et al. The Third International Consensus Definitions for sepsis and septic shock (Sepsis-3). *JAMA*. 2016;315(8):801–810.

Spahn DJ, Bouillon B, Cerny V, et al. The European guidelines on management of major bleeding and coagulopathy following trauma: 5th edition. *Criti Care*. 2019;23(98):1–74.

Stratton SJ. *BMJ Best Practice: Shock*. London: BMJ Publishing; 2017. http://bestpractice.bmj.com/topics/en-gb/1013.

Stratton SJ. *BMJ Best Practice: Shock*. London: BMJ Publishing; 2022. https//bestpractice.bmj.com/topics/en-gb/1012.

Suh GJ, Lee JH. Introduction to shock. In: Suh GJ, ed. *Essentials of Shock Management: A Scenario-Based Approach*. Singapore: Springer Nature; 2018;pp 3–5.

Tait D. The patient in shock. In: Tait D, James J, Williams C, Barton D, eds. *Acute and Critical Care in Adult Nursing*. 2nd ed. London: Learning Matters/Sage; 2016.

Tait D, Williams C, Barton D, James J. *Acute and Critical Care in Adult Nursing*. 3rd ed. London: Learning Matters – SAGE Publishing Company; 2022.

Resuscitation Council (UK). *Advanced Life Support*. 5th ed. London: Resuscitation Council (UK); 2021.

UK Resuscitation Guidelines. Resuscitation Council UK. Resuscitation Guidelines. 2021. https://www.resus.org.uk/library/2021-resuscitation-guidelines.

UK Sepsis Trust. Toolkit: emergency department management of sepsis in adults and young people over 12 years. 2022a. https://sepsistrust.org/education/clinical-tools/.

UK Sepsis Trust. The Sepsis Manual. 4th ed. 2017–2018. 2022b. https://sepsistrust.org/product/sepsis-manual/.

Vahdatpour C, Collins D, Goldberg S. Cardiogenic Shock. *J Am Heart Assoc*. 2019;8:e011991.

Van Diepen S, Katz JN, Albert NM, et al. Contemporary management of cardiogenic shock: a scientific statement from the American Heart Association. *Circulation*. 2017;136(00–00):e1–e37.

Useful Websites

National Institute for Health and Care Excellence (NICE), www.nice.org.uk

Resuscitation Council (UK), www.resus.org.uk/resuscitation-guidelines/

UK Sepsis Trust, https://sepsistrust.org

20

Pain Management

ANTHONY WHEELDON

CHAPTER OUTLINE

Introduction

Pain from a worldwide perspective is a major clinical, social and economic problem and the economic cost in terms of loss of productivity, loss of income and burden of pain to the individual is significant. Pain affects all populations globally regardless of age, gender, race, ethnicity and social class. Therefore pain management presents a major challenge to healthcare providers globally that requires a collective response. The major causes of pain include cancer pain, osteo- and rheumatoid arthritis, surgery, traumatic injuries and spinal problems, making the aetiology of pain a complex transdisciplinary phenomenon. Pain is a subjective and ambiguous experience that is difficult to quantify, which can lead to clinicals underestimating its impact (Wheeldon 2021).

The Global Pain Index (GSK Consumer Healthcare 2020) summarises the global pain experience, stating that globally 93% of the world population experienced 'body pain' in the previous 12 months and 50% of the world population experience 'back pain' once a month. Beyond the economic impact, pain touches the very fabric of people's lives, as reported by approximately two in three individuals who suffer pain stating that it impacts upon their ability to enjoy life and three in four wishing they could better control their pain.

Chronic pain affects at least 10% of the world's population, approximately 60 million people, with estimates of chronic pain prevalence closer to 20%–25% in some countries and regions, and an additional 1 in 10 people develop chronic pain every year worldwide. However, akin to the general global burden of disease, there are inequalities between high- and low-income countries in terms of risk factors for persistent pain, with those most disadvantaged bearing higher burdens of persistent pain and lesser likelihood of effective treatment.

Chronic pain is a health crisis and 'silent epidemic' (McCabe 2017) and is the most common reason an individual will seek medical care. Hanley et al. (2022) established that 51% of surgical patients remained in pain 30 days after surgery, with 42% reporting pain a year later. Chronic pain therefore presents a significant disease burden. Indeed, it is estimated that chronic pain is prevalent in between one-third and one-half of adults in the UK. The incidence of chronic pain increases with age, with 53% of people aged 75 years and older reporting pain in comparison with 16% of people aged between 16 and 24 years. The most common cited causes being back pain, headache and joint pain (National Institute for Health and Care Excellence [NICE] 2021b).

Pain is a critical component, and at times the only element, of disease processes. Pain management and subsequent nursing interventions entail a moral, humanitarian, ethical and legal obligation to ensure that people in our care have their pain relieved. This requires competent and knowledgeable practitioners who are 'fit for purpose'. Pain is also a critical ethical issue because it has the capacity to dehumanise the human person. Effective pain management as a fundamental human right is a widely regarded moral imperative, but pain on a global scale remains inadequately treated because of cultural, attitudinal, educational, legal and system-related ideologies (Brennan et al. 2019). Today the best available evidence indicates a gap between an increasingly sophisticated understanding of the pathophysiology of pain, and the widespread inadequacy in its treatment.

It was a series of high-profile cases and reports (Berwick 2013, Bubb 2014, Care Quality Commission 2015, Department of Health 2012a, 2012b, Keogh 2013, Willis 2013, 2015) that provided the watershed for change and galvanised collective action. Recommendations from the Francis (2013) report highlighted multiple failings of frontline care delivery, such as staff routinely neglecting their patients, patients feeling humiliated and patients left in pain. Patients experience compassion whenever they experience their basic needs being met in gentle, respectful ways that acknowledge their unique humanity, paying attention to what really matters to them. Francis stated that what was required was a real change in culture and refocus upon the recommitment of all who work in the National Health Service (NHS), from top to bottom of the system. In 2004, the International Pain Society and Global Health Community concluded that 'failure to treat pain is viewed worldwide as poor medicine, unethical practice, and an abrogation of a fundamental human right'. Since that time, pain management has become enshrined in international law as a basic human right, with countries ethically mandated to provide pain treatment as part of their core obligations under the right to health (Brennan et al. 2019). Furthermore, adequate pain management is part of each healthcare professional's duty of care. Values and ethics embraced within The Code: Professional Standards of Practice and Behaviour for Nurses, Midwives and Nursing Associates (Nursing and Midwifery Council [NMC] 2018) reflect the duty of care that nurses have towards those in their care. Every person, irrespective of age, deserves to be pain free.

Nurses working within a multidisciplinary team (MDT) need up-to-date evidence-based knowledge and understanding of pain to competently prevent and minimise pain. Nurses must therefore be aware of the following:

- the causes of pain and major influences on the perception of pain
- the effects of unrelieved pain on the individual
- appropriate methods of pain assessment
- pharmacological interventions according to the needs of the person
- complications of pharmacological interventions
- the use of appropriate nonpharmacological interventions (Wheeldon 2021).

This chapter outlines the key issues relating to pain and the challenge of defining and describing pain due to its elusive, complex and subjective nature. It will also explore how historical perspectives, pain myths and misconceptions have helped to shape contemporary practice and policy. The chapter will conclude with a description of the tools available for pain assessment and the pharmacological and nonpharmacological therapies used in pain management.

Defining Pain: Competing Perspectives

Historically, pain has often been attributed, in differing cultures, to 'wrongdoing', suffering and punishment. Pain is multidimensional,

embracing physical, psychosocial, emotional and spiritual components (Chary 2021). Furthermore, the multidimensional nature of pain makes it possible to be with an individual who is in pain and be unaware of its impact. It is therefore increasingly recognised that pain is a complex phenomenon, and it is difficult to assign a simple single definition. The International Association for the Study of Pain (IASP) (2022) describe pain as:

An unpleasant sensory and emotional experience associated with actual or potential tissue damage or described in terms of such damage.

Whilst this definition describes both the sensory and emotional aspects of pain, it has limitations because it fails to account for other peripheral nervous system (PNS) activity and stimuli within the central nervous system (CNS), and the variable way in which the nervous system can respond to injury. Moreover, this definition disregards the sociocultural aspects of an individual's life, which recognises that body, mind and culture also influence pain. Over 50 years ago, McCaffery (1968) proposed a simple definition which has become accepted within nursing and has encouraged nurses to focus upon the patient/client's pain perspective.

Pain is whatever the patient says it is and exists when he [sic] says it does.

This definition embraces the subjective nature of pain and has encouraged nurses and others to value the person's reporting of their pain. Despite a lack of consensus on the definition of pain, ongoing research has expanded our understanding of the pain experience. Therefore healthcare professionals must be aware of and responsive to an individual's pain, taking account of the variables that influence the individual's lived-in experience of pain (Reflection 20.1).

Historical Perspectives and Contemporary Thinking About Pain

The history of pain treatment is extensive: ample literature and documentary evidence describes the pervasive influence and intrusive nature of pain on every facet of life since the earliest human experience (Brennan et al. 2007, p. 207). The treatment and management of pain have evolved over the centuries from early treatments with herbs to modern day pain management with drugs and nonpharmacological methods. The antecedents of pain theories and treatments originate from early civilisations which had quite different views of pain; often, the commonly held belief was that pain was the consequence of, or the punishment for, sins committed, or the magical influence of spirits of the dead. Every religion

---

REFLECTION 20.1

Factors Influencing the Pain Experience

Reflect upon your own pain experiences, and how the intensity of pain may have been influenced by other factors. The pain you experienced may have hindered your daily living activities. These factors may include position, noise, stress, tiredness, hunger, frustration, a fast-approaching assignment deadline, not having enough information or an impending big occasion.

Activity

Discuss your thoughts with colleagues and list the factors that reduce pain intensity, and what might increase pain intensity.

has addressed the issue of pain, and religion, philosophy and folklore have saturated pain with meaning (Brennan et al. 2007).

History recounts that 4500 years ago, the Chinese had a well-developed system of pain management based upon acupuncture. They also used herbal remedies, and evidence from early in their history suggests that they used opioids or other narcotics. The Egyptians appear to have believed that gods or disincarnate spirits inflicted pain on people, and, as in India, the Egyptians also believed the heart to be at the centre of sensation. The Indian culture attached more significance to the emotional roots of pain. It was the ancient Greeks who introduced the concept of the brain as the main organ of pain sensation. However, Aristotle refuted this theory and considered the heart as the main organ for pain sensation instead. Hippocrates (the 'father of medicine') held a view that was like the Chinese theory of the 'elements' or 'humours': blood, phlegm, yellow bile and black bile. The humours were traditionally associated with the causation of disease, whereby an imbalance of the humours caused pain.

Eventually, philosophy accepted that brain was the centre for the recognition and sensation of pain. The ancient Greeks established an intimate connection between the brain and peripheral nerves. Galen demonstrated that both CNS and PNS components were collectively involved in pain sensation. Even so, Galen continued to hold the view that pain was a 'passion of the soul'. Pain is the oldest medical problem. However, an understanding of its pathophysiology is a recent phenomenon.

Theories of Pain

This section of the chapter outlines pain theories, historical and contemporary, including the specificity theory, the pattern or summation theory, the gate control theory, the neuromatrix theory of pain, brain plasticity and pain and allostatic load theory.

Specificity Theory

Descartes (1596–1650) proposed the classic specificity theory. This traditionally held theory proposed a direct channel for pain from the periphery of the body to the brain, proposing that when there is exposure to a painful stimulus, a specified pain pathway transports pain messages to the brain. This is of historical significance as proposals for new, refined and accepted pain theories that demonstrate the inherent inadequacies of specificity theory are recent concepts. According to MacMahon et al. (2013), its biggest flaw is that it cannot account for how a single stimulus can create different responses, including emotional and cognitive.

Pattern or Summation Theory

According to Field and Smith (2019), the pattern theory was dominant from the end of the 19th century until the early 1960s. Goldscheider, at the end of the 19th century, proposed the pattern or summation theory which was based upon the excitatory effects of converging stimuli. He claimed that the summation of the skin impulses had a sensory input at the dorsal horn cells and produced patterns of nerve impulses that produced pain. When receptors normally activated by nonnoxious heat or touch were subject to excessive stimulation or pathological conditions, these would enhance the summation of impulses and eventually produce acute pain, and prolonged periods of summation would produce chronic pain. Livingston (1943) first proposed a central summation theory asserting that a central neural mechanism was responsible for pain

syndromes such as phantom limb pain. However, this is contentious because surgical lesions of the spinal cord, in most cases, do not eliminate pain for any sustained length of time, indicating that a mechanism operates at a higher level than the dorsal horns.

Gate Control Theory

Melzack and Wall (1965) developed the gate control theory of pain. According to this theory, a gating mechanism situated in substantia gelatinosa cells in the dorsal horn of the spine can modify potential pain stimuli. This mechanism can increase or decrease the flow of nerve impulses from the periphery to the CNS. If the gate is open, impulses pass through unimpeded; if it is partially open, fewer impulses pass through; and if the gate shuts, no impulses get through and the individual experiences little or no pain. Melzack and Wall argued that whether the gate is open or closed is determined by:

- activity in small-diameter fibres (A-δ and C fibres, which transmit pain)
- activity in large-diameter fibres (A-β fibres, which transmit touch)
- descending influences from higher centres, including those concerned with motivational and cognitive processes.

Melzack and Wall proposed that large A-β fibres activate the substantia gelatinosa, which subsequently closes the gate. Small A-δ and C fibres have the opposite effect and open the gate. This activity then influences the information sent to the brain, which in turn initiates descending inhibitory controls depending on the information from other areas such as the cortex (Fig. 20.1).

Understanding of the physiology of pain has developed since the gate control theory was first proposed, such as the discovery of endogenous opioid neurotransmitters (e.g. endorphins). Chemicals, such as prostaglandins, released in response to a painful stimulus also influence whether the gate closes or remains open. However, the inherent fundamental principles have stood the test of time and influenced pain management. The principles of gate control theory influence nursing care decisions, such as the application of heat/cold, or massage. The use of touch and massage stimulates the skin, increasing large fibre (A-β) activity and thereby closing the gate at the spinal cord level and relieving pain. This rationale also explains the benefit of advice to 'rub it better'. Closing the gate at the brain stem level can sometimes be achieved by ensuring sufficient sensory input, for example by using distraction. Similarly, at the level of the cortex/thalamus, reducing anxiety can close the gate, for example by providing accurate information about the cause, prognosis and relief of pain and thereby increasing the person's confidence and sense of control. Factors that may exacerbate pain (i.e. opening the gate) may include injury, anxiety, low mood, fatigue or boredom and focusing too much upon the pain (Wheeldon 2021).

Interestingly, Descartes originally observed that the nervous system could regulate the intensity of the pain experience, and Melzack, Wall and others such as Beecher later took the credit (Grady et al. 2007).

The Neuromatrix of Pain

The theory relating to the concept of a pain neuromatrix suggests that modulation of pain perception has multiple simultaneous influences. Melzack developed this theory which represents an expansion beyond the original 'gate control' theory of pain proposed in 1965. Whilst the neuromatrix theory does not negate the original gate control theory, it describes the effects of nonpharmacological effects upon the individual. Individuals have an innate network of neurones (self neuromatrix), and each person's matrix is unique and affected by all elements of that

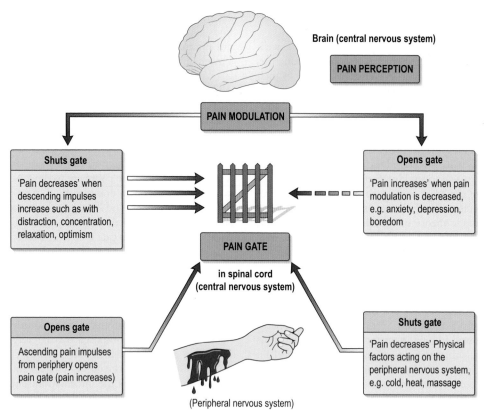

Figure 20.1 Gate-control theory. (Reproduced from Brooker C, Waugh A, eds. *Foundations of Nursing Practice: Fundamentals of Holistic Care*. Edinburgh: Mosby; 2007 with permission.)

individual's physiological, physical, psychological and emotional traits. Melzack (2001) states that sensory inputs and cognitive events, such as psychological stress, can modulate the neuro-signature pattern. It may also occur because stressors, physical as well as psychological, act on stress-regulation systems, which may produce lesions of muscle, bone and nerve tissue, thereby contributing to the neuro-signature patterns that give rise to chronic pain. Therefore this theoretical proposition relating to the neuromatrix of pain explains that the nature of pain represents a change in thinking (McAllister 2017). The neuromatrix model stands in contrast to the widely held belief which associates pain with tissue damage and resultant detection by the PNS. Furthermore, this model places the 'placebo affect' in new light.

Neuroplasticity and Pain

The concept of neuroplasticity refers to the capacity of the brain to change and adapt and is a physiological response to experience. The shift in neuroplasticity changes the structure in the brain and with every thought, emotion or new experience we reinforce the neural pathway. This 'neuroplasticity' is described as the muscle-building part of the brain and repeated thoughts and actions lead to physiological changes. Moreover, neuroplasticity is active throughout life and neural connections are constantly weakening or strengthening dependent upon activity. Furthermore, evidence supports the theory that neurogenesis (generation of new brain cells) does continue into and throughout adult life, although only in specific areas of the brain. Sibille et al. (2016) state that neuroplastic changes in the brain structure and function are associated with pain and the consequence of chronic pain can be responsible for the maintenance of pain symptoms. Furthermore, they suggest that evidence has identified a wide range of methods which can 'reopen', and stimulate neuroplastic responsiveness and enhance plasticity of the brain. Therefore treatments and rehabilitation programmes, tailored to the individual's needs, can enhance neuroplasticity and optimise the brain's ability to adapt, learn and interpret added information and improve treatment outcomes and quality of life.

Allostatic Load Theory

Sterling and Eyer (1988) proposed the 'allostatic load theory (allostosis)'. It describes an additional process of reestablishing homeostasis, but more recently the theory extends to suggest that persistent exposure to deleterious social and economic conditions activates the human body's fight–flight–fight response in perpetuity. The response to stress highlights that the brain dramatically adapts between the interface of the biological self and the changing environment; thus, there is a convergence between a biological and a psychosocial model. The core emotional regions of the brain constitute the primary mediator of the well-established association between stress and health, as well as the neural focus of 'wear and tear' due to the ongoing adaptation. The persistent exposure to stress hormones such as when an individual is experiencing persistent pain leads to negative health outcomes (Sibille et al. 2017).

Pain Physiology and Functional Anatomy – An Overview

The physiology of pain is complex and not fully understood. However, in summary the generation of pain follows a basic three-step process.
1. Injury occurs and special nerve cells called nociceptors detect the damage.

2. When nociceptors detect tissue damage, pain impulses travel towards the central nervous system.

3. The brain then establishes the extent and significance of the tissue damage.

Nociceptors (noxious sensation receptors) are specialised neurones found throughout the body, especially in the skin. The speed that nociceptors transmit pain messages varies and is dependent on the diameter of the axon and whether it is myelinated. Larger axons can conduct pain messages faster than small axons. Myelin acts as an electrical insulator, which also increases transmission velocity. Nociceptors may be mechanoceptors or polymodal nociceptors, which are responsible for diverse types of impulses and have distinctive characteristics. For example, mechanoceptors respond to pressure over a wide skin area, whereas polymodal receptors respond to tissue damage caused by mechanical stimuli, chemicals released in response to damaged tissue, for example kinins, histamine, 5-hydroxytryptamine (5-HT, serotonin), substance P and prostaglandins, or thermal insults. Silent nociceptors, which are inactive or in a resting state, are refractory to mechanical or electrical stimuli. However, in the presence of tissue damage or inflammation, the nociceptors 'switch on' and become active (Wheeldon 2022).

Once a nociceptor detects tissue damage, an electrical impulse is conducted along an afferent (sensory) neurone. The impulse travels in the dorsal columns of the spinal cord to the brain. The impulse may be modified by the gate control mechanism within the spinal cord. Impulses can also be modified by descending control from the brain. Further modification in the spinal cord and brain stem prevents pain impulses ever reaching consciousness. The brain stem then processes and integrates pain sensations, and endogenous opioid neurotransmitters capable of reducing pain perception are released from brain tissue, for example endorphins and enkephalins.

CLASSIFICATION OF PAIN

For nurses to provide evidence-based care, it is crucial to understand the person's pain experience, which in its broadest sense is classified according to timescale (Chamley and James 2013) (Fig. 20.2). However, timescale may be too simplistic for the complex spectrum of the pain experience. Pain can also be classified according to factors such as the presumed origin that may include related pathology and type of pain or clinical specialty and client group. Historically, pain has been considered as being either acute or chronic, but clear distinctions or the transition between the two are not easily discernible (Finnerup et al. 2022).

Acute Pain

This is often described as being short lived, that is, less than 6 weeks' duration, and is commonly nociceptive pain associated with surgery, trauma or acute disease. Acute pain will usually diminish as healing occurs before ceasing completely. Acute pain may occur suddenly, or the onset may be slower. It can be of any intensity ranging from a mild headache to agonising chest pain with a major heart attack (see Chapter 2, Nursing Patients With Cardiovascular Disorders). Acute episodes of pain occur throughout life. These episodes are usually self-contained and sometimes predictable, for example in people who experience migraine or sickle cell disease episodes, but in between these episodes, the individual is pain free. Ongoing time-limited pain (chronic–acute) may last for a prolonged period but usually it will cease once the cause is removed or treated, such as with burns pain. Four processes participate in acute nociceptive pain: transduction, transmission, modulation and perception (MacMahon et al. 2013).

Transduction occurs when nociceptors of C fibres and A-δ fibres of afferent neurones respond to painful stimuli causing the release of inflammatory chemicals including prostaglandins, kinins, histamine and 5-HT, forming an 'algesic (pain causing) soup'. The categories of noxious stimuli include:

- mechanical – pressure, swelling, abscess, incision and tumours
- thermal – burns and scalds
- chemical – including inflammation/infection, ischaemia and toxins.

The effects of inflammatory chemicals released from damaged tissue can be modified by nonsteroidal anti-inflammatory drugs (NSAIDs), for example ibuprofen.

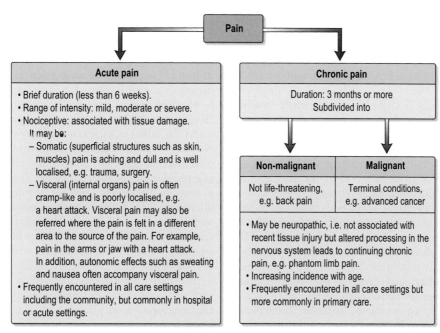

Figure 20.2 Types of pain. (Reproduced from Brooker C, Waugh A, eds. *Foundations of Nursing Practice: Fundamentals of Holistic Care.* Edinburgh: Mosby; 2007 with permission.)

Transmission. The pain impulse is transmitted from the site of transduction along the nociceptor fibre to the dorsal horn of the spinal cord and onwards to the brain stem, thalamus, the cerebral cortex and higher centres. As there is no dedicated pain centre, impulses that arrive in the thalamus are directed to multiple areas within the brain for processing. Opioid pharmacological treatments for pain interfere with the transmission of pain impulses along the pathway between the site of tissue injury and the cerebral cortex, for example topical anaesthetic and analgesic (against pain) products.

Modulation. This occurs when the pain impulse is inhibited or changed (modulated) by chemical or neural influences on the 'pain gate'. The complex and multiple pathways involved in pain modulation are described as the descending modulatory pain pathways, and activities within these pathways can either increase transmission of pain impulses (excitatory) or inhibit or decrease transmission. Nerves descending from the brain stem to the spinal cord close the gate by releasing endogenous opioids, and this may be the reason nociceptive pain is responsive to opioids and accounts for the variation in pain perception seen in clinical practice. That is, a proportion of patients have more effective modulation than others (MacMahon et al. 2013). Chamley and James (2013) draw our attention to the 'placebo effect', which has been identified in individuals who have an analgesic response to a masked inert substance (such as a sugar pill) in a double-blind trial of inert substance versus an active drug. Some individuals respond to the placebo whilst others have a poor or no response. Placebo responders may be those with a well-developed endogenous opioid system.

Perception is the result of neural activity where pain becomes a conscious multidimensional experience. As there is no 'pain centre' in the brain, pain perception occurs through an 'action system'. Opioid-binding sites have been identified in several parts of the brain, indicating that they have a role in pain perception. When painful stimuli are transmitted to the brain stem and thalamus, multiple cortical areas are activated, and a response is elicited. The first aspect of pain perception is warning and protection, and the individual would rapidly assess what has occurred and initiate action (Melzack and Wall 2005), but psychological factors also have an important role, for example anxiety, emotional distress and helplessness are known to increase pain perception. The person's previous experiences of pain will influence their response.

The perception of pain is complex and dynamic involving sensory impulses relayed from the pain gates and activation of pain responses mediated through the reticular system, somatosensory cortex and the limbic system (Wheeldon 2021).

The neurophysiology of acute pain is complex. and intense acute pain is often accompanied by physiological effects, for example tachycardia and sweating, as the body responds to the potent stressor. Initially, these are activated by the sympathetic division of the autonomic nervous system and are referred to as 'flight or fight' responses which are automatic, primitive survival mechanisms. It is important for nurses to understand the physiological and behavioural effects of pain (Information 20.1). This is crucial when caring for people who have difficulties in communication or are unable to articulate their pain, such as preverbal children, individuals who have learning disabilities and associated communication problems or people with dementia.

INFORMATION 20.1

Physiological and Behavioural Responses to Pain

Physiological responses include:
- Sweating
- Increased heart rate, respiratory rate and blood pressure
- Vomiting due to gastric stasis
  Behavioural responses include:
- Anxiety
- Withdrawal and lack of cooperation
- Aggression, abusiveness, swearing, agitation
- Attention seeking
- Quietness
- Poor concentration (focused on pain)
- Grimacing, frowning
- Rubbing or holding the painful part
- Thrashing about, pacing, adopting a particular position, keeping very still
- Moaning, shouting, screaming, crying
- In children, fractiousness, food refusal, withdrawal
  People who have learning disabilities may exhibit changes in their behaviour, but it is important that the pain is recognised and changes in behaviour are not just attributed to personality/disability.

Adapted from Chamley C, James G. Pain management – minimizing the pain experience. In: Brooker C, Waugh A, eds. *Foundations of Nursing Practice: Fundamentals of Holistic Care.* 2nd ed. Edinburgh: Mosby; 2013:653-679.

Referred Pain

Referred pain occurs when acute nociceptive pain originates in an internal organ such as the heart and the pain is experienced away from the chest, that is, in the arms (particularly the left arm) or the back, neck and jaw. This is due to sensory impulses from the left arm and the heart entering the spinal cord at the same level. Normally, few sensory impulses are processed from the heart, so when more impulses than normal are received to be processed, this results in the perception of pain in the arm. The pain is usually referred to a structure developed from the same embryonic structure or sclerotome (Tortora and Derrickson 2016).

Chronic Pain

Chronic pain is pain with no clear underlying cause or pain (or its impact) that is out of proportion to any observable injury or disease (National Institute for Health and Care Excellence 2021, p. 40). Increasingly, the term 'persistent pain' is used to describe chronic pain and to classify pain by pathophysiological mechanisms including nociceptive and neuropathic pain (see later). Nociceptive pain is caused by tissue damage, whereas neuropathic pain describes pain that persists beyond the original cause, such as a nerve injury or infective cause. These pain types are defined as non-life-threatening (benign) or nonmalignant. Pain may be intermittent, for example irritable bowel syndrome (IBS), rheumatoid arthritis or back pain. The pain has not responded to conventional treatment and may last for life. Low back pain affects around 33% of the UK population, with 1 in 15 people needing to consult with their GP (Reflection 20.2).

The exact mechanisms involved in the pathophysiology of chronic persistent pain are complex and to date remain unclear. Even after the original acute painful episode has healed, chronic pain may manifest, and in some instances presents with no initial physiological assault. Chronic pain may follow injury or disease with rapid long-term changes occurring within the CNS, particularly if the acute

REFLECTION 20.2

Chronic Pain and Trauma

Chronic pain after trauma is associated with serious clinical, social and economic burden. Due to limitations in trauma registry data and previous studies, the current prevalence of chronic pain after trauma is unknown, and little is known about the association of pain with other long-term outcomes. We sought to describe the long-term burden of self-reported pain after injury and determine its association with positive screen for posttraumatic stress disorder (PTSD), functional status and return to work (Herrera-Escobar et al. 2018).

Activity

Access the study by Herrera-Escobar et al. (2018). Reflect upon the outcomes from this study and consider the implications that follow a traumatic event and how this can impact the lives of individuals daily.

Resource

Herrera-Escobar JP, Apoi M, Weed C, et al. Association of pain after trauma with long-term functional and mental health outcomes. J Trauma Acute Care Surg. 2018;85(4):773-779.

episode was not effectively managed. Within the spinal cord a central mechanism exists known as 'wind-up', which has links to physiological hypersensitivity and hyperexcitability. Wind-up occurs when there are repeated, prolonged and sustained noxious stimuli which cause the dorsal horn cells to fire and transmit progressively increasing numbers of pain impulses (Mendell 2022).

During episodes of chronic pain, sensitisation can occur. There is also amplification and distortion of pain messages, and the pain sensed is out of proportion to the original injury (Field and Smith 2019). Furthermore, spinal cord sensitisation can result from chemical reactions which increase pain messages being forwarded to the brain. PNS sensitisation can result from inflammation which causes nociceptors to fire with greater intensity.

Chronic pain is subdivided into:
- chronic nonmalignant pain (nociceptive and neuropathic pain); NB both types may coexist
- malignant (life-threatening) pain
- chronic nonmalignant pain.

There is persuasive evidence which suggests that chronic pain is a widespread public health issue (NICE 2021a). Across Europe for example, it is estimated that around 18% of people live with chronic pain (Scottish Intercollegiate Guidelines Network [SIGN] 2019). Chronic nonmalignant pain can be caused by persistent tissue injury where a degenerative condition exists and between 35% and 51% of the UK population experience chronic pain in one form or another (Fayaz et al. 2016). It is thought that chronic nonmalignant pain involves physiological changes to pain processing in the CNS which results in pain memories and leads to conditions such as phantom pain following amputation.

See Evolve website Critical thinking question 20.1

Chronic nonmalignant pain can be as destructive as malignant pain, as eventually it impacts on the individual's family and social life and employment and it leads to sleep deprivation, feelings of helplessness and depression (Chary 2021). *Chronic malignant pain* is associated with life-threatening conditions and most frequently with cancer in which there may be progressive spread of the disease, which contributes to the chronicity of pain.

Pain associated with cancer is rarely a presenting feature, but the person's 'cancer journey' may begin with acute pain (nociceptive) resulting from diagnostic procedures, including surgery. If the cancer metastasises, the pain becomes chronic, involving nociceptive and neuropathic elements but also psychoemotional ones. There needs to be regular assessment and readjustment of treatment to meet the needs of the individual; this requires the skills of an MDT (see Chapter 31, Nursing the Patient With Cancer, and Chapter 32, Nursing Patients Who Need Palliative Care). The prevalence of cancer increases with age, and pain is one of the most distressing symptoms. Unfortunately, for older people, it is more likely that pain will be underreported and undertreated.

Depression may occur concomitantly as chronic pain may exacerbate depression and vice versa. The link between chronic pain and depression is well established (IsHak et al. 2018) and it is estimated that around 85% of patients living with chronic pain will also suffer from depression (Sheng et al. 2017). Given that chronic pain impacts on around one-third of the population, the burden on mental health should not be underestimated (Howarth and Poole 2019). Pain disorder or the chronic pain syndrome is a specific syndrome characterised by:
- Pain as the predominant presenting complaint.
- Pain causing significant distress or impairment in social, occupational or other aspects of life.
- Psychological factors that are considered to play a significant role in the onset, severity exacerbation and/or maintenance of pain.
- No malingering.
- No alternative explanation such as depressive disorder, including anxiety or mood disorders.

There are advantages in the recognition and acceptance of pain disorder – there is the recognition that affective factors need to be addressed for there to be a chance of improvement for the person. There is the need to acknowledge that chronic pain is an illness and that it warrants holistic management embracing the wholeness of the individual.

Nociceptive Pain

Nociceptive pain is the most common type of pain seen in clinical settings and may be somatic or visceral (see Fig. 20.2). Pain results from stimulation of nociceptors following tissue damage or inflammation, for example surgery, infection or trauma. Intense and ongoing stimulation of nociceptors increases the excitability of neurones in the spinal cord leading to central sensitisation.

Neuropathic Pain

Neuropathic pain is initiated or caused by a primary lesion or disease of the somatic nervous system (IASP 2022). The damage to the PNS and CNS can be due to stroke, spinal cord injury, brachial plexus avulsion, herpes zoster (shingles) leading to postherpetic neuralgia or following amputation. Damage leads to the development of central sensitisation causing reorganisation of synapses in the spinal cord and hyperexcitability in the peripheral nerves, and as a result the individual experiences symptoms that are characteristic of neuropathic pain. This definition has attracted criticism, being described as vague, particularly in relation to the term 'dysfunction' which blurs the distinction between neuropathic pain and other pain types that may arise from different underlying mechanisms. It has been observed that pain and other neurological symptoms due to PNS or CNS disease/injury present in very similar ways, and this observation has led to a group designation of neuropathic pain (Dimos-Dimitrios et al. 2022).

This definition is based upon the presence of neurological disease; however, it is important to note that most disorders that involve the nociceptors responsive to thermal stimuli do not present with pain and would suggest that these people have conditions that are genetic in origin. Affected individuals can experience increased sympathetic activity including sweating and changes to skin colour, texture and temperature. Pain in an area of sensory loss may be described as spontaneous, paroxysmal, sharp, shooting or stabbing. Depending on the exact cause, it may manifest as:

- Phantom (limb) pain/syndrome – feeling that a limb is still part of the body following amputation. The pain felt appears to originate from the amputated limb. It is caused by altered pain processing in the CNS, due to earlier nerve or tissue damage. Effective pain relief before amputation can minimise the risk of this occurring. If phantom pain does become chronic, treatment with nerve blocks and adjuvant drugs, and/or various nonpharmacological therapies such as ultrasound, relaxation or transcutaneous electrical nerve stimulation (TENS), may be helpful.
- Allodynia – sensation of pain in response to a nonnoxious stimulus, such as touch.
- Hyperalgesia – extreme sensitivity to a stimulus that is normally painful.
- Dysaesthesia – abnormal sensations, e.g. tingling, burning or numbness.
- Neuropathic pain may respond poorly to opioids.

🌐 **See Evolve website Critical thinking question 20.1**

Psychological (Soul) Pain

Psychological pain described as nonbiological in origin is also referred to as 'algopsychalia' and 'psychalgia' and refers to psychological states described as mental pain, emotional suffering, soul pain, social pain, spiritual pain or psychic pain. The term was coined by Shneidman in the field of suicidology in 1996 (Shneidman 1996) and more recently it is suggested that physical pain and psychological pain potentially may share underlying neurological mechanisms. Regions of the brain that are suggested as being consistently found to be implicated in both types of pain are the anterior cingulate and prefrontal cortices of the brain. Soul pain may result from a traumatic event such as bereavement, divorce or another life event and is a deep visceral pain which is all-consuming at times. Simington (2011) describes it as:

> *The sum of the physical, mental, emotional, and social distress experienced following a tragic life event. ….Soul pain is a crisis of the human spirit. It is suffering of the deepest kind. It is a plague deep within. It is a wrestling with the imponderable questions of life and death, of heaven and hell, of resurrection and reincarnation.*

Simington (2011) outlines the three phases of soul pain as a journey:
1. We come to the journey struggling and questioning the meaning of this experience, and we might attempt to obliterate the discomforting effects of the situation which may also have physical manifestations.
2. We succumb to the exhaustion and struggle, which at times is all-consuming and we start to become absorbed in our attempts to find answers.
3. During this phase, we become keenly aware that through the pain of the experience we have become something/someone different because of our journey. The experience of this life event/tragedy has moulded and reshaped us.

KEY CONCEPTS

This section of the chapter outlines the concepts of pain threshold and pain tolerance – terms often confused and used erroneously. Pain myths/misconceptions and individual differences in pain tolerance (related to gender and cultural influences) are discussed.

Pain Threshold

The pain threshold is 'the minimum intensity of stimulus that is perceived as painful' (IASP 2022). Laboratory studies of pain have demonstrated that pain thresholds are constant across the population. In other words, most people agree on the point at which a sensation becomes painful.

Pain Tolerance

Pain tolerance is 'the maximum intensity of a pain-producing stimulus that a subject is willing to accept in a given situation' (IASP 2022). Pain tolerance must be distinguished from drug threshold. Pain tolerance differs widely amongst people and is a far more important concept than pain threshold in medicine and nursing, as it usually means that the pain has gone beyond an acceptable tolerance level, and at this point the individual will seek professional help (Field and Smith 2019).

Advancing age is known to be associated with a greater prevalence of pain, with people between the ages of 75 and 85 at greatest prevalence. Thereafter, pain prevalence decreases with age (Schofield 2018) (Evidence-Based Practice 20.1). Moreover, older adults are more likely to have comorbidities and polypharmacy. There is little evidence to suggest that neonates, infants and children have a different pain tolerance from adults and the previously held belief that infants were incapable of experiencing pain is now completely accepted to be a myth (Alotaibi et al. 2019).

Pain Myths

Pain management may be subject to traditional and ill-informed prejudice which sometimes holds sway over evidence and a common-sense approach to pain management. There are enduring myths, misconceptions, false judgements, mistaken beliefs and misunderstandings which reflect outmoded beliefs and lack of knowledge and understanding in relation to the pain experience of another (Information 20.2). Children have been disadvantaged over time, as it has only been since the 1970s that child pain assessment and management have attracted any interest. The lack of scientific evidence encouraged poor practice: children, in particular infants, were operated upon, sutured, injected and subjected to intense levels of procedural pain. Advances in science and technology have provided evidence that refutes many of these myths and increasingly evidence-based practice is used to provide effective pain management across the lifespan.

A barrier to effective pain relief was linked to misconceptions relating to medications, particularly opioids, among healthcare professionals. There was concern regarding opioid addiction, tolerance and hyperalgesia, including correct dosage, escalation and physical dependence. Fear of opioids among healthcare professionals is compounded by their ignorance of opioids (Volkow and Thomas-McLellan, 2016). At the heart of these concerns are inadequate education and training among healthcare professionals and

EVIDENCE-BASED PRACTICE 20.1

Assessment of Pain in Older Adults: UK National Guidelines 2018 (Schofield 2018)

Millions of people who live in the UK experience chronic pain and as we go into older age, it is suggested that up to 93% of people have pain which is often 'expected to be part of ageing' or something that they must 'learn to live with'. One of the fundamental issues regarding pain management in any age group is assessment of pain. This can be particularly challenging in older adults due to the age-related changes in vision, hearing and cognition. Literature has suggested in the past that we have around 50% of the older population who live in the community experiencing uncontrolled chronic pain. This guidance highlights the problems in assessing and managing pain in an ever-increasing older population. The prevalence of pain has been established to be in the order of one in four of the adult population, with between 25% and 30% having pain that leads to other comorbidities, resulting in a very poor quality of life. These problems become more frequent with advancing years and are often associated with difficulty in conveying the intensity and quality of the pain, as well as the impact that it has on the patient's life. As we describe pain as the 'fifth vital sign', a fundamental principal underpinning this is that we should measure the pain alongside routine observations. Just because someone does not have the ability to tell us that they have pain in a language that we can understand, does not mean that we should not measure it, as we would with any other adult or patient in our care. These guidelines provide a range of tools which demonstrate good validity and reliability for clinical practice in assessing pain in older people. There is permission to use them and so they should be implemented from this formal documentation by all healthcare providers in every care setting across the UK (Schofield 2018).

Activity

Access the full article by Schofield (2018). Consider how these guidelines may be implemented in your area of practice and discuss with your mentor or Practice Facilitator.

Resource

Schofield P. The assessment of pain in older people: UK guidelines. *Age Ageing*. 2018;47:i1-i22. Available from the Institute for Chronic Pain and online at https://www.ncbi.nlm.nih.gov/pmc/articles/PMC5888957/pdf/afx192.pdf.

INFORMATION 20.2

Pain Myths: Explained

Pain is the earliest symptom of cancer. A myth, except in cancers involving nerve tissue or bone. Pain is usually a late symptom of advanced cancer.

Older adults and health professionals may believe that chronic pain is inevitable during ageing. This myth is firmly embedded in sociocultural beliefs and poses significant barriers to pain relief for older people. Pain may be overlooked as part of the ageing process. It is a common symptom associated with comorbidities of old age. The ability of the older person to withstand chronic illness and pain may also depend upon their circumstances and coping mechanisms.

Pain medication always causes heavy sedation. People with chronic and enduring pain will have had problems sleeping. Therefore opioid analgesics may produce some initial sedation for 24 hours which allows them some rest and sleep.

Infants cannot feel pain due to their immature nervous system. Complete development of nerves is not required for pain perception, and neonates exhibit both behavioural and physiological responses to pain.

Infants and children experience less pain than adults. Younger children may perceive a greater intensity of pain than older children and adults.

A person's behaviour accurately reflects their level of pain. Children and adults who are sleeping, or who are active, playing or working may still be experiencing pain but are coping with it.

Psychological dependence and respiratory depression are common side-effects of opioid analgesics. These are uncommon side-effects but fear of them can hamper effective pain management.

Some types of pain cannot be treated. Some types of pain require combined approaches (multimodality) for effective pain relief. The recent advances in pain management ensure that all types of pain can be controlled.

People need to be in hospital to receive effective pain management. It is easier to provide safe and effective pain relief at home than it is in the average hospital.

Treating depression in older people with chronic illness has negligible effect on coping with pain. Depression in older people enhances coping with the pain associated with chronic illnesses and improves quality of life.

Complementary and alternative therapies do not have a key role in pain management. Various techniques can be used by people as coping strategies for managing pain.

---

patients who express concerns about opioids, particularly with advancing age. Known as 'opiophobia', this is common among palliative care patients (up to 50%) treated with strong opioids. Furthermore, NICE guidelines recommend that a physician first discuss with the patient the potential concerns about opioid analgesics before prescribing them (Graczyk et al. 2018).

Research conducted over the past 20 years suggests that nurses still lack adequate information about pain management and often underestimate the patient's pain intensity (Cousins et al. 2022). Opioids remain the drug of choice for the treatment of moderate to severe pain regardless of aetiology, but fear of opioid misuse and addiction continues to shape policy and prescription of these drugs (Volkow and Thomas-McLellan, 2016).

Individual Differences in Pain Perception

The way in which an individual perceives and responds to pain is unique to the individual and is the culmination of variables that include gender, past pain experiences and social and cultural factors. Furthermore, it is recognised that pain experiences early in life can influence pain processing over the rest of the lifespan, as is illustrated in children who remember their early pain experiences but can learn to modify their responses. The interrelationship between pain, anxiety and fear has been extensively investigated and the evidence would suggest that anxiety and fear magnify pain, particularly in children. Therefore the person's emotional state is important, and several factors contribute to that state, including diagnosis, prognosis, coping ability and their social support networks coupled with their own beliefs and meanings they assign to pain (Field and Smith 2019).

Locus of control testing indicates how people will respond and adapt to pain. People with an internal locus of control believe that through their own behaviour they more readily exert control over their own health; the perception of lack of control can result in increased anxiety. Those with an external locus of control believe that they have little or no influence over the outcomes of their pain experience and that their health is in the 'hands of others', fate or chance. They may therefore appear to be very dependent upon others.

Contemporary thinking has moved away from the idea that personality and overt pain behaviours are interrelated and places greater emphasis upon the mental processes such as memory, locus of control, self-efficacy and comprehension that help to mediate individual pain behaviour (Chamley and James 2013).

Gender

The perceived wisdom is that men are more stoical and more able to tolerate pain than women. This is associated with their reluctance to report pain or seek medical help. When compared to men, women are often thought of as being more sensitive to pain and more willing to vocalise their discomfort and seek medical help. Furthermore, conditions in which pain is the only symptom are more common in women than men. Such conditions, however, tend to be viewed with less concern by medical professionals. There is, therefore a cultural paradox in which women are more likely to experience pain and to seek help, yet their pain experiences are taken less seriously by medical professionals, with female pain experiences often dismissed as being psychological or nonexistent (Samulowitz et al. 2018). While these differences are well documented, they are cultural rather than biological and it is important that nurses recognise them as such.

Cultural Influences on Pain Expression

Each cultural group is considered to have its own behaviours, beliefs, values and meaning 'scripts' that shape responses to pain, as well as help-seeking activities and receptivity to healthcare interventions. For example, British people are thought to value the control of their pain, often referred to as 'maintaining a stiff upper lip', whereas in other cultures, it is acceptable to vocalise pain and be seen to be visibly upset and disturbed. As with gender, observed cultural differences in pain expression are not biological, rather they are social and based on upbringing and life experience. The influence of culture on the experience and expression of pain has more recently been explored through narrative research, and cultural attitudes towards the pain experience remain prevalent, and still influence pain management decisions (Puntillo et al. 2021). Therefore it remains essential for nurses to seek to understand the influence of culture on the pain experience and to take a non-judgemental approach to pain assessment and management (Wheeldon 2022).

Pain in the Older Person

It is estimated that around 50% of older people experience chronic pain. In residential homes and care facilities, chronic pain incidence rises to around 80% (Miaskowski et al. 2020). As we age, chronic pain increases in complexity, complainants highlighting multiple sites of pain and different types of pain at any one time (Butera et al. 2019, Thakral et al. 2016). Chronic pain in older adults is further complicated by social attitudes towards pain and pain management. Nurses may find that older people are reluctant to report their discomfort or accept or take analgesics. This could be due to a desire not to be a burden or that people view pain as an inevitable consequence of aging. Anxiety and trepidation could also be a factor. Older people often express fears of addiction, for example, or they may be concerned that their pain signifies mortally (Veal et al. 2018).

MANAGEMENT OF PAIN

Pain assessment and measurement are critical to the holistic care and management of the individual's pain: one of the most challenging and commonly undertaken tasks for nurses. Pain assessment is complex and depends upon the interaction of several variables, not least the therapeutic relationship between the nurse and the person with pain. Objective and systematic assessment of pain is a fundamental right of everyone and Article 3 of the Human Rights Act (1998) states that 'No one shall be subject to torture or to inhumane or degrading treatment or punishment'.

The NMC states that to provide optimal care nurses require appropriate knowledge, skills and attitudes towards pain and the associated assessment and management of the patients' pain journey. This must be based upon the best available evidence to prevent patients from suffering (NMC 2018). It is unacceptable for people to experience unmanaged pain, or for nurses to have inadequate knowledge about pain and poor understanding of their professional accountability in this aspect of care (Dimond 2016). Furthermore, pain has been identified as the fifth vital sign to facilitate and engender greater accountability for pain assessment and management (Campbell 2016). The 'gold standard' is to ask and believe the person about their pain experience and assessment should not be based upon, for instance, the expected pain associated with a particular surgical procedure or a medical condition, which will underestimate the pain.

There is no single test for pain, and to date, there is no single evidence-based document for pain management. There are, however, a variety of measures that can inform the overall pain assessment, including biomedical, psychosocial and behavioural responses.

Pain Assessment

Pain assessment also encompasses pain measurement (see later). Assessment is the overall appraisal of the factors that are influencing the experience and expression of pain. This is the comprehensive process of describing the pain and its effect upon the person's function based upon a systematic process of assessment, measurement and reassessment or evaluation. Melzack and Katz (2013) outline the aims of assessment, including to:
- determine the intensity, quality and duration of pain
- aid diagnosis
- determine the most appropriate therapy
- evaluate the relative effectiveness of different treatment modalities
- monitor the standards of clinical practice.

Field and Smith (2019) suggest four main approaches to pain assessment:
1. Talk to the person.
2. Observe the person's behaviour.
3. Record physiological signs.
4. Use appropriate pain assessment tools.

Talking with the person and discussing their pain are the most fundamental ways to assess the pain – after all, only the person with the pain knows how much it hurts. This aspect of pain assessment is often undervalued and studies report that few patients were asked about their pain and consequently experienced unnecessary pain (Wooldridge and Banning 2020). The interplay of variables can influence this process. In the first instance the person may be reluctant to report pain because they do not want to worry family or interrupt the work of busy nursing staff. Children may lack either the language or cognitive ability, and adults with learning disabilities or cognitive impairment such as dementia may not be able to articulate their pain. Furthermore, personal biases, myths and prejudices of the nurses, who may believe that pain should be managed according to their own views of pain, may influence the assessment.

Pain Measurement

Measuring pain enables the nurse to assess the amount of pain the person is experiencing. Where possible the person's self-report of their pain is regarded as the highest standard of pain assessment measures by providing the most valid pain measurement (Ford 2019). Pain measurement enables appropriate intervention, evaluation and understanding of the individual's pain. Measurement refers to pain on a scale, which is the application of a metric to a specific element, usually pain intensity. Therefore pain should be measured using an appropriate pain assessment tool that identifies both quantitative and/or qualitative dimensions of the person's pain. However, an assumption may be made that pain measurement is subjective and therefore will be of little value. Furthermore, some nursing staff distrust patients' self-reporting of pain, which suggests that some nurses may have their own personal benchmarks of what is deemed acceptable as to when and how people should express their pain (Wooldridge and Banning 2020). The reality is that if measurements are conducted properly, sensitive and consistent results can be obtained. However, there are circumstances when it may not be possible to measure pain or when reports are likely to be unreliable. Most acute pain analgesic studies include measurements of pain intensity and/or pain relief and the commonest tools are categorical and visual analogue scales (VASs) (see later).

❖ Nursing Management and Health Promotion: Assessing and Measuring Pain

Pain assessment, which includes pain measurement, is the responsibility of every nurse – not just those nurse specialists working within pain teams.

Pain is measured on a scale without taking into consideration any other component related to pain, such as mood (Chamley and James 2013). A valid pain assessment is one that involves the person in pain, meaning that the nurse should not assess the patient's pain in isolation from the patient (Field and Smith 2019). Always asking the person about their pain ensures that they can verbalise (if able) their unique pain experience (Gregory 2019).

Therefore communication skills are essential for effective pain assessment and the nurse must consider how she/he frames questions. Questions that may help to understand and characterise the person's pain include:

- When did your pain start?
- How long does it usually last?
- Is there anything which makes the pain worse (such as movement or eating/drinking)?
- Where does it hurt?
- Does the pain stop you from doing anything?
- What do you do to relieve your pain?
- Does the pain occur at certain times of the day or night?
- Does the pain stop you from sleeping?

Nurses need to be aware of potential barriers and individual differences in the expression of pain, such as age, cognitive ability, gender and culture. Also, nurses should not be influenced by their own beliefs, prejudices, first-hand experiences, attitudes and values (Field and Smith 2019). Equally, it is crucial to acknowledge that for some people, verbal communication may be absent or difficult because of coexisting pathology, for example after a stroke, or other language difficulties, or when the language is not understood or fully developed. This is because during assessment of the individual's pain, the nurse is not only measuring pain intensity but asking what this experience means to the person and how it affects their activities of living.

The essential issues of pain assessment are:

- Ask about the pain but appreciate that people may not use traditional descriptors for their pain (see later).
- Accept and respect what they have to say about their pain – they know it best.
- Intervene appropriately to relieve the pain.
- Ask them after intervention about their pain.

Many words are used to describe the sensation of pain. The following box contains the words most often used.

Aching	Cutting	Heavy	Pressing	Stinging
Agonising	Discomfort	Hurting	Punishing	Takes my breath away
Biting	Dragging	Irritation	Scalding	Tearing
Boring	Drawing	Lancing	Sharp	Tender
Burning	Dull	Penetrating	Shooting	Throbbing
Bursting	Exhausting	Piercing	Smarting	Tingle
Colicky	Gnawing	Pinching	Soreness	Twinge
Cramping	Grinding	Pins and needles	Spasms	Torture
Crushing	Gripping	Pounding	Stabbing	Wearing

Pain assessment is cyclical (assess–plan–intervention–evaluation) involving the MDT working interprofessionally to secure positive outcomes for the person.

Observation alone is difficult and unreliable but should not be dismissed. People who are in pain may articulate this in their behavioural responses, especially infants and children who do not have the language skills and people with cognitive impairment.

Pain Maps

Pain maps are increasingly used during assessment to help identify or locate the person's pain. These comprise a picture of a body outline (anterior and posterior) combined with other forms of evaluation; the person marks or identifies the areas of pain and records other information, such as intensity, nature of the pain(s) and what makes it worse or better.

🌐 **See Evolve website Fig. 20.1**

The maps are an important way for the person to retain 'ownership' of their pain management, empowering carers and patients, particularly those with chronic pain. Pain maps are useful tools for evaluating pain.

Pain Diaries

Keeping a pain diary can be an effective means of identifying patterns of pain and this can be useful especially for people who experience chronic pain. Pain diaries can also inform the assessment and management process because people may document the complex components associated with the pain experience, such as the emotional, social and financial effects, as well as the physical.

Pain Assessment Tools

Pain assessment tools must be dependable and valid. Reliability refers to consistency, stability and the reproducibility of measurements made by different nurses. Validity refers to the appropriateness, applicability and the representativeness of measurements which reflect the true findings of an individual's pain at any given time.

A further consideration is that assessing different pain types requires different pain assessment tools that are appropriate for the age and cognitive ability of the individual. To assess acute pain the nurse may use a tool that is quick and easy to use, for example a VAS, numerical rating scale (NRS) or a verbal/descriptive scale. However, the assessment of types of chronic pain, including pain associated with cancer, may require a more detailed assessment tool that can be used to provide a more comprehensive analysis of the person's pain and how it might be relieved (Field and Smith 2019).

Pain assessment tools may be unidimensional or multidimensional. Unidimensional tools collect and measure one dimension of the pain experience, for example pain intensity. They are accurate, quick and easy to use and understand, for example body map, numerical scales, picture scales or verbal rating scales (VRSs). Multidimensional tools capture both qualitative and quantitative pain data. They are useful for neuropathic pain, but they do require that the person be able to communicate effectively, and they take longer to complete. Examples include the Hospital Anxiety and Depression Questionnaire (HAD), Brief Pain Inventory, McGill Pain Questionnaire (MPQ), Pain Disability Index, cognitively impaired/dementia pain scales and Multidimensional Pain Inventory.

Observational tools are useful for people with altered consciousness or who are sedated or cognitively impaired. These tools assess physiological responses and behavioural responses, such as grimace or restlessness. Global scales are useful to rate the effectiveness of patient-controlled analgesia (PCA) for acute pain management, or TENS in chronic pain management. Pain assessment tools are classified as:

- self-report
- observational
- physiological measurement
- self-report pain assessment tools.

Self-report scales include a variety of simple methods to collect data relating to the person's pain (Reflection 20.3). These include VAS, NRS and VRS. Other scales in this category may also include questionnaires and interviews. Self-reporting can be adapted for children by modifying the scale, for example using a 'pain thermometer' scale, or children can use their own words on a scale of no pain to worst hurt. Moreover, Chamley and James (2013) suggest that the pain thermometer with a scale of 0–10/100 has been well received by older people. However, patient preference is all important with acceptability and engagement with a tool.

Visual Analogue Scale (VAS) is usually a 10-cm line (usually horizontal but can be vertical) with 'no pain' at one end and 'worst pain possible' at the other end (Fig. 20.3A). The person marks the position on the scale which best reflects their pain. The assessor measures the mark in centimetres from the left-hand side or the foot of a vertical scale to obtain the 'score'. The advantages of this scale include the absence of numbers or words; the person in pain is not required to assign a precise numerical value to the pain or to choose a word that may not exactly represent their pain. Furthermore, these tools can be modified to use with children (9–10 years) who have the cognitive ability to understand proportions and translate their experience into an analogue format (Chamley and James 2013).

Numerical Rating Scale (NRS) is like the VAS but is calibrated with the numbers 0–10 (Fig. 20.3B). The person selects a number on the scale which best describes their pain intensity.

Verbal Rating Scale (VRS) provides graded categories: 'no pain', 'slight pain', 'moderate pain', 'very bad pain' and 'agonising pain' (Fig. 20.3C). People often find this scale easy to use although it has the disadvantage of fewer assessment points compared to a 0–10 scale and therefore is not as sensitive.

The visual, numerical and verbal pain scales rate pain intensity, which is only one aspect of pain experience and therefore do not provide a holistic pain assessment. This was borne out by a participant in Whelan's (2003) study who commented on the difficulty of expressing the meaning of the pain when using a numerical scale: 'I wanted to put a meaning next to those numbers, so that if I said to my doctor "I'm having pain that's about a seven" what I mean is, it's really bad, it's incapacitating enough that I'm not able to do my daily duties, but it's not so bad that I'm not able to get out of bed'.

Detailed coverage of assessing children's pain is not within the scope of this chapter; however, all nurses will have contact with children even if only occasionally, such as in emergency departments or health centres, and resources are available to support this, including NICE guidelines. Children have the right to feel secure and to be nursed in an atmosphere where compassion, trust and caring are at the heart of all decisions. Accurate pain assessment in children and

REFLECTION 20.3

Pain Assessment Tools

With your mentor, discuss the pain assessment tools used in your practice area and consider the rationale for choice.

Activities

- Have there been any problems with implementation of the tools? If so, what were the main reasons for this?
- Reflect on how existing pain assessment tools could be adapted further to capture pain assessment data more effectively.
- Consider your patient group. Are there any barriers such as sociocultural or language barriers which could interfere with using self-report tools?
- How does pain audit in your area help to improve the pain experience of patients?

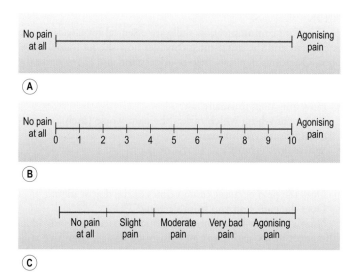

Figure 20.3 Self-report pain scales. (A) Visual analogue scale. (B) Numerical rating scale. (C) Verbal rating scale.

young people is complex and challenging and despite the significant impact of pain on the child, it is still reported as inadequately assessed and managed, particularly in areas such as learning disabilities and children who require palliative care (Warlow and Hain 2018).

Children and young people need careful consideration because of age, cognitive and developmental ability. However, several self-report scales are available and in current use for children, for example Faces Scale, Pain Thermometer, Colour Scale used together with a body map.

Groups With Special Needs

Whilst the assessment of pain is recognised as an essential component of quality care, the assessment and management of pain for certain groups need special consideration. Visually impaired individuals may not be able to use a VAS and may benefit from using a VRS which is adapted to their individual needs. Older adults may use a range of words other than pain to describe their pain, and cognitively impaired individuals may have problems using a range of pain measurement tools, but self-report tools have been reported as more effective. For people with marked cognitive impairment there is a range of NICE guidelines (see Useful Websites).

The British Pain Society has produced a series of pain scales to assist in the assessment of individuals whose first language is not English; for example, scales are available in Albanian, Arabic, Bengali, Chinese (simple and traditional), Greek, Gujarati, Hindi, Polish, Punjabi, Somali, Swahili, Turkish, Urdu, Vietnamese and Welsh (see Useful Websites).

Observation

Observation includes:

- pain behaviours
- verbal and motor responses
- sleep and rest patterns.

Observation of pain is difficult and unreliable but is usually based on verbal clues such as direct statements, as well as moaning, crying and sighing, and nonverbal clues such as grimacing, guarding, bracing and lying perfectly still. However, these clues do not have to be present for someone to be in pain. Indeed, such clues are frequently absent. Thus, caution should be exercised in the interpretation of nonverbal signals. However, they remain an important source of assessment for people who cannot respond verbally, such as those who have altered consciousness or are disorientated and confused. Ford (2019) stresses the importance of selecting the best available pain-behaviour assessment tool for use in nursing home residents who have dementia.

Physiological Measurements

The usefulness and reliability of physiological measurements continue to be debated and in part the difficulty is because physiological responses can be also attributed to competing stressors. It is also important to note that ongoing pain leads to adaptation, which may result in pain not presenting through physiological assessment. Physiological measurements relate to the objective measurement of pain. The parameters that are usually measured are vital signs such as heart rate, respiratory rate and oxygen saturation, and endocrine and metabolic responses. Although these measures have their limitations, they have been used in the assessment of neonatal pain as there are few reliable measures for this group. See the website for more information on biomedical, psychosocial and behavioural responses.

❖ Nursing Management and Health Promotion: Pain

Nurses have an incredibly significant role to play in pain management. Effective pain management depends upon the therapeutic relationship developed between the nurse and the person and, in part, therefore pain assessment is so important, as it sets the 'spirit' of that relationship, whether the person's concerns will be taken seriously and how they will be responded to (Francis 2013). The importance of this kind of therapeutic relationship, and of the nature of the characteristics required to achieve it, can be drawn from several studies that represent the 'patient view'. Ali (2017) states that competing demands coupled with lack of privacy and a noisy environment may be potential barriers to effective communication between the patient and nurse, coupled with their illness, pain and/or anxiety and the effect of medication. Moreover, the cultural values and belief of the nurse or patient may lead to lack of understanding or interpretation of key messages. Ali (2017) cites a good example in relation to effective communication in Evidence-Based Practice 20.2.

Social Networking

Platforms such as Twitter can be used as a medium to debate professional issues, and share information or ideas, although it is vital that nurses also understand and adhere to local policies and NMC (2017) guidance when engaged in using any form of social media use. For example, Swift (2018) led a Twitter Chat on pain management in the acute hospital setting on the BMJ Evidence-Based Nursing Blog. In her blog post, Swift (2018) suggests that nurses feel disempowered when unable to help someone who is in pain, citing a study by Slatyer et al. (2015). Among the many barriers to providing effective healthcare, poor knowledge, poor communication and lack of shared team goals are key themes (Table 20.1).

Swift (2018) highlights the role of the pain resource nurse (PRN) model in the management of pain, pointing to a review by Crawford et al. (2016) which suggested that PRN education had the following benefits for pain management practice:

- Improved comfort of nurses with opioid administration
- Improved documentation
- Increased assessment and reassessment of pain
- Increased analgesia administration/pain interventions/appropriate use of analgesia
- Improvements in patient and nurse knowledge
- Improved patient perception of control over pain
- Increased local pain education and use of protocols
- Improved collaboration between physicians and nurses
- Reduced postoperative complications
- Enhanced job satisfaction/reduced staff turnover
- Improved ability to advocate for patients

EVIDENCE-BASED PRACTICE 20.2

Making Time for Communication

Nurse Amy Green was allocated a bay of four patients and two side wards for her shift. Halfway through the morning, one of her patients in a side ward became ill and Amy realised that she needed to spend quality time with him. She quickly visited her other patients to explain what was happening and reassured them that she had not forgotten about them. She checked that they were comfortable and not in pain, asked them to ring the call bell if they needed her and explained that she would return as soon as she could. The patients understood the situation and were reassured that their immediate needs had been assessed and they were not being neglected (Ali 2017).

From Swift A. Pain resource nurses: do they help to improve pain management in the acute hospital setting? EBN Twitter Chat. 2018. https://blogs.bmj.com/ebn/2018/06/03/pain-resource-nurses-do-they-help-to-improve-pain-management-in-the-acute-hospital-setting.

TABLE 20.1 Examples of Barriers That Obstruct the Provision of Effective Healthcare

Nurse	Patient	Other
Poor knowledge	Fear of side effects	Poor communication
Reluctance to assess pain	Fear of toxicity/overdose	Unhelpful ward ethos/hierarchy
Fear over use of pain drugs	Fear of addiction	Workload
Suspicion over patient motives	Anxiety about cause of pain	Lack of staff (medical and nursing)
Other priorities/workload	Stoical nature	Poor prescribing practices
Lack of awareness of patient needs	Anxious to be a good patient	Institutional constraints

Slatyer et al. (2015) suggest that hospital in-patients can experience significant pain, which can delay healing and potentially increase the risk of developing chronic pain. Their study used a grounded theory approach to develop a theory to explain the perspective of hospital nurses when caring for patients in severe pain. Their results indicated that nurse participants experienced psychosocial problems of feeling disempowered when their patients experienced persisting severe pain. Slatyer et al. (2015) concluded that their theory proposed a link between the disempowerment experienced by nurses and the development of coping responses which gave direction to support nurses' practice. Slatyer et al. (2015) recommend that further research is warranted to verify and extend this theory to other settings and nursing populations.

The patient's family, or significant others, is fundamental to the patient's journey. Therefore within their pain management role, the nurse must include these others as part of the wider relationship with the patient and recognise that family members have information needs of their own, particularly if they are the key carers.

The next section of the chapter discusses the strategies for managing pain, both pharmacological and nonpharmacological modalities. However, we should remember that relieving pain and enhancing the patient's experience can also depend upon the simplest of nursing measures. These might include ensuring analgesia is given before movement; skilful positioning with use of pillows, wedges or a bed cage/cradle; a warm bath; and other initiatives that give comfort. Nurses should ensure that people have sufficient rest and sleep, as this too will enhance coping abilities.

Pharmacological Pain Management

Most pain can be managed with drugs, and effective relief can be achieved using nonopioids (e.g. paracetamol), including the NSAIDs (e.g. ibuprofen), or opioids (e.g. codeine, morphine) and sometimes with adjuvants for certain types of pain. Problems can be overcome with most standard interventions and protocols, but there are certain groups that will require special consideration to prevent predictable problems including:

- older people with comorbidities
- people with learning disabilities
- people unable to speak and/or understand English
- people living chronic disease
- people with speech problems, e.g. following a stroke
- those with a recent brain injury or impaired consciousness
- people who abuse opioid drugs
- people already prescribed opioid drugs
- people living with sickle cell disease
- infants and preverbal children.

Patient understanding of the pain experience is important as people may feel reluctant to request pain relief, seeing it as a sign of weakness, or not wanting to bother busy nursing staff (Field and Smith 2019). Furthermore, people may be reluctant to take 'strong' medication because of the myths and misconceptions relating to opioid addiction. It is important that people are given the information needed to empower them to make informed decisions about their pain relief in partnership with the medical and nursing staff, that is, concordance.

Pain algorithms, for example for postoperative pain relief, are increasingly being developed and used in clinical practice. These are based upon the best available evidence and aim to expedite recovery and enhance the quality of the patient's pain journey. An algorithm is any set of detailed instructions that results in a predictable end state, for example in assembling flatpack furniture. Applied to the management of pain, it is regarded as a recommended patient management strategy that has been developed to direct decision-making, such as a flow chart, decision grid or a decision tree.

Pharmacological Therapies for Pain

Analgesics are a large and diverse group of drugs that act upon the CNS and PNS to relieve pain. They can be divided into nonopioids (including the NSAIDs) and opioids. Nonopioids include over-the-counter (OTC) medications such as paracetamol and ibuprofen. Opioids range from mild drugs such as codeine which are available OTC and strong morphine. In addition, a variety of adjuvant drugs such as amitriptyline are used with analgesics to relieve pain.

Readers should always consult their national formulary, for example the British National Formulary (BNF), for authoritative information relating to analgesics (see Useful Websites). The person's age, pain type and intensity, health problems and the setting are important considerations when determining the appropriate type of analgesic. It is especially important to be aware that the action of analgesic drugs may be affected by individual pharmacokinetics and metabolism, for example in older people or those with renal or hepatic dysfunction.

Nonopioid Analgesics

Nonopioid analgesic drugs include paracetamol and NSAIDs.

Paracetamol. This has both analgesic and antipyretic properties but has no antiinflammatory action. Paracetamol is commonly used for mild pain and is thought to work centrally (in the CNS) and peripherally at the point of the pain by inhibiting the production of pain mediators, for example kinins or histamine (Field and Smith 2019). Paracetamol can cause liver and less commonly kidney damage taken in even moderate amounts.

NSAIDs. Common NSAIDs include ibuprofen, diclofenac and naproxen. Weaker NSAIDs can be bought OTC, for example ibuprofen. They are used to relieve mild to moderate pain and inflammation. Most NSAIDs are absorbed quickly and act at the point of pain. They too inhibit the production of inflammatory chemicals such as prostaglandins. Gastrointestinal side-effects include discomfort, bleeding and ulceration.

Aspirin (acetylsalicylic acid) is another NSAID that is commonly used for mild to moderate pain and to relieve inflammation. Aspirin acts by inhibiting prostaglandin production. Aspirin must be used with caution as it can cause gastrointestinal bleeding. It should not be given to children under the age of 16 years, except in certain conditions, as there is a link between aspirin and Reye's syndrome. Reye's syndrome is most likely to affect children under 5 years but can also, in rare cases, affect older children and can be fatal (see Useful Websites, e.g. BNF). Aspirin in small doses (e.g. when used as an antiplatelet drug – see Chapter 2, Nursing Patients With Cardiovascular Disorders) is not considered a NSAID.

Opioid Analgesics

Opioid analgesics may be derived from the opium poppy or synthetic analgesics which mimic the action of the natural substance. They act upon the opioid receptors in the CNS to block pain transmission by mimicking the effects of naturally occurring endorphins at the receptor sites, thereby minimising pain. Examples of opioids include codeine, buprenorphine, diamorphine, dihydrocodeine, fentanyl, pethidine, methadone, morphine, oxycodone and tramadol. They vary in efficacy and strength, ranging from codeine (a mild opioid used for moderate pain) to morphine (a strong opioid used for severe pain). Opioids cause constipation, may cause nausea, vomiting and sleepiness, and can depress respiration (see Chapter 32, Nursing Patients Who Need Palliative Care).

Adjuvants. Adjuvant agents or drugs act to modify or enhance the effects of pharmacological agents or other treatments. They may be needed in the management of neuropathic pain. Examples include:

- Antidepressants, e.g. amitriptyline, prevent the reuptake of noradrenaline (norepinephrine) from the synaptic cleft after its release by the neurone to transfer chemically an action potential, thus depleting available neurotransmitters.
- Corticosteroids, e.g. dexamethasone, are used to reduce swelling. They are used in nerve compression and to reduce cerebral oedema.
- Antiepileptics (anticonvulsants), e.g. gabapentin, carbamazepine and sodium valproate, act in a variety of ways to decrease the effects of neuropathic pain.
- Antispasmodics, e.g. hyoscine butyl bromide.
- Capsaicin, an irritant chemical present in sweet peppers, is used topically for postherpetic neuralgia.

Delivery Frameworks

There coexist a plethora of frameworks to guide the use of analgesics which have in common the principle that safe and effective analgesia can be provided by titrating the dose of analgesics to gain a balance between therapeutic effect and potential side-effects. Aneka and Cascella (2022) suggest that the World Health Organisation (WHO) pain relief ladder is just as applicable today not only for cancer patients but also for all patients with either acute or chronic enduring pain. The ladder rests upon five simple recommendations for the correct and effective use of prescribed treatments. However, it is noteworthy that the analgesic ladder has been adapted and modified, but the modifications are not intended to negate or advise against the use of the original ladder (Aneka and Cascella 2022).

The World Health Organisation Pain Relief Ladder

The WHO pain relief ladder, first proposed in the 1980s and developed in 1996, was originally a three-step ladder that guided analgesic decision-making. The WHO developed the ladder following recommendations from an international group of experts and served as a catalyst for increasing awareness worldwide relating to the critical importance of treating cancer pain. The underpinning principle of this framework is that the right drug should be given, at the right dose, at the right time. In persistent pain, titration should be done by moving from nonopioids, for example paracetamol, and NSAIDs through to mild opioids, for example codeine, and then to strong opioids, for example morphine, that is, moving up the ladder. In surgical or trauma pain, titration will move in reverse order, from strong opioids to weak opioids to nonopioids and NSAIDs (Fig. 20.4). In both cases, analgesics should be given regularly to maintain a constant analgesic plasma concentration (Fig. 20.5). For example, if a patient needs morphine, this will require to be given 4-hourly unless given as a modified-release preparation such as MST 12-hourly or MXL 24-hourly. The right dose of analgesic is that which provides pain relief with the lowest side-effect profile. When moving from strong opioids to weak opioids, or vice versa, it is important to consider the equipotency of the drugs involved. If the person has been having 60 mg oral codeine 6-hourly and still has pain, the starting dose of oral morphine needs to be equivalent to more than this dose, to increase analgesia.

See Evolve website Critical thinking question 20.2

Opioids are central to cancer pain management, either used alone or in combination with other medication. Some people will require more intensive measures and/or mixed modalities of treatment. Other treatments may include nerve blocks or spinal analgesia (epidural or intrathecal). Associated neuropathic pain may be opioid-responsive but may require specific antineuropathic medication, and pain can also be treated using drugs that specifically target the pathological processes responsible for cancer pain (Phillips et al. 2021).

Opioids are often the first-line treatment for severe acute pain, including postoperatively, and there is no compelling evidence that one opioid is better than another. The key message for safe and effective use of opioids is to titrate the dose against the desired effect (pain relief) and minimise the unwanted side-effects. If the person is asking for more pain relief, then it is usually a sign of inadequate pain control which may be due to:
- too little drug administered
- too much time between doses
- inadequate pain assessment
- too rigid an application of protocols.

Routes and Modes of Delivery

The age of the person is an important consideration when analgesic drugs are prescribed. Infants, young children, adults and older people all have different body compositions, and the metabolism and elimination of drugs are influenced by their life stage. Also, a child's age, weight and height are important in calculating doses. In older people, reduced metabolism and drug excretion can result in an accumulative effect and polypharmacy

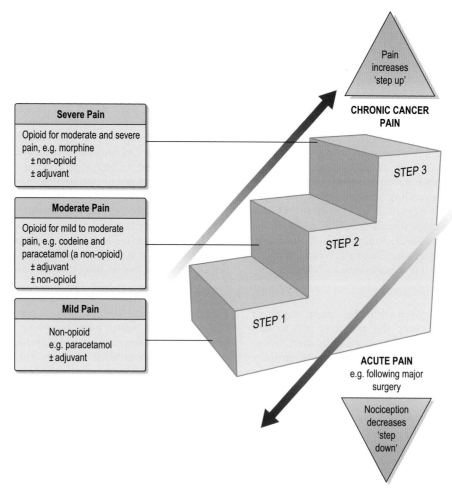

Figure 20.4 Pain relief (analgesic) ladder. (Based on WHO 2005; reproduced from Brooker C, Waugh A, eds. *Foundations of Nursing Practice: Fundamentals of Holistic Care.* Edinburgh: Mosby; 2007 with permission.)

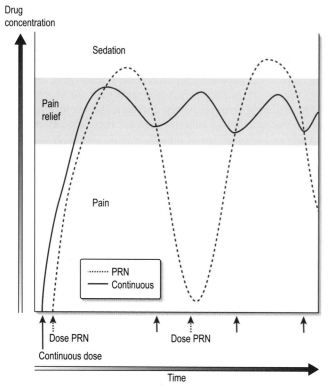

Figure 20.5 Pro re nata *(PRN)* as and when required versus around-the-clock administration of analgesics.

may cause drug interactions. There is a general saying that if the person is cooperative and can swallow, it is best to give the drug orally, but this is not always possible or desirable. Routes of administration include:

- oral
- sublingual or buccal
- intranasal
- inhalation
- subcutaneous
- intramuscular
- epidermal
- intravenous
- intrapleural
- transdermal
- rectal
- intraspinal.

It is important that nurses are familiar with the advantages, disadvantages and effectiveness of each route, and this been improved by the availability and use of algorithms and staff must adhere to local policy. The more commonly used routes are outlined in the following sections.

Oral. Tablets or liquids are typically easy to administer and place no restrictions on a person's mobility. However, their effectiveness is dependent on patient adherence. Sustained-release preparations can enhance adherence by limiting the number of tablets needed each day and have the advantage of attaining consistent drug plasma levels. However, absorption will be compromised if nausea and vomiting are present. In addition, this route has the disadvantage that it is susceptible to the first-pass effect in the liver and intestine, by which a proportion of the drug is metabolised and thus less enters the circulation. The oral route can be used for both mild nonopioids and oral opioids such as morphine.

Intramuscular. This route was often used to relieve postoperative pain but has mostly been superseded by PCA. It has the advantage that it enables the rapid absorption of drugs, although morphine may be more slowly and erratically absorbed than water-based drugs such as diamorphine. Intramuscular injections can be painful, particularly so if the volume of drug exceeds 4 mL. Moreover, people may have to move to expose an injection site, thus causing additional pain.

Intravenous. The action of analgesics administered by this route is rapid in onset but of short duration, and therefore a continuous infusion rather than bolus injection may be more effective in maintaining the level of analgesic in the bloodstream.

Rectal. Analgesics, for example diclofenac and morphine, given as a suppository are absorbed across the rectal mucosa, and opioid availability when given rectally is at least equivalent to oral administration. However, absorption is affected in the presence of hard faeces in the rectum. The rectal route is useful for people who have nausea and vomiting or dysphagia. Rectal preparations may not be suitable for people who are neutropenic or in danger of being so. Minor trauma from insertion of the drug may allow entry of gastrointestinal commensals into the bloodstream resulting in septicaemia. Rectal administration can be used at home and is useful in palliative care. However, people often find rectal administration unacceptable (Stannard and Booth 2004).

Sublingual and Buccal. Medication is placed under the tongue or between the upper lip and gum or between the cheek and gum. These routes may avoid the first-pass effect and are rapid in onset of action. However, there is the disadvantage that the person may inadvertently swallow the drug, and buccal administration may be difficult for people with upper dentures. An example of an analgesic drug administered by this route is buprenorphine.

Transdermal. A drug-containing patch is placed directly onto the skin, where absorption occurs. The opioid fentanyl provides effective pain relief by this route. Patches need to be changed, usually every 3 days (follow local policy), and have the advantage of continuous pain relief without the need to remember to take tablets throughout the 24 hours. This route is dependent on the patch being in contact with the skin and on the availability of oral morphine to control 'breakthrough' pain. NSAIDs such as diclofenac are available as gels/creams OTC for mild pain.

Subcutaneous Infusion is used for administration of opioids and NSAIDs for people with chronic disorders when oral medication is not possible. It offers a simple, safe and effective alternative to intravenous or intramuscular injections and can be used safely at home.

Inhalation enables rapid absorption of gaseous, volatile and atomised substances. For example, nitrous oxide and oxygen (Entonox) administered via mask or mouthpiece can help with intermittent pain, as in labour, or during minor procedures, dressings. However, it can be difficult to administer an exact dose and there may be airway irritation (National Institute for Health and Clinical Care Excellence 2022).

Spinal. Medications given directly into the epidural or subarachnoid space have rapid onset of effect and can provide effective pain relief in a variety of situations (McLaren et al. 2020). Typically, opioids and anaesthetic agents are given by this route. The direct access to the CNS means that much smaller doses are required. Whilst this route has advantages, including a reduction in postoperative complications and neuromodulation of persistent pain, using opioids to reduce wind-up in neuropathic pain, it has important and potentially serious complications – respiratory depression and sudden dramatic hypotension. Despite the need for caution, people with persistent pain can be managed at home for lengthy periods of time, with spinal analgesics administered via a small portable syringe pump or through a medication pump implanted under the skin.

Patient-Controlled Analgesia (PCA)

PCA is increasingly recognised as an ideal approach for postoperative pain management. It minimises pharmacokinetic and pharmacodynamic variability in individual patients and provides significantly better analgesia and patient satisfaction (Luo and Min 2017). PCA refers to the administration of analgesics by any appropriate and safe route over which the person has control. When they feel pain, pressing a button delivers a prescribed dose of medication, usually an opioid. Usual routes include intravenous, subcutaneous or epidural (see also inhaled Entonox earlier). Regular assessment of the patient is important, as is monitoring for nausea and vomiting, which are common side-effects of opioids (see Chapter 25, Nursing the Patient Undergoing Surgery). The pump is set with 'lock-out' intervals and doses to regulate the amount of drug administered. This method is typically used postoperatively but can be used in other painful situations. The person must be able and willing to use it, and therefore meeting the person's information needs is important, for example explaining potential side-effects and reassurance that it is safe, and that overdose and addiction are not possible. Multiple PCAs can be chosen, including IV PCA, patient-controlled epidural analgesia (PCEA), patient-controlled regional analgesia (PCRA), patient-controlled intranasal analgesia (PCINA), patient-controlled transdermal analgesia (PCTA) and patient-controlled sublingual analgesia (PCSA). Different agents, techniques and/or their combinations enable more options of PCA. There is evidence that PCA offers improved pain relief and quicker recovery following surgery. Current evidence suggests that regional analgesic techniques are effective in the reduction of pain. The most frequently purported psychological benefit of PCA is the person's specific control over pain. Acute postoperative pain potentially delays recovery and increases morbidity and mortality. PCA eliminates the need to wait for traditional nurse-administered analgesia, which is often cited as being inefficient for many reasons (Wiraz et al. 2017). To assess the influence and potential benefits of PCA, Wiraz et al. (2017) undertook a pilot feasibility study to evaluate the safety, efficacy and usability of a novel, patient-controlled analgesic dispenser, the PCoA (Acute). Two groups of patients scheduled for elective surgery, both taking oral analgesics, were enrolled into either a control group, who received opioids dispensed by nurses, or a test group, opioids dispensed via the PCoA (Acute). Results showed no severe adverse events were recorded. Average pill intake time was reduced in the PCA group (from 8:58 minutes in the control group to 1:17 minutes in the test group). The PCA group took 67% more pills than the control group, indicating enhanced compliance, and pain scores were significantly lower for patients in the test group. The study concluded that over 90% of PCoA Acute users were satisfied with its use and that patients and medical staff accepted it was safe and effective and served to optimise pain medication administration.

Other Medical Interventions

Local Anaesthesia and Regional Nerve Blocks are achieved with the injection of local anaesthetic, sometimes together with a corticosteroid, near to or in a peripheral nerve or major nerve plexus or into the spine. Although there can be adverse reactions and complications, the pain-relieving effects often outlast the duration of the local anaesthetic.

Surgery. Nerve transection can reduce or eliminate intractable pain. Although this may work initially, pain often returns and may be worse than it was presurgery. For this reason, other techniques, such as spinal cord stimulation, are more common. Implanted epidural electrodes are controlled either via an external radiofrequency transmitter or an implanted pulse generator. Pulse generators implanted subcutaneously are used to stimulate the brain.

Radiotherapy, Chemotherapy and Specific Drug Therapy. Radiotherapy and chemotherapy may be used to relieve pain, for example in metastatic cancer. Bisphosphonates such as pamidronate are effective in relieving pain from bone metastases (see Chapter 31, Nursing the Patient With Cancer, and Chapter 32, Nursing Patients Who Need Palliative Care).

Specialised Pain Services

Acute Pain Services

In response to evidence of inadequate postoperative pain relief and a recommendation by the British Pain Society in collaboration with the Royal College of Anaesthetists, multiprofessional acute pain services are now well established in many hospitals in the UK and the multiprofessional team can assist in:

- formalising staff and patient education
- organising and monitoring acute pain management
- safely introducing new techniques and maximising the potential of existing ones
- standardising pain assessment
- formulating and introducing practice guidelines
- auditing service efficacy.

The Core Standards for Pain Management Services in the UK give comprehensive details in their guidelines which reinforce The British Pain Society recommendations in their Pain Management Services: Good Practice and include all the above plus further provisions for acute pain services:

- Provision of specialist care and advice for difficult acute pain problems such as occur in people who misuse opioids.
- Seamless liaison with other healthcare teams responsible for the shared care of people with acute pain.
- Back-up arrangements, education programmes and appropriate guidelines or protocols to ensure that there is continuous cover for acute pain management around the clock, 7 days a week.

Hospice/palliative care teams have a wealth of expertise in pain and symptom control and can be a valuable resource (see Chapter 32). Such teams are usually multidisciplinary and situated in a variety of care settings. The key functions of such teams are to provide support to other professionals in caring for people with life-threatening illness.

Chronic or 'Persistent' Pain Services

These offer a service to people with persistent pain. Clinics are usually multidisciplinary and may be staffed by anaesthetist nurses, psychologists, physiotherapists, occupational therapists and pharmacists with the aim of increasing the person's ability to function and lead a more fulfilled life. This aim incorporates the belief that persistent pain is the result of multiple interrelating physical, psychological and social or occupational factors.

Non-pharmacological Pain Management

Over recent years the use of nonpharmacological methods of pain control has received greater acceptance in conventional healthcare systems. Although there is still a paucity of robust evidence, these methods have become more acceptable and more widely available.

Nonpharmacological methods include complementary and alternative medicine (CAM) therapies, which nurses have incorporated into their practice. Nursing staff who provide CAM therapies are subject to The Code: Professional Standards of Practice and Behaviour for Nurses, Midwives and Nursing Associates (NMC 2018). Complementary and alternative therapies and registrants must have successfully undertaken training and be competent to practise the administration of complementary and alternative therapies. The nurse must have undertaken an approved course or programme of study that deems the practitioner competent to administer such treatments. Furthermore, the nurse must work within the framework of clinical governance which aims for continuous quality improvement to provide safe and effective patient care. An employed nurse must first have authority from the NHS Trust or other employer to practice CAM and must ascertain that the employer's vicarious liability covers such activity. Self-employed nurses should have professional indemnity insurance that includes CAM, such as the schemes offered by professional organisations.

This section of the chapter outlines nonpharmacological methods, including CAM therapies used in pain management. Nonpharmacological methods can be classified into two broad types: physical (counter-irritation) and psychological. However, methods such as massage have both physical and psychological benefits.

Physical methods:

- acupuncture
- aromatherapy
- chiropractic
- herbal medicine
- homeopathy
- hot/cold
- low-level laser therapy (LLLT)
- photobiomodulation (PBM)
- massage
- osteopathy
- reflexology
- therapeutic touch
- TENS
- ultrasound
- yoga.

Psychological methods:

- art therapy
- behavioural therapy
- biofeedback
- distraction
- drama therapy
- hypnosis
- imagery
- music therapy
- relaxation.

Hot or Cold Therapy. The application of superficial heat promotes vasodilation, thereby increasing blood flow to an area, and pain-inducing chemical mediators are 'diluted'. Equally, the application of cooling measures reduces the metabolic rate and lowers cellular activity and the consumption of oxygen. If the cooling is sufficiently intense, pain and cold sensations are suppressed. Caution must be exercised in using these therapies if there is existing reduction in skin sensation or if this therapy is contraindicated by the patient's condition, for example impaired blood supply to an area.

Massage is an ancient form of pain relief often used in conjunction with oils or creams. The evidence for the effectiveness of massage is sparse. It is thought that massage activates certain elements of the gate-control mechanisms and releases endorphins. The pain relief achieved when rubbing an area after a knock or a bump is an example of this, and massage not only provides healing but also relaxes tight muscles that may be associated with stress.

Acupuncture treats the person and not the disease. It is based upon a technique whereby fine needles are inserted and manipulated in specific points (approximately 365) along meridians. The meridians are channels through which energy known as Qi is said to flow. The effects of such treatment are still subject to scientific scrutiny. A similar technique using pressure without needles can be used on the acupuncture points, which may be more acceptable to people who are needle phobic.

Distraction relies on distracting attention away from the painful stimulus. This may involve asking the person to breathe deeply, the aim of which is to shield the sensation of pain by increasing sensation via another sensory route (Field and Smith 2019). The list of distracters includes those for adults and children. They include:

- company and conversation
- humour and laughter
- reading
- television
- listening to music
- hobbies
- companion animals
- exercise, activity and sport if applicable
- e-mailing friends and 'surfing' the internet
- computer games
- blowing bubbles
- therapeutic play
- storytelling, reading to children
- music and singing, shouting and yelling
- visits by well-known people and role models.

Transcutaneous Electrical Nerve Stimulation (TENS) is a method of pain relief in which a controlled level of low-voltage electricity is applied to the body via electrodes. This is understood to relieve pain by stimulating the release of endorphins. It may be useful during labour and for chronic pain.

⊕ **See Evolve website Fig. 20.2**

Low-Level Laser Therapy (LLLT) or Photobiomodulation (PBM). LLLT and PBM use a different type of laser from the heat-generating lasers used in surgery (Grady et al. 2007). The nonthermal application of red and infrared laser light has selective stimulatory effects at cellular level. According to the evidence the laser light action in managing pain is multifaceted. It includes a reduction in inflammatory and pain chemicals and normalisation of nerve outputs and their membrane function which reduces pain transmission at the spinal gate. It is now suggested that with advancing research and greater understanding of PBM, different disease types and conditions are now becoming amenable to its beneficial effects (Hamblin 2016). Adrenocorticotrophic hormone (ACTH) and endorphins are released as a secondary response. LLLT has been used in the treatment of conditions such as failed back surgery, musculoskeletal pain, chronic postsurgical pain and posttraumatic pain of the spine and limbs. LLLT is not associated with serious adverse reactions and has a high benefit-to-risk ratio.

Support and Self-Help Groups

A detailed account of CAM therapies is beyond the scope of this book; readers requiring more information can access NHS resources available from Child and Adolescent Mental Health Services (see Useful Websites). Pain is isolating, particularly so in chronic pain where the person and their carers may withdraw from social interactions. Contact with appropriate self-help and support groups can help to reduce the isolation of pain. The chance to share experiences and feelings provides emotional support, encourages hope and promotes empowerment and control. Sharing information about coping strategies can be especially useful. Nurses can discuss the potential benefits of self-help groups (see Useful Websites) with the person, but the importance of close family support, emphasised in diverse cultures, should be respected.

Mindfulness and Pain Management

Mindfulness is based on ancient Eastern meditation practices. It facilitates an attentional stance of detached observation, and over the past three decades, mindfulness-based interventions (MBIs) have gained increasingly wide use for the treatment of painful conditions including cancer pain (Feng et al. 2022). Early mindfulness studies in pain patients showed promising outcomes on pain symptoms, mood disturbance, anxiety and depression, as well as pain-related drug utilisation and systematic reviews on the effects of mindfulness meditation have been published in recent years. Of those that report pain outcomes, there has been a focus on specific types of pain such as low back pain, fibromyalgia or somatisation disorder (Hilton et al. 2016).

For more on mindfulness, see Useful Websites.

Clinical Governance in Pain Management

Clinical governance is a systematic approach to maintaining and improving the quality of care within health systems. It is also a doctrine whereby the practitioner is responsible to the employing authority as well as their professional body for aspects of professional and ethical conduct. Scally and Donaldson (1998) defined clinical governance as 'a framework through which the NHS organisations are accountable for continuously improving the quality of their services and safeguarding high standards of care by creating an environment in which excellence in clinical care will flourish'.

Clinical governance involves at least the following elements:

- risk assessment
- risk management
- clinical audit
- clinical effectiveness
- transparency and openness
- education and training
- research and development.

It can be argued that all these elements are applicable to pain management. The NICE guidance and the SIGN ensure that services and clinical standards are delivered through local systems of clinical governance. Furthermore, Core Standards for Pain Management Services in the UK have established guidelines and standards of the principle driving these standards is to have an acceptable level of care in pain management which is consistent, both geographically and from initial to escalating levels of care (Faculty of Pain Medicine of The Royal College of Anaesthetists 2021).

Role of Guidelines and Policies in Pain Management

Despite the increasing numbers of initiatives to improve pain management, powerful myths can cloud rational actions, and entrenched perceptions can spread with ease, independent of logic and professional acumen. Combating these myths and outmoded ideals has been made easier by the availability of government-endorsed clinical practice guidelines and local initiatives. Guidelines and recommendations relating to pain management have been published by professional bodies (British Pain Society, CSPMS, NHS England, NICE, RCN, WHO). Common to all is a clear commitment to quality pain management achieved through the highest professional standards and that the person has the right to ethical and appropriate pain management, but most importantly the individual has the right to be believed in their expression of pain and the right to appropriate pain assessment and management strategies that take account of individual differences. However, it is worth mentioning that recommendations alone do not change professional attitudes or behaviour, but collectively, they provide professionals with the clarity, structure and rationale of pain management that has been sadly lacking in previous decades (Brennan et al. 2007).

Practice guidelines are systematically developed recommendations that assist practitioners and those in their care in making informed decisions about healthcare. In turn, recommendations can be adopted, modified or rejected according to the needs of the client population and clinicians' needs and constraints and should be based upon current best evidence. However, practice guidelines cannot guarantee specific outcomes, or revision subject to advances in professional knowledge, technology and practice – only people can do that.

Summary: Key Nursing Issues

- 'Pain is whatever the patient says it is and exists when he [sic] says it does' (McCaffery 1968).
- Nurses are part of the MDT who use up-to-date evidence-based knowledge and understanding of pain to competently prevent and minimise pain.
- Pain is a complex, subjective and multidimensional experience that has physical, psychosocial, emotional, cultural and spiritual influences.
- Pain assessment and measurement are critical to the holistic care of a person with pain.

- Relieving pain and enhancing the patient's experience can also depend upon the simplest of nursing measures.
- Holistic pain management involves both pharmacological and nonpharmacological approaches.
- Nurses empower people with chronic pain by encouraging independence and coping skills.
- Ineffective pain management impedes recovery after surgery/trauma and may lead to unrelieved chronic pain.
- Effective pain management is a quality issue for all nurses.

Reflection and Learning – What Next?

- **Test** your knowledge by visiting the Evolve website 🌐 and answering the multiple-choice questions and critical thinking questions.
- **Consolidate** your learning by looking at some of the further reading suggestions, references and specialist websites.
- **Revisit** some of the additional material on the Evolve website.

- **Consider** what you have learnt and how this will help your professional development.
- **Reflect** on how you can apply this knowledge to the care of your patients.
- **Discuss** your learning with your mentor/supervisor, lecturer and colleagues.

References

Ali M. *Communication skills 2: overcoming barriers to effective communication.* Nursing Times; 2017. https://www.nursingtimes.net/clinical-archive/assessment-skills/communication-skills-2-overcoming-the-barriers-to-effective-communication/7022518.article.

Alotaibi K, Higgins I, Chan S. Nurses' knowledge and attitude toward pediatric pain management: A cross sectional study. *Pain Manag Nurs.* 2019;20(2):118–125.

Aneka AA, Cascella M. WHO Analgesic Ladder. National Library of Medicine. 2022. https://www.ncbi.nlm.nih.gov/books/NBK554435/.

Barrie J, Loughlin D. Managing chronic pain in adults. *Nurs Stand.* 2014;29(7):50–58.

Berwick D. *A Promise to Learn – A Commitment to Act: Improving the Safety of Patients in England.* London: Department of Health; 2013.

Brennan F, Carr D, Cousins M. Pain management: a fundamental human right. *Anesth Analg.* 2007;105(1):205–221.

Brennan F, Lohman D, Gwyther L. Access to pain management as human right. *Am J Public Health.* 2019;109(1):61–65.

British Pain Society. Participant information for pain management programs. https://www.britishpainsociety.org/people-with-pain/. Accessed 24 November 2022.

Bubb S. *Winterbourne View – Time for Change: Transforming the Commissioning of Services for People with Learning Disabilities and/or Autism.* London: Department of Health; 2014.

Butera KA, Roff SR, Buford TW, et al. The impact of multisite pain on functional outcomes in older adults: biopsychosocial considerations. *J Pain Res.* 2019;12:1115–1125.

Campbell JN. The fifth vital sign revisited. *Pain.* 2016;157(1):3–4.

Chamley C, James G. Pain management – minimizing the pain experience. In: Brooker C, Waugh A, eds. *Foundations of Nursing Practice: Fundamentals of Holistic Care.* 2nd ed. Edinburgh: Mosby; 2013:653–679.

Chary S. What do we need to consider for pain management?. In: Waisundara VY, Banjari I, Balkic J, eds. *Pain Management Practices, Novel Therapies and Bioactives.* London: Intechopen; 2021.

Care Quality Commission. *The State of Health Care and Adult Social Care in England 2014/2015.* London: TSO; 2015.

Cousins M, Lane-Krebs K, Matthews J, et al. Student nurses' pain knowledge and attitudes towards pain management over the last 20 years: a systematic review. *Nurse Educ Today.* 2022;108:1–7.

Crawford CL, Boller J, Jadalla A, Cuenca E. An integrative review of pain resource nurse programs. *Crit Care Nurs Q.* 2016;39(1):64–82.

Department of Health. *The NHS Constitution.* London: DH; 2012a.

Department of Health. *Compassion in Practice.* London: DH; 2012b.

Dimond B. *Legal Aspects of Pain Management.* 2nd ed. London: Pearson International; 2016.

Dimos-Dimitrios M, Moka E, Orillo E. Neuropathic pain in neurological disorders: a narrative review. *Cureus.* 2022. doi:10.7759/cureus.22419.

Faculty of Pain Medicine of The Royal College of Anaesthetists. Core Standards. 2021. https://fpm.ac.uk/standards-guidelines/core-standards

Fayaz A, Croft P, Langford RM, et al. Prevalence of chronic pain in the UK: a systematic review and meta-analysis of population studies; 2016. https://bmjopen.bmj.com/content/bmjopen/6/6/e010364.full.pdf.

Feng B, Hu X, L WW, et al. Are mindfulness treatments effective for pain in cancer patients? A systematic review and meta-analysis. *Eur J Pain.* 2022;26(1):61–76.

Field L, Smith B. Pain management. In: Field L, Smith B, eds. *Nursing Care: An Essential Guide for Nurses and Healthcare Workers in Primary and Secondary Care.* 3rd ed. Harlow: Pearson Education; 2019:207–250.

Finnerup NB, Nikolajsen L, Rice A. Transition from acute to chronic pain: a misleading concept? 2022; 163(9): e985–e988.

Ford C. Adult pain assessment and management. *Br J Nurs.* 2019;28(7): 421–423.

Francis R. *Report on the Mid Staffordshire NHS Foundation Trust Public Inquiry.* London: TSO; 2013.

Graczyk M, Borkowska A, Krajnik M. Why patients are afraid of opioid analgesics: a study on opioid perception in patients with chronic pain. *Pol Arch Intern Med.* 2018;128(2):89–97.

Grady K, Severn A, Eldridge P. *Key Topics in Pain Medicine.* 3rd ed. Hampshire: Thompson Publishing; 2007.

Gregory J. Use of pain scales and observational pain assessment tools in hospital settings. *Nurs Stand.* 2019. doi:10.7748/ns.2019.e11308.

GSK Consumer Healthcare. *Global Pain Index Report,* 4th ed.; 2020. Available at https://www.gsk.com/media/6351/2020-global-plain-index-report.pdf.

Hamblin M. Photobiomodulation or low-level laser therapy. *J Biophotonics.* 2016;11-12:122–1124.

Hanley C, Ladha KS, Clarke HA, Cuthbertson BC, et al. Association of postoperative complications with persistent post-surgical pain: a multicentre prospective cohort study. *Br J Anaesth.* 2022;128(2):311–320.

Herrera-Escobar JP, Apoi M, Weed C, et al. Association of pain after trauma with long-term functional and mental health outcomes. *J Trauma Acute Care Surg.* 2018;85(4):773–779. Available at: https://www.ncbi.nlm.nih.gov/pubmed/30020227.

Hilton L, Hempel S, Ewing BA, et al. Mindfulness meditation for chronic pain: systematic review and meta-analysis. *Ann Behav Med.* 2016;51(2). www.researchgate.net/publication/308548195_Mindfulness_Meditation_for_Chronic_Pain_Systematic_Review_and_Meta-analysis.

Howarth A, Poole D. Assessment and management of chronic pain. *Nurs Stand.* 2019. doi:10.7748/ns.2019.e11395.

Human Rights Act. 1998. https://www.legislation.gov.uk/ukpga/1998/42/contents.

International Association for the Study of Pain. Terminology. 2022. https://www.iasp-pain.org/resources/terminology/.

IsHak WW, Wen R, Naghdechi L, et al. Pain and depression: a systematic review. *Harv Rev Psychiatry.* 2018;26(6):352–363.

Keogh E. *Review into the Quality of Care and Treatment Provided by 14 Hospital Trusts in England: Overview Report.* NHS England; 2013. https://www.nhs.uk/NHSEngland/bruce-keogh-review/Documents/outcomes/keogh-review-final-report.pdf.

Livingston WK. *Pain Mechanisms.* New York: Macmillan; 1943.

Luo J, Min S. Post operative pain management in a post anesthesia care unit: an update. *J Pain Res.* 2017;10:2687–2698.

MacMahon S, Koltzenburg M, Tracey I, et al. *Wall & Melzack's Textbook of Pain.* 6th ed. Philadelphia: Elsevier; 2013.

McAllister MJ. *What is the neuromatrix of pain?.* Institute for Chronic Pain; 2017. Available at: http://www.instituteforchronicpain.org/understanding-chronic-pain/what-is-chronic-pain/neuromatrix-of-pain.

McCabe C. Effective pain management in patients in hospital. *Nurs Stand.* 2017;31(29):42–46.

McCaffery M. *Nursing Practice Theories Related to Cognition, Bodily Pain and Man–Environmental Interactions.* California: UCLA Students Store; 1968.

McLaren S, Hughes M, Sheehan C. A guide to epidural management. *Br J Hosp Med.* 2020;81(1). https://doi-org.ezproxy.herts.ac.uk/10.12968/hmed.2019.0174.

Melzack R. Pain and the neuromatrix in the brain. *J Dent Educ.* 2001; 65(12):1378–1382.

Melzack R, Katz J. Measurement in persons in pain. In: Wall P, Melzack R, eds. *Textbook of Pain.* 6th ed. Edinburgh: Churchill Livingstone; 2013.

Melzeck R, Wall P. Pain mechanisms: a new theory. *Science.* 1965;150:971–979.

Melzack R, Wall PD. *The Challenge of Pain (Updated).* 2nd ed. Harmondsworth: Penguin Books; 2005.

Mendell LM. The path to discovery of windup and central sensitization. *Front Pain Res.* 2022;3:1–5.

Miaskowski C, Blythe F, Nicosia F, et al. A biophysical model of chronic pain for older adults. *Pain Med.* 2020;21(9):1793–1805.

National Institute for Health and Care Excellence. British National Formulary (BNF). https://bnf.nice.org.uk/. Accessed 24 November 2022.

National Institute for Health and Care Excellence. Chronic pain: how prevalent is it? 2021a. https://cks.nice.org.uk/topics/chronic-pain/background-information/prevalence/.

National Institute for Health and Care Excellence. *Chronic pain (primary and secondary) in over 16s: assessment of all chronic pain and management of chronic primary pain.* NICE guideline [NG193]; 2021b. www.nice.org.uk/guidance/ng193.

Nursing and Midwifery Council (NMC). Guidance on the use of social media; 2017. http://www.nmc-uk.org.

Nursing and Midwifery Council (NMC). The Code: Professional Standards of Practice and Behaviour for Nurses, Midwives and Nursing Associates; 2018. https://www.nmc.org.uk/globalassets/sitedocuments/nmc-publications/nmc-code.pdf.

Phillips C, Contreras E, Oswald J. NSAIDs, opioids, and beyond. In: Waisundara VY, Banjari I, Balkic J, eds. *Pain Management Practices, Novel Therapies and Bioactives.* London: Intechopen; 2021.

Puntillo F, Giglio M, Paladini A, et al. Pathophysiology of musculoskeletal pain: a narrative review. *Ther Adv Musculoskelet Dis.* 2021;13:1–12.

Samulowitz A, Gremyr I, Eriksson E, et al. "Brave men" and "emotional women": a theory-guided literature review on gender bias in health care and gendered norms towards patients with chronic pain. *Pain Rese Manag.* 2018;2018:1–14.

Scally G, Donaldson LJ. The NHS's 50th anniversary. Clinical governance and the drive for quality improvement in the new NHS in England. *Br Med J.* 1998;317(7150):61–65.

Scottish Intercollegiate Guidelines Network. Management of Chronic Pain A National Clinical Guideline. 2019. https://www.sign.ac.uk/assets/sign136.pdf.

Shneidman ES. *The Suicidal Mind.* Oxford: Oxford University Press; 1996.

Schofield P. The assessment of pain in older people: UK guidelines. *Age Ageing.* 2018;47:i1–i22. https://www.ncbi.nlm.nih.gov/pmc/articles/PMC5888957/pdf/afx192.pdf.

Sheng J, Liu L, Wang Y, et al. The link between depression and chronic pain: neural mechanisms in the brain. *Neural Plast.* 2017;2017:1–10.

Sibille KT, Bartsch F, Reddy D, et al. Increasing neuroplasticity to bolster chronic pain treatment: a role for intermittent fasting and glucose administration. *J Pain.* 2016;17(3):275–281.

Sibille KT, McBeth J, Smith D, et al. Allostatic load and pain severity in older adults: results from the English longitudinal study of aging. *Exp Gerontol.* 2017;88:51–58.

Simington S. Soul pain, grief and transformation; 2011. https://www.opentohope.com/soul-pain-grief-and-transformation/.

Slatyer S, Williams AM, Michael R. Seeking empowerment to comfort patients in severe pain: a grounded theory study of nurse's perspective. *Int J Nurs Stud.* 2015;52(1):229–239.

Stannard CF, Booth S. *Churchill's Pocketbook of Pain.* 2nd ed. Edinburgh: Churchill Livingstone; 2004.

Sterling P, Eyer J. Allostasis: a new paradigm to explain arousal pathology. In: Fisher S, Reason JT, eds. *Handbook of Life Stress, Cognition, and Health.* Chichester: Wiley; 1988.

Swift A. Pain resource nurses: do they help to improve pain management in the acute hospital setting? EBN Twitter Chat; 2018. https://blogs.bmj.com/ebn/2018/06/03/pain-resource-nurses-do-they-help-to-improve-pain-management-in-the-acute-hospital-setting.

Thakral M, Shi L, Foust JB, et al. Pain quality descriptors in community-dwelling older adults with nonmalignant pain. 2016:157(12); 2834-42.

Tortora GJ, Derrickson B. *Principles of Anatomy and Physiology.* 15th ed. New York: John Wiley & Sons; 2016.

Veal F, Williams M, Bereznicki L, et al. Barriers to optimal pain management in aged care facilities: an Australian qualitative study. *Pain Manag Nurs.* 2018;19(2):177–185.

Volkow DMD, Thomas-McLellan A. Opioid abuse in chronic pain – misconceptions and mitigation strategies. *N Engl J Med.* 2016;374(3):1253–1263.

Warlow TA, Hain RDW. 'Total pain' in children with severe neurological impairment. *Children (Basel).* 2018;5(1).

Wheeldon A. Pain and pain management. In: Peate I, ed. *Fundamentals of Applied Pathophysiology: An Essential Guide for Nursing and Healthcare Students.* 4th Ed. Chichester: Wiley-Blackwell; 2021.

Wheeldon A. The principles of pain management. In: Peate I, Mitchell A, eds. *Nursing Practice: Knowledge and Care.* 3rd ed. Chichester: Wiley-Blackwell; 2022.

Whelan E. Putting pain to paper: endometriosis and the documentation of suffering. *Health (N Y).* 2003;7(4):463–482.

Willis P. *Quality with Compassion: The Future of Nursing Education. Report of the Willis Commission.* London: RCN; 2013.

Willis PJ. *Raising the Bar: Shape of Caring Review.* London: RCN; 2015.

Wiraz S, Conrad S, Shtrichman R, et al. Clinical evaluation of a novel technology for oral patient-controlled analgesia: the PCoA acute device for hospitalized patients with postoperative pain in pilot feasibility study. *Pain Res Manag.* 2017. https://doi.org/10.1155/2017/7962135 Article ID 7962135.

Wooldridge S, Banning J. Congruence between nurses' and patients' assessment of postoperative pain: a literature review. *Br J Nurs.* 2020;29(4):212–220.

Further Reading

Blyth FM, Huckel Schneider C. Global burden of pain and global pain policy – creating a purposeful body of evidence. *Pain.* 2018;159:S43–S48.

Doidge N. *The Brain's Way of Healing: Remarkable Discoveries and Recoveries From the Frontiers of Neuroplasticity.* Updated Edition Harmondsworth: Penguin Books; 2016.

Hilton L, Hempel S, Ewing BA, et al. Mindfulness meditation for chronic pain: systematic review and meta-analysis. *Ann Behav Med.* 2016;51(2). www.researchgate.net/publication/308548195_Mindfulness_Meditation_for_Chronic_Pain_Systematic_Review_and_Meta-analysis.

Rastogi KS, McCarthy FK. Complex pain in children and young people: part I – assessment. *BJA Education.* 2017;17(10):317–322.

Schofield P. The assessment of pain in older people: UK guidelines. *Age Ageing.* 2018;47:i1–i22. Available from the Institute for Chronic Pain and online at: https://www.ncbi.nlm.nih.gov/pmc/articles/PMC5888957/pdf/afx192.pdf.

Smith HS. *Current Therapy in Pain.* St Louis: WB Saunders; 2010.

Stannard C, Kalso E, Ballantyne J. *Evidence-Based Chronic Pain Management.* Oxford: Wiley–Blackwell; 2010.

Tortora GJ, Derrickson B. *Principles of Anatomy and Physiology: Maintenance and Continuity of the Human Body.* 15th ed. Hoboken, NJ: Wiley; 2017.

Useful Websites and Resources

Websites

Aromatherapy Council, www.aromatherapycouncil.org
British Acupuncture Council, www.acupuncture.org.uk/
Bandolier Oxford Pain Internet Site, www.bandolier.org.uk/booth/pain-pag/index.html
British National Formulary (BNF), www.bnf.org
British Pain Society, www.britishpainsociety.org
British Pain Society, Guidelines for pain management programmes for adults, www.britishpainsociety.org/british-pain-society-publications/professional-publications/
CAMHS (Child and Adolescent Mental Health Services), www.nhs.uk/using-the-nhs/nhs-services/mental-health-services/child-and-adolescent-mental-health-services-camhs/
Complementary and Natural Healthcare Council, www.cnhc.org.uk/
Faculty of Pain Medicine, Opioids aware: a resource for patients and healthcare professionals to support prescribing of opioid medicines for pain, www.rcoa.ac.uk/faculty-of-pain-medicine/opioids-aware
Healthcare Improvement Scotland (chronic pain), www.healthcareimprovementscotland.org/our_work/long_term_conditions/chronic_pain_services.aspx
International Association for the Study of Pain, www.iasp-pain.org
Migraine Action, www.migraine.org.uk
MIND: For Better Mental Health (mindfulness), www.mind.org.uk/information-support/drugs-and-treatments/mindfulness/#.W1NoKdJKjIU
Mindfulness free resources, www.freemindfulness.org/download
NHS, Healthy Body (chronic pain), www.nhs.uk/live-well/healthy-body/ways-to-manage-chronic-pain/.
NICE (National Institute for Health and Care Excellence) (pain guidance), www.nice.org.uk/guidance/published?q=pain
NICE (National Institute for Health and Care Excellence) (patients with learning disabilities), www.nice.org.uk/guidance/published?q=learning+disabilities
Pain Assessment and Management Initiative (PAMI), free access resources: com-jax-emergency-pami.sites.medinfo.ufl.edu/files/2016/07/PAMI-Module-1-Basic-Principles-of-Pain-Management.pdf
com-jax-emergency-pami.sites.medinfo.ufl.edu/files/2016/07/Acute-Pain-Managment.pdf
com-jax-emergency-pami.sites.medinfo.ufl.edu/files/2016/07/PAMI-Module-3-Procedural-Sedation-and-Analgesia-10_31_2017.pdf
PainHEALTH (mindfulness), painhealth.csse.uwa.edu.au/pain-module/mindfulness-and-pain/
Pain scales in multiple languages, www.britishpainsociety.org/british-pain-society-publications/pain-scales-in-multiple-languages/
Pain-Talk (UK discussion forum for healthcare professionals), www.pain-talk.co.uk
Royal College of Nursing, www.rcn.org.uk/library/subject-guides/pain
Royal College of Nursing, Pain knowledge and skills framework for the nursing team, www.rcn.org.uk/professional-development/publications/pub-004984
Scottish Intercollegiate Guideline Network (SIGN), Guideline 136 Management of chronic pain, www.sign.ac.uk/our-guidelines/management-of-chronic-pain/
Tame the Beast, www.tamethebeast.org/resources/
Understanding neuroplasticity impact on chronic pain management (video), www.youtube.com/watch?v=lRu2hdVmFao

Podcasts

Podcasts are a useful adjunct to aid learning in the form of digital audio files which are available widely on the Internet for downloading to a computer or mobile device. There are a variety of podcasts available across the spectrum of pain. A small sample is listed here:

Pain concern – hosts a podcast called Airing Pain, which explores a range of pain related topics, www.painconcern.org.uk/airing-pain/

The Faculty of Pain Medicine – hosts podcasts on pain and pain management, www.fpm.ac.uk/fpmlearning/podcasts

Arthritis Foundation – hosts a podcast called Live Yes! With Arthritis, which explores pain management as well as guidance and advice for people living with arthritis, www.arthritis.org/liveyes/podcast

TED Talks

The TED talks website hosts videos on living with pain, www.ted.com/search?q=pain

21

Maintaining Fluid, Electrolyte and Acid–Base Balance

NOLEEN PATRICIA JONES

CHAPTER OUTLINE

Introduction

Monitoring and manipulating body fluid and electrolytes form a crucial aspect of nursing care. For a lean adult male, about 18% of the body weight is protein, 15% fat and 7% minerals; 60% is water. For health, body water and electrolytes must be maintained within a limited range. Homeostatic mechanisms regulate parameters such as body fluid volume, acid–base balance (pH) and electrolyte concentrations, maintaining a delicate, dynamic balance which can be destabilised during illness. In extreme cases, the fluid or electrolyte deficit or excess can lead to death. Consequently, nurses must have a clear understanding of fluid and electrolyte homeostasis (autoregulatory processes that maintain fluid and electrolyte levels, e.g. pH, blood glucose, within set parameters) so that they can assess fluid and electrolyte status, anticipate and recognise deterioration and implement corrective interventions.

Nursing interventions in relation to fluid therapy may range from encouraging the patient to drink an afternoon cup of tea to managing a complicated intravenous fluid regimen. Ill-defined terms, such as 'encourage fluids', and instructions to record fluid intake/output or daily weight, are commonly encountered. However, without a knowledgeable appreciation of the physiology and pathophysiology of fluid and electrolyte balance, there is a real risk that these activities will be performed in a somewhat mechanistic fashion, without sufficient thought or understanding.

This chapter reviews the normal mechanisms which regulate body fluid and electrolytes and outlines some of the basic adaptive responses to imbalances. The regulation of acid–base balance is also considered, along with basic principles in the management of fluid and electrolyte disorders. Within the chapter, typical clinical situations where fluid and electrolyte control may be compromised are identified. Students who are unfamiliar with the physiology of fluid, electrolyte and acid–base balance or need to refresh their understanding are advised to read this chapter in conjunction with their physiology textbooks.

Nursing goals in the care of patients with existing or potential fluid and electrolyte problems include:

- the promotion and maintenance of a healthy pattern of fluid intake/output appropriate to the patient's lifestyle and wishes
- the detection of existing or potential fluid and electrolyte imbalances
- the reestablishment of fluid and electrolyte balance when homeostasis is disturbed
- the development of educational programmes for the maintenance of fluid and electrolyte balance.

This chapter will provide some of the essential knowledge necessary to achieving these goals.

Fluid in the Body

Water is essential to life and has a range of functions within the body, including giving form to body structures and acting as a transport medium for nutrients, electrolytes, blood gases, metabolic wastes, heat and electrical currents. Water makes up nearly three-quarters of the body's active tissues and homeostatic regulation of body fluids is essential to normal function and health.

An average male in his 40s has a total body water (TBW) of about 60% of their body weight, or approximately 42 L in a 70-kg man (Tobias et al. 2020). The percentage of body weight represented by the TBW varies from one individual to another depending on factors such as age, gender and build. Most of this variation is due to fat (adipose tissue). Adipose tissue contains only about 10% of water and so contributes little towards TBW. A 70-kg woman of average build would have a TBW of about 52% (36 L) due to the greater proportion of adipose (fatty) tissue. In both genders, the percentage of body water decreases with age.

Fluid Compartments

Body water is distributed between two major compartments: approximately two-thirds as intracellular fluid (ICF) and one-third extracellular fluid (ECF) (Fig. 21.1). The volume of ICF is around 28 L in a 70-kg male. The ECF has a volume of approximately 12 L. It comprises the *intravascular fluid* (about 2.5 L within the heart and vessels) and the *interstitial fluid* (about 9.5 L) surrounding the cells and forming a relatively constant environment. In addition,

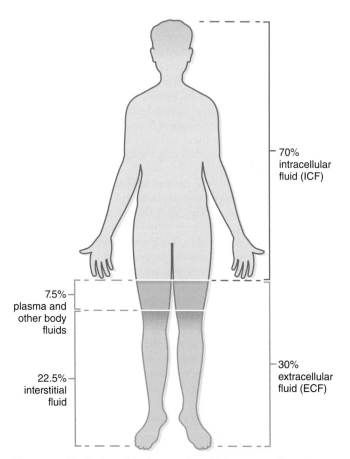

7.5% plasma and other body fluids

22.5% interstitial fluid

70% intracellular fluid (ICF)

30% extracellular fluid (ECF)

Figure 21.1 Distribution of body water in a 70-kg person. (Reproduced from Waugh A, Grant A. *Ross and Wilson Anatomy and Physiology in Health and Illness*. 12th ed. Edinburgh: Elsevier; 2014, with permission.)

there are very small quantities of transcellular fluid (e.g. within the eye, cerebrospinal fluid, glandular secretions) and water in bone.

The distinction between the different fluid compartments is maintained by the selective permeability of cell membranes. The membrane is freely permeable to water and the movement of other solutes is influenced by amongst other things the size of molecule, concentration gradient and electrical charge. Large proteins which are synthesised by the cell remain inside as they are too big to pass through the membrane. Distribution of electrolytes and water is influenced by selective membrane transport processes.

Electrolytes in the Body

Fluid in the body cannot be equated simply with water, as it also contains dissolved substances or solutes as well as larger particles in suspension (colloids). Solutes may be complete molecules (non-electrolytes) or parts of molecules (electrolytes). An electrolyte is a chemical compound that, when in solution, dissociates into electrically charged particles called *ions*. These ions can be positively charged (cation) or negatively charged (anion). The main electrolytes found within the body are sodium (Na^+), chloride (Cl^-), potassium (K^+), magnesium (Mg^{2+}), calcium (Ca^{2+}), phosphorus as phosphates ($H_2PO_4^-$ and HPO_4^{2-}) and bicarbonate (HCO_3^-). In solution, a molecule of sodium chloride dissociates into a positively charged sodium ion Na^+ (cation) and a negatively charged chloride ion Cl^- (anion). Sodium is the dominant cation in the ECF. Chloride and bicarbonate (HCO_3^-) are the major extracellular anions. Inside the cell, potassium (K^+) is the dominant cation. Glucose is a good example of a nonelectrolyte in that it dissolves in body water but does not dissociate into ions.

Electrolytes are essential for cellular activity and need to remain within a specific range for optimal function. In clinical practice, serum electrolytes are measured by a simple blood test, urea and electrolytes, often known as 'U&Es'. Nurses should be aware of normal ranges and factors that may cause electrolyte imbalances in patients for whom they are caring, for example patients with cardiovascular disease or renal disease or those receiving diuretic medication. This knowledge will assist nurses and other health professionals to respond with appropriate care interventions. Information 21.1 provides a more detailed description of the common electrolytes.

Water and Electrolyte Homeostasis

Maintaining Fluid and Electrolyte Balance

Maintaining normal, healthy fluid intake and the constancy of the internal environment is essential for efficient cell function. Fluid balance in the body is maintained by a number of physiological mechanisms. These mechanisms help to ensure that water gain and water loss are balanced (Table 21.1) and prevent the consequences of imbalances such as dehydration and possible death. The main stimulus for increasing intake of fluid is the thirst mechanism.

Fluid and electrolyte balance are inextricably linked and in health the volume and composition of the different fluid compartments are finely regulated, with daily fluctuations in TBW of less than 0.2%. Water and electrolytes are ingested and absorbed through the gastrointestinal (GI) tract, although a small volume of water is produced through the oxidation of hydrogen in food. Excess water, electrolytes and waste products are excreted via the kidneys and in faeces. Additional water and salt loss occurs via the skin and respiratory tract, known as insensible loss. Since losses

INFORMATION 21.1

Common Electrolytes: Functions and Features

Sodium (Na⁺) – Normal Range 135–143 mmol/L

- Most abundant cation in ECF
- Provides plasma with up to half its osmotic pressure
- Required for action potential in neurones and muscle
- Levels regulated by the hormones aldosterone, antidiuretic hormone and atrial natriuretic peptide (ANP)
- Exchanged for K⁺ ions when Na⁺ crosses cell membrane
- Average dietary intake usually exceeds daily requirements
- Kidney can conserve sodium if necessary
- Sweating increases loss of sodium.

Potassium (K⁺) – Normal Range 3.3–4.7 mmol/L

- Most abundant cation in ICF
- As the majority of K⁺ is intracellular, serum levels do not accurately reflect total K⁺ in the body
- Plays a key role in resting membrane potential, repolarisation of neurones and muscle cells
- Maintains ICF volume
- Exchanged for Na⁺ ions when K⁺ crosses cell membrane
- Levels regulated by the hormone aldosterone
- K⁺ mainly lost in urine with small amount in faeces and sweat
- Kidneys cannot conserve K⁺ in the same way as they conserve Na⁺.

Calcium (Ca²⁺) – Normal Range 2.1–2.6 mmol/L

- Most abundant mineral in the body
- Majority combined with phosphate as salts
- Essential for blood clotting
- Controls release of neurotransmitters

- Essential for excitability of nerves and muscles
- In its ionised form (Ca²⁺) is mainly extracellular
- Levels in the blood are controlled by parathyroid hormone and calcitonin.

Magnesium (Mg²⁺) – Normal Range 0.75–1.0 mmol/L

- Magnesium is a cofactor required for enzyme action
- Required for the sodium–potassium pump
- Half of body magnesium found in bone matrix as magnesium salts
- Remainder is ionised (Mg²⁺) and found mainly in ICF.

Chloride (Cl⁻) – Normal Range 97–106 mmol/L

- Most common extracellular anion (Cl⁻)
- Crosses cell membrane freely in exchange for bicarbonate.

Phosphate – normal range 0.8–1.4 mmol/L

- Ionic forms of phosphate ($H_2PO_4^-$ and HPO_4^{2-}) have a role in phosphate buffer system
- Found as a salt in bones and teeth
- Present in nucleic acids and ATP
- Principally found in ICF
- Levels controlled by parathyroid hormone and calcitonin.

Bicarbonate (HCO_3^-) – Normal Range 22–28 mmol/L

- Essential for homeostasis of blood pH through the bicarbonate buffer system
- Second most abundant extracellular anion
- Levels regulated by kidneys in response to pH of blood

Adapted from Waugh (2003) with permission.

TABLE 21.1 Water Balance: Water Gain and Water Loss (Adult)

Input – Water Gain	Output – Water Loss
Beverages: 1500 mL	Urine: 1500 mL
Food: 750 mL	Faeces: 100 mL
Water produced during metabolism: 250 mL	Sweat: 200 mL
	Skin and respiration: 700 mL (insensible loss)
Total: 2500 mL	Total: 2500 mL

from the GI and respiratory tract are not subject to fine regulation, the kidney is the main regulator of fluid and electrolyte balance (see Chapter 10, Nursing Patients With Urinary Disorders). The flow of blood through the kidney is known as the glomerular filtration rate (GFR) and a normal GFR is 125 mL/min (Kaufman et al. 2020). In 24 hours, the total blood flow through the kidneys is approximately 180 L; this means that the plasma contained within the body is filtered and reabsorbed about 60 times a day. The kidney regulates not only fluid volume, but also electrolyte composition, pH and osmolality. Central to the renal regulation of body fluid osmolality and volume is the kidney's role in handling of sodium and water.

The osmotic pressure of a solution is expressed as the osmolality (the number of particles present per kilogram of solvent). Osmolality is a standard measure used in medicine and in the very simplest of terms could be considered a measure of the concentration of a solution. Each of the constituents within the ECF and plasma, for example the principal ions (sodium, potassium, chloride, etc.) and other nonionic substances such as glucose and amino acids, exerts a different osmotic pressure. The total sum of these is the measure of the osmolality of the ECF and plasma within 1 kg of the principal solvent within the body, water. The ECF and plasma are said to have an osmolality of around 300 mOsm/kg. The osmotic pressure produced by the proteins, although small, plays an important role in the exchange of fluid between body compartments (Pocock et al. 2017).

Fluid Exchange Between the Intracellular and Extracellular Compartments

The movement of body fluids and their constituents between the different compartments is dynamic and involves the following processes:
- diffusion
- osmosis
- facilitated diffusion
- active transport
- filtration.

These processes take place through the selectively permeable membrane separating the different fluid compartments, that is, the cell membrane and the capillary wall (single-cell layer of endothelium). The cell membrane separates the ICF from the ECF, and the capillary wall represents the boundary between the intravascular and interstitial compartments of the ECF.

Diffusion is the movement of solutes from an area of higher concentration to an area of lower concentration, which results in an equal concentration in both areas. Diffusion is a form of passive transport because no energy is required and the solutes just move or flow across the membrane.

Osmosis is the passive movement of fluid from an area of lower concentration (of solutes) to an area of higher concentration, in an attempt to dilute the 'stronger' solution and achieve an equal balance on both sides of the membrane. The capillary wall is selectively permeable to substances of a molecular weight less than 69,000 Daltons (69.0 kDa) and to lipid-soluble molecules. Lipid-soluble substances diffuse directly through the cell membrane, while water and electrolytes utilise channels formed by membrane proteins. The membrane is freely permeable to water but is only selectively permeable to electrolytes. Permeability is affected by the size and charge of the hydrated ion; for example, the membrane is 50–100 times more permeable to potassium than to sodium.

Some substances move through *facilitated diffusion* or *active transport*, for example, glucose moves under the influence of insulin. The most important example of active transport is the sodium–potassium pump. This pump is a membrane protein that couples the active transport of sodium out of the cell with the active transport of potassium inwards. It requires energy derived from the hydrolysis of adenosine triphosphate (ATP) to function.

The exchange of water, electrolytes, metabolites and waste products between the plasma and interstitial fluid occurs in the capillary bed. The capillary endothelium is freely permeable to water and solutes but the larger plasma proteins are retained. The movement of fluid through the capillaries relies on a process called capillary filtration. At the arterial end, fluid is forced out of the capillary by hydrostatic pressure. As water is lost from the capillary, the plasma proteins become more concentrated and the colloid osmotic or oncotic pressure exerted by the plasma proteins increases. At the venous end, the hydrostatic pressure, now lower than the rising osmotic pressure, results in fluid being drawn back into the capillary.

The lymphatic system is central to maintaining interstitial fluid volume. Blind-ended lymphatic capillaries in the interstitium are more permeable than the capillaries and easily take up and remove any plasma proteins that have leaked out and fluid from the interstitial space. The fluid formed in these vessels – lymph – is carried through the lymphatic system, eventually returning to the circulation via the central lymphatic and the thoracic duct.

Disturbances in Fluid Exchange

As approximately 20% of body fluid is found in the interstitial or tissue spaces, the maintenance of fluid volume in this compartment plays a key role in homeostasis. Normally, a dynamic equilibrium exists which maintains the extracellular fluid content of both the plasma and the tissue spaces. However, this delicate balance can easily be disturbed by the following factors and the resulting clinical picture for many of them will be oedema (Reflection 21.1). Further information about oedema is available on the website.

- *Alterations in capillary pressure* – changes in pressure at either end of the capillary bed will alter net movement of fluid. Increased arterial pressure or venous congestion both tend to favour the loss of fluid to the interstitial space. Examples include hypertension, hypotension, heart failure and arterial or venous obstruction.

REFLECTION 21.1

Oedema

Think back to a patient you have cared for who had peripheral oedema.

Activity

- What had caused their oedema? What clinical manifestations did they have?
- How was their oedema being managed and what nursing care did they require?
- Reflect upon the effectiveness of the care given in terms of patient comfort.

- *Alterations in the plasma proteins* – a reduction in plasma proteins due to malnutrition, liver or renal disease, loss of circulating plasma or leakage of proteins into the tissue fluids will alter the osmotic pressure gradient and prevent fluid being reclaimed from the tissue spaces. Failure of the lymphatics to remove this fluid will increase the osmotic pressure of the interstitial fluid and favour fluid retention.
- *Changes in the integrity of the capillary endothelium* – factors that alter the normal mechanisms regulating the permeability/pore size of the capillary endothelium also change the osmotic or hydrostatic pressures. These effects may be local or systemic. Examples include membrane damage from burns, anoxia, pressure, sepsis and the presence of inflammatory mediators such as bradykinin or histamine.
- *Accumulation of metabolites* – an accumulation of metabolites within the tissue fluid can alter the hydrostatic and colloidal osmotic pressures with consequent changes in fluid movement. For example, in some states of shock or tissue hypoxia, the cumulative effects of lactic acid and carbon dioxide when combined with vasoactive substances may result in oedema.

Regulation and Adjustments of ECF Volume, Osmolality and Sodium

The circulatory system comprises the arterial system of high pressure and low volume and the venous system which operates with a lower pressure and higher volume. Approximately 55% of the plasma volume is in the venous system, 10% in the arterial system and the remaining 35% distributed in the heart, lungs and capillaries (see Chapter 2, Nursing Patients With Cardiovascular Disorders). Thus changes in volume are usually accommodated by the venous system. The effect of gravity upon fluid in the circulatory system is marked, causing pooling of blood in the venous system with a consequent reduction in the arterial blood volume. If an individual stands for a prolonged period, particularly in a warm environment, there is a reduction in arterial flow to the cells; inadequate venous return then leads to a fall in end-diastolic volume and hence cardiac output. Inadequate perfusion of the brain can then lead to fainting.

The tissue spaces can accommodate large volumes of fluid, but the process is slow and causes fewer disturbances to the ICF or plasma. Adults can usually tolerate changes of about 2 L in the tissue spaces before there are noticeable signs of a volume shift. This 'hidden' accumulation of fluid may, however, be noticed by changes in body weight, 1 L of water (pure) being equivalent to 1 kg.

Volume and osmolality regulation of the ECF involves a series of homeostatic mechanisms. Although the plasma compartment is small, it is dynamic, with shifts in volume and pressure occurring in response to internal and external stimuli. Sodium is also a major factor in the regulation of ECF. The kidney regulates sodium and water ingestion/excretion under the influence of two hormones, aldosterone and antidiuretic hormone (ADH; also known as arginine vasopressin (AVP) or vasopressin).

Influence of Antidiuretic Hormone

Within the hypothalamus are specialised cells called osmoreceptors which monitor and respond to changes in plasma osmolality (see earlier). They are very sensitive and respond to changes of as little as ±3 milliosmoles (mOsm). Plasma osmolality is normally in the range of 300 mOsmL/kg water. The osmoreceptors respond to variations in plasma osmolality by stimulating or inhibiting two mechanisms: thirst and ADH release.

As plasma osmolality rises, the stimulation of the thirst centre will make the active, independent individual seek fluid to drink, thus attempting to correct any dehydration or shortage of water. ADH will act on the epithelial cells of the nephron collecting ducts and latter part of the distal convoluted tubule to increase/decrease tubular permeability to water. If there is fluid loss, or excess ingestion of salt, plasma osmolality is increased and registered by the osmoreceptors and the individual should begin to feel thirsty. The release of ADH (from the posterior pituitary gland) affects the permeability of the nephron collecting ducts and latter section of the distal convoluted tubule, and water will be reabsorbed into the blood to dilute the hypertonic plasma. This will result in a decrease in urine volume and increase in urine osmolality – urine produced will have a darker, more concentrated appearance. Conversely, if a large volume of water is ingested, the plasma sodium is diluted, causing a fall in the plasma osmolality. This fall is registered by the osmoreceptors, with a resultant decrease in ADH release. Lowered plasma ADH then results in decreased tubular permeability, less water is reabsorbed and water is excreted in the form of a more dilute urine.

The presence of a nonabsorbable solute in the renal tubular lumen will also increase water loss. For example, when plasma glucose levels are raised, as in poorly controlled diabetes mellitus (see Chapter 5, Nursing Patients With Endocrine and Metabolic Disorders), and filtered glucose exceeds the ability of the nephrons to reabsorb it, urine production is increased. The glucose exerts an osmotic force, keeping water in the tubule. Osmotic diuresis can also be induced therapeutically by the intravenous administration of a non-absorbable molecule such as the sugar mannitol.

Other Factors Affecting ADH Regulation of Osmolality

ADH release may be altered by some drugs, including nicotine and alcohol. Alcohol inhibits the release of ADH, with a resulting diuresis. Nicotine and morphine are drugs which may increase ADH release. Adrenal insufficiency alters the renal response to water loading. Deficiency in adrenal glucocorticoids (e.g. cortisol) causes an increase in distal tubular permeability to water. Water reabsorption is increased and dilute urine cannot be produced. Tubular response to ADH is decreased and, even in the absence of ADH, permeability to water remains high.

Influence of Aldosterone

ECF volume is principally determined by sodium, and body sodium is regulated by the kidney, mainly under the influence of aldosterone. Aldosterone is a mineralocorticoid, released from the adrenal cortex, and is essential for sodium (with associated water) reabsorption. Aldosterone release is stimulated by changes in ECF volume, plasma sodium concentration and plasma potassium concentration. Increases in serum potassium levels of as little as 0.2 mmol/L can cause a marked increase in aldosterone release.

The release of aldosterone is part of a physiological mechanism often known as the *renin–angiotensin–aldosterone* system. Renin is a proteolytic enzyme released from the kidney, more specifically from the juxtaglomerular apparatus (JGA) situated near the afferent arteriole of the glomerulus. It is released in response to changes in plasma sodium and effective circulating volume. Renin acts on a circulating plasma protein (angiotensinogen) to form angiotensin I. Angiotensin I is in turn altered by a converting enzyme found in the lungs to its active form angiotensin II. Angiotensin II has two key actions: it is a potent vasoconstrictor and it stimulates the release of aldosterone. This release of aldosterone will then result in an increase in sodium (and water) reabsorption within the distal tubule of the nephron. The increase in sodium reabsorption is in direct exchange for potassium. A rising serum potassium will directly stimulate the production of aldosterone, which in turn will increase sodium reabsorption from the kidney tubule in exchange for potassium which will be lost in the urine.

Hypovolaemia (reduced volume of circulating blood), which reflects a fall in sodium content (as opposed to concentration), will increase aldosterone secretion via the renin–angiotensin system. The resulting vasoconstriction and reabsorption of sodium and water reflect the body's attempt to correct the intravascular volume and thereby maintain blood pressure.

In certain types of hypertension, this mechanism malfunctions and is managed by medication such as angiotensin-converting enzyme inhibitors (ACE inhibitors) and angiotensin II receptor blockers (ARBs).

Fluid and Electrolyte Disturbances

Water volume and sodium imbalances frequently occur in combination with other electrolyte problems, although occasionally they occur alone. Principal causes of disturbance can be related to:
- insufficient or excessive intake or output
- problems in the regulation of intake and output which may be associated with disease states, e.g. heart failure, renal or endocrine disorders
- problems related to fluid shifts within the body.

Assessment of fluid and electrolyte balance is covered later (including Tables 21.4 and 21.5 that outline some of the signs associated with fluid and electrolyte disturbances and measurable parameters and their significance).

Fluid Imbalances

Fluid imbalances may be *isotonic* or *osmolar* in nature depending upon the composition of the fluid lost and the resulting balance of water and electrolytes in relation to the ECF. Isotonic imbalances result from the loss of water and electrolytes in proportion to their normal levels in the ECF. Osmolar imbalances are the result of water loss (hyperosmolar) or water gain (hypo-osmolar) which affects the concentration of electrolytes in the ECF and changes the serum osmolarity. Most fluid imbalances are often a combination of both isotonic and osmolar disturbances. This next section considers the effects of fluid imbalances such as dehydration (fluid deficit) or overhydration (water intoxication) of the body and tissues.

Fluid Deficits

An ECF volume deficit will arise when fluid loss exceeds fluid intake. Fluid losses may be related to a number of factors, and the National Institute for Health and Care Excellence (NICE) (2013) has produced a helpful diagram summarising these potential ongoing losses. Some of the causes of fluid deficits are discussed here.

Hyperosmolar Losses

Dehydration

Strictly speaking, dehydration refers only to water losses from the body that exceed intake, leaving the person with a corresponding accumulation of sodium (a hyperosmolar state). This might be seen for example in someone with delirium or cognitive impairment such as dementia who does not drink adequately and over a period of days becomes dehydrated. This shortage of water results in a rise in sodium and an increase in serum osmolality. Water will then shift from the cells (ICF) into the ECF and vascular compartment to try to correct the imbalance, although this will result in the cells themselves becoming dehydrated.

Pure water losses are unusual and it is more common for water to be lost in conjunction with sodium (and other electrolytes), as is seen in vomiting and diarrhoea.

Initially, compensatory mechanisms will maintain blood pressure and heart rate and the kidneys will reduce output, but as the dehydration continues, blood pressure falls, pulse volume weakens and heart rate and packed cell volume (PCV) (also known as haematocrit) rise. Haemoconcentration (relative increase in the volume of red blood cells to that of plasma) also causes apparent rises in haemoglobin and albumin levels. This can lead to hypovolaemic 'shock' and eventually the obligatory volume necessary to maintain renal function and excrete waste products in the urine will be inadequate – known as acute kidney injury. The sequelae of acute kidney injury can result in metabolite accumulation, acidosis (the processes that result in the build-up of excess acid in the body), electrolyte imbalances and fluid accumulation – any of which may lead to death if left untreated.

Dehydration can be categorised according to the approximate percentage of body water that is lost; in the adult, this may be defined as follows:
- mild: 4% (3 L)
- moderate: 5%–8% (4–6 L)
- severe: 8%–10% (7 L).

The management of dehydration is often complex, especially in severe states where there is gross derangement of body chemistry. In mild to moderate dehydration, fluid losses should be replaced slowly to prevent sudden shifts of water and/or electrolytes between fluid compartments, which would aggravate ionic balance. However, in cases of severe dehydration, as seen in diabetes insipidus or severe heat exhaustion, this may lead to fatal hypovolaemia and so aggressive therapy is required (see Chapter 5, Nursing Patients With Endocrine Disorders). The effects of hyponatraemia (decreased sodium concentration in the blood) and hypernatraemia (increased sodium concentration in the blood), which may accompany dehydration, are summarised in Table 21.2.

Urinary Loss

A number of disease states may result in an excessive production of urine. Patients who have incurred head injury, have undergone hypophysectomy (removal of the pituitary gland) or who have a primary diagnosis of diabetes insipidus may excrete excessive volumes of water and electrolytes due to a disruption in the release of ADH from the pituitary gland. Diabetes insipidus occurs when there is either a deficiency in the manufacture and release of ADH, or an inability of the kidney tubules to respond to ADH.

Isotonic Losses

Gastrointestinal Losses

Within the GI tract, there is a continuous exchange of fluids, with most of the fluid produced being absorbed. Illnesses that present with diarrhoea or vomiting, or conditions in which fistulae, drainage tubes or GI suction are present, can result in excessive fluid and electrolyte losses, potentially up to 8–9 L/day. Continuous GI or fistula drainage will have the same consequences for a patient as severe diarrhoea and vomiting.

🌐 **See Evolve website Critical thinking question 21.1**

Third Space Losses

The concept of the *third space* is used to describe the presence of fluids in areas of the body where they are usually absent, or present only in small quantities. This may occur in patients with sepsis, burns or major trauma. Although not lost from the body, the fluid is physiologically unavailable and thus the patient presents as if they are deficient in fluid.

Skin Losses

The loss of sodium and water from the skin increases dramatically during excessive sweating or if large areas of the skin have been damaged. For example, in extreme hot weather, as much as 1.5–2.0 L/h can be lost through sweat. In the patient with fever, water loss may be up to 3 L/24 hours. Burns patients suffer excessive fluid losses; evaporation losses can be 3 to 4 times greater than in people with healthy skin (Alonso-Fernandez and Lopez-Pablo 2021) and total loss of fluid from severe burns can be as much as 6–8 L/24 hours (see Chapter 29, Nursing the Patient With Burn Injury).

Osmotic Diuresis

In osmotic diuresis, polyuria (excretion of excessive volume of urine) results from the presence of large quantities of solutes in the blood which enter the glomerular filtrate and are not reabsorbed. The high osmolality of the filtrate in the renal tubules inhibits the action of ADH and prevents reabsorption of water. This principle can be used to produce an osmotic diuresis therapeutically, for example when mannitol is administered to reduce intracranial pressure. In people with diabetes mellitus, an excess of glucose, leading to hyperglycaemia (too much glucose in the blood) or diabetic ketoacidosis, results in a level of glucose that exceeds the kidney's ability to reabsorb it. This causes polyuria, a common presenting symptom of diabetes mellitus.

Fluid Volume Excess

The retention of fluid and electrolytes results in a fluid volume excess. Such an imbalance can be caused by overloading with fluids or by reduced functioning of the body's homeostatic mechanisms responsible for maintaining fluid and electrolyte balance. The most likely scenario is retention of sodium accompanied by the retention of water as seen in congestive heart failure, renal disease and inappropriate administration of intravenous fluids containing sodium. Isotonic fluids such as 0.9% sodium chloride (physiological saline) or sodium lactate compound (Hartmann's

TABLE 21.2	Common Electrolyte Disturbances – Deficits and Excesses of Sodium, Potassium and Calcium		
Electrolyte Disturbance	Reasons	Clinical Examples	Typical Signs and Symptoms
Hyponatraemia (serum sodium <135 mmol/L)	a. Excess sodium loss b. Sodium dilution c. Hormone-induced water gains	a. GI losses, exercise b. Excessive fluid intake c. Renal tubule dysfunction, increased ADH secretion	Muscle cramps, weakness, headache, mood changes, depression, lethargy, altered consciousness, tachycardia, hypotension, oedema
Hypernatraemia (serum sodium >143 mmol/L)	a. Excess sodium intake b. Decreased extracellular water c. Water deprivation and decreased water intake d. Hormone related	a. Diet, near drowning, excessive intravenous administration of solutions containing sodium b. Dehydration c. Confusion, impaired thirst sensation, communication difficulties d. Diabetes insipidus	Confusion, lethargy, twitching, convulsions, polydipsia (excessive thirst), hypertension, weight gain
Hypokalaemia (serum potassium <3.3 mmol/L)	a. Inadequate intake b. Excessive GI losses c. Excessive renal losses d. Intercellular movement	a. Starvation, anorexia b. Diarrhoea, vomiting, excessive nasogastric tube aspiration c. Diuretic therapy, hyperaldosteronism d. Muscular weakness, cardiac dysrhythmias and cardiac arrest, alkalosis, mental confusion, fatigue and hypoventilation	Side-effect of some beta-blockers, insulin therapy, e.g. diabetic ketoacidosis
Hyperkalaemia (serum potassium >4.7 mmol/L)	a. Excessive intake or gain b. Inadequate renal losses c. Release from cells (intracellular compartment)	a. Oral or intravenous potassium b. Renal failure, renal tubule dysfunction, side-effects of ACE inhibitors c. Tissue trauma, burns, crush injuries	Anxiety, confusion, cardiac dysrhythmias, bradycardia and cardiac arrest, twitching, muscle weakness, nausea, vomiting and other GI disturbances
Hypocalcaemia (serum calcium <2.1 mmol/L)	a. Impaired ability to mobilise calcium from bone b. Abnormal calcium binding c. Abnormal losses d. Renal failure, liver disease	a. Hypoparathyroidism b. Increase in blood pH (more alkaline), such as with hyperventilation, rapid transfusion of citrated blood c. Pancreatitis d. Reduced absorption or intake	Paraesthesia, spasms, cramp, tetany, hypotension, ventricular dysrhythmias, bone pain
Hypercalcaemia (serum calcium >2.6 mmol/L)	a. Excessive gains b. Increased bone resorption c. Increased level of parathyroid hormone d. Inadequate losses e. Renal insufficiency	a. Increased vitamin D or calcium in the diet, excessive use of calcium-containing medicines, or nutritional supplements b. Metastatic tumours of bone, paraneoplastic syndrome, Paget's disease c. Hyperparathyroidism d. Thiazide diuretics, lithium therapy e. Altered calcium and phosphate absorption or binding	Polyuria, polydipsia Vague symptoms of anorexia, abdominal pain, nausea, vomiting, constipation, muscle weakness/pain and lethargy. Cardiac disturbances

ACE, Angiotensin-converting enzyme; *ADH,* antidiuretic hormone; *GI,* gastrointestinal.

solution) contain large amounts of sodium. With some patients, for example older people or those who have a history of heart or renal disease, careful attention must be given to intravenous fluid therapy (Stickel et al. 2019). Other sources of sodium gain include some over-the-counter (OTC) drugs that contain significant amounts of sodium salts.

Hypo-Osmolar Imbalance or Water Excess

When a large volume of water is ingested, it begins to be absorbed within about 15 minutes, in consequence of which the osmolality of the blood decreases. This causes an inhibition of the production and secretion of ADH. Absence of ADH makes the distal convoluted tubule and collecting duct impermeable to water and so more urine is excreted by the kidney, thus producing a more dilute urine and a water diuresis. Following a single large intake of oral fluid, the maximum effect upon diuresis will be noticed about 40 minutes later. A similar effect is achieved if a bolus or fluid challenge of intravenous fluid is administered.

Water Intoxication

The kidney has a maximum rate at which it can excrete fluid. If water ingestion, or a hypotonic intravenous fluid administration, exceeds this capacity, then the ECF remains hypotonic. The hypotonic ECF results in fluid moving into the ICF, with a subsequent swelling and bursting of cells. This is most serious in the brain, causing raised intracranial pressure (RIP), convulsions and death. Another significant cause of death from water intoxication occurs as a consequence of the use of illegal drugs, that is, 3,4-methylenedioxymethamphetamine (MDMA) (also known as ecstasy). MDMA can reduce or suppress the thirst sensation with a resultant risk of dehydration, and as it is often taken in an environment of high-energy dancing (and sweating), to minimise harm and prevent the likelihood of dehydration, users are advised to drink approximately a litre of water an hour if they become hot and/or expend energy. The danger occurs when the person misjudges or loses awareness how to compensate their fluid intake.

Risk Factors and Disorders Associated With Fluid and Electrolyte Imbalance

This section outlines some areas in which patients commonly experience difficulties with fluid and electrolyte control. Some patients may be at risk for a number of reasons and older people in particular are at increased risk. Nurses in many areas of practice will encounter patients whose fluid and electrolyte balance has been challenged, with potentially dire consequences, for example patients with burns, cardiac failure or respiratory problems. Some important risk factors associated with fluid and electrolyte imbalances include:

- *Shortage of water* – in developing countries, water is often in short supply or involves long journeys to obtain it. Drinking the required daily amount to maintain hydration (especially in hot climates) may be very difficult for some to achieve.
- *Fasting or restricted intake* – many medical procedures or the need for surgery require a period of 'nil by mouth' and it is important that this be no longer than necessary. For patients who are repeatedly starved it may be necessary to commence intravenous fluids. Some religious practices involve fasting and may put some members of the population, e.g. older people or those with renal impairment, at risk. Adjustments to strict practices are possible for those with underlying health conditions, and advice can be sought.
- *Inability to respond to thirst* – people with delirium or cognitive impairment, and those who are depressed, frail or debilitated may not be able to obtain their own fluid/drinks independently. It is important to identify such patients and ensure appropriate measures are taken for them to obtain adequate fluid.
- *Vomiting or loss of GI fluid*, e.g. via nasogastric aspirate, if not replaced with appropriate fluid can cause dehydration. If prolonged or severe, it may also lead to metabolic alkalosis and malnutrition (see Chapter 22, Nutrition and Health). The loss of gastric juices, which contain hydrochloric acid and potassium ions, initially leads to metabolic alkalosis due to a surplus of bicarbonate ions. In severe, prolonged vomiting without adequate nutritional replacement, the body begins to metabolise fats as an energy source, producing ketone bodies and the potential for further acid–base disturbance. Patients who have had abdominal surgery may develop paralytic ileus and the gastric fluid produced is drained via a nasogastric tube rather than being reabsorbed. This will result in a fluid deficit if not appropriately replaced by intravenous fluids.

🌐 **See Evolve website Critical thinking question 21.1**

- *Diarrhoea* – worldwide, diarrhoea is a serious problem and the most important indication for fluid and electrolyte replacement. It occurs when the body is unable to reclaim/absorb the fluids in the intestinal tract and the peristaltic contractions of the gut expel the intestinal contents. Generally, intestinal fluids are isotonic with the ECF until the colon is reached, at which point the contents gradually become hypotonic due to the colon's role in water reabsorption. Severe and prolonged diarrhoea, as seen in cholera or in some forms of infant gastroenteritis, can lead to severe electrolyte imbalance, dehydration and, ultimately, death if treatment is unsuccessful or delayed. Fluid and electrolyte replacement is an essential component in the management of the effects of diarrhoea, with accompanying management of the causative agent. Oral rehydration solution is frequently employed in cases of gastroenteritis and dehydration, providing the gut is able to absorb ingested fluids.

🌐 **See Evolve website Critical thinking question 21.1**

- *Problems associated with the mouth and throat* – patients who have had a stroke (cerebrovascular accident – CVA) and have dysphagia (difficulty in swallowing) will find taking oral fluids and food difficult and sometimes distressing. Full assessment by the speech and language therapist (SLT) will be essential before oral fluids are given to assess their ability to swallow without choking or risk aspirating fluid into the lungs. Other patients at risk include those who have facial trauma or have had extensive oral or dental surgery.
- *Reduced mobility and dexterity* – many people will fit into this category. It may be a patient who has undergone a hip replacement; it could be someone who has a new disability such as following stroke, or someone with severe rheumatoid arthritis. For these patients, it is important to ensure that they can reach and easily access fluid so that they can drink independently, or the nurse should ensure that the patient is given fluids at regular intervals.
- *Cardiovascular and renal problems* – people with these problems often present with retention of sodium and water. This is the result of physiological mechanisms not functioning correctly, e.g. the renin–angiotensin–aldosterone mechanism. It is often necessary to restrict fluid intake to prevent fluid overload, and restriction of salt and potassium is also required for some patients.
- *Diuretic therapy* – diuretic medication increases urine output, and therefore influences fluid and electrolyte loss. It is important to monitor that the diuresis is not too far in excess of the patient's intake so that they risk becoming dehydrated. Patients who are required to take this medication may choose to omit it if they find they have to make repeated trips to the lavatory in the night (hence it is often prescribed first thing in the morning) or if they are afraid of falling whilst hurrying to the lavatory.
- *Loss of continence* – people with continence problems may sometimes restrict their fluid intake in a hope that it will reduce their need to pass urine or soil their underwear. This situation may also arise in hospital when patients may similarly reduce their fluid intake so that they do not have to ask for the commode/bedpan or ask to be taken to the lavatory too frequently.

Disorders of Electrolyte Balance

As stated earlier, electrolytes are essential for cellular activity and their concentration in the blood must remain within a specific range for optimal function. There are many clinical situations which may result in disorders of electrolyte balance, some of which are life-threatening. Nurses should be aware of the normal biochemical ranges (Information 21.1) and factors that may cause electrolyte imbalances in patients they are caring for (see earlier). Table 21.2 outlines a range of commonly encountered electrolyte disorders, including possible causes and the effects on bodily function. By fully understanding the implications of electrolyte disturbances, the nurse can respond with appropriate care interventions.

Maintaining Acid–Base Balance

Body fluids are normally slightly alkaline (basic), within a pH range of 7.36–7.44 (hydrogen ion concentration ($[H^+]$) 35–45 nmol/L). Blood has an H^+ concentration of 40 nmol/L, or a pH of 7.4. Acidaemia occurs when the arterial blood pH is less than 7.36

(greater than 44 nmol/L H⁺). An arterial pH greater than 7.44 (or less than 36 nmol/L H⁺) is alkalaemia. The body enzymes which control most physiological processes are optimally active within the normal pH range, and variations from this range can rapidly result in severe physiological dysfunction or death. It is therefore essential to understand the basis of acid–base balance in health and the effects of disease on this balance. A pH outside the range 6.9–7.7 is incompatible with life; variations outside 7.36–7.44 are serious and may be difficult to rectify. Whilst the blood pH is maintained at a slightly alkaline level, the pH of urine is frequently acidic as the body seeks to excrete surplus acids which have been produced by both metabolic and respiratory processes.

The medium- and long-term regulation of pH occurs through the lungs and kidneys, whilst chemical buffers in the blood provide an immediate response to changes in pH. With adjustments in respiratory rate, carbon dioxide levels and hence pH can also change. The response, involving the kidney, is slower and sometimes referred to as the 'renal lag'. The kidney's ability to regenerate bicarbonate ions whilst excreting hydrogen ions enables it to aid the regulation of pH. Crucial to the management of acid–base imbalance is the identification and reversal or removal of the causative factor.

Disorders of Acid–Base Balance

Homeostatic mechanisms within the body ensure that the environment for cellular activity is maintained within important limits to allow them to function effectively. One of these mechanisms is regulation and balance of acids and bases (see earlier). Slight imbalances in the pH of body fluids can result in significant effects on body metabolism and essential functions. There are many potential causes of acid–base imbalances, for example infection, respiratory disease, renal disease or dysfunction and some medications. The resulting states may be:

- Acidosis – the process that results in the build-up of excess acid (hydrogen ions) in the body. It leads to acidaemia in which the pH of the blood is below normal (i.e. the pH shifts further towards the neutral point).
- Alkalosis – the process that results in low levels of acid (excess of alkali) in the body. It leads to alkalaemia in which there is a low level of acid (hydrogen ions) and an above normal pH.

Because the lungs and the kidneys are ultimately responsible for the maintenance of acid–base balance, imbalances are categorised as having a respiratory or metabolic cause, that is, respiratory or metabolic acidosis and respiratory or metabolic alkalosis. The four key disturbances of acid–base balance are outlined in Information 21.2. Sometimes, however, patients have a mixed disorder of acid–base balance. Any of these states may be life threatening. In the acute or critically unwell patient, the pH of the blood and other parameters are assessed via arterial blood gas measurements. The normal values of arterial blood gases are outlined in Table 21.3.

❖❖ Nursing Management and Health Promotion: Fluid and Electrolyte Balance

Water is essential for life, and healthy living messages constantly advise people to drink 'plenty' (6–8 glasses) of fluid throughout the day (British Dietetic Association 2020). Inadequate fluid intake can quickly result in functional and long-term health problems (Wilson 2014). For older adults, a reduction of as little as 1% of body water has been shown to lead to a decrease in

Acid–Base Disturbances

Respiratory Acidosis
- Respiratory acidosis is caused by an excess of carbon dioxide due to hypoventilation.
- It is most frequently caused by primary disorders of the respiratory tract, or by conditions which affect the respiratory centre, e.g. drug overdose and central nervous system problems.
- Faults in the management of mechanical ventilation may also lead to respiratory acidosis.
- Compensation is through the renal system which retains bicarbonate ions to counter the high level of $PaCO_2$ (the partial pressure of carbon dioxide in arterial blood).
- People with chronic respiratory problems such as chronic obstructive pulmonary disease (COPD) may have well-established compensatory mechanisms.

Respiratory Alkalosis
- The most common cause of respiratory alkalosis is hyperventilation, which may occur in a panic/anxiety attack (see also hypocalcaemia).
- The subsequent removal of carbon dioxide leads to a raised pH and eventually a fall in the bicarbonate level when renal compensation has occurred.

Metabolic Acidosis
- Common causes include renal failure, lactic acidosis (occurring in severe shock with poor tissue perfusion causing hypoxia, sepsis, cardiac and respiratory dysfunction), diabetic ketoacidosis, diuretic therapy with carbonic anhydrase inhibitors and excessive loss of GI fluid such as through a fistula or diarrhoea.
- Characterised by a low pH and low levels of bicarbonate ions.
- The lowered pH leads to a compensatory respiratory drive to hyperventilate, thus causing a transitory fall in the $PaCO_2$.
- Renal compensation is made through the excretion of excess hydrogen ions.
- If the acidosis is severe, cardiac contractility may be affected resulting in bradycardia with a consequent reduction in cardiac output.

Metabolic Alkalosis
- Caused by a loss of hydrogen ions, e.g. through vomiting, gastric aspiration or a gain of alkali, as in excess intake of sodium bicarbonate. It may also be caused by some diuretic therapy, or excessive secretion of adrenal cortical hormones – Cushing's syndrome or hyperaldosteronism.
- Characterised by high pH and a high concentration of bicarbonate ions.
- Respiratory response seeks to compensate by raising the $PaCO_2$ through a decreased respiratory effort.
- Renal compensation can occur through the conservation of hydrogen ions.

TABLE 21.3	Normal Arterial Blood Gases (ABGs)
Parameter	Normal Range
pH	7.36–7.44
[H+]	35–45 nmol/L
PaCO$_2$	4.6–5.6 kPa (35–42 mmHg)
PaO$_2$	11.3–14 kPa (90–105 mmHg)
HCO$_3$	23–31 mmol/L
Standard HCO$_3^-$	22–28 mmol/L
Base excess	–2 to 2 mmol/L
Saturation O$_2$	97%

Note: Slight variations occur between laboratories.

cognitive performance (Merhej 2019). Despite this clear need for an adequate fluid intake, there is evidence to suggest that patients in hospital are not always being helped to meet this requirement (Davidson et al. 2020). Furthermore, 25% of those admitted to hospital from nursing homes are found to be dehydrated (Hooper et al. 2016). This led, in 2007, to the Nursing and Midwifery Council (NMC) identifying Nutrition and Fluid Management as one of the essential components of preregistration nursing programmes. The 'Future Nurse' standards state that a qualified nurse must 'Use evidence-based, best practice approaches for meeting needs for care and support with nutrition and hydration, accurately assessing the person's capacity for independence and self-care and initiating appropriate interventions' (NMC 2018, p. 34). They go on to identify seven specific areas of competency, directly related to hydration that must be achieved by students from all fields.

One of the main reasons for an inadequate fluid intake is the lack of access to a drink when desired (Reflection 21.2). Whilst this is unlikely to be a problem for fit healthy adults, for those with reduced cognitive ability, mobility and/or dexterity, it may be a significant obstacle. This may be as a result of age, illness or other mobility difficulties. The thirst sensation is diminished in older people and so they are less likely to seek hydration. Also, older adults living alone may be unable to prepare a drink for themselves, or carry it to where they wish to sit. The same could apply to individuals convalescing after surgery or debilitated by ill-health. Therefore a fundamental role of the nurse is to ensure that whoever is caring for the individual is aware of the need for

---

REFLECTION 21.2

Helping People to Access Sufficient Oral Fluids

Reports have highlighted that people in hospital, care facilities or at home do not always have access to adequate oral fluids.

Activities

- When you are next on a placement, look around to see what percentage of the patients/clients have a drink within their reach. Ask if they were given a choice of drink and if the drink available is what they really want.
- Reflect on your findings and consider how oral fluids could be made more accessible and acceptable. Discuss your findings with your mentor or lecturer.

---

fluids to always be both available and accessible. This may include pouring a drink for someone who is unable to do so and making sure that it is within reach and in a suitable drinking vessel. Safety is paramount and the use of specialised cups and/or straws may mean that an individual is able to maintain their independence without the risk of injury. For those for whom help is only available at certain times of the day, equipment such as an insulated jug, preferably with a pushbutton dispenser, will allow the person easy access to hot or cold drinks for several hours.

A poor fluid intake may also be a result of a reduced desire to drink. Lukewarm water which has sat in a jug all day is unlikely to encourage anyone to drink. It is important that the nurse identifies what types of drink the individual likes and, unless medically contraindicated, tries to make these available. Simple measures such as providing cold, fresh water, perhaps with the addition of ice, if available, will make drinks much more palatable than lukewarm stale water.

Failure to meet a patient's need for adequate fluid can have catastrophic effects on their health and well-being. In two early reports, the signs of potential deterioration, often linked to inadequate fluid intake, were not being recognised and subsequently patients experienced delays in receiving appropriate treatment (National Confidential Enquiry into Patient Outcome and Death (NCEPOD) 2005, National Patient Safety Agency (NPSA) 2007). In the NPSA report, out of the 576 deaths reported to them, 11% or 66 deaths were attributed to signs of deterioration not being recognised or acted upon. The need for comprehensive assessment is therefore paramount. Despite these reports, more recent studies continue to demonstrate that there is still room for improvement in meeting the hydration needs of vulnerable people in care services (Davidson et al. 2020, Hooper et al. 2016).

Assessment – Fluid and Electrolyte Status

The effects of a fluid/electrolyte loss or gain depend to a large extent on the volume involved and the rate at which it occurs. Effects are more acute when loss or gain develops rapidly, when the person is at the extremes of age and when the person is debilitated. Signs and symptoms observed by the nurse will depend upon the effects of the fluid loss or gain on the serum osmolality. A major problem in the assessment of fluid and electrolyte imbalance is that significant changes occur before they can be detected by clinical measurements such as blood pressure or central venous pressure. The nurse therefore needs to be able to use a wide range of skills to detect early changes. These include the following:

- *Knowing what to look for* – using a sound knowledge of physiology, the nurse will know what early and late clinical signs may be present. Recognition of signs of compensation, as the body attempts to restore homeostasis, is also essential as this will help highlight an underlying imbalance.
- *Knowing how often to look* – the nurse will be able to assess the severity of the situation and assess/monitor the patient accordingly.
- *Knowing what the anticipated effects of a variety of medical interventions are* – in order to assess effectiveness of treatment and plan further care.

Changes in tissue fluid volume are noticed mainly through observation of mucous membranes and skin elasticity, the latter being more easily observed over bony prominences. Skin turgor is a less reliable indicator of dehydration in an older person, due to the natural loss of elasticity of the skin. With an infant, the anterior fontanelle provides a good indication of hydration status.

The nurse's frequent contact with the patient should enable detection of any disturbances of features which may be related to fluid and electrolyte status. Unfortunately, nursing management of patients' needs for food and fluid is often neglected or delegated. In addition, the recording of fluid status is notoriously inaccurate. In illness, certain groups, such as older people, infants/children and pregnant women, are particularly susceptible to fluid and electrolyte problems. Others are at risk by virtue of an underlying pathological problem and/or as a result of nursing or medical interventions. In light of this, regular evaluation of fluid and electrolyte status should be undertaken by an experienced and knowledgeable practitioner.

A number of parameters may indicate changes in fluid or electrolyte status, but minor changes are often only recognised by those familiar with the person. Thus effective communication is crucial between nurses, for example at handover reports, and with relatives and carers who may notice subtle changes. The rapid detection of patterns and trends can be important in identifying deterioration or improvement in the patient's condition.

A structured approach to nursing assessment should facilitate the identification of actual and potential patient problems. Indeed, the initial assessment may not be completed until a 24-hour observation of the patient has been undertaken. Assessment of the patient's fluid and electrolyte status involves a four-stage process, some of which may run concurrently:

- Stage 1: Consider observable and reported parameters
- Stage 2: Consider measurable parameters
- Stage 3: Consider the underlying pathophysiology
- Stage 4: Consider the effects of medications

Many changes in tissue volume can be noticed through sensory observation or by the patient reporting symptoms. When this information is combined with the measurable data, it can give a reliable indicator of the patient's fluid status (Tables 21.4 and 21.5). For further details of the physiological processes that influence fluid and electrolyte status (see Further Reading suggestions, e.g. Norris 2019). Underlying pathological processes and the effect of medications frequently distort clinical signs and therefore must also be considered. A Cochrane review exploring traditional assessment methods including a dry mouth, feeling thirsty, heart rate, urine colour and urine volume found that these were not reliable indicators of dehydration in older adults. For this age group, all individual assessments had limited diagnostic ability but a combination of the individual having missed some drinks between meals and expressing fatigue had a high level of sensitivity (detecting problems) and specificity (not giving false-positives) (Hooper et al. 2015).

Monitoring Fluid Balance

The two most important components of monitoring a patient's fluid balance are measurements or estimations of fluid intake/output and weight. Insensible fluid losses are estimated according to standard norms and often account for a much larger volume than is usually estimated in clinical practice (Marieb and Hoehn 2018). It is therefore important to make adjustments for the following factors:

- body temperature
- ambient temperature
- basal metabolic rate (BMR)
- respiratory rate
- respiratory assistance, e.g. use of oxygen, humidification

- other pathologies
- fluid content in stools
- internal losses due to fluid movement
- losses through skin trauma.

Whilst some losses and gains have to be estimated, in appropriate circumstances others can be measured, for example:
- volume of oral fluid intake and fluid in foods
- intravenous fluids
- GI gains through enteral feeding
- GI losses from gastric aspiration, fistulae and drains
- urine: volume and concentration, i.e. an output <0.5 mL/kg body weight per hour
- central venous pressure.

Unfortunately, the volume of oral fluid intake or fluid in food is usually estimated rather than measured. Indeed, some fluid-containing foods such as soups and custards are not necessarily included in fluid recording. This is particularly important in patients who are restricted to a liquid diet or whose fluid intake is restricted, as in renal failure.

Fluid Balance Charting: Possible Sources of Error

Nurses should be aware of the many ways in which the accuracy of fluid intake/output calculations may be compromised. Examples include:
- duplication or omission of items
- use of estimations rather than measurements (consider weighing wet sheets to calculate output)
- arithmetical errors
- intravenous fluids administered in theatre and not correctly accounted for
- staff shift change errors, i.e. in carrying forward from the previous shift
- not specifying whether fluid is colloid or crystalloid in calculations
- recording wrong intravenous bag – confusion between treatment chart and fluid chart
- failure to observe patterns in consecutive daily balance
- the patient is unable to accurately recall events and forgets their fluid or food intake
- unmeasurable loss, e.g. vomit over the floor.

Measurement errors also arise when inappropriate utensils are used (Reflection 21.3). To reduce the margin of error, low volumes of urine should be measured in containers with gradations designed for low volumes. Large volumes measured from catheter drainage bags may prove to be different if the bag is emptied and then measured in a rigid measuring jug. Similarly, intravenous fluid bags may contain more than the actual amount specified. In the clinical setting, it is possible to use scales to measure body fluids; subtracting the weight of the empty receptacle, for example vomit bowl or urinal, from the total weight. A very approximate conversion of weight to volume is straightforward, for example 250 g = 250 mL, but this simple conversion relates to pure water and further allowances must be made, for instance when vomit contains undigested food.

Understanding the relative acceptable margins of error is an essential but neglected aspect of fluid monitoring. In a fit, healthy person, small errors may not be significant, but in a vulnerable person, they can lead to inappropriate treatment regimens with consequent problems. Due to the problems associated with estimating and measuring fluid intake and output volumes, many view the use of daily weight recordings as a more reliable indicator of fluid status. However, for these measurements to be accurate and meaningful, the weight should be

TABLE 21.4   Observable/Reportable Signs of Fluid and Electrolyte Disturbance and Their Possible Significance

Clinical Signs/Symptoms	Clinical Significance	Cautions in Interpretation
Mucous membranes will appear dry and the patient will complain of thirst	Decreased saliva production will result in a dry mouth and sensation of thirst. Osmoreceptors detecting hypovolaemia will also trigger a feeling of thirst. This acts as a useful backup, as effective oral hygiene often disguises the decreased saliva production	Mouth breathing Oxygen administration Anticholinergic drugs, e.g. dicycloverine hydrochloride
Tongue furrows	A normal tongue has one long longitudinal furrow, but in dehydration additional furrows will be present and the tongue will appear smaller due to fluid loss	–
Sunken eyes	The result of decreased intraocular pressure	–
Increased jugular venous pressure (JVP). With a patient positioned at 45 degrees, venous distension should not exceed 2 cm above the sternal angle	Distended veins indicate fluid overload; flat veins indicate decreased plasma volume	Assessing the right internal jugular vein gives a more reliable reading than on the left as it is the most anatomically direct route to the right atrium
Reduced capillary refill time	Capillary refill taking 2–3 seconds indicates a mild fluid deficit Refill times in excess of 3 seconds signify severe fluid deficits	Peripheral shutdown due to cold will slow capillary refill irrespective of fluid status
Reduced skin turgor	Reduction in interstitial and intracellular fluid will reduce skin elasticity	In an older person, it is difficult to detect changes in skin turgor due to the gradual loss of skin elasticity with age
Cool peripheral temperature and pale skin colour	As a result of the renin–angiotensin cycle, hypovolaemia will result in peripheral vasoconstriction and therefore reduced temperature and colour	Patients with poor circulation, e.g. peripheral vascular disease or Raynaud's disease, will normally have cool peripheries Certain antihypertensives including vasodilators and ACE inhibitors will disguise the body's normal compensatory mechanism
Dark urine	Hypovolaemia will trigger release of ADH, leading to more concentrated urine	Patients with liver disease may have bilirubin present in their urine giving it a very dark colour. Diuretic therapy will override the body's production of ADH
Peripheral oedema	Oedema occurs with the movement of fluid into interstitial spaces as a result of fluid excess and/or reduced levels of plasma proteins A consequent decrease in intravascular fluid may lead to a reduction in blood pressure	–
Pulmonary oedema (fluid within the lung alveoli), observable through frothy, pink-stained sputum and/or dyspnoea (shortness of breath)	Pulmonary oedema will result in decreased gaseous exchange, with a reduction in oxygen saturation and arterial oxygen levels	–

ACE, Angiotensin-converting enzyme; *ADH,* antidiuretic hormone.

taken at the same time each day and with the patient wearing the same clothes and shoes. Lean body mass changes do not occur quickly and the measurement of daily weight is particularly useful when assessing the older person and those with renal or cardiac impairment.

Finally, measurement of bioimpedance analysis (BIA) may be a way forward in the assessment and treatment of fluid volumes within the body (Chung and Kim 2021). The extent to which the body conducts electricity can be used to estimate intra- and intercellular water. This involves attaching a surface electrode to the patient's hand and foot before passing an imperceptible electrical current through their body fluids. Despite the speed and simplicity of this technique, it is still not commonly seen in practice. Further studies into its value continue, to assess if it could help overcome the problems associated with inaccurate fluid balance charts.

Managing Fluid and Electrolyte Therapy

The aims of all fluid and electrolyte therapy are to:
- Regulate, where possible, the patient's fluid and electrolyte balance by controlling the content and volume of fluids taken by the oral/enteral route. When the oral/enteral route is inadequate, venous access is required.
- Control excessive losses and gains, such as by means of surgical intervention to prevent blood loss or by the use of diuretics to regulate fluid balance.

Both the medical and nursing management of the patient's fluid and electrolyte status will be derived from the initial assessment. The patient may require one or more of the following interventions:
- Assistance with the maintenance of normal fluid and electrolyte requirements; this usually occurs for a short period of time

TABLE 21.5	Measurable Parameters and Their Significance in Fluid and Electrolyte Imbalance	
Clinical Parameters/ Measurements	Clinical Significance	Cautions in Interpretation
Pulse	If there is a reduction in circulating volume and therefore stroke volume, the heart rate will increase to compensate and maintain cardiac output (see Chapter 2) Initial assessment of rhythm, based on the regularity of the pulse, may be useful and indicate a need for an electrocardiogram (ECG) recording	Cardiac drugs, e.g. beta blockers, such as atenolol, celiprolol, will inhibit the body's compensatory mechanism and therefore block an increase in heart rate
Blood pressure	Measurement of blood pressure will give an indication of circulating volume. Pulse pressure, the difference between systolic and diastolic pressure, will give an indication of vasoconstriction, i.e. compensation by the body	As a result of numerous compensatory mechanisms, blood pressure is maintained by the body for as long as possible. A 'normal' blood pressure in the presence of compensation must be acted upon immediately
Central venous pressure (CVP)	Will be reduced as a result of hypovolaemia and/or vasodilatation An increase in CVP does not necessarily indicate fluid overload as CVP is influenced by numerous other factors including cardiac competence, systemic vascular resistance (SVR), intrathoracic and intraabdominal pressure	For further information, see Chapter 19, The Deteriorating Patient, Recognising and Managing Shock
Urine volume	In health, the body produces 1 mL urine/kg of body weight per hour Acceptable urine output in the critically ill patient is equal to 0.5 mL urine/kg per hour	Knowledge of the patient's weight and calculation of desired urine output based upon that is essential Administration of diuretics will override normal physiological processes. Their use must be noted when assessing volume of urine produced
Specific gravity (SG) of urine	Demonstrates the body's ability to concentrate urine as an indicator of kidney function and/or response to ADH production	Administration of diuretics will override normal physiological processes. Their use must be noted when assessing urinary SG

REFLECTION 21.3

Reducing Errors in Recording Fluid Balance

Reflect on your experience of recording fluid balance in practice and identify potential sources of error.

Activities

- Measure out 100-mL quantities of water using an accurate measure (e.g. a syringe) and transfer them into the following containers, observing the water levels: urinal, catheter drainage bag, a measuring jug and a standard glass, cup and cereal/soup bowl used in your placement.
- Determine how much liquid is contained in the standard glass, cup and bowl used, when full to the brim, about half full or filled to the level usually served by the catering staff.
- Consider the implications of your findings with regard to a patient's/client's hydration status and discuss them with your mentor or lecturer.
- Think about how the ward/unit team could reach a consensus about recording the exact volume of oral fluids.

in a previously well-nourished person, e.g. following surgery or during a brief period of altered consciousness.
- Correction of fluid/electrolyte imbalances.
- Parenteral nutrition (PN) (see Chapter 22, Nutrition and Health, Chapter 27, Nursing the Unconscious Patient).

Occasionally, a person will require all three measures simultaneously; for example, someone with a major abdominal injury may need immediate correction of fluid loss (including blood loss) and electrolyte disturbances, followed by a need to ensure that normal fluid and electrolyte requirements are met, with consideration being

given to changes in demand due to the injury. If oral/enteral feeding is unlikely to be resumed, then the introduction of parenteral feeding will be urgently considered by the multidisciplinary team (MDT).

In deciding on the most appropriate plan for a patient, consideration is given not only to the type and constituents of the fluid replacement therapy, but also to the resources available, the patient's coexisting problems, for example diabetes mellitus, and the particular hazards associated with the respective methods of administration. The timing, rate and duration of the therapy can also determine which route will be most effective.

Determining the Volume and Content of the Therapy

The regimen prescribed for the patient will be based on the following essential considerations of what needs to be:
- replaced – measured and insensible or hidden losses from the body
- removed – where there is excess production or excretory failure
- adjusted – where there is translocation of fluids or electrolytes
- resolved – the cause of the problem, e.g. vomiting, haemorrhage.

Routes for Fluid and Electrolyte Therapy

The routes discussed include oral, enteral, subcutaneous and parenteral.

Oral Route

Replacing fluids via the oral route is without doubt the safest method and one that maintains normality. In a healthy adult who has no circulatory or renal insufficiency, the need for fluid is 1500–3000 mL/24 hours. Replacing fluids orally will involve identifying the person's preferred drinks and then making these available, where reasonable, in the desirable quantity.

In some situations the patient may be prescribed 'restricted fluids', the amount usually being stated. For example, a person with renal failure may have a restricted fluid intake of 1000 mL/24 hours (usually based on the previous day's urine output plus an amount for insensible loss). In other circumstances the nurse may be instructed to 'encourage fluids', especially when the goal is to prevent urinary stasis in the catheterised patient.

Two key points for the nurse to bear in mind when caring for patients requiring replacement of fluid and electrolytes by the oral route are:

- Ascertain the exact meaning of vague orders (verbal or written) concerning fluid replacement, e.g. 'push fluids', 'encourage fluids', 'taking sips'. Remember that fluid and electrolyte balance is vital and that the nurse has a key role to play in preventing further problems.
- If at all possible, know exactly how much fluid a person is required to have over a 24-hour period. Medical orders can easily be written to identify appropriate daily fluid intake targets, e.g. 2000–2500 mL/24 hours.

Sometimes, patients having fluid replacement therapy still complain of thirst. The patient troubled by thirst may appreciate the nurse:

- providing frequent oral hygiene
- applying lubricant to lips
- giving mouth rinses with fresh water
- choosing carefully the type and temperature of fluids
- offering ice for the patient to suck.

Enteral Route

A tube may be inserted into the stomach (nasogastric) or the small intestine (nasoenteral) to administer fluids and electrolytes; this may be as part of nutritional support (see Chapter 22, Nutrition and Health). A nasogastric tube is used short-term, but for long-term therapy a percutaneous endoscopic gastrostomy (PEG) tube is inserted, or a jejunostomy is performed.

Subcutaneous Route

Subcutaneous fluid replacement is known as hypodermoclysis. In older patients in whom venous access may be difficult, in patients who are confused or find it difficult to tolerate an alternative route, or in the terminally ill patient, the use of subcutaneous fluid administration can be the most appropriate route for hydration needs (Specialist Palliative Audit and Guideline Group 2018). The sites of choice include the anterior or lateral aspects of the chest wall, the abdominal wall, the anterolateral aspects of the thigh and the scapula. The site of the subcutaneous administration should be regularly inspected and changed every 24 hours.

Parenteral Route

For a number of patients, fluid and electrolyte therapy must be administered via the parenteral route (a route other than the alimentary tract). Most commonly, this is administered intravenously. Parenteral fluid administration enables solutions to enter the extracellular compartment directly, enabling a rapid and controlled method of delivery. Fundamental to safe effective administration of intravenous fluids/electrolytes is the selection of an appropriate route and site for administration and the type and quantity of fluid to be administered.

Managing an intravenous therapy regimen has become a common nursing responsibility, with some practitioners being qualified to initiate specified therapies under specified authority or using Patient Group Directions. There are several different ways of achieving parenteral access in patients who are unable meet their fluid requirements with oral intake alone. A Cochrane Review attempted to determine the value of each, but due to poor quality evidence was unable to draw definitive conclusions (Ker et al. 2015). The authors did identify peripheral intravenous access as the preferred route, however, as this allows infusion of larger volumes of fluid than by other routes. Where this is not possible, they suggest that the intraosseous route is a viable alternative. Finally, for patients who are not severely dehydrated but in whom ongoing fluid losses cannot be met by oral intake, they propose the subcutaneous route as a potential method of fluid administration.

Due to advances in technology, intravenous therapy is now relatively safe; however, it is still possible for serious complications to arise. The introduction of Visual Infusion Phlebitis (VIP) scoring as an evidence-based method of determining when a cannula should be removed, and has helped reduce incidence of phlebitis (Tzolos and Salawu 2014) and VIP scoring is the recommended tool for the assessment and maintenance of peripheral cannula (Royal College of Nursing 2022).However, cannula-related complications do still occur and are all too often regarded by some as routine occurrences or merely a 'nuisance', when they can have serious consequences. The most common complications are:

- occlusion
- infiltration, i.e. leakage of nonirritant or vesicant fluid into the tissues surrounding the vein
- extravasation, i.e. infiltration of irritants or vesicants that cause tissue damage and in the worst instances loss of a limb
- phlebitis.
  Factors associated with an increased incidence of phlebitis include:
- cannula location – lower extremities or proximity to joints presents an increased risk
- duration of therapy – increasing time raises the incidence, especially over 24 hours
- blood flow problems in the region of the cannula site
- inadequate cleaning of the cannula site
- pre-existent infection
- pH and osmolality of the fluid – acidic infusates in particular
- particulate matter which may contaminate the delivery system.

Selecting the Site

Patients who are particularly vulnerable to complications are those with existing infections or immune suppression and those whose restlessness or mental state may lead them to traumatise the cannula site. In their seminal work, Maki et al. (1976) pointed out that the cannula site is similar to an open surgical wound containing a foreign body and should be treated as such.

Some practical considerations are involved in site selection, namely:

- the nature and anticipated duration of the therapy
- situational and environmental factors
- patient and safety factors
- availability of products
- staff expertise.

Insertion of intravenous cannulae is often undertaken by medical staff but is now more commonly undertaken by a competent healthcare practitioner who has undertaken appropriate training. Standardised education for intravenous drug administration is outlined by eLearning for Healthcare (2022). Tackling the reduction of infection associated with peripheral venous cannulae was addressed as part of the Saving Lives initiative and more directly through High Impact Intervention no. 2 – peripheral venous cannula care bundle (Department of Health [DH], 2007). In life-threatening circumstances, the selection of the intravenous site is largely dependent upon the expertise of the staff available, the products to hand and the purpose of the intravenous line. Whilst infection control measures are important, at the scene of a disaster or accident environmental contaminants may be inevitable and speed may take priority. The more invasive the procedure, the greater is the importance of environmental control. Central venous catheters must also be inserted under strict aseptic conditions, and the Department of Health High Impact Intervention no. 1 – central venous catheter care bundle (DH 2007) provided further guidance for appropriate care and management. Local factors that may be controlled during the time of insertion include the elimination of airborne contaminants and the avoidance of debris or bacteria entering via the insertion site.

Patient Factors. Patient mobility and comfort may be enhanced or hindered by site selection. It is wiser, and causes less discomfort, to site the intravenous cannula away from joints or sites where clothes may rub. Skin areas that are vulnerable to breakdown should also be avoided, including areas that are burned, oedematous, otherwise traumatised, inflamed or affected by conditions such as eczema or psoriasis. The integrity and state of the veins themselves should also influence selection.

The safety of intravenous lines in patients who are restless often poses a practical problem for nurses. Stability of the line may be enhanced by the method of attachment to the patient, and applying principles of countertraction, through the use of loops, may prevent unnecessary trauma. Modern dressings may also help tackle this problem.

Central Lines (Central Venous Catheters)

Central lines are used to measure central venous pressure (see Chapter 19, The Deteriorating Patient, Recognising and Managing Shock) and for the long-term administration of infusates, for example PN and chemotherapy (cytotoxic and antibiotic) (see Chapter 8, Nursing Patients With Disorders of the Breast and Reproductive System, 9, Nursing Patients With Disorders of the Male Reproductive System, Chapter 13, Nursing Patients With Blood Disorders, Chapter 22, Nutrition and Health, and Chapter 31, Nursing the Patient With Cancer). However, the greatly increased incidence of complications associated with the use of central lines necessitates a very cautious and competent approach to their management. Young and You (2020) remind healthcare professionals of the dangers associated with central line insertion and maintenance, namely pneumo- or haemothorax, arterial puncture, atrial fibrillation, venous embolism on insertion, during maintenance or upon withdrawal, infection and thrombosis.

Intravenous Fluid Therapy

In 2013 as a result of concerns surrounding ongoing errors in intravenous fluid administration, the NICE published guidelines related to intravenous fluid administration for adults within hospital settings (updated 2017). They estimated that as many as one in five patients receiving intravenous fluids experience complications or increased morbidity as a result of inappropriate administration. This was largely as a result of a poor level of recording and monitoring of intravenous fluids, with staff failing to reassess and respond to changes in a patient's fluid status. Furthermore, a lack of evidence from randomised control studies, or even large scale cohort studies, and the subsequent ongoing debate surrounding the best type of intravenous fluid to administer, meant that patients did not always receive the optimum regime. The guidelines stress the importance of a comprehensive assessment of the patient's fluid and electrolyte requirements taking into account their history, clinical examination, current medications, clinical monitoring and laboratory investigations.

- History should include any previous limited intake, thirst, the quantity and composition of abnormal losses and any comorbidities.
- Clinical examination should include an assessment of the patient's fluid status, including:
  - pulse
  - blood pressure
  - capillary refill and jugular venous pressure
  - presence of pulmonary or peripheral oedema
  - presence of postural hypotension.
- Clinical monitoring should include current status and trends in:
  - National Early Warning Score (NEWS 2) (Royal College of Physicians 2017)
  - fluid balance charts
  - weight.
- Laboratory investigations, again measuring current status and trends, in full blood count and urea, creatinine and electrolytes.

Following an initial assessment, the NICE guidelines propose a series of algorithms to aid management of the 5Rs, which are:

- Resuscitation
- Routine maintenance
- Replacement
- Redistribution, and finally
- Reassessment

The importance of ongoing reassessment cannot be underestimated. This will help to quickly detect signs of deterioration, perhaps as a failure of compensatory mechanisms, and help to determine the patient's response to interventions. The frequency of observation will be determined by clinical need but should form part of the ongoing fluid management plan (NICE 2017).

The algorithms contained within the guideline identify both the type and quantity of fluid to be infused, whilst recognising the importance of individualised regimes where necessary. The type of fluid administered remains the subject of intense clinical debate.

Types of Intravenous Therapy

Broadly speaking the infusates commonly used in intravenous therapy may be categorised as:

- crystalloids – balanced salt solutions which are commonly used as maintenance
- colloids – blood and blood products; plasma and plasma substitutes; starch-based products.

Colloids contain a more complex molecular structure and are frequently used to maintain haemodynamic stability. Infusates can also be categorised with respect to their tonicity:

- Isotonic solutions have the same osmolarity (tonicity) as serum or other body fluids and expand the intravascular compartment without affecting the intracellular and interstitial compartments; 0.9% saline is an isotonic fluid with respect to plasma.
- Hypotonic solutions have a lower osmolarity than serum and cause body fluids to shift away from the intravascular compartment and into the intracellular and interstitial spaces to areas of higher osmolarity. Hypotonic solutions may be used in the case of cellular dehydration due to diabetic ketoacidosis.

Hypertonic solutions have a higher osmolarity than serum and cause fluid to move from the interstitial and intracellular compartments towards the intravascular compartments (see Chapter 19, The Deteriorating Patient, Recognising and Managing Shock).

Problems Associated With Fluid and Electrolyte Imbalance

This section outlines some areas in which patients/clients experience difficulties with fluid and electrolyte balance – dehydration and hydration at the end of life, vomiting, diarrhoea and the special needs of the person undergoing surgery. This information is supported by additional material on the website and the opportunity to complete critical thinking questions.

Dehydration and Hydration in End-of-Life Care

The debate continues as to whether, and when, to withhold or withdraw intravenous, subcutaneous or nasogastric hydration in the days or hours before an expected death. Nurses may well be presented with situations where a decision regarding hydration of their patients must be made. The most recent guidelines from NICE (2015) relating to care of dying patients in the last days of life advocate supporting the dying person to drink if they wish to and are able to. The need to check for difficulties with swallowing to prevent aspiration is reinforced, as is the importance of communication with the individual and those close to them. It is essential that the risks and benefits of either oral or 'clinically assisted hydration' are discussed fully and that all involved have the opportunity to have any concerns addressed. If individuals do not have the capacity to make decisions for themselves, procedures must be guided by the Mental Capacity Act 2005 (Ministry of Justice 2005).

Vomiting

Fluid loss caused by vomiting can rapidly cause dehydration and electrolyte imbalance; if prolonged or severe, it may lead to metabolic alkalosis and further acid–base disturbance (see Disorders of Acid–Base Balance). The fluid and electrolyte losses caused by vomiting may be summarised as follows:
- depletion of the ECF volume
- hypochloraemia (low serum chloride level caused by loss of Cl^-)
- alkalosis
- hypokalaemia
- possible acidosis.

See Evolve website Critical thinking question 21.1

Diarrhoea

Worldwide, diarrhoea is a serious problem and the most important indication for fluid and electrolyte replacement. The fluid losses from diarrhoea may cause:
- depletion of ECF volume
- hyponatraemia
- hypokalaemia
- metabolic acidosis (loss of bicarbonate in the digestive juices)
- severe water dehydration (if the colon is involved).

See Evolve website Critical thinking question 21.1

Special Needs of the Person Undergoing Surgery

The person undergoing surgery, whether elective or emergency, is particularly vulnerable to several disturbances of fluid and electrolyte balance. Disturbances in the composition and placement of the body fluids and electrolytes accompany many procedures and include blood loss, dehydration from preoperative fasting, bowel preparation and surgical exposure (see Chapter 25, The Care of a Person Undergoing Surgery).

See Evolve website Critical thinking question 21.2

Summary: Key Nursing Issues

- Homeostasis of water, electrolytes and acid–base balance is vital to cellular function.
- Fluid and electrolyte imbalance is associated with too little (caused by reduced intake and/or increased loss) or too much (caused by increased intake and/or decreased loss).
- Disturbances of fluid balance may be isotonic or osmolar.
- Nurses need a clear understanding of fluid, electrolyte and acid–base balance and the common disorders in order to assess fluid and electrolyte status, anticipate and recognise deterioration and implement corrective interventions.
- Awareness of potential risk factors for fluid and electrolyte imbalance is vital.
- Nurses are key to the early recognition of disturbances and therefore need to be able to use a wide range of skills to detect early changes, such as monitoring fluid balance.
- Nursing interventions in relation to fluid therapy range from providing appropriate oral fluids to managing a complicated intravenous fluid regimen.
- Safe management of the person with a fluid, electrolyte or acid–base disturbance is complex and requires skilful and knowledgeable nursing practice.

Reflection and Learning – What Next?

- **Test** your knowledge by visiting the Evolve website and answering the multiple-choice questions and critical thinking questions.
- **Consolidate** your learning by looking at some of the further reading suggestions, references and specialist websites.
- **Revisit** some of the additional material on the website.
- **Consider** what you have learnt and how this will help your professional development.
- **Reflect** on how you can apply this knowledge to the care of your patients.
- **Discuss** your learning with your mentor/supervisor, lecturer and colleagues.

References

Alonso-Fernandez JM, Lopez-Pablo C. Body temperature and heating temperature in major burns patients' care. *Enfermeria Global*. 2021;61:476–486.

British Dietetic Association. *Fluids (Water and Drinks): Food Fact Sheet*; 2020. Available at: https://www.bda.uk.com/resource/fluid-water-drinks.html.

Chung YJ, Kim EY. Usefulness of bioelectrical impedance analysis and ECW ratio as a guidance for fluid management in critically ill patients after operation. *Sci Rep*. 2021;11:1–10.

Davidson J, Folkard S, Hinkley M, et al. A multicentre prospective audit of bedside hydration in hospital. *Br J Nurs*. 2020;29(1):50–54 9.

Department of Health (DH). *Saving Lives: Reducing Infection, Delivering Clean and Safe Care*. London: DH; 2007. Archived at: https://tinyurl.com/y5ajqgun.

eLearning for Healthcare. About the IV Therapy Passport programme; 2022. https://www.e-lfh.org.uk/programmes/iv-therapy-passport/.

Hooper L, Abdelhamid A, Attreed NJ, et al. Clinical symptoms, signs and tests for identification of impending and current water-loss dehydration in older people (Cochrane review). *Cochrane Library*. 2015;2015(4):CD009647.

Hooper L, Bunn D, Downing A, et al. Which frail older people are dehydrated? The UK DRIE Study. *Br Med J (Clin Res Ed)*. 2016;71(10):1341–1347.

Kaufman DP, Basit H. and Knohl SJ. *Physiology, Glomerular Filtration Rate*; 2020. https://www.ncbi.nlm.nih.gov/books/NBK500032/.

Ker K, Tansley G, Beecher D, et al. Comparison of routes for achieving parenteral access with a focus on the management of patients with Ebola virus disease. *Cochrane Database*. 2015(2):CD011386.

Maki DG, Rhame FS, Mackel DC, Bennett JV. Nationwide epidemic of septicemia caused by contaminated intravenous products: I. Epidemiologic and clinical features. *The American Journal of Medicine*. 1976;60(4).

Marieb EN, Hoehn K, eds. *Human Anatomy and Physiology*. 12th ed. New York: Pearson; 2018.

Merhej R. Stigma on mental illness in the Arab world: beyond the sociocultural barriers. *International Journal of Human Rights in Healthcare*. 2019;12(4);285–298.

Ministry of Justice. Mental Capacity Act: making decisions; 2005. http://www.justice.gov.uk/guidance/mental-capacity.htm.

National Confidential Enquiry into Patient Outcome and Death (NCEPOD). An acute problem 2005? http://www.ncepod.org.uk/2005aap.htm.

National Institute for Health and Care Excellence (NICE). Intravenous fluid therapy in adults in hospital: diagram of ongoing losses; 2013. https://www.nice.org.uk/guidance/cg174/resources/diagram-of-ongoing-losses-191664109.

National Institute for Health and Care Excellence (NICE). *Care of dying adults in the last days of life of life*. NICE guideline [CG31]; 2015. https://www.nice.org.uk/guidance/ng31.

National Institute for Health and Care Excellence (NICE). *Intravenous fluid therapy in adults in hospital*. Clinical guideline [CG17], 2017. https://www.nice.org.uk/guidance/cg174.

National Patient Safety Agency (NPSA). Safer care for the acutely ill patient: learning from serious incidents; 2007. http://www.npsa.nhs.uk/nrls/alerts-and-directives/directives-guidance/acutely-ill-patient/.

Nursing and Midwifery Council (NMC). Future Nurse: Standards of Proficiency for Registered Nurses; 2018. https://www.nmc.org.uk/globalassets/sitedocuments/education-standards/future-nurse-proficiencies.pdf.

Pocock G, Richards CD, Richards DA. *Human Physiology*. 5th ed. Oxford: Oxford University Press; 2017.

Royal College of Nursing. *Standards for Infusion Therapy*. 5th ed. London: RCN; 2022.

Royal College of Physicians. National Early Warning Score (NEWS2): standardising the assessment of acute-illness severity in the NHS; 2017. https://www.rcplondon.ac.uk/projects/outputs/national-early-warning-score-news-2.

Specialist Palliative Audit and Guideline Group. Guideline for the use of subcutaneous hydration in palliative care; 2018. https://www.palliativedrugs.com/download/180214_Subcutaneous_hydration_in_palliative_care_v2.4_Final.pdf. Accessed 12 April 2022.

Stickel S, Gin-Sing W, Wagenaar M, et al. The practical management of fluid retention in adults with right heart failure due to pulmonary arterial hypertension. *Eur Heart J Suppl*. 2019;21(Supplement_K): K46-K5.

Tobias A, Ballard BD, Mohiuddin SS. Physiology, Water Balance; 2020. https://www.ncbi.nlm.nih.gov/books/NBK541059/.

Tzolos E, Salawu A. Improving the frequency of Visual Infusion Phlebitis (VIP) scoring on an oncology ward. *BMJ Qual Improv Rep*. 12,3(1):u205455.w2364; 2014. https://bmjopenquality.bmj.com/content/3/1/u205455.w2364.

Waugh A. Problems associated with fluid, electrolyte and acid-base balance. In: Brooker C, Nichol M, eds. *Nursing Adults: The Practice of Caring*. Edinburgh: Mosby; 2003:135–136.

Wilson L. *Hydration and older people in the UK: addressing the problem, understanding the solutions. (On behalf of the Parliamentary Hydration Forum)*. London: International Longevity Centre-UK; 2014. www.scie.org.uk/publications/guides/guide15/files/hydration-and-older-people-in-the-uk.pdf.

Young MP, You TH. *Overview of complications of central venous catheters and their prevention in adults*. UpToDate; 2020. https://www.uptodate.com/contents/overview-of-complications-of-central-venous-catheters-and-their-prevention-in-adults.

Further Reading

British National Formulary. No. 82; 2022. www.bnf.org.

Nursing Fundamentals Open Resources. 15.2 Basic fluid and electrolyte concepts; 2022. https://wtcs.pressbooks.pub/nursingfundamentals/chapter/15-2-basic-fluid-and-electrolyte-concepts/.

Department of Health. Essence of Care; 2010. http://www.dh.gov.uk.

Dougherty L, Lister S. *The Royal Marsden Hospital Manual of Clinical Nursing Procedures Online*. 10th ed; 2020. https://www.rmmonline.co.uk/.

National Institute for Health and Care Excellence. *Intravenous fluid therapy in adults in hospital*. Clinical guideline [CG174]; 2017. https://www.nice.org.uk/guidance/cg174.

Nursing and Midwifery Council (NMC). The Code: Professional Standards of Practice and Behaviour for Nurses, Midwives and Nursing Associates; 2018. https://www.nmc.org.uk/globalassets/sitedocuments/standards-of-proficiency/nurses/future-nurse-proficiencies.pdf.

Norris TL. *Porth's Essentials of Pathophysiology: Concepts of Altered Health States*. 5th ed. Philadelphia: Wolters Kluwer; 2019.

Royal College of Nursing Standards for infusion therapy; 2022. https://www.rcn.org.uk/clinical-topics/Infection-prevention-and-control/Standards-for-infusion-therapy

Useful Websites

The Eat Well Guide, https://www.nhs.uk/live-well/eat-well/food-guidelines-and-food-labels/the-eatwell-guide/

National Library of Medicine (US) MedlinePlus, www.nlm.nih.gov/medlineplus/fluidandelectrolytebalance.html

National Patient Safety Agency, https://www.npsa.org.uk/

NHS National Library for Health, www.library.nhs.uk/

National Institute for Health and Care Excellence (NICE), www.nice.org.uk

Scottish Intercollegiate Guidelines Network (SIGN), www.sign.ac.uk

Visual Infusion Phlebitis (VIP) scoring, www.vipscore.net

22

Nutrition and Health

SUE M. GREEN

CHAPTER OUTLINE

Introduction

Good nutrition and hydration are essential for health. An adequate intake of nutrients and water is required to maintain physiological function, to allow for growth and maintenance of tissues, and to provide energy to meet the demands of daily living. Although a biological necessity, eating and drinking have significance beyond the merely physiological, forming an important part of social and psychological well-being. Meals are used as a time for people to come together, food or drink may be offered to make a guest feel welcome and formal meals are a feature of many family, religious and national ceremonies.

The importance of the role of the nurse in ensuring nutritional needs are met is well recognised. The Nursing and Midwifery Council (NMC) Standards of Proficiency for Registered Nurses (NMC 2018a) include outcomes focused on nutritional care. The responsibilities of the nurse concerning nutritional care are extremely varied and range from promoting health to caring for the malnourished. Nurses play a more minor role in the preparation and serving of food to individuals in their care than they have done in previous years. Changes in food delivery and serving

methods have acted to reduce the nursing input required at mealtimes. In many areas, there is a necessary delegation of responsibility concerning mealtime care to healthcare assistants or other staff. However, it must be remembered that it is the registered nurse (RN) who is responsible for ensuring food is provided, as appropriate, to the patient in their care and this is clearly stated in the NMC Code (NMC 2018b).

This chapter will consider principles of nutritional science, public health nutrition and nutritional care by nurses. The principles of nutritional science are only briefly considered in this chapter and the reader is advised to obtain a good understanding of the form and function of macronutrients and micronutrients in a human anatomy and physiology textbook (e.g. Waugh and Grant 2023).

Principles of Nutritional Science

To maintain health, an adequate supply of nutrients is required. The foods that make up the diet can vary considerably but the nutritive constituents of the diet fall into two main groups: the energy-yielding macronutrients (carbohydrates, protein and fat) and micronutrients (vitamins and minerals). Alcohol (in the form of ethanol) may also be considered a form of macronutrient in that it is energy-yielding. However, it is not an essential nutrient and does not lead to a deficiency condition if not consumed.

Table 22.1 outlines the key vitamins required by the body, and gives details of rich food sources, at-risk groups and signs and symptoms of deficiency, and Table 22.2 provides similar information for some minerals.

Some components of foods, such as nonstarch polysaccharides (NSPs) (or dietary fibre) and water, provide few if any nutrients but are important for physiological function. The diet may also contain other substances such as food colourings, food preservatives and caffeine, which have little or no nutritional value but can enhance the quality of the diet.

Nutrients have a complex role in physiological function and most have a number of functions in the body. Nutrients are required to form the structural components of the body, for example, protein is the major constituent of muscles. Nutrients are also important in metabolic pathways and enzyme systems that enable the body to function appropriately. They can either form a part of the pathway or assist in the enzymatic reactions in that pathway (a cofactor). For example, vitamin C is required in the pathway that forms collagen. Nutrients also provide energy for metabolism. Metabolic demand needs to be met by an effective supply of nutrients.

Nutrients come from two sources: the food eaten and the breakdown of body tissues. There is a dynamic process between food eaten, body tissues and metabolism. Carbohydrate and fat

TABLE 22.1	Vitamins: Rich Food Sources, At-risk Groups and Signs and Symptoms of Deficiency		
Nutrient	Examples of Rich Food Sources	Groups at Risk of Dietary Deficiency	Common Signs and Symptoms of Deficiency
Vitamin A (retinol)	Cheese, eggs, oily fish, fortified margarine, some green, yellow and red fruits and vegetables, liver and liver products	Deficiency rarely seen in high-income countries. At risk of deficiency: people with diseases of the gastrointestinal tract affecting absorption (e.g. coeliac disease), young children and pregnant women in low-income countries due to poor dietary intake At risk of excessive intake: pregnant women should avoid supplements containing vitamin A (unless advised otherwise by their General Practitioner or Midwife) and liver or liver products Postmenopausal women and older men who are more at risk of osteoporosis are advised to avoid more than 1.5 mg of vitamin A day from food and supplements in the UK (National Health Service 2020) In the UK the government recommends that all children aged 6 months to 5 years be given vitamin supplements containing vitamins A, C and D, except for babies having more than 500 mL infant formula a day	Signs and symptoms can include impaired dark adaptation (night blindness), xeropthalmia, skin changes, impaired immune function and decreased growth rates Leading cause of childhood blindness and increases risk of disease and death from severe infections in low-income countries
Vitamin B$_1$ (thiamine)	Found in many types of foods, good sources include whole grains, nuts and fortified breakfast cereals.	At risk of deficiency: people with alcohol dependence, people who have impaired absorption or low intake due to gastrointestinal disease or surgery	Early symptoms can include fatigue, irritability, anorexia and muscle weakness Deficiency of thiamine can cause Beriberi and Wernicke's encephalopathy.
Vitamin B$_2$ (riboflavin)	Found in many foods, good sources include milk, eggs and fortified grains and cereals	At risk of deficiency: people with alcohol dependence, people who have low intake due to poor diet	Symptoms can include sore throat, lesions of the lips and mucosa of the mouth and skin problems
Vitamin B$_3$ (niacin: generic term for nicotinic acid and nicotinamide)	Meat, wheat flour, eggs, and dairy products	At risk of deficiency: people with alcohol dependency, people taking the antibiotic isoniazid, people who have impaired absorption	Early symptoms include anorexia, dermatitis, depression and insomnia Severe deficiency leads to pellagra characterised by dermatitis, diarrhoea and dementia
Pantothenic acid (B$_5$)	Widely distributed in foods particularly meat, eggs, milk and whole grains	Deficiency is considered very rare but can be present due to a genetic disorder	Deficiency is considered rare
Vitamin B$_6$ (pyridoxine)	Found in many foods including poultry, chickpeas, bananas and some nuts	At risk of deficiency: people with alcohol dependency, people with renal disease, people who have impaired absorption, people taking the antibiotic isoniazid	Symptoms can include microcytic anaemia, dermatitis, depression and confusion
Biotin (B$_7$)	Widely distributed in foods, particularly meat, fish, nuts and seeds	Deficiency is very rare but can be present due to a genetic disorder and in people with alcohol dependency	Deficiency is considered rare
Vitamin B$_{12}$ (cyanocobalamin)	Almost all foods of animal origin and some fortified breakfast cereals	At risk of deficiency: people who have impaired absorption, vegans and vegetarians, people taking some medications such as metformin	Signs and symptoms can include tiredness, depression, muscle weakness, numbness and tingling (paraesthesia) and megaloblastic anaemia
Folate (folic acid)	Widely distributed in foods, particularly leafy green vegetables, brown rice, fortified flour and breakfast cereals	At risk of deficiency: people with alcohol dependency, pregnant women, women of childbearing age, people with malabsorption disorders and people with alcohol dependency Women thinking of becoming pregnant and those in the first trimester of pregnancy are advised to take a daily supplement in many countries	Signs and symptoms can include folate deficiency anaemia, gastrointestinal symptoms, skin changes and sore tongue Folic acid supplementation during the early stages of pregnancy may reduce the risk of the fetus developing neural tube defects
Vitamin C (ascorbic acid)	Fresh vegetables and fruit, particularly peppers, broccoli, strawberries and citrus fruits	At risk of deficiency: people who smoke, people who eat a restricted diet and people with malabsorption disorders In the UK the government recommends that all children aged 6 months to 5 years be given vitamin supplements containing vitamins A, C and D, except for babies having more than 500 mL infant formula a day	Early signs and symptoms can include joint and bone pain, loose teeth, bleeding gums and poor wound healing Scurvy is caused by severe deficiency

TABLE 22.1	Vitamins: Rich Food Sources, At-risk Groups and Signs and Symptoms of Deficiency—cont'd		
Nutrient	Examples of Rich Food Sources	Groups at Risk of Dietary Deficiency	Common Signs and Symptoms of Deficiency
Vitamin D (calciferol)	Most vitamin D is obtained through the action of sunlight on skin. Dietary sources include oily fish, liver, eggs and fortified fat spreads and some breakfast cereals	At risk of deficiency: people with limited sun exposure (e.g. nursing home residents and people who habitually cover their skin), older adults, people with dark skin and people with malabsorption disorders. In many countries the government advises supplementation for infants, young children and other groups considered at risk. In the UK the government recommends that all children aged 6 months to 5 years be given vitamin supplements containing vitamins A, C and D, except for babies having more than 500 mL infant formula a day. The UK government also advises that everyone should consider taking a daily vitamin D supplement during the autumn and winter	Signs and symptoms can include bone pain or ache, depression, fatigue and hair loss. Prolonged deficiency leads to rickets in children and can lead to osteomalacia in adults. Vitamin D deficiency also increases the risk of some chronic diseases, e.g. osteoarthritis and heart disease
Vitamin E	Vegetable oils, nuts and seeds	Deficiency is rare but may occur in people with malabsorption disorders. Vitamin E supplements may interact with some medications (e.g. anticoagulants)	Deficiency is considered rare
Vitamin K	Green leafy vegetables, cereal grains and vegetable oils	Deficiency is rare but may occur in people with malabsorption disorders. Vitamin K supplements may interact with some medications (e.g. anticoagulants). A single dose of vitamin K is given to newborns in many countries to prevent vitamin K deficiency bleeding	Deficiency is considered rare

TABLE 22.2	Minerals: Rich Food Sources, At-risk Groups and Effects of Deficiency		
Nutrient	Rich Food Sources	Groups at Risk of Dietary Deficiency	Effects of Deficiency
Calcium	Milk, yoghurt, calcium-enriched milk alternatives, cheese, small fish, e.g. sardines, tofu set with calcium sulphate, fortified breakfast cereals	Groups at risk of deficiency include postmenopausal women and people who avoid dairy products. Calcium can interact with some medications for example lithium and levothyroxine	Deficiency reduces bone strength and can cause rickets in children and osteoporosis and osteomalacia in adults. Low intake of calcium has been associated with some cancers and cardiovascular disease
Magnesium	Found widely in foods, particularly grains, nuts and seeds	Groups are risk of deficiency include people with alcohol dependency, people with type 2 diabetes mellitus, older adults and people with gastrointestinal disease. People at risk of excessive intake include people taking high doses of magnesium from medications (e.g. magnesium-containing laxatives and antacids). Magnesium status can be influenced by some medications for example some antibiotics, loop diuretics and proton pump inhibitors	Signs and symptoms of deficiency include anorexia, fatigue, nausea, numbness, tingling, cramps and abnormal heart rhythms. Low intake of magnesium has been associated with osteoporosis, type 2 diabetes mellitus and cardiovascular disease
Phosphorus	Found in most foods, particularly dairy products, fish, poultry, meat and grains	Deficiency is rare. Groups at risk may include preterm infants, people with genetic disorders affecting phosphate regulation and people with severe malnutrition. Those at risk of high phosphorus levels include people with chronic kidney disease. Phosphorous status can be influenced by some medications, e.g. some antacids and laxatives	Signs and symptoms of low levels of phosphorus in the blood (hypophosphatemia) include anorexia, muscle weakness, bone pain, rickets, osteomalacia and confusion
Sodium chloride	Found widely in foods particularly table salt and salty foods	Deficiency can occur following excessive loss of body fluids, e.g. sweating and vomiting	Common symptoms of low blood sodium (hyponatraemia) include weakness, headache, nausea, muscle cramps, confusion and irritability

Continued

TABLE 22.2	Minerals: Rich Food Sources, At-risk Groups and Effects of Deficiency—cont'd		
Nutrient	Rich Food Sources	Groups at Risk of Dietary Deficiency	Effects of Deficiency
Potassium	Found widely in foods particularly fruit (e.g. bananas), vegetables, dairy products and meat	Groups at risk include people with inflammatory bowel disease and people who take some diuretics and laxatives Those at risk of high potassium levels include people with chronic kidney disease and people who take some medications such as ACE inhibitors and potassium-sparing diuretics	Low levels of potassium in the blood (hypokalaemia) are associated with muscle weakness, fatigues, polyuria, vomiting and arrhythmias Low intake of potassium has been associated with hypertension and type 2 diabetes mellitus
Iron	Red meat, pulses, fortified breakfast cereals, nuts, dried fruit and dark chocolate Animal-based sources are more easily absorbed	Groups at risk of deficiency include pregnant women, infants and young children, menstruating women, people with some cancers, people with inflammatory bowel disorder and people with heart failure People at risk of high iron levels include people with haemochromatosis Iron status can be influenced by some medications, e.g. levodopa, levothyroxine and proton pump inhibitors	Iron deficiency anaemia is common, and signs and symptoms include weakness, fatigue, difficulty concentrating, impaired immune function and gastrointestinal disorders
Zinc	Meat, fish, seafood, red meat, eggs, dairy products and fortified breakfast cereals	Groups at risk of deficiency include people with gastrointestinal disorders, people with alcohol dependency, children with sickle cell disease, vegans, pregnant and breastfeeding women Zinc status can be influenced by some medications. For example, some antibiotics and thiazide diuretics	Sign and symptoms of zinc deficiency in adults include changed sense of taste and smell, change in cognitive ability and delayed wound healing Zinc status has been associated with type 2 diabetes mellitus, age-related macular degeneration and pneumonia in children
Selenium	Present in many foods including fish, meat, brazil nuts and dairy products	Groups at risk of deficiency include people undergoing kidney dialysis, people living in remote areas where there are low levels of selenium in the soil and people with HIV.	Deficiency is associated with Keshan disease and male fertility Selenium status has been associated with some cancers, cardiovascular disease and thyroid disease
Iodine	Marine fish, eggs, seaweed and iodised salt	At risk of deficiency: deficiency is endemic in some areas of the world where the soil contains little iodine (further reading: https://www.who.int/data/nutrition/nlis/info/iodine-deficiency) At risk of excessive intake: people exposed to excess iodine for example contrast media and topical iodine	Deficiency effects arise from reduced thyroid activity (hypothyroidism) Sign and symptoms include goitre, effects on fetal growth and development including the congenital form where fetal and infant growth and development is affected
Fluoride	Generally obtained from fluoridated drinking water and dental products Rich food sources include tea and fish	Fluoride is widely distributed in the environment with no risk of deficiency described At risk of excessive intake: people exposed to too much fluoride	Fluoride use is associated with dental caries prevention and no specific deficiency syndrome has been described

are the body's predominant energy sources, but protein may be used if these are not readily available. If food intake is inadequate, fat and muscle tissues will be used to supply the energy needed for metabolic demand.

Estimated nutritional requirements for different groups of people within populations have been established. These are usually termed 'dietary reference values' in Europe with values varying between countries. Nutritional requirements vary across the lifespan. Infants and children require sufficient nutrients to grow and develop. Requirements for some nutrients are increased during pregnancy and whilst breast feeding, and also change with ageing. It is important to recognise that dietary reference values are not recommendations for intake by individuals but are estimates for healthy populations only; within a clinical setting the advice of a healthcare professional experienced in clinical nutrition must be sought.

Nutritional requirements of individuals will vary depending on a person's basal metabolic rate (BMR), activity level and response to certain factors such as cold exposure and ingestion of food. BMR is the metabolic rate of the body at rest and is influenced by several factors, including genetic makeup, gender and body mass. Illness can increase the requirement for nutrients; however, this may be counteracted by a reduction in physical activity level during the period of the illness. If an individual has an inadequate intake of energy for a period of time, the body can adapt by reducing BMR.

If intake of a particular nutrient or range of nutrients affects physiological function adversely, then the person can be said to be malnourished. Malnutrition can refer to both overnutrition, that is, intake of energy and nutrients in excess of requirements, and undernutrition, that is, intake of insufficient energy and nutrients to meet requirements. Malnutrition may jeopardise health status and increase morbidity and mortality.

It is important to understand the different nutrients required by the body, what the nutrients are used for and the consequence of a poor nutritional intake and use this understanding when working with people to enable them to achieve a nutritional intake that meets their body's needs.

Public Health Nutrition

Public health nutrition refers to the promotion of good nutritional health and the prevention of diet-related illness in groups of people, rather than the nutritional care of individuals. Public health nutrition can be an important aspect of the nurse's role, for example school nurses may work to improve the nutritional health of a group of school children. It is important to consider the wider aspects of nutritional care, for example why people choose to eat certain foods.

The Diet

The diet consists of the foods people eat from day to day. Although foods containing all known nutrients can be formulated, no single naturally occurring food can meet all the daily nutritional demands. Different types of food contain different proportions of macro- and micronutrients, and therefore a range of foods is necessary to provide the daily requirement of individual nutrients. The diet should supply all the necessary nutrients in sufficient quantity, whilst avoiding excessive intake.

Government dietary guidelines in the United Kingdom (UK) recommend a food and fluid intake which is thought to promote maximum health for the population. These guidelines are shown pictorially in the Eatwell Guide (Fig. 22.1). The Eatwell Guide (National Health Service [NHS] 2022) is based on five main food groups and indicates what percentage of the diet should come from each group. It includes guidance on fluid intake. The UK NHS website also provides advice on vitamin and mineral intake for the general population (NHS 2023c).

It is important to consider factors which influence food intake of both individual and populations. At a global level, government policies influence what a population eats because food supply and legislation are essentially determined by government policy. For example, the fortification of foods or water with particular nutrients is a feature in many countries and is usually managed at a central government level, for example fortification of flour with calcium. The policy for food labelling which can influence individuals' choice is determined centrally. Within a country, there are generally regional, temporal and socioeconomic differences in dietary intake which can influence individuals' health. For example, decreases in fruit and vegetable intake during the COVID-19

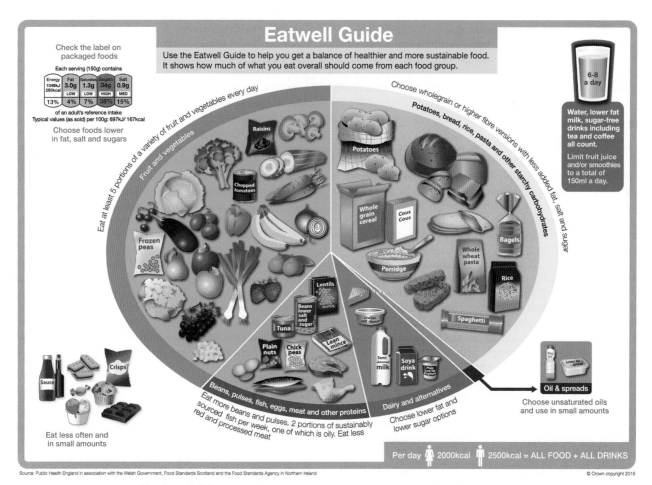

Figure 22.1 The Eatwell Guide shows five main food groups and their recommended contribution to the daily diet. It is intended as a tool for use with most adults. (Public Health England in association with the Welsh government, Food Standards Scotland and the Food Standards Agency in Northern Ireland. Guidance. The Eatwell Guide. Gov.UK. 2018. https://www.gov.uk/government/publications/the-eatwell-guide.)

pandemic were greater in women than men and those considered most deprived (Braithwaite et al. 2022).

At an individual level, people choose to eat a particular type of diet for a variety of reasons which include sociological, psychological, economic and behavioural factors. Sociological factors include age, culture, religion, income, food availability and cooking facilities. Psychological factors encompass a variety of factors ranging from aversions to particular foods to overeating particular food types. Economic factors influence both the quality and quantity of dietary intake. If a type of food, such as fruit, is not available to buy or if there is insufficient money to buy a range of foods in appropriate amounts, dietary intake will be reduced in quality and quantity. Behavioural elements of food choice can also influence dietary intake. For example, toddlers can be very particular about the type of food that they will eat.

When food is available, the amount eaten is determined by appetite. Appetite is controlled by many factors, including the presence of nutrients in the gastrointestinal (GI) tract, levels of GI hormones, levels of nutrients in the blood and the response of the central nervous system to hunger signals from the rest of the body. Emotional factors may also influence what is eaten, for example some people eat particular foods to 'cheer themselves up' or a celebratory meal may be eaten. The environment also affects appetite, for example the smell of freshly baked bread when passing a bakery may instigate feelings of hunger. Conversely, smelling a very unpleasant odour when eating tends to diminish appetite. People tend to eat more when eating with other people in a social setting, although this is not always the case.

As outlined earlier, there are many factors to consider when developing strategies to improve the diet of a group of people. In addition to the nutritional value to foods, the quality of foods is also an important factor and issues of food safety need to be considered.

Obesity

Obesity is the condition of excessive accumulation of fat in the body, leading to an increase in weight beyond that considered desirable. Obesity quite simply results when intake of energy is greater than energy usage. However, the reasons why this happens are complex (Jackson et al. 2020). Although many people have the genetic propensity to develop obesity, the propensity does not mean the person will become obese; customary diet and lifestyle play a major role.

Obesity is considered a major world health problem as the number of people who are obese is rapidly escalating (World Health Organisation [WHO] 2023). Obesity is associated with many common disorders such as coronary heart disease, hypertension and type 2 diabetes mellitus (WHO 2023). Individuals with obesity may also be subject to psychological distress and social penalties. Supporting people with obesity and involvement with obesity prevention and treatment approaches are important components of nursing activity. For example, nurses may deliver primary care-based interventions for the treatment of obesity, support weight loss efforts and care for people undergoing surgery to support weight loss. Losing weight can be very difficult to achieve particularly for some groups, for example people taking antipsychotic medication as this is associated with clinically significant weight gain. People who are obese can feel stigmatised in healthcare environments and it is important that nurses reflect on their approach to people with obesity to address this. A negative attitude towards a person's weight can lead people to feel ashamed and avoid future healthcare encounters (Talumaa et al. 2022).

REFLECTION 22.1

Malnutrition and the Nurse's Role

Florence Nightingale said in 1859, 'thousands of patients are annually starved in the midst of plenty from want of attention to the ways which make it possible for them to take food. I say to the nurse, have a rule of thought about your patient's diet'.

Activities

Reflect on this statement.
    In your placement experience has this situation changed?

Undernutrition

Protein–energy malnutrition (PEM) affects large numbers of the world's population and contributes significantly to mortality and morbidity. Certain groups are at particular risk, including older adults, people with a low income, institutionalised people and people with acute or chronic conditions affecting nutrient intake (Reflection 22.1).

Undernutrition can occur as a result of reduced food intake or increased nutritional requirements as well as an impaired ability to digest, absorb or metabolise nutrients. Illness and long-term conditions can reduce food intake by causing anorexia (loss of appetite), pain, nausea, dysphagia, dyspnoea, fatigue and a reduction in the ability to obtain and eat food. Illness can increase the need for nutrients; for example, pyrexia results in an increased metabolic rate and, therefore, increased energy demands. Infection and the process of tissue repair can increase the need for specific nutrients. However, some conditions can also result in a reduction in the need for some nutrients as physical activity level may be reduced. Some illnesses and conditions can cause changes in the function of the GI tract, resulting in altered digestive and absorptive processes and can also affect the body's ability to metabolise nutrients.

There is evidence of significant undernutrition in hospitalised patients in the UK (Malnutrition Task Force 2023) and concerns have been raised about the incidence of malnutrition in community settings. Hospitalisation or moving into residential care may predispose to undernutrition for a variety of reasons. The change in environment can cause anxiety which reduces food intake and the condition the patient has been admitted for may make them unable to eat well. Hospitals may serve food and fluids that are unfamiliar to individuals and may not serve it at a time at which they are used to eating and drinking. The environment in hospitals may not be conducive to eating and investigations and treatments may interrupt normal eating patterns. The role of the nurse is key in planning interventions that promote food and drink intake both at a group level (e.g. implementing protected mealtimes) and at an individual level.

Food Safety

Food safety is a topic encompassing a wide range of factors in food preparation, handling and storage to prevent foodborne harm. These include the use of plastic to wrap food, allergens, food fraud, pesticide residues, natural toxins and food-borne illness. Food-borne illnesses are a topic of nursing concern due to their impact on the health of individuals. Serving high-risk food, food which has not been heated appropriately and poor food hygiene in food preparation areas and by food handlers can all contribute to foodborne illness.

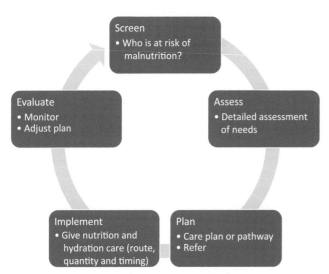

Figure 22.2 Process of nutritional care of individuals by nurses.

Healthcare-associated foodborne outbreaks can occur and have significant consequences because of their effects on vulnerable groups. Three pathogens have been associated with many outbreaks in Europe: *Salmonella*, norovirus and *Listeria monocytogenes* (Boone et al. 2021). *L. monocytogenes* caused the most deaths.

Nurses must ensure that food hygiene policy and guidelines in their practice area are followed (see Reflection 22.2 for reflective activity).

Nutritional Care by Nurses

Nutritional care by nurses in the context of this chapter refers to the nutritional care given to individuals. Nutritional care is a process that involves screening, assessment, planning, intervention and evaluation (Fig. 22.2). The Code (NMC 2018b) outlines that the nurse needs to ensure that those receiving care have adequate access to nutrition and hydration and provide help for those unable to feed or drink fluid unaided. Likewise, national health and care regulators often specify the need for health and social care providers to make sure people in their care eat and drink sufficient to meet their needs (e.g. the Care Quality Commission 2022a).

Nutritional Screening and Assessment

Nutritional screening and assessment is the first step to ensuring people are supported to eat and drink sufficient to meet their needs. This process allows for identification of nutritional status and needs. In many countries, healthcare guidance on nutritional care supports the use of screening tools as a quick and easy process to identify those at risk of malnutrition (Green 2018). Nutritional screening tools use risk factors that may lead to or be associated with malnourishment and are similar in format to a pressure injury risk assessment tool (see Chapter 23). They are typically in questionnaire format and are useful as an aide-mémoire for screening and as a record of information. An appropriate plan of action is identified by some. Of the many nutritional screening tools published, only a few have undergone rigorous testing of reliability and validity (Green 2018). The British Association for Parenteral and Enteral Nutrition (BAPEN) has introduced a valid and reliable screening tool for use by nurses in all areas of clinical practice (BAPEN 2023): the Malnutrition Universal Screening Tool (MUST). Other tools include the Short Nutritional Assessment Questionnaire tools which include assessment of appetite (Dutch Malnutrition Steering Group 2023).

Nutritional screening aims to identify those with, or at risk of, malnutrition and can highlight potential causes. If an individual is considered to be at risk of, or to have malnutrition, then nutritional assessment should be undertaken. Nutritional assessment is a 'systematic process of collecting and interpreting information about the nature and causes of nutrition related health conditions' (BAPEN 2022). A variety of healthcare professionals may undertake this assessment depending on the type of problem identified at screening. The majority of patients will be referred to the dietitian if malnutrition is suspected. However, referral to another healthcare professional may also be appropriate, for example referral to the speech and language therapist (SLT) if a swallowing deficit (dysphagia) is identified.

National Institute for Health and Care Excellence (NICE 2017) guidance outlines that hospital inpatients, outpatients, people in care homes and general practice surgeries should be screened for malnutrition (guidelines for those >18 years). They should be screened on admission or registration and subsequently assessed weekly for inpatients or more frequently if there is clinical concern.

Specific guidelines concerning screening and assessing for eating disorders (NICE 2019) and obesity (NICE 2014) are also available.

Screening and assessment allow identification of needs, planning of interventions and setting of goals (Green 2018). Following this, interventions can be implemented. As always, interventions should be recorded and regularly evaluated and modified as required. Screening and assessment can also establish a baseline from which to monitor changes in status. There are five principal methods of screening or assessing nutritional status:

- dietary history and intake
- clinical examination
- anthropometric measures
- biochemical tests.

Dietary History and Intake

The type of diet a person consumes is influenced by many factors, particularly in a home environment. Elementary assessment by nurses of dietary history and intake is essential to determine the risk of malnutrition and support the development of a plan of care if needed. Factors such as change in appetite, reduced food intake and absorption, the use of supplements and other issues, for example dietary adherence, should be considered. Dietary habits, food preferences and economic factors affecting food intake are also important to explore. In care environments, food charts can be used to record food intake over a period of time to assess whether dietary needs are being met. Asking a person to recall what they have eaten over the previous day or to describe what they generally eat is also a useful way of assessing dietary intake and to identify food that may have caused a reaction.

Assessment of food intake over a longer period of time, for example 7 days, by the use of a food diary can be useful in some circumstances, for example when working to promote dietary change in a person with obesity. This involves the person writing down everything that they have eaten and drunk for several days and can help to increase a person's awareness of their dietary intake and highlight aspects that can be modified to help achieve an intake that follows healthy eating guidelines (Fig. 22.1). The nurse is able to carry out an elementary dietary assessment, but more comprehensive dietary analyses should be undertaken by a dietitian as thorough dietary assessment is a complex process.

Clinical Examination

Nurses carry out a clinical examination of patients on admission to care and as required following the initial examination. As part of the clinical examination, assessment of how medical conditions and treatment may influence intake, digestion and absorption of nutrients can be undertaken. For example, a patient who feels nauseated is likely to have a reduced dietary intake. Other aspects of the clinical examination also give information about nutritional status and can help to inform a plan of care. Assessment of drug and alcohol use, appetite, taste and smell changes and dental issues should be considered in relation to dietary intake. Observation of general appearance, cognitive ability, activity level, fit of clothes and skin condition are also important factors to consider. It is also essential to assess a person's functional ability to eat; for example, are there physical or mental factors that might impair the process of eating? Finally, issues such as literacy and visual impairment need to be considered if written dietary advice is to be given. If the person is unable to understand and read the language in which the advice is given, it is likely to be ineffective.

Anthropometric Tests

Simple anthropometric measures can be used by nurses to screen and assess nutritional status. Anthropometry refers to the measurement of the human body. It is important to weigh individuals on admission to care and periodically thereafter to identify any subsequent losses or gains. To ensure accuracy, the person should, if possible, be weighed on the same scales at the same time each day, preferably in the same clothes, and after emptying their bladder and bowel. Single measurements of weight are of limited value, but serial measurements permit trends in weight loss or gain to be identified.

Percentage weight change can be calculated using the equation:

$$(\text{previous weight} - \text{current weight} / \text{previous weight}) \times 100$$

Unintentional weight loss of 10% or more in the previous 3 to 6 months suggests an individual may require nutritional support (NICE 2017). If a person is underweight and loses more than 5%, they may require nutritional support (NICE 2017). However, caution is required when interpreting weight changes as factors such as dehydration, oedema or tumour growth can complicate the picture. Further, even when weight loss is intentional, a loss of more than 10% in 3 to 6 months may result in poor nutritional status.

Weight considered in relation to height gives a more accurate assessment of the degree to which a person is under- or overweight than weight alone. Body mass index (BMI) is commonly used to assess weight in relation to height. This is simply the body weight in kilograms (kg) divided by the height in metres squared (m^2). For example, a person with a body weight of 57 kg and a height of 1.62 m has a BMI of $57/1.62^2 = 21.7$ kg/m^2. Height can be difficult to determine, due to factors such as spine curvature and inability to stand. An estimation of height can be made, for example by using ulna length (BAPEN 2023).

The WHO (2010) has defined the following BMI categories:
- <18.5 underweight
- 18.5–24.9 normal range
- 25.0–29.9 overweight
- 30.0–34.9 obese (class 1)
- 35.0–39.9 obese (class 2)
- >40.0 obese (class 3)

When using BMI with older people, the resulting plan and intervention need to be carefully considered. A higher BMI may provide a protective effect in older age as a result of various factors such as bone protection following a fall and nutritional reserve when dietary intake is poor during illness (Ramel and Stenholm 2021).

Waist circumference can be used to assess the amount of fat located in the abdominal region. Adults with high waist circumferences are at increased adverse health risk. Measurement of waist circumference and BMI is recommended to guide patient management to reduce risks associated with obesity and monitor the effectiveness of healthy eating and activity weight management approaches with individuals (Ross et al. 2020).

Anthropometric measures that assess fat levels or muscle mass (lean tissue) of the body can be used by dietitians or doctors in clinical environments. Nurses may use these measures in specialist units following training in their use. These measures include skinfold measures to estimate body fat and midarm muscle circumference to estimate skeletal muscle mass. Electrical bioimpedance is a method of assessing the fat mass of the body which is being used increasingly in some environments such as health clubs. Functional tests of nutritional status are usually performed by the doctor or dietitian and include tests such as handgrip strength (using a dynamometer).

Regular checks of accuracy and, if necessary, recalibration are essential for all equipment used to measure individuals, including weighing scales. In addition, equipment must be designed for healthcare rather than personal use.

Biochemical Tests

Biochemical measures to assess nutritional status include measurement of a nutrient or metabolite in blood, urine, stool or other tissues. These include measurement of vitamins and minerals as well as other macronutrients. Other measures commonly undertaken include measures associated with deficiency disease, for example full blood count to assess for anaemia.

Measurement of proteins present in the serum, such as albumin and pre-albumin, is sometimes undertaken but the interpretation of what the level means needs to be considered carefully. Serum protein levels are an indicator of inflammation and can be changed as a result of treatments, such as administration of blood products. They are, therefore, not reliable measures of total body protein or muscles mass in acute and chronic illness (Evans et al. 2021).

Nitrogen balance reflects the intake or loss of whole body protein. Nitrogen balance is determined by estimating protein intake and subtracting urinary nitrogen excretion with an allowance for nitrogen loss via hair, skin and faeces. Additionally, losses from wound drainage or GI fistulae are considered. Nitrogen balance can be used to assess whether protein intake is adequate. A positive nitrogen balance indicates that the patient is in an anabolic state, whereas a negative balance indicates catabolism.

Information about nutritional status from only one source can be open to misinterpretation due to the many factors, such as disease processes, that can influence individual parameters. A combination of two or more measures obtained from dietary history and intake, clinical examination, functional tests, anthropometric measures and biochemical tests is required to gain an accurate picture of an individual's nutritional status. The methods described previously may be used by nurses in the context of a busy clinical environment. Other methods are employed by dietitians and other healthcare professionals in the clinical environment and research settings.

Refeeding Syndrome

If the patient is very malnourished, problems can arise from sudden feeding, known as refeeding syndrome. This is caused by a rapid shift of electrolytes, glucose and water between extracellular and intracellular compartments. As the syndrome can be life threatening, it is crucial that anyone at risk of refeeding syndrome is identified before nutritional support is given so that appropriate intervention can be planned. The NICE (2017) outlines several criteria used to determine those at risk. These criteria include BMI of less than 16 kg/m^2, unintentional weight loss of greater than 10% within 3 to 6 months, little or nothing to eat for more than 5 days, a history of alcohol or drug use disorder and low potassium, phosphate or magnesium levels. If patients meet these criteria, then they must be referred to the dietitian and doctor before food or fluid is given to determine a plan of nutritional care. This will usually be focused on giving nutritional support at no more than 50% of requirements initially and correcting electrolyte deficiencies (De Silva and Nightingale 2020).

Drug–Nutrient Interactions

Medication absorption and metabolism can be influenced by some foods or nutrients. This can also occur with herbal supplements. Drug–nutrient interactions are considered to be common in clinical practice, but healthcare professionals may lack knowledge to identify them (Osuala and Ojewole 2021). The interaction may potentiate or inhibit the activity of the medication or result in side-effects. The type of interaction will vary depending on the medication and the nutrient or herbal supplement. For example, the effect of warfarin can be reduced by vitamin K found in food supplements and St John's wort can decrease digoxin concentration.

This is an important issue for the nurse to consider when involved in the administration of medications and providing advice to patients, clients or carers. The nurse should be aware of the potential of commonly prescribed medications to interact with nutrients and highlight any problems that could potentially arise following drug administration with the prescriber or pharmacist. The nurse should also undertake assessment carefully to identify if the patient takes any herbal supplements. The British National Formulary provides comprehensive information on drug–nutrient interactions and can be referred to during medication administration (Joint Formulary Committee 2023). The hospital or community pharmacist can also provide advice on the potential effect of the herbal supplement on the patient's medication.

Care Planning and Intervention

Following screening and assessment of an individual, the nurse will plan and deliver appropriate interventions. The following sections outline interventions that may be planned by the nurse, usually in association with other healthcare professionals such as the dietitian. These include advising on a 'healthy diet', promoting oral intake and enteral and parenteral nutrition (PN). Obesity and undernutrition are also discussed. In many situations, referral to the dietitian is a necessary part of the nutritional plan of care. However, in some circumstances, for example giving advice concerning healthy eating to an individual who is overweight, this can be given by the nurse.

Local guidelines should outline when referral to a dietitian is appropriate. Individuals who require therapeutic diets, for example those with diabetes mellitus type 2, renal disease, coeliac disease and food allergy, should always be referred to the dietitian. Nurses may then follow through a plan of care prescribed by the dietitian.

Healthy Eating Advice

The diet which is currently recommended to promote the health of the general population in the UK is shown in Fig. 22.1 as outlined in the Diet section. This pictorial representation is termed the 'Eatwell Guide' and is designed to be used as a health promotion tool. Such a diet is sometimes termed a 'healthy' or 'balanced' diet. This diet consists of 40% vegetables and fruit, 38% complex carbohydrate foods, 12% protein-containing foods, 8% dairy products or similar foods and 1% oils and spreads (this adds up to 99% as the figures are rounded to whole numbers). The proportions shown are representative of food consumption overall rather than a specific time period such as one meal. Current recommendations suggest that individuals eat at least five portions of a variety of fruit and vegetables a day (NHS 2023a). The type of diet outlined earlier is not suitable for those under 2 years of age or those following a diet prescribed by the dietitian.

The UK national food and diet advice (NHS 2022) also includes eight 'tips for healthy eating'. These are:
- Base your meals on higher fibre starchy carbohydrates
- Eat lots of fruit and veg
- Eat more fish, including a portion of oily fish
- Cut down on saturated fat and sugar
- Eat less salt: no more than 6 g a day for adults
- Get active and be a healthy weight
- Do not get thirsty
- Don't skip breakfast

Public Health England encourages organisations and individuals to use the Eatwell Guide to ensure consistent messages about what constitutes a healthy diet. Therefore nurses working with patients should use the Eatwell Guide and associated NHS resources when supporting people to follow healthy eating guidelines (NHS 2023a).

Obesity Management

Approaches to the treatment of obesity include diet, activity, behavioural, pharmacological and surgical interventions. Behavioural interventions aim to modify behaviour to increase physical activity level and improve dietary habits and quality. Multicomponent interventions are recommended (NICE 2014), for example increasing activity and reducing energy intake. Nurses should provide information, advice and support about healthy lifestyle and refer to weight management services as required (Office for Health

Improvement and Disparities 2022). This requires knowing which services are available and identifying and using appropriate resources and approaches, such as the Eatwell Guide and the Making Every Contact Count programme (Health Education England 2023).

Diet, Activity and Behavioural Interventions

Changes to diet and activity level can be supported by a wide variety of interventions which aim to reduce energy intake and increase physical activity. Changing diet and activity level requires a change in behaviour. Behavioural interventions include self-monitoring of behaviour and progress, stimulus control, goal setting, ensuring social support, problem solving and modifying thoughts.

In terms of diet, current UK national guidance focuses on making small changes to eating and drinking habits to promote weight loss (NHS 2023b). There are many types of weight loss diets advocating various types and combinations of food. Low-energy diets promote weight loss because energy intake is less than energy expenditure, so body stores of energy are used. Low-energy diets can include meal replacement products, such as soups and shakes. Very-low-energy diets (about 800 kilocalories a day) may be appropriate for some people in the short-term (12 weeks or less) (Muscogiuri et al. 2021). However, they can be difficult to follow, unsuitable for some groups (for example teenagers and pregnant women) and it can be a challenge to ensure nutritional requirements (other than energy) are met.

Increased physical activity can facilitate weight loss and improve aspects of health independent of weight loss (Pojednic et al. 2022). The WHO (2022) recommends that adults aged 18 to 65 should undertake at least 150 to 300 minutes of moderate or 75 to 150 minutes of vigorous intensity aerobic physical activity (or a combination of the two). In addition to this, muscle-strengthening activities two or more days a week are recommended. Recommendations for adults aged 65 and over include activities to enhance functional capacity. Activity can be promoted by integrating it into lifestyle, for example taking the stairs instead of using a lift and walking instead of driving if travelling short distances. Exercise referral schemes are in place in many areas of the UK to support sedentary adults to return to become active. Some individuals may have conditions that limit physical activity level and advice on activity will need to be modified.

Generally, interventions aimed at weight loss usually include dietary, activity and behavioural components. For example, the free NHS Weight Loss Plan app includes goal setting, planning food choice and activity advice and recording progress (NHS 2023b). A number of commercial organisations provide weight loss plans and support for weight loss.

Pharmacological Interventions

In the UK, medication may be prescribed for the treatment of obesity if dietary and physical activity interventions have been evaluated and they form part of the approach to obesity management (NICE 2014). Several antiobesity medicines can be prescribed for use by NHS healthcare professionals. Orlistat is a drug that inhibits the actions of lipases in the GI tract, thus limiting the absorption of fat, which is consequently excreted in the stools. It has been shown to be useful in promoting weight loss and supporting weight maintenance. Liraglutide and semaglutide are drugs which activate glucagon-like peptide-1 receptors to increase insulin secretion, suppress glucagon secretion and slow gastric emptying. Other drugs may be prescribed for rare forms of obesity, such as setmelanotide. The field of obesity research is rapidly evolving so other types of medication are likely to be available in the future.

Surgical Interventions

Obesity can be treated by surgical means if other methods of obesity management have not supported a person to lose weight (NICE 2014). The decision to undertake surgical treatment is not taken lightly as there are risks involved and a change to eating behaviour is required. Weight loss surgery, sometimes called bariatric surgery, is undertaken within NHS services if specific criteria are met. These include a person having a BMI of 40 or more, or a BMI between 35 and 40 and an obesity-related condition such as hypertension (NICE 2014).

Surgical treatments involve reducing the size of the stomach so less food can be eaten and include gastric band placement, sleeve gastrectomy and gastric bypass. A gastric bypass can also reduce the number of kilocalories absorbed. It is important that anyone undergoing surgical treatment for obesity is referred to the dietitian. Surgical treatment for obesity will not automatically result in the consumption of a healthier diet and may actually lead to a poorer quality of diet being consumed. The nurse must be aware that, following surgery, whilst the patient may be pleased with a very fast weight loss, a poor diet may be the cause, which can lead to a risk of malnutrition. As with any method of weight loss, weight loss maintenance is important, and diet and lifestyle changes are essential factors in this.

Prevention of Obesity

Globally the number of people who are obese is continuing to rise. To address this, with the aim of both preventing and reducing obesity, many countries and regions within countries have developed strategies focused on healthy lifestyle promotion. Examples of these include regional plans to create built and natural environments to promote physical activity, such a cycle lanes and creating safe routes to schools. Where appropriate, health promotion and education strategies by nurses should promote adherence to healthy eating guidelines and increased activity levels, not only for individuals but also for their families. Nurses who work with communities, such as school nurses and occupational health nurses, usually work to prevent obesity in their communities as well as working with individuals who are obese.

Food and Drink Intake in Care Settings

Nurses are ideally placed to help individuals, whether at home or in hospital, to meet their nutritional needs through diet and fluid intake (van den Berg et al. 2021). In addition to meeting nutritional needs, it is important for the nurse to acknowledge that food and drink have a number of other roles, such as expressing beliefs and culture. Following screening and assessment, if a patient is identified as malnourished or at risk of malnutrition, the nurse should identify with the patient ways in which oral nutritional requirements can be met, considering all the factors which affect their intake, and produce a plan of care. The plan of care should include appropriate interventions and be evaluated at regular intervals. The next section discusses factors to consider when planning and delivering oral nutritional intake.

Factors Influencing Food and Drink Acquisition

For an individual to eat an adequate oral diet at home, a number of activities are required and need to be considered:

- Is the person able to shop (online or in person) and to choose and purchase appropriate foods and drink?
- Does the person have financial resources to purchase the required foods and drink?
- Once purchased, can food and drink be transported home or delivered to the home?

- Are there adequate facilities for storing food and drink at home, e.g. a refrigerator?
- Are adequate cooking facilities available and can the person use them safely?

If there are issues of concern in any of these areas, ways to address them need to be outlined in the plan of care. Ordering shopping online, mobile shops and delivery services may help some people to shop independently. Some people may require support from family, informal carers, volunteer services or social services as appropriate to procure food and drink. The home environment may need to be modified to enable independent food and drink storage and preparation. If this is considered necessary, the person should be referred to the occupational therapist (OT) for assessment.

Factors Influencing Eating and Drinking

To eat and drink without support requires the ability to transfer food and fluids to the mouth, the ability to retain food in the mouth, to chew and to swallow. Sensory function is also important as appetite is improved if a person can see, smell and taste their food and drink. As people age, the ability to detect sweetness and saltiness generally diminishes and more highly seasoned and sweeter foods and drinks may be preferred by older adults. Some illnesses, conditions and treatment cause taste and smell changes resulting in a change in the types of foods and drinks liked by an individual or a reduction in appetite. Conditions such as upper respiratory tract infections can cause a temporary reduction in the sense of smell, which makes eating and drinking less appealing. Reduced oral sensitivity or confusion may cause the temperature of foods and drinks to be misjudged, resulting in a greater risk of burn injury from hot food and drinks.

Reduced mobility may cause problems in attaining a comfortable and safe eating and drinking position. Some patients or clients are required to maintain a supine or prone position for eating and drinking. Individuals may have difficulty with arm or hand movement or hand–eye coordination, making transferring food to their mouth difficult. The person may need to be offered specific food types and textures sometimes termed 'finger foods to enable eating (Heelan et al. 2020). Referral to the OT is required when it is considered that eating is restricted by reduced dexterity. The OT will be able to identify which eating and drinking aids, such as modified cutlery and plate guards, are appropriate for the person and advise on positioning.

The state of the teeth and mouth is important. Teeth are needed for effective chewing and tooth loss has been associated with changed dietary habits, for example reduced vegetable and dairy products intake and lower vitamin intake (Ke-hui et al. 2023). People with tooth loss or poor oral health may require food of a softer texture or food cut into smaller pieces. Poor oral health can alter the taste and consequently enjoyment of a meal. If oral tissues are dry, inflamed or painful, a person may be reluctant to eat.

Meals and drinks that look unappetising or are poorly presented can reduce appetite and enjoyment of a meal. People with visual impairment may appreciate knowing where different foods are positioned on the plate by the server advising them when the food is served. People who have experienced a stroke or other brain injury may only perceive a portion of the plate and, therefore, need to be reminded about the remainder.

The texture of food is important. The person who has few natural teeth, poor oral health or dentures may choose not to eat particular food types. Some medical conditions cause difficulty chewing, closing the mouth or swallowing resulting in food dribbling from the mouth. This can cause the person to feel self-conscious and result in them avoiding eating. Food texture may need to be modified for individuals who have dysphagia. Dysphagia can be caused by a number of conditions which affect neurological function (such as stroke or motor neurone disease) or cause anatomical changes (such as head and neck cancers). The degree of dysphagia must be assessed by the SLT and local guidelines for the referral of patients with swallowing difficulties followed. It may be that no oral intake or texture modified and thickened drinks can be tolerated. If oral intake is problematic or impossible, then enteral feeding must be considered. The International Dysphagia Diet Standardisation Initiative Framework provides a common terminology to describe food textures and drink thickness (The International Dysphagia Diet Standardisation Initiative 2023) and the SLT will assess the patient and prescribe the appropriate diet and fluid modification. The role of the nurse is then to ensure the healthcare team support the patient to adhere to the prescription and the patient themselves is able to tolerate the prescribed diet and fluid modification. Any issues with adherence must be discussed with the SLT, who can then support staff with education and review the patient's prescription with them.

Culturally Appropriate Nutritional Care

People may follow a particular type of diet or pattern of food intake as part of their cultural values. It is important that the nurse asks a person or their carers what they require to support them to meet their cultural needs, so a plan of care can be put into place, for example providing a Kosher or Halal diet and serving it in an appropriate way, providing a vegan menu, providing appropriate cutlery or offering food or drink several times before it is accepted (Care Quality Commission 2022b). It is particularly important that the nurse is aware of dietary requirements and ensures appropriate food and drink is offered when people are not able to express their cultural needs due to their condition. For example, people with dementia may not recognise a food item that they would not usually find acceptable to consume. It is the role of the nurse to ensure that food and drink offered meets their cultural needs.

Access to Nutrition

Some groups that nurses care for have limited access to food and drinking water to support them to eat a diet that promotes their health. Access to food can be affected by low income, mental health issues, drug and alcohol use and inability to store, prepare and cook food. Low income and poor living conditions can result in people relying on food donations and take-away food. Groups particularly as risk are people experiencing homelessness, who are more likely to have a BMI outside of the healthy range and have low blood levels of nutrients such as iron, folate, vitamins C, D, and B$_{12}$ and haemoglobin (Huang et al. 2022). Nurses working with people with limited access to nutrition need to be aware of local resources so they can refer people to food banks or other organisations that provide support for people to achieve a healthy dietary intake.

People in prisons may have limited choice of food or poor-quality food. Food has the potential to enhance prisoner health and involving prisoners in food preparation can improve life skills and mental wellbeing (Woods-Brown et al. 2023). Nurses working in the prison environment can work to promote healthy eating (Leach and Goodwin 2014).

Organising Effective Mealtimes

Mealtimes are often the focal point of the day for patients or clients. Ensuring a supply of nutritious food, at the right temperature and in an attractive and hygienic manner, is the responsibility of both nursing and catering services. Food preparation is not usually a nursing task, but the nurse is responsible for ensuring that food is ordered and should act as advocate between the patient/client and the centralised catering services. Meals are often delivered to patients or clients preplated in heated trolleys at fixed times. Some patients or clients may need or prefer more frequent and smaller amounts of food so snacks should be offered between meals. When a patient or client does miss a meal, it is the nurse's responsibility to ensure an alternative is offered. NHS organisations should have suitable 24-hour food service provision where appropriate (NHS England 2022). 'Protected Mealtimes', where ward activity other than eating and drinking activities is limited during a mealtime, has been implemented in many areas, although the value of this approach has been questioned (Porter and Hanna 2020).

In continuing care settings, some flexibility over meal timing is preferable and it is important that an effort is made to enable people to follow their normal pattern of eating. In a continuing care environment, there is often a dining room or large table for people to sit at to eat meals. Eating with others in a dining room or at a table can encourage food intake, although it must be recognised that some individuals may prefer to eat alone. If a dining room is available for residents or patients, it should be pleasantly decorated and provided with small tables to allow people to eat in their natural groupings. If a person has visitors during meals, this can be helpful, as relatives can be involved in assisting with eating or enjoy a meal with them.

Food Selection and Presentation

Although RNs do not always serve meals, it is important for them to make sure that each person receives the right food in sufficient quantities. Patients and clients need to be active in food selection where possible by filling in a menu card or choosing from a bulk trolley. Foods should be attractively served. Small portions should be offered to those with a small appetite as large portions can be daunting. For those requiring a texture modified diet, food moulds can enhance the presentation of a meal.

The temperature of food is another factor that affects appetite; care should be taken to ensure hot foods are served hot and cold foods are served cold. It is also important that food is served using a no-touch technique. Chipped or cracked crockery should not be used as it will not clean properly and can become a source of cross infection.

Assisting a Person to Eat

When someone has difficulty eating, it becomes the RN's responsibility to assist with this activity of living. Before preparing for the meal, the person should be offered toilet facilities, followed by the opportunity to wash their hands. It is generally easier to eat sitting in a chair, but the person confined to bed can be assisted to sit upright (if this is not contraindicated). An appropriate table is required so that the food can be set out, allowing the person to see the food and indicate preferences. The patient or client should be offered protection for their clothing. Where possible, independence should be promoted by preparing food and drink for an individual, so it is ready to eat. Sitting with a person and using verbal and non-verbal prompts as required may enable them to eat the meal independently. Where a person is unable to transfer food or drink into their mouths, it is necessary to do this for them. This requires considerable skill, and the consent of the patient or client is required. It should be recognised that having to be fed by someone can be a threat to the individual's integrity and self-esteem, so every effort

should be made to minimise the negative aspects. The nurse should sit level with the person and encourage a relaxed social atmosphere. The rate and manner of assistance with eating and drinking should be at the person's normal pace and pattern. The pace of eating can be controlled by the person if their hand is placed on the nurse's forearm during assistance with feeding and drinking. Plenty of time is essential to allow the person to chew, to pause between mouthfuls and to have a drink when desired. The nurse should check that plates and food are at an appropriate temperature and ensure that any bones or fruit pips are removed. Fluid should be offered periodically as this will facilitate swallowing. Mouth care should be offered when the meal is finished, and the person should remain sitting for a period of time after the meal to promote digestion. It is important to stop giving food and fluid to a patient/client if their voice sounds gurgly, they show signs of choking or food is pocketing in their mouth as this suggests that the swallow reflex is compromised and referral to the SLT may be appropriate. (See Further Reading, e.g. Brooker and Waugh 2007, for information about mealtime environment and feeding patients/clients.)

Between meals a drink should be within the patient's/client's reach. If appropriate, snacks can also be positioned so the person can help themselves as required.

Supplementing the Diet

If an individual's intake is poor, it is important to 'make every mouthful count'. This can be achieved through strategies such as encouraging the person to choose high-energy foods to eat and increasing the nutritional value of foods by adding butter or cheese to vegetables and ice cream to puddings and milk drinks.

People with a poor appetite or dysphagia may not be able to ingest enough food to meet nutritional needs, and oral nutritional supplements between meals may be prescribed. These consist of drinks, puddings or powders that are mixed with milk or water that have added kilocalories and other nutrients. Supplements can be presented in a range of ways: frozen to the consistency of a mousse or ice cream or warmed to resemble soup. They should be served at the temperature recommended by the manufacturers. Once opened, they should be considered to be similar to a glass of milk and discarded promptly if not consumed. Patients/clients may prefer them served in a glass or cup rather than the container in which they are packaged. The short-term use of oral nutritional supplements has been shown to be a cost-effective way of improving nutritional intake (Thomson et al. 2022).

In addition to oral nutritional supplement drink and puddings, a prescription for vitamin and mineral supplements may be required to correct specific micronutrient deficiencies or generally increase the intake of micronutrients.

Enteral Feeding by Tube

Enteral feeding by tube refers to the delivery of nutrients directly to the patient's stomach or small intestine via a tube. If a patient is not able to eat or drink sufficiently adequately to maintain nutritional status, enteral feeding should be considered and can be used as the sole form of nutrition or as a supplement to oral intake.

If a person has a functioning gut, enteral nutrition should always be considered before PN (NICE 2017). Enteral nutrition is less costly, safer and easier to manage and has fewer side-effects than PN. Compared with PN, it is thought to preserve intestinal mucosal structure and function and allow for the absorption and utilisation of nutrients in a more physiologically normal way.

Enteral nutrition is contraindicated in some conditions, for example obstruction or incompleteness of the GI tract. The decision as to whether a person is enterally or parenterally fed should be informed by the Nutrition Support Team if present in the clinical setting or made with the input of a dietitian if not. When deciding whether enteral nutrition is appropriate for an individual, ethical and legal issues need to be considered. For further reading on this complex and important area of clinical practice, see Cardenas (2020).

It is essential that a person receiving enteral feeding has a written plan of care so that all involved with the care of that person are aware of the goals of care, interventions planned and the evaluation strategies. It is also important that the plan of care is made in partnership with the patient/client where possible and that carers are informed where appropriate. Often it seems there is a lack of clarity in care settings as to what the overall plan of care is for an individual, for example why a particular type of tube is used, when it has been placed and the duration of any side-effects.

The major enteral route via the nose is to the stomach (nasogastric (NG) tube), although a tube may also be inserted from the nose to the duodenum (nasoduodenal tube) or jejunum (nasojejunal tube). Postpyloric placement is indicated when the risk of aspiration (into the respiratory tract) is considered high or when the patient's medical condition, for example obstruction by tumour, or treatment, for example oesophageal surgery, indicates this. Less commonly, a tube may be passed via the mouth to the stomach (orogastric tube). Tubes may also be inserted through the abdominal wall into the stomach (gastrostomy) or jejunum (jejunostomy). For short-term feeding, enteral feeding tubes are usually inserted via the nose, but if a tube is required in the longer term, a gastrostomy is the preferred route of choice. As NG and gastrostomy tubes represent the most common approaches to tube feeding, they will be the focus of the rest of this section.

Nasogastric Tube Insertion and Care

NG tube feeding is indicated when short-term nutritional support is required. As the NG route interferes minimally with oral function, it can be used to supplement oral intake. The tube used should be EnFit compliant, narrow in diameter and flexible. Tubes that have a wide diameter are poorly tolerated as they are uncomfortable, can cause pressure necrosis in the nose and oropharynx and may encourage gastro-oesophageal (cardiac) sphincter/valve incompetence, thus increasing the risk of gastro-oesophageal reflux and aspiration. As fine-bore tubes (6 to 8 FG) are flexible, a wire introducer may be required when the nurse is inserting the tube. The length of time the tube can be in place before it is replaced is detailed in the manufacturer's guidelines.

Insertion of the tube must follow guidelines approved by the clinical setting (please see a clinical procedure guide for information on how to insert enteral tubes, for example The Royal Marsden Manual for information). Nurses may insert tubes safely and effectively in most individuals; however, the insertion of fine-bore tubes on patients with fractures in the base of the skull, maxillofacial and oesophageal disorders or following surgery in these regions is not straightforward and in these situations a nurse or doctor with advanced clinical skills in this procedure should place the tube. Local guidelines on which patients/clients RNs may insert an NG tube should be followed.

Once the tube is in place, its position may be checked by pH testing of aspirate using the appropriate pH range indicator strips or by X-ray. However, no method is foolproof; gastric aspirate may be obtained from the trachea if the person has aspirated, and an X-ray is only accurate at the time it was taken. Guidelines approved by the clinical setting must be followed when ascertaining the placement

of a tube and the patient carefully observed for signs of respiratory distress or general discomfort once feeding has commenced.

Following insertion, the position of the tube should be checked before administration of any solution or medication, if the patient complains that the tube feels uncomfortable, if feed is seen in the mouth and following episodes of vomiting, coughing or suctioning. Regular flushing of the tube with water is essential to reduce the chance of blockage. Syringes designed specifically for use with enteral tubes (EnFit compliant) should only be used to flush the tube to avoid any potential confusion with venous access ports. A 50-mL syringe is recommended by some practice areas as the most appropriate size of syringe to use for flushing or aspirating, as use of a smaller syringe is thought to generate a higher pressure within the tube. Excessive pressure should not be used to force fluids down the tube as this may split the tube wall. Many practice guidelines suggest that the tube should be flushed with 30 mL of water at the beginning and end of each feed and before and after giving medication. For some patients, fluid intake may be limited due to their medical condition, in which case advice from the Nutrition Nurse Specialist (NNS) or pharmacist should be sought.

Premature removal of NG tubes by patients is common. An NG tube should be secured to the nose and side of the face to prevent the tube from being displaced.

The act of eating and drinking cleanses and hydrates the oral mucosa. For patients/clients who are tube fed, frequent mouth care is a priority to keep the mouth in a clean and comfortable condition.

Gastrostomy Tube Insertion and Care

Gastrostomy feeding is used if enteral feeding is likely to continue for longer than a month (NICE 2017). This has become a relatively common nutritional intervention. The procedures most commonly used to place a gastrostomy tube are termed 'percutaneous endoscopic gastrostomy' (PEG) and 'radiologically inserted gastrostomy' (RIG) although tubes may also be inserted surgically. Prior to the procedure the patient will require preoperative preparation (see Chapter 25).

Gastrostomy placement is contraindicated in some medical conditions such as ascites. The doctor in charge of the patient's medical care or the Nutrition Support Team will assess the patient's suitability for gastrostomy placement prior to the procedure and obtain the patient's written consent. A gastrostomy is normally performed after the patient has received a sedative medication; therefore, postoperative care should follow the general guidelines following an operative procedure under sedation (see Chapter 25). Complications of gastrostomy insertion can occur, such as bleeding and pneumoperitoneum (air/gas in the peritoneal cavity), and the nurse should carefully observe the patient's condition in the postoperative period.

Following the procedure, tube feeding can usually commence within 4 hours of insertion of a PEG tube (NICE 2017). Local guidelines should be followed after insertion of one of the other types of gastrostomy tube. Until the gastrostomy tract has granulated, the site can be dressed with a dry dressing which is changed daily using an aseptic technique. Once the tract has healed and the stoma formed, the site should be washed daily with water and dried thoroughly. Some types of gastrostomy tube need to be rotated at least weekly once the tract is healed to prevent skin from growing around the tube. The frequency with which this should be carried out is variable, therefore local clinical guidelines must be followed. It is suggested that the tube should be gently pushed in by 1 cm and then returned to its original position whilst rotating it through 360 degrees. The fixation plate should be approximately 5-mm distance from the abdomen and should be undone and pulled back to facilitate cleaning. The patient with a gastrostomy tube can swim or bathe once the tract has healed. Gastrostomy tubes retained by balloons need the balloon integrity checked at frequent intervals. The guidance provided by the manufacturers should be followed.

If the gastrostomy tube is removed accidentally, then immediate action must be taken as the tract will close over within a matter of hours. If the tube cannot be reinserted by the NNS or doctor within a short period of time, then a replacement may be inserted to keep the stoma patent; fluid should never be infused until the position of the tube has been confirmed by a healthcare professional experienced in the care of gastrostomy tubes.

Complications as a result of gastrostomy formation are reported to be common and may include infection and leakage (Green et al. 2019). Overgranulation of the stoma may also occur; advice on this may be sought from the NNS or in some situations from the Tissue Viability Nurse (see Chapter 23).

The procedure for the removal of a gastrostomy tube varies according to the type of tube placed. Some tubes can be withdrawn through the stoma, following deflation of the retainer in the stomach; some tubes may be cut and the portion remaining in the stomach removed endoscopically or allowed to pass through the GI tract. If a tube is to be removed, local guidelines should be followed or the advice of the NNS or unit personnel who have placed the tube should be obtained.

Administration of Medications via Enteral Tube

The pharmacist should be consulted if medication is to be given via an enteral tube as there are risks associated with this route of administration such as tube blockage, drug toxicity and a reduction in drug efficacy. The pharmacist is able to advise on the appropriate route, formulation, timing and monitoring.

The location of the enteral tube needs to be considered before medication is given as some drugs are not absorbed effectively when delivered directly into the small intestine rather than to the stomach. Medications in the form of oral liquid and dispersible tablets are most easily administered via an enteral tube. However, some liquids may be hyperosmolar and cause diarrhoea, especially if directly administered further down the small intestine. Some viscous oral liquids may be diluted with water to ease administration. Tablets may be crushed, but the advice of the pharmacist must be sought. Medication which is coated (film or enteric) is rarely suitable for administration via an enteral tube. Tablets or capsules of cytotoxic, hormonal, steroidal or antibiotic medications should not be crushed or opened because of the potential risk of exposure to staff and others. (See Further Reading, e.g. The Royal Marsden Manual of Clinical Nursing Procedures guidelines for the administration of medication via enteral feeding tubes.)

The pharmacist is also able to advise on the potential for drug–nutrient interactions; for example, the drug phenindione should not be administered with feed as this can affect the amount of drug absorbed from the GI tract. If several medications are to be given at one time, the tube should be flushed with at least 10 mL of water between each medication. Two drugs may interact with each other, and their effects may change as a result.

Selection of Enteral Solution

There is a wide range of commercially prepared enteral solutions ('feeds') that may be prescribed. Commercially prepared feeds are of a known nutritional content, are sterile and are designed for ease of administration. The dietitian will choose the most appropriate feeding regimen for the patient, basing such choice on assessment of the patient's needs and medical condition. Generally, the dietitian will

also order the feed and ensure it is available for the nurses to administer. Feeds may cause GI disturbances when feeding is being initiated or if they are infused too rapidly. Enteral solutions should be administered at room temperature, as administration of a cold feed can cause the patient to experience abdominal discomfort. Enteral solution should be stored according to the manufacturer's instructions. 'Use by' dates should always be checked prior to administration.

Method of Administration of Enteral Solution

The equipment for feeding consists of a reservoir, the NG tube, and usually a giving set that connects to the reservoir and a pump. The reservoir may be a bottle or soft pack and may require filling or may be filled with feed at the manufacturing stage. NG feeds can be delivered intermittently or continuously. Intermittent feeding is the administration of a 'bolus' of feed periodically. Continuous feeding involves the delivery of a feed over a period of many hours. In clinical settings, enteral feeding pumps are commonly used to deliver a steady flow of solution over a period of time. Feeding intermittently reflects more closely the normal eating pattern and permits free movement between feeds; however, it may be more likely to result in feelings of nausea, intestinal distension, cramps and diarrhoea. There may also be an increased risk of reflux and aspiration. The dietitian will prescribe the rate at which a solution should be administered following assessment of the individual. During feeding and for 1 hour after, unless contraindicated, the patient should sit up at 30 degrees or higher to reduce the risk of aspiration (NICE 2017). The amount of feed remaining in the stomach (gastric residue) can be checked if the individual complains of nausea or gastric distension. In some clinical settings, for example intensive care units, checking the amount of feed in the stomach should be carried out periodically; local guidelines should be consulted on this issue.

Monitoring and Complications of Enteral Feeding

Monitoring of a patient on enteral feeding is essential to observe for signs of complications and to ensure nutritional goals are being met. Monitoring should include assessment of fluid and food intake, vital signs, weight, GI function, stool frequency, tube position and leakage and general clinical condition. Biochemical monitoring is carried out, the frequency determined by the patient's condition. For further details, see the NICE guidelines on nutrition support for adults (NICE 2017).

Complications of enteral feeding can be categorised into three broad groups: mechanical, biochemical and GI/infectious (Table 22.3). The serious complication of refeeding syndrome is discussed earlier.

The psychological effects of tube feeding should also be considered, since food has a profound influence on psychosocial well-being. One study highlighted that having a gastrostomy has a major impact on the lifestyle of patients and their carers (Green et al. 2019). Effective symptom management and support are identified as important factors in enabling patients to cope (Green et al. 2019). The nurse should ensure that the nursing care recognises and meets the patient's and carer's needs.

If a patient is likely to be discharged from hospital with an enteral feeding tube in situ, then it is essential that appropriate discharge arrangements are made for the continuation of nutritional care (NICE 2017). Patients and carers should receive training and education concerning their enteral feeding regimen before discharge and appropriate support by community services following discharge. NICE (2017) outlines that the patient should have the support of a coordinated multidisciplinary team and an individualised care plan and that the patient and their carers should receive training and relevant information.

TABLE 22.3   Complications Associated With Enteral Feeding

Potential Complications	Prevention/Management
Mechanical Complications	
Tube blockage	• Flush tube with water regularly according to local guidelines • Maintain continuous flow of feed according to feed prescription • Replace tube as required • Consult pharmacist concerning appropriate medications • Clear tube blockage using solution detailed in local guidelines; these may include warm water or enzymes
Knotted tube	• Note any pain on tube withdrawal • Consult Nutrition Nurse Specialist or doctor if pain is present
Tube displacement	• Use correct procedure to reinsert tube or arrange for tube to be reinserted • Use appropriate type and length of tube • Secure tube firmly • Explain need for tube to patient and assess whether they consent to having the tube
Aspiration of feed	• Elevate head and shoulders by 30 degrees or more whilst feeding and for 1 hour after • Confirm position of tube prior to use • Check gastric residual volume as indicated by local guidelines
Discomfort	• Give mouth care regularly • Lubricate lips • Use smallest appropriate bore of tube • Use alternate nostril for tube insertion
Excessive or inadequate feed flow	• Use an enteral feeding pump and appropriate giving set and reservoir to administer feeds or follow dietitian's instruction concerning bolus feed administration • Give feed at rate indicated by feed prescription. Do not interrupt feed unless clinically indicated and do not increase the feed rate beyond the prescribed amount
Biochemical Complications	
Changes in electrolyte levels and hydration status	• Monitor electrolyte levels according practice area guidelines and act promptly if changes detected • Record fluid input and output daily and weigh at least weekly • Consider refeeding syndrome • Follow dietitian's instructions concerning rate and type of feed • Monitor clinical condition (e.g. temperature, blood pressure, pulse and respiration) daily initially or more frequently if clinical condition unstable
Gastrointestinal and Infectious Complications	
Abdominal discomfort	• Avoid administering high-osmolality fluids by ensuring medications are given in appropriate forms • Avoid rapid infusion rates by adhering to prescribed feed rate • Administer fluids at room temperature • Check residual gastric volume if nausea is experienced and consult dietitian and doctor • Stop feed if vomiting is experienced and consult dietitian • Consider antiemetic or antispasmodic administration • Review procedures used to administer feeds and ensure giving set is changed according to local guidelines
Diarrhoea	• Establish cause of diarrhoea: consider medications used, e.g. antibiotic therapy, laxatives and high-osmolality fluids, and medical diagnosis • Consult dietitian as feed type and rate may need reviewing • Administer feed at room temperature • If diarrhoea persists, send a stool sample for culture • Review procedures used to administer feeds and ensure giving set is changed according to clinical setting guidelines
Constipation	• Monitor frequency and consistency of stool • Contact dietitian, as feed type may need reviewing • Encourage mobility • Give laxatives as prescribed • Ensure adequate fluid intake
Stoma site inflammation	• Clean site daily • Ensure fixation device is in the appropriate position to avoid external pressure at stoma site • Avoid the use of a dressing around the site • Rotate tube according to local guidelines • Consult Nutrition Nurse Specialist for advice if inflammation persists or is severe • Send swab from site for microbiological examination • Observe for signs of systemic infection

Parenteral Nutrition

In parenteral feeding, nutrients in solution are infused directly into the venous system. PN may be used as a supplement to oral or enteral feeding, or it can be the sole form of feeding. Appropriate early intervention by PN can prevent or reduce the likelihood of malnutrition developing. This invasive technique is associated with several hazards and problems and should be used only when other methods of nutritional support have been excluded. The term 'TPN' (total parenteral nutrition) is commonly used, but 'PN' is preferred.

Indications for PN

The risks and expense associated with PN are significant, and the key factor to consider when deciding to use this form of feeding is the availability of the GI system. PN will be the method of choice if the GI system is unavailable. In addition, patients may not be able to tolerate the oral or enteral intake required to rectify their nutrition deficits, and supplementary parenteral feeding may be considered. Conditions in which PN may be indicated include intestinal obstruction, GI stasis and pancreatitis.

Many people will require only short-term PN (less than 2 weeks) until GI function has improved sufficiently. Some, however, with prolonged GI failure, will need long-term PN. In order to support and maintain a patient with PN successfully, a team approach is needed, involving not only the nursing and medical staff, but also the biochemist, pharmacist and dietitian, and a primary care team if the patient is to receive PN at home. Specialist primary care nutrition teams assist patients and their carers to manage PN successfully at home, giving advice on such things as storage of PN bags, management of the regimen and equipment use.

Delivery of PN

PN can be administered through a peripheral or central vein. Central venous catheterisation with a long-term catheter is the route of choice for long-term PN. Infusion into the central venous system promotes rapid dilution of the fluid infused which avoids irritation of the veins. Administration of PN via a peripheral venous catheter can be considered for patients who are receiving PN in the short term (e.g. less than 14 days) and who do not require a central venous catheter for another reason (NICE 2017). Careful insertion site management is essential as the site and catheter are at high risk of infection that can quickly spread to the systemic system (see Chapter 18).

All nutrient solutions should be administered through a dedicated feeding line, using volumetric pump/controllers with occlusion and air in line alarms (NICE 2017). This is important and will help to avoid complications associated with PN such as air embolism, catheter occlusion and metabolic and fluid complications as a result of a rapid infusion rate.

PN is prescribed and must be checked carefully before administration. Nutrient solutions are prepared in pharmacy or by or a licensed manufacturer to ensure stability of solutions and minimise the risk of microbial contamination.

The general complications of IV therapy are discussed elsewhere, for example Chapter 21. The particular risks of PN in terms of IV therapy are those related to the administration of large quantities of fluid rich in nutrients which increases the risk for catheter blockage, tissue damage in extravasation and microbial growth. Therefore, the complications of PN can be very serious and so generally the management of PN is an extended role of the nurse and therefore beyond the scope of this textbook.

Observation of the patient's general condition is important however, and basic clinical observations need to be performed regularly and if there is any cause for concern.

Management of patients by Nutrition Support Teams or NNSs has been suggested to reduce the complications experienced with PN (NICE 2017).

The psychosocial impact of PN must also be considered. People who receive PN are usually either not able to eat or can eat but what they can eat is limited. The impact on normal daily life of drastically changing eating habits should not be underestimated. Eating and drinking is part of our everyday life and enables us to express our cultural and religious beliefs. Removing or reducing the ability to eat and drink normally will have a psychological and social impact on the person and the people with which they share their life. In addition, a person who is receiving PN at home will have to adapt their home and lifestyle to deal with bag changes and PN infusion. Their work and social life will also be affected. The psychosocial impact will depend on the length of time nutritional support is given and a person's cognitive ability to appraise the situation. For example, if a person receives PN for 14 days when acutely ill, the psychosocial impact is likely to be much less than for a person who is informed that they will require PN for the rest of their life. It is important to support the patient and their family by providing appropriate information and enabling them to express their concerns. It is very difficult for healthcare professionals to really understand what people and their carers experience when they are prescribed long-term PN. They can be informed about the registered charity Patients on Intravenous and Nasogastric Nutrition Therapy (PINNT). This charity aims to support both adults and children who require nutrition therapy, to provide understanding and contact between patients and to eliminate some of the problems which come with treatment (PINNT 2023).

Evaluation

The final stage of the process of nutritional care of individuals is evaluation. Nutritional plans of care must be evaluated to ensure that the nutritional plan is effective. The evaluation process should use the screening and assessment methods outlined earlier. If the patient's plan of care is not effectively improving their nutritional status or other identified goal, then the plan of care needs to be reviewed. It is vital that interventions are evaluated to ensure that they are effective, and that the evaluation process is appropriately recorded.

The Nutrition Support Team and the Nutrition Nurse Specialist

An expert, multidisciplinary nutrition team within acute care can coordinate nutritional care across the setting. Such a team is usually termed a Nutrition Support Team. Membership of a Nutrition Support Team varies between hospitals, but at a minimum usually includes a senior medical doctor, an NNS, a dietitian and a pharmacist. The team may also include biochemistry and microbiology laboratory staff members. The responsibilities of a team vary according to setting but usually include ensuring that enteral nutrition and PN are administered appropriately, providing nutritional education and training, conducting audit and setting standards of clinical practice in nutritional support through the development of policies and procedures. The team can also ensure that the nutritional care of patients within each care setting is standard and follows local and national policy and guidelines. The presence of a Nutrition Support Team leads to a reduction in complications and costs associated with nutritional care (Reber et al. 2019). Home Enteral Nutrition teams have a similar function to the Nutrition Support Team but focus on supporting people with enteral tubes in the community. In the UK, such teams are dietetic led and may include an NNS. Increasingly enteral nutrition homecare companies are contracted to provide supplies and support from people living with enteral tubes at home, in association with the Home Enteral Nutrition team or community dietetic service.

The NNS is a clinical nurse specialist who works with the Nutrition Support Team. NICE (2017) recommends that all acute Trusts should employ at least one NNS. The NNS acts to ensure nursing practice concerning nutritional care is appropriate, follows policy and guidelines and is patient/client centred. The role of the NNS varies according to the practice setting but generally includes clinical practice, education and training, management, audit and provision of advice and guidance. Research activity may also form part of the role of the NNS.

Future Directions in Nutritional Care

New ideas about dietary provision that may influence the way nurses provide nutritional care are evolving. The use of functional foods, that is, those foods that have ingredients that offer health benefits beyond their nutritional value, is likely to develop. Examples of functional foods include cereals fortified with folic acid and eggs enriched with omega 3. In healthcare, probiotics in foods such as yoghurt are being increasingly used to treat diarrhoea and may be used to in the clinical treatment of constipation (He et al. 2022).

Sustainable nutrition that considers the impact on the environment is becoming a key aspect in food and drink policy. This includes reducing waste, packaging, transport costs and other aspects of the food cycle. NHS Organisations are required to monitor, manage and actively reduce production waste, plate waste and unserved meals (NHS England 2022). Nurses play an important role in this by ordering judiciously and ensuring food and drink are consumed by patients rather than wasted.

Personal robotic eating devices are assistive eating designed for people with motor impairment which affects their ability to eat. They enable a person to eat independently without the support of a carer or nurse. These devices are rapidly developing and becoming more common in a range of settings.

Summary: Key Nursing Issues

- Nurses are involved in aspects of public health nutrition by enabling groups of individuals to achieve a diet that meets their nutritional requirements.
- The nutritional care of individuals is a fundamental part of good nursing practice.
- The role of the nurse is to ensure nutritional care is carried out appropriately and in accordance with the patient's wishes.
- The nurse does not act independently to ensure nutritional needs are met – the involvement of the entire healthcare team is crucial.

Reflection and Learning – What Next?

- **Test** your knowledge by visiting the Evolve website 🌐 and answering the multiple-choice questions and critical thinking questions.
- **Consolidate** your learning by looking at some of the further reading suggestions, references and specialist websites.
- **Revisit** some of the additional material on the Evolve website.
- **Consider** what you have learnt and how this will help your professional development.
- **Reflect** on how you can apply this knowledge to the care of your patients.

References

Boone I, Rosner B, Lachmann R, et al. Healthcare-associated foodborne outbreaks in high-income countries: a literature review and surveillance study, 16 OECD countries, 2001 to 2019. *Euro Surveill.* 2021;26(41).

Braithwaite VS, Sharp SJ, Koulman A, Wareham NJ, Rennie KL. An investigation of factors affecting changes in health behaviours during the COVID-19 pandemic in a UK population-based cohort study. *Public Health.* 2022;212:46–54. doi:10.1016/j.puhe.2022.08.005.

British Association for Parenteral and Enteral Nutrition. (2022, November 2). Nutritional Assessment. https://www.bapen.org.uk/nutrition-support/assessment-and-planning/nutritional-assessment

British Association for Parenteral and Enteral Nutrition. (2023). 'MUST' calculator. https://www.bapen.org.uk/screening-and-must/must-calculator.

Cardenas D. Ethical issues and dilemmas in artificial nutrition and hydration. *Clin Nutr ESPEN.* 2020;41:23–29.

Care Quality Commission. (2022a). Regulation 14: meeting nutritional and hydration needs. https://www.cqc.org.uk/guidance-providers/regulations-enforcement/regulation-14-meeting-nutritional-hydration-needs.

Care Quality Commission. (2022b). Examples of culturally appropriate care. https://www.cqc.org.uk/guidance-providers/adult-social-care/examples-culturally-appropriate-care.

De Silva A, Nightingale JM. Refeeding syndrome: physiological background and practical management. *Frontline Gastroenterol.* 2020;11:404–409. doi:10.1136/flgastro-2018-101065.

Dutch Malnutrition Steering Group. Summary of screening tools; 2023. https://www.fightmalnutrition.eu/toolkits/summary-screening-tools.

Evans DC, Corkins MR, Malone AM, et al. The use of visceral proteins as nutrition markers: an ASPEN position paper. *Nutr Clin Pract.* 2021;36(1):22–28.

Green SM. Nutritional screening. In: Hickson M, Smith S, Whelan K, eds. *Advanced Nutrition and Dietetics in Nutrition Support.* Oxford: John Wiley & Sons Ltd; 2018:43–49.

Green SM, Townsend K, Jarrett N, Westoby C, Fader M. People with enteral tubes and their carers' views of living with a tube and managing associated problems: a qualitative interview study. *J Clin Nurs.* 2019;28(19-20):3710–3720.

He Y, Zhu L, Chen J, Tang X, Pan M, Yuan W, Wang H. Efficacy of probiotic compounds in relieving constipation and their colonization in gut microbiota. *Molecules.* 2022;27(3):666.

Health Education England. About the Making Every Contact Count programme. elearning for healthcare; 2023. https://www.e-lfh.org.uk/programmes/making-every-contact-count/.

Heelan M, Prieto J, Roberts N, Gallant C, Barnes S, Green S. The use of finger foods in care settings: an integrative review. *J Hum Nutr Diet.* 2020;33(2):187–197.

Huang C, Foster H, Paudyal V, Ward M, Lowrie R. A systematic review of the nutritional status of adults experiencing homelessness. *Public Health.* 2022;208:59–67.

Jackson SE, Llewellyn CH, Smith L. The obesity epidemic – nature via nurture: a narrative review of high-income countries. *SAGE Open Med.* 2020;8:1–11.

Joint Formulary Committee. *British National Formulary*. London: British Medical Association and Royal Pharmaceutical Society of Great Britain; 2023. https://bnf.nice.org.uk/.

Ke-hui X, Ling L, Shuai-lin J, Qihong L, et al. Association of tooth loss and diet quality with acceleration of aging: evidence from NHANES. *Am J Med*. 2023. doi:10.1016/j.amjmed.2023.04.008.

Leach B, Goodwin S. Preventing malnutrition in prison. *Nurs Stand*. 2014;28(20):50–56. doi:10.7748/ns2014.01.28.20.50.e7900.

Malnutrition Task Force. Malnutrition in England factsheet; 2023, January. https://www.malnutritiontaskforce.org.uk/malnutrition-england-factsheet.

Muscogiuri G, El Ghoch M, Colao A, Hassapidou M, Yumuk V, Busetto L. Obesity Management Task Force (OMTF) of the European Association for the Study of Obesity (EASO). European guidelines for obesity management in adults with a very low-calorie ketogenic diet: a systematic review and meta-analysis. *Obesity Facts*. 2021;14(2):222–245. doi:10.1159/000515381.

National Health Service. Overview; 2020. Vitamins and minerals. https://www.nhs.uk/conditions/vitamins-and-minerals/.

National Health Service. The Eatwell Guide; 2022a. https://www.nhs.uk/live-well/eat-well/food-guidelines-and-food-labels/the-eatwell-guide/.

National Health Service. The Eatwell Guide; 2022b. https://www.nhs.uk/live-well/eat-well/food-guidelines-and-food-labels/the-eatwell-guide/.

National Health Service. Eat well; 2023a. https://www.nhs.uk/live-well/eat-well/.

National Health Service. Lose weight. Better Health; 2023b. https://www.nhs.uk/better-health/lose-weight/.

National Health Service. Overview. Vitamins and minerals; 2023c. https://www.nhs.uk/conditions/vitamins-and-minerals/.

National Institute for Health and Care Excellence (NICE). *Obesity: identification, assessment and management*. London: National Institute for Health and Care Excellence; 2014. https://www.nice.org.uk/guidance/cg189.

National Institute for Health and Care Excellence. *Nutrition support for adults: oral nutrition support, enteral tube feeding and parenteral nutrition*. Clinical guideline [CG32]; 2017, February 22. https://www.nice.org.uk/guidance/cg32.

National Institute for Health and Care Excellence (NICE). *How should I assess a person with a suspected eating disorder?*. Clinical Knowledge Summaries (CKS); 2019, July. https://cks.nice.org.uk/topics/eating-disorders/diagnosis/assessment/.

NHS England. *National Standards for Healthcare Food and Drink*. London: NHS England; 2022.

Nursing and Midwifery Council (NMC). *Future Nurse: Standards of Proficiency for Registered Nurses*. London: Nursing and Midwifery Council; 2018.

Nursing and Midwifery Council (NMC). *The Code: Professional Standards of Practice and Behaviour for Nurses, Midwives and Nursing Associates*. London: Nursing and Midwifery Council; 2018.

Office for Health Improvement and Disparities. *Guidance. Adult obesity: applying All Our Health*. Gov.UK; 2022, February 11. https://www.gov.uk/government/publications/adult-obesity-applying-all-our-health/adult-obesity-applying-all-our-health.

Osuala EC, Ojewole EB. Knowledge, attitudes and practices of healthcare professionals regarding drug–food interactions: a scoping review. *Int J Pharm Pract*. 2021;29(5):406–415.

PINNT. (2023). Friendship and support for patients receiving artificial nutrition. https://pinnt.com/Home.aspx. Accessed April 21, 2023.

Pojednic R, D'Arpino E, Halliday I, Bantham A. The benefits of physical activity for people with obesity, independent of weight loss: a systematic review. *Int J Environ Res Public Health*. 2022;19(9):1–14.

Porter J, Hanna L. Evidence-based analysis of Protected Mealtime policies on patient nutrition and care. *Risk Manag Healthc Policy*. 2020;13:713–721.

Public Health England in association with the Welsh government, Food Standards Scotland and the Food Standards Agency in Northern Ireland. *Guidance. The Eatwell Guide*. Gov.UK; 2018. https://www.gov.uk/government/publications/the-eatwell-guide.

Ramel A, Stenholm S. Obesity and health in older adults. In: Geirsdottir OG, Bell JJ, eds. *Interdisciplinary Nutritional Management and Care for Older Adults*. Cham: Springer; 2021:207–214.

Reber E, Strahm R, Bally L, Schuetz P, Stanga Z. Efficacy and efficiency of Nutritional Support Teams. *J Clin Med*. 2019;8(9):1281.

Ross R, Neeland IJ, Yamashita S, et al. Waist circumference as a vital sign in clinical practice: a consensus statement from the IAS and ICCR Working Group on Visceral Obesity. *Nat Rev Endocrinol*. 2020;16:177–189. doi:10.1038/s41574-019-0310-7.

Talumaa B, Brown A, Batterham RL, Kalea AZ. Effective strategies in ending weight stigma in healthcare. *Obes Rev*. 2022;23(10):e13494. doi:10.1111/obr.13494.

The International Dysphagia Diet Standardisation Initiative. The IDDSI Framework; 2023. https://iddsi.org/Framework.

Thomson KH, Rice S, Arisa O, et al. Effectiveness and cost-effectiveness of oral nutritional supplements in frail older people who are malnourished or at risk of malnutrition: a systematic review and meta-analysis. *Lancet Healthy Longev*. 2022;3(10):e654–e666.

van den Berg GH, Huisman-de Waal GG, Vermeulen H, de van der Schueren ME. Effects of nursing nutrition interventions on outcomes in malnourished hospital inpatients and nursing home residents: a systematic review. *Int J Nurs Stud*. 2021;117:103888. doi:10.1016/j.ijnurstu.2021.103888.

Waugh A, Grant A. *Ross and Wilson Anatomy and Physiology in Health and Illness*. Edinburgh: Elsevier; 2023.

Woods-Brown C, Hunt K, Sweeting H. Food and the prison environment: a meta-ethnography of global first-hand experiences of food, meals and eating in custody. *Health Justice*. 2023;11(23). doi:10.1186/s40352-023-00222-z.

World Health Organisation. *A healthy lifestyle – WHO recommendations*. World Health Organisation Europe; 2010, May 6. https://www.who.int/europe/news-room/fact-sheets/item/a-healthy-lifestyle—who-recommendations.

World Health Organisation. Physical activity; 2022, October 5. https://www.who.int/news-room/fact-sheets/detail/physical-activity.

World Health Organisation. Obesity; 2023. https://www.who.int/health-topics/obesity#tab=tab_1.

Useful Websites

British Association for Parenteral and Enteral Nutrition (BAPEN), www.bapen.org.uk

British Nutrition Foundation, www.nutrition.org.uk

Office for Health Improvement and Disparities, www.gov.uk/government/organisations/public-health-england

The Scottish Public Health Observatory, www.scotpho.org.uk

Patients on Intravenous and Nasogastric Nutrition Therapy, pinnt.com/Home.aspx

World Health Organization (WHO) Nutrition, www.who.int/health-topics/nutrition#tab=tab_1

23

Tissue Viability and Managing Chronic Wounds

JACQUI FLETCHER, IRENE ANDERSON

CHAPTER OUTLINE

Introduction

For most people, the word 'wound' conjures up thoughts of a cut, a graze or a surgical incision that heals without difficulty. For nurses, however, wound management is a complex aspect of patient care, requiring knowledge and expertise. Nurses and other healthcare professionals care for patients with wounds in many settings, including patients with surgical incisions nursed in hospital or at home, those with chronic leg ulcers nursed at home and patients with industrial injury or trauma treated at their workplace.

The impact of a wound on an individual can be considerable. Pain, fear and scarring are the most obvious, but individuals vary in their response to having a wound. For some, restriction in social activity, or the loss of earnings, should also be considered alongside the psychological effects of altered body image (Kapp and Santamaria 2017).

The presence of a wound will inevitably have some effect on wellbeing. There may be no difficulty when a wound is small and heals rapidly, but many patients experience anxiety relating to the wound irrespective of size (Woo 2015). This can disrupt sleep, increase pain perception and impair immune function. In more serious wounds, a disturbance of body image may also cause lasting distress, particularly if the patient is unprepared for this (Kapp and Santamaria 2017).

The healing process comprises a complex series of events that depend on a number of factors, and in order for it to proceed at its optimal rate, the individual concerned should be in good health. In caring for patients with wounds, nurses have an important role in promoting health.

Clinical effectiveness and the delivery of evidence-based care are key to wound management.

Wound Definition, Types and Classification

A wound is a defect or breach in the continuity of the skin. This is an injury to the skin or underlying tissues/organs caused by surgery, a blow, a cut, chemicals, heat/cold, friction/shear force, pressure or as a result of disease, such as leg ulcers and cancers.

There is no clear-cut method of classifying wounds. Some practitioners refer to wounds by anatomical site, for example abdominal wall wounds. Others classify wounds by their depth, for example epidermal loss and progression into or through the dermis. In the first group, there are wounds with little or no tissue loss where the skin edges can be brought together and sutured or clipped. In the second, there may be substantial tissue loss and the skin edges cannot be brought together. A further description may be to group wounds by their potential to heal, with wounds being described as acute or chronic (Raziyeva et al. 2021, Wounds UK 2022). More recently, it has been acknowledged that the language we use to describe the potential for healing can impact on both the patient and the individual delivering care and use of terms such as hard to heal should be avoided as it sets up a negative mind set which makes healing seem unachievable (Wounds UK 2022).

Epidemiology

The epidemiology of wounds is not clearly documented. Because people with wounds can be found in almost every specialty, information relating specifically to wounds is not consistently collected. Extrapolated data from The Health Improvement Network (THIN) database identified that 3.8 million people with wounds were being managed in 2017/2018 at a cost of £8.3 billion (Guest et al. 2020); only 70% of these patients healed within a year. Annual levels of resource use attributable to wound management included 54.4 million district/community nurse visits, 53.6 million healthcare assistant visits and 28.1 million practice nurse visits; from these, 81% of the cost was incurred in the community.

Physiology of Wound Healing

A number of cell types are involved in the healing process (Table 23.1).

Tissue Repair

The wound healing process comprises a complex series of events whereby the continuity and strength of damaged tissues are restored by the formation of connective tissue and regrowth of epithelium. The process can be divided into four phases (Fig. 23.1), but since wound healing is a continuous biological process, there is some overlap between them.

Phase I – Haemostasis

As soon as a wound occurs, it bleeds and blood initially fills the wound defect. Platelets aggregate and degranulate, resulting in clot formation and haemostasis. A fibrin clot forms as a result of prothrombin being converted to thrombin which in turn converts fibrinogen to fibrin. The blood coagulates and acts as a preliminary matrix or scaffold within the wound into which cells can migrate.

Phase II – Inflammation

The fibrin clot begins to degrade and the surrounding capillaries dilate and become permeable, allowing fluid into the wound site. This activates the complement system, several interacting soluble

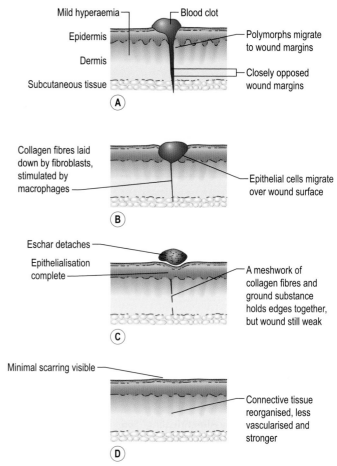

Figure 23.1 Wound healing by primary intention. (A) Haemostasis. (B) Inflammation. (C) Proliferation/reconstruction phase. (D) Maturation phase.

proteins found in serum and extracellular fluid that induce lysis and destruction of target cells, such as bacteria. Cytokines and proteolytic fragments are also found in the wound space (Hassan-shahi et al. 2022) which initiate a massive influx of other cells. The two main inflammatory cells are neutrophils and macrophages:

- Neutrophils flood into the wound shortly after injury and reach peak numbers within 24–48 hours. They destroy bacteria through ingesting and destroying unwanted materials, phagocytosis. Neutrophils also kill bacteria by releasing substances such as proteases which are toxic to bacteria. Neutrophils have a very short lifespan and their numbers reduce rapidly 3 days post injury, provided there is no infection.
- Tissue macrophages, like neutrophils, destroy bacteria and debris through phagocytosis. However, the macrophage is also a rich source of biological regulators, including cytokines and growth factors, bioactive lipid products and proteolytic enzymes, elements essential for the normal healing process.

This phase is one of biological 'cleansing'. It does, however, make considerable metabolic demands on the body. Much heat and fluid can also be lost. The shorter the duration of this phase, the better, because as it nears completion, proliferation or formation of new tissue can begin. Following the inflammatory phase, the wound site is prepared for the repair process to begin.

Phase III – Proliferation/Reconstruction

Tissue repair takes place during this phase. It usually begins at around day 3 and lasts for some weeks. Proliferation is characterised by the

TABLE 23.1	Important Cells in Wound Healing
Cell	**Function**
Endothelial cells	Help to achieve haemostasis
Polymorphonuclear leucocytes ('polymorphs')	Take part in the initial inflammatory response
Macrophages	Digest debris and stimulate other cells to function; orchestrate wound healing processes
Fibroblasts	Produce collagen
Myofibroblasts	Aid wound contraction by producing mature collagen

formation of granulation tissue in the wound space. This new tissue consists of a matrix of fibrin, fibronectin, collagens, proteoglycans and glycosaminoglycans and other glycoproteins. Fibroblasts move into the wound space and proliferate. Their function is to synthesise and deposit extracellular proteins, producing growth factors and angiogenic factors that regulate cell proliferation and angiogenesis (DesJardins-Park et al. 2018). Fibroblasts will multiply rapidly in the well-nourished individual and, to be most effective, need adequate amounts of vitamin C, iron, oxygen and nutrients. Granulation tissue also contains elastin, providing the wound with elasticity and resilience.

Angiogenesis is the formation of new blood vessels in the wound space which are essential for the delivery of oxygen and other nutrients. Angiogenesis is triggered by the platelets as they release growth factors which stimulate the repair of damaged blood vessels. The key cells involved in angiogenesis are the vascular endothelial cells, which arise from the damaged end of vessels and capillaries (Morton and Phillips 2016). New vessels sprout from existing small vessels at the wound edge, endothelial cells detaching from these small vessels and penetrating the wound space. These sprouts are then extended in length until they meet other capillaries, connecting together to form new vascular loops and networks.

Re-epithelialisation begins a few hours after injury and continues as the wound begins to fill with granulation tissue. At the wound edges, epithelial cells divide and, gradually, epithelium migrates from the edges towards the middle of the wound. Epithelialisation of larger areas is achieved not only by migration, but also by rapid division of epithelial cells near hair follicles, which might be present deep in the dermis. Islands of epithelium appear wherever a follicle is present. Cells migrate from these islands to meet each other, while cells from the edges of the wound grow inwards to cover the raw surface.

The final feature of proliferation is wound contraction, beginning around day 5. Wound contraction is a dynamic process where cells reorganise the surrounding connective tissue, reducing the amount of granulation tissue. This effect is mostly due to the activity of fibroblasts and myofibroblasts which, under the influence of cytokines, contract to pull the wound edges together.

Phase IV – Maturation/Remodelling

Maturation usually begins around 7 days post injury and continues for many months or years, long after the wound looks to be closed or healed. The immature collagen laid down earlier is gradually replaced by a mature collagen. The formation of new collagen and the lysis of immature collagen are balanced so that the amount of collagen present remains constant. The immature collagen is laid down in a random, haphazard fashion, its function being to fill the wound defect as quickly as possible. The remodelling process involves the balance between synthesis and degradation of collagen, where the cells producing the different types of collagen are subjected to apoptosis (programmed cell death) (Xue and Jackson 2015). Mature collagen is laid down following lines of tension within the wound and is cross-linked to give strength. Tensile strength at 14 days in sutured wounds is approximately 10% of the original strength of the skin. Within 3 weeks, this increases to 20%, gradually reaching a maximum of 70%–80% about 1 year later.

Healing by Primary/First Intention

Following wounding, treatment aims to effect complete healing as quickly as possible with minimal scarring. To achieve this, the method of choice is healing by primary intention, which occurs when wound edges are in apposition. There is minimal formation of granulation tissue and, once the wound has healed, only a thin scar remains. Healing by primary intention is only possible where there is adequate, mobile tissue and no complicating bacterial contamination. In situations where contamination is suspected, wound closure is accompanied by the use of prophylactic systemic antibiotics. For healing to take place by primary intention, the wound edges need to be closely approximated and held together until the wound has healed sufficiently. The skin may be closed by using tapes, clips, continuous or interrupted sutures or glue (Fig. 23.2).

Healing by Secondary Intention

Where there is significant tissue loss and/or bacterial contamination, wounds are usually left open to heal by secondary intention through the formation of granulation tissue and, later, wound contraction (Fig. 23.3), a process of repair. Due to the amount of tissue excised or lost during injury, wound healing by secondary intention is a longer process, taking weeks or even months to complete. The healing process proceeds in much the same way as for healing by primary intention. The proliferative phase is much extended, as this is when granulation tissue forms and fills the wound defect. It was established many years ago (Marks et al. 1983) that, for some wounds, the length of time taken to heal depends on the original size; that is, small wounds heal more quickly than larger ones, and it is therefore possible in some wound types (pilonidal sinus, abdominal and axillary wounds) to predict when wounds of a given size that are free from infection will heal.

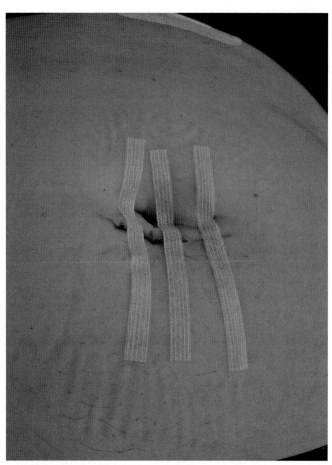

Figure 23.2 Wound healing by primary intention – wound edges in apposition, held by Steristrips.

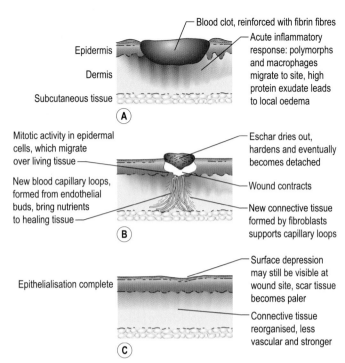

Figure 23.3 Wound healing by secondary intention. (A) Haemostasis/inflammation. (B) Proliferation phase. (C) Maturation phase.

Scar Tissue

A scar is the mark that may remain after healing. It consists of relatively avascular collagen fibres covered by a thin layer of epithelium.

Most scars fade with time and the resultant cosmetic effect is generally acceptable, but abnormal scarring can lead to problems, as follows:

⬤ **See Evolve website Fig. 23.1**

- Stretching of scar tissue – can occur where sutures have been removed prematurely, especially over areas that are under tension, e.g. the skin over the scapula and back.
- Hypertrophic scar tissue – collagen lysis and collagen production are out of synchrony and excessive tissue lies within the boundaries of the scar.
- Keloid – a protuberant, prominent scar resulting from excessive dermal collagen formation during connective tissue repair.

Hypertrophic scarring and keloidal scarring are examples of excessive scar formation. Such scarring is more common in young people, especially during puberty and pregnancy, and also in dark skins, the peristernal area being particularly susceptible.

Information 23.1 outlines factors influencing scarring.

Factors That Adversely Affect Healing

Many factors can adversely affect the normal rate of healing, slowing it down and, in severe cases, impairing it altogether. These factors can be described as pathophysiological (see next section), psychological or practical (Wounds UK 2022).

⬤ Pathophysiological Factors

This section outlines intrinsic and extrinsic pathophysiological factors. These can be systemic factors such as malnutrition, or

local wound factors including the presence of clot, devitalised tissue, foreign bodies, local hypoxia or infection.

Intrinsic Factors

Advanced Age

With advanced age the dermis gradually thins and the underlying structural support, collagen, reduces (see Chapter 33, Nursing Care for Older People). Reduced collagen production results in loss of skin elasticity and its ability for elastic recoil, leading to creases and wrinkles. The amount of subcutaneous fat reduces, and there is less of a cushion for underlying bone. The natural moisture from sebum secretions lessens, leading to increasing dryness of the skin. The consequence of ageing is dry, thin, inelastic skin that is susceptible to damage, with a reduced metabolic rate and prolonged healing.

⬤ **See Evolve website Fig. 23.2**

These factors, together with poor circulation associated with older age, affect the tensile wound strength.

Malnutrition

Malnutrition may result in delayed wound healing and the production of weak, poor quality scars.

Protein–Energy Malnutrition (PEM) is caused by an absolute or relative deficiency of energy and protein that affects between 19% and 50% of hospitalised patients (Avelino-Silva and Jaluul 2017). Several factors contribute to PEM, including a reduced intake of nutrients, reduced digestion and absorption of nutrients and increased metabolic use. Malnutrition can impede healing by reducing tensile strength, increasing wound dehiscence and the likelihood of infection. Malnutrition also leads to poorer outcomes for patients and greatly increases the cost of healthcare. A study into the nutritional management of older patients with pressure ulcers identified that an improvement in the nutritional care of patients is required as few receive screening for malnutrition, referral to a registered dietician enriched food or snacks or oral nutritional supplements (ONSs) (Egsleer et al. 2019).

Nutrient Deficiency. Caloric needs are ideally met by a healthy diet; however, some individuals are unable or unwilling to consume an adequate diet. Overly restricted diets may make food unpalatable and unappealing, and therefore reduce intake. Fortified foods and/or high-calorie, high-protein ONSs can be offered between meals if nutritional requirements cannot be achieved by dietary intake, and ONSs, enhanced foods and food fortifiers can be used to combat unintended weight loss and malnutrition.

The International Pressure Ulcer Guidelines (European Pressure Ulcer Advisory Panel [EPUAP], National Pressure Injury Advisory Panel [NPIAP], Pan Pacific Pressure Injury Alliance [PPPIA] 2019) recommend a minimum daily intake of 30–35 kilocalories per kg body weight for adults at risk of a pressure ulcer who are assessed as being at risk of malnutrition, and additional intake for people assessed as underweight. Oral, enteral and parenteral supplements should be considered if the person is unable to maintain an adequate intake. Some people may have difficulty in maintaining adequate nutrition, for example, an older person living alone may lose interest in cooking or a patient having chemotherapy may be unable to eat due to nausea. The importance of diet cannot be overemphasised, and wherever possible the nurse should ensure that the patient receives all the nutrients required for healing. The advice of a dietitian may be sought in an attempt to improve or supplement the nutritional status of vulnerable individuals (see Chapter 22, Nutrition and Health). Ideally, adult patients at risk of, or with, pressure ulcers should aim to have 1.25 to 1.5 g protein/kg body weight daily which should be reassessed as the patient's condition changes (EPUAP, NPIAP, PPPIA 2019)

Dehydration. The normal metabolic processes of an individual require approximately 2500 mL of water every 24 hours. Dehydration disrupts cell metabolism and this will adversely affect wound healing.

Disease
Many disease processes can delay healing, for example anaemia, cardiovascular disorders, diabetes mellitus, cancer, inflammatory disease, immune disease and organ failure, as in any other disease that impairs immune function. Importantly, some patients, particularly older people, have comorbidities.

Impaired Blood Supply to the Area (Ischaemia)
Where the blood supply to the wounded area is impaired, insufficient nutrients and oxygen are supplied and the healing is prolonged, for example in patients with peripheral arterial disease and lower limb ulcers. Slower healing is to be expected anywhere where gross oedema is present.

Smoking
Smoking adversely affects the healing process in a number of ways. Smoking and the absorption of nicotine have a vasoconstricting effect. The main influences of nicotine and carbon dioxide relate to the effects on peripheral tissues, with a reduction in tissue oxygen tension and the formation of thrombi. Nicotine has been demonstrated to inhibit epithelialisation (McDaniel and Browning 2014) and the healing of abdominal wounds, the overall cosmetic effect of a scar being poorer in patients who were smokers.

Extrinsic Factors
Poor Surgical Technique. Excessive handling of tissues during surgery can cause damage, resulting in haematoma formation.

This can lead to an infection as the haematoma is broken down. A void (dead space) may also occur if tissues are not correctly approximated during surgery, again encouraging the development of infection. In addition, where sutures are inserted too tightly, the tissue becomes damaged and necrosis can occur.

Medication. Several medications affect healing. Cytotoxic chemotherapy can destroy healthy as well as cancer cells. Ideally, its use is withheld until any wound healing is complete, usually a period of 4 weeks. Glucocorticosteroids also delay, or prevent, healing taking place and their use is closely monitored in individuals with wounds.

Inappropriate Wound Management. The healing process may be adversely affected by the use of poor dressing technique, the wrong dressing material or unnecessary antiseptics. It is essential that the nurse is aware of what is required from a dressing material in order to ensure that each product is used cost-effectively.

Infection of all the factors that can delay or prevent healing, infection is the most important (see later and Chapter 18, Infection Prevention and Control).

Psychosocial Factors
There is a close association between psychological and physical well-being. Stress and anxiety can impair immune function through elevation of stress hormones glucocorticoids and catecholamines (e.g. adrenaline, noradrenaline). The same authors describe the effects of increased levels of stress hormones including reduced lymphocyte proliferation and reduced antibody production. Sleep disturbances are linked to stress, and sleep is thought to be essential for healing and tissue repair (Bartolo and Hill 2023, House 2015).

Wound Infection
It is inevitable that most wounds contain microorganisms, but it is only pathogenic organisms, usually bacteria, which delay healing and cause systemic illness (Wounds UK 2020). Established infection in a healing wound often delays healing and may cause a range of surgical wound complications including surgical wound dehiscence (SWD), hypergranulation, seroma, haematoma, peri-wound maceration, delayed healing, poor quality or abnormal scar formation, incisional hernia and surgical site infection (SSI) (Sandy-Hodgetts et al. 2022 Wounds UK 2020). These have been shown to delay healing and result in significant morbidity, mortality and related socioeconomic costs. The clinical signs and symptoms of a wound infection are summarised in Information 23.2. Despite all the technological advances that have been made in surgery and wound management, the problem of wound infection persists, with SSI being one of the six most common healthcare-associated infections accounting for 15.7% (Health Protection Agency 2017). The incidence of SSI varies by operative site, with the highest incidence being bowel surgery (9.2%) and the lowest in hip and knee prosthetic surgery (0.6% each). SSI also accounts for a high proportion of readmissions in surgical patients (Public Health England (PHE) 2017).

It is suggested that at least 5% of patients undergoing surgery develop a SSI. This relates to advances in surgical and anaesthetic techniques which have allowed patients with many comorbidities and therefore greater risk levels to be considered for surgery (National Institute for Health and Care Excellence [NICE] 2020, https://www.nice.org.uk/guidance/ng125).

The wound environment itself can encourage bacterial growth. Anaerobic microorganisms, for example, thrive in wounds with a

INFORMATION 23.2

Signs of Wound Infection

Acute Wounds, e.g. Surgical or Traumatic Wounds, or Burns

Localised Infection
Classic signs and symptoms:
- new or increasing pain
- erythema
- local warmth
- swelling
- purulent discharge

Pyrexia – in surgical wounds, typically 5–7 days post surgery
Delayed (or stalled) healing
Abscess
Malodour

Notes:
Burns – also skin graft rejection, pain is not always a feature of infection in full-thickness burns.
Deep wounds – induration, extension of the wound, unexplained increased white cell count or signs of sepsis may be signs of a deep wound infection. Immunocompromised patients – signs and symptoms may be modified and less obvious.

Spreading Infection
As for localised infection plus
Further extension of erythema
Lymphangitis
Crepitus in soft tissue
Wound breakdown/dehiscence

Chronic Wounds, e.g. Diabetic Foot Ulcers, Venous Leg Ulcers, Arterial Leg/Foot Ulcers, Pressure Ulcers

Localised Infection
New, increased or altered pain*
Delayed or stalled healing*
Periwound oedema
Bleeding or friable (easily damaged) granulation tissue
Distinctive malodour or change in odour
Wound bed discolouration
Increased or altered/purulent exudate
Induration
Pocketing
Bridging

Notes:
In patients who are immunocompromised and/or who have motor or sensory neuropathies, symptoms may be modified and less obvious. For example, in a diabetic patient with an infected foot ulcer and peripheral sensory neuropathy, pain may not be a prominent feature.
Arterial ulcers – previously dry ulcers may become wet when infected.
Clinicians should also be aware that in the diabetic foot, inflammation is not always indicative of infection. For example inflammation may be associated with Charcot's arthropathy.
*Individually highly indicative of infection. Infection is also highly likely if the patient has two or more of the other signs listed.

Spreading Infection
As for localised infection plus
Wound breakdown*
Erythema extending from the wound edge
Crepitus, warmth, induration or discolouration spreading into periwound area
Lymphangitis
Malaise or other nonspecific deterioration in patient's general condition

poor oxygen supply. A wound bed or area that is free from haematoma and dead tissue and is clean reduces the risk of infection.

The way in which the wound is managed can also affect infection. Bacterial contamination, through poor technique by the nurse, poor hygiene or loss of continence, can all increase the risk of wound infection. The consequences of wound infection vary depending upon the patient's condition and the environment in which they are being nursed: in hospital, a patient with a surgical wound infection poses a considerable risk to other patients with wounds on that ward; at home, that patient is less of a risk to the family and community, who are unlikely to be vulnerable.

Factors That Predispose to Wound Infection

Factors can be described as major, moderate or minor – see the following table.

Category	Modifiable Patient Related	Preoperative	Perioperative	Postoperative
Major	• BMI ≥35.0 kg/m² • Diabetes mellitus • Current or recent smoking	• Emergency surgery • Age >65 years	• Extended duration of surgery • Inadequate surgical closure • Peri-operative hypothermia	• Mechanical pull on incisional wounds • Patient/family touching the wound
Moderate	• COPD • Malnutrition: hypoalbuminaemia (serum albumin <3.0 g/dL) • Anaemia • BMI 30.0–35.0 kg/m² • Alcohol use disorder	• Male gender • ASA Physical Status ≥2 • Previous wound healing problems • Immunosuppression • Long-term steroid use • Malignant disease • Chemotherapy • Radiotherapy • Uraemia • Peripheral vascular disease • Suboptimal timing or omission of prophylactic antibiotics	• Blood transfusion • High wound tension closure • Tissue trauma/large area of dissection and/or undermining	• Failure to wean from ventilator • One or more other surgical complications • Premature suture removal
Minor	• BMI 25.0–29.9 kg/m² • Congestive cardiac failure • Cardiovascular disease	• Extended pre-operative hospitalisation or residency in a nursing home	• Failure to obliterate dead space	• Trauma across the incision

Main risk factors for SSI, which may vary depending on surgery type (adapted from WUWHS 2018).
ASA, American Society of Anaesthesiologists; *BMI*, body mass index; *COPD*, chronic obstructive pulmonary disease.
Reproduced with permission from Wounds UK (2020).

Modifiable Patient-Related Factors

Several factors, in addition to delayed healing (see earlier), can predispose a patient to wound infection. These can be identified on first assessment:

- Poor nutritional status – PEM has been linked to hospitalisation and impacts on all aspects of patient care, including developing pressure ulcers and influencing SSI, and a hypoalbuminaemia (serum albumin <3.0 g/dL) is classified as a moderate risk factor.
- Immunosuppression – with cancer treatments, diabetes mellitus, glucocorticosteroid therapy, etc., can lead to increased risk of infection.
- Excessive body weight
- Advanced age
- Smoking
- Anaemia
- Alcohol use disorder
- Cardiovascular disease

Other Risk Factors

- Adverse spatial arrangements – when too many patients are nursed in close proximity to each other, especially in an open ward, the wound infection rate increases. An increase occurs when more than 25 patients are being nursed in an open ward (NHS Estates 2002).
- Length of preoperative hospital stay – the wound infection rate is linked to the length of time a patient spends in hospital prior to operation. The longer this period, the more likelihood there is of the individual being colonised by the pathogenic bacteria found in hospitals.
- Inappropriate preoperative care – it is not usually necessary to shave the site preoperatively (Williams and Leaper 1998). Where shaving is required, it should occur immediately prior to surgery to reduce the risk of bacterial growth on newly shaved skin (see Chapter 25, The Care of a Person Undergoing Surgery). These precautions should result in a wound infection rate of less than 1%.
- Prolonged operative procedure – longer surgeries usually occur in more complex cases and in patients with multiple comorbidities, increasing the patient-related risk factors. In addition, the longer the surgical site is exposed to the air (i.e. the wound is not closed), the more opportunity there is for natural ingress of bacteria into the wound.
- Surgery type – in elective surgery, e.g. excision of breast lump, the rate of infection should be less than 5%, and with effective surveillance and control, this can be reduced to less than 2% (NICE 2020). For emergency surgery, complete pre- and perioperative infection prevention strategies or risk factor management may not be possible due to time constraints. These patients are often very physiologically unwell (i.e. acidosis, hypoxia), which interrupts the normal immune cell response postsurgery. Colorectal surgery is associated with a high rate of SSI due to frequency of bowel flora; vascular surgery is associated with a high rate of SSI due to frailty and multiple comorbidities of the patient group (PHE 2019).
- Use of drains – used to close or minimise dead space in a wound or to evacuate haematomas or body fluids, in order to reduce infection risk (NICE 2020). They should be used with caution, as all drains are foreign bodies and may cause tissue reactions.

As a wound infection develops, localisation of the infection leads to the formation of a wound abscess. This may drain through the suture line or into the wound in the case of cavities. Occasionally, if deep seated, the abscess will need surgical incision to drain it properly. Where partial wound breakdown occurs, some wounds will be assessed as suitable for healing by secondary intention.

The National Wound Care Strategy (2021) has produced guidance on the care of surgical wounds(see Useful Websites).

Sources of Wound Infection

Endogenous

Organisms found on the patient's own skin are endogenous sources of wound infection. These organisms, usually *Staphylococcus aureus* or gut commensals, are either present under normal circumstances or are hospital pathogens that colonise the body after admission to hospital. Shortening the time between admission and surgery reduces the possibility of skin contamination by hospital-acquired bacteria (NICE 2020).

S. aureus is found on the skin and sometimes in the upper respiratory tract. This organism does not normally affect the patient adversely, but when a wound has been created, *S. aureus* can invade the wound from adjacent skin or from the nose during exhalation.

Exogenous

Exogenous infections occur following contamination of the wound from a source external to the patient. This may happen in theatre or later in the ward when pathogens are allowed to fall onto the wound and penetrate it. Bacteria such as *Pseudomonas aeruginosa* can be found in wet areas or where moisture is present, for example in water, other fluids or ventilators. *P. aeruginosa* is also found in flower vases, sinks and drains.

Accidental injuries are highly likely to have been contaminated by bacteria. *Clostridium tetani* and *C. perfringens* present in the soil can be hazardous. People who receive minor injuries whilst gardening are at risk and the status of their tetanus immunity should be checked in case further treatment is required. Insect bites and stings can lead to cellulitis (diffuse, acute inflammation affecting the skin and subcutaneous tissue).

⊕ See Evolve website Critical thinking question 23.1

❖ Nursing Management and Health Promotion: Holistic Wound Care

All patients should have access to a minimum standard of care, regardless of where that care is provided or by whom, in order to optimise the chance of achieving a straightforward, uncomplicated and timely healing process. This should be a systematic process which is adapted to best suit the local circumstances, for example the National Wound Care Strategy (https://www.nationalwound-carestrategy.net/wp-content/uploads/2021/05/Shared-Care-for-Wounds 30.03.20.pdf).

Although functioning best as a multidisciplinary specialty, wound care is frequently seen as the responsibility of nurses, with community nurses spending on average 50% of their time on wound care.

Research has been undertaken using different study designs to answer a diverse range of clinical questions, and to explore patients' views. Best available evidence is used not only to inform practice but also to develop clinical guidelines (NICE 2014, 2017, EPUAP, NPIAP, PPPIA, 2019).

Patient Assessment

This should be patient centred and comprehensive and should consider the physical and social environment.

Whether the patient is being cared for at home, other community setting or hospital, or is young or old, assessment of the patient's general condition should be undertaken. This is done to identify any of the factors that might impair the wound-healing process for those factors seen as reversible, treatment should be sought; for those factors where no treatment is possible, some degree of delay in healing should be anticipated and allowed for in the care plan.

The patient's social environment can affect the treatment options. For example, when caring for a frail older person living alone, the nurse may need to select a dressing that is waterproof, in order that carers who come in to bathe the person need not disturb the wound unnecessarily.

Wound Assessment

In assessment of the wound and surrounding skin, a range of wound criteria are considered which can help ensure that the patient receives the most appropriate care for their needs. A range of theoretical frameworks exist to guide this assessment for example: TIME – focuses on Tissue type, Infection/Inflammation, Moisture balance and Edge/Epithelialisation Applied Wound Management which utilises the wound healing continuum, the wound infection continuum and the wound exudate continuum. In practice, these are translated into wound assessment charts which may vary from area to area but usually collect information around key parameters which suggest if the wound is healing/deteriorating or static. More recently, wound assessment has been the subject of a quality improvement payment in the NHS which has driven community organisations to review their assessment practice and follow a minimum data set (NHS England 2017).

The minimum data set (Coleman et al. 2017) includes:
- general health information
- wound baseline information
- wound assessment parameters
- wound symptoms.
  Key parameters to consider include:
- cause of the wound
- wound location
- measurements (e.g. length × width or surface area)
- description of the tissue type and percentage present, e.g. necrotic tissue, slough, granulation, epithelialisation
- volume of exudate
- odour
- pain
- condition of surrounding skin.

Where wound-specific assessment tools are used, for example a leg ulcer assessment chart, other data such as the ankle brachial pressure index would also be included. Once a thorough assessment has been completed, objectives of care can be set in conjunction with the patient's needs and wishes.

Cause of the Wound. For many wound types, identifying and addressing the cause of the wound will be the major factor in progressing a wound to healing; for example, removing the cause of pressure damage is the most important factor in healing a pressure ulcer.

Wound Location. This is important to record not only because it makes it easier for successive practitioners to find but also because it may impact on treatment choices; for example, sacral wounds are at high risk of contamination from urine and faeces, and wounds on the foot are difficult to dress because of high shear forces and limited space within footwear if the patient needs to remain mobile.

Wound Measurement. There are a variety of ways of measuring wounds; most commonly a simple length × width is recorded using a ruler. It is possible to convert this into a surface area; however, unless the wound is square or rectangular, this is a very inaccurate

measurement (Nicholls 2015). A simple and more accurate practice is to trace the wound outline onto an acetate sheet with grid squares; these can then be counted and the area calculated.

🌐 See Evolve website Fig. 23.3

In some areas, this may be calculated digitally using a hand-held digital tablet or converted via a computer programme. Weekly measurement is often sufficient and steady progress should be evident.

Description of the Tissue Type. Tissue types in a wound may be described in relation to colour (e.g. red, black, yellow) or terms such as granulating, necrotic, sloughy or epithelialising. It is important to recognise that in most wounds, there may be a combination of tissue types and for this reason the descriptor is usually accompanied by an approximate percentage.

🌐 See Evolve website Fig. 23.4

Necrotic (black) tissue is dead (devitalised). It indicates the presence of hypoxia in the area and should be removed (unless there are other more pressing objectives) as its presence can encourage the development of infection.

Sloughy tissue, which may present from cream through to yellow, is a fibrinous covering which occurs as the dead cells from the wound healing process rise to the surface of the wound. Although it is generally removed, its presence does not particularly indicate a problem in the healing process.

Granulation tissue is usually red and moist with an uneven granular appearance. It is formed by the creation of new capillary loops, which give the uneven, bumpy texture, and the laying down of ground substance and extracellular matrix. If the granulation tissue is a deep unhealthy red, friable (bleeds easily) or appears dehydrated, this may be a sign of infection in the wound.

Epithelial tissue (pale pink) is the formation of new skin over the surface of the wound. Epithelial tissue can only be generated from epidermal cells which occur at the wound margin and from around any surviving hair follicles. This type of tissue is particularly fragile and requires protection and appropriate moisture balance.

Occasionally, the wound may appear green in colour. This is a clear sign of clinical infection and wound swabs should be taken (Information 23.3).

Volume of Exudate. Recording the volume of exudate is difficult as it cannot be accurately captured in routine practice. Typically, wound assessment charts record the volume as +, ++, +++ or use a range of subjective descriptors such as minimal, moderate, heavy. Being very subjective, they do not assist in planning care. A more objective description is to record the frequency of dressing change, so if a dressing had previously needed changing twice daily and was now only requiring changing every other day, it can be seen that the volume of exudate has reduced. Exudate can also be combined with other fluid; for example, in a patient with gross oedema of the lower leg and a leg ulcer, it is not possible to determine what is truly exudate and what is leakage of the protein-rich fluid from the leg. Where water-based dressings such as hydrogels are used, a similar situation occurs. In wounds that are progressing normally, such as uncomplicated surgical wounds, exudate levels decrease normally with time. In chronic wounds, exudate levels may remain high due to a prolonged inflammatory phase. A sudden increase in exudate level in any wound, especially if accompanied by a change or increase in pain, is a strong indicator of the presence of infection.

Odour. As with exudate, odour is difficult to assess/measure and is frequently recorded with +s or simply as 'malodour present'.

Patients and inexperienced clinicians may consider the presence of malodour as a sign of infection; however, most wounds have a distinctive odour, as do some dressings, so care should be taken to distinguish what is normal but unpleasant from an indicator of infection. Several systems suggest evaluating the odour level by identifying when it can be detected, for example on entering the room, when close to the patient or only on dressing removal; this allows for a degree of objectivity. Consideration should also be given to the impact of the odour – for many patients a strong odour is the reason that they become increasingly isolated as visitors stop coming or the patient themselves chooses to withdraw from embarrassment.

Pain. Pain should be assessed both to address patient comfort and also as an indicator of what may be happening in the wound. Several assessment tools exist to allow the patient to rate the severity of the pain. These may be numerical, for example how bad is the pain, when 0 is no pain and 10 is the worst pain imaginable, or be based on images of smiling/grimacing faces (see Chapter 20, Pain Management). Consideration should also be given to:
- pain location
- duration

- what it feels like
- what initiates or worsens pain
- what relieves pain (Gardner et al. 2017).

Changes in pain type and intensity may be related to a developing infection. Pain relating to dressing changes should trigger a review/evaluation of the management.

Condition of Surrounding Skin. This is an indicator of general health, for example dry skin in a dehydrated patient, but may also reflect the efficiency of the wound management, for example the appearance of macerated skin when a dressing does not adequately control exudate levels.

Creating an Environment for Healing

Principles of Moist Wound Healing

Healing proceeds at its optimal rate when the wound is enclosed in a warm, moist environment (Fig. 23.4). Under these conditions, cellular activity is maximised; the benefits of such an environment have been recognised since the early 1960s (Winter 1962). This is true for the whole spectrum of wounds encountered, from superficial cuts and grazes to large, extensive granulating wounds. Exposure of a wound to the air precipitates drying out of the wound surface and scab formation. Nurses should consider the importance of providing a suitable environment for wound healing when choosing a wound management material. There are hundreds of dressings available and local formularies and protocols should be used to guide the selectin. See (Wound Care Handbook, 2024) for an overview of dressing categories and products.

Principles of Cleansing

Sutured wounds rarely need cleansing unless leakage has occurred. In this situation the suture line can be gently, aseptically cleansed with sterile 0.9% sodium chloride solution. With open wounds, strict asepsis is not always required. Patients can bathe or preferably shower to irrigate the wound with warm water after 48 hours (NICE 2017). For patient comfort, wound cleansing fluids should be warmed to body temperature. The main reason for cleansing open cavity wounds is to remove any loose debris and excess wound secretions (International Wound Infection Institute [IWII] 2022). A shower is particularly useful as gentle flushing with the spray will remove any particles that are loose and flushing for 10–15 seconds is usually sufficient. If bathing, the wound should be flushed by splashing water into it. Lower limb wounds can be bathed in a

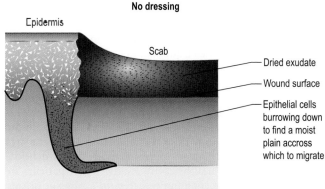

Figure 23.4 Healing of skin wounds with and without a semi-permeable membrane dressing. (Adapted from Winter GD. Formation of the scab and rate of epithelialization of superficial wounds in the skin of the young domestic pig. *Nature*. 1962;193:293-294.)

bucket (lined with a commercial bin liner) or bowl, gently splashing the wound to remove loose debris. A lining protects the bucket from contamination and makes cleaning of the bucket much easier, thus reducing the potential risk of cross-infection.

The Role of Antiseptics and Topical Agents. Antiseptics are rarely used for cleaning wounds unless they are heavily contaminated, for example a dirty traumatic wound, or at very high risk of infection, for example a sacral pressure ulcer when the patient has uncontrollable diarrhoea. For an overview of the role of antimicrobials in wound care see Useful Websites, for example IWII.

Wound Cleansing. The purpose of wound cleansing is to gently remove loose debris and other surface contaminants, so providing an optimal healing environment prior to applying a dressing (IWII 2022). However, wound exudate bathes the surface of wounds and provides nutrients and cytokines essential for healing. Cleansing the surface of a wound removes exudate and in some cases this inhibits the healing process. Nurses need to consider carefully why they are cleansing a wound and to balance the need to remove exudate because of harmful effects, against leaving it in place to enhance healing. Exudate needs to be removed if:

- it is causing maceration to the wound bed and/or surrounding tissues
- there are signs of infection
- foreign bodies are present
- devitalised tissue is present
- it has an unpleasant odour, which is embarrassing and making the patient feel nauseous
- it is excessive and is oozing through dressings and onto clothing/bedding/furniture.

Removal of Devitalised Tissue – Debridement

Debridement, the removal of devitalised (dead) tissue, is most commonly achieved clinically by autolytic debridement, surgical and sharp debridement and biosurgical debridement which is outlined in Table 23.2.

Autolytic Debridement is the most commonly used method. Dressings are used which facilitate autolysis (the body's natural ability to remove devitalised tissues by leucocytes and lytic enzymes). These work best under moist conditions. Several types of wound dressing provide this moist environment that facilitates removal of devitalised tissue from the wound bed. These dressings can effectively remove devitalised and necrotic tissue without damaging either the skin surrounding the wound or healthy tissue within the wound. Included in these are the hydrogels and hydrocolloids (Table 23.2).

Surgical Debridement is usually carried out in theatre where the surgeon removes devitalised tissue back to healthy bleeding tissue.

Sharp Debridement is the removal of devitalised tissue using a scalpel and scissors. It is sometimes possible to excise devitalised tissue with or without local anaesthesia depending on the site and depth of the problem. If general anaesthesia is not indicated, then careful consideration is needed to ensure that the patient has no pain or discomfort, and that the area is not painful. The advantages of this method are that debridement is instant and a healthy cavity results. Where patients are being cared for in the community, access to a surgeon or specialist nurse may be limited and this is not always a practical alternative for many patients. This procedure should not be carried out without specialised training and achievement of clinical competency.

Excessive Granulation

From time to time, epithelialisation fails to take place due to the presence of excessive granulation tissue or 'proud flesh'. Treatment is needed to flatten the granulation tissue to a level with the epithelial edge, as new epithelium cannot migrate up over proud flesh. Silver nitrate (75%) stick should not be used to cauterise the tissue. A less traumatic method is the use of a cream containing a corticosteroid, although this should be used under medical supervision. Careful assessment is paramount in the successful treatment of cavity wounds. When planning a wound care programme, consideration of these factors should provide the nurse with an accurate picture of the needs of each patient and also provide some assistance with the dressing selection process.

Dressing Techniques

Throughout the UK, there are many different policies, procedures and protocols for dressing changes (Table 23.2). Standard infection control procedures must be adhered to when changing dressings (Gould et al. 2020). This involves either clean or aseptic technique depending on the wound type, clinical setting and clinical considerations (Gould et al. 2020). Wound dressing packs no longer contain cotton wool to avoid fibres from the material becoming incorporated into wound tissue and perhaps causing an inflammatory reaction. Nor do the packs contain forceps, which were sometimes difficult to manoeuvre and risked causing trauma to the delicate wound bed. The sterile packs contain gauze to cleanse periwound skin and to dry around the wound after cleansing. The pack may contain a receptacle for cleansing fluid and a disposal bag for contaminated dressings and procedure debris. After handwashing the pack is opened and laid out using a nontouch technique. The disposal bag can act as a glove for the removal of the soiled dressing. Once the dressing has been removed, the person carrying out the procedure washes and dries their hands and applies gloves prior to the dressing procedure.

A dressing needs to be changed when:

- There is a specific purpose, e.g. to remove sutures or when the maximum wear time for the dressing has been reached (see pack insert for individual dressings).
- Clinical signs of infection are present.
- Wound discharge has leaked, or is about to leak, through the dressing (ideally a dressing should be changed before leakage occurs to reduce the risk of infection).
- Special treatments are needed, e.g. burns dressings.

Clinical Setting

Any differences in technique depend on the clinical setting. In hospitals, clinics or nursing homes for instance, there may be an element of control over the environment in terms of cleanliness, equipment such as trolleys and clean surfaces and space. In this kind of environment, there are many patients in close proximity to each other and often several members of staff moving around. This increases the risk of cross-contamination (cross-infection) and procedures need to take this risk into account. In a patient's home, there are fewer people moving around but the nurse has to be mindful of cross-infection when moving from house to house, and equipment, space and cleanliness may be more of a challenge. However, many patients and their families go to great lengths to create a clean and safe working environment for wound care.

The two main methods of dressing change are aseptic or clean procedure techniques. Both require a sound knowledge of infection control principles including the use of aprons and gloves,

| TABLE 23.2 | Dressings and Topical Wound Products | | | |

Material	Presentation	Action	Indications for Use	Special Considerations
Alginates (fibres of calcium or sodium alginate derived from seaweed)	Flat sheets, ropes and packing	Absorbent; gels in contact with exudate Nonadhesive, nonocclusive	Partial- and full-thickness wounds Moderate to heavily exuding wounds	Can be packed into cavities and sinuses Can be rinsed from wound bed, cavity or sinus Usually require a secondary dressing
Antimicrobial dressings (impregnated with iodine, silver, honey or other antimicrobials)	Flat sheets and packing	Have an antimicrobial effect on the wound bed	Heavily contaminated or infected partial- and full-thickness wounds Moderate to heavily exuding wounds as these products usually need exudate to activate the antimicrobial effect	Usually require a secondary dressing Silver products can cause staining of surrounding skin and clothing if not contained
Foams (hydrophilic polyurethane/polymer)	Flat sheets and cavity dressings Some are adhesive, some are semi-occlusive	Absorbent; some can retain exudate in foam	Partial and full-thickness wounds Moderate to heavily exuding wounds	Removed in one piece Some can be cut to shape if necessary
Films (polyurethane or copolymers)	Adhesive sheets	Transparent dressing Maintain a moist environment Impermeable to fluids and microorganisms	Superficial, dry or lightly exuding wounds as a primary dressing	Removed in one piece Can be used as a primary wound contact dressing or to hold other dressings in place (e.g. hydrogels or absorbent pads)
Hydrocolloids (hydrophilic colloid particles derived from cellulose, gelatines and pectins (constituents vary according to manufacturer) bound to a polyurethane foam backing)	Adhesive flat sheets in different thicknesses and shapes Also in gel or paste forms	Maintain a moist environment Provide an environment for autolysis Adhesive sheets are impermeable to fluids and microorganisms	Partial- and full-thickness wounds Dry to moderately exuding wounds	Sometimes leave a residue that can be malodorous Can be cut to shape
Hydrofibres (fibres of carboxymethyl-cellulose)	Flat sheets and packing	Absorbent product that gels on contact with exudate	Partial- and full-thickness wounds Moderately to heavily exuding wounds	Require a secondary dressing
Hydrogels (water- and glycerine-based cross-linked hydrophilic polymers)	Sachets of gel Sheet forms and packing available	Maintain a moist environment Provide an environment for autolysis	Partial- and full-thickness wounds Dry to lightly exuding wounds Provide an environment for autolysis	Usually require a secondary dressing to hold gel in contact with wound bed May cause maceration of skin surrounding wound and so often not recommended for heavily exuding wounds
Low adherent dressings (woven mesh or net of polyamide)	Sheets often silicone-coated to help reduce risk of adherence to the wound	Wound contact layers that wick exudate onto a retention dressing	Partial- and full-thickness wounds Moderately to heavily exuding wounds	Used under compression bandaging systems and in situations where a secondary dressing absorbs exudate
Skin substitutes or equivalents (bioabsorbable matrix containing fibroblasts and/or keratinocytes)	Single or multilayers of living cells, transported on a mesh or medium	Replaces skin and provides wound coverage with cellular activity	Partial- and full-thickness wounds Usually indicated for chronic and slow or non-healing wounds such as diabetic foot ulcers and venous leg ulcers Have been used extensively in burns patients	Usually require specialist skills and facilities Require special transportation and storage as some products are provided frozen and others are incubated Some wound bed preparation is needed prior to application
Negative pressure therapy	Gauze or foam material placed in wound bed and attached to a sealed unit that exerts a negative pressure continuously or intermittently	Removes excess exudate, removes wound debris and microorganisms Stimulates granulation tissue	Full- or partial-thickness wounds, acute or chronic	Special techniques and precautions for some complex wound situations Appropriate training is necessary before using the device

N.B.: This table provides examples of the main groups of dressings and topical wound products. However, it is not an exhaustive list and other products are available as combinations or variations of these main groups.

INFORMATION 23.4

Principles of Aseptic Technique

- Perform the procedure in an area which is closed, clean and well ventilated at least 1 hour after periods of activity where possible. Bed making and cleaning, for example, increase the circulation of dust particles and airborne microorganisms.
- Use a clean trolley – this should be thoroughly cleaned daily and wiped with an alcoholic solution before and after use.
- Wash hands (see Chapter 18, Infection Prevention and Control) before, after and at any point during the procedure should they become contaminated. The use of an alcoholic hand-rub can sometimes be substituted.
- Wear a clean plastic apron to protect the patient from bacteria on the nurse's clothing and to protect your clothing from wound debris and fluids.
- Use sterile equipment for the procedure – be aware of how your health trust/authority/board identifies equipment which is sterile and therefore safe to use.
- Discard equipment which has broken or damaged packaging.
- Use sterile fluids and dressing materials.
- Prepare equipment before dressings are removed.
- Use gloves to remove any dressings and dispose of both immediately. Alternatively, insert your hand into the disposal bag using it like a glove. When turned the right way out it becomes a disposal bag for the rest of the procedure.
- Carry out the procedure using clean or sterile gloves depending on the procedure, discarding equipment as it becomes contaminated.
- Dispose of used equipment in the appropriate bin.

cleansing of working surfaces, the careful washing and drying of hands and disposal of contaminated material. The practitioner must ensure that clinical protocols in relation to procedure clothing, hair and jewellery are strictly adhered to.

Aseptic Technique

In some acute wounds or for particularly vulnerable patients, an aseptic technique may be indicated (Information 23.4). The aseptic technique adopts a nontouch technique; the practitioner wears sterile gloves for the procedure and sterile fluids are used if the wound requires cleansing.

Clean Procedure

This technique involves cleansing with tap water and the use of clean gloves. It is most commonly used for chronic wounds such as leg or pressure ulcers. People with leg ulceration may wash the wound in a container or use a shower. The leg and the skin surrounding the wound are dried carefully using paper roll or a clean towel. This ensures the patient is socially clean and helps to ensure their skin is cared for. This type of cleansing is also beneficial from a psychological perspective, especially for people with long-term conditions. There is no evidence to suggest that the use of tap water from a clean source puts the patient at any higher risk of infection (Evidence-Based Practice 23.1, Fernandez and Griffiths 2008).

Involving Patients in Wound Care

Wherever patients are cared for (home, community settings or hospital), there are many opportunities for the nurse to involve patients in wound management. This is important in empowering patients with a sense of independence and will help promote a return to normality.

EVIDENCE-BASED PRACTICE 23.1

Wound Cleansing

Fernandez and Griffiths (2008) in a Cochrane Review on using water for cleansing suggest that there is little benefit in cleaning wounds with sterile solutions such as 0.9% sodium chloride solution (normal saline), particularly in the community setting.

Activity

- Access the review by Fernandez and Griffiths (2008) and consider the evidence.
- With your colleagues, discuss why you think sterile saline continues to be the cleansing solution of choice for many nurses. You may want to consider the views of both the healthcare professional and the patient.
- Identify occasions when you would feel that tap water would be a better option and also times when you would only use sterile saline.

Resources

Fernandez R, Griffiths R. Water for wound cleansing. *Cochrane Database Syst Rev.* 2008;(1):CD003861. http://www.cochrane.org/reviews/en/ab003861.html.

Patients with sutured wounds can be taught to monitor themselves for clinical signs of infection and in self-care areas such as nutrition, fluid intake, rest and avoidance of excessive movement of the affected area. In addition, they can be taught about the appearance of the wound surface and what to expect during the healing phase. In the community, patients and families can be taught the basic dressing-change technique where asepsis is not necessary, and the community nurse can assume a supervisory role. This obviously depends on individual circumstances and the patient's level of understanding, but certainly many patients with open wounds are able to play a major role in wound management. This is important as the patient begins to resume a more normal lifestyle and it also avoids the need for routine frequent visits by the community nurse (Reflection 23.1).

Diverse Populations and Wound Care

People with wounds reflect a diverse population therefore individual needs and settings must be taken into account when planning

REFLECTION 23.1

Involving Patients in Wound Care

Whilst you are caring for a patient with a wound, and if it is appropriate to do so, talk to them about their wound and how it impacts on their activities of daily living.

Activities

- Find out what they know about the cause and progress of their wound.
- What information have they been given about their treatment plan?
- Ask how easy is it for them to follow the plan and what they find challenging.
- Reflect on the areas of their treatment plan that they find challenging and discuss with your assessor/supervisor how this could be addressed.
- Find out what wound care related information is available in your clinical area (e.g. information leaflets, DVDs, etc.).

care and the person's involvement in that care. For instance, in children with wounds, or older people with severe learning difficulties, it is advantageous to keep the assessment and wound dressing process as brief and straightforward as possible to help minimise upset and trauma of the wound management process on top of an already traumatic experience of the wounding (Resch et al. 2021). People who are homeless may have limited access to healthcare and this may be compounded by chaotic lifestyles. People in prison have access to healthcare but this may be disrupted due to the confines of the prison system and safety concerns for prisoners and staff (Hankins et al. 2022). Regardless of such factors, people with wounds should have the opportunity to be part of their wound care management plan and their needs and wishes taken into account as much as possible.

Patients with chronic wounds, such as leg ulcers and pressure ulcers, need specific help and support, but it is very important to gain their cooperation. Patients with venous leg ulcers require advice on leg elevation techniques and calf pump muscle exercises, which stimulate the circulation and aid drainage of the lower limb. Carers of patients with pressure ulcers need advice and training on manual handling, that is, turning and repositioning the patient. Carers also need to know how the pressure-reducing aids work, so that these are used correctly at all times. Concordance is where patients and practitioners reach agreement on management regimens through open discussion and negotiation about what is desirable and what is manageable. Patient compliance is commonly referred to in the literature but often leads to conflict and is not easily sustainable in long-term conditions (De Mauri et al. 2022). The patient, and where appropriate their carers, need to be involved in decisions and helped to feel that they have some control about what happens; this is concordance.

Wound Management Policies and Guidelines

Most healthcare providers in the UK have developed wound treatment and prevention policies as well as wound selection formularies to help guide their staff towards safe and standardised care. Ideally, these are based on the best available evidence sourced from systematic reviews of the literature covering randomised controlled trials, but other sources of evidence need to be included to ensure that patients' perspectives and experiences form part of the evidence base. The National Wound Care Strategy Programme for England (https://www.nationalwoundcarestrategy.net/lower-limb/) has produced clinical pathways and clinical recommendations for lower limb wounds and pressure ulcers, and similar is in process for surgical wound complications. These documents set out what good care looks like and should be adopted by all organisations.

National and international guidance for wound care is produced by organisations including:
- Scottish Intercollegiate Guidelines Network (SIGN)
- National Institute for Health and Care Excellence (NICE)
- National Wound Care Strategy Programme (NWCSP)
- Department of Health (DH)
- Cochrane Collaboration
- European Pressure Ulcer Advisory Panel (EPUAP)
- European Wound Management Association (EWMA)
  See Useful Websites.

Care delivery and wound outcomes seem to vary significantly depending on wound aetiology. There is good evidence of healing rates for those patients with venous leg ulcers but little at all for patients with pressure ulcers; there is significant effort towards the prevention of pressure ulcers but little towards the prevention of venous leg ulcers. Patients who have diabetes and a foot ulcer will have access to rapid assessment and treatment from a multidisciplinary team, whereas those with an equally at risk foot but without diabetes face a lottery in terms of the quality of their care including who they will be seen by and how quickly. Pathways of care for all patients with wounds should follow a standard format beginning with primary prevention, identifying and where possible modifying risks and then applying evidence-based care and secondary prevention. Only by considering all of these steps can the total burden of wounds be reduced.

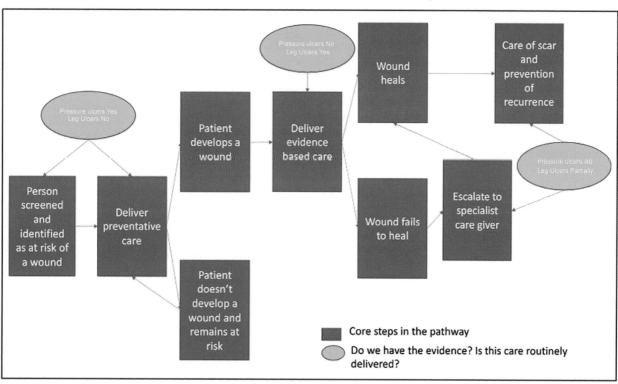

Reproduced with permission (Fletcher 2022)

Expectations of Outcome and Effectiveness of Treatment

Following individual patient and wound assessment, the nurse should have reasonable expectations regarding the prospects of achieving complete healing. In some wounds, complete healing is expected rapidly, as in primary wound closure following appendicectomy in a healthy young person. For others, the prognosis for healing is less good, for example an older woman with arthritis and a venous leg ulcer. The expected outcome affects the choice of treatment for individual patients. For patients with a poor prognosis for healing, treatment is often directed towards minimising symptoms and preventing further wound breakdown, such as in terminally ill patients with superficial pressure ulcers where the aim is to prevent the ulcer from penetrating into deeper tissues. Patient comfort and convenience become the priorities and provide some measure of the effectiveness of the treatment. Where healing is expected, effectiveness means complete healing occurring in the minimum number of days with the fewest complications.

Cost-Effectiveness

Efficacy is also measured by the cost of treatments. Hospital doctors, GPs, practice nurses or district nurses and the pharmacists who supply materials for wound management can be misled into believing that, because the initial cost of a material is high, then it follows that the total treatment costs will also be high. Modern wound dressing materials can be relatively expensive to buy per unit. However, these dressings can often be left on the wound for several days and, in some cases, for a full week.

It is important, when comparing the costs of dressing materials, to consider:

- How long the product can be left on the wound
- The nursing time needed to change and apply dressings
- The benefits of using interactive products that stimulate tissue growth to achieve rapid healing or stimulate healing in chronic wounds
- How the dressing prevents damage to skin surrounding the wound, helping to reduce pain and discomfort, reducing ancillary product and analgesia costs
- The reduction of unnecessary pain, suffering and disruption for patients
- The cost to the environment and contribution to Net Zero targets

The consideration of sustainability as a cost is a relatively new concept however, the delivery of evidence-based care that promotes faster healing can have significant benefits. When a patient heals more quickly or requires less visits, savings can be made in terms of travel (less fuel usage), product use (consider the dressing pack, cleansing agents, dressing product, retention system, possibly debridement products, tapes, gloves, aprons) and therefore also less waste generated, delivering multiple eco benefits.

Specific Wound Types

This section covers pressure ulcers, leg ulcers, sutured wounds, traumatic wounds and malignant wounds (burn injuries are covered in Chapter 29).

❖ Nursing Management and Health Promotion: Pressure Ulcers

A pressure ulcer is localised damage to the skin and/or underlying tissue, usually over a bony prominence (or related to a medical or other device), resulting from sustained pressure (including pressure associated with shear). The damage can be present as intact skin or an open ulcer and may be painful.

(NHS Improvement 2018a)

Pressure ulcers develop most commonly on the sacral area. Tissue damage ranges from superficial epidermal loss to damage to underlying structures, including muscle and bone (see later).

The prevention and management of pressure ulcers present major challenges for nurses. The pressure ulcer problem is widespread and persistent, affecting patients of all ages and with a range of illnesses. It reduces quality of life and causes distress to patients and carers and makes major financial demands on health services. Particular difficulties arise in trying to identify patients who might develop a pressure ulcer, and when they are at risk of doing so.

Nurses have a basic responsibility to:

- Use a structured approach to risk assessment to identify people at risk of pressure ulcer development.
- Conduct a structured risk assessment on admission, and repeat as regularly and as frequently as required by patient acuity. Reassessment should also be undertaken if there is any change in patient condition (NICE 2015).
- Document all risk assessments.
- Develop and implement a prevention plan when individuals have been identified as being at risk of pressure ulcer development (EPUAP, NPIAP, PPPIA 2019)

Aetiology

Pressure ulcers result from areas of previously healthy tissue becoming devitalised, resulting in localised tissue death. Pressure ulcers develop primarily due to cell deformation which can occur due to the application of external mechanical forces which include:

- Direct, unrelieved pressure of soft tissues against bone or another hard surface such as a catheter.
- From shear forces that frequently accompany both direct pressure and friction; shear forces develop in tissues that are distorted and pulled and cause maximum cellular distortion. Shear forces can also be caused by the direct application of pressure.
- From friction occurring between the patient and the surface of a bed or chair, such as when the patient is moved and the skin is dragged over a sheet.

Classification

In order to assess the extent or degree of damage, a range of categorisation systems have been developed. Most recently, the NPIAP (2016) has classified six categories of damage which have been adopted by NHS Improvement (2018a). The wording of these definitions is currently under review to ensure that they represent a more diverse population as not all skin tones demonstrate skin reddening. For people with dark skin tones, other early signs of pressure damage should be considered; these include change in skin colour, temperature and texture and also patient-reported pain, discomfort, itching or tenderness (Wounds UK 2021).

Category 1 Pressure Ulcer: Non-blanchable erythema of intact skin

Intact skin with a localized area of non-blanchable erythema, which may appear differently in darkly pigmented skin. Presence of blanchable erythema or changes in sensation, temperature, or firmness may precede visual changes. Colour changes do not include purple or maroon discoloration; these may indicate deep tissue pressure injury.

Category 2 Pressure Ulcer: Partial-thickness skin loss with exposed dermis

Partial-thickness loss of skin with exposed dermis. The wound bed is viable, pink or red, moist, and may also present as an intact or ruptured serum-filled blister. Adipose (fat) is not visible and deeper tissues are not visible. Granulation tissue, slough and eschar are not present. These ulcers commonly result from adverse microclimate and shear in the skin over the pelvis and shear in the heel. This stage should not be used to describe moisture associated skin damage (MASD) including incontinence associated dermatitis (IAD), intertriginous dermatitis (ITD), medical adhesive related skin injury (MARSI), or traumatic wounds (skin tears, burns, abrasions).

Category 3 Pressure Ulcer: Full-thickness skin loss

Full-thickness loss of skin, in which adipose (fat) is visible in the ulcer and granulation tissue and epibole (rolled wound edges) are often present. Slough and/or eschar may be visible. The depth of tissue damage varies by anatomical location; areas of significant adiposity can develop deep wounds. Undermining and tunnelling may occur. Fascia, muscle, tendon, ligament, cartilage and/or bone are not exposed. If slough or eschar obscures the extent of tissue loss this is an Unstageable Pressure Ulcer of at least category 3.

Category 4 Pressure Ulcer: Full-thickness skin and tissue loss

Full-thickness skin and tissue loss with exposed or directly palpable fascia, muscle, tendon, ligament, cartilage or bone in the ulcer. Slough and/or eschar may be visible. Epibole (rolled edges), undermining and/or tunnelling often occur. Depth varies by anatomical location. If slough or eschar obscures the extent of tissue loss this is an Unstageable Pressure Ulcer.

Unstageable Pressure Ulcer: Obscured full-thickness skin and tissue loss

Full-thickness skin and tissue loss in which the extent of tissue damage within the ulcer cannot be confirmed because it is obscured by slough or eschar. If slough or eschar is removed, a category 3 or Category 4 pressure ulcer will be revealed. Stable eschar (i.e. dry, adherent, intact without erythema or fluctuance) on the heel or ischemic limb should not be softened or removed. At least a category 3 pressure ulcer.

Deep Tissue Injury: Persistent non-blanchable deep red, maroon or purple discoloration Intact or non-intact skin with localized area of persistent non-blanchable deep red, maroon, purple discoloration or epidermal separation revealing a dark wound bed or blood-filled blister. Pain and temperature change often precede skin colour changes. Discoloration may appear differently in darkly pigmented skin. This injury results from intense and/or prolonged pressure and shear forces at the bone-muscle interface. The wound may evolve rapidly to reveal the actual extent of tissue injury, or may resolve without tissue loss. If necrotic tissue, subcutaneous tissue, granulation tissue, fascia, muscle or other underlying structures are visible, this indicates a full thickness pressure ulcer.

Additional pressure ulcer definitions.

Medical Device Related Pressure Ulcer:

This describes an aetiology. Medical device related pressure ulcers result from the use of devices designed and applied for diagnostic or therapeutic purposes. The resultant pressure ulcer generally conforms to the pattern or shape of the device. The ulcer should be categorized as per the categorisation system.

Mucosal Membrane Pressure Ulcer: Mucosal membrane pressure injury is found on mucous membranes with a history of a medical device in use at the location of the injury. Due to the anatomy of the tissue these ulcers cannot be categorized as the mucosa does not have the layers of tissues described in the categorization system.

A poster illustrating the categories can be found here: https://www.nationalwoundcarestrategy.net/wp-content/uploads/2021/07/Pressure-ulcer-categorisation-poster.pdf.

Assessment of Risk

In an acute illness, even the most unlikely individual may become 'at risk' of developing a pressure ulcer; therefore, all patients should be assessed on admission to hospital, care/nursing home or a community nurse's caseload. A combination of disease and/or drug therapies or surgery, for example, can quite suddenly put an individual into an 'at risk' category.

The following are at risk of developing pressure ulcers:
- the very old or very young
- the immobile, e.g. paraplegic or after some orthopaedic surgery
- those with sensory loss, e.g. altered consciousness or diabetic sensory neuropathy
- those with systemic diseases, e.g. anaemia, peripheral vascular disease, cancer
- those having medication including anti-inflammatories, cytotoxics or corticosteroids
- those with loss of continence
- poorly nourished individuals
- those with body mass index (BMI) <20 or BMI >30.

Several scales and scoring systems have been devised for assessing risk; the most widely used in the UK is currently the Waterlow score Fig. 23.5A), although NHS Wales has used the PURPOSE T screening and assessment tool (see Fig. 23.5B) since 2019 and this will be adopted by NHS England and NHS Ireland from 2023. This system was developed based on a systematic review of risk factors and has been designed to lead to three outcomes which are presented based on traffic light system (red, amber, green) which leads to a plan of care (Coleman et al. 2018). Patients in the red category have a 'pressure ulcer category 1 or above' or scarring from previous pressure ulcers; patients in the amber category have 'no pressure ulcer but are at risk'; and those in the green category are deemed as 'no pressure ulcer, not currently at risk'. The PURPOSE T tool can be downloaded free of charge from https://ctru.leeds.ac.uk/purpose/purpose-t/. A series of videos about using PURPOSE T can be found here: https://www.youtube.com/watch?v=36EXz8Dmr3o&list=PLoKuDJo_vt6DIoqOEzteffvMWaf_j_84B.

There are other risk assessment scores available, although only some – the Norton Scale, the Braden Scale and the Central Begeleidings Orgaan (CBO) – have undergone validity testing (Braden 1997, Schoonhoven et al. 2002). National (NICE 2014) and international (EPUAP, NPIAP, PPPIA 2019) guidelines have

WATERLOW PRESSURE ULCER PREVENTION/TREATMENT POLICY
RING SCORES IN TABLE, ADD TOTAL. MORE THAN 1 SCORE/CATEGORY CAN BE USED

BUILD/WEIGHT FOR HEIGHT		SKIN TYPE VISUAL RISK AREAS		SEX AGE		MALNUTRITION SCREENING TOOL (MST) (Nutrition Vol.15, No.6 1999 - Australia
AVERAGE BMI = 20-24.9	0	HEALTHY	0	MALE	1	A - HAS PATIENT LOST WEIGHT RECENTLY / B - WEIGHT LOSS SCORE
ABOVE AVERAGE BMI = 25-29.9	1	TISSUE PAPER	1	FEMALE	2	YES - GO TO B / 0.5 - 5kg = 1
OBESE BMI > 30	2	DRY	1	14 - 49	1	NO - GO TO C / 5 - 10kg = 2
BELOW AVERAGE BMI < 20	3	OEDEMATOUS	1	50 - 64	2	UNSURE - GO TO C AND / 10 - 15kg = 3
BMI=Wt(Kg)/Ht (m)²		CLAMMY, PYREXIA	1	65 - 74	3	SCORE 2 / > 15kg = 4, unsure = 2
		DISCOLOURED GRADE 1	2	75 - 80	4	C - PATIENT EATING POORLY OR LACK OF APPETITE 'NO' = 0; 'YES' SCORE = 1 / NUTRITION SCORE If > 2 refer for nutrition assessment / intervention
		BROKEN/SPOTS GRADE 2-4	3	81 +	5	

CONTINENCE		MOBILITY		SPECIAL RISKS
COMPLETE/ CATHETERISED	0	FULLY	0	**TISSUE MALNUTRITION** / **NEUROLOGICAL DEFICIT**
URINE INCONT.	1	RESTLESS/FIDGETY	1	TERMINAL CACHEXIA 8 / DIABETES, MS, CVA 4-6
FAECAL INCONT.	2	APATHETIC	2	MULTIPLE ORGAN FAILURE 8 / MOTOR/SENSORY 4-6
URINARY + FAECAL INCONTINENCE	3	RESTRICTED	3	SINGLE ORGAN FAILURE (RESP, RENAL, CARDIAC,) 5 / PARAPLEGIA (MAX OF 6) 4-6
		BEDBOUND e.g. TRACTION	4	PERIPHERAL VASCULAR DISEASE 5 / **MAJOR SURGERY or TRAUMA**
		CHAIRBOUND e.g. WHEELCHAIR	5	ANAEMIA (Hb < 8) 2 / ORTHOPAEDIC/SPINAL 5, ON TABLE > 2 HR# 5
				SMOKING 1 / ON TABLE > 6 HR# 8

SCORE
10+ AT RISK
15+ HIGH RISK
20+ VERY HIGH RISK

MEDICATION - CYTOTOXICS, LONG TERM/HIGH DOSE STEROIDS, ANTI-INFLAMMATORY MAX OF 4

\# Scores can be discounted after 48 hours provided patient is recovering normally

© J Waterlow 1985 Revised 2005*
Obtainable from the Nook, Stoke Road, Henlade TAUNTON TA3 5LX
* The 2005 revision incorporates the research undertaken by Queensland Health. www.judy-waterlow.co.uk

REMEMBER **TISSUE DAMAGE MAY START PRIOR TO ADMISSION, IN CASUALTY. A SEATED PATIENT IS AT RISK** ASSESSMENT (See Over) IF THE PATIENT FALLS INTO ANY OF THE RISK CATEGORIES, THEN PREVENTATIVE NURSING IS REQUIRED A COMBINATION OF GOOD NURSING TECHNIQUES AND PREVENTATIVE AIDS WILL BE NECESSARY **ALL ACTIONS MUST BE DOCUMENTED**

PREVENTION PRESSURE REDUCING AIDS
Special Mattress/beds: 10+ Overlays or specialist foam mattresses. 15+ Alternating pressure overlays, mattresses and bed systems 20+ Bed systems: Fluidised bead, low air loss and alternating pressure mattresses Note: Preventative aids cover a wide spectrum of specialist features. Efficacy should be judged, if possible, on the basis of independent evidence.
Cushions: No person should sit in a wheelchair without some form of cushioning. If nothing else is available - use the person's own pillow. (Consider infection risk) 10+ 100mm foam cushion 15+ Specialist Gel and/or foam cushion 20+ Specialised cushion, adjustable to individual person.
Bed clothing: Avoid plastic draw sheets, inco pads and tightly tucked in sheet/sheet covers, especially when using specialist bed and mattress overlay systems Use duvet - plus vapour permeable membrane.

NURSING CARE
General HAND WASHING, frequent changes of position, lying, sitting. Use of pillows
Pain Appropriate pain control
Nutrition High protein, vitamins and minerals
Patient Handling Correct lifting technique - hoists - monkey poles Transfer devices
Patient Comfort Aids Real Sheepskin - bed cradle
Operating Table Theatre/A&E Trolley 100mm(4ins) cover plus adequate protection

Skin Care General hygene, NO rubbing, cover with an appropriate dressing

WOUND GUIDELINES
Assessment odour, exudate, measure/photograph position

WOUND CLASSIFICATION - EPUAP
GRADE 1 Discolouration of intact skin not affected by light finger pressure (non-blanching erythema) This may be difficult to identify in darkly pigmented skin
GRADE 2 Partial thickness skin loss or damage involving epidermis and/or dermis The pressure ulcer is superficial and presents clinically as an abrasion, blister or shallow crater
GRADE 3 Full thickness skin loss involving damage of subcutaneous tissue but not extending to the underlying fascia The pressure ulcer presents clinically as a deep crater with or without undermining of adjacent tissue
GRADE 4 Full thickness skin loss with extensive destruction and necrosis extending to underlying tissue.
Dressing Guide Use Local dressings formulary and/or www.worldwidewounds

IF TREATMENT IS REQUIRED, FIRST REMOVE PRESSURE

A

Figure 23.5 (A) The Waterlow pressure ulcer prevention/treatment policy.

Pressure Ulcer Risk Assessment – PURPOSE T (V2)

Patient name	DOB	Hospital / NHS number	Ward

Step 1 – screening

Mobility status – *tick all applicable*
- Needs the help of another person to walk ☐
- Spends all or the majority of time in bed or chair ☐
- Remains in the same position for long periods ☐
- Walks independently with or without walking aids ☐

If **ONLY** blue box is ticked

If **ANY** *yellow boxes are ticked,* **go to Step 2**

Skin status – *tick all applicable*
- Current PU category 1 or above? ☐
- Reported history of previous PU? ☐
- Vulnerable skin ☐
- Medical device causing pressure/shear at skin site e.g. O_2 mask, NG tube ☐
- Normal skin ☐

If **ONLY** blue box is ticked

If **ANY** *yellow or pink boxes are ticked,* **go to Step 2**

Clinical Judgment – *tick as applicable*
- Conditions/treatments which significantly impact the patient's PU risk e.g. poor perfusion, epidurals, oedema, steroids ☐
- No problem ☐

If **ONLY** blue box is ticked

If **ANY** *yellow boxes are ticked,* **go to Step 2**

No pressure ulcer **not** currently at risk

Tick if applicable ☐

Not currently at risk pathway

Step 2 – full assessment   Complete ALL sections

Analysis of independent movement

Tick the applicable box (where frequency and extent categories meet)

		Extent of all independent movement / Relief of all pressure areas		
		Doesn't move	Slight position changes	Major position changes
Frequency of position changes	Doesn't move	☐	N/A	N/A
	Moves occasionally	N/A	☐	☐
	Moves frequently	N/A	☐	☐

Sensory perception and response – *tick as applicable*
- No problem ☐
- Patient is unable to feel and/or respond appropriately to discomfort from pressure e.g. CVA, neuropathy, epidural ☐

Moisture due to perspiration, urine, faeces or exudate – *tick as applicable*
- No problem / Occasional ☐
- Frequent (2–4 times a day) ☐
- Constant ☐

Diabetes – *tick as applicable*
- Not diabetic ☐
- Diabetic ☐

Perfusion – *tick all applicable*
- No problem ☐
- Conditions affecting central circulation e.g. shock, heart failure, hypotension ☐
- Conditions affecting peripheral circulation e.g. peripheral vascular / arterial disease ☐

Nutrition – *tick all applicable*
- No problem ☐
- Unplanned weight loss ☐
- Poor nutritional intake ☐
- Low BMI (less than 18.5) ☐
- High BMI (30 or more) ☐

Medical device – *tick as applicable*
- No problem ☐
- Medical device causing pressure/shear at skin site e.g. O_2 mask, NG tube ☐

Vulnerable skin (precursor to PU) e.g. blanchable redness that persists, dryness, paper thin, moist.
NPUAP / EPUAP Pressure Ulcer Classification System (2009)
Cat 1 Non-blanchable redness of intact skin
Cat 2 Partial thickness skin loss or clear blister
Cat 3 Full thickness skin loss (fat visible/ slough present)
Cat 4 Full thickness tissue loss (muscle/bone visible)
Cat U (Unstageable/Unclassified): full thickness skin or tissue loss - depth unknown

Current Detailed Skin Assessment – *tick if pain, soreness or discomfort present at any skin site as applicable.*
For each skin site tick applicable column – either vulnerable skin, normal skin or record PU category

Skin site	Pain	Vulnerable skin	PU category	Normal skin	Skin site	Pain	Vulnerable skin	PU category	Normal skin	Skin site	Pain	Vulnerable skin	PU category	Normal skin
Sacrum	☐	☐		☐	R Hip	☐	☐		☐	R Elbow	☐	☐		☐
L Buttock	☐	☐		☐	L Heel	☐	☐		☐	Other as applicable *(may be medical device site)*				
R Buttock	☐	☐		☐	R Heel	☐	☐		☐					
L Ischial	☐	☐		☐	L Ankle	☐	☐		☐					
R Ischial	☐	☐		☐	R Ankle	☐	☐		☐					
L Hip	☐	☐		☐	L Elbow	☐	☐		☐					

Previous PU history – *tick as applicable*
- No known PU history ☐
- PU history – *complete below* ☐
- Number of previous pressure ulcer(s)
- Detail of previous PU (if more than 1 previous PU give detail of the PU that left a scar or worst category).

Approx date	Site		PU cat	Scar	No scar
				☐	

Other relevant information (if required):

Step 3 – assessment decision

If **ANY pink boxes** are ticked/completed, the patient has an existing pressure ulcer or scarring from previous pressure ulcer.

If **ANY orange boxes** are ticked (but no pink boxes), the patient is at risk.

If only **yellow and blue boxes** are ticked, the nurse must consider the risk profile (risk factors present) to decide whether the patient is at risk or not currently at risk.

PU Category 1 or above or scarring from previous pressure ulcers
Tick if applicable ☐
Secondary prevention and treatment pathway

No pressure ulcer but at risk
Tick if applicable ☐
Primary prevention pathway

No pressure ulcer not currently at risk
Tick if applicable ☐
Not currently at risk pathway

Nurse printed name	Nurse signature	Date	Time

B

PURPOSE T Version 2.0 – Copyright © Clinical Trials Research Unit, University of Leeds and Leeds Teaching Hospitals NHS Trust, 2017 (Do not use without permission)

Figure 23.5 (B) The PUROSE T screening and assessment tool. (A, reproduced by permission of Judy Waterlow, MBE, SRN, RCNT, http://www.judy-waterlow.co.uk/.)

Waterlow Risk Assessment

EPUAP, NPIAP and PPPIA (2019) produced new guidelines on pressure ulcer prevention and treatment. Following a systematic review of the literature and consideration of the methodological adequacy of the studies, they presented a list of factors which they felt were important in increasing patients' risk of developing pressure ulcers.

The unvalidated Waterlow risk assessment is one of several risk assessment tools available for use in clinical practice. It is a commonly used tool in the UK.

Activities

- Access the guideline from EPUAP, NPIAP and PPPIA (2019) and compare the evidence they present for inclusion of the individual risk factors to those used within the Waterlow Pressure Ulcer Prevention/Treatment Policy chart (Fig. 23.5A) and the PURPOSE T screening and risk assessment tool (Fig. 23.5B).
- Discuss with the trained staff how accurate they feel the Waterlow score is and what factors they feel are important in clinical practice. Consider how easy staff find each tool to use.

Resources

European Pressure Ulcer Advisory Panel, National Pressure Injury Advisory Panel and Pan Pacific Pressure Injury Alliance. *Prevention and Treatment of Pressure Ulcers: Clinical Practice Guideline. The International Guideline.* Haesler E, ed. EPUAP/NPIAP/PPPIA; 2019.

been produced to guide nurses towards an evidence-based approach to caring for patients (Evidence-Based Practice 23.2).

The National Wound Care Strategy on behalf of NHS England has produced a pressure ulcer clinical pathway and accompanying recommendations to guide best practice.

As part of guideline recommendations, risk assessment tools are designed to support nurses' clinical judgement and not to replace it; the PURPOSE T tool specifically includes clinical judgement as part of the decision-making process. They are useful only if used regularly – on admission and again each time the patient's condition changes (NICE 2015). The scores need to be accurately documented and then used to determine the most appropriate plan of care for the patient.

Prevention of Pressure Ulcers

Once patients have been identified as being 'at risk', it is recommended that a 'bundle of care' is put into place; this bundle is known as aSSKINg and includes consideration of

- Assessment of risk
- Skin assessment and care
- Support surface selection and use
- Keeping the patient moving
- Incontinence assessment and management
- Nutrition and hydration
- Giving of information
  (NHS Improvement 2018b)

Managing Patients With Established Pressure Ulcers

In addition to providing a suitable surface on which to nurse the patient and ensuring adequate nutrition and using good handling techniques when moving a patient, local care of the pressure ulcer needs to be considered. The wound should be fully assessed and appropriate dressing applied to manage the presenting symptoms.

Removal of the cause of the damage is the most critical factor. Clear documentation of both the assessment and care within the clinical record ensures both good communication with the multidisciplinary team and also facilitates data capture without the need for additional documents. Guidance on good record keeping is available from the Professional Records Standards Body (PRSB 2023)

The management of patients with established pressure ulcers is costly in both economic and personal terms. Prevention of pressure ulcers is often far cheaper than management. Health service managers are able to cost the treatment of pressure ulcers more accurately (NHS Improvement 2018c).

Staff and Patient Education

In the prevention and management of pressure ulcers, patients have an important role to play. All patients, including young people with chronic disabilities, can be taught methods of regularly relieving pressure by changing position (EPUAP, NPIAP, PPPIA 2019). Patients who are not able to take such an active part in their own management can be taught the value of and need for the changes of position that nurses and other carers carry out for them. Concordance increases when patients understand why intervention is necessary.

Education leaflets, websites, etc., can also be useful. An extract from a typical patient information leaflet demonstrates how the nurse and the patient share in the prevention of pressure ulcers (Information 23.5).

As pressure ulcer prevention is such a core element of care, a national curriculum in relation to pressure ulcer prevention has been developed by NHS Improvement (2018b). Many resources can also be obtained from the National Wound Care Strategy website (see Useful Websites) and a series of powerful videos from patients discussing their own experiences (https://www.national-woundcarestrategy.net/pressure-ulcer/).

Throughout the UK and mainland Europe, guidelines for the prevention and treatment of pressure ulcers are produced in different languages for professionals, carers and patients (see Useful Websites, e.g. EPUAP).

Extract From an Education Leaflet: Preventing Pressure Ulcers

As most pressure ulcers are the result of staying in one position for too long, the answer is to:

Relieve the Pressure by Changing Position

Ideally, you should get up out of bed or your chair at least once every 2 hours during the day and take a short walk. This activity also helps your blood circulation and stops your muscles getting lax.

If you are confined to a chair, you should lift your bottom off the seat for a few moments every half an hour by pushing up on the arms of the chair.

If you have to stay in bed, then your bed may be fitted with a 'monkey pole' or rope ladder – the nurse will show you how to use this to lift yourself off the bed.

If your pressure ulcer is extensive or deep, or your movement is very restricted, a special movement chart will be devised for you by the nursing staff to keep you off the ulcer as much as possible, and you may be given a special bed or mattress.

Reproduced with permission from Morison M, Moffatt C, Bridel-Nixon J, Bale S, eds. *A Colour Guide to the Nursing Management of Chronic Wounds.* 2nd ed. London: Mosby; 1997.

❖ Nursing Management and Health Promotion: Leg Ulcers

Leg ulceration is a common problem, affecting between 1% and 2% of the population (Lim et al. 2018). Essentially a community-based problem, the day-to-day care of patients with these wounds is usually undertaken by district and general practice nurses, supported by GPs, although there are an increasing number of specialist leg ulcer clinics in the community. The major cause of leg ulceration in the UK is chronic venous insufficiency associated with venous hypertension (70%–75%). Between 20% and 30% of patients with a leg ulcer have some degree of ischaemia, with diabetes, vasculitis and trauma accounting for other causes of leg ulceration (Lim et al. 2018).

One of the most important stages in the assessment of patients is to diagnose the aetiology of the ulcer, as this dictates the most appropriate method of management. Data demonstrate that many people do not have their ulcer aetiology diagnosed and that significantly adds to cost and poorer outcomes for patients (Guest et al. 2018). Such diagnosis is achieved by conducting a full patient assessment and a lower limb assessment in conjunction with the use of hand-held Doppler to ascertain the arterial flow to the lower limb (Partsch and Mortimer 2015). In order to address issues of suboptimal wound care, the National Wound Care Strategy was launched in 2018 in England. A part of this initiative is the Lower Limb Strategy (https://www.nationalwoundcarestrategy.net/lower-limb/), which aims to support the care of people with any wound of the lower limb.

Venous Ulcers

This is the most common leg ulcer aetiology. Damage to the valves within the deep veins of the lower leg allows venous blood to flow the wrong way towards the foot. Because of this backflow the veins become congested with increased blood volume. This means that venous blood flows backwards through the perforator veins which sit between and join the deep and superficial system (Fig. 23.6). Extra blood volume results in the superficial veins having to expand to deal with this extra capacity. As the vein walls are stretched, they leak plasma and red cells into the tissue of the lower leg which is visible as oedema and red/brown staining from blood pigments that are broken down in the tissue (Anderson 2018). Poor venous return affects the integrity of the skin and skin changes occur. As well as staining, the skin becomes dry and may become very sensitive to anything applied to it such as moisturisers, cleansing products and dressings, so extra care must be taken (Anderson 2018). Any knock or minor injury to the lower leg leads rapidly to breakdown of the skin and ulceration. Most commonly, ulceration occurs around the medial malleolus.

🌐 **See Evolve website Fig. 23.5**

The ulcers are shallow and can be painful, especially if there is ankle oedema and damage to the surrounding skin from exudate leakage. A typical past history reveals phlebitis, deep vein thrombosis (DVT), leg fracture or severe leg injury or varicose veins (SIGN 2010). It can take weeks or many months for venous ulcers to heal. Due to the poor condition of the tissues, ulceration can recur and patients need to wear compression hosiery, even after healing, to help maintain drainage of the affected limb.

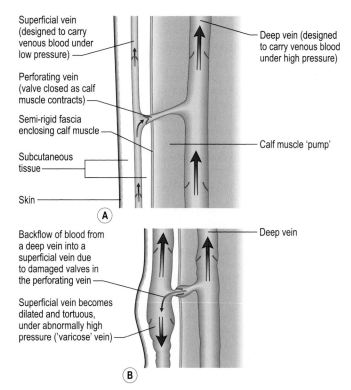

Figure 23.6 (A) Healthy, intact valves prevent backflow of blood from the deep to the superficial veins. (B) An incompetent valve in a perforating vein allows backflow of blood from the deep to the superficial venous system.

Assessment

One of the primary aims of assessing a patient with a leg ulcer is to determine the cause. Nurses are the main healthcare professionals who carry out this assessment, but input from other members of the healthcare team is important to ensure a full assessment with appropriate clinical investigations. There is concern that people with leg ulcers are not being assessed and managed in a skilled and evidenced-based way. This is not satisfactory for patients and their lives and is extremely costly for health services (Guest et al. 2018). Assessment includes:

- A comprehensive medical history which might indicate the presence of venous disease, e.g. previous DVT, vein surgery or pelvic trauma.
- A thorough clinical examination to support the medical history.
- Appropriate investigations, e.g. a Doppler assessment to ascertain the ankle pressure index which is used to detect the presence of significant arterial disease (Vowden and Vowden 2018) (Information 23.6). Other investigations may include full blood count to exclude anaemia, erythrocyte sedimentation rate (ESR) to indicate inflammation, blood glucose to exclude diabetes mellitus and wound swab where infection is suspected.

Sometimes further vascular investigations are indicated such as a Duplex scan to investigate arterial blockages, to identify venous disease if surgery is an option or when the aetiology may be in doubt. A biopsy may be performed, particularly where malignancy is suspected.

Management

Bandaging. The most important component in the treatment of venous ulcers is the use of compression therapy. This is normally in the form of compression bandages, wrap systems or hosiery. Therapy continues after healing normally with hosiery or wrap systems

INFORMATION 23.6

How to Take the Ankle Brachial Pressure Index (ABPI)

- Lay the patient flat and allow the patient to rest quietly for 20 minutes. This is necessary to reduce the effects of gravity on the legs.
- Place the sphygmomanometer cuff on the upper arm, and apply gel over the brachial artery. Hold the Doppler probe at a 45–60-degree angle and measure the systolic pressure. Repeat for the other arm and write down the highest of the two arm pressure readings.
- Place the sphygmomanometer cuff around the malleolus (should the ulcer be sited here, cover the ulcer with protective material such as plastic film). Apply gel on at least two of the pulse points on the foot and take a systolic pressure reading from at least two of these points. Write down the highest reading.
- The ABPI is calculated by dividing the highest ankle pressure reading by the highest brachial pressure reading.
- Do the same for the other leg, again using the highest brachial reading for the calculation.
- Normal ABPI ≥1 (1.3 is the upper limit of normal) – full compression therapy may be applied.
- Abnormal ABPI ≤1 (this indicates a degree of arterial disease is present) – if the patient assessment is satisfactory then full compression therapy may be applied.
- ABPI ≤0.8 and equal to or above 0.6 (arterial impairment is likely to be significant) – reduced compression therapy may be used under specialist supervision.
- ABPI 0.5 or less (the patient has critical ischaemia) – no compression is to be used.

to control oedema to help reduce the risk of ulcer recurrence. Compression therapy is designed to give graduated compression providing more support at the ankle and less at the knee to squeeze the veins and help the valves to close, thus preventing venous backflow. Compression eases venous congestion, reduces oedema and allows improved blood flow to tissues. As the ulcer heals and the venous disease is controlled, the skin condition should improve (Dini et al. 2020). The venous disease remains when the ulcer heals, so it is important that the patient continues compression therapy even after healing. Bandages are most often multilayer systems using elastic materials or inelastic material (short stretch), or a combination of materials (Fig. 23.7). In the elastic system, bandages are applied in a spiral with a 50% stretch and 50% overlap. Layer 3 (of 4) is applied as a figure of eight. In the inelastic system the bandage is unrolled onto the skin at a 100% stretch with a 50% overlap and application techniques can vary according to the size and shape of the leg. Two-layer systems combine elements of elastic and inelastic materials. The principles of compression therapy are:

- Ensure the lower leg is graduated in shape, i.e. a smaller circumference at the ankle than the calf (if this is not the case padding material is used to form the correct shape).
- The therapy is applied from toes to just below the knee (otherwise oedema will be pushed into the foot).
- When bandaging keep the tension of the bandage the same while the bandage is applied. The graduated shape of the leg will mean that more pressure is applied to the ankle and less as the circumference of the leg increases to the knee – 30–40 mmHg of pressure may be required at the ankle, graduating to 15–20 mmHg below the knee (Partsch and Mortimer 2015).
- Ensure that the bandage, hosiery or wrap does not slip, causing constriction of the limb.

Exercise and Leg Elevation. are very important in managing venous disease. The most effective exercise to aid lower leg

Figure 23.7 Compression bandaging. (A) Padding. (B) Short stretch bandage. (C) Multilayer bandage.

venous return is walking. If this is difficult then the patient must be taught and encouraged to rotate and flex the ankle joint as much as possible to create movement in the calf muscle. When the patient is sitting or lying, they should be encouraged to have their feet higher than their hips to aid drainage of fluid from the lower leg. This can be uncomfortable when sitting and may be easier lying on a bed or couch.

Dressings. Dressing management should be carefully considered once the factors outlined previously have been successfully tackled. The ulcer should be assessed as for wounds and the appropriate material then selected . Caution should be exercised with dressings and lotions as these patients quickly develop sensitivities to many of the commonly used products (Dini et al. 2020). The simplest treatments should be used first, for example non- or low-adherent textile dressings, as the most important part of management is compression. However, more interactive dressings may be selected depending on patient preference and clinical indications. For instance, an antimicrobial, absorbent or pain-reducing dressing may be particularly indicated. A comprehensive patient assessment should aim to result in a complete treatment package. A suitable wound contact dressing and skin care combined with adequate compression therapy, exercise and leg elevation combined with patient education are most likely to produce the best patient outcomes.

🌐 **See Evolve website Critical thinking question 23.2**

Arterial Ulcers

These are often the result of atherosclerosis (John et al. 2022) affecting the arterial supply to the lower leg. The underlying disease processes are different from venous disease (Table 23.3). Damage to the arteries supplying the leg can occur and they gradually become occluded. Additionally, infarction of smaller arteries is caused by embolus formation, which causes ischaemia in the area of skin normally supplied by that artery. What follows is a very rapid breakdown of the skin.

The characteristics of these ulcers are a history of intermittent claudication and rapid onset of a deep ulcer that is often extremely painful. Relief may be gained by lowering the affected limb and hanging it over the edge of the bed or chair. These patients rarely go to bed to sleep, or if they do, they have to get up in the night because of the pain. They tend to sleep in a chair, which allows the affected limb to hang down, optimising the arterial blood supply as gravity aids the arterial blood flow to the foot.

Arterial ulcers can occur anywhere on the lower leg, but usually present on the foot and lateral aspect of the lower leg. Foot pulses are often absent or very difficult to palpate. Doppler assessment reveals that the ankle brachial pressure index (ABPI) is significantly <0.8. There may also be a history of cardiovascular disease, typically hypertension, myocardial infarction, transient ischaemic attacks or stroke (NICE 2012).

Management

Surgical intervention may be necessary to improve the circulation or debridement of the ulcer, and skin grafting may be considered. Compression must be avoided as this would further impede an already poor blood supply to the area. Healing of these wounds is slow and the prognosis for eventual healing often poor. Treatment aims to keep the patient as comfortable as possible, to relieve pain and to achieve debridement and cleansing where necessary. Useful dressings include alginate or hydrofibre sheets if the wound is wet, hydrogel sheets for pain reduction if necessary (where the exudate level is not significant) and topical antimicrobial dressings if necessary. The Lower Limb Strategy (2021) has a useful summary (https://www.nationalwoundcarestrategy.net/wp-content/uploads/2023/07/Leg-Ulcer-Recommendations-Summary-27.07.23.pdf) which guides initial management of wounds on the lower limb until a comprehensive assessment can be carried out. This includes the use of mild graduated compression to manage oedema until a diagnosis is reached as long as there are no overt signs of significant arterial insufficiency. It is important to note however that the recommendation is for assessment to be completed within 14 days.

Mixed Aetiology Ulcers

Around 20% of venous ulcers also have a poor arterial blood supply (Anderson 2018). This further complicates management, as oedema control is needed but without restricting the already compromised blood supply. Reduced levels of compression may be indicated to control oedema but if the arterial disease is progressing then optimising arterial flow must take precedence over managing venous disease. In some cases, a support bandage with sufficient underpadding can be used to control oedema, but this must be under the direction of local protocols and a specialist nurse or doctor to ensure the patient is not harmed. Other types of leg ulcers are outlined in Information 23.7.

Patient Education

Individual education regarding wound management can have a dramatic effect on progress. This aspect of care is particularly appropriate in patients with leg ulcers, especially venous leg ulcers. Patients who understand the cause of their ulcer and the rationale for the treatment and activities they are asked to engage with are much more likely to have a concordant relationship with their practitioner. However, leg ulcers are long-term conditions and patients will need much support and encouragement to continue with treatment. Education can be helped by providing patients with appropriate information to be read at home (Information 23.8).

TABLE 23.3   Characteristics of Venous and Arterial Disease of the Lower Limb

Characteristic	Venous Disease	Arterial Disease
Site of ulcer	Around the 'gaiter' area, commonly above the medial malleolus	Anywhere on the lower limb including the foot, but commonly affecting the toes
Depth of ulcer	Shallow and spreading	Deep, with a punched-out appearance
Presence of oedema	Common, due to poor venous return	Often not detected
Onset	Gradual, unless precipitated by trauma	Rapid
Pain	Often uncomfortable, nagging in character, often worse if oedema increases. Related skin conditions can cause pain, discomfort and itching	Pain, sometimes made worse by elevation of limb relieved by lowering it (the blood flow is increased when the limb is in the dependent position). The pain of ischaemia can be unremitting
Temperature of foot	Warm and well perfused	Cool or cold and poorly perfused
Condition of the skin surrounding the ulcer	Varicose eczema, lipodermatosclerosis	Often shiny and hairless
ABPI	>0.8 (ABPI does not indicate venous disease)	<0.8 (indicates progressive arterial disease as index decreases)

N.B.: It is possible that a combination of both disease processes is present. It is important that a full assessment is conducted.
ABPI, Ankle brachial pressure index.

INFORMATION 23.7

Other Types of Leg Ulcer

The following types of leg ulcer account for between 2% and 5% of lower limb ulcers:

- Vasculitic ulcers – these are due to connective tissue disease, e.g. rheumatoid arthritis and scleroderma, and also occur on the lower leg. They are unusual and extremely difficult to manage due to the underlying disease process and the medication that these patients require.
- Diabetic ulcers – these occur most commonly on the foot (see Chapter 6). Again, due to the general condition of the patient, they heal slowly. It is worth noting that people with diabetes mellitus may give a falsely high reading on Doppler assessment due to peripheral hypertension.

  The management of rheumatoid and diabetic ulcers is generally under specialist care and treatment is prescribed by the individual consultant.

- Miscellaneous causes – neoplastic and tropical ulcers are examples in this category.

Based on data from Moffatt et al. (2007).

INFORMATION 23.8

Leg Ulcer Forum: Patient Information (Leaflet Number 9)

How Can I Help My Venous Leg Ulcer to Heal?

You will be given a lot of information about wearing bandages and doing exercises. Your nurse will have discussed options with you so that you are involved in decisions which affect you. There are lots of things you can do to help your ulcer heal and make you feel better while this is happening.

Wear Your Bandages or Compression Hosiery

You have a problem with the circulation of blood in your veins. When the blood flow slows down, it can cause your ankles to swell. Wearing bandages or hosiery keeps the blood moving efficiently and helps to reduce the swelling in your ankles. This is why you are asked to wear them all the time.

Do Your Exercises

Put your hand on the back of your calf and move your foot up and down. You will feel the muscle move and it is this movement which helps to keep the blood flowing in your legs. This happens when you walk but some people are not able to do this and everyone needs to do a little more exercise. The exercises are simple, you move your feet up and down and rotate your ankle. It is good to do this a few times every hour especially if you have been sitting down for a while. You may have been given a leaflet explaining exercise in more detail. If not ask your nurse or the person prescribing your care for a copy.

Put Your Feet Up

Your ankles swell because of the slow blood flow. You will find that your ankles are less swollen when you have been in bed and it gets worse when you are sitting or standing. If you put your feet up so that they are higher than your hips, the swelling should be reduced.

Some people put their feet on the arm of the settee when they are sitting down, or put a cushion on a coffee table or footstool to rest their feet on. It does not matter as long as your feet are higher than your hips.

If you have stiffness in your hips it may be uncomfortable to sit with your feet up. It may be better to lie on the bed with a couple of pillows or cushions under your ankles. It is helpful to get into a routine for your rest time, perhaps when there is something you enjoy on the radio or television. It is best to have your feet up at least three times a day. When you do not have your feet up remember to do your exercises. It is important to do both.

Eat a Healthy Diet

As your ulcer heals it uses a lot of goodness from the food you eat. It is important that your diet contains protein, vitamins and minerals. These are found in a varied diet of meat, fish, eggs and cheese, as well as fruit and vegetables. Please ask your nurse for information on healthy eating.

It is important to watch your weight. If you are overweight you are putting an extra load on the veins in your legs.

Drink Plenty of Fluids

It is important to drink plenty of fluid during the day (unless you have been told not to by the doctor). This helps your ulcer to heal and helps to keep your skin healthy. Don't worry that this will add to the swelling in your ankles, the fluid here is different. Water is the best drink but you can have other drinks, but be careful not to have too many caffeine drinks or those high in sugar.

Take Your Medication

You may have been given medicine to help reduce the swelling in your ankles. It is important to take this and to wear your bandages or hosiery as well. If you have any questions about medicine you have been given, please discuss this with your doctor, nurse or pharmacist.

Skin Care

The skin on your leg is very delicate. You may already apply cream to your face and you need to look after your legs just as carefully. While you are wearing your bandages the nurse will help you to wash your legs and apply a moisturiser. Only very gentle products should be used on your skin. Avoid using anything with lanolin (wool fat) or perfume. Some baby products contain these.

Keep in Touch

When you have an ulcer you will see your nurse often. When the ulcer has healed, you will still be advised to see the nurse from time to time. If you are worried about your legs, it is important to tell the nurse as soon as possible. Problems might be a sore spot, itching or swelling. It is easier to sort problems out if they are found early.

Do Other Things

You might feel uncomfortable and that your ulcer is taking over your life. Try to do other things that you enjoy and discuss your worries with your nurse. It is important to get the ulcer healed as quickly as possible, but any pain, discomfort or practical difficulties can also be dealt with along the way. This is much easier to do if you and your nurse work together.

Leaflets in the Range

- Venous disorders of the lower leg explained
- What is a venous leg ulcer?
- Arterial disorders of the lower leg explained
- What is a Doppler ultrasound scan?
- I am going for a Duplex scan
- Understanding compression bandaging
- Understanding compression hosiery
- Exercises to improve ulcer healing and help prevent recurrence
- How can I help my venous leg ulcer to heal?
- Care of your skin

Contact Details of the Person Prescribing/Providing Your Care

This leaflet is provided to offer advice but does not intend or claim to cover all eventualities.

If you are concerned you must seek professional help from your nurse or doctor or the person providing your care.

Reproduced with permission from the Leg Ulcer Forum.

Sutured Wounds

Common methods of wound closure are sutures, staples or adhesive glue. The decision which to use is often based on the extent, depth and site of the wound as well as patient circumstances. For instance, there may be a risk of sensitivity to the material used, or the area may be subject to movement and flexion which may make adhesives less useful. A Cochrane Review which considered the merits of different closure methods concluded that each method has benefits in different circumstances and a holistic patient assessment must guide choice (Dumville et al. 2014). Although the vast majority of sutured wounds heal without complication, there is a need for observation of both the patient and their wound for signs of infection by:

- Monitoring changes in vital signs, pulse, temperature or malaise.
- Observing the wound for signs of infection after the initial inflammatory response has passed, i.e. redness, swelling, pain, discharge, heat.
- The best time for removal of sutures depends upon:
  - Wound site – wounds on the head and neck usually heal within 2 days due to the rich blood supply to the area, whereas wounds on the back may take 10–14 days to heal. The skin here is thicker and less vascular.
  - Patient variation – if, during suture removal, the wound begins to gape, then the nurse should stop and refer to the surgeon or a nurse specialist for advice. The skin edges can be pulled back together and held for a few more days with paper sutures.
  - Cosmetic considerations – leaving sutures in for too long can cause excessive scarring.

In general, the principles for managing sutured wounds are to leave the wound undisturbed and the theatre dressing intact unless either the patient or the wound area shows signs that indicate the presence of infection (Bale and Leaper 2000). Disturbing dressings unnecessarily can lead to the entry of bacteria into the wound or disturb newly forming epithelium. Local wound infection can slow down the rate of healing and also increase the amount of scar tissue produced. Careful postoperative observation is important. Ultimately, a severe wound infection can spread into the tissues and also the bloodstream, causing life-threatening septicaemia (Williams and Leaper 1998).

Traumatic Wounds

Patients presenting to the emergency department with traumatic wounds need special consideration. These patients may be shocked or have other injuries and their wounds are often contaminated due to the nature of the trauma (see Chapter 19, The Deteriorating Patient, Recognising and Managing Shock, Chapter 26, Nursing the Patient Who Experiences Trauma).

These wounds are frequently irregular, with varying degrees of tissue loss (Nagle et al. 2022). Due to contamination, wound closure is often not attempted (Bale and Leaper 2000). Mechanical cleansing of the wound is undertaken to remove debris such as glass, wood or tarmac. Where wound closure is attempted, antibiotic cover may be given to prevent infection where thorough exploration or irrigation of the wound is not possible, or in the case of animal bites (Bonham 2016) and the patient also needs to have prophylactic tetanus protection if they are not already covered (Bonham 2016). Patients with extensive injuries are admitted for inpatient treatment. However, the majority of patients with wounds are discharged into the community. They may be instructed to care for the wound themselves or asked to return to the emergency department for any dressing changes, or the community nurse may be asked to manage wound care.

Malignant Wounds

This is one group of wounds where healing is not always the expected outcome of wound management. Carcinomas and sarcomas are most likely to result in ulceration and fungation in the latter stages of the disease (Qui and Good 2021). Such lesions may be associated with advanced breast cancer or malignant melanoma where the cancer ulcerates through the epithelium. The growth of tumours is a complex process that controls blood flow and tissue oxygenation. Tissue hypoxia causes tissue breakdown and encourages anaerobic and aerobic bacterial growth, producing malodour (Adderley and Holt 2014).

Problems encountered with malignant wounds include:

- Wound site – often present in areas which are extremely difficult to dress in terms of keeping the dressing in place, e.g. the chest wall, groin and lower limb.
- Wound size and bulk – it may be difficult to find a dressing sufficiently large to cover the wound. The wound dimensions, shape and high exudate levels mean that dressings have to be bulky, which adds to the difficulties patients have in managing both practically and psychologically (Lister et al. 2019).
- Exudate production – the exudate tends to be thick and sticky. Many dressings that do not adhere to other wound types will do so in the presence of this particularly viscous exudate. Hydrogel sheets and gel are very useful dressings for these wounds.
- Malodour – see Gethin et al. (2023).
- Pain – where nerve endings are exposed, changing dressings and rubbing from dressings can be painful. Keeping the wound covered reduces the irritation to the nerve endings, and using gel dressings may help to reduce pain at dressing changes.

Where healing is not the ultimate aim, wound management should maximise convenience and minimise distress.

Summary: Key Nursing Issues

- Chronic and acute wounds have costs in terms of disruption to patients' lives, reduced quality of life and a huge financial cost in providing care.
- Nurses are key to the effective support and management of people with wounds; however, holistic wound care depends on the skills of many health professionals through interdisciplinary working.
- Evidence-based wound care requires an understanding of wound types and causes.

- Nurses must understand the physiology of wound healing in order to assess wounds.
- The prevention of problems by dealing with underlying factors such as nutritional assessment and optimal nutrition, maintaining continence, pressure relief, compression therapy, etc., are vital aspects of wound management.
- Developments in tissue viability and the management of chronic wounds proceed at a rapid pace and nurses have a professional responsibility to update their knowledge.

Reflection and Learning – What Next?

- **Test** your knowledge by visiting the Evolve website 🌐 and answering the multiple-choice questions and critical thinking questions.
- **Consolidate** your learning by looking at some of the Further Reading suggestions, and specialist websites.
- **Revisit** some of the additional material on the Evolve website.

- **Consider** what you have learnt and how this will help your professional development.
- **Reflect** on how you can apply this knowledge to the care of your patients.
- **Discuss** your learning with your assessor/supervisor, lecturer and colleagues.

References

Adderley UJ, Holt GS. Topical agents and dressings for fungating wounds. Cochrane Database Syst Rev. 2014;2014(5). https://doi.org/10.1002/14651858.CD003948.pub3.

Anderson I. Assessing and managing venous leg ulcers. *Nurs Residential Care.* 2018;20(4):145–148.

Avelino-Silva TJ, Jaluul O. Malnutrition in hospitalized older patients: management strategies to improve patient care and clinical outcomes. *Int J Gerontol.* 2017;11:56–61.

Bale S, Harding DJ, Leaper KG. *An introduction to wounds.* London: Emap Healthcare; 2000.

Bale S, Jones V. *Wound Care Nursing: A Patient-Centred Approach.* Edinburgh: Mosby Elsevier; 2006.

Bartolo K, Hill EA. The association between obstructive sleep apnoea and wound healing: a systematic review. *Sleep Breath.* 2023;27(3):775–787. doi:10.1007/s11325-022-02660-9.

Bonham J. Assessment and management of patients with minor traumatic wounds. *Nurs Stand.* 2016;31(8):60–71. doi:10.7748/ns.2016.e10573.

Braden BJ. Risk assessment in pressure ulcer prevention. In: Krasner D, Kane D, eds. *Chronic Wound Care.* Wayne, PA: Health Management Publications; 1997.

Coleman S, Nelson EA, Vowden P, et al. Improving Wound Care Project Board, as part of NHS England's Leading Change Adding Value Framework. Development of a generic wound care assessment minimum data set. *J Tissue Viability.* 2017;26(4):226–240.

Coleman S, Smith IL, McGinnis E, et al. Clinical evaluation of a new pressure ulcer risk assessment instrument, the Pressure Ulcer Risk Primary or Secondary Evaluation Tool (PURPOSE T). *J Adv Nurs.* 2018;74(2):407–424.

De Mauri A, Carrera D, Vidali M, et al. Compliance, adherence and concordance differently predict the improvement of uremic and microbial toxins in chronic kidney disease on low protein diet. *Nutrients.* 2022;14(3):487.

DesJardins-Park HE, Foster DS, Longaker MT. Editorial: fibroblasts and wound healing: an update *Regen. Med.* 2018;13(5):491–495.

Dini V, Janowska A, Oranges T, De Pascalis A, Iannone M, Romanelli M. Surrounding skin management in venous leg ulcers: A systematic review. *J Tissue Viability.* 2020;29(3):169–175.

Dumville JC, Coulthard P, Worthington HV, et al. Tissue adhesives for closure of surgical incisions. *Cochrane Database Syst Rev.* 2014(11):CD004287.

Egsleer D, Hödl M, Lohrmann C. Nutritional management of older hospitalised patients with pressure injuries. *Int Wound J.* 2019;16(1):226–232. doi:10.1111/iwj.13016.

European Pressure Ulcer Advisory Panel, National Pressure Injury Advisory Panel and Pan Pacific Pressure Injury Alliance. In: Haesler Emily, ed. *Prevention and Treatment of Pressure Ulcers: Clinical Practice Guideline. The International Guideline.* EPUAP/NPIAP/PPPIA; 2019.

Fletcher J. Why do we prevent pressure ulcers and treat a leg ulcers? *Wounds UK.* 2022;18(1). https://www.wounds-uk.com/journals/issue/657/article-details/why-do-we-prevent-pressure-ulcers-and-treat-leg-ulcers.

Gethin G, Murphy L, Sezgin D, Carr PJ, Mcintosh C, Probst S. Resigning oneself to a life of wound related odour- a thematic analysis of patient experiences. *J Tissue Viability..* 2023;32(4):460–464. https://doi.org/10.1016/j.jtv.2023.07.004.

Guest JF, Fuller GW, Vowden P. Venous leg ulcer management in clinical practice in the UK: costs and outcomes. *Int Wound J.* 2018;15:29–37.

Guest JF, Fuller GW, Vowden P. Cohort study evaluating the burden of woundsto the UK's National Health Service in 2017/2018: update from 2012/2013. *BMJ Open.* 2020;10:e045253. doi:10.1136/bmjopen-2020-045253.

Gardner SE, Abbott LI, Fiala CA, Rakel BA. Factors associated with high pain intensity during wound care procedures: a model. *Wound Repair Regen.* 2017;25(4):558–563. doi:10.1111/wrr.12553.

Gould LJ, Liu J, Wan R, Carter MJ, Dotson M, Driver VR. Evidence supporting wound care end points relevant to clinical practice and patients' lives. Part 3: The Patient Survey. *Wound Repair Regen.* 2020;29:60–69. doi:10.1111/wrr.12872.

Hankins F, Charlesworth G, Hearty P, Wright N, Sheard L. What are the sources of patient experience feedback in the UK prison setting, and what do patients and healthcare staff think about giving and receiving feedback in prison? A qualitative study. *Patient Experience J.* 2022;9(1):138–145. doi:10.35680/2372-0247.1603.

Hassanshahi A, Moradzad M, Ghalamkari S, Fadaei M, Cowin AJ, Hassanshahi M. Macrophage-Mediated Inflammation in Skin Wound Healing. *Cells.* 2022;11:2953. https://doi.org/10.3390/cells11192953.

Health Protection Agency. Healthcare associated infections (HAI): point prevalence survey. 2017. England. https://assets.publishing.service.gov.uk/government/uploads/system/uploads/attachment_data/file/1123846/SSI-annual-report-2021-to-2022.pdf.

House SL. Psychological distress and its impact on wound healing. *J Wound Ostomy Continence Nurs.* 2015;42(1):38–41.

International Wound Infection Institute. IWII Wound Infection in Clinical Practice consensus document: 2022 update. *J Wound Care. (WUWHS Supplement).* 2022;31(12):S10–S21.

John J, Tate S, Price A. Non-surgical treatment for arterial ulcers: a narrative review. *J Wound Care.* 2022;31(11).

Kapp S, Santamaria N. The financial and quality-of-life cost to patients living with a chronic wound in the community. *Int Wound J.* 2017;14:1108–1119.

Lim CS, Baruah M, Bahia SS. Diagnosis and management of venous leg ulcers. *BMJ.* 2018;362:k3115.

Lister S, Hofland J, Grafton H, Wilson C. (Eds). *The Royal Marsden manual of clinical nursing procedures.* John Wiley & Sons; 2012.

Marks J, Hughes LE, Harding KG, et al. Prediction of healing time as an aid to the management of open granulating wounds. *World J Surg.* 1983;7:641–645.

McDaniel JC, Browning KK. Smoking, chronic wound healing, and implications for evidence-based practice. *J Wound Ostomy Continence Nurs.* 2014;41(5):415–423.

Morton LM, Phillips TJ. Wound healing and treating wounds: differential diagnosis and evaluation of chronic wounds. *J Am Acad Dermatol.* 2016;74:589–605.

Nagle SM, Stevens KA, Wilbraham SC. Wound Assessment. *StatPearls [Internet].* Treasure Island (FL): StatPearls Publishing; 2022 2023 Jan–. PMID: 29489199.

NHS England. 2017/19 CQUIN. CQUIN Guidance. 2017. https://www.england.nhs.uk/nhs-standard-contract/cquin/cquin-17-19/.

NHS EstatesInfection Control in the Built EnvironmentNorwich. TSO; 2002.

NHS Improvement. Pressure ulcers: revised definition and measurement. 2018a. https://www.england.nhs.uk/pressure-ulcers-revised-definition-and-measurement-framework/.

NHS Improvement. Pressure ulcer core curriculum. 2018b. https://www.england.nhs.uk/pressure-ulcer-core-curriculum/.

NHS Improvement. Pressure ulcers: productivity calculator. 2018c. https://www.england.nhs.uk/pressure-ulcers-productivity-calculator/.

National Institute of Health and Clinical Excellence (NICE). *Peripheral arterial disease: diagnosis and management.* Clinical guideline [CG147]; 2012. https://www.nice.org.uk/guidance/cg147/resources/peripheral-arterial-disease-diagnosis-and-management-pdf-35109575873989.

National Institute for Health and Care Excellence (NICE). *Pressure ulcers: prevention and management of pressure ulcers.* Clinical guideline [CG179]; 2014. Available at: https://www.nice.org.uk/guidance/cg179/chapter/1-recommendations.

National Institute for Health and Care Excellence (NICE) (2015). *Pressure ulcers.* Quality standard [QS89]; 2015. https://www.nice.org.uk/guidance/qs89.

National Institute for Health and Care Excellence (NICE). *Surgical site infections: prevention and treatment.* Clinical guideline [CG74]; 2017. https://www.nice.org.uk/guidance/CG74/chapter/1-Guidance#preoperative-phase.

National Institute for Health and Care Excellence (NICE) (2020)

Surgical site infections: prevention and treatment NICE guideline [NG125]. 2020. https://www.nice.org.uk/guidance/ng125.

Nicholls E. Wound assessment part 1: How to measure a wound. *Wound Essentials.* 2015;10(2):51–55.

National Pressure Injury Advisory Panel (NPIAP) (2016). NPIAP pressure injury stages. https://cdn.ymaws.com/npiap.com/resource/resmgr/online_store/npiap_pressure_injury_stages.pdf.

National Wound Care Strategy (2021). Surgical wound recommendations. https://www.nationalwoundcarestrategy.net/wp-content/uploads/2021/05/Surgical-Wound-Recommendations-WEB-25Feb21-1.pdf.

Partsch H, Mortimer P. Compression for leg wounds. *Br J Dermatol.* 2015;173(2):359–369.

Public Health England. Surveillance of surgical site infections in NHS Hospitals in England April 2016 to March 2017. 2017. https://assets.publishing.service.gov.uk/government/uploads/system/uploads/attachment_data/file/666465/SSI_annual_report_NHS_hospitals_2016–17.pdf.

Public Health England. *Surveillance of surgical site infection in NHS hospitals in England 2018/19.* London: Public Health England; 2019. https://assets.publishing.service.gov.uk/government/uploads/system/uploads/attachment_data/file/854182/SSI_Annual_Report_2018_19.pdf.

PRSB (2023). Wound care standard. https://theprsb.org/standards/wound-care-standard/.

Qui JM, Good MD. Making the best of multidisciplinary care for patients with malignant fungating wounds: A qualitative study of clinicians' narratives. *Palliat Med.* 2021;35(1):179–188.

Raziyeva K, Kim Y, Zharkinbekov Z, Kassymbek K, Jimi S, Saparov A. Immunology of acute and chronic wound healing. *Biomolecules.* 2021;11(5). doi:10.3390/biom11050700.

Resch A, Staud C, Radtke C. Nanocellulose-based wound dressing for conservative wound management in children with second-degree burns. *Int Wound J.* 2021;18(4):478–486. doi:10.1111/iwj.13548.

Sandy-Hodgetts K, et al. *Optimising Prevention of Surgical Wound Complications: Detection, Diagnosis and Prediction.* London: Wounds International; 2022. www.woundsinternational.com.

Schoonhoven L, Haalboom JR, Buskens E, et al. Prognostic ability of risk assessment scales. *EPUAP Rev.* 2002;4(1):17–18.

Scottish Intercollegiate Guidelines Network (SIGN). *Management of chronic venous leg ulcers.* A national clinical guideline [SIGN120]; 2010. https://www.sign.ac.uk/assets/sign120.pdf.

Vowden P, Vowden K. The importance of accurate methodology in ABPI calculation when assessing lower limb wounds. *Br J Community Nurs.* 2018;23(Suppl 3):S16.

Williams NA, Leaper DJ. Infection. In: Leaper DJ, Harding KG, eds. *Wounds: Biology and Management.* Oxford: Oxford Medical Publications; 1998.

Winter GD. Formation of the scab and rate of epithelialization of superficial wounds in the skin of the young domestic pig. *Nature.* 1962;193:293–294.

Woo KY. Unravelling nocebo effect: the mediating effect of anxiety between anticipation and pain at wound dressing change. *J Clin Nurs.* 2015;24:1975–1984.

Wounds UK. *Best Practice Statement: Post-Operative Wound Care – Reducing the Risk Of Surgical Site Infection.* London: Wounds UK; 2020. https://www.wounds-uk.com.

Wounds UK. *Best Practice Statement: addressing skin tone bias in wound care: assessing signs and symptoms in people with dark skin tones.* UK, London: Wounds; 2021. https://www.wounds-uk.com/resources/details/addressing-skin-tone-bias-wound-care-assessing-signs-and-symptoms-people-dark-skin-tones.

Wounds UK. *Best Practice Statement: active treatment of non-healing wounds in the community.* London: Wounds UK; 2022. https://www.wounds-uk.com.

Xue M, Jackson CJ. Extracellular matrix reorganization during wound healing and its impact on abnormal scarring. *Adv Wound Care (New Rochelle).* 2015;4(3):119–136.

Useful Websites

Aseptic Non Touch Technique (ANTT), www.antt.org

Cochrane Reviews (systematic reviews of evidence related to wound care and infection control), www.cochrane.org/reviews/en/topics/96_reviews.html

Cochrane Wounds Group, http://wounds.cochrane.org/

Diabetic Foot Study Group, www.dfsg.org

European Pressure Ulcer Advisory Panel (EPUAP) (e.g. resources/guidelines related to the prevention and management of pressure ulcers), www.epuap.org/glprevention.html

European Wound Management Association (EWMA) (resources and position documents related to wound care, including leg ulcer management), www.ewma.org/english/publications.html

International Wound Infection Institute, www.woundinfection-institute.com

Leg Ulcer Forum, www.legulcerforum.org

NHS Diabetes (e.g. foot care guidance), www.diabetes.nhs.uk

National Wound Care Strategy, https://www.nationalwoundcarestrategy.net

Scottish Intercollegiate Guidelines Network (SIGN) (e.g. The diagnosis and management of peripheral arterial disease), www.sign.ac.uk/pdf/sign89.pdf

Society of Tissue Viability, https://www.youtube.com/watch?v=36EXz8Dmr3o&list=PLoKuDJo_vt6DIoqOEzteffvMWaf_j_84B

Stop the Pressure You Tube Channel, https://www.youtube.com/channel/UC0AJoyu_5kZxO1aOTItK7WA

Nursing Times series on the aSSKING bundle, https://www.nursingtimes.net/clinical-archive/clinical-series/#21

Wound Care Handbook, https://www.woundcarehandbook.com/

24

Maintaining Continence

SUSAN WALKER

CHAPTER OUTLINE

Introduction

Having control over urinary and faecal elimination is an expected norm within every society. In all but the very young, loss of continence is generally not viewed with sympathy and the real suffering it causes to individuals and their carers has not received the attention it deserves. Epidemiological research has shown that the number of people suffering from loss of continence in some form or other far exceeds the number of cases reported to health professionals. An underlying theme of this chapter is the need to acknowledge the extent of the problem and to promote continence by improving screening practices and raising public and professional awareness of preventive measures against incontinence and of the range of treatments available.

Loss of continence is a symptom that is often wrongly labelled as a disease. This chapter describes the underlying conditions that can prevent the acquisition of continence or provoke its loss. It is argued that a sound understanding of the causes and types of loss of continence is essential for its proper investigation, nursing management and treatment and that diagnostic assessment must recognise the individuality of each person. Similarly, where incontinence is intractable, assessment for aids and equipment must be sensitive to the values, needs and priorities of each person in order to ensure that an optimal quality of life (QoL) is achieved.

Throughout the chapter the emphasis is on a positive, problem-solving approach towards this often hidden problem, to reflect upon personal attitudes towards the subject of loss of continence, and to provide evidence-based care based on up-to-date research. Health promotion activities and nursing management are key in assisting people to maintain continence. However, if continence is impaired, then the purpose is to assist individuals to regain continence whenever possible. Should incontinence be intractable, it is necessary for the nurse and other health professional to work in partnership with the individual to find solutions to problems that enhance the person's QoL. Nurses working within an interdisciplinary team (IDT) fulfil a central role in the prevention of loss of continence.

CONTINENCE

The acquisition of continence in early childhood is a much-valued developmental milestone. In the adult, the ability to control urinary and faecal elimination is largely taken for granted, and a loss of continence will have profound implications for the individual's ability to participate fully within society. While it may be deemed acceptable for a child to have an occasional 'accident', this is not generally the case for adults. The issue of loss of continence is one that many people find difficult to discuss openly, and one that is poorly understood.

The onus is on health professionals to foster a change in social attitudes by acquiring a clear understanding of how continence is attained and how loss of continence can develop. Nurses can make an important contribution to the promotion of continence among particularly vulnerable groups.

Defining Continence

Continence may be defined in terms of the actions and abilities necessary for the appropriate management of urinary and faecal elimination. These include:

- recognising the need to pass urine or faeces
- identifying the correct place to pass urine or faeces
- delaying elimination until the appropriate place is reached
- reaching the correct place
- passing urine or faeces appropriately once a suitable place is reached.

Acquiring Urinary Continence

Urinary continence cannot be acquired until the nerve pathways necessary for micturition have matured. Once this has taken place, becoming continent is a matter of imitation, skill attainment and social conditioning.

The bladder acts as a reservoir for urine and it contracts to expel urine at the volition of the individual. Urine remains in the bladder as long as the intravesical (within the bladder) pressure does not exceed the urethral resistance.

In normal micturition, the contraction of the detrusor (expelling) muscle of the bladder induces the bladder neck to open while the pelvic floor muscles and the external urinary sphincter relax. For a child to obtain continence, they must acquire control of the mechanisms that prevent the bladder from automatically emptying when it is full; this is usually achieved by the age of 3 years.

The neurological control of the bladder at birth involves a simple sacral reflex arc whereby automatic filling and emptying of the bladder are under the control of some sacral segments of the spinal

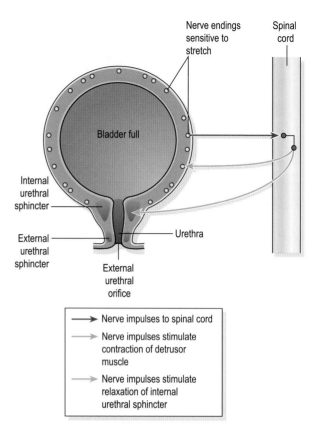

Figure 24.1 Reflex control of micturition when conscious effort cannot override the reflex action. (Reproduced from Waugh A, Grant A. *Ross and Wilson: Anatomy and Physiology in Health and Illness*. 13th ed. Edinburgh: Churchill Livingstone; 2018, with permission.)

cord. Nerve endings in the bladder wall are activated by stretch as urine accumulates. These relay impulses with increasing frequency through the parasympathetic nerves to the spinal cord until the motor parasympathetic nerve impulses cause the bladder muscle to contract and the urethral sphincters to open, whereupon reflex emptying occurs (Fig. 24.1).

In order to achieve continence, a child needs to become aware of the sensation of bladder filling and through trial and error attempt to overcome the reflex emptying mechanism by using the pelvic floor muscles to keep the urethral sphincter closed. Sensory impulses from the bladder travel in the spinal cord to the cerebral cortex, whereupon motor impulses from the cerebral cortex travel to the bladder to inhibit the bladder contractions; this requires practice as well as maturation of the central nervous system. Continence thus involves the active inhibition of nerve impulses. When micturition is initiated, the brain ceases to initiate inhibitory impulses, allowing the spinal reflex arc to be completed. Fig. 24.2 illustrates the control of micturition once bladder control is established.

Normal patterns of micturition can vary markedly from one individual to another. Normally, the adult bladder contains around 200–400 mL of urine before the urge to pass urine becomes too great. Most adults empty their bladder four to six times a day and have a bladder capacity of up to 600 mL (or more); this is influenced by age, fluid intake, medication, perspiration, body temperature, activity and stress. People who are anxious generally feel the need to empty their bladders more often; in the event of acute emotional distress or sudden shock, it is possible for involuntary bladder emptying to occur.

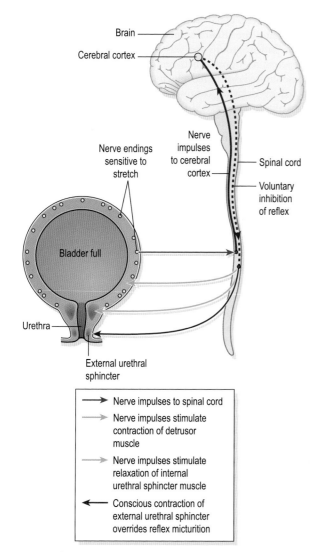

Brain

Cerebral cortex

Nerve impulses to cerebral cortex

Nerve endings sensitive to stretch

Spinal cord

Voluntary inhibition of reflex

Bladder full

Urethra

External urethral sphincter

→ Nerve impulses to spinal cord

→ Nerve impulses stimulate contraction of detrusor muscle

→ Nerve impulses stimulate relaxation of internal urethral sphincter muscle

← Conscious contraction of external urethral sphincter overrides reflex micturition

Figure 24.2 Control of micturition after bladder control has been established. (Reproduced from Waugh A, Grant A. *Ross and Wilson: Anatomy and Physiology in Health and Illness*. 13th ed. Edinburgh: Churchill Livingstone; 2018, with permission.)

Acquiring Faecal Continence

Defecation is the expulsion of faecal matter from the rectum with the aid of peristaltic movements of the muscular walls of the intestine. As with urination, involuntary or autonomic reflex defecation occurs in the infant and young child, until voluntary control of the external sphincter is gained. Children usually gain this control in the second or third year of life.

The rectum is stimulated to empty by strong peristaltic waves (mass movements) in the colon; these are initiated by the gastrocolic reflex (a sensory stimulus that happens when food enters the stomach). The need for defecation is felt as a response to distension of the sigmoid colon and the stimulation of the receptors.

Anxiety can produce an urge to defecate more often, and in situations of extreme crisis, faecal control can be temporarily lost.

Attitudes Towards Loss of Continence

In the UK, attitudes towards loss of continence are slowly changing. Loss of continence is becoming an acceptable subject for open discussion and began to be addressed openly in the media from 1985 onwards. Today, advertisements for absorbent products fill many magazine pages and television commercials. Nevertheless, certain myths still persist, such as the notion that incontinence is an inevitable consequence of old age, or that wearing pads is the only solution. Such myths must be dispelled in favour of seeking the underlying cause of incontinence in each individual case.

The psychosocial implications of incontinence are far-reaching and have a severe impact on QoL. Social exclusion is common, as individuals with incontinence are often afraid to leave home, afraid they may be unable to access a lavatory in time or experience an episode of incontinence in the presence of others. Avoiding everyday activities such as work, exercising and enjoying the company of others often leads to social isolation (Bladder Interest Group 2021). For those who rely on others for assistance to the toilet, risk of incontinence is increased, in particular, for those living with dementia who are at significant risk of developing urinary and/or faecal incontinence (Edwards et al. 2021). Difficulty in reaching the toilet in time and lack of ability to manipulate clothing may lead to an episode of incontinence leading to embarrassment and, often in the long-term, depression. It is important for nurses to examine their own attitude towards bladder, bowel and continence care (see Evidence-Based Practice 24.1).

The Royal College of Physicians (RCP) in 2010 published findings of a national audit about the quality of care and services for people with bladder and bowel incontinence in England, Wales and Northern Ireland. The report detailed the care given to 18,253 people, in a variety of National Health Service (NHS) settings, including wards, clinics, mental health hospitals and care homes. The audit findings were shared with all who contributed and showed a real need for improvement in continence care for people with bladder and bowel problems. The results highlighted that 'Overall, adherence to national guidance (NICE) for urinary and faecal incontinence is very variable' and that 'Quality of care (assessment, diagnosis and treatment) is worse in older people (patients aged 65 years and over as compared with those aged <65)' (RCP 2010, p. 6).

Based on the 2010 audit, the RCP published in 2011 a document 'Keeping control: What you should expect from your NHS bladder and bowel service'. This document worked to inform both the public and NHS staff of the level of care and service to be expected. Further guidance published by NHS England continues to support the need for better continence care. NHS England's (2018) 'Excellence in Continence Care' indicates minimum standards of competence and knowledge for those involved in continence care. The Nursing and Midwifery Council's (NMC) (2018b) 'Future Nurse: Standards of Proficiency for Registered Nurses' makes clear that registered nurses must use evidenced-based, best practice approaches for meeting the needs of individuals requiring care and support with bladder and bowel health, accurately assessing the individual's capacity for independence and self-care and initiating appropriate interventions

IMPACT OF COVID-19 ON CONTINENCE SERVICES

As part of the EPICCC-19 national survey, Palmer at al. (2022) conducted an online survey of 65 community continence services in England to establish the professional perspectives on impacts, benefits and disadvantages of changes made to community continence services during the COVID-19 pandemic. In response to the COVID-19 pandemic, changes were made to the organisation

'We Tend to Get Pad Happy': A Qualitative Study of Health Practitioners' Perspectives on the Quality of Continence Care for Older People in Hospital

Bladder and bowel control difficulties are particularly prevalent in those aged 65 and over. However, according to Percival et al. (2021) the quality of continence can often be poor, impacting on the general health and wellbeing of the person and increasing the risk of infection. Incontinence in the older population is a key factor leading to admission to nursing or residential care home placement. Percival et al. (2021) conducted 27 qualitative interviews with nursing, medical and allied health practitioners in three hospitals, using purposive sampling and thematic analysis in order to identify factors that help or hinder good continence care for those aged 65 and over in hospital, medical ward settings.

Results

Good continence care was said to be promoted and delivered through person-centred care, robust assessment, monitoring and a proactive approach to encourage self-care and independence.

Barriers were identified as oversight, automatic use of incontinence products and pressures due to low staffing levels.

Suggested improvements included partnership working in continence care, a more person-centred approach, open communication and greater emphasis when care planning on bladder and bowel health.

Conclusions

Findings give some explanation for the persistence of barriers in the provision of good-quality care to those aged over 65 in the hospital medical ward setting. Greater emphasis on continence promotion and throughout the NHS would reduce reliance on containment products and the risk of catheter associated gram-negative bacteraemia. Robust nursing assessment, planning, implementation and evaluation of continence, with regular training updates for staff, may mitigate resource limitations and aid delivery of person-centred time-efficient continence care.

Activity

- Access Percival et al. full paper. Discuss the main findings of their study with your practice supervisor, practice assessor or a colleague.
- Which continence assessment tools have you seen used?
- Consider how you explore the views of older patients in your care with regard to their continence status.
- Have you been in a clinical area when the continence nurse specialist/advisor was consulted?

Resources

Percival J, Abbott K, Allain T, et al. 'We tend to get pad happy': a qualitative study of health practitioners' perspectives on the quality of continence care for older people in hospital. *BMJ Open Qual.* 2021;10:e001380. doi:10.1136/bmjoq-2021-001380.

investigation/tests could lead to missed diagnosis or initiation of inappropriate care. Remote/online consultation posed difficulties for some patient groups and was also seen to limit the building of a therapeutic relationship between professionals and patients. Staff were also limited due to redeployment during the pandemic which impacted by delaying continence care provision. Results overall from participants indicated that continence care was perceived to have been deprioritised and undervalued.

The survey concluded that whilst efficiency and convenience may be achieved for some, through utilisation of remote/online consultations, physical 'in-person' consultation is preferable and much valued for best-quality, person-centred community continence care.

Continence services are working to resume and restore pre-COVID services to meet the needs of the communities they serve.

Equality and diversity in access to services are key in ensuring fairness. Those with physical disability may need home visits, and those with a learning disability may require support from a family member or a support worker to ensure they receive information in a way they are able to understand and respond to. Those from certain ethnic, religious or cultural backgrounds may prefer to be examined by a same-sex health professional.

According to Parker and Crabtree (2017), there is growing apathy to care and support in the UK. This makes the most vulnerable at risk. The continuing ageing population also has impact on health and social care needs and the financial implications of meeting health and social care costs within a changing demography.

Reaching out to marginalised groups such as the homeless who are in poverty and socially excluded to encourage them to access healthcare services is very difficult. Estimates from 2018 suggest that 280,000 people experienced homelessness in England, with over 4000 people classed as 'unsheltered or 'rough sleepers' (Ministry of Housing, Communities and Local Government 2018).

Many of these people may be affected by bladder and bowel issues which contribute to a decline in their overall health status, which is already compromised through homelessness. Within the UK there is a drive, to meet the healthcare needs of this marginalised group, supported by the Care Quality Commission (CQC) (2022) and their standard of care for homeless people. GPs have a responsibility to register people who are homeless, or of no fixed abode. A homeless person may register under a friend's name, a day centre or the GP practice address itself. The CQC (2022) also gives examples of good practice which include longer timed appointments for the homeless person, keeping prescriptions short, ensuring clear boundaries (which applies for all patient's), giving fast access and waiving charges for housing letters and medical reports.

Healthcare professionals within the UK, often working alongside charities, actively take healthcare services out to the homeless, offering the homeless person an opportunity to speak to a healthcare professional and seek advice, treatment and referral if necessary.

INCONTINENCE

This section of the chapter outlines the prevalence, types and causes of urinary and faecal incontinence and medical management.

Urinary Incontinence

The National Institute for Health and Care Excellence (NICE) (2015) defines urinary incontinence in line with the International Continence Society as 'the complaint of involuntary leakage of urine'.

and delivery of NHS community continence services for adults and children experiencing bladder and bowel problems. The benefits of continence services for those who use them, on both physical and mental health and QoL, are well known. The survey explored professional perspectives on the impact of changes in continence services in relation to practice, care provision and patient experience. A thematic analysis of open and closed question responses was conducted. Results indicated that the use of remote/online consultations enabled continuation of continence care, and increased access as time efficient, which was favoured by some patients however, physical examination and investigation/tests were not possible. There were raised concerns that lack of physical assessment and

NHS England (2018) estimates that 14 million men, women, young people and children are living with bladder problems.

It is recognised that although urinary incontinence affects all age groups, male and female, its prevalence is greatest amongst women, particularly older women (NICE 2015).

It is only when the specific type and cause of the person's incontinence are known that appropriate treatment can be offered.

Types and Causes of Urinary Incontinence

Stress Urinary Incontinence (SUI) results from a failure of the urethral sphincter to remain closed when a sudden increase in abdominal pressure on the bladder occurs, for example on effort or exertion, during coughing, sneezing or laughing. The weak pelvic floor allows the urethra to descend and the sphincter to open, releasing urine.

Urge Incontinence results from the contraction of the detrusor muscle of the bladder as if to void, although the bladder may not be full. This may be caused by overactive detrusor function (motor urgency) or by hypersensitivity (sensory urgency).

Mixed Incontinence is the involuntary leakage of urine associated with both urgency and exertion, effort, sneezing or coughing.

Overflow Incontinence occurs as a consequence of urinary retention, which may in turn result from:
- obstruction, e.g. tumour, faecal impaction or prostatic enlargement
- underactive detrusor muscle, resulting in a flaccid bladder and thus failure to generate enough pressure to open the urethra
- failure of the urethra to open.

Reflex Incontinence may occur as a result of damage to the spinal cord and loss of sensation associated with the desire to micturate, leading to failure to inhibit the simple reflex arc.

Enuresis refers to any involuntary loss of urine during the day or night time. Nocturnal enuresis is the term for urinary incontinence that occurs during sleep, in the absence of organic disease or infection (not to be confused with nocturia, which is being woken at night by the urge to pass urine). Enuresis may be primary or secondary. Nocturnal enuresis is most common in children. Education and Resources for Improving Childhood Continence (ERIC) a national charity dedicated to improving bladder and bowel health for children, indicates that 12% of 7- to 9-year-olds regularly wet the bed, with up to 2% continuing into their teenage years. Some children gain continence and then begin bed wet again. This is referred to as secondary enuresis, and causes may be psychological/psychosocial, including insecurity and bullying (ERIC 2017, www.eric.org). The number of adults afflicted with nocturnal enuresis is uncertain, due to the hidden nature of the problem.

There are three conditions that may contribute to enuresis, often in combination:
- a reduced bladder capacity
- an inability to concentrate urine at night
- difficulty in waking when the bladder is full.

Functional incontinence. An individual with this type of incontinence would, in favourable circumstances, be able to remain continent but is prevented by pre-existing disease or disability from gaining access to an appropriate place at an appropriate time to pass urine. Conditions that may affect mobility and dexterity, and therefore continence, include multiple sclerosis (MS), spina bifida, arthritis and spinal cord injury. In addition, conditions associated with ageing, such as slowness of movement, pain, joint stiffness, inability to climb stairs or difficulty in manipulating fastenings, may all contribute to incontinence.

Faecal Incontinence

According to NICE (2007), faecal incontinence is a not a diagnosis but is a symptom or sign. Reaching a consensus on a definition of faecal incontinence is difficult. NICE (2014) offers the definition as 'involuntary loss of faeces that is a social or hygiene problem, in adults (18 years or older) in the community and the hospital'. The Royal College of Nursing (RCN) (2019) concurs with this definition, but adds 'passive soiling (liquid or solid) which occurs when an individual is unaware liquid or solid stool is leaking from the anus; this may be after a bowel movement or at any time'. The prevalence of faecal incontinence in the UK is difficult to ascertain as it remains a taboo subject and people are reluctant to discuss their problems or seek help, due to embarrassment, anxiety and fear. It is estimated that faecal incontinence is experienced by 10% of the adult population, with 1%–2% reporting major symptoms (Royal College of Surgeons [RCS] 2017). It is known that faecal incontinence is more common in older people, particularly frail older women, increasingly so in those with cognitive impairment and reduced or lost functional ability and mobility. Prevalence rates for older people living in UK care homes are much higher than the general population (Goodman et al. 2015). As previously mentioned, faecal incontinence is an associated symptom to disease and illness such as MS; according to Dibley (2017), faecal incontinence occurs in 50% of people with MS, causing significant distress.

While urinary incontinence is more prevalent in the population than faecal incontinence, the latter is the more distressing problem. Faecal incontinence is socially even less acceptable than urinary incontinence and raises strong emotions among carers who have to deal with it. It is a source of discomfort and acute embarrassment for the sufferer, and contributes to feelings of helplessness, loss of self-esteem and social isolation.

Types and Causes of Faecal Incontinence

The causes of faecal incontinence must be determined before treatment is instigated. Other than simple constipation, faecal impaction with overflow diarrhoea (spurious diarrhoea), the main cause of faecal incontinence, is usually damage to the pelvic floor and anal sphincters (such as during childbirth, rectal prolapse or surgery), resulting in an inability to recognise that the rectum is full or to distinguish between flatus and faeces.

Causes of faecal incontinence in adults include:
- Faecal impaction with overflow diarrhoea in very frail older people and often those with dementia and physical disability.
- Diarrhoea/intestinal hurry caused by gastroenteritis, inflammatory bowel disease (IBD) (see Chapter 4, Nursing Patients With Gastrointestinal, Liver and Biliary Disorders) and medications such as antibiotics, excessive use of laxatives and some foods.
- Neurological disease which may include spinal nerve injury, spina bifida, stroke and diseases such as Parkinson's and MS.
- Anal sphincter damage due to direct trauma caused during childbirth or surgery.

Rao (2004) states that many people who experience faecal incontinence refer to themselves as having diarrhoea or urgency as this seems more tolerable. Rao refers to faecal incontinence being graded in relation to its severity:

- Passive – involuntary discharge of faecal matter or flatus without awareness. The person may have impaired perception or impaired reflexes. There may also be sphincter dysfunction.
- Urge – involuntary discharge of faecal matter or flatus, in spite of active attempts to retain the bowel contents. This is usually related to sphincter disruption.
- Seepage – undesired leakage after a normal bowel movement. Mostly, this is due to incomplete evacuation of the bowel contents and/or impaired rectal sensation. The sphincter function and the pudendal nerve are mostly intact.

Faecal incontinence or soiling in children is termed 'encopresis' and is defined as the passage of a normal consistency stool in a socially unacceptable place. Involuntary defecation, also known as reflex defecation, occurs in infants as they have not developed control over the external anal sphincter. A child by the age of 2 or 3 years can normally override this reflex. Should a child not have gained control by the age of 4 years, the term encopresis is used. Encopresis occurs in 2.8% of 4-year-olds, 1.9% of 6-year-olds and 1.6% of 10-year-olds (Philichi 2008), with 1% of teenagers suffering from bowel incontinence (www.eric.org).

Often, the most common reason for faecal incontinence in children is constipation, as an overloaded bowel cannot empty as required.

Epidemiology of Incontinence – Prevalence Studies

Seminal research into the prevalence of incontinence by Thomas et al. (1980) found that whilst incontinence was most prevalent among older women, its occurrence was significant across all age groups. Stress incontinence was reported less often by nulliparous than by parous women of all ages, and was especially prevalent among those who had borne four or more children. Urge incontinence also occurred more commonly among parous than nulliparous women. No significant class differences were found among men or women, but individuals of African Caribbean or part African Caribbean descent were more likely to have some form of incontinence than those of Asian descent.

The most important finding of the study, however, was the ratio of known to unknown cases of incontinence. This suggests that for every incontinent person who is known to health or social services professionals, there are 10 others who are unidentified. As further in-depth interviews revealed, many people try to 'cope' with moderate to severe problems of incontinence without professional support. These findings identify the need for healthcare workers to take advantage of all appropriate opportunities in all care settings to identify those who require assessment and treatment for incontinence.

The *Essence of Care Benchmark for Bladder, Bowel and Continence Care* recommended that nurses use a 'trigger' question to initiate conversation that may lead to further assessment of a person's continence, bladder and bowel status (Department of Health (DH) 2010). The Minimum Standards for Continence Care in the UK report of 2015 reflects the importance of skilled and sensitive assessment by healthcare staff. The standards indicate that staff should be trained to assess, treat and refer individuals as required. This includes having knowledge of the anatomy and physiology relevant to continence status and an understanding of the impact of impaired continence on the individual affected. The healthcare professional must be able to 'red flag' signs and symptoms, and understand and initiate any conservative treatment, knowing when to refer onwards if necessary.

The NMC (2018) state that nurses must prioritise people, practice safely, preserve safety and promote professionalism and trust. Platform 1 of the 'Future Nurse: Standards of Proficiency for Registered Nurses' (NMC 2018) states, 'It is the nurses responsibility to act as an accountable professional, always acting in the best interest of people, putting them first and providing care that is person centred and compassionate'.

It is recognised that the nurse asking a question provides an opportunity for the person to talk about this sensitive subject. An open question offers the opportunity for an in-depth answer, for example 'Tell me about any difficulties you have maintaining continence or with your bladder or bowel function'.

Ostle (2016) indicates that past evidence suggests that nurses have often focused on containment rather than assessment and treatment for incontinence (Francis 2010, Harari et al. 2013). The Francis Report of 2010 identified failings in continence care, which impacted greatly on individual patients. NHS England (2018) indicates that nurses should have the relevant skills to provide an initial assessment of continence, and treatment where appropriate with onwards referral to a continence specialist for all patients. Improvements in continence care will improve QoL and reduce care home admissions, which are known to increase when an individual has the complication of incontinence with other comorbidities (Livesley et al. 2011, Yates 2021). Commissioning continence services for dignity and value to improve continence care will reduce personal cost, both physical and emotional, to the individual but will also reduce NHS costs (NHS England 2018).

Sociological Factors in Underreporting of Incontinence

That incontinence remains to such a large extent a hidden problem among the general population can be attributed in part to the embarrassment felt by many people, leading to reluctance to admit to incontinence and seek treatment (Yates 2021). Rantell (2015) indicates that there is often a misconception that incontinence is inevitable with ageing. Individuals who experience incontinence may often have low expectation of successful treatment (Stewart 2018). Severity of symptoms and the impact of these on daily living are often the triggers for an individual to seek support from a healthcare professional. Other factors may be related to culture and embarrassment when discussing intimate problems. Many Muslim women will only be examined by a female healthcare professional, and will often not discuss continence issues with a male healthcare worker, or in the presence of their husbands (Galanti 2014). An episode of incontinence during prayer would cause great stress to someone of Muslim faith, as they would be considered unclean by others of the same faith (Galanti 2014). This adds to the stress they experience through incontinence.

It may also be true that, in women, the private nature of and, to some degree, secretiveness surrounding menstruation give an easily transferable model of management to follow should incontinence develop. Many women conceal the leakage of urine as they have concealed menstruation previously.

For any individual of any faith, continence assessment must be carried out with sensitivity and consideration to individual need.

For many people, incontinence is a source of embarrassment or shame rather than a signal to seek medical help. The dysfunction is seen mainly in terms of its social consequences rather than as a symptom of a possible underlying illness or disease process.

Incontinence may restrict employment, and educational and social activities, which in turn may compromise both physical and mental well-being.

Personal and social attitudes towards incontinence are not, however, the only factors that account for the underreporting of this widespread health problem. The way that particular health services are marketed or presented can also influence an individual's decision whether to seek help or cope on their own. It is therefore important that continence services reflect positive attitudes and approaches to promoting continence, and progress on this is demonstrated in the setting of standards by nurses and monitoring of services and treatment. It is vital that people and carers affected by incontinence are given every opportunity to regain their continence, to be empowered and to be involved in the development of targeted services.

The United Kingdom Continence Society (UKCS) have developed minimum standards for continence care, covering all aspects of adult care and including specific services for children and young people; the Paediatric Continence Forum together with the UKCS has also developed minimum standards for children and young people (see Useful Websites).

The participation of those most affected by incontinence has been further strengthened by the inclusion of patients/carers on all the working parties for national publications, since the publication of the findings of the National Audit of Continence (2010), which audited services and quality of care for people with bladder and bowel incontinence in England, Wales and Northern Ireland.

Factors Contributing to Incontinence

Incontinence is basically due either to a delay in achieving continence, or loss of established continence.

Delay in Achieving Continence

In childhood, the acquisition of the skills necessary to achieve continence may be delayed. Nocturnal enuresis may present as a primary or secondary feature; its cause is not known. Although it often spontaneously resolves, it is sometimes not resolved during childhood. In such cases, if it remains untreated, it may be a problem throughout life (Hjalmas et al. 2004).

Learning disability may also prevent a person from attaining continence. Professionals working with people who have learning disabilities should base their interventions on the assumption that, although the process of toilet training may be slow, continence will eventually be achieved provided interventions are tailored to the individual and their family's requirements (Keenan et al. 2018). Physical difficulties can hinder the acquisition of continence. Some children cannot become continent without medical intervention, such as in some types of spina bifida. An infant or child who is continuously wet should always be investigated for either congenital fistula or failure to empty the bladder. Such symptoms should be taken seriously as failure of bladder emptying (with stasis of urine) can lead to vesicoureteric reflux (VUR). There is reflux of urine up the ureters following a rise of pressure within the bladder during voiding. The urine later runs back to the bladder and is not immediately voided, which in turn increases the risk of urinary tract infection (UTI). The constant reflux of infected urine into the ureters can lead to chronic pyelonephritis (reflux nephropathy) (see Chapter 10, Nursing Patients With Urinary Disorders).

Factors Affecting Existing Continence

A number of factors can affect continence. These include:

Physical Factors

Age. While incontinence is more prevalent among older people (especially women), it is not an inevitable consequence of growing older. However, with normal ageing comes a decline in renal function; it is reduced by up to 50% by the age of 80 years, thus impairing the ability of the kidney to concentrate urine. Bladder capacity and urethral pressure also decline with age (Thirugnanasothy 2010).

Ageing may also have some effect on the cerebral control of micturition; changes in cortical neurones can reduce their effectiveness in inhibiting the sacral reflex arc, so that involuntary emptying of the bladder occurs.

Ignoring the Urge to Urinate or Defecate. Ignoring the need to empty the bladder may lead to an episode of incontinence of urine, whilst ignoring the need to defecate may lead to constipation. Constipation is a common contributing factor to urinary incontinence and also retention of urine. Because of the anatomical proximity of the rectum and the urethra, it is possible for the urethra to be closed off by a faecal mass. This can result in incomplete voiding and stasis of urine, which in turn can encourage growth of bacteria and UTI.

Immobility. Reduced mobility or a lack of mobility may mean that an individual is unable to get to the lavatory, or is dependent upon assistance. Should assistance not be available, or an individual be unable to manoeuvre themselves, they may be incontinent. Undoing zips or pulling down underwear may be difficult if manual dexterity is impaired. People may misguidedly attempt to reduce the need to micturate or defecate by reducing fluid and food intake, leading to dehydration and constipation.

Fluid/Diet. Eating and drinking play a significant part in the process of elimination. A lack of nonstarch polysaccharides (NSPs or fibre) can cause constipation; fruit eaten in excess can result in diarrhoea. Increased fluid intake may increase the need to urinate, whilst reduced fluid intake leads to dehydration and constipation.

Hormones. Constipation can occur during pregnancy.

Medications and Other Substances. Diuretics, sedatives, laxatives, opioids, antibiotics, alcohol, etc., may influence elimination. For example, antibiotic-induced diarrhoea may lead to faecal incontinence.

Environmental/Social/Economic
- *Lack of facilities* – no toilet tissue or handwashing facilities.
- *Poor facilities* – cold, dirty, dark, too far away.
- *Lack of privacy/change in environment* – admission to hospital and having to use a bedpan/commode. Having to use communal facilities.
- *Costs* – need for adaptations to the home environment or aids to facilitate and promote independence with maintaining continence.

Psychological
- *Anxiety and stress* – can lead to diarrhoea.
- *Low mood, depression and dementia* – can be associated with constipation.
- *Life events* – bereavement and loss, a new sibling, change in a relationship, etc., can affect bowel habit.

Pre-Existing Conditions
- *Bladder or bowel disease* – UTIs (see Chapter 10, Nursing Patients With Urinary Disorders) may cause frequency and urgency resulting in an episode of incontinence. IBD (see

EVIDENCE-BASED PRACTICE 24.2

Living With Inflammatory Bowel Disease: A Review of Qualitative Research Studies

IBD is a chronic condition representing both Crohn's disease and ulcerative colitis. The cause is not known and many patients have unmanaged symptoms which include abdominal pain, weight loss, chronic fatigue and diarrhoea. Fourie et al. (2018) state that despite high incidence in well-developed countries, the significant impact of symptoms on QoL is little known. Fourie et al. (2018) completed a qualitative systematic review to explore the patient's experience of living with IBD. The review focused on studies published in English between 2000 and 2017. Thematic analysis was used to identify key themes from 23 studies.

Results

Patients living with IBD were reluctant to disclose their illness and a lack of information from healthcare professionals dominated their experiences. Their ability to disclose was impacted by a perceived lack of awareness amongst the community and stigma surrounding symptoms. Symptoms included fatigue, incontinence, concerns about body image and worries about an uncertain future. The main theme referred to as 'overarching' by Fourie et al. was 'Living in isolation and exclusion'.

Conclusions

The priorities for those living with IBD often differ from the priorities of the healthcare professional. More evidence is needed for healthcare professionals to provide holistic care for those living with IBD. The disease is estimated to become a global disease, which may make long-term care unsustainable.

Activity

- Access the full paper by Fourie et al. (2018) and consider how their results and conclusions could be used to enhance your practice.
- Consider the information given to patients regarding IBD and management of symptoms in your clinical/community area.
- Are leaflets with health-promoting advice, useful websites and contact telephone numbers available to give to patients and carers?
- Using Useful Websites in the chapter, or by contacting your health promotion unit, find out what information on IBD is available for members of the public.

Resources

Fourie S, Jackson J, Aveyard H. Living with inflammatory bowel disease: a review of qualitative research studies. *Int J Nurs Stud.* 2018;87:149-156. https://crohnsandcolitis.org.uk/.

Chapter 4, Nursing Patients With Gastrointestinal, Liver and Biliary Disorders) may cause diarrhoea with incontinence (Evidence-Based Practice 24.2). Functional bowel disorders may cause a number of problems, including faecal incontinence and constipation.

- *Painful anorectal conditions* – e.g. haemorrhoids, fissure (see Chapter 4) cause people to 'put off' defecation, leading to constipation which compounds the problem as it will cause even more pain on defecation.
- *Neurological conditions* – MS, paraplegia, stroke (see Chapter 11, Nursing Patients With Disorders of the Nervous System). Urinary and faecal incontinence is common following a stroke. Urinary incontinence affects up to 60% of patients following a stroke (Slark and Stewart 2018). All patients following a stroke should have a management plan to promote continence. If loss of bladder control is still present after 2 weeks, the patient should be reassessed to identify cause and ongoing treatment

(Slark and Stewart 2018). Continence can be regained through individualised nursing and rehabilitation.

- *Systemic conditions* – thyroid disease can change bowel habit (see Chapter 5). Serious infection can lead to incontinence. Hyperglycaemia or hypercalcaemia can also lead to urinary incontinence.
- *Acute confusional state* – can precipitate urinary incontinence.

Medical Management

Incontinence is best managed by a multidisciplinary team (MDT) comprising a specialist continence nurse, physiotherapist, pharmacist, GP, specialist doctor and the person/carers. Many interventions that were previously the domain of the medical staff are now initiated or undertaken by specialist continence nurses. However, for clarity, medical history, examination, investigations and nonsurgical and surgical interventions are outlined here.

History and Examination

A full medical history is taken and the person is asked to describe the problem and how it affects their QoL. Listening to the person's lived experience is vital to reaching the correct diagnosis and ensuring acceptable outcomes. The person is examined by a health professional who has developed the appropriate knowledge and expertise (Hunter 2016). Explicit consent is required. In women, a vaginal examination can determine whether atrophic vaginal changes, vaginitis or painful excoriation are a problem, and whether cervicovaginal or uterovaginal prolapse is present. Examination in both men and women will determine whether rectal prolapse, painful anorectal conditions or constipation is present. An assessment of pelvic floor contraction strength should be undertaken before initiating a pelvic floor muscle re-education programme. Men should be examined for prostatic enlargement and to determine whether the bladder is palpable. If the bladder is palpable or the history suggests inability to empty the bladder completely, it may be necessary to ask the person to pass urine, after which a catheter can be introduced, or a portable bladder scanner used to assess the residual volume of urine.

If digital rectal examination is undertaken, it also requires explicit consent and must be documented in the person's medical and nursing records. The RCN provides guidance on all aspects of digital rectal examination (RCN 2019).

Assessment of a person with faecal incontinence should include a history of the complaint and the person's normal bowel habit prior to the incontinence in order to establish the specific type of incontinence. Bleeding, loss of sensation, feeling that defecation is incomplete, pain with defecation and the presence of mucus should all be investigated. A full description of the incontinence and its frequency is also important to the diagnosis. Liquid faecal leakage is quite different from true diarrhoea. Following a rectal examination by an appropriately trained and competent health professional other investigations may be necessary (see later).

Investigations

Investigations ordered will depend on the person's particular type of incontinence and situation. Those for urinary incontinence may include:

TABLE 24.1	Urodynamic Investigations	
Test	To Establish	Indications
Post void residual urine (PVR)	The volume of urine remaining in the bladder after voiding	Should be done in all patients to exclude incomplete emptying and consequent recurrent infections, or damage to the upper urinary tract
Uroflowmetry	The rate of urine flow via the urethra	Advised for all patients to exclude voiding difficulties
Pressure/flow studies	Voiding pressures (related to voiding, not incontinence)	Follow-up from abnormal PVR or uroflowmetry, to distinguish between possible causes, e.g. poor bladder contraction or urethral obstruction
Cystometry	The pressure/volume relationship within the bladder, detrusor activity, bladder capacity and bladder compliance	Basic urodynamic evaluation for patients experiencing incontinence to assess bladder function, especially prior to considering surgery
Urethral pressure profile	The closure pressure within the urethra available to counteract increase in bladder pressure	Suggested, although not proven, for individuals in whom urethral dysfunction is suspected
Leak point pressure	The bladder pressure at which involuntary leakage of urine from the urethra is observed (the rise in bladder pressure may be from detrusor contraction or increased abdominal pressure)	Detrusor leak point pressure estimations allow assessment of risk to the upper urinary tract. Abdominal leak point pressure assesses the increase in abdominal pressure that causes stress incontinence, and thus assesses the urethral contribution to continence
Surface electromyography	The efficiency of the pelvic floor muscles during the filling and voiding phases	Limited value in routine urodynamics
Video urodynamics	The simultaneous measurement of pressure and visualisation of anatomy	Useful in patients with a complex history, for example individuals with neurological disease
Ambulatory urodynamic monitoring	Leakage, flow rates and bladder and abdominal pressure while the individual is ambulant	Useful to assess therapeutic effects of medication or to establish patterns that cannot be exhibited in a clinic

- *Urine testing* – observation for dark, cloudy or malodorous urine, and dipstick urine testing for protein, blood, glucose, etc., to exclude UTI and detect the possibility of other urinary pathology such as cancer or diabetes (see Chapter 5, Nursing Patients With Endocrine Disorders, and Chapter 10, Nursing Patients With Urinary Disorders). NICE (2015) recommends that a urine dipstick test should be used for those presenting with urinary incontinence and/or symptoms that indicate infection. In people with symptoms of UTI and a positive urine dipstick test for blood, leucocytes and nitrites, infection is likely.
- *Midstream urine (MSU)* sent for microscopy, culture and sensitivity.
- *Frequency volume charts*.
- *Urodynamic investigations* measure the pressure and flow relationships in the bladder and urethra (Table 24.1). They can aid diagnosis of the type of incontinence by showing sphincter incompetence, detrusor instability, urethral instability and problems with voiding due to obstruction or an underactive detrusor. Clement et al. (2013) following a systematic review concluded that while urodynamic testing can change clinical decision making, there is some evidence that better outcomes in terms of continence are not always achieved. The procedures are invasive, and time consuming.
- *Cystoscopy* allows inspection of the bladder and urethra, observing for tumours, stones, strictures and the condition of the mucosa.
- *Imaging*
  - Intravenous urogram (IVU), ultrasound scanning (USS) or magnetic resonance imaging (MRI) – used to detect structural abnormalities of the urinary tract, stones or cancer and the extent of faecal impaction in the colon and to show any bowel narrowing or obstruction.
  - Cystography and cystourography – a urinary catheter is introduced and the bladder is filled to capacity with contrast medium and X-rayed, revealing any bladder abnormalities. The catheter is then removed to observe the function of the bladder and upper urethra during micturition – a micturating cystourogram.
- Those for faecal incontinence may include:
  - abdominal X-ray
  - faecal occult blood (FOB)
  - stool culture
  - endoscopic examination – proctoscopy, sigmoidoscopy or colonoscopy to rule out serious pathology
  - barium enema (used less often)
  - specialist ultrasound investigations.

Nonsurgical Intervention

An outline of nonsurgical interventions is provided here, some of which are discussed in more detail in the nursing section later.

Urinary Incontinence
- Prevention of constipation
- Sufficient fluid intake
- Drugs including:
  - antimuscarinics, e.g. oxybutynin hydrochloride, propiverine, fesoterodine; for urge incontinence
  - desmopressin, an antidiuretic analogue of vasopressin; for nocturnal enuresis
  - tricyclic antidepressants, e.g. amitriptyline; for nocturnal enuresis
  - duloxetine, an antidepressant that inhibits serotonin and noradrenaline reuptake; licensed for moderate/severe stress incontinence in females
  - oestrogen pessaries/creams vaginally, or hormone replacement therapy if appropriate for atrophic vaginal changes.
- Pelvic floor training
- Biofeedback

- Electrical stimulation
- Bladder retraining
- Clean intermittent self-catheterisation (ISC)

Faecal Incontinence
- Prevention of constipation
- Pelvic floor training
- Electrical stimulation
- Biofeedback
- Bowel retraining
- Retrograde rectal irrigation (self-care).

McWilliams (2010) suggests that if biofeedback used alone has not improved the passage of faeces in people with functional bowel disorders, then rectal irrigation may be an option.

Surgical Intervention

There are several surgical interventions that may be used when other modalities fail to alleviate the problem (NHS 2017).

Urinary Incontinence
Depending on the type of incontinence and the underlying cause, surgical interventions include:
- Procedures used for stress incontinence in women that prevent descent of the urethra:
  - retropubic mid-urethral tape procedures
  - colposuspension.
- Sacral nerve stimulation.
- Increasing bladder capacity – augmentation cystoplasty.
- Urinary sphincter surgery.
- Urinary diversion (see Chapter 10).
- Transurethral resection of the prostate (TURP) may be required (see Chapter 9) or prostate artery embolisation, usually under local anaesthesia, under X-ray guidance.

Benign prostatic hyperplasia is common in older men, leading to an increase in prostate size, causing compression on the urethra. Symptoms include hesitancy during micturition, interrupted or decreased urine volume and flow rate, nocturia, incomplete voiding and urinary retention. See NICE (2010, 2018b) for further information.

Faecal Incontinence
Depending on the type of incontinence and the underlying cause, surgical interventions include:
- Sacral nerve stimulation
- Repair of anal sphincter
- Artificial sphincter
- Appendicostomy (used for anterograde rectal irrigation), or continent colonic conduit
- Stoma formation (last resort)
  See NICE (2007) for further information.

❖ Nursing Management and Health Promotion: Promoting Continence

Nurses working in many different settings will meet people who have continence problems. The aim is always to promote continence and to look for ways to improve the problems experienced.

'Nurses support and enable people at all stages of life and in all care settings to make informed choices about how to manage health challenges in order to maximise their QoL and improve health outcomes'

NMC 2018b, Annexe B, p. 31

It is important that nurses work with the person with a continence problem and carers, using their experiences and input from members of the IDT to inform the problem-solving approach – assessment, planning care and setting goals, implementation of care and evaluation of outcomes – to ascertain that the goals have been achieved.

Involving the person is empowering and increases their understanding, motivation and self-esteem. This encourages independence, control and effective coping skills.

'Where people have special communication needs or a disability it is essential that reasonable adjustments are made in order to communicate, provide and share information in a manner that promotes optimum understanding and engagement and facilitates equal access to high quality care'.

NMC 2018b, Annexe A, p. 27

This part of the chapter concentrates on urinary incontinence and outlines some issues concerning faecal incontinence.

Assessment

Assessment should be carried out in a manner that respects the person's privacy and dignity (Social Care Institute for Excellence [SCIE] 2020). It is vital that this assessment is conducted with a view to ascertaining the cause of any incontinence, for only then can the correct type of treatment be instigated. In collecting information from individuals, the nurse must have a clear understanding of the rationale behind the questions asked and of the implications for diagnosis and treatment of the person's responses (Table 24.2).

A full assessment should include:
- the person's/carer's account of the problem
- a detailed history
- recording of micturition and bowel movements, and incontinence over a few days.

See earlier discussion for medical history, examination and investigations.

Assessment should take place in a private setting and allow adequate time for the person to air concerns and ask questions. In order to establish a good rapport with the person, it is important to meet their own agenda when discussing the potentially embarrassing topic of incontinence. Open questions such as 'Tell me about the problems with wetting that you have been having' will provide the person with a greater opportunity to relate the problem in detail than will closed questions requiring a 'yes/no' response. Sometimes, however, yes/no questions are useful with people who are embarrassed and cannot find a comfortable vocabulary to describe their problems.

The nurse's choice of language and sensitivity to the person's preferred terminology will be important to help to relax the person. People generally use terms such as 'passing water' or 'peeing' rather than 'micturition' or 'voiding' and many find words such as 'accidents', 'wetting' or 'leaking' more acceptable than 'incontinence'. Where the person uses a euphemism or is vague, the nurse should seek clarification if there is any danger of misunderstanding, for example 'What do you mean by "*a little*"?'

More specific questions may be indicated when the person has a preexisting illness, or where bleeding, pain or discharge has occurred. Obviously, some questions, such as those concerning childbirth or prostate problems, will be gender specific. Supplementary questions can be asked by means of a written assessment form.

TABLE 24.2	Urinary Incontinence Assessment Questions
Question	**Rationale**
How long have these symptoms been present?	The symptoms may have begun at a life crisis or on taking a new medication, or they may have had a long-standing problem, but some new development has prompted the person to ask for help
Are you wet every time?	It is important to establish the degree and frequency of wetting
How many times do you pass urine each day?	A baseline needs to be established in order for progress to be charted
Are you wet at night as well as by day?	This gives an indication of the degree of the problem as well as the type of incontinence
Are you aware of the need to go to the lavatory before you are wet?	This will determine whether signals are normal or absent
Do you have feelings of urgency to go to the lavatory?	This indicates whether signals are present and their degree of urgency
Do you lose urine if you laugh, cough, jump or run?	A positive response often indicates genuine stress incontinence
Do you pass small amounts of urine?	Passing small amounts of urine may be due to urge, stress or overflow incontinence. It may also be indicative of reduced fluid intake
Does the stream of urine seem normal or has it changed?	Passing a full stream suggests the bladder capacity is normal
Is the stream of urine poor?	The flow rate may indicate a degree of obstruction or the bladder's inability to contract
Does passing urine sting?	Stinging urine usually indicates infection or a sore or broken area
Is your urine dark and has it a strong smell?	Concentrated urine is often dark with a strong smell
Is your urine cloudy, does it contain blood or have an unpleasant smell?	Cloudy urine with blood and an unpleasant smell may indicate UTI
Does it hurt/burn when you pass urine?	Pain on micturition (dysuria) may indicate UTI
Do you have difficulty in starting to pass urine?	Hesitancy may be caused by an obstruction, e.g. prostatic enlargement
Do you dribble urine before or after going to the lavatory?	Dribbling before suggests overflow; dribbling after suggests a failure to completely empty the bladder or an incompetent sphincter
Do you need to use pads or other aids, and if so how many and how often?	The answer may indicate the degree of urine loss
How often do you pass faeces? Are you constipated?	Constipation is a common cause of urinary incontinence
Have you had any abdominal, gynaecological or urinary surgery?	Surgical trauma may be significant
Have you difficulty in getting to the lavatory, problems with undoing clothes or any sight problems?	If the person has problems with mobility or dexterity, clothes may need to be adapted and toilet seats raised. Supports to steady patients and aids to help them locate the toilet may be required
Are you taking any medication?	Many medications can affect the functioning of the urinary tract
Is the person mentally aware?	Dementia may be the cause of incontinence due to a failure to remember the routines of the day
Gender-Specific Questions	
Women should be asked about the number of children they have had and the type of labour and delivery	Stress incontinence is associated with childbirth
Men should be asked further specific questions to ascertain if they have prostatic enlargement, such as 'Do you find it difficult to start passing water?' (see Chapter 10)	An enlarged prostate gland is associated with several urinary problems, e.g. overflow incontinence

N.B.: Some of the routine questions will also be helpful.
UTI, Urinary tract infection.

It is important that the nurse listens to the person's own account of their symptoms before asking specific questions.

Charting Information

The person's history may yield enough information to determine the probable type and cause of the incontinence. A baseline chart, recorded over a few days, can confirm the accuracy of the history by supplying information indicating frequency of micturition and incontinence and, where required, the volume of urine passed. Charting such information again at intervals of a few weeks or at the end of treatment can be used to evaluate the intervention. Any chart provided should be straightforward and easily understood so that the person is encouraged to use it, as the success of any future treatment will depend upon their motivation. Lucas et al. (2012) refer to the European Association of Urology (EAU) 2012 Guidelines, which state that voiding diaries of 3–7 days' duration are reliable for quantifying voided volume and day- and night-time frequency. NICE (2019) support the use of bladder diaries for a minimum of 3 days noting variations in their usual activities, on both working and days of leisure.

The before and after weighing of pads may also be considered for some patients.

The Bristol Stool Form Scale

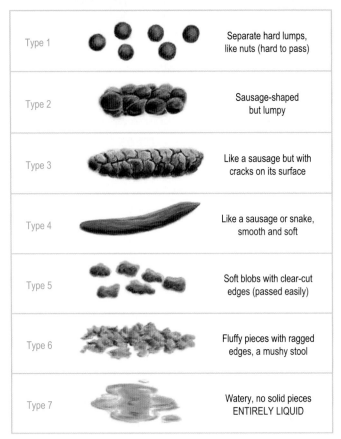

Type 1	Separate hard lumps, like nuts (hard to pass)
Type 2	Sausage-shaped but lumpy
Type 3	Like a sausage but with cracks on its surface
Type 4	Like a sausage or snake, smooth and soft
Type 5	Soft blobs with clear-cut edges (passed easily)
Type 6	Fluffy pieces with ragged edges, a mushy stool
Type 7	Watery, no solid pieces ENTIRELY LIQUID

Figure 24.3 Bristol Stool Form Scale. (© 2000 Rome Foundation, Inc. All Rights Reserved.)

Charts and diaries are also useful for those with bowel problems, to establish patterns. The Bristol Stool Form Scale (Fig. 24.3) is the 'gold standard' resource for assessing and recording types of bowel movements, and is particularly useful as part of a bowel retraining programme.

For most people, it is possible for the healthcare professional to diagnose the type of incontinence without the need for complex and invasive investigations. A thorough assessment will indicate the likely type, or cause, of the incontinence and a care/treatment plan can be devised.

Planning Care Strategies for Promoting Continence: An Overview

Effective treatment can be implemented only when the type of incontinence has been correctly diagnosed. This may seem obvious, but people report instances where their continence problem has been dismissed as trivial, something they have 'to live with' rather than a symptom to be thoroughly investigated (NICE 2019, RCP 2010, 2011).

Strategies include advice on diet, fluid and caffeine intake, pelvic floor muscle training, biofeedback and other techniques,

bladder retraining, medication, clean ISC and relieving underlying medical conditions and surgical interventions.

Advice on Diet, Fluid and Caffeine Intake

Diet should be reviewed in relation to establishing and maintaining a regular bowel habit. The avoidance of constipation is critical in preventing faecal incontinence and also will benefit urinary continence as an overfull rectum can distort the anatomical position of both the bladder and the pelvic floor. Many people are unclear about what constitutes appropriate fluid intake. Some will mistakenly restrict fluids in the hope of minimising incontinent episodes; others continually top up their cup or glass, generating such large volumes of urine that the bladder is unable to cope. Six to eight cups or glasses of fluid in 24 hours is appropriate for most adults (British Nutrition Foundation 2021). It is accepted that a reduction in caffeine intake will reduce over activity of the bladder (NICE 2019).

⊕ **See Evolve website Critical thinking question 24.1**

Pelvic Floor Muscle Training

Stress incontinence in men or women is the main problem for which pelvic floor muscle training may be used. Stress incontinence occurs when the pelvic floor muscles (Fig. 24.4) are unable to counteract a sudden rise in abdominal pressure and allow the urethral sphincter to open; that is, the intravesical pressure overcomes the intraurethral pressure.

Pelvic floor muscle training can also be useful for people with frequency and urge incontinence. Sitting down when strong 'signals' occur and carrying out pelvic floor muscle contraction can help to overcome the feeling of urgency and encourage the bladder to fill a little more before being emptied in a controlled way.

It is recommended that pelvic floor muscle training should be offered to women during their first pregnancy as a strategy to prevent urinary incontinence. According to Price et al. (2010), women reduce the chances of postpartum leakage of urine, in the first year after child birth, if they actively undertake pelvic floor exercise whilst pregnant. It is also useful following prostate surgery or other pelvic surgery in which the pelvic floor muscles may

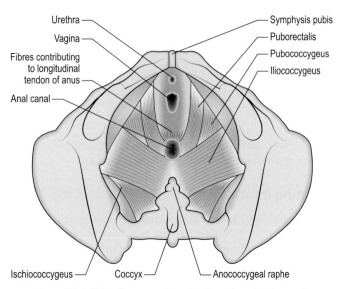

Figure 24.4 Pelvic floor muscles – levator ani, perineal aspect.

Pelvic Floor Muscle Training

The inability of the pelvic floor to maintain urinary continence can affect a wide spectrum of people, ranging from a 'new mum' to a person with a persistent cough associated with chronic obstructive pulmonary disease (COPD) (see Chapter 3, Nursing Patients With Respiratory Disease) or someone who does heavy lifting at work.

Activities

Access the publication *Personal Training for Your Pelvic Floor Muscles* produced by the Chartered Society of Physiotherapy. This can be accessed from https://www.csp.org.uk/system/files/personal_training_for_your_pelvic_floor.pdf
- Find out the causes of weak pelvic floor muscles.
- Reflect on the problems experienced by people with weak pelvic floor muscles.
- Discuss with your supervisor/assessor or lecturer how you could use the information in your own practice.

Resource
- Chartered Society of Physiotherapy (CSP). Pelvic floor exercises. 2021. https://www.csp.org.uk/conditions/incontinence/exercise-advice-incontinence.

be weakened (Chartered Society of Physiotherapy [CSP] 2021) (Reflection 24.1).

Nurses work closely with specialist continence physiotherapists who provide pelvic floor muscle training. The first step is to ensure that the person can identify the pelvic floor muscles – levator ani (keeps the anal sphincter closed) and its anterior part the pubococcygeus (which stops the flow of urine). The CSP (2021) suggests that people imagine that they need to stop themselves passing 'wind' and at the same time to stop passing urine; they describe it as a feeling of 'squeeze and lift', and that men should notice a slight rise of the scrotum.

Once the physiotherapist has provided advice about pelvic floor muscle training, the nurse should ensure that the person has understood the programme. Importantly, the nurse offers support and encouragement for the person to continue with the training. They should understand that, like all training, it will be some months before any benefit is evident so sustained motivation is needed. An individual exercise regimen should be developed related to the person's current muscle strength and situation. An unrealistic regimen will be demotivating. The person should aim to do their training three times a day and should be reminded that they will need to continue with the exercises to prevent loss of muscle strength (CSP 2021).

Other Techniques

Physiotherapists employ a range of equipment and techniques to help people to overcome stress incontinence besides pelvic floor exercises. These include biofeedback and neuromuscular electrical stimulation. For women, weighted vaginal cones can be used to aid exercise of the pelvic floor (Pelvic Obstetric and Gynaecological Physiotherapy [POGP] 2014).

The person can be provided with biofeedback by a variety of methods, for example digital palpation, manometry or electromyography, which will demonstrate evidence of muscle strength and illustrate any improvement, providing positive reinforcement of the benefit of the training programme.

Neuromuscular electrical stimulation can be used to initiate muscle contractions, in the absence of a nerve impulse, by stimulating the muscle with a mild electric current. This is beneficial where a person is unable to perform a voluntary muscle contraction.

Nurse-led clinics providing treatment for faecal incontinence using electrical stimulation have been very successful (Dueland-Jackson et al. 2015).

Positive outcomes may be measured objectively by reviewing diary and chart recordings, and subjectively by the person's perceived improvement in continence or the number of visits to the lavatory for successful micturition or a bowel movement, or the number of pad changes required per day.

Bladder Retraining

For urge incontinence, bladder retraining, in conjunction with antimuscarinic medication, is the main treatment. The aim of this treatment is for the bladder to 'learn' to increase its capacity and for the urethral sphincter to remain closed as the bladder fills, thereby lengthening the intervals between voiding.

Initially, a baseline measurement is obtained of working bladder capacity, that is, the amount of urine passed, and frequency of voiding at the time of assessment. In stages, the person learns to hold on for a few minutes more between the bladder signal and going to the lavatory. As each lengthened interval is achieved and maintained, new objectives are set for the next few days.

Antimuscarinic medication such as oxybutynin hydrochloride is a useful adjunct to bladder retraining, as it reduces the initial urge to void and thereby helps to increase bladder capacity. However, there are side-effects such as dry mouth, constipation (which may exacerbate incontinence) and sometimes difficulty in micturition. Modified-release oxybutynin has fewer side-effects. Newer antimuscarinics are available such as propiverine and fesoterodine.

When an acceptable social interval between visits to the lavatory and an adequate bladder capacity are reached, the medication is reduced and eventually discontinued. The person then aims to maintain the same regimen as when taking the medication. Success is judged to be maintaining the same interval between voiding.

Timed and prompted voiding is referred to as habit training, and is a behavioural technique to improve continence status.

Whatever the degree of success of the treatment, toileting regimens will remain individual to each person. In order to evaluate progress, a further continence chart should be completed after a few weeks' treatment and again towards the end of treatment. Comparison of the charts, showing both voiding intervals and quantities, will allow an objective evaluation to be made as to the success of the treatment.

Specific Strategies for Nocturnal Enuresis

It is important to chart the pattern of enuresis before treatment is commenced. Often, a form of bladder training is tried initially, whereby the person learns to hold onto urine longer during the day, thus leading to an increased bladder capacity and increased ability to hold urine at night.

The main treatment for nocturnal enuresis for teenagers and adults is the use of an alarm system to assist with learning to wake in time to void. A small electrode attached to a battery alarm system about the size of a matchbox is attached to a region of the person's nightwear likely to become wet if enuresis occurs. When the first drop of urine touches the electrode, a signal is activated and wakes the person. The alarm system may be combined with short-term use of desmopressin (an antidiuretic analogue of vasopressin) given sublingually or orally. The antidepressant amitriptyline may be prescribed short-term.

Some people may benefit from a combination of an alarm and medication to begin the treatment programme and then gradually withdraw both as control is established (see Useful Websites, e.g. ERIC).

Clean Intermittent Self-Catheterisation

Clean ISC can be used by people with voiding difficulties caused by conditions such as an atonic bladder or detrusor–sphincter dyssynergia, in which bladder contraction does not synchronise with opening of the urethral sphincter. It has also been of particular benefit to individuals with conditions that include MS, spina bifida and paraplegia.

Clean ISC is a relatively simple strategy for incomplete bladder emptying, or for urinary incontinence that has not responded to other techniques. Assessment for ISC must include identification of the specific type of incontinence and an evaluation of the person's manual dexterity, mental ability and their motivation; there is a requirement that the person is able to identify the urethral opening. Children as well as adults have been successful in learning the technique. A small-gauge catheter without a balloon is introduced into the bladder several times a day, dependent on individual requirements for assisted bladder emptying.

The procedure of self-catheterisation simulates normal voiding: the bladder is allowed to fill, the clean catheter is introduced and the bladder is then completely emptied. This prevents the buildup of residual urine in the bladder, which otherwise may cause:

- proliferation of bacteria in the bladder and UTI
- nerve damage
- overflow incontinence
- VUR of infected urine into the ureters and kidneys with the potential to cause chronic pyelonephritis (reflux nephropathy).

Unlike long-term indwelling catheterisation, in which aseptic technique is of paramount importance, ISC may seem unhygienic. However, the clean technique is not associated with bladder infection, as the bladder is, and should be, completely emptied each time a catheter is passed. NICE (2012) guidance on infection control, updated in 2017, recommends that if ISC is a clinically appropriate and practical choice for the patient, then as it is associated with less risk of infection, if should be a preferable option to an indwelling urinary catheter.

Catheters are available as prelubricated and nonlubricated. Prelubricated catheters are for single use only. Nonlubricated catheters can be used with or without separate lubrication depending on the person's preference. Nonlubricated catheters can be rinsed and reused, for a single person, for up to a week.

Most people find that inserting the catheter becomes easier with each attempt. Success can be measured in terms of the improved QoL it offers to people who previously were continually wet or who had to visit hospital emergency departments to seek relief from pain caused by failure to empty their bladder.

Managing Symptoms Related to Conditions That Exacerbate Incontinence

The impact of some types of incontinence can be reduced by managing or preventing underlying conditions such as constipation

and confusional states (UTI is discussed in Chapter 10, Nursing Patients With Urinary Disorders).

Constipation

Constipation can be defined as 'the infrequent and difficult passing of hard stools'. It is a causative factor in urinary retention and subsequent incontinence. An investigation of the cause of the constipation must be undertaken to exclude serious pathology such as colorectal cancer, including a review of medication and concurrent conditions. Diet, fluid intake and exercise/mobility should also be assessed.

Constipation may be associated with headache, general malaise and lack of appetite, abdominal discomfort, rectal fullness and cramps (NHS 2020). During physical examination, the abdomen can be measured for signs of increasing distension.

In people with a normal bowel, constipation may be caused by any of the following:

- insufficient NSP intake
- insufficient fluid intake
- inactivity
- ignoring the urge to defecate
- anorectal pain, e.g. from haemorrhoids, etc., which may lead the person to avoid defecation
- immobility/inability to position oneself comfortably on the lavatory, leading to avoidance of defecation
- orodental problems, leading to intake of soft foods only
- the use of pads for urinary incontinence, leading to neglect of faecal elimination by person or staff where assistance is required
- opioid drugs (prescribed and illegal, see Chapter 32, Nursing Patients Who Need Palliative Care), sedatives or hypnotic medication
- unacceptable facilities – upstairs, outside, dirty, cold, used by others, lack of privacy, dependent on others such as asking for the commode
- unfamiliar surroundings or circumstances, leading to loss of habit
- inability to recognise social expectations, as in some cases of learning disability, dementia or substance misuse including alcohol.

Where no obvious cause is found for the constipation, the problem may be due to damage to the pelvic floor and anal sphincter or to some other pathology, such as loss of rectal sensation resulting from surgery, injury or tumour. Other contributing conditions include dehydration resulting from endocrine or metabolic disorders, and neurological damage.

Preventing Constipation

People who are prone to constipation should be encouraged to be as active as possible. Requests by people to go to the lavatory should always be responded to as quickly as possible, in order to ensure that the gastrocolic reflex is never ignored. Once on the lavatory the person should be encouraged to sit for as long as is required. Structural adaptations may be necessary to make the lavatory more accessible, such as a raised seat.

A lack of privacy, time or comfort in a care setting can easily interfere with the maintenance of good bowel habits. Nurses must apply standards that maintain dignity and privacy when determining the need for support and intervention to assist with toileting, and to effectively manage the use of appropriate aids (NMC 2018). Constipation can be prevented by the introduction of adequate NSP into the diet, in conjunction with a fluid intake of eight cups/glasses a day. A dental check-up may be necessary to ensure that patients will be able to manage the raw or chewy food typical of a high-NSP diet. Individuals who are forced by dental problems to eat only soft foods will be susceptible to constipation, and therefore particular attention should be paid to their NSP intake, with addition to the diet as required.

A suitable laxative (oral or rectal) may be required to deal with the initial constipation and to prevent its recurrence (Perry 2021).

Nurses must be alert to the possibility of spurious diarrhoea that can occur in severe constipation when liquid faeces leak around a hard mass of faeces causing faecal soiling/incontinence. It is essential that the exact cause is identified as it would be disastrous to treat faecal soiling with anti-diarrhoeal medication, thus exacerbating the constipation.

Confusional States

For people with dementia or other confusional states, adherence to a regular routine will help to reinforce the need to go to the lavatory at particular times during the day. If an adequate intake of NSP and sufficient fluids is encouraged and usual patterns of defecation maintained, usually 30 minutes after breakfast, a hot drink or other meal, it should be possible to prevent constipation. It is preferable for people with dementia to be assisted to the lavatory at normal intervals rather than to be asked to adapt to new regimens such as using a commode (Kyle 2012).

Referring Patients

The nurse is responsible for investigating the cause of a person's incontinence through assessment and knowledge application. Nurses in all areas of practice should take responsibility for their patients' continence assessments as part of a holistic care plan. The findings from history taking can be supplemented with a baseline chart that records the times of elimination of urine and/or faeces. Having fully assessed the person's continence problem, the nurse should be in a position to initiate a plan of care aimed at restoration of continence. People with continence problems are best managed by the IDT, and the nurse who lacks specialist experience should liaise with a specialist continence nurse, continence advisor or specialist continence physiotherapist who can assist in interpreting the data obtained from the person's history and baseline elimination chart.

Should the person present with a complex history or be unresponsive to the treatment plan, the nurse should arrange referral to the appropriate professional. This may be a specialist continence nurse, specialist continence physiotherapist, occupational therapist (such as for home adaptations, ways of achieving specific tasks, etc.) gynaecologist, urologist, consultant in medicine for older people, neurologist or the mental health team.

'Registered nurses provide leadership by acting as a role model for best practice in the delivery of nursing care. They play an active role in the inter-disciplinary team, collaborating and communicating effectively with a range of colleagues.'

NMC 2018b, Platform 3, p. 13

In a busy setting, the significance of the person's incontinence may not be fully appreciated. The nurse, as their advocate, should make a case for further investigation, as the individual often feels embarrassed by the problem and may be unable to convince the doctor of its impact on their QOL.

Continence Advisory Services

Over two decades ago, *Good Practice in Continence Services* recommended models of good continence services. People with continence problems and their carers are entitled to access professional organisations and specialist charities to ensure their needs and rights are met, in relation to accessing education, continence aids, services and support, both financial and practical (RCP 2011).

Many people with continence problems are cared for in the community. The continence needs of older people in the community are often different from those of older residents in care homes. It should be noted that palliative approaches to continence, for example containment management, should not be instigated without careful consideration of continence promoting activities, for example timed voiding, medication review and a reduction of fluid intake in the early evening. Standards for continence care apply to all (DH 2010).

Most hospitals and primary care trusts provide the support of a specialist team including a specialist continence nurse and continence physiotherapists who work between the hospital and community to offer seamless care.

For further information on continence care in palliative care, see https://www.mariecurie.org.uk/professionals/palliative-care-knowledge-zone/symptom-control/continence-care.

❖ Nursing Management and Health Promotion: Intractable Incontinence

For some, the loss of continence will unfortunately be intractable. The key to successful management of their requirements for toileting programmes, aids and equipment is, as always, to determine individual needs and priorities with a view to improving QoL. The problem-solving approach should again be applied, taking into account:
- personal preference
- lifestyle
- home conditions
- family support
- the degree and frequency of micturition or defecation
- financial considerations.

Aids and Equipment

The type of aid that should be recommended for an individual will depend upon the specific type of incontinence experienced. The assessment of a person's requirements for aids or equipment must be informed by an understanding of the cause of the incontinence.

Aids to enhance mobility and stability, raised lavatory seats, portable bidets or commodes and clothes that have been chosen or adapted for ease of access may be helpful to many individuals. Aids to personal cleansing can also be made available to help the person maintain independence and dignity.

Urinals can be used by both men and women. These are particularly useful for women who are, for example, confined to a wheelchair, have arthritis or are taking diuretics, for whom incontinence may result from an inability to get to the lavatory in time.

Additional equipment designed to enable men to contain urinary incontinence is available on prescription. Sheaths (urodomes) with varying types of adhesive fixings and drainage systems are continually being modified. Urethral occlusive devices are available but should be used with caution. Y-front pants with a padded, waterproof-backed gusset are particularly useful for men with a retracted penis and dribbling problems.

A wide range of pads, pants and appliances is available for people who cannot achieve urinary control. The Association for Continence Advice (2017) published guidance for the provision of containment products for adult incontinence. The person's local NHS continence service will be able to provide information on the availability of containment products in their locality. A range of absorbent products is provided through local health services. The availability of aids and collection or delivery service varies for each area. Whatever the local arrangements, the person and carers must be assured about continuity of supply (NICE 2015) and be provided with contact numbers in case of problems.

The choice of absorbent product for an individual will be influenced by factors such as the laundry facilities available, the role of any carer and the time available to that carer. During assessment for such aids, the nurse should balance the person's wishes and the availability of laundry facilities, such as a washing machine, home help or laundry service, with the problems of soiled waste disposal, for example a limited weekly volume of waste collected by the local authority. A lack of supplies or aids will add to a person's anxiety, and may impact upon their ability to maintain continence. It is recognised that in the community, incontinence is a prime reason for many people moving into nursing homes as relatives and carers feel unable to cope. During assessment for aids and equipment, it is advisable to consult an occupational therapist, physiotherapist or continence advisor on the range of supplies available in a particular health area. The person may also wish to investigate aids to daily living on view in regional centres or in specialist outlets. Accurate advice and support regarding continence products and services are essential for anyone living with loss of continence.

Long-Term Catheterisation

Long-term indwelling catheterisation is used in the management of incontinence only after all other treatment possibilities have been eliminated. It is associated with several complications, not least UTI.

It should not be undertaken without due consideration of the person's lifestyle, preferences and likely level of concordance. The possible effects of long-term catheterisation on sexual relationships must be considered and discussed. Whilst sexuality is acknowledged as part of any patient holistic assessment, it is often a neglected area in all adults, particularly older people (Baker-Green 2017, Farell and Belza 2012).

Insertion of a suprapubic catheter may be preferable for some people. The person/carer should be made aware of what catheter management will entail before the procedure is carried out.

Catheter care is an important part of the nurse's role in all care settings; an understanding of the principles of catheter selection and closed drainage system management, together with skill in educating people/carers, are prerequisites for this. Leg drainage bags are provided for people with a catheter or a sheath who are up and about during the day. A care plan for teaching catheter management is provided on the website.

Emergency Help and Contact Numbers

All catheterised patients in the community should be given a 24-hour contact number through which to gain help in an emergency. Practical advice on what constitutes a real problem and what to do in certain emergencies should be given in writing to patients and carers.

Chapter 9 provides detailed information about the management of an indwelling urinary catheter.

Preventing Urinary Tract Infection

Healthcare-associated infections (HCAIs) develop as a direct result of contact with a healthcare setting, or as a result of an invasive intervention such as surgery. A UTI is the most common HCAI. Patients with an indwelling device such as a long-term indwelling urinary catheter are more likely to develop a HCAI (NICE 2012). However, infection following urinary catheterisation is not inevitable and can be prevented when the potential entry points of microorganisms are properly managed (see Chapter 10, Nursing Patients With Urinary Disorders, and Chapter 18, Infection Prevention and Control). Bladder washouts should not be part of prophylaxis for UTIs; they do not prevent catheter-associated urinary tract infection (CAUTI) (NICE 2020).

Supplying Catheter Equipment

Community nurses who have undertaken the required training may prescribe items, including catheters, drainage bags and sheaths, from the *Nurse Prescribers' Formulary for Community Practitioners* (British National Formulary 2017) for people in the community with an indwelling catheter (https://bnf.nice.org.uk/nurse-prescribers-formulary/).

The person and carers should be given a list of all of their equipment, including sizes, types and capacity, as well as the name of a reliable pharmacist, retailer or mail order supplier.

Relationships – Expressing Sexuality

The impact of incontinence on self-esteem and the fear of wetting or soiling during intercourse can understandably have a negative effect on an individual's sex life. Esparza et al. (2018) conducted a phenomenological study into the experiences of men and women with urinary incontinence. Six categories emerged; these were normalisation of incontinence, verbalisation of the problems, social isolation, feelings and emotions, impact on daily routine and adaptation self-care strategies to address their problems. There is reluctance to discuss continence difficulties for most people, even during a nursing assessment. Feelings and emotions related to incontinence are often concerned with the impact of incontinence on the activities of daily living, for the individual and those around them. The reluctance to discuss continence problems coupled with an avoidance of intimacy for fear of urinary leakage or faecal leakage will inevitably lead to relationship difficulties. Urinary incontinence is a predictor of sexual function and QoL incontinence. There are links between incontinence and depression, which affect QoL (Esparza et al. 2018).

Although many professionals may not see the aspect of maintaining sexuality as a priority, people who have been sexually active and are suddenly faced with incontinence caused by injury, childbirth or disease, or those who are facing progressive incontinence as a result of chronic disease, will have to make difficult adjustments to changes in their sexual life. Problems of sexuality and incontinence affect both genders regardless of age. Counselling with regard to the implications of incontinence for the individual's sexuality should be initiated only when the person signals that they are ready to address the issue. However, the nurse may need to introduce the subject and thereby give the person 'permission' to voice any concerns (Evidence-Based Practice 24.3). Reluctance to discuss questions of sexuality may be due to the nurse's own inexperience or lack of self-awareness.

There is no justification in encouraging a person to divulge such personal and sensitive information if the nurse is not able to offer help or referral to the appropriate specialist.

EVIDENCE-BASED PRACTICE 24.3

Nurses' Experiences of Discussing Sexuality With Urinary Catheter Patients

Indwelling urinary catheters provide artificial drainage of urine. Community nurses support those living with an indwelling urinary catheter. The community nurses support patients to adapt to living with an indwelling urinary catheter, through education and practical advice. They support patients with individual management issues, they advise on products and services, and offer much needed psychological support. Living with an indwelling urinary catheter can impact on a person's QoL and sexual relationships. Ongoing assessment of the patient and their ability to cope and adapt to an indwelling urinary catheter is essential. However, expressing sexuality is often overlooked as an activity of daily living and is a neglected part of the assessment process.

Baker-Green (2017) conducted a qualitative research study which aimed to 'establish registered nurses experiences of discussing sexuality with urinary catheter patients'. Nine community nurses participated in the study and semistructured interviews were used to collect data. From the interview, four themes emerged:

- The importance of the nurse–patient relationship
- Peer support and role models
- Maintaining professionalism
- Lack of experience and knowledge
  Nurses reported barriers that discouraged them from discussing sexuality with patients. These included their own lack of knowledge, their own embarrassment causing patient embarrassment and discussing sexuality with older people.

Nurses at all levels were reluctant to discuss issues relating to a patient's sexuality, and when they did, they were uncomfortable doing so.

Recommendations from the Baker-Green (2017) study were for further training for nurses to allow them to offer better support regarding sexuality for those living with an indwelling urinary catheter. Greater use of nursing assessment models and documentation that reflect the importance of expressing sexuality and the impact of this on QoL.

Baker-Green (2017) concludes that it is the responsibility of the nurse to ensure that sexuality is assessed as an integral part of any holistic nursing assessment.

- Access the full paper by Baker-Green (2017) and consider how you would use the findings from this paper to enhance your practice.
- Discuss with your or a colleague how they approach sexuality as part of holistic assessment for patients with an indwelling urinary catheter.
- Find the contact details of the Continence Nurse Specialist for your area and find out how you would make a referral if necessary for a patient who may wish to discuss the impact of incontinence/urinary catheterisation on their sexual health and wellbeing.

Resource

Baker-Green R. Nurses' experiences discussing sexuality with urinary catheter patients. *J Urol Nurs.* 2017;11(1):6-12.

Certain issues concerning sexuality and incontinence may be dealt with in a practical manner. For many women who are incontinent, orgasm produces further episodes of urine loss. Passing urine before sexual intercourse may help. Protecting the bed and discussing the problem with one's partner can help to make the wetting less of an issue. However, for people in a new relationship such a discussion is likely to be difficult.

People with a urinary catheter need not avoid intercourse. For men, the catheter may be strapped to the underside of the penis and, in some individuals with a degree of erectile dysfunction, may also help with rigidity (see Chapter 9). In women, the catheter may be strapped to the inner thigh or up onto the abdomen. If clinically appropriate, sexually active people may opt for a urinary catheter which is inserted suprapubically.

The nurse should be able to provide the person with contact details for specialist sexual counselling should it be required.

Summary: Key Nursing Issues

- The number of people suffering from incontinence far exceeds the number of cases reported to health professionals.
- Loss of continence is embarrassing and affects every aspect of the person's life.
- Many factors affect a person's ability to gain continence and remain continent throughout life.
- The nurse's role in promoting urinary and faecal continence is critical.
- Incontinence is best managed by an MDT comprising a specialist continence nurse, physiotherapist, pharmacist, GP, specialist doctor and the person/carers.
- Over recent years, many interventions that were previously the domain of medical staff are now initiated or undertaken by specialist continence nurses.

- Positive communication and interpersonal skills are vitally important when assessing and assisting a person with continence, bladder or bowel problems.
- In all settings the nurse delivers care that is individual and considerate of a person's lifestyle, attitudes, beliefs and culture.
- Privacy and dignity should be promoted at all times during nursing interventions for continence, bladder and bowel care.

🌐 **See Evolve website Critical thinking question 24.2**

- Continence service provision is available to offer advice to those with continence, bladder and bowel problems. This service exists to ensure equity and quality in the service offered. The nurse has a responsibility to ensure that those who need it are aware of continence service provision and how it can be accessed.

Reflection and Learning – What Next?

- **Test** your knowledge by visiting the Evolve website 🌐 and answering the multiple-choice questions and critical thinking questions.

- **Consolidate** your learning by looking at some of the further reading suggestions, references and specialist websites.
- **Revisit** some of the additional material on the website.

- **Consider** what you have learnt and how this will help your professional development.
- **Reflect** on how you can apply this knowledge to the care of your patients.

References

Association for Continence Advice. *Guidance for the Provision of Containment Products for Adult Incontinence. A Consensus Document.* Association of Continence Advice; 2017.

Baker-Green R. Nurses' experiences discussing sexuality with urinary catheter patients. *J Urol Nurs.* 2017;11(1):6–12.

Bladder Interest Group (2021). The cost of poor bladder management report. https://bladderinterestgroup.co.uk/wp-content/uploads/2021/12/Cost-of-Poor-Bladder-Management-Report-2021.pdf.

British National Formulary (BNF). Nurse Prescribers' Formulary for Community Practitioners 2017–2019; 2017. https://bnf.nice.org.uk/nurse-prescribers-formulary/.

British Nutrition Foundation. Hydration. 2021. https://www.nutrition.org.uk/healthy-sustainable-diets/hydration/?level=Health%20professional.

Care Quality Commission. GP mythbuster 29: looking after homeless patients in general practice. 2022. https://www.cqc.org.uk/guidance-providers/gps/gp-mythbusters/gp-mythbuster-29-looking-after-homeless-patients-general-practice.

Chartered Society of Physiotherapy (CSP). Pelvic floor exercises. 2021. https://www.csp.org.uk/conditions/incontinence/exercise-advice-incontinence.

Clement KD, Lapitan MCM, Omar M I, Glazener CMA. Urodynamic studies for management of urinary incontinence in children and adults. *Cochrane Database Syst Rev.* 2013(10):CD003195. doi:10.1002/14651858.CD003195.pub3.

Department of Health (DH). Essence of Care. The Stationary Office. London; 2010.

Dibley L, Coggrave M, McClurg D, et al. 'It's just horrible': a qualitative study of patients' and carers' experiences of bowel dysfunction in multiple sclerosis. *J Neurol.* 2017;264(7):1354–1361.

Dueland-Jackson J, Haas S, Buntzen S, et al. Nurse-led clinics can manage faecal incontinence effectively. *Colorectal Dis.* 2015(17):710–717.

Education and Resources for Improving Childhood Continence (ERIC). 2017. www.eric.org.uk.

Edwards D, Harden J, Jones A, Featherstone K. Understanding how to facilitate continence for people with dementia in acute hospital settings: a mixed methods systematic review and thematic analysis. *Syst Rev.* 2021;10:199. https://systematicreviewsjournal.biomedcentral.com/articles/10.1186/s13643-021-01743-0.

Esparza AO, Tomas MAC, Pina-Roche F. Experiences of women and men living with urinary incontinence. *Appl Nurs Res.* 2018;40:68–75.

Farell J, Belza B. Are older patients comfortable discussing sexual health with nurses? *Appl Nurs Res.* 2012;61(1):51–57.

Francis R. Independent inquiry into care provided by Mid Staffordshire NHS Foundation Trust. January 2005–March 2009, Volume 1; 2010.

Galanti G. *Caring for Patients From Different Cultures.* 5th ed. Philadelphia: University of Pennsylvania Press; 2014.

Goodman C, Rycroft Malone J, Norton C, et al. Reducing and managing faecal incontinence in people with dementia who are resident in care homes: protocol for a realist synthesis. *BMJ.* 2015;5(7):e007728. doi:10.1136/bmjopen-2-15-007728.

Harari D, Rogers J, Eustice S, Colley W, 2013 for All Party Parliamentary Group for Continence Care. Continence Care Services England 2013 Survey Report; 2013. http://tinyurl.com/lavb6hx.

Hjalmas K, Arnold T, Bower W, et al. Nocturnal enuresis: an international evidence-based management strategy. *J Urol.* 2004;171(6):2545–2561.

Hunter K. ICS Updates in continence care: the role of the nurse continence specialist in continence services. *Urol News.* 2016;21(1).

Keenan P, Fleming S, Horan P, et al. Urinary continence promotion and people with an intellectual disability. *Learn Disabil Pract.* 2018. doi:10.7748/ldp.2018.e1878.

Kyle G. *The importance of assessing constipation.* Independent Nurse for Primary Care and Community Nurses; 2012. www.independentnurse.co.uk/clinical-article/the-importance-of-assessing-constipation/63629.

Livesley N, Crosby S, Bowman C. Bupa Centre for Policy on Ageing: the changing role of care homes; 2011. www.cpa.org.uk/information/reviews/changingroleofcarehomes.pdf.

Lucas MG, Ruud J I, Burkhead FC, et al. EAU guidelines on assessment and non-surgical management of urinary incontinence. *Eur Urol.* 2012;62(2012):1130–1142.

Ministry of Housing, Communities & Local Government. Rough Sleeping Statistics: Autumn 2018, England (Revised). MHCLG, 2019. https://assets.publishing.service.gov.uk/government/uploads/system/uploads/attachment_data/file/781567/Rough_Sleeping_Statistics_2018_release.pdf.

McWilliams D. Rectal irrigation for patients with functional bowel disorders. *Nurs Stand.* 2010;24(26):42–47.

National Institute for Health and Clinical Excellence (NICE). *Faecal incontinence: the management of faecal incontinence in adults.* Clinical guideline [CG49]; 2007. Quick reference guide. http://www.nice.org.uk/nicemedia/pdf/CG49QuickRefGuide.pdf.

National Institute for Health and Clinical Excellence (NICE). *Lower urinary tract symptoms in men; management.* Clinical guideline [CG97]; 2010. http://www.nice.org.uk/guidance/cg97.

National Institute for Health and Clinical Excellence (NICE). *Infection: prevention and control of healthcare-associated infections in primary and community care.* Clinical guideline [CG139]; 2012. http://www.nice.org.uk/guidance/cg139.

National Institute for Health and Care Excellence (NICE). *Faecal incontinence in adults.* Quality standard [QS54]; 2014. http://www.nice.org.uk/guidance/QS54.

National Institute for Health and Care Excellence (NICE). *Urinary incontinence in women: management.* Quality standard [QS77]; 2015. http://www.nice.org.uk/guidance/QS77.

National Institute for Health and Care Excellence (NICE). *Urinary tract infections in adults.* Quality standard [QS90]; 2015. https://www.nice.org.uk/guidance/qs90.

National Institute for Health and Care Excellence (NICE). *Surgery for stress urinary incontinence in women.* NICE Pathways; 2018. http://www.nice.org.uk/pathways/urinary-incontinence-in-women.

National Institute for Health and Care Excellence (NICE), Prostate artery embolization for lower urinary tract symptoms caused by benign prostatic hyperplasia (IPG 691). 2018b. https://www.nice.org.uk/guidance/ipg611/resources/prostate-artery-embolisation-for-lower-urinary-tract-symptoms-caused-by-benign-prostatic-hyperplasia-pdf-1899873917137861.

National Institute for Health and Care Excellence (NICE). *Urinary incontinence and pelvic organ prolapse in women: management.* NICE guideline [NG123]; 2019. https://www.nice.org.uk/guidance/ng123.

National Institute for Health and Care Excellence (NICE). *Preventing Infection Related to Long-Term Urinary Catheters.* London: NICE; 2020.

NHS England. *Synthetic Vaginal Mesh Tape Procedure for the Surgical Treatment of Stress Urinary Incontinence in Women. Patient Information Leaflet.* London: NHS England; 2017.

NHS England. *Excellence in Continence Care. Practical Guidance for Commissioners, and Leaders in Health and Social Care.* London: NHS England; 2018. https://www.england.nhs.uk/wp-content/uploads/2018/07/excellence-in-continence-care.pdf.

Nursing and Midwifery Council (NMC). *The Code: Professional Standards of Practice and Behaviour for Nurses.* Midwives and Nursing Associates; 2018. https://www.nmc.org.uk/globalassets/sitedocuments/nmc-publications/nmc-code.pdf.

Nursing and Midwifery Council (NMC). Future Nurse: Standards of Proficiency for Registered Nurses. 2018b. https://www.nmc.org.uk/globalassets/sitedocuments/standards-of-proficiency/nurses/future-nurse-proficiencies.pdf.

- **Discuss** your learning with your assessor/supervisor, lecturer and colleagues.

Ostle Z. Assessment, diagnosis and treatment of urinary incontinence in women. *Br J Nurs.* 2016;25(2):84–91.

Palmer C, Richardson D, Rayner J, Drake MJ, Cottrill N. Professional perspectives on impacts, benefits and disadvantages of changes made to community continence services during the COVID-19 pandemic: findings from the EPICCC-19 national survey. *BMC Health Serv Res.* 2022;22:783.

Parker J, Crabtree S. A (2017) Social work with disadvantaged and marginalised people. Google Books. https://books.google.co.uk/books?hl=en&lr=&id=5uk7DwAAQBAJ&oi=fnd&pg=PT8&dq=Continence+outreach+for+the+homeless+uk+articles+2018+onwards&ots=2ajTCx8sZ9&sig=NF5k9Mm2VIhNqmGoBFgW1O8o1yk&redir_esc=y#v=onepage&q&f=false.

Pelvic Obstetric and Gynaecological Physiotherapy (POGP). *A Common Problem for Men and Women: Promoting Continence With Physiotherapy.* Excellence Matters; 2014. https://pogp.csp.org.uk/system/files/promoting_continence_2015.pdf.

Percival J, Abbott K, Allain T, et al. 'We tend to get pad happy': a qualitative study of health practitioners' perspectives on the quality of continence care for older people in hospital. *BMJ Open Qual.* 2021;10:e001380. doi:10.1136/bmjoq-2021-001380.

Perry M. Understanding constipation in adults. *Gastroenterol Health Clinical.* 2021;32(12). https://www.practicenursing.com/content/clinical/understanding-constipation-in-adults.

Philichi L. When the going gets tough: pediatric constipation and encopresis. *Gastroenterol Nurs.* 2008;31:121–130.

Price N, Dahwood R, Jackson SR. Pelvic floor exercise for urinary incontinence: a systematic literature review. *Maturitas.* 2010;67(4):309–315.

Rantell A. Understanding urinary incontinence in women. *Pract Nurs.* 2015;26(6):275–281.

Rao SS. Practice guideline. Diagnosis and management of fecal incontinence. *Am J Gastroenterol.* 2004;99(8):1585–1604.

Royal College of Nursing (RCN). *Bowel care. Management of Lower Bowel Dysfunction, Including Digital Rectal Examination and Digital Removal of Faeces. Guidance for Nurses.* London: RCN; 2019.

Royal College of Physicians (Clinical Standards Department). *National Audit of Continence Care. Combined Organisational and Clinical Report.* London: RCP; 2010.

Royal College of Physicians. *Keeping Control: What You Should Expect From Your NHS Bladder and Bowel Service.* London: Healthcare Quality Improvement Partnership/RCP; 2011.

Royal College of Surgeons. *Commissioning Guide: Faecal Incontinence.* London: Royal College of Surgeons of England; 2017.

Slark J, Stewart J. Advances in nursing assessment and management of urinary incontinence for stroke survivors. *Br J Neurosci Nurs.* 2018;13(suppl 5).

Social Care Institute for Excellence (2020). Dignity in care. https://www.scie.org.uk/dignity/care/privacy.

Stewart E. Assessment and management of urinary incontinence in women. *Nurs Stand.* 2018;33(2):75–81.

Thirugnanasothy S. Managing urinary incontinence in older people. *BMJ.* 2010;341:c3835.

Thomas TM, Plymet KR, Blannin J, et al. Prevalence of urinary incontinence. *BMJ.* 1980;281:1243–1245.

Waugh A, Grant A. *Ross and Wilson: Anatomy and Physiology in Health and Illness.* 13th ed. Edinburgh: Churchill Livingstone; 2018.

Yates A. Faecal incontinence: a healthcare taboo. *Br J Nurs.* 2021;30(4). www.britishjournalofnursing.com/content/comment/faecal-incontinence-a-healthcare-taboo.

Further Reading

Royal College of Physicians (Clinical Standards Department). *National Audit of Continence Care. Combined Organisation and Clinical Report.* London: RCP; 2010.

Steggall M. Elimination of urine: care and promotion of continence. In: Brooker C, Waugh A, eds. *Foundations of Nursing Practice: Fundamentals of Holistic Care.* 2nd ed. London: Mosby Elsevier; 2013:491–515.

Walker S. Continence, bowel and bladder care. In: Iggulden H, Macdonald C, Staniland K, eds. *Clinical Skills: The Essence of Caring.* Maidenhead: Open University Press/McGraw-Hill Education; 2009:167–187.

Walker S. Elimination of faeces: care and promotion of continence. In: Brooker C, Waugh A, eds. *Foundations of Nursing Practice: Fundamentals of Holistic Care.* 2nd ed. London: Mosby Elsevier; 2013:517–540.

Walker S. Eliminating. In: Holland K, Jenkins J, eds. *Applying the Roper, Logan and Tierney Model in Practice.* 3rd edition Edinburgh: Churchill Livingstone; 2019:235–266.

Useful Websites

Association for Continence Advice (ACA), www.aca.uk.com
British National Formulary for Community Nurse Prescribers, bnf.nice.org.uk
Bladder and Bowel UK (BBUK), bbuk.org.uk
Chartered Society of Physiotherapy (CSP), www.csp.org.uk
Education and Resources for Improving Childhood Continence (ERIC), www.eric.org.uk
Marie Curie, https://www.mariecurie.org.uk
National Association for Continence; Bladder and Bowel Health (NAC), www.nafc.org
NHS Knowledge and library services (formerly National Library for Health), www.library.nhs.uk
Healthcare Improvement Scotland, www.healthcareimprovementscotland.org
Outsiders (an organisation that supports social inclusion), https://the-outsiders.org.uk/
Paediatric Continence Forum, http://www.paediatriccontinenceforum.org/wp-content/uploads/2016/07/minimum-standards-for-paediatric-continence-care.pdf
Relate, www.relate.org.uk
United Kingdom Continence Society, www.ukcs.uk.net

Nursing Specific Patient Groups

25

The Care of a Person Undergoing Surgery

RUTH MAGOWAN

CHAPTER OUTLINE

Introduction

In this chapter the care of a person undergoing surgery is considered based on current evidence and guidelines, prompting health professionals to consider an individual's priorities and the best possible care experience. Person-centred care is about ensuring that people who require healthcare are at the centre of everything we do, and this is arguably most important when the stakes are highest, such as with surgery. This person-centred care is best delivered when health and social care professionals work collaboratively with people to support what matters to them. It ensures that care is personalised, coordinated and enabling so that people can make informed choices, manage their own health and, where possible, live independent lives (National Education Scotland [NES] 2021).

Preoperative Care

The Decision to Operate and Consent

The only certainty with surgery is that there will be 'injury' to the patient, but this is in the hope, in the longer term, of providing the patient with a longer or better life. The decision to operate, therefore needs to carefully consider the pros and cons of the operation, and it is the patient who must make the final decision as to what treatment is accepted. Knowing what patients hope to gain from an operation, how complications might impact on their overall quality of life and what they would consider an acceptable compromise are all crucial factors in the decision process. Nurses have a valuable role in ensuring the person can make an informed decision and understand the procedure fully (Reflection 25.1).

REFLECTION 25.1

Nursing People Presenting for Surgery: Stop and Think

Ask a person who has recently experienced surgery what signs and symptoms first brought the illness to their attention.

    What made them seek treatment?

    What was the part of their surgical journey that concerned them most?

People have the right to be involved in discussions and make informed decisions about their care, as described in national guidelines and policy (National Institute for Health and Care Excellence [NICE] 2020). All clinical staff must respect, support and document a person's right to accept or refuse care and treatment, and encourage and empower people to share decisions about their treatment and care. An important aspect of this is also an understanding of patient advocacy which includes protecting patients, being the patients' voice, provision of quality care and interpersonal relationship as well as educating patients (Nursing and Midwifery Council [NMC] 2018).

For most healthcare decisions, like a chest X-ray or inserting a suppository, it is reasonable to rely on a patient's verbal consent if clinical staff are satisfied they have had the opportunity to consider any relevant information and decided to go ahead. When a patient is to undergo surgery, particularly if a general anaesthetic is required, it is advisable and standard practice to obtain written consent. With this, it is essential to ensure that:

- The patient understands the information, and not just that it has been given and received.
- The extent of the information is sufficient for that patient to make the decision.

Nurses can consent to patients for procedures in which they are directly involved and have a valuable role in providing the medical team with their knowledge of the individual's need for information when medical consent is specifically required.

In some situations, a patient may be too ill to comprehend what is proposed and thus to give informed consent. Also, within society, there are groups of individuals unable to make decisions for themselves or who cannot communicate. This inability is known as 'mental incapacity'. In Scotland, any issue relating to the welfare of an 'incapable adult' is governed by the Adults With Incapacity Act (Scotland) (2000). Similar legislation was introduced in England and Wales in the Mental Capacity Act 2020 (Office of the Public Guardian 2020). When an adult patient is unconscious or mentally incapacitated, it is necessary to find out whether a family member or friend has been given Power of Attorney, that is, allowed to make decisions on the patient's behalf, or if the patient has previously indicated their wishes in an advance statement. An 'advance statement' is an expression of the patient's preference for treatment or care, given when they are legally competent. This may include the refusal of certain treatments such as surgical intervention or cardiopulmonary resuscitation. If there is no power of attorney, the court of protection may appoint a person, called a 'deputy', to make decisions on behalf of the patient.

In some cases, an Anticipatory Care Plan (ACP) will be developed by the patient, their relatives and their care provider. An ACP is a dynamic record which consists of a summary of 'Thinking Ahead' discussions that should be developed through conversation, collaborative interactions and shared decision making. The ACP is a record of the actions, interventions and responses that care providers should make should the patient ever deteriorate in their care. It should be regularly reviewed and updated in accordance with the patient's condition or personal circumstances. The patient's relatives have no legal right to give or, more importantly, to refuse consent. Lifesaving procedures can be performed without consent using the doctor's clinical privilege. A doctor has the power to take such action as is necessary, but only the minimal amount of treatment should be undertaken to alleviate the emergency and should follow established practice; good practice would suggest that the relatives are consulted, and a decision is made in the patient's best interests (Reflection 25.2). Similarly, relatives have no legal rights in determining whether information should be given to or withheld from the patient. In fact, the doctor or nurse would be in

---

REFLECTION 25.2

Decision-Making

How can nursing staff clarify where decision-making responsibility lies in the following cases?

- A 25-year-old man with Down syndrome is admitted to the ENT ward for elective tonsillectomy.
- An 81-year-old woman is admitted from a nursing home to the vascular ward with an ischaemic left foot. She has a 5-year history of dementia and is very confused. An embolectomy under local anaesthetic and sedation is proposed.
- A young motorcyclist is admitted to the emergency department following a motorcycle accident. He is unconscious and the CT scan reveals a subdural haematoma which requires emergency surgical evacuation.

breach of confidentiality if they were to tell the relatives first, or to tell them at all, without the patient's expressed consent.

When a patient is too ill to be told, or cannot give informed consent, nursing and medical staff must carry out their professional duty to act in the patient's best interests, whilst considering the wishes of the relatives. The NMC Code: Professional Standards of Practice and Behaviour for Nurses, Midwives and Nursing Associates (NMC 2018) provides further guidelines on professional practice.

Assessment

Most patients undergoing surgical procedures are now seen in advance of surgery, often in a preoperative assessment clinic, to highlight any problems there might be and to minimise the risks of these. A common model is where patients are assessed by a nurse, doctor and anaesthetists are also involved. Investigations often include a full blood count in case the patient is anaemic, urea and electrolytes to assess renal function, glucose or HbA1c in case there is diabetes and any relevant cardiac or respiratory tests, for example an electrocardiogram (ECG) or pulmonary function tests. Blood may also be sent for group and save in case a blood transfusion is needed.

Using these results and the patient's history, is it often possible to evaluate the risks of the anaesthetic, and this can be more accurately achieved by using a classification scale, for example the American Society of Anesthesiologists (ASA) Physical Status Classification System; see Table 25.1 or the American College of Surgeons Risk Calculator (https://riskcalculator.facs.org/RiskCalculator/). If any unexpected problems are found, it may be necessary to delay the operation until remedial treatment has been offered, or even cancel the operation if the risks are felt to outweigh the benefits. It is essential that the patient is involved in all of these decisions with regards to surgery.

The preoperative assessment appointment is an important time in which to give the patient more information about the operation and offering emotional support, and nurses are ideally placed for this. For some patients, too much information may become confusing and lead to heightened anxiety, while others may wish minimal information, and some sensitivity is required to pitch the advice appropriately. Verbal, written, video and online resources may be of value. Advice is often given about the person being in optimum health prior to the operation. For example, lifestyle advice in terms of diet and weight optimisation in line with NICE guidelines is given and this may be aided by a nutritional assessment tool, for example the Malnutrition Universal Screening Tool (MUST). MUST is a screening tool used to detect patients who

TABLE 25.1 ASA Physical Status Classification System

Classification	Definition	Example
ASA I	A normal healthy patient	Healthy, nonsmoking, no or minimal alcohol use
ASA II	A patient with mild systemic disease	Mild diseases only without functional limitations. Examples include current smoker, social alcohol drinker, pregnancy, obesity (30 > BMI < 40), well-controlled DM/HTN, mild lung disease
ASA III	A patient with severe systemic disease	Substantive functional limitations; one or more moderate to severe diseases. Examples include poorly controlled DM or HTN, COPD, morbid obesity (BMI ≥40), active hepatitis, alcohol dependence or alcohol abuse, implanted pacemaker, history (>3 months) of MI, CVA, TIA or CAD/stents
ASA IV	A patient with severe systemic disease that is a constant threat to life	Examples include recent (<3 months) MI, CVA, TIA, or CAD/stents, ongoing cardiac ischaemia or severe valve dysfunction, sepsis, DIC, ARD or ESRD not undergoing regularly scheduled dialysis
ASA V	A moribund patient who is not expected to survive without the operation	Examples include ruptured abdominal/thoracic aneurysm, massive trauma, intracranial bleed with mass effect, ischaemic bowel in the face of significant cardiac pathology or multiple organ/system dysfunction
ASA VI	A declared brain-dead patient whose organs are being removed for donor purposes	

ARD, Allergic respiratory disease; *ASA,* American Society of Anesthesiologists; *BMI,* body mass index; *CAD,* coronary artery disease; *COPD,* chronic obstructive pulmonary disease; *CVA,* cerebrovascular accident; *DIC,* disseminated intravascular coagulation; *DM,* diabetes mellitus; *ESRD,* end-stage renal disease; *HTN,* hypertension; *MI,* myocardial infarction; *TIA,* transient ischaemic attack.
Adapted from American Society of Anesthesiologists (ASA). ASA Physical Status Classification System. Updated 2020. https://www.asahq.org/standards-and-practice-parameters/statement-on-asa-physical-status-classification-system.

are at risk from malnutrition. It also includes management guidelines which can be used to develop a care plan. The MUST score is calculated using five steps including: body mass index (BMI), percentage weight loss in the past 6 months and disease effect (BAPEN 2013). In 2013, NICE recommended the use of BAPEN's interactive e-learning resource on nutritional screening using 'MUST' for staff working in all healthcare settings.

Bowel Preparation

While bowel preparation (e.g. with a laxative) is important for patients undergoing colonoscopy, there is debate about whether this (in conjunction with antibiotics) is helpful in major bowel surgery. NICE currently recommends against the routine use of bowel preparation before major bowel surgery (NICE 2019). Bowel preparation is not recommended for non-gastrointestinal (GI) surgery.

Venous Thromboembolic (VTE) Prophylaxis

Current national guidelines and standards recommend that all patients are routinely assessed for their level of mobility on admission to hospital (NICE 2015, 2021). All surgical patients with reduced mobility should be considered at risk of developing a VTE and treated accordingly (NICE 2019).

VTE events consist of deep vein thrombosis (DVT) and pulmonary embolism (PE). DVT is the formation of a clot in the deep leg veins (femoral or popliteal veins), or in the deep veins above the leg (iliac veins or the inferior vena cava) that typically develops between days 3 and 14 postoperatively. A proportion of DVTs dislodge and travel to the pulmonary artery or one of its branches, potentially compromising lung function and sometimes causing death. This is called pulmonary embolism (PE) (Routhier et al. 2023).

Patients undergoing surgery are at increased risk of clot formation due to stasis from immobility, any trauma to the veins and increased coagulability with dehydration. Prevention of DVT is an important part of preoperative nursing care. It is now generally accepted that all patients should use anti-embolism stockings

(TED stockings) as these reduce the risk of developing DVT. Intermittent pneumatic compression stockings can also be during the operation. Although it is not fully understood how anti-embolism stockings work, these stockings create decreasing pressure gradient in the leg from approximately 18 mmHg at the ankle to 8 mmHg at the thigh (full length) or create a calf pressure of 14–15 mmHg (NICE 2019). The gradient increases blood flow in the femoral vein, inhibits stasis of the venous circulation, stops build-up of any nidus of thrombosis formation and prevents the venous distension that causes endothelial damage.

The nurse's role is to ensure that a well-designed and well-fitting stocking is applied. Nurses should ensure that patients understand the importance of wearing anti-embolism stockings appropriately. Stockings are fitted according to calf size and leg length and are available in a wide variety of sizes, ensuring the manufacturer's instructions are carefully followed. There are two lengths of stocking commonly available: thigh and knee length (Lister et al. 2020). Thigh-length stockings are suggested to be more effective (NICE 2019), but below-knee stockings are more comfortable and concordance with therapy may be better.

Some patients should not be offered anti-embolism stockings if they are suspected or proven to have peripheral arterial disease, peripheral arterial bypass grafting, peripheral neuropathy or other causes of sensory impairment, any local conditions in which anti-embolism stockings may cause damage (e.g. fragile skin, dermatitis and recent skin graft), major limb deformities and severe leg oedema (NICE 2019). If there are any concerns about correct fitting, the legs should be remeasured and new stockings applied. Patients should wear stockings prior to surgery and postoperatively until fully mobile.

Other measures that should be encouraged where possible are early activity and hourly leg exercises. The patient should be taught to dorsiflex the foot preoperatively. This will assist venous return by the action of the calf muscle compressing blood in the deep veins. Deep breathing exercises will also aid the respiratory pump, as deep inspiration reduces intrathoracic pressure and hence increases venous return. In addition, ensuring adequate hydration will reduce hypercoagulability. Low-molecular-weight heparin will also be prescribed prophylactically to minimise hypercoagulability. These anticoagulants are given daily subcutaneously (NICE 2019). As full anticoagulation does not occur, the risk of increased intraoperative bleeding complications is minimal.

Minimising Infection

There is a strong association between infection and surgery (NICE 2019). Patients may develop infection at the site of their surgery (surgical site infection – SSI) which may include wound infections, infection of body cavities (e.g. peritonitis), bones, joints, meninges or any of the soft tissues involved in the operation. Infection can also occur at sites away from the operation, for example chest infection associated with hypoventilation at general anaesthesia, urinary tract infection from bladder catheterisation or systemic sepsis following the bacteraemia of any invasive procedure. Attention to hygiene, aseptic nontouch technique (ANTT), physiotherapy and antibiotics can help to minimise the risk of infection. Advice about appropriate preoperative antibiotic prophylaxis is available (NICE 2019). Specific issues that health professionals should be aware of are considered in the following.

The risk of respiratory infection is increased in patients who receive a general anaesthetic or who have prolonged periods of immobility. Smokers, those who vape and patients with preexisting respiratory disease are also more likely to develop perioperative respiratory problems such as pneumonia or bronchospasm (Carrick et al. 2019).

All patients, regardless of whether they are smokers or not, should be taught deep breathing exercises and coughing. It can be difficult to teach a patient to contract the diaphragm to breathe deeply preoperatively, let alone postoperatively. The tendency is to use intercostal and accessory muscles to lift the rib cage and draw the abdomen in. Although instruction may be the responsibility of the physiotherapist, it will still require reinforcement from the nursing staff.

Deep breathing exercises taught preoperatively should include encouraging the patient to practice the following routine:

- Sitting upright, carefully position a pillow over the incision or wound for abdominal support
- Start with gentle and slow breaths in through the nose and out through the mouth
- After 5–10 normal breaths focusing on slow and deep breathing
- Take a deep breath and hold for 2–5 seconds.

The need for early mobilisation can also be described to the patient.

Patients who are undergoing a local anaesthetic, general anaesthetic or heavy sedation are all at risk of aspiration pneumonitis. When a patient is anaesthetised or unconscious, the swallowing reflex is absent. From the point of induction of the anaesthetic, there is a risk that stomach contents may reflux and be inhaled through the open larynx into the lungs. This leads to the development of pneumonitis (lung inflammation) induced by stomach acid, which may become secondarily infected to become pneumonia. Risks can be minimised, partly through the administration of

---

Preoperative Fasting in Adults Undergoing Elective Surgery – 'The 2 and 6 Rule'

'2' – Patients should be encouraged to drink clear fluids (including water, pulp-free juice and tea or coffee without milk) up to 2 hours before elective surgery.

'6' – Solid food should be prohibited for 6 hours before elective surgery in adults.

The anaesthetic team should consider further interventions for patients at higher risk of regurgitation and aspiration.

From Smith et al. 2011.

---

certain drugs, but also by fasting the patient of both diet and fluids according to national guidelines and local policy and procedure.

In younger and healthy individuals, pulmonary aspiration is a rare complication of anaesthesia. However, elderly patients, those who receive opioids and those with diabetes (both type I and type II) may have reduced gastric motility (NICE 2022). Patients with gastro-oesophageal reflux disease are also more at risk of aspiration, particularly when in a prone position. Gastric emptying is usually complete for most meals in 4–5 hours but even fasting patients may still have residual fluid in the stomach. Considering this, the recommended minimum preoperative fasting period is 2 hours for water and 6 hours for food. This is known as the '2 and 6' rule (Liddle 2022, NICE 2020) (Information 25.1).

Premedication

The term 'premedication' (often abbreviated to 'premed') is used to describe medications given to preoperative patients before the operation. Premedication can be used to relieve anxiety, induce a state of analgesia, reduce bronchial and salivary secretions, prevent vasovagal stimulation (mainly bradycardia) and make the patient less aware and drowsy (see Table 25.2). If the medication is likely to make the patient drowsy, it is wise to ensure that the consent form has been signed, the patient has emptied their bladder and that all other preoperative checks are complete before giving the medication.

Intraoperative Care

Theatre Safety

Environmental Safety

The environment in the operating theatre is designed to minimise the risk of exogenous infection to the patient. It is the nurse's role to ensure a safe environment for the patient at all times.

TABLE 25.2	Common Premedication			
Drug A Benzodiazepine Is Used, e.g.		**Usual Adult Dose**	**Route**	**Effects**
Temazepam		10–20 mg	Oral	Sedative: reduces tension and anxiety. Induces drowsiness
Lorazepam		1–3 mg	Oral	Sedative: reduces tension and anxiety. Decreases muscle tone and potentiates nondepolarising muscle relaxants. Induces mental detachment and amnesia

For preemptive analgesia, oral preparations are commonly used instead of IM/SC, e.g. paracetamol and ibuprofen, or oxycodone hydrochloride (long-acting opiate) 10 mg every 12 hours.
From NICE British National Formulary. Pre-medication and peri-operative drugs. 2023. https://bnf.nice.org.uk/treatment-summaries/pre-medication-and-peri-operative-drugs/.

1. Clean, filtered air is pumped into clean areas. Air pressure is higher inside the theatre than outside to maintain air flow from the theatre to the outside. This prevents potentially contaminated air from the rest of the hospital moving into the theatres. Waste anaesthetic gases are also removed via a scavenging system.
2. Temperature is controlled through the ventilation system. This is to provide a comfortable working environment for staff and to prevent patients from developing intraoperative hypothermia.
3. Humidity is maintained at 50%–55%. This is to prevent a build-up of static electricity and the risk of sparks if flammable anaesthetic gases are used. It also suppresses bacterial growth.
4. Clean and dirty areas are delineated by doors or a line on the floor. All personnel moving into clean areas should be clean and appropriately dressed (see later). All items brought into clean areas should be clean. All dirty items leaving the theatre should do so via dirty areas. Staff must be aware of the dirty and clean areas and corridors.
5. The numbers and movements of staff inside theatres should be kept to a minimum to reduce the number of skin scales shed, mixing of air, contamination rate of surgical wounds and prevent SSIs (Anderson et al. 2017).
6. All staff entering clean areas should be appropriately dressed. Clean theatre 'scrubs' are worn, and hair should be completely covered by a theatre cap. Acrylic or gel nails should not be worn as these have been shown to harbour microorganisms such as fungi and Gram-negative bacteria even after hand washing; they can also inhibit hand washing (Association for Perioperative Practice [AfPP] 2020).

A sterile field is created around the patient. The patient and trolleys in this area are all covered with sterile drapes. The surgeon and scrub nurse (or health professional assisting with surgery) wear sterile gloves and gowns to work within the sterile field.

Patient Safety

The nurse must carry out preoperative checks before the administration of the premed, as the results of the checks may cause a delay in going to theatre. Many hospitals have created their own checklists. Examples of criteria for preoperative checklists are given in Table 25.3.

During the immediate preoperative period, the patient may feel extremely vulnerable and anxious. They will wear only a gown, their dentures may have been removed, they may be unable to see well without glasses and may feel drowsy from the premed. Anxiety about the impending operation can be high, especially among patients placed in the later part of the operating list. Reassurance by the nurse and, for some patients, distraction can be helpful. A family member or designated staff member offering support to the patient at this time may have a calming effect (NICE 2020).

If able, patients may walk to the theatre, otherwise they will be brought on a trolley or on a bed, and are usually transferred to a bed at the end of the operation.

The theatre nurse or operating department practitioner (ODP) receiving the patient goes through the preoperative check again (see Table 25.3) and, if possible, asks the patient to confirm details. All patients must be supervised by a healthcare professional in this preinduction time, as the patient may have received premedication and is in a stressful and unfamiliar environment.

The roles of nurses and other theatre staff are summarised in Information 25.2. Traditionally, a surgeon performs the surgery, although it is now common for advanced nurse practitioners and ODPs to perform minor surgical procedures. The anaesthetist will usually visit the patient preoperatively in the ward or clinic to assess the patient's ability to tolerate the anaesthetic, give information and reassurance and prescribe a premedication if needed.

The emphasis of all roles in theatre is on patient safety and teamwork, and each professional has an important part to play in the patient's passage through theatre (Information 25.3. In reality, nurses need to have the ability with other theatre practitioners to be

TABLE 25.3	Preoperative Checklist	
Criteria	**Action**	**Rationale**
Identification	Prepare two name bands with the patient's full name, hospital unit number, date of birth, home address (as a minimum), plus ward and consultant Clearly note allergies on the anaesthetic sheet and on wrist bands as well as the prescription chart Ensure site is correctly marked with indelible ink	Correct identification of patient Avoidance of all allergens Correct identification of site
Documentation	Ensure that medical notes, nursing notes, signed consent form, X-rays and anaesthetic sheet accompany patient to theatre Ensure the complete set of observations for baseline has been documented	Ready availability of all necessary information
Fasting	Document when the patient last had anything to eat or drink	Prevention of aspiration pneumonia
Empty bladder	Ask the patient to pass urine prior to administering premedication	To prevent damage to full bladder during surgery To enable complete bed rest after premed To prevent postoperative discomfort due to a full bladder
Risk of diathermy burns	Ask the patient to remove all jewellery, hair pins and other items containing metal (wedding rings may be covered with tape)	To remove all metal that may concentrate the diathermy current
Prostheses	Ask the patient to remove all prostheses, e.g. dentures, hearing aids, contact lenses, false eyes, glasses, etc.	To prevent harm caused by prostheses To prevent loss
Care of valuables	Offer to receive valuables into safekeeping for the patient	Patient will be away from the ward and unfit to be responsible for these valuables
Circulatory assessment	Ask the patient to remove all makeup, lipstick and nail varnish	To facilitate observation of colour of skin, lips and nail beds

INFORMATION 25.2

Theatre Roles and Responsibilities of Nursing Staff/Theatre Practitioners

Although some roles are outlined here with specific responsibilities, in reality, nurses need to have the ability with other theatre practitioners to be interchangeable and adaptable to many roles, and this may change from day to day and case to case.

The Anaesthetic Nurse/Practitioner

- Receives the patient in the reception area of the anaesthetic room.
- Checks patient in, deals with any irregularities.
- Helps to relieve patient anxiety.
- Initiates routine monitoring of patient and assists with insertion of invasive monitoring devices if needed.
- Assists in the induction (and maintenance) of anaesthesia.
- Performs emergency preparation of patients for theatre.
- Uses and checks anaesthetic equipment.
- Maintains patient safety and comfort.

The Circulating Nurse/Practitioner

- Performs the surgical checklist and surgical pause.
- Assists with the provision of equipment.
- Maintains nursing records.
- Positions the patient.
- Ensures safety regarding instruments and swabs.
- Cleans and sterilises equipment.
- Observes, measures and records vital signs.

The Scrub Nurse/Practitioner

- Positions the patient.
- Provides appropriate sterile equipment.
- Assists the surgeon.
- Protects the patient's dignity and changes drapes to avoid pooling of cleansing agents (e.g. povidone-iodine)
- Prevents diathermy and pressure injuries, and ensures no equipment is rubbing.
- Ensures safety regarding instruments and swabs.
- Manages the high-risk patient.

The Recovery Room Nurse/Practitioner

- Maintains patency of the airway
- Observes patient for level of consciousness and safety.
- Monitors vital signs: colour, respiration, temperature (core and peripheral), pulse, blood pressure, fluid intake and output, wounds and drainage.
- Assesses pain and nausea and administers analgesics and antiemetics.
- Reassures the patient and provides a quiet environment.
- Provides total patient care.
- Provides documentation and facilitates communication.
- Ensures patient meets discharge criteria prior to transfer from recovery room.

---

interchangeable and adaptable to many roles, and this may change from day to day and case to case Information 25.2). Communication problems leading to information loss could compromise patient safety in the operating room (Espin et al. 2020).

Most theatres have a prelist and postlist team briefing, and all theatres use preoperative World Health Organization (WHO) surgical safety checklists (WHO 2022). This list decreases errors and adverse events and improves teamwork and communication in surgery.

Surgical Safety Checklist

World Health Organization | Patient Safety
A World Alliance for Safer Health Care

Before induction of anaesthesia	Before skin incision	Before patient leaves operating room
(with at least nurse and anaesthetist)	(with nurse, anaesthetist and surgeon)	(with nurse, anaesthetist and surgeon)

Before induction of anaesthesia

Has the patient confirmed his/her identity, site, procedure, and consent?
- ☐ Yes

Is the site marked?
- ☐ Yes
- ☐ Not applicable

Is the anaesthesia machine and medication check complete?
- ☐ Yes

Is the pulse oximeter on the patient and functioning?
- ☐ Yes

Does the patient have a:

Known allergy?
- ☐ No
- ☐ Yes

Difficult airway or aspiration risk?
- ☐ No
- ☐ Yes, and equipment/assistance available

Risk of >500ml blood loss (7ml/kg in children)?
- ☐ No
- ☐ Yes, and two IVs/central access and fluids planned

Before skin incision

- ☐ Confirm all team members have introduced themselves by name and role.
- ☐ Confirm the patient's name, procedure, and where the incision will be made.

Has antibiotic prophylaxis been given within the last 60 minutes?
- ☐ Yes
- ☐ Not applicable

Anticipated Critical Events

To Surgeon:
- ☐ What are the critical or non-routine steps?
- ☐ How long will the case take?
- ☐ What is the anticipated blood loss?

To Anaesthetist:
- ☐ Are there any patient-specific concerns?

To Nursing Team:
- ☐ Has sterility (including indicator results) been confirmed?
- ☐ Are there equipment issues or any concerns?

Is essential imaging displayed?
- ☐ Yes
- ☐ Not applicable

Before patient leaves operating room

Nurse Verbally Confirms:
- ☐ The name of the procedure
- ☐ Completion of instrument, sponge and needle counts
- ☐ Specimen labelling (read specimen labels aloud, including patient name)
- ☐ Whether there are any equipment problems to be addressed

To Surgeon, Anaesthetist and Nurse:
- ☐ What are the key concerns for recovery and management of this patient?

This checklist is not intended to be comprehensive. Additions and modifications to fit local practice are encouraged.   Revised 1 / 2009   © WHO, 2009

INFORMATION 25.3

Top Tips for Students on a Theatre Placement

- Be aware of the specialist area you are going to be working in. Having a good general knowledge of the physiology relating to the specialised area, for example orthopaedics or cardiothoracic, is an advantage as it means you have increased understanding of the surgical procedures taking place.
- Get to know the daily routine and layout of the theatres. Each theatre will differ slightly, but being aware of the patient pathway is helpful in learning when to get equipment ready for a procedure, whether as circulating nurse or scrub nurse.
- Know the dress code, even when socialising in the staff room. Scrubs, hat and clean shoes (which are only for theatre purposes) are essential. This is to prevent infection. When entering the theatre, a mask is also needed, and a lead overcoat may be necessary if X-rays are being taken. When scrubbed up, a sterile overcoat, gloves, mask and glasses are essential.
- Work with different people – everyone will have differing experiences of working in theatres in terms of specialised areas, length of work time and trauma or elective theatre work.
- Be aware of the different stages of each procedure so that you can predict what implements may be needed, for example sutures or dressings.
- Participate in maintaining the theatre environment – cleaning after each patient, changing suction, wiping the whiteboard which contains information in relation to swab/suture counts, making sure correct equipment is available.
- If you are given the opportunity to scrub up, familiarise yourself with the basic trays and common sutures, alcoholic washes and dressings, so you are more likely to be aware of each of the instruments and their uses. Knowing the stages of the differing procedures is helpful here as you can predict which supplementary implements may be needed and what instruments the surgeon is likely to require. Knowing the basics can also help reduce anxiety when participating as the scrub nurse.

INFORMATION 25.4

Patient-Related Risk Factors for Venous Thromboembolism

- Immobility
- Active cancer or cancer treatment
- Dehydration
- Known thrombophilias
- One or more significant medical comorbidities (e.g. heart disease; metabolic, endocrine, or respiratory pathologies; acute infectious diseases; inflammatory conditions)
- Personal history or first-degree relative with a history of VTE
- Use of hormone replacement therapy
- Use of oestrogen-containing contraceptive therapy
- Varicose veins with phlebitis
- Pregnancy or <6 weeks postpartum (see NICE guidance for specific risk factors)
- Age >60 years
- Obesity (body mass index >30 kg/m^2)

Adapted from National Institute for Health and Care Excellence (NICE). Perioperative care in adults. NICE guideline [NG180]. 2020. https://www.nice.org.uk/guidance/ng180.

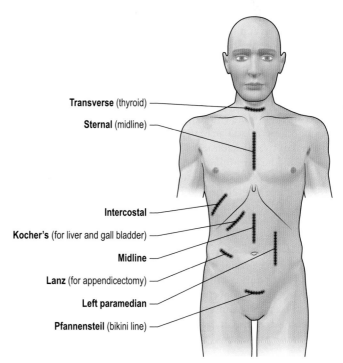

Transverse (thyroid)
Sternal (midline)
Intercostal
Kocher's (for liver and gall bladder)
Midline
Lanz (for appendicectomy)
Left paramedian
Pfannensteil (bikini line)

Figure 25.1 Some incision sites used in surgery.

It is also important to ensure that:

1. There is careful positioning on the operating table to minimise the risk of developing pressure ulcers and the risk of VTE (Information 25.4). Patients who have regional anaesthesia (e.g. spinal, or epidural) have reduced sensation in the lower extremities and impaired leg movement because of the effects of the anaesthetic mixture on the motor nerve pathways in the spinal cord. These patients are especially at risk of heel pressure ulcers because they may fail to change the position of their legs in bed or feel the sensation of discomfort. Pressure-relieving padding, mattresses or overlays can be used in high-risk patients to protect vulnerable areas such as elbows, heels and sacrum. Once patients are anaesthetised, they may lose muscle tone. Care should be taken with all limbs, as nerve damage can occur from compression or traction of a limb whilst the patient is anaesthetised. A nurse must also be aware when positioning patients on the operating table of limitations in movement that may result from previous joint replacement surgery; for example, hip flexion may be restricted in patients with a total hip replacement prosthesis. Patient position will depend on the requirements of the surgical procedure. Common surgical positions are supine, prone and lithotomy.

2. The diathermy pad is carefully positioned. A self-adhesive pad may be used, and the pad is usually placed on the thigh to ensure good contact over the entire surface. Poor contact by only part of the surface may concentrate the current, causing it to leave a burn.

3. Swabs, needles and instruments used during the operation are counted and checked throughout and at the end of the operation by the scrub nurse and circulating nurse. This ensures that all items used are accounted for and none left inside the patient.

4. The patient's skin is cleaned at the start of the procedure with an antiseptic skin preparation. The most common antiseptics are chlorhexidine gluconate, alcohol-based solutions and iodophors like povidone-iodine and this will depend on the site of the incision (see Fig. 25.1). Current evidence suggests that 2% chlorhexidine gluconate in 70% isopropyl alcohol should be used for skin preparation as it is quick acting, produces a rapid reduction in bacterial counts on the skin and its action is longer lasting in comparison

to iodine. Once applied, alcohol-based solutions must be allowed to dry completely lest they ignite on contact with diathermy. Prophylactic antibiotics may be administered (usually intravenously) during the operation, or the site of the surgery may be irrigated with an antibiotic solution. These measures are usually taken only if there is a specific risk of contamination, or if contamination from an abscess or the GI tract is already present. Individual patient assessment is essential.

5. Bleeding during surgery is minimised by the use of clamps and ligatures, local pressure and diathermy to seal small vessels. To facilitate the surgeon's vision, the site of operation is kept free of blood by swabbing or suctioning. The circulating nurse may weigh the swabs and note the volume of blood in the suction bottle to estimate 'total blood loss'. Suction can also be used in laparoscopic and robotic surgery for fluid and blood removal.

6. Particular care must be taken in the use of sharps, especially in the transfer between the surgeon and the scrub nurse in case of needlestick injury to prevent cross-infection and to reduce risks involved with cleaning and spillages, disposable equipment is used where possible (Lister et al. 2020).

Anaesthesia

An anaesthetic is used to block any sensations of pain during surgery. It may be applied locally or regionally for surgery, or generally throughout the body.

Local Anaesthesia

Local anaesthesia blocks transmission of pain from the region operated upon. In some cases, only the sensory receptors may be blocked; this is more correctly termed 'local analgesia'. Types and common uses of local anaesthetics are summarised in Table 25.4. Epidural or spinal anaesthetics may be used when a general anaesthetic could be harmful or undesirable, for example older patients with arteriosclerosis or diabetes, patients with respiratory disorders and those with hypertension. Some patients, if suitable, may be offered a choice. An infusion of epidural anaesthetic agents can also be continued after surgery to provide effective postoperative analgesia. The procedure causes hypotension and so should be avoided in patients with this condition.

Care must be taken to prepare the patient psychologically for what to expect during a procedure using local anaesthetic to reduce anxiety and ensure cooperation. Psychological and emotional support and reassuring conversation should continue throughout the operation if appropriate, and the nurse should ensure the patient's vision of the procedure is adequately screened.

TABLE 25.4	**Types and Common Uses of Local Anaesthetics**	
Method of Administration	**Effect**	**Example of Drugs and Their Uses**
Topical: solution or cream applied to skin or mucous membranes	Blocks local sensory nerve receptors	Lidocaine Amitop cream (topical) Minor ENT procedures Insertion of cannulae
Infiltration: injection into surgical site	Blocks local sensory nerve receptors	Lidocaine, bupivacaine E.g. removal of skin moles, insertion of Hickman line

ENT, Ears, nose, throat.

General Anaesthesia

General anaesthesia is characterised by loss of consciousness, analgesia and muscle relaxation. These effects occur according to the stage of anaesthesia, as follows:

Stage 1

The pain is reduced or relieved, but the patient is still conscious. Heavy sedation can produce 'dissociative anaesthesia' and some muscle relaxation, while local analgesics supplement pain control, as necessary. The patient may remain drowsy but conscious throughout the procedure. Entonox (50% oxygen with 50% nitrous oxide) may be self-administered during childbirth or painful procedures such as large wound dressings to achieve stage 1 anaesthesia for pain control.

Stage 2

Consciousness is lost, but the patient may still show movements and irrational behaviour. With intravenous induction of anaesthesia, this stage is passed through very quickly; it may be more in evidence when the patient is recovering from anaesthesia.

Stage 3

Breathing becomes regular and there is relaxation of the muscles along with loss of reflexes. This is the level of surgical anaesthesia. The degree of muscle relaxation needed to facilitate surgery can be achieved by deepening this stage, but this has undesirable side-effects such as a fall in cardiac output, respiratory depression and liver damage. To overcome this problem, muscle relaxants can be administered to enable a relatively light anaesthetic to be used and so reduce the risks in older people and those with cardiovascular and respiratory complications.

The induction of anaesthesia is usually achieved with a short-acting intravenous agent administered with a short-acting muscle relaxant. This rapidly produces surgical anaesthesia in which the patient is unable to maintain their own airway (due to lack of reflexes) and the breathing muscles are paralysed. The airway is maintained usually with either a laryngeal mask (LMA) over the vocal cords or an endotracheal tube passed through the relaxed cords. Artificial ventilation will be required in those who are paralysed. For those patients who require emergency surgery, who have not fasted, the anaesthetist may decide to use rapid sequence induction with cricoid pressure – as the patient becomes unconscious, pressure is applied to the cricoid cartilage in the throat, which mechanically occludes the oesophagus and is thought to reduce the likelihood of aspiration of any regurgitated gastric contents.

Anaesthesia can be maintained during surgery, usually by means of inhaled anaesthetics and a longer-acting muscle relaxant. At the end of the operation, the anaesthetic gas is discontinued, and the effects of the muscle relaxant are reversed with an appropriate drug. The patient gradually regains consciousness, passing through stages 2 and 1 of anaesthesia and regaining muscle tone, which enables independent breathing. During this time, the patient is transferred to the recovery room. The anaesthetist will hand over care of the patient to a recovery room nurse who will monitor the patient closely.

Recovery

The patient will normally be nursed in the recovery room until the immediate effects of the anaesthetic have worn off. Regular and careful assessment of the patient is important for early detection of any problems and to instigate immediate treatment. Recovery room nurses may follow the ABCDE approach and follow on actions (airway, breathing, circulation, disability, exposure) to structure their assessment (Resuscitation Council UK 2021).

Assessment and close observations of the patient should be recorded on a National Early Warning Scale (NEWS) 2 chart. NEWS 2 is an evidence-based tool that supports recognition, escalation and communication of acute illness, which includes sepsis (Royal College of Physicians 2017).

Airway

A patient airway can be achieved by placing the patient in a lateral or semiprone position, tilting the head backwards and pulling the mandible forwards, or inserting a Guedel (oropharyngeal) airway. If a Guedel airway is used, it can be left in position until, as reflexes return, the patient expels it spontaneously. Anaesthetic drugs, muscle relaxants, narcotics and severe pain itself can cause nausea and vomiting and so there is a risk of upper airway obstruction and aspiration pneumonia should the patient vomit while regaining consciousness. Therefore working suction equipment must be available.

Breathing

Patients are usually prescribed supplementary oxygen until fully awake, in order to maintain PO_2 while there is still some respiratory depression due to anaesthesia. A recovery room nurse should observe the patient's respiratory rate, rhythm and depth closely for signs of hypoventilation due to secretions or uncontrolled pain, or respiratory depression due to opiates, supported by pulse oximetry monitoring. It should be noted that SpO_2 may be overestimated in hypoxia in those with darker skin (NHS Race and Health Observatory 2021).

Circulation

Close and frequent observation of pulse and blood pressure is required for the early detection of changes in the patient's condition. During surgery and anaesthesia the patient's blood pressure may have been reduced due to the effects of anaesthesia and blood loss. Hypotension is often induced during surgery due to anaesthetic agents and during the recovery period patients are especially at risk of reactionary haemorrhage as their blood pressure rises – a suture or clot may become dislodged, leading to haemorrhage and hypovolaemic shock. Observation of wound dressings and drains will also aid assessment of any continued blood loss in the recovery period. A patient who is bleeding may appear pale but natural skin tone should be considered before determining the degree of pallor. Skin colour is particularly important when observing the patient for cyanosis. Central cyanosis (cyanosis of the lips, mucous membranes and tongue) occurs when arterial oxygen saturation falls below 85% in patients with normal haemoglobin levels. In light-skinned or paler patients, cyanosis usually presents as a dark bluish tint to the skin and mucous membranes (indicating the bluish tint of unoxygenated haemoglobin). But in dark-skinned patients, cyanosis will present as grey or whitish (not bluish) skin around the mouth, and the conjunctivae may appear grey or bluish. In patients with yellowish skin, cyanosis may cause a greyish-greenish skin tone (Sommers 2011).

During surgery, the patient may have had a large surface area exposed, leading to loss of body heat. A high risk of hypothermia (a core temperature of less than 35°C) exists in surgery, particularly when the peritoneal cavity has been opened or when large amounts of unwarmed irrigation fluids are used. Shivering will have been suppressed due to skeletal muscle relaxants.

Extra blankets, forced air system and warming of intravenous fluids can be used, but it is important to be aware that warming the patient too quickly can lead to peripheral vasodilation and a consequent fall in blood pressure.

Disability

A nurse should observe the patient's level of consciousness and be aware that a stage of excitement (stage 2 anaesthesia) may occur. Close observation and the use of side rails may be required. Opioid analgesics may cause a fall in blood pressure and respiratory depression, and severe pain can lead to shock and shallow breathing.

As the patient regains consciousness, the nurse should bear in mind that hearing is usually one of the first senses to return. Verbal reassurance that the operation is over should be given. It is appropriate to return hearing aids and glasses to the patient at this point. The patient should be allowed to rest as quietly as possible during this period and will usually fall asleep after regaining consciousness. Most patients will require attention to their mouth, as mucous membranes will be dry due to oxygen therapy, fasting and perhaps dehydration, as potential pressure areas should be monitored.

The patient should be fully conscious, able to maintain a clear airway and be considered haemodynamically stable before transfer back to the ward (Lister et al. 2020). Pain should also be controlled, and appropriate medication regimens prescribed. In some cases, the patient will be transferred directly to the intensive therapy unit (ITU) while continuing to be intubated and their respiration is maintained by artificial ventilation. Alternatively, the patient may be ventilated in the recovery room overnight, hereby avoiding unnecessary admission to ITU.

The recovery room nurse will document the care given and provide a summary to the ward nurse who collects the patient so that continuity of care can be achieved. The role of the recovery room nurse is summarised in Information 25.2. Anaesthetic and surgical staff should document clear instructions for postoperative treatment and highlight possible complications.

For more excellent resources, please see the perioperative toolkit produced by the AfPP (Perioperative Toolkit, theatre etiquette educational session. https://www.afpp.org.uk/careers/educationhub/toolkit).

Postoperative Care

The postoperative phase of care is from when patients have regained stable vital functions in recovery until they are ready for discharge. All patients require close observation during the immediate postoperative period to detect complications. Close observation may be continued for hours or days for the patient requiring intensive nursing care or, in day surgery, for less than a few hours.

Rehabilitation will be achieved at a different pace and to differing levels by each patient. The patient with a hip replacement may find that their joint pain is almost immediately reduced postoperatively and that their functional ability is far better than before the operation. Some patients may not be able to achieve the desired level of recovery and others may be seeking palliation rather than cure.

Assessment

The most common general postoperative complications include postoperative fever, haemorrhage, atelectasis, wound infection, embolism and DVT.

Airway and breathing problems, for example, may occur with oversedation or excess intravenous fluids; intraabdominal or intrathoracic bleeding may not be apparent, particularly if there has been no drain inserted; untreated sepsis may lead to multiorgan failure; cardiac shock may result from a pulmonary embolus or ischaemic heart disease; irreversible acute kidney injury may occur secondary to hypoperfusion; raised intracranial pressure can occur following intracranial procedures; and limb ischaemia from compartment syndrome can develop rapidly, and can easily be missed. All of these are correctable, but only if identified early, and correct interpretation of deteriorating clinical observations is key to this correction and recovery. Escalation and documentation of findings are key to avoiding deterioration.

The frequency of the recordings is determined by the patient's condition and in accordance with local policies and guidelines. Early warning scores, or track and trigger score (TTS) systems such as NEWS2 (RCP 2017), can be used to identify early deterioration. The exact details of these early warning scoring systems are frequently updated as new evidence arises and are often specific to different specialties, for example obstetrics, but usually include a variety of physiological measurement such as pulse, blood pressure, temperature, oxygen saturation, blood results and neurological parameters. Evidence suggests that outcomes are improved but this will only happen when the scoring systems are used alongside clinical knowledge and experience to separate truly deteriorating patients from those who are well and do not need to be escalated (Grant and Crimmons 2018).

Many surgical units have standard postoperative protocols in place which prescribe the frequency of routine recordings in the immediate postoperative period, for example every 15 minutes for the first hour, decreasing to 30 minutes over the next hour and hourly thereafter. It is important that nurses consider each patient's observations carefully, as the frequency of recordings may need to be escalated in response to changes in the patient's condition, for example if the patient has uncontrolled pain or becomes increasingly confused. Nursing and medical staff should agree acceptable parameters for the monitoring of postoperative patients and actions to be taken if the parameters being monitored change (Lister et al. 2020). A table of the key postoperative nursing considerations in the immediate postoperative period is provided on the website. See also Reflection 25.3.

Haemostasis and Hypovolaemic Shock

The consequences of poor tissue perfusion include single or multiple organ failure, breakdown of surgical anastomoses, cerebral damage and death. The most common cause of shock immediately postoperatively is primary haemorrhage in the first 24 hours, but particularly in the first few hours, causing hypovolaemic shock. The patient may collapse suddenly and will usually need to return to theatre. Hypovolaemic shock may also occur due to a slow, continuous loss of fluid; this might be a slowly bleeding vessel or the pooling of fluid in the GI tract during the paralytic ileus that occurs as a consequence of surgery. The loss of fluid may be detected as soakage on the dressing or blood in the wound drains, but if the patient is bleeding into a body cavity or losing fluid into the gut, it may be less obvious. Secondary haemorrhage can occur 1–7 days postoperatively due to vessel erosion by infection or from a long, slow bleed.

REFLECTION 25.3

Postoperative Monitoring: Deviation of Vital Signs

What causes of tachycardia would you need to consider in a postoperative patient?

INFORMATION 25.5

Signs and Symptoms of the Initial Compensation and Failing Compensation

Initial Compensation
- Appears clammy, pale
- Peripheral cyanosis
- Appears restless; may complain of feeling generally unwell
- Falling urine output but may remain above 0.5 mL/kg per hour
- Increase in pulse rate
- Slight rise in systolic blood pressure
- Increased soakage of blood on wound dressings and in wound drains

Failing Compensation
- Appears cold, clammy
- Central cyanosis
- Appears confused, often agitated, and then increasingly drowsy
- Urine output falls below 0.5 mL/kg per hour
- Tachycardia
- Fall in blood pressure
- Capillary refill >2 seconds
- Large volumes of blood may be lost

Activities
- Access the literature and current guidelines relating to perioperative nutrition.
- Reflect on the practices you have observed in placement regarding the postoperative nutrition of patients following abdominal surgery.
- Consider the ways in which you can discuss recent evidence about safety and tolerability of early feeding with members of multidisciplinary surgical teams to improve nutritional care.

The aim of nursing observations in the first 24 hours following surgery is to detect changes that might indicate the initial stages of compensation to hypovolaemic shock (Information 25.5). As the circulating volume falls, the nurse may see increased loss of blood on dressings or in wound drainage bags or bottles. There will be a slight rise in heart rate to maintain cardiac output, but systolic blood pressure may remain unchanged, or even rise slightly. Peripheral vasoconstriction to conserve blood supply to vital organs (brain, heart and lungs) and secretion of sweat from the eccrine glands on the palms and forehead may lead to a pale, clammy appearance. The brain is extremely sensitive to hypoxia resulting in confusion; the respiratory rate may also be increased, and the patient may also appear restless. In an average adult weighing 70 kg, the body can compensate for blood losses up to 750 mL, and changes in physiological signs can be difficult to detect at this early stage. Blood pressure may be maintained because of the combination of vasoconstriction and increased cardiac contractility brought about by the sympathetic nervous system response. Vasoconstriction of the veins maintains diastolic (end) volume and therefore preserves stroke volume. This, along with increased cardiac contractility, can maintain blood pressure to at least preshock levels. It is not until fluid losses exceed 750 mL that changes in vital signs will occur as the body's compensation mechanisms deteriorate. Action should be taken immediately when hypovolaemic shock is suspected. If nurses wait until the patient displays the classic signs of tachycardia and profound hypotension, then blood loss may already be significant.

If the blood or fluid loss continues, then these mechanisms will eventually fail to compensate effectively, leading to further vasoconstriction of the arterioles to increase peripheral resistance. There is also reduced parasympathetic activity to increase heart rate and stroke volume, resulting in increased cardiac output. At this point, the heart rate increases further, and blood pressure begins to fall. Urine output decreases rapidly, due to decreased renal perfusion over and above the effects of increased antidiuretic hormone (ADH) and aldosterone (see Chapter 10, Nursing Patients With Urinary Disorders), as blood flow is conserved to maintain the brain, heart and lungs as a priority.

Less common causes of postoperative shock are cardiogenic, septic, anaphylactic (usually from drug reactions) and neurogenic (from severe pain). Cardiogenic shock is caused by failure of the heart to pump and maintain adequate cardiac output. Possible causes following surgery may be pulmonary embolus, causing massive resistance to the output from the right side of the heart, fluid overload and concomitant heart failure, anaesthetic depression of cardiac output or myocardial infarction. Careful patient assessment may reveal dilatation of neck veins and a 12-lead ECG will detect arrhythmias and myocardial ischaemia.

Oxygen therapy is essential to reduce hypoxia. In hypovolaemic shock the lost fluid must be replaced or returned to the circulation – initially crystalloid, but also blood (ideally through a warmer) if there is haemorrhage. Some patients may have large amounts of fluid available in the body, as in paralytic ileus or peripheral oedema, but in the wrong body compartment. This fluid can be drawn back into the circulation by treating the cause and by raising the osmotic pressure of the circulation. If there is a urinary catheter in situ, the measurement of hourly urine volumes will allow the nurse to monitor renal perfusion, and a central venous catheter may be inserted in those whose shock proves difficult to manage.

Reflection – what are the signs of shock and sepsis and the important first nursing priorities in the deteriorating patient?

Fluid and Electrolyte Balance

Most patients experience some loss of fluid during surgery which may be compounded by electrolyte disturbances resulting from the illness itself or trauma during surgery. Nurses should also account for other potential fluid losses such as GI fluid loss through vomit, nasogastric (NG) tube or fistula. Patients having a general anaesthetic will be fasted postoperatively until they are fully conscious and cough and swallowing reflexes have returned. Some may be required to fast for longer than this if there is paralytic ileus or after facial or laryngeal surgery. These patients may require fluid and electrolyte replacement via the intravenous route to meet normal demands and some require over and above this volume to replace fluid lost during surgery. Many surgical patients complain of thirst and a dry mouth postoperatively. This is due partly to dehydration, to the drying effects of oxygen therapy and to the anticholinergic effects of drugs given during anaesthesia. Thirst is therefore an unreliable measure of hydration.

Fluid and electrolyte balance can be significantly affected by the body's physiological response to surgical stress. Glucocorticoid secretion increases reabsorption of sodium and water in the renal nephrons with a reciprocal loss of potassium and hydrogen ions. Elevated levels of ADH also increase water reabsorption and high aldosterone levels increase sodium reabsorption further. The net effect is to increase the extracellular fluid volume and reduce urine output. It would not be unusual for a well-hydrated patient to retain fluid and have a high positive fluid balance for the immediate postoperative period. The careful monitoring of urinary function is thus a key element of nursing observations in the postoperative period.

Surgery by its very nature causes trauma to the tissues during surgery, such that cells are damaged and their intracellular potassium is released. This may, in major surgery, lead to hyperkalaemia (high potassium) which is cardiotoxic; potassium levels should therefore be closely monitored in patients who have undergone major surgery and fluid replacement adjusted accordingly and, occasionally, treatment given to reduce potassium levels.

Pain

The aim for managing pain postoperatively is to reduce or diminish pain and discomfort with a minimum of side-effects (see Chapter 20, Pain Management). Being in pain is the major preoperative concern of many patients. Patients may have little knowledge of the nature of postoperative pain or the methods available to treat it. While major thoracic and abdominal operations tend to cause most pain, pain management is also a considerable issue for day surgery patients in the first 24 hours postoperatively. More than 80% of patients who undergo surgical procedures experience acute postoperative pain and approximately 75% of those with postoperative pain report the severity as moderate, severe or extreme (Chou 2017).

Macintyre and Schug (2021) identify several barriers to effective nursing management of pain including:
- Perception that it is normal and acceptable for patients to have pain after surgery.
- Misconception that patients will become addicted to opioid analgesics.
- Underestimation of the severity when patients report pain and therefore failure to administer adequate analgesics to control pain.
- Failure to undertake regular assessment of pain and reassessment following administration of analgesics.
- Reluctance of some patients to ask for analgesics.
- Reluctance/lack of knowledge on behalf of the nurse.

Good pain control allows for early activity, so minimising problems of immobility such as constipation, chest infection, urinary tract infection, DVT, pressure ulcers and muscle wasting. Ineffective pain relief in the postoperative period can also have serious psychological consequences for patients facing subsequent surgery and is also associated with the development of chronic pain.

Nurses have two specific roles in the management of postoperative pain: pain assessment and provision of the means to alleviate the pain. Assessment is the cornerstone of care and accurate and systematic assessment of pain is essential. Opioid analgesics are the mainstay of postoperative pain control. Some commonly used analgesics are given in Table 25.5. Opioid analgesics can be given via intramuscular, subcutaneous, intravenous or epidural routes. The patient should be advised not to wait until the pain is unbearable (experiencing the ill-effects of this pain) as they may continue to experience pain for a further 15–20 minutes until the injection takes effect. Analgesia can be administered before painful stimulus occurs and may prevent or substantially reduce subsequent pain or analgesic requirements; this is known as preemptive analgesia. There is substantive evidence that the use of preemptive analgesia reduces postoperative pain, opioid consumption and postoperative nausea or vomiting, and delays rescue analgesia (Xuan et al. 2022).

Nonsteroidal antiinflammatory drugs (NSAIDs) are very effective for the management of postoperative pain. These medications are often used in combination with opioid analgesics and local

TABLE 25.5	Analgesics Commonly Used in Postoperative Pain Control	
Method of Administration	**Example of Drug Used**	**Example of Types of Surgery**
Epidural infusion	Bupivacaine and lidocaine, fentanyl and bupivacaine mixture, diamorphine	Major pelvic or lower abdominal, e.g. colectomy
Intravenous infusion, e.g. PCA	Diamorphine, morphine sulphate, fentanyl, tramadol	Major surgery where moderate to severe pain expected
Intravenous or subcutaneous injection	Diamorphine, morphine sulphate, fentanyl, oxycodone	Major pelvic or abdominal, e.g. gastrectomy
Subcutaneous injection	Morphine, oxycodone	Many types of surgery, as for IM injection
Intramuscular injection	Morphine sulphate, tramadol Codeine	Many types, e.g. total hip replacement Specifically used in neurosurgery
Nerve blocks and local anaesthetic	Lidocaine with adrenaline Ropivacaine	Thoracic surgery, wound areas can be infiltrated after surgery Total knee arthroplasty
Oral	Diclofenac sodium (Voltarol), tramadol, co-codamol, paracetamol	Many products are available Used in continued recovery and rehabilitation or alone after minor surgery
Per rectum	Diclofenac sodium (Voltarol), paracetamol	Commonly used following minor surgery or as part of multimodal approach to pain relief following major surgery

PCA, Patient-controlled analgesia.

anaesthetics for the relief of severe postoperative pain. The combination results in reduced narcotic requirements and improved analgesia compared with opioids and/or local anaesthetics (Macintyre and Schug 2021).

It should be noted that these NSAIDs inhibit platelet aggregation and are associated with bleeding from any site, but there is an additional risk of bleeding from the upper GI tract because of inflammation, erosions, ulcers or perforation. These drugs may also be associated with renal failure and gastric ulceration. The role of one of the most common analgesics, paracetamol, should not be overlooked. Paracetamol can be used alone to treat mild pain, or in combination with opioids, because of its morphine-sparing properties. It can be given orally, via the rectal route and intravenously (British National Formulary (BNF) 2023).

Patient-Controlled Analgesia (PCA)

PCA allows the patient to control the administration of small boluses of intravenous analgesic (see Chapter 20). A special infusion pump is set to give a specific volume of solution (and therefore a set dosage according to the dilution of the drug) when the patient presses a hand-held button. The machine is programmed to provide a bolus only after a certain length of time has elapsed (lockout) and a maximum total number of boluses over a specified time period.

PCA can be highly effective and many studies comparing PCA with conventional intramuscular or subcutaneous administration highlight better analgesic effects from PCA and enhanced patient satisfaction. Therapeutic levels of opioid can fall while the patient is sleeping, leading to awakening in pain. Some patients experience unpleasant side-effects such as nausea and itching and antiemetic medication should be prescribed and administered appropriately. It should be explained to the patient prior to theatre about how to use the device and its benefits. (Macintyre and Schug 2021).

Epidural Analgesia (EA)

EA is common following major surgery, for examplee.g., following radical prostatectomy or open abdominal surgery. EA is an effective form of postoperative pain relief for this group of patients because a solution of local anaesthetic and/or opiate is infused

into the epidural space in the spine. This blocks the dermatomal nerves supplying the area of the wound. Such patients may have little or no sensation of pain at all in the immediate postoperative period and are able to carry out breathing exercises and get out of bed shortly after surgery, thus minimising the risk of complications (Sawhney 2012). EA is also associated with decreased levels of postoperative anxiety. There are, however, several complications associated with EA, including hypotension and urinary retention, pressure ulcers and DVT from reduced mobility in the lower limbs, and infection such as dural abscess formation.

Postoperative Nausea and Vomiting (PONV)

PONV is common and, in those without a paralytic ileus, most frequent in the first 24 hours following surgery. Its causes are multifactorial but include patient-related factors, the length and nature of surgery and the anaesthetic agent used (Table 25.6).

PONV is exacerbated when patients have pain and inadequate pain relief reported that relief of postoperative pain is usually associated with relief of nausea. Unfortunately, PONV is also a common side-effect of opioid analgesics. A period of prolonged starvation can cause PONV but so can also inadequate preoperative fasting and the collection of secretions in the stomach. Paralytic ileus can lead to the accumulation of a large quantity of GI secretions. Following some surgery, for example partial gastrectomy, patients may have some bleeding into the stomach postoperatively which can induce nausea. Postoperative hypotension is another common cause of PONV which can be avoided by helping patients to move in bed or sit up slowly.

Treatment of established PONV is less effective than prevention. The cause of PONV should be identified and an appropriate antiemetic administered prophylactically and regularly. Caution must be taken with the administration of metoclopramide as this promotes gut motility and should be avoided in patients with bowel obstruction. It is important, however, that patients are aware preoperatively that PONV is not an inevitable outcome of anaesthesia, and that medication can and should be provided (Pierre and Whelan 2013).

TABLE 25.6	Risk Factors for Postoperative Nausea and Vomiting (PONV)
Risk Factor	**Explanation**
Increased age	Older adults experience less PONV than younger adults
Female gender	Women are three times more likely to experience PONV than men
Prior history of travel sickness	A history of motion sickness is associated with an increased incidence of PONV
High preoperative anxiety	Anxiety related to previous experience of PONV or general fears about a hospital admission can increase the likelihood of PONV occurring
Type of surgery	Abdominal gynaecological procedures have an increased risk because of disturbance to the gut during surgery. Pain PONV is exacerbated when patients have pain and inadequate pain relief (In orthopaedic procedures the use of extradural infusions has been linked to the high incidence of PONV; Alexander and Fenelly 1997) Any surgical procedure of longer than 30 minutes places the patient at increased risk of PONV
Anaesthetic agent used	Patients receiving thiopental as an induction agent are more likely to experience PONV than those who receive propofol PONV is also a common side-effect of opioid analgesics Spinal and regional blocks are less likely to cause PONV than general anaesthetics
Smoking	Smokers are less at risk than nonsmokers, although the exact mechanism for this is not understood (Whalen et al. 2006)
Obesity	Obesity may be a risk factor for PONV, but the causes are not clearly understood. Jolley (2001) suggests that fat-soluble anaesthetic agents accumulate in adipose tissue and the anaesthetics are slowly released. Therefore individuals with more adipose tissue will experience side-effects for longer

From Pierre S, Whelan R. Nausea and vomiting after surgery. *BJA Educ.* 2013;13(1):28–32.

Patient-Controlled Analgesia (PCA)

PCA allows the patient to control the administration of small boluses of intravenous analgesic (see Chapter 20). A special infusion pump is set to give a specific volume of solution (and therefore a set dosage according to the dilution of the drug) when the patient presses a hand-held button. The machine is programmed to provide a bolus only after a certain length of time has elapsed (lockout) and a maximum total number of boluses over a specified time period.

PCA can be highly effective and many studies comparing PCA with conventional intramuscular or subcutaneous administration highlight better analgesic effects from PCA and enhanced patient satisfaction. Therapeutic levels of opioid can fall while the patient is sleeping, leading to awakening in pain. Some patients experience unpleasant side-effects such as nausea and itching and antiemetic medication should be prescribed and administered appropriately. It should be explained to the patient prior to theatre about how to use the device and its benefits (Macintyre and Schug 2021).

Epidural Analgesia (EA)

EA is common following major surgery, for example following radical prostatectomy or open abdominal surgery. EA is an effective form of postoperative pain relief for this group of patients because a solution of local anaesthetic and/or opiate is infused into the epidural space in the spine. This blocks the dermatomal nerves supplying the area of the wound. Such patients may have little or no sensation of pain at all in the immediate postoperative period and are able to carry out breathing exercises and get out of bed shortly after surgery, thus minimising the risk of complications (Sawhney 2012). EA is also associated with decreased levels of postoperative anxiety. There are, however, several complications associated with EA, including hypotension and urinary retention, pressure ulcers and DVT from reduced mobility in the lower limbs, and infection such as dural abscess formation.

Paralytic Ileus

Surgical trauma to the GI tract causes temporary paralysis of the smooth muscle known as postoperative or temporary paralytic ileus. This is manifest by cessation of peristalsis and hence the absence of bowel sounds (high-pitched gurgling noises caused by liquid and air moving through the GI tract), bowel distension (which may cause tension on any bowel anastomosis) and consequent bowel distension. Nurses should be vigilant for any symptoms, particularly abdominal distension, nausea and vomiting. The condition usually resolves with minimising oral intake and intravenous fluid support, although an NG tube may need to be inserted to drain the stomach contents particularly if vomiting is a problem. Accurate fluid balance charting is important to document the drainage from the NG tube as losses can be substantial. If paralytic ileus continues for approximately 1 week, it will be necessary to consider parenteral nutrition.

Infection and Sepsis

If a local infection is suspected (redness, swelling or production of pus), a wound swab should be obtained immediately and sent for culture and sensitivity. Signs of systemic infection such as elevated temperature, tachypnoea and tachycardia should be identified early and antibiotic treatment instigated depending on the cause (e.g. abdominal, chest, urinary, wound). Sepsis should be treated as a medical emergency, that is, be treated as quickly and efficiently as possible as soon as it has been identified. The Sepsis Six 'bundle' was developed to reduce the risk of death from sepsis. It involves six steps which, when implemented within an hour of diagnosis, improves the patient's chance of survival. These steps are:
- Give high flow oxygen.
- Take blood cultures.
- Give IV antibiotics.
- Give IV fluids.
- Measure lactate levels.
- Monitor urine output (The UK Sepsis Trust 2022).

Nutrition

Early oral feeding after surgery is the best practice among adult, noncritically ill patients, even after GI surgery. Evidence recommends commencing liquid and solid feeding within 24 hours of surgery to improve patient (e.g. reduced morbidity) and hospital (e.g. reduced length of stay) outcomes (Rattray et al. 2017).

VTE Diagnosis and Treatment

Around three-quarters of DVTs are asymptomatic but signs are unilateral leg swelling (typically calf or thigh), tight erythematous, shiny skin and pain at site particularly exacerbated dorsiflexion of the foot. Investigation of a suspected DVT is initially with ultrasound of the femoral or popliteal veins, and PE with either a CT scan of the pulmonary artery (CTPA) or a ventilation/perfusion (V/Q) scan. Both are treated with low-molecular-weight heparin, usually subcutaneously, moving onto oral therapy as appropriate, with treatment usually lasting at least a few months (Routhier et al. 2023).

Wound Care

The aim of wound care is to promote healing and minimise the risk of infection. Adverse patient factors are increased BMI, comorbidities like diabetes, prolonged hypoxia, dehydration, local pressure and protein-calorie malnutrition. Factors to be considered in all patients regarding wound healing are discussed in Chapter 23. The mainstay of preventing hospital-acquired infection is handwashing (WHO 2020). Nursing staff must wash their hands before any patient contact. In addition to this, prevention of infection begins in the preoperative period with skin cleansing and reduction of anxiety.

The use of wound drains and aseptic nontouch technique, along with precautions against haematoma formation, will help to reduce wound infections postoperatively (Information 25.6). In the immediate postoperative period, the wound and any drains in the operation site must be checked as part of the post-operative observations for signs of bleeding. Volume markings on drainage bottles and bags can indicate the amount of blood or fluid lost. Large volumes of bloodstained fluid may be due to the fluid used to wash out a cavity, but this should still be reported. There is some debate about whether early (<48 hours) or late dressing removal is the most appropriate (Toon et al. 2015).

Wound drains may be used to drain blood and inflammatory exudate, prevent haematoma formation and infection and to give an indication of blood loss. Some drains may have suction applied to collapse the space left in the tissues after an operation. Drains can also indicate when an anastomosis has broken down by discharging blood, digestive or faeculent fluid and, when an abscess has resolved, the cessation of discharge of pus. Some examples of the more common types of wound drain are given in Fig. 25.2.

Figure 25.2 Common types of wound drains. (A) Vacuum drain (prongs come together as vacuum is lost). (B) Concertina-type drain. (C) Simple tube/Penrose drain. (D) Corrugated drain: secured by a suture and then a safety pin as the drain is shortened to prevent it from falling back into the patient. Fluid drains down the channels and into a bag.

INFORMATION 25.6

Patient Factors That Increase Risks of Postoperative Infection

- Immune compromise (e.g. steroid use, cancer)
- Contamination of peritoneum (e.g. perforated bowel)
- Malnutrition
- Low cardiac output prior to surgery
- Increased age
- Diabetes

Resource

National Institute of Health and Care Excellence (NICE). Surgical site infections: prevention and treatment. Clinical guideline [CG74]. 2017. https://www.nice.org.uk/guidance/cg74/chapter/1-Guidance.

Elimination

Postoperative constipation is a common problem arising from immobility, opioid analgesics and dehydration. Conversely, diarrhoea can occur as postoperative temporary ileus resolves, but normal bowel function should resume spontaneously in a few days. Patients may experience colicky pain due to flatus and muscle spasm; this can be reduced by increasing mobility, and anecdotally (although there is no evidence), offering warm water or peppermint water can be soothing. Ensuring adequate hydration and early activity helps prevent constipation before it becomes necessary to use oral laxatives.

All patients should be monitored to ensure that they pass urine in the hours following surgery to ensure return of normal bladder function and urine production. Urinary retention may occur due to immobility, the relaxation of bladder muscle tone caused by anaesthesia, or as the result of temporary ileus following abdominal or pelvic surgery. When urinary retention is anticipated, the patient should be catheterised in theatre to minimise discomfort. Otherwise, patients should be given the opportunity for privacy and assistance to assume a normal position to pass urine where possible. If retention leads to distension of the bladder and discomfort, or is a cause for concern, urinary catheterisation may be required. If the catheter is required for monitoring urine output in haemodynamic shock, or retention due to immobility, it can be removed when monitoring is no longer required, or the patient is sufficiently active to pass urine independently.

Sleep

Sleep and rest are essential, not only for a feeling of well-being, but also for anabolism and tissue repair. Surgical inpatients often have very disrupted sleep patterns. In addition to factors affecting the sleep of all hospital patients, surgical patients are exposed to pain, general discomfort, frequent observations and restricted positioning. Opioids can alter normal sleep patterns, with patients reporting dropping off to sleep and feeling they have slept for hours, only to find that just a few minutes have passed. Delirium is also likely to affect sleep patterns. Reassurance, reduced night-time lighting and keeping observations to a minimum are helpful (NICE 2020).

Communication

When a patient recovers from a general anaesthetic, the first sense to return is that of hearing. Care of the patient in the recovery room can be enhanced by having aids to communication, such as their hearing aid and glasses, made quickly available. A number of patients, especially older people or the very ill, may become and remain confused postoperatively; this may be due to the change in their environment, anxiety, the effects of the anaesthetic, prescribed medication, a history of alcohol and drug use, the presence of comorbidities and uncertainty about their prognosis. Efforts must be made to identify and treat the cause, and nursing measures to reorientate and minimise confusion should be taken. Effective communication among professionals in the postoperative period is essential, especially around diagnosis, discharge, follow-up and ongoing care (NICE 2020).

Discharge Planning and Education

Planning for discharge from hospital should begin on admission if an emergency or if the person is admitted for elective surgery this should be discussed preadmission, with plans reviewed before discharge. Health and care professionals who are facilitating hospital discharges should work in close partnership with individuals, and – where relevant – families and unpaid carers, to discharge people to the setting that best meets their needs. This process should be person centred, strengths based and driven by choice, dignity and respect. This will ensure that people are supported to be discharged to the right place, with the correct support that will lead to maximise their independence and quality of life (NICE 2015).

This will enable the person and their family or carers to be involved with the planning, ask questions and receive timely information to make informed choices about the discharge pathway that best meets the person's needs. Unpaid carers may benefit from signposting to local carers' support services, and they should also be made aware of their right to an assessment for their own needs by their local authority.

A person who does not have family or friends to help, or who may find it difficult to understand, communicate or speak up, should be informed of their right to an independent advocate.

Discharge planning aims to provide a smooth transition from hospital to either home or the place of ongoing care for continued patient care and should be considered from the time of preadmission clinics, or as soon as the decision for surgery has been made. The growth of day surgery and decreasing lengths of hospital stay for major surgery have reduced the time available for nurses to meet patients' postdischarge needs. Inadequate discharge planning can lead to patients being readmitted because they are unprepared for self-care or developing postoperative complications such as wound infections.

Most patients are referred to their GP on discharge from hospital. Nurses will decide whether the patient needs to be referred to the community nursing team. Referrals can be made for nursing interventions ranging from wound care to providing end-of-life support for the patient and family where there is a poor prognosis.

Discharge from hospital especially after surgery is often a traumatic experience. This is especially acute for people without a fixed address, and surveys suggest that 30%–70% of homeless inpatients are 'discharged to the street' (i.e. sleeping rough or sofa-surfing immediately after discharge). Homelessness is a persistent social problem that is associated with poor health outcomes, with cohort studies showing mortality rates of three to six times the general population. Although the size and structure of the homeless population are difficult to estimate, UK data suggest steep increases in recent years. The number of people sleeping rough in England increased from 1353 in 2010 to 4266 in 2019, with actual numbers likely to be greater than this. The same period also saw a steep increase in hospital attendances for people with 'no fixed abode'. In addition, access to ongoing community healthcare may be poor.

Qualitative research has identified barriers including stigmatisation when accessing health services, primary healthcare practitioners refusing to register homeless people, and priorities that compete with health such as arranging accommodation. These inequalities mean that outcomes after hospital discharge may be poor, and homeless inpatients are more likely to be readmitted than housed inpatients.

Communication is fundamental to the process of collaborative discharge planning. A personal telephone call to the relevant community nurses and a discharge summary outlining the patient's care can be useful in enhancing continuity. The role of a discharge coordinator who implements a discharge protocol can facilitate this process by providing consistent advice and initiating referrals to all relevant members of the multidisciplinary team. Information is essential; this should be both written and verbal, and should include advice about pain, wound care and resumption of activities – particularly work, exercise and driving. It should also inform the patient about symptoms that might suggest that complications are developing.

Patients and their carers should be aware that patients usually should not drive home from hospital and should be accompanied for the first 24 hours after surgery. Advice should include:

- Do not drink alcohol.
- Do not drive a motor vehicle.
- Have a responsible adult stay overnight with you.
- Do not make important decisions for 24 hours following a general anaesthetic, regional anaesthetic and/or intravenous sedation.

In summary, to implement best practice in discharge planning, National Health Service (NHS) bodies and local authorities should work together to:

- Determine what an individual needs and wants after discharge, if anything, so that they are discharged onto the pathway that best meets their needs.
- Appropriately refer qualifying individuals to independent advocacy services on admission, so their voice is heard during the discharge planning process.
- Plan, commission and deliver appropriate care and support that meets population needs and is affordable within existing budgets available to local NHS services and authorities.
- Understand the quality, cost and effectiveness of local treatment, care and support to inform people of their options.

- Understand the role that each organisation has in safeguarding and put appropriate safeguarding policies and procedures in place.
- Take joint responsibility for the individual's and unpaid carer's, including young carer's, welfare when making decisions about discharge and postdischarge support.
- Transfer people seamlessly and safely from hospital to their own home or new care setting with joined up care, via clear, evidence-based and accurate assessments that fully represent the medical and psychological needs and social preferences of the person.
- Transfer information between settings in a clear, timely and appropriate way.
- Identify any carers, including young carers, and determine whether any carer is willing and able to provide care and, if so, what support they might need.

Adapted from NICE (2015) Guideline Transition between inpatient hospital settings and community or care home settings for adults with social care needs.

Rehabilitation

Rehabilitation can be a lengthy process, requiring continued support by community nurses, or a short event with minimal professional intervention. Successful rehabilitation has been shown to include minimising impairment and disability and maximising well-being, social participation and recovery. Postoperative recovery requires energy, as the patient returns to preoperative levels of dependence or independence and regains control over physical, psychological, social and habitual functions. Increased numbers of day surgery mean that more patients are recovering from surgery at home. However, older and frailer patients may require additional time in hospital for specific tailored programmes of rehabilitation, for example following major surgery such as amputation, orthopaedic surgery and cardiac surgery. Also, patients with comorbidities may have delayed recovery as the acute care episode complicates pre-existing conditions.

Summary: Key Nursing Issues

- People undergoing surgery have the right to be fully included in all decision making.
- Patients undergoing surgery require a range of care from nurses in the hospital and community settings, in both the pre- and postoperative periods.
- Whilst care may appear to be focused on performing tasks in a standardised manner, nurses are ideally placed to deliver, coordinate and humanise the surgical experience, but also to facilitate a safe and speedy recovery in a person-centred manner.
- The increasing average age of surgical patients means that they often have more complex underlying medical problems including diabetes, obesity and cardiorespiratory disease.
- Careful preassessment and planning are important in selecting the most appropriate surgical pathway and ensuring patients are physically and psychologically prepared.

- In the preoperative period, nurses have a vital role in helping to anticipate problems and minimise complications, through effective physical and psychological preparation of patients.
- In an operating theatre, patient safety is essential. This includes meticulous preoperative checks and coordinated intraoperative teamwork.
- Patient care in the recovery room includes careful assessment and management of airway, breathing and circulation.
- In the postoperative period the early identification of the deteriorating patient and complications such as hypoxia, haemorrhage, ileus, sepsis and shock can be life-saving.
- The patient's overall experience is likely to be very much better if the symptoms of pain and nausea are proactively managed.
- Discharge planning should begin at, or even prior to, admission and should be individualised to the person, their condition and their specific circumstances.

Reflection and Learning – What Next?

- **Test** your knowledge by visiting the Evolve website 🌐 and answering the multiple-choice questions and critical thinking questions.
- **Consolidate** your learning by looking at some of the references and specialist websites.
- **Revisit** some of the additional material on the website and the useful websites listed later.

- **Consider** what you have learnt and how this will help your professional development.
- **Reflect** on how you can apply this knowledge to the care of people undergoing surgery and how you can deliver person-centred care.
- **Discuss** your learning with your assessor/supervisor, a critical friend, lecturer and colleagues.

References

Adults With Incapacity Act (Scotland); 2000. https://www.legislation.gov.uk/asp/2000/4/contents.

Alexander R, Fenelly M. Comparison of ondansetron, metoclopramide, and placebo as premedicants to reduce nausea and vomiting after major surgery. *Anaesthesia.* 1997;52(7):695–698.

Anderson T, Walls M, Canelo R. Day case surgery guidelines. *Surgery.* 2017;35(2):85–91.

American Society of Anesthesiologists (ASA). ASA Physical Status Classification System. Updated 2020. https://www.asahq.org/standards-and-practice-parameters/statement-on-asa-physical-status-classification-system.

Association for Perioperative Practice (AfPP). *Theatre Attire Poster in Standards and Recommendations for Safe Perioperative Practice.* 3rd ed. Harrogate: AfPP; 2020. https://theatre-attire-a2-poster-v5-final.pdf.

BAPEN (2013). Malnutrition Universal Screening Tool. https://www.bapen.org.uk/pdfs/must/must_full.pdf.

British National Formulary. 2023. British Medical Association and the Royal Pharmaceutical Society. https://bnf.nice.org.uk/.

Carrick MA, Robson JM, Thomas C. Smoking and anaesthesia. *BJA Educ.* 2019;19(1):1–6. doi:10.1016/j.bjae.2018.09.005 Published online 2018 Nov 6.

Chou R. Management of postoperative pain: a clinical practice guideline from the American Pain Society, the American Society of Regional Anesthesia and Pain Medicine, and the American Society of Anesthesiologists' Committee on Regional Anesthesia, Executive Committee, and Administrative Council. *J Pain.* 2017;17(2):131–157.

Espin S, Indar A, Gross M, Labricciosa A, D'arpino M. Processes and tools to improve teamwork and communication in surgical settings: a narrative review. *BMJ Open Quality.* 2020;9:e000937.

Grant S, Crimmons K. Limitations of track and trigger systems and the National Early Warning Score. Part 2: sensitivity versus specificity. *Br J Nurs.* 2018;2(12).

Jolley S. Managing post-operative nausea and vomiting. *Nurs Stand.* 2001;15(40):47–52; quiz 53–5.

Liddle C. Preoperative fasting: exploring guidelines and evidence to ensure consistent, high-quality care. *Nurs Stand.* 2022;37:77–82. doi:10.7748/ns.2022.e12033.

Lister S, Hofland J, Grafton H. *The Royal Marsden Manual of Clinical Nursing Procedures, Professional Edition (Royal Marsden Manual Series).* Wiley; 2020.

Macintyre E, Schug SA. *Acute Pain Management: A Practical Guide.* 5th ed. Boca Raton, FL: CRC Press; 2021.

National Education Scotland (NES) (2021). Person centred care. https://www.nes.scot.nhs.uk/our-work/person-centred-care.

National Institute for Health and Care Excellence (NICE). *Venous thromboembolism: reducing the risk of venous thromboembolism (deep vein thrombosis and pulmonary embolism) in patients admitted to hospital. NICE clinical guideline [CG92].* London: National Institute for Health and Clinical Excellence; 2015. http://www.nice.org.uk/guidance/CG92.

National Institute for Health and Care Excellence (NICE). *Surgical site infections: prevention and treatment.* Clinical guideline [CG125]; 2019. https://www.nice.org.uk/guidance/ng125.

National Institute for Health and Care Excellence (NICE). *Perioperative care in adults.* NICE guideline [NG180]; 2020. https://www.nice.org.uk/guidance/ng180.

National Institute for Health and Care Excellence (NICE). *Venous thromboembolism in adults.* Quality standard [QS201]; 2021. https://www.nice.org.uk/guidance/qs201.

National Institute for Health and Care Excellence (NICE). Smoking cessation. Clinical knowledge summary. 2018. Updated 2023. https://cks.nice.org.uk/smoking-cessation.

NHS Race and Health Observatory. Pulse oximetry racial bias report. 2021. https://www.nhsrho.org/wp-content/uploads/2021/03/Pulse-oximetry-racial-bias-report.pdf.

Nursing and Midwifery Council (NMC). The Code: professional standards of practice and behaviour for nurses, midwives and nursing associates. 2018. https://www.nmc.org.uk/standards/code/.

Pierre S, Whelan R. Nausea and vomiting after surgery. *BJA Education.* Vol. 2013;13(1):28–32.

Rattray E, Roberts S, Marshall A, Desbrow B. A systematic review of feeding practices among postoperative patients: is practice in-line with evidenced-based guidelines? *J Hum Nutr Diet.* 2017;31. doi:10.1111/jhn.12486.

Resuscitation Council UK. Resuscitation guidelines. 2021. https://www.resus.org.uk/library/abcde-approach.

Routhier N, Tagalakis V, Zarka F. *BMJ Best Practice.* Venous thromboembolism (VTE) prophylaxis; 2023. Available at: https://bestpractice.bmj.com/topics/en-gb/1087.

Royal College of Physicians. National Early Warning Score (NEWS) 2. 2017. https://www.rcplondon.ac.uk/projects/outputs/national-early-warning-score-news-2.

Sawhney M. Epidural analgesia: what nurses need to know. *Nurs Manage.* 2012;42(8):36–41.

Sommers M. Color awareness: a must for patient assessment. *Am Nurse.* 2011. https://www.myamericannurse.com/color-awareness-a-must-for-patient-assessment/.

Smith I, Krinke P, Murat I, Smith A. Perioperative fasting in adults and children: guidelines from the European Society of Anaesthesiology. *Eur J Anaesthesiol.* 2011;28(8):556–569.

The UK Sepsis Trust (2022). Sepsis treatment; 2018. https://sepsistrust.org/professional-resources/.

Toon CD, Lusuku C, Ramamoorthy R, Davidson BR, Gurusamy K. Early versus delayed dressing removal after primary closure of clean and clean-contaminated surgical wounds. *Cochrane Database Syst Rev.* 2015(9):CD010259. doi:10.1002/14651858.CD010259.pub3.

Whalen R, Sprung J, Burkle CM, et al. Recent smoking behavior and postoperative nausea and vomiting. *Anesth Analg.* 2006;103(1):70–75.

World Health Organization (WHO). The evidence for clean hands; 2020. http://www.who.int/gpsc/country_work/en/.

World Health Organization (WHO). WHO Surgical Safety Checklist. 2022. https://www.who.int/teams/integrated-health-services/patient-safety/research/safe-surgery/tool-and-resources.

Xuan C, Yan W, Wang D, Chin V, Coule T, Wang J. Efficacy of preemptive analgesia treatments for the management of postoperative pain: a network meta-analysis. *Br J Anaesth.* 2022. doi:10.1016/j.bja.2022.08.038.

Useful Websites

Association of Anaesthetists, www.aagbi.org/
Association for Perioperative Practice (AfPP), www.afpp.org.uk/home
National Institute for Health and Care Excellence (NICE), www.nice.org.uk
Royal College of Nursing (RCN) Perioperative Forum, www.rcn.org.uk/get-involved/forums/perioperative-forum
Royal College of Anaesthetists, www.rcoa.ac.uk
Royal College of Surgeons, www.rcseng.ac.uk

Useful Tools

The American Society of Anesthesiologists (ASA) Physical Status Classification System, see Table 25.1 or the American College of Surgeons Risk Calculator (https://riskcalculator.facs.org/RiskCalculator/).

National Institute for Health and Care Excellence (NICE). Nutrition support in adults. Quality standard [QS24]. 2012. https://www.nice.org.uk/guidance/qs24/chapter/quality-statement-1-screening-for-the-risk-of-malnutrition.

NICE British National Formulary. Premedication and peri-operative drugs. 2023. https://bnf.nice.org.uk/treatment-summaries/pre-medication-and-peri-operative-drugs/.

NICE Guidelines on diet. https://www.nice.org.uk/guidance/lifestyle-and-wellbeing/diet-nutrition-and-obesity.

26

Nursing the Patient Who Experiences Trauma

TRISH BURTON

CHAPTER OUTLINE

Introduction

The Centre for Trauma Sciences (C4TS) describes traumatic injury which result in a blunt or penetrating force impacting on a person. Injuries can be sustained from falls, road traffic collisions, stabbings. However, the word trauma is often used in a number of ways; for example, trauma can relate psychological effects of a disturbing or frightening event, or series of events, for example natural disasters, wars, etc. For the purposes of this chapter, trauma relates to the injuries caused by sudden application of an external force (TCAR 2020). Trauma is not a new disease; according to the World Health Organisation (WHO), trauma-related deaths account for 8% of all deaths worldwide (WHO 2021).

Historically, people have suffered traumatic injuries caused by modes of transport (the horse and cart for example), assaults, falls and work-related incidents. Conflict also causes death and disability due to traumatic injury.

Trauma patients are now cared for by a variety of practitioners in many clinical settings – from the paramedic and/or the prehospital teams at the roadside to the nurse in a rehabilitation unit; trauma is a relatively new specialty in its own right. In fact, the past 30 years has evidenced that with the development of organised trauma systems and improved public health initiatives in high-income countries, survival rates in trauma patients have greatly improved (Gabe and Beck 2021). However, survival is not the end of the trauma patient experience; disability following major trauma has a significant impact not only on trauma patients but also on their families, the wider community and healthcare systems themselves, and indeed globally the overall impact of trauma on individuals and the wider community has remained largely unchanged (GBD 2019, Diseases and Injuries Collaborators 2020).

Much of the trauma literature focuses on the care that the patient receives in the emergency department (ED). This is the area of the hospital where patients with potentially life-changing injuries or illnesses are assessed and treated. However, this is a very small part of the patient's journey and does not really reflect the reality of contemporary trauma nursing. This chapter will outline the principles of care needed for the trauma patient, from prehospital care through to definitive care. Reflection boxes will help you to consider a trauma case history and reflect on the care needed. Contemporary evidence-based practice will be discussed, with links to web-based critical thinking exercises and further reading material.

Trauma: Epidemiology and the Need for Injury Prevention

Traumatic injury can be unintentional or intentional and continues to be a significant health problem. Trauma does not capture the public attention in the same way as other diseases such as cancer, cardiac disease or, more recently, COVID-19; however, traumatic injury *is* a disease. It has a host (the patient) and a mode of transmission (a vehicle, fire, knife) (American College of Surgeons [ACS] 2018) and the statistics are shocking. Trauma affects all age groups and it is the main cause of death in young people under the age of 40. Annually in the UK, up to 16,000 deaths occur as a result of trauma (Trauma Audit Research Network [TARN] 2022), with 24,000 patients being admitted to hospital each year as a result of a serious road traffic collision (Department of Transport 2018). According to NHS Digital (2022), there were just over 250,000 emergency trauma and orthopaedic hospital admissions in 2020–2021. The average age of major trauma patients has increased over the past 20 years, and is now 53.8 years of age. Major trauma patients are older than ever before and falls of less than 2 m are increasingly considered a significant mechanism of injury (MOI) (Alshibani et al., 2021, Kehoe et al. 2015).

However, this is not always the case. Traumatic injury should not be thought of as an accident – this word implies a random circumstance, whereas injuries occur in specific, usually preventable patterns. Individuals in high-risk situations or environments, such as children playing near a busy road, adults driving a car at speed or following alcohol consumption, working without protective equipment or carrying a knife, provide a chain of events that results in traumatic injury. Legislation such as seatbelt laws, environment modifications such as road-calming measures, implementation of dedicated bicycle routes and health promotion campaigns by organisations such as the Royal Society for the Protection of Accidents (RoSPA) have all helped to reduce death and disability, however more needs to be done. Trauma nurses who care for the injured are ideally placed to practise health promotion and injury prevention strategies, either during interactions with patients or by supporting injury prevention strategies such as the Fall Fighter Programme (RoSPA 2022).

Mechanism of Injury

Following a traumatic event, information about the MOI may help identify up to 90% of a patient's injuries (ACS 2018). MOI can be classified into four main groups (Greaves et al. 2001, TCAR 2020):
- blunt – such as a road traffic collision, assault, fall or sporting injury
- penetrating – such as a stab wound or impalement
- blast – caused by an explosive element, which may be intentional (a bomb) or accidental (an industrial incident)
- thermal – caused by extreme heat, such as a fire, or extreme cold, such as frost bite.

In general, 98% of the trauma in the UK is blunt, caused by injury, and other mechanisms make up the rest. However, this picture is changing in urban settings, with penetrating injury becoming more prevalent – in 2019, NHS England reported almost 5000 hospital admissions were related to penetrating injuries in 10–19-year-olds.

According to TARN (2022), falls are the leading most common MOI leading to hospital admission.

Death Following Trauma

Death due to traumatic injury occurs in one of three time periods, described as the trimodal death distribution (ACS 2018) (Fig. 26.1). This has significance for trauma nurses working throughout all the areas of trauma care.

The first period is where death occurs within seconds to minutes of sustaining the injury. Deaths are caused by very severe injuries such as major vessel (aorta, vena cava) disruption, severe traumatic brain injury, high spinal cord injury or apnoea. Arguably, this period can only be significantly reduced by preventing the incident occurring in the first place.

The second period is where death occurs minutes to hours following the injury. Deaths are caused by injuries resulting in overwhelming hypoxia and hypovolaemia or a rapidly accumulating intracranial haematoma pressing on the brain. Nurses and practitioners working in prehospital and emergency care settings must carry out prompt assessment and resuscitation to recognise problems, seek expert help early and minimise death in this period.

The third period is where death occurs days or weeks after the initial injury. This is usually due to multifactorial complications that have arisen such as multiorgan failure, coagulopathy (failure of normal clotting mechanisms), acute respiratory distress syndrome or overwhelming sepsis. Nurses working in definitive trauma care settings are responsible for assessment, monitoring and support of patients, in order to detect potential complications and maximise recovery.

Disability

It must be remembered that death is not the only outcome following traumatic injury. Worldwide, large numbers of people are left permanently disabled following intentional or unintentional injury, causing a huge financial and social burden on society (Hatchimonji et al. 2022, WHO 2008). Disabilities following injury include:
- physical and/or cognitive limitations due to neurotrauma
- paralysis due to spinal cord trauma
- partial or complete amputation of limbs
- physical limb deformation or nerve damage resulting in mobility impairments
- psychological trauma
- sensory disability such as blindness and deafness.

The National Institute for Health and Care Excellence (NICE) (2021) stated that 45,000 people in England alone are affected by major trauma every year. A combination of increased injury prevention awareness, better patient care and post-traumatic injury rehabilitation can help to reduce the number of disabilities and provide better outcomes for not only for the patient, but also their families and wider communities.

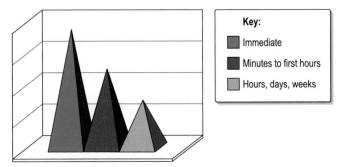

Trimodal death distribution in trauma

Figure 26.1 Trimodal death distribution in trauma.

Prehospital Care

Prehospital care is defined as the provision of skilled medical help at the scene of an accident, medical or other clinical emergency and during transport of the patient to hospital (Noble-Mathews 2005). Wibring et al. (2020) describe how care has adapted to provide early assessments and interventions that support the patient transfer to a hospital setting. In most UK settings this will involve specialised staff from an ambulance service, using road vehicles or possibly helicopters to assess, resuscitate and then transport trauma patients to hospital. Currently in the UK, there are only a few prehospital care nurses working in the field of trauma, in comparison to the United States and other European countries.

As well as good clinical knowledge, prehospital care doctors, paramedics and nurses need specialist skills, such as ensuring scene safety or extrication of patients trapped in vehicles. This is achieved through education and training and also collaboration with other emergency services such as the police and fire and rescue teams HEMS teams.

Advanced Notification

Prehospital care staff provide essential information from the scene to the hospital teams waiting to receive the patient in the ED. This advanced notification allows the receiving hospital to prepare the necessary equipment and personnel to ensure the best clinical care and outcome (Cole and McGinley 2005, The Royal College of Emergency Medicine [RCEM] 2023). Advanced notification may differ between ambulance services; however, it will generally include the following:

- age
- gender
- MOI
- cardiovascular observations
- respiratory rate and oxygen saturations
- Glasgow Coma Scale (GCS) (or level of consciousness)
- obvious and predicted injuries
- treatment given at scene or en route
- numbers of patients if more than one person is involved.

Handover

Once in the ED, the prehospital care staff will 'hand over' the patient to the hospital staff. This will involve the clinical aspects of the patient's injuries and care thus far. If possible, it should also involve information about the patient's relatives or next of kin (NOK) (if known) and any police liaison that may be involved. Handover will be given verbally but the prehospital care staff will also provide a written and/or electronic summary of their care that should form part of the patient's notes.

Emergency Department

Many EDs use a variety of protocols to assess (or triage) the patients on arrival to determine the severity of their injury, and then streaming (or directing) them to the appropriate clinical area (Adulwahid et al. 2016, Bickerton et al. 2005). The ED is usually divided into clinical areas where patients with minor injuries can be seen and treated in a designated area away from those who are more seriously ill or injured. The minor injuries section is where single system traumatic injuries such as ankle or wrist fractures, soft tissue injuries or uncomplicated wounds can be seen and treated.

Once the major trauma patient has arrived at the hospital, they should be assessed in a resuscitation area. This is a clinical area which is designed to have the necessary equipment and space readily available to enable a trauma team to care for the patient efficiently and effectively. In the ED, it is vital that there is a predetermined system, such as the Advanced Trauma Life Support (ATLS) protocols (ACS 2018), to guide personnel through the initial assessment of the patient. Using a systematic approach (C, A, B, D, E) helps the trauma team to identify life-threatening conditions quickly and to treat them appropriately (Information 26.1).

The Trauma Team

The trauma team is made up of clinicians (including nurses, specialty doctors, radiographers, blood bank) who carry out preassigned roles so that several interventions can occur simultaneously (Cole and Crichton 2006, Tiel Groenestege-Kreb et al. 2014). The aim of the trauma team is to promptly stabilise the patient, identify injuries and initiate a definitive management plan. It has been shown that the most efficient resuscitation will occur if a 'horizontal organisation' approach is adopted. This is when each member of the team carries out individual tasks simultaneously rather than sequentially (vertical organisation). This reduces the time taken to resuscitate a patient and initiate life-saving procedures, which will improve the patient's chances of survival. All members of the team should have received training in trauma care to ensure that they have the appropriate level of clinical knowledge and skills. Here in the UK, nurses working as part of the trauma team are expected to achieve core competencies, to ensure best practice and researched based care is exercised (NICE 2016).

Trauma teams are usually alerted following the advanced notification information from the prehospital team. If the MOI and/or the status of the patient are suggestive of serious traumatic injury, the NICE (2016) suggests that trauma patients be brought to either a trauma unit (TU) or a major trauma centre (MTC). This is dependent on the MOI, severity of injury or instability of the patient. Whether a TU or MTC, the trauma team should be called for:

- trauma patients with any of the following:
  - actual or potential airway compromise
  - signs of a pneumothorax (respiratory distress)
  - SpO_2 <90%
  - heart rate >100 beats per minute (adults)
  - GCS score <14 associated with a head injury
  - penetrating wound anywhere from the neck to the thighs
  - any gunshot wound
  - fall from >25 feet/8 m
  - ejection from a vehicle;
- children involved in a traumatic incident:
  - with an altered level of consciousness
  - with a capillary refill time of >3 seconds
  - with tachycardia
  - a pedestrian or cyclist hit by a vehicle.

INFORMATION 26.1

Advanced Trauma Life Support (ATLS) Primary Survey Assessment

- Airway with cervical spine control
- Breathing and ventilation
- Circulation and haemorrhage control
- Disability and dysfunction
- Exposure and environment control

Initial Assessment and Management of the Patient: The Primary and Secondary Surveys

Initial assessment and management of the trauma patient are usually performed in two stages: the primary survey and later the secondary survey (ACS 2018, Cole 2008).

Haemorrhage Control – Circulation

Major haemorrhage is the leading cause of death in major trauma (ACS 2018). Therefore control of bleeding is paramount. This can be either from direct pressure, tourniquets, surgical intervention – damage control surgery or embolisation in interventional radiology (McCullough et al. 2014, Spahn et al. 2019). Fluid resuscitation is a complex and dynamic element of trauma care, especially in the prehospital and assessment phase of care (Spahn et al. 2019).

The Primary Survey

The initial assessment (primary survey) has six components – 'C, A, B, C, D, E':

- Circulation – haemorrhage control
- Airway with cervical spine control
- Breathing and ventilation
- Circulation and haemorrhage control
- Disability and dysfunction
- Exposure and environmental control

If any life-threatening condition is identified during the process, it is treated before moving on to the next stage. For example, if the patient is found to have a compromised airway, this is stabilised before the patient's breathing and ventilation are assessed. Each component is now discussed in detail.

Airway With Cervical Spine Control

The first step of this assessment is to find out if the patient has a patent airway (Reflection 26.1). Following a traumatic event the airway can become obstructed by bleeding in the mouth; swelling of the face, mouth or oropharynx; a reduced level of consciousness or vomiting and aspiration. Expert anaesthetic help should be sought immediately if there is any doubt about the patient's ability to maintain their own airway.

All nurses working with trauma patients should be able to perform a systematic approach to airway management. This is essential, as simple manoeuvres may be all that is required to keep the airway patent until anaesthetic help arrives. The sequential approach to airway assessment involves:

1. *Talking to the patient* – this helps to provide psychological support but also assesses the airway. If the patient is talking freely in a normal voice (i.e. no grunting or hoarseness), then it can be assumed that the airway is patent (Resuscitation Council UK (RCUK) 2021). If there is no response or the patient is making noises from the airway, then the next step should be followed.
2. *Look in the mouth* for signs of obstruction, such as vomit or blood. Suction with a rigid suction catheter attached will help to remove any foreign bodies, which once carefully removed may allow the patient to maintain their own airway.
3. *Open the airway* using a jaw thrust technique to pull the tongue and soft palate forward. This is used instead of the head tilt/chin lift because the neck must be kept still whilst the airway is opened as trauma patients are always at risk of a cervical spine injury.
4. *Insert an airway adjunct.* Airway adjuncts should be used in conjunction with an airway opening manoeuvre (jaw thrust) as they will not keep the airway open on their own in the unconscious patient lying supine (Cole 2008). The choice of airway is either an oropharyngeal airway (Guedel) in the unconscious

REFLECTION 26.1

Emergency Airway Management

A 35-year-old man has been knocked off his bicycle by a motor vehicle. He appears to have sustained injuries to both legs and is very pale. On arrival to the ED, he is drowsy but has a gag reflex. He does not appear to have had a head or face injury.

Activity

- Why are airway assessment and management so important and which airway adjunct should be used to maintain his airway?

Figure 26.2 How to size an oropharyngeal airway.

patient without a gag reflex or a nasopharyngeal airway if a gag reflex is present (RCUK 2021).

(a) Oropharyngeal airway. To ensure the correct size, an oropharyngeal airway is measured from the tragus of the ear to the corner of the mouth ('soft to soft') (see Fig. 26.2). It is inserted upside down, rotated 180 degrees and then pushed into position. The flange should sit flush with the lips. If the patient gags or coughs during insertion, the airway should be removed and a nasopharyngeal airway used instead.

(b) Nasopharyngeal airway. The size of a nasopharyngeal airway is chosen by ensuring that the diameter of the tube is smaller than the diameter of the nostril. The airway should be lubricated prior to introduction and inserted into the nose with a slight twisting motion. Nasopharyngeal airways extend from the nostril to the nasopharynx, with the wider end sitting at the nostril (Cole 2008).

5. *Definitive Airway.* For patients who have more serious injuries or are unable to maintain their own airway, it may be necessary to protect the airway definitively; this means a secure airway that can remain in place until the patient is able to maintain their own airway, usually endotracheal (ET) intubation. This is done by an anaesthetist who will intubate the patient using a laryngoscope and ET tube. It is important to sedate and paralyse the patient to facilitate this process. The anaesthetist will require a range of drugs and the nurse assisting with the procedure should be familiar with these and have them ready for immediate use. Once the ET tube is in place, a mechanism for ventilation will be required which must be attached to a high percentage of oxygen

Figure 26.3 Cervical spine immobilisation.

via a piped oxygen supply. Ideally, all this equipment should be preprepared for rapid use. For patients who have sustained massive facial injuries, a surgical airway may be the only way to oxygenate them adequately. This requires specialist equipment (e.g. a scalpel, tracheal dilators, a small tracheostomy tube or ET tube that can be attached to a catheter mount), which should be readily available for immediate use in the ED (Royal College of Anaesthetists [RCoA] 2021) Ideally, a preintubation patient safety checklist should be completed. This is to ensure the trauma team have accounted for the risks involved, that the intubation is systematic, thorough and optimises the patient given their injuries (Dattatri et al. 2021, Smith et al. 2015, WHO 2009).

For any trauma patient, it is vital that the cervical spine is protected with in-line immobilisation until a senior clinician can rule out a cervical spine injury. This requires a correctly sized semirigid collar to be applied to the neck and manual immobilisation. Alternatively, head blocks and tape (attached to an immovable part of the trolley) can be applied to immobilise the head and neck (Fig. 26.3).

It is important to recognise factors that may influence the use of collars, for example body habitus, comorbidities and age (NICE 2016). Elderly or frail patients may not be able to tolerate c-spine immobilisation and/or lie flat due to chronic lung disease and kyphosis and therefore c-spine immobilisation may have to be individualised for patient safety and long-term management (Peck et al. 2018).

The nurse assisting with maintenance of the patient's airway must be vigilant in observing the patient for any signs of nausea or vomiting. With the cervical spine immobilised, the patient is unable to move. If vomiting is likely, the team will have to log roll the patient to protect the spine (Fig. 26.4) and assist the patient with suction apparatus. In this case, an antiemetic may be prescribed and administered urgently.

Breathing and Ventilation

The patient's respiratory rate must be measured and recorded to observe for the efficacy of ventilation, that is, effective gaseous exchange taking place at the alveolar capillary membrane. Assessment should include the rate, depth and use of any accessory muscles (see Chapter 3, Nursing the Patient With Respiratory Disorders). All patients who have a faster than expected respiratory rate (tachypnoea) should be considered to have had chest injury until proven otherwise. All patients who have sustained traumatic injuries are at risk of hypoxia and should receive a high flow of oxygen. This can be delivered via a mask with a reservoir bag (nonrebreathe mask) with a flow rate of 15 L/min (ACS 2018). By the addition of a reservoir bag, the patient will receive up to 90% oxygen concentration compared to only 50% oxygen concentration with an ordinary oxygen mask (RCUK 2021). Pulse oximetry assists with monitoring of the patient's oxygenation saturation of arterial blood. An arterial blood gas sample may be taken if the patient is hypoxic or hypoventilating so that the clinician can gain an accurate picture of the patient's ventilatory status (Cole 2008).

Trauma patients must have their respiratory observations monitored regularly to detect any deterioration.

Major chest injuries can be divided into those that are immediately life-threatening and those that are life-threatening

Figure 26.4 The log roll technique. (Courtesy of the Advanced Trauma Nursing Course [ATNC], UK.)

TABLE 26.1	Classification of Major Thoracic Injury
The Lethal Six	**The Hidden Six**
Airway obstruction	Traumatic aortic disruption
Massive haemothorax	Tracheobronchial tree injury
Tension pneumothorax	Oesophageal perforation
Open pneumothorax	Cardiac contusion
Cardiac tamponade	Pulmonary contusion
Flail chest	Diaphragmatic tear or rupture

TABLE 26.2	Changes in Observations in Response to Haemorrhage
Pulse rate	Tachycardia due to adrenaline and noradrenaline release *(tachycardia is an early sign!)* N.B.: Patients who are on beta-blockers or patients who are very athletic will not appear to be tachycardic, although they may be hypovolaemic
Respiratory rate	Tachypnoea (increased respiratory rate) due to increased oxygen demand and compensatory mechanisms
Level of consciousness	Anxiety or confusion due to the reduction in oxygen delivery to the brain
Capillary refill time	Delayed >2 seconds due to systemic vasoconstriction
Blood pressure	Normal or raised due to compensation: systemic vasoconstriction *(hypotension may be a late sign!)*
Skin colour	Pale, cool peripheries due to systemic vasoconstriction
Urine output	Reduced urine output and increased urine concentration due to antidiuretic hormone and aldosterone production (part of the compensation process)

but are less obvious and often difficult to diagnose. The two groups of injuries have been described as the Lethal Six and the Hidden Six (Cole 2008) (see Table 26.1). In most cases, the life-threatening chest injuries will need a chest drain inserted as part of the initial treatment. The nurse should be familiar with the equipment and assistance needed for chest drain insertion (see Chapter 3, Nursing Patients With Respiratory Disorders).

Circulation and Haemorrhage Control

Haemorrhage is the main cause of early trauma deaths (ACS 2018) and can contribute to problems such as clotting disorders or organ failure once the patient has reached definitive care. In severely injured patients, hypovolaemia is common and it is the nurse's role to closely assess and monitor for signs of hypovolaemic shock (see Chapter 19, The Deteriorating Patient, Recognising and Managing Shock). This includes regular measurement and recording of the patient's heart rate, blood pressure, capillary refill time and, where possible, urine output (catheterisation may be necessary to monitor this). Table 26.2 summarises the changes to observations in response to haemorrhage.

Shah et al. (2023) describe how definitions in major trauma have varied in previous years. However, 50% blood loss in less than 3 hours or bleeding more than 150 mL a minute can be regarded as massive haemorrhage (Shah et al. 2023).

Common sites of haemorrhage following traumatic injury include the chest, the abdomen, the pelvis, the shaft of femurs and external haemorrhage from deep wounds including the scalp. Internal haemorrhage can be difficult to detect by clinical examination and plain X-ray alone. Increasingly, diagnostic imaging such as ultrasound scans (known as FAST: Focused Assessment with Sonography in Trauma) and computerised tomography (CT) scans are performed in the ED (or as close as possible) so that the source of bleeding can be found quickly. Trauma patients who are bleeding will need to be seen urgently by a senior surgeon to decide whether surgical, interventional radiology or conservative treatment is necessary (ACS 2018, Cole 2008). Interventional radiology is becoming more common in the management of trauma patients where clinically indicated, and can lead to the avoidance of open surgery, thus decreasing the known risks that open surgery can attract (McCabe 2016).

Fluid Resuscitation in Early Trauma

The injured patient needs two wide-bore cannulae inserted into large veins, such as those found in the crease of the elbow joint (antecubital fossa). At this point, blood is taken for full blood count, clotting, urea and electrolytes and blood grouping (and

if necessary cross-matching for a transfusion). Intravenous fluid therapy may be necessary if the patient is hypovolaemic. The goal of any trauma fluid resuscitation is to control the bleeding, support/supplement circulating volume and adequate tissue and organ perfusion (Ramesh et al. 2019)

The European Guidelines (Spahn et al. 2019) on management of major haemorrhage include the following recommendations:

- Fluid therapy using isotonic crystalloid solutions be initiated in the hypotensive bleeding trauma patient.
- Excessive use of 0.9% NaCl solution be avoided.
- Hypotonic solutions such as Ringer's lactate be avoided in patients with severe head trauma.
- The use of colloids be restricted due to the adverse effects on haemostasis (Ramesh et al. 2019).

The volume of intravenous fluids required will depend not only on the cardiovascular status of the patient and the injuries that they have sustained, but also on their age and comorbidities (Ramesh et al. 2019). Traditionally, if a patient is bleeding, intravenous fluids are given to keep their blood pressure at a normal level. However, modern trauma practice suggests that if the patient is given a lot of fluids to maintain the blood pressure, then there is a risk of causing clotting problems, hypothermia and further bleeding (Cole 2008, Rossaint et al. 2016). Therefore fluids need to be prescribed and administered following careful consideration of the patient's haemodynamic status and potential injuries. Should intravenous fluids be commenced, it is vital that cardiovascular observations (respiratory rate, heart rate, blood pressure, oxygen saturations and temperature) are recorded every 5 minutes to determine whether the patient is responding. A patient who improves following intravenous fluids may not need urgent surgery, whereas a patient who only improves transiently or not at all is unstable and is likely to require an urgent blood transfusion. If the patient's own blood group and rhesus match is not available, O Rh-negative blood (the universal donor) will be used.

Disability and Dysfunction: Neurological Assessment

If the patient has sustained a head injury or has a reduced level of consciousness, a neurological assessment should be carried out. This can be done using two methods: ACVPU and the GCS.

ACVPU. This is a simple acronym used to categorise the patient's response and level of consciousness:

- Is the patient Alert?
- Are they acutely Confused?
- Is the patient responding to your Voice?
- Is the patient only responding to Pain?
- Is the patient Unresponsive?

If the patient is anything less than Alert or new-onset Confusion, further investigation should be carried out using the GCS and may trigger a prompt reassessment and clinical review (Williams 2019).

Glasgow Coma Scale. The GCS is an international scale used to assess and score level of consciousness. The patient's eye opening, verbal response and motor function are assessed and given a numerical rating between 3 (the worst score) and 15 (the best score). The nurse should also use a torch to assess the patient's pupils to see if they are equal in size and react to light. This should be documented as a baseline for future comparison. For more information about the GCS, see Chapter 11, Nursing Patients With Disorders of the Nervous System.

Blood Glucose Level. At this point, if not already done, a blood glucose measurement should be taken in order to rule out hypoglycaemia or hyperglycaemia as a cause of reduced level of consciousness.

Exposure and Environmental Control

Whilst the patient's dignity must be preserved as much as is possible, it is essential that all clothing is removed so that the entire body can be examined, front and back, to ensure that no injuries are missed. It is important to remember that exposure can cause rapid body heat loss, so the resuscitation room temperature should be warm enough to preserve the patient's body temperature. Blankets should be replaced between any procedure or examination, to help prevent further temperature drop. The log roll technique (see Fig. 26.4) should be used to enable full examination of the patient's spine, and a rectal examination will be performed to assess sphincter tone (which may be altered with a spinal injury) and for signs of pelvic injury.

The Secondary Survey

The secondary survey is only started when the primary survey is complete and the patient's condition is stabilised. If the patient is critically injured, this secondary survey may not take place in the ED, as the patient is likely to require surgical intervention to stabilise their condition. However, if the patient's condition does permit, then the secondary survey involves a full head-to-toe examination and gives the nurse the opportunity to complete a thorough assessment, documenting wounds (location, surface area and depth), skin integrity, tetanus status, allergies and others. Any simple wounds should be thoroughly irrigated. This may be with 0.9% NaCl or povidone iodine; however, current evidence suggests that potable (drinking) water is just as effective in cleaning traumatic wounds and removing contaminants (Milne and Penn-Barwell 2023, Svoboda et al. 2008). Once clean, the wound should be covered with a sterile dressing until closure or exploration can be completed (Cole 2008, Milne and Penn-Barwell 2023). Local policies should be referenced and adhered to when managing wounds. Fractured limbs may need to be splinted or immobilised until treatment of more urgent injuries has been carried out.

Pain Management

Patients who have suffered traumatic injury will usually experience a great deal of pain. This can occur post injury, during the initial assessment, post operation or whilst recovering in definitive care. Pain is a physiological response to the injury and the stress response to this can have negative effects on the physical well-being of the patient including their ability to engage with nurses and the wider multidisciplinary team (MDT). In turn, this can have lasting ill effects on their overall rehabilitation and recovery (Dattatri et al. 2021). Additionally, the emotional response to pain can cause altered behaviour which may be affected by previous experiences of pain, culture, fear and so forth. It is essential that the nurse asks the patient if they are in pain, and observes for signs of pain such as groaning, facial expressions or a reluctance to move.

In the acute stages of trauma care, an intravenous analgesic such as morphine, fentanyl or oxycodone is effective and may be given as a bolus, as an infusion or as patient-controlled analgesia. Once able to tolerate oral medication, the patient may be prescribed a weak opioid such as co-codamol and/or a nonsteroidal anti-inflammatory such as naproxen. As well as observing for pain and monitoring the effect of the analgesic, nurses caring for the trauma patient should be aware of the side-effects of opiates, such as respiratory depression, nausea and constipation, and ensure that these are prevented or relieved (Reflection 26.2).

Diagnostic Imaging: The Nurse's Role

Most trauma patients need diagnostic imaging in the early stages of their care, and consequently, radiographers and radiologists are key members of the trauma service. Diagnostic imaging usually involves X-rays of the cervical spine, chest and pelvis; however, CT scans are increasingly being used to obtain more in-depth images.

At any stage of trauma care, accompanying an unstable or unwell trauma patient to the CT scan needs careful planning and preparation. Moving a patient to, from and within the CT scan is a high-risk procedure, especially if the patient's condition is unstable due to hypovolaemia, a head injury or overwhelming infection. Resuscitation equipment must be taken to and from imaging with the patient, and should include:

- oropharyngeal airways (unless the patient is intubated)
- oxygen – cylinder and masks

REFLECTION 26.2

Care of Patients With Nausea and Vomiting

A 27-year-old woman has been admitted to the trauma ward following a fall from a ladder. At the scene of the incident, she sustained a head injury and lost consciousness for a couple of minutes. In the ED, her assessment included a CT scan of her brain, which showed no injury. However, as she is drowsy and lives alone, she has been admitted for neurological observations. Shortly after arriving on the ward, she starts to complain of a 'terrible headache' and nausea, requesting a vomit bowl. The patient has been prescribed codeine phosphate for analgesia however, no antiemetics have been prescribed.

Activity

- Reflect on the care of a nauseated or vomiting patient following a head injury – what do these symptoms signify?
- Can you think of the names and doses of antiemetic medication that you know? Look them up in the British National Formulary (BNF).

- bag-valve – mask device
- cardiac and blood pressure monitoring equipment
- fluids/blood products or medications as prescribed
- patient documentation (notes, charts) to enable observation recording throughout the procedure.

The nurse should explain to the patient and family about the need for movement from one area to another and what the CT scan will involve. Privacy, dignity and warmth must be maintained by ensuring that the patient is properly covered. It is also important to ensure that the correct number of staff is available to assist with a log roll (see Fig. 26.4) or sliding manoeuvre to move the patient to and from the imaging table.

Definitive Care

Definitive care refers to the inpatient areas that the patient will be admitted to from the ED or theatres. Definitive care includes intensive care, the high-dependency unit (HDU) or a ward. Transfer between departments can be challenging and resuscitation equipment must accompany the patient (as discussed earlier). Furthermore, clear communication is essential between the nurses working in each area that the patient may pass through. This will help to ensure that the receiving area has time to prepare for the patient's admission.

Theatres and Operative Care

Definitive treatment of traumatic injuries often involves surgery depending on patient presentation, blood results, imaging results – X-rays, FAST and CT scans – and senior clinical acumen. The decision to take a patient to theatre or indeed interventional radiology, and indeed the timing of such interventions, is ultimately the decision of the trauma surgeon. As trauma patients can present to the hospital at any time, it is essential that there is an operating theatre available 24 hours a day for trauma emergencies. Trauma surgery, such as an emergency laparotomy to investigate internal bleeding, can be extremely challenging and requires a trauma consultant presence within the operating theatre (Findlay et al. 2007, NICE 2016). van Maarseveen et al. (2022) found that having a senior trauma surgeon present during trauma calls improves adherence to policies and protocols including ATLS guidelines. Skilled theatre staff are essential to care for the patient before, during and after operative procedures, from checking the patient, their identity, vital signs, allergy status, vascular access and others, as they arrive until discharge to the care of a unit or ward nurse. A trauma patient may need to return to theatre on more than one occasion if revision of surgery is needed. The theatre staff can do much to relieve the anxiety of these patients by providing a reassuring presence and clear communication.

When collecting the patient following trauma surgery, it is once again essential that the accompanying nurse has the necessary resuscitation equipment available (as discussed earlier) to ensure a safe transfer.

Critical Care

Many seriously injured patients will need to spend the first part of their definitive care in a critical care setting. This may be in an intensive care unit (ICU) or an HDU, depending on the patient's needs and the resources available. Critical care nurses need to be skilled and knowledgeable about caring for trauma patients in a high-technology environment. The remit of critical care in trauma is to provide (Cole and McGinley 2005):

- airway and ventilatory support (including physiotherapy)
- invasive monitoring (e.g. respiratory, cardiovascular, neurological, fluid balance)
- support for organ function when the patient cannot manage independently (e.g. the heart, the kidneys)
- delivery of powerful medication through central intravenous routes, such as inotropic drugs or antiarrhythmics
- pain management
- nutritional management
- maintenance of skin integrity and wound care
- psychosocial support
- care of the dying patient.

In general, a patient requiring intubation and ventilation and having multisystem problems will go to ICU for a period of one-to-one care and support. Surgical HDUs will generally admit patients who are not intubated (usually problems with only one system), but who may require invasive monitoring and organ support with inotropic drugs such as noradrenaline. These drugs help to maintain blood pressure and preserve renal function in critically ill patients. Patients may also be admitted to the HDU after being 'stepped down' from the ICU as their condition improves. For more on critical care, see Chapter 28.

Trauma Ward

It may be assumed that trauma patients are only cared for in the ED and ICU; however, the trauma patient will often spend the largest amount of their hospital admission on a ward. Trauma ward nurses care for patients with a range of problems including:

- orthopaedic injuries (such as fractures and postoperative care)
- plastics injuries (such as deep wounds, skin loss, postoperative care and burn management)
- head and face injuries (such as head injury observation following concussion or postoperative care)
- vascular injuries (primary damage to blood vessels, postoperative care or following angiography)
- spinal, nerve or musculoskeletal (MSK) injuries
- a combination of these injuries – polytrauma patients.

Detecting Patient Deterioration

Considering this, trauma ward nurses need to have excellent assessment and nursing skills to look after a large number of injured patients with differing needs. Patients may deteriorate at any time, days or even weeks following the initial injury, for example following an infection, secondary haemorrhage or clotting problem.

⊕ **See Evolve website Critical thinking question 26.1**

In a busy ward environment, it can be difficult to identify the deteriorating patient because signs of serious problems developing are often very subtle in the early stages. Therefore early warning systems (sometimes known as Early Warning Scores) need to be in place to assist the nurse in detecting such problems (Reflection 26.3), and to gain access to senior or specialist help as needed (Royal College of Physicians [RCP] 2017). Early detection of any deterioration is vital to enable timely treatment and prevention of further deterioration. Early identification has been shown to help nurses and medical staff intervene when patients are at high risk of deterioration or death (Goldhill and McNarry 2004, Williams 2019). However, it is also recognised that EWS should not be relied upon in isolation. Looking at the patient as a whole and being mindful of their MOI along with the EWS should ensure a detailed meaningful assessment of the patient (Carberry et al. 2014).

Care of the Elderly Trauma Patient (Over 65 Years)

The Older Adult Trauma Patient

The shift in aging population is having an impact on trauma presentations. In 1990, the mean age of major trauma patients was just over 36 years; by 2013, it had risen to almost 54 years (Kehoe et al. 2015). According to Raymond et al. (2021), 2.6 million people in the UK will be aged 85 years and over in the next 25 years. Therefore our trauma patient population can be expected to age accordingly. The TARN (2017) goes further to describe how low-level falls often result in severe injury in older adults. Traditionally, low-level falls have not been regarded as attracting high-impact/severe injuries, but certainly for this older cohort of patients, this belief is being rebuked.

Challenges to caring for older trauma patients aged 65 years and older include a lack of appreciation of age on trauma, including premorbid state, aging physiology, frailty and polypharmacy. The introduction of the Comprehensive Geriatric Assessments (CGA) along with dedicated older adult trauma pathways and increased surveillance in the management of elderly trauma patient should serve to provide more evidence supporting improved patient care, safety and outcomes throughout their admission (London Major Trauma System 2021).

Frailty, according to the British Geriatrics Society (2018), is 'a state of increased vulnerability to poor resolution of homoeostasis after a stressor event'. This is especially true in elderly trauma patients, where falls, delirium, limited mobility due to injury itself, pain or loss of confidence put this cohort of patients at further risk of deterioration and, in extreme cases, death.

Bryant et al. (2019) found that a multidisciplinary approach with frail elderly patients resulted in fewer episodes of delirium and reduced 30-day readmission rate. Such evidence-based practice, in an ever increasing population, further underpins how a whole team approach in trauma care optimises patient outcomes.

As the bedside nurse, your role is crucial; from basic physiological observations, to delirium screening and management, appreciating behavioural changes, appropriate, timely pain management along with engaging in therapeutic conversations all help inform your practice in the care of these patients and that of the wider team. Nurses often have the most oversight on their patients and are best placed to advocate for the patient with the wider team.

There is a long way to go in appreciating the impact of traumatic injuries on our aging population. Here in the UK, steps have already taken towards recognising that older adults do need increased screening and surveillance, including adapted trauma calls 'silver trauma'. In some centres, for example, these trauma calls recognise that low-level/low-energy falls or collisions can result in older adults sustaining significant major injuries, and therefore require the same level of response as higher-impact trauma. Frailty scoring, detailed medical and social history and delirium screening all help to support the patient in maximising their recovery and/or recognising that trauma may be life limiting or life ending. Should the injuries be deemed to be unsurvivable, this should be discussed within the MDT, the patient and their NOK. End-of-life protocols should then be initiated.

Discussions around end of life, death and dying can present their own unique set of challenges, and for trauma patients, there can be the added distress of the MOI. Such conversations may have to be taken slowly and layered; patients and family may need time to appreciate not only the injuries, but also the impact of the injuries on outcomes. It is important to have clear, open, honest and compassionate conversations with the patient and their families at this time. Such conversations are often led by senior doctors and nurses however, bedside nurses also need to be included or briefed so that all members of the team are up to date with care planning.

Rehabilitation

An important part of trauma ward care is to help with the process of rehabilitation, which starts soon after the injury has occurred as the treatment is commenced. This usually involves a multidisciplinary approach with physiotherapists to assist with mobilisation, occupational therapists to assist with functional and cognitive needs, speech and language therapists, dietitians who assist with functional and calorific support and possibly social workers for financial/social support. The trauma ward nurse's role in rehabilitation may include administering analgesics prior to mobilisation or exercise, ensuring that appropriate nutrition, hydration and elimination needs are met or working with the other disciplines to help the patient regain independence and confidence prior to discharge. Crucially, it is the nurse's role to keep the patient in the centre of their care planning, motivated and engaged with teams. Nurses are crucially placed to empower the patient to have their voices heard and understood. The nurse is often the one constant throughout their hospital stay; they see them at their lowest ebb and their highest ascent. Early links with community support teams are essential to ensure that the patient receives nursing, social care and rehabilitation input on leaving hospital. For more on nursing and rehabilitation, see Chapter 30.

Trauma-Informed Care

The vast majority of trauma patients sustain their injuries completely unexpectedly. How they react to a sudden, potentially violent and unforeseen event is based on many factors which can include previous trauma – either physical or psychological – previous health experiences and any adverse childhood experiences (domestic violence, neglect, caregiver substance misuse, etc.). According to the UK government, trauma-informed practice aims to reduce the impact of traumatic experiences on physical and mental health outcomes (Office for Health Improvement and Disparities 2022). For a working definition of trauma-informed practice, see www.gov.uk.

The six key principles of trauma-informed practice are safety, trust, choice, collaboration, empowerment and cultural consideration. In nursing, these principles should be embedded in the caring and compassionate care we extend to our patients and their families. However, if we evolve our practice so that we can appreciate the patient's own life experiences, in turn this can have a huge impact on how they interact with health professionals and external agencies, their perception of pain, their understanding of injury and rehabilitation and overall engagement in their health and wellbeing. If we, as nurses can appreciate that patients come with their own set of beliefs and values that need to be acknowledged and understood in order to establish how their current needs are best met. This is an emerging area of innovation, not only in nursing but also across health and social care. It will be interesting to see if and how trauma-informed practice becomes part of our everyday practice in nursing.

Psychological Care

Traumatic injury, by the very nature of its mechanism, is nearly always an unexpected event. This means that the patient and family have no time to prepare for the ill-health, incapacity and hospitalisation that will usually ensue. Many trauma patients are in the first four decades of life, and often this is the patient's first experience of inpatient healthcare, surgery and many other investigations and examinations. Trauma is a very stressful, frightening experience and patients need psychological support and care from the outset (Falkenberg et al. 2017, Mohta et al. 2003, Olive et al. 2022). In the early stages of trauma care, the patient may be unconscious, or intubated and sedated. Despite this, it is essential that nurses and other members of the healthcare team talk to the patient and family, explaining and reassuring as if the patient was conscious. Some patients report flashbacks or nightmares of the events surrounding the injury and delirium which can be psychologically debilitating (Cole and McGinley 2005, Jarman et al. 2023). Conversely, patients' previous life experiences can impact on how they understand and engage with health professionals – this is now commonly known as trauma-informed care, as previously discussed.

Once fully conscious, patients may find it difficult to comprehend what has happened or why they are in hospital; this may be due to their injuries or medication such as sedatives and antianxiolytics. Again, clear, supportive communication is necessary and, if appropriate, nonverbal reassurance such as holding the patient's hand or touching the patient's arm to provide extra reassurance when talking to them. Some trauma patients will need extensive rehabilitation to try to gain either full or partial return to their preinjury state. Injuries may leave the patient unable to carry out 'normal functions' such as walking, talking and defaecating unaided. They may also be cognitively impaired, and this can be psychologically devastating (Kellezi et al. 2017). Here, the contribution of occupational, physio and speech and language therapists cannot be underestimated. Moreover, many patients (and possibly their relatives) may need counselling or support from the mental health team or support groups to help them cope and come to terms with what has happened and what the future holds for them.

Post-Traumatic Stress Disorder

Post-traumatic stress disorder (PTSD) is a common outcome for patients who have suffered psychological or physical trauma. PTSD causes the patient to suffer from overwhelming anxiety and it is hard for the person to get the trauma out of their mind (ptsduk.co.uk). If left unrecognised and untreated, PTSD can have

devastating consequences for the patient and the family. Patients can suffer from flashbacks of the injury (or hospital stay), insomnia, nightmares and terror of facing the cause of the injury (e.g. getting into a car again or travelling on a train after a train crash). Whilst in the first 4–6 weeks this reaction is completely normal as the brain tries to process the events, memories and stimulus the patient has suffered, symptoms usually resolve; but for some, they do not, and it is then that professional advice and support should be sought. It is difficult to predict who will suffer from PTSD. A recent study looked at severity of injuries compared to development of PTSD (Evidence-Based Practice 26.1) and suggested that careful community follow-up helps to identify these patients.

Care of Relatives of the Trauma Patient

It is important from the beginning of the trauma patient's care that relatives or NOK are considered. In the ED and during an operation, it is often necessary for the relatives to be separated from their loved one. This can add to an already distressing situation and it is important that trauma nurses use calm, caring and sensitive communication skills when talking to and supporting relatives. Open, honest, clear information is essential, and if the nurse caring for the relatives does not have the answers to questions, then a senior member of trauma team should be sought. If the patient is in the critical care setting or a trauma ward, the relatives may want to participate in their care, and this should be encouraged and supported by the nursing team. The patient's relatives and friends play an important part in recovery and rehabilitation. If patients are in hospital for a prolonged period of time, having regular multidisciplinary meetings including the patient and family, where possible, is one way to ensure all parties are aware of the progress made and the challenges that may lie ahead, and how they can all work together to maximise rehabilitation and recovery. The nurse should be at the heart of these discussions. Nurses are often best placed to support and implement goals that have been made with and for their patients.

Care of Relatives of the Dying or Deceased Trauma Patient

A difficult situation for the trauma nurse may arise when resuscitative or treatment measures are not going to succeed. If staff know that the resuscitation attempts are likely to be futile and the family is present, it is important that the relatives are gently and sensitively made aware of the situation by the clinical teams caring for them, who can outline the gravity of the situation. This provides the family with time, even just a few minutes, to internalise the seriousness of the situation. The decision to stop resuscitation or treatment efforts is a difficult one, and one that should be made after considering individual team members' views with the consultant in charge of the patient's care making the ultimate decision. If the relatives are present, it may be possible to offer them the option of seeing their loved one to say goodbye before the resuscitation efforts are stopped. Traumatic injuries can be visually distressing and therefore it is important that a nurse or other healthcare professional stays with the relatives to support them during the process. However, although the research is limited for witnessed resuscitation after trauma, initial studies highlight it does not have a deleterious impact on the family (Leske et al. 2017). Where the patient has been in hospital for a longer period of time, there is often a layering of conversations explaining injuries, patients' response to interventions, management plans and

EVIDENCE-BASED PRACTICE 26.1

Post-Traumatic Stress Disorder

PTSD is a common outcome following major traumatic injury; however, it is difficult to predict who will suffer from this condition.

A study by Harris et al. (2008) aimed to examine the role of physical and psychosocial factors in the development of PTSD following major trauma. During the study period, all adult patients presenting to one MTC in New Zealand with major trauma were identified. Their injury characteristics and clinical data were recorded from the hospital records and the hospital trauma database.

A questionnaire was posted to the patients at intervals between the first and the sixth year following the injury, asking them to complete a PTSD checklist (see later) and supply other data – employment, income, etc. Multiple linear regression (looking at the relationship between variables) was then used to identify significant independent associations with PTSD.

Three hundred and fifty-five patients (61%) responded to the questionnaire. Of those, 129 (36.3%) were classed as having PTSD. Symptoms of PTSD were not significantly related to how severe the injury had been, the time since the injury, education level, household income or employment status at the time of injury. PTSD was significantly associated with younger age, the presence of chronic illnesses, unemployment at the time of follow-up, use of a lawyer to try to settle a claim, blaming others for the injury and having an unsettled compensation claim. The authors concluded that PTSD following major trauma was not related to measures of injury severity, but was related to other factors, such as blaming others for the accident and the processes involved in claiming compensation.

Significance for Practice

Any trauma patient may go on to develop PTSD. As a result, two factors play an important role in their care. First, all major trauma patients who are to be discharged from hospital need to be taught about recognising the signs and symptoms of PTSD, and where to seek help if this occurs. Follow-up clinics should be offered, not only for the review of physical injuries, but also for a review of patients' psychological health and well-being.

Secondly, this study suggests that there is a role for community health and social care teams to provide follow-up for all major trauma patients, with a specific remit of carefully monitoring those patients in the identified high-risk groups. Neither of these initiatives is currently offered as a routine to all trauma patients in the UK.

Organisations such as www.ptsduk.co.uk can offer support and guidance for patients who are at risk of or who have developed PTSD.

For other useful information see: www.nhs.uk/Conditions/Post-traumatic-stress-disorder/Pages/Introduction.aspx?url=Pages/what-is-it.aspx

PTSD Checklist – Civilian Version

Patient's name: _____

Instruction to patient: Below is a list of problems and complaints that people sometimes have in response to stressful life experiences. Please read each one carefully, and, using the scale below, put a figure in the box to indicate how much you have been bothered by that problem in the past week.

Not at all (1)
A little bit (2)
Moderately (3)
Quite a bit (4)
Extremely (5)

1. Repeated, disturbing *memories, thoughts, or images* of a stressful experience from the past? ☐
2. Repeated, disturbing *dreams* of a stressful experience from the past? ☐
3. Suddenly *acting* or *feeling* as if a stressful experience *were happening* again (as if you were reliving it)? ☐
4. Feeling *very upset* when *something reminded* you of a stressful experience from the past? ☐
5. Having *physical reactions* (e.g. heart pounding, trouble breathing, or sweating) when *something reminded* you of a stressful experience from the past? ☐
6. Avoid *thinking about* or *talking about* a stressful experience from the past or avoid *having feelings* related to it? ☐
7. Avoid *activities* or *situations* because they *remind you* of a stressful experience from the past? ☐
8. Trouble *remembering important parts* of a stressful experience from the past? ☐
9. Loss of *interest in things that you used to enjoy?* ☐
10. Feeling *distant* or *cut off* from other people? ☐
11. Feeling *emotionally numb* or being unable to have loving feelings for those close to you? ☐
12. Feeling as if your *future* will somehow be *cut short?* ☐
13. Trouble *falling* or *staying asleep?* ☐
14. Feeling *irritable* or having *angry outbursts?* ☐
15. Having *difficulty concentrating?* ☐
16. Being *"super alert"* or watchful or on guard? ☐
17. Feeling *jumpy* or easily startled? ☐

Resource

Harris IA, Young JM, Rae H, et al. Predictors of post traumatic stress disorder following major trauma. ANZ J Surg. 2008;78(7):583–587.

---

expected outcomes. In this way the family may begin to appreciate the limits of modern trauma care, and indeed its limitations, that death is a process best facilitated in collaboration of local policies including reducing or eliminating certain medications and support; comfort, dignity and pain relief are paramount. The religious and cultural beliefs of the patient and their family should be accommodated as much as is practical – visits from the chaplaincy or faith leaders may be offered for example.

Following the death, if relatives wish to see their loved one, nurses can do much to help. If possible, those parts of the body that are exposed should be washed. One or (if possible) both of the deceased's hands should be left outside the sheets. The head of the trolley/bed should be slightly raised; otherwise, the face may seem distorted or discoloured when the family first sees the body. False teeth should be replaced if possible and the hair combed or smoothed. Where there are external injuries, bandages or dressings should be left in place and perhaps covered with a clean outer layer. A nurse should initially accompany the relatives and, if they seem hesitant, can indicate that it is all right for them to touch the body, perhaps by doing so personally or by asking the family members if they wish to hold the loved one's hand. The nurse should then offer to withdraw. Not everyone will want to be left alone or indeed want to see their loved ones after death, but some may have private words of parting to say and should be given the opportunity to do so. Where a whole family is present, this chance should be given to each person individually. One family member may not feel able to ask for this for themselves, but when it is suggested by the nurse, they may gratefully accept. Relatives should also feel free to hug or kiss the body; in the case of a dead child, the parents should be able to take the child in their arms, should they wish to do so. This seems to help people to cope with the denial stage of grieving, especially in cases of sudden or traumatic death

(Hackett et al. 2022, Kubler-Ross 1984). Before bereaved relatives see or touch the deceased, it is crucial that the nurse ensure they are allowed to do so. There may be a legal reason, for example unexplained death or murder. In such cases, close liaison with police and coroner is crucial to ensure ongoing investigations are not put at risk.

Death at any stage of the patient's care in hospital is a difficult and sad time for relatives. Death related to traumatic injuries can be even more distressing for relatives and friends of the deceased. This may be due to the suddenness of events, the MOI and perceived injustice of the death itself. This combined with the complexity of grief, personal circumstances and previous life experiences can often mean nurses need to be especially compassionate and patient with families and friends. It can be incredibly distressing for all involved. Ensuring that the relatives and also the nursing and wider MDTs have support throughout this part of the patient journey is crucial. Bereaved people sometimes have difficulty in remembering information so the nurse should consider writing information down or providing preprepared information about what has happened and what will happen next (e.g. the potential need for a post mortem or when the body can be released from hospital). In the UK, trauma-related deaths need to be reported to the coroner to determine the exact cause of death (Ministry of Justice [MoJ] 2022).

It is also important that the nurse is aware of the individual's religious and cultural beliefs, following a trauma death. Each healthcare trust should have direct access to faith leaders from different faiths who can offer advice or, if the family members request it, be present to support them during this difficult period. For more information on trauma-related deaths, see MoJ (2022) Guidance for Registered Medical Practitioners on the Notification of Deaths Regulations (publishing.service.gov.uk).

Organ and Tissue Donation Following Trauma Death

Following a trauma-related death in the ED or critical care, a family member may indicate to the nurse that the patient carried a donor card or had registered as a donor. It would at that point be appropriate for the consultant in charge of care to be informed and contact made with the Specialist Nurse – Organ Donation (SNOD). The SNOD can then give advice and guidance, and can liaise with NHS Blood and Transplant regarding would-be recipients.

Organs are most usually taken from patients who have been diagnosed with brain stem death by two senior doctors in the ICU where the potential for donation is recognised and the transplant coordinator is informed while the patient is being ventilated. These are called beating-heart donors. In some EDs, patients who die in the department can donate kidneys, tissue and cells. The kidneys are preserved by inserting a femoral cannula and perfusing the kidneys with a preservative fluid. This allows time for family to be contacted and the deceased's wishes to be established. These are called non-heart-beating donors (Meisner 2008). Many nurses find the concept of talking to relatives about donation challenging, especially at a time of grief and distress. It is essential that trauma nurses who are involved in this process have been trained to use the appropriate language and have the correct information to give the family. If the nurse or any member of the trauma team has not been trained, the SNOD can offer support and will liaise with the family directly. A family should not be approached by untrained staff.

There are only two conditions where organ donation is completely ruled out: a person who has had cancer that has spread in the last 12 months and patients who have Creutzfeldt–Jakob disease (CJD) (NHS Blood and Transplant).

Staff Stress and Grief

It is very difficult for staff (including students and support staff) to have worked hard to save a patient's life but without success. Feelings of inadequacy and failure may arise, especially when the patient is young or when the circumstances of the traumatic incident seem senseless. Repeatedly caring for patients and relatives in these circumstances may take its toll, both emotionally and physically, which means that the caregivers themselves may become casualties. It is important, therefore to consider the distress and/or grief that will be felt by staff who have been involved with the patient and/or the relatives. There should be a forum for expressing feelings and anxieties within the department. One method is a 'defusing' session which can be described as a short type of crisis intervention for staff involved in such an incident (Hallet and Dickens 2017). It allows staff to talk with one another about the experience in a relaxed atmosphere and provides an opportunity to give all staff the key information relating to the whole episode of the incident. This ventilation of feelings and rerun of events can be of benefit in two ways: it can allow staff to express their emotions, and it can highlight defects in the system or ways of improving practice in the future (Bloomer et al. 2022).

For particularly distressing incidents, a more formal type of debriefing may be required. Critical incident stress debriefing (CISD) (Ireland et al. 2008) is a session which may be facilitated by someone who has knowledge of counselling skills. It usually takes place 24–72 hours after the event and follows a structured format that focuses on the emotional consequences for staff involved in these types of incidents. Knowledge about stress and coping mechanisms will help staff and students recognise their own limitations and know when they themselves need help. Staff counselling should be offered for those who feel it necessary. Health and well-being of staff are crucial, and compassion fatigue is a recognised reaction to constant exposure to end-of-life care. However, so too is compassion satisfaction, that is, when the nurse feels satisfaction from a job well done, a family and patient supported through their trauma and all that that entails (Hinderer et al. 2014). These two emotional responses are not distinct and nurses can experience both. What is important is that nurses, and indeed all staff, are supported through education, debriefing, supportive rota management/allocation as well as access to external support if needed. The past few years have had a significant impact on staff; the COVID pandemic saw nurse education and work practices change in ways previously thought to be impractical and even unimaginable. Staff welfare and burnout, school leavers inspired to join the profession and vast numbers of experienced staff leaving the profession have created a mismatch in nursing that will need careful managing in the years to come, to safeguard not only the nurses themselves but also the patients. In 2020, Bateman et al. went further and found that running Death Cafes for staff in a systematic and formalised manner over a number of weeks helped all staff involved in the death of patients and helped address burnout prevention in critical care environments.

Medico-Legal Aspects of Trauma Care

Due to the nature of traumatic injury (e.g. road traffic collisions and assault), nurses are often required to work in close collaboration with the police. In order to investigate a traumatic incident or a trauma-related death, the police may require information about the patient or clothing/blood samples for forensic evidence. This sometimes creates a conflict in the nurse's professional practice. All patients are entitled to confidentiality in respect of information pertaining to them and it is the nurse's responsibility to ensure that this right is respected (Nursing and Midwifery Council [NMC] 2018).

There are exceptions where patient confidentiality may be broken because disclosure of information is required by the law, and this affects the public, not just nurses (Meisner 2008). This includes:

- Following a road traffic collision, the Road Traffic Act 1991 requires any person to provide the police, when requested, with information that may identify the vehicle driver involved in a collision. The nurse must be sure of the facts as it is not always clear once the patient has arrived in hospital who was the driver.
- Under the Prevention of Terrorism Act 2000, any person who believes a person may have been involved in a terrorist act and has information to support this belief should inform the police.
- A court may order disclosure of information.
- Whilst injury involving firearms does not mandate disclosure, information may be given to the police in the public interest.

The nurse may be required to make a statement about the patient's care or injuries which will form part of the police investigation. It should be noted, however, that it may be several years before a case, whether criminal or civil, comes before the courts and the nurse is asked to write the statement. For this reason, it is important that careful attention is paid to accurate documentation within the patient's nursing and medical records.

In the ED, it is not uncommon for police officers to ask for a pretransfusion blood sample to be taken and then given to them. However, unless the hospital has predetermined protocols allowing this, *blood samples must not be handed to police officers without a court order from a judge* (Meisner 2008). In some areas of the UK, a police doctor, a forensic medical examiner, may come to the hospital to take blood from the patient.

The police may also ask for patient's clothing or any weapons that may have been brought to hospital. Anything that is handed to the police must be clearly documented in the patient's notes, with the police officer's name and number recorded.

Challenging Behaviour

A minority of patients (and/or their relatives) who have been involved in a traumatic incident may appear to be aggressive or threatening. It is important that nurses remember that aggression is seldom directed towards them personally. Many factors can contribute to the feelings of aggression towards a situation or person. These include frustration about the injury and a lack of information either about the condition of a relative or about the excessive waiting times. Waiting rooms in all clinical areas that have poor facilities can contribute to an individual's level of frustration, for example shabby decor, uncomfortable seating and an unwelcoming decor. The attitude of staff to patients, particularly if it appears judgemental and unsympathetic, may contribute to the development of a confrontation between patient or relative, nurse and the wider team.

Sometimes, the aggression is a result of physiological processes which cause acute confusional or combative states, for example pain, hypoxia or a head injury. In these situations the patient has little or no control over their actions and the cause of the altered mental state should be recognised and, if possible, treated.

It is essential that nurses are able to recognise when a patient is becoming aggressive if they are to prevent the situation escalating. Strategies that help to defuse difficult situations include the use of good verbal and nonverbal communication and the adoption of a calm, nonthreatening, nonpatronising approach. Other strategies include:

- Adopt an open appropriate body posture, arms unfolded, standing or sitting at arm's length away from the patient.
- Listen carefully, demonstrating a genuine interest in what the individual has to say. It is difficult not to shout back when being shouted at, but it is more effective if the pitch, tone and volume of the nurse's voice remain within a normal conversational range.
- Be sympathetic; offer clear explanations and an apology where necessary.
- Try to agree a plan. It is unwise to give false information or agree on solutions that are unachievable, as this will result in trust being lost and may cause further aggression at a later stage.
- Avoid physical risk. Ensure that you are talking in a private yet open environment where escape can be made if necessary.

It is important that, following any incident of aggression or violence, whether verbal or physical, an incident form is completed and that this is reviewed by the trust risk management team in accordance with local policy and procedure. This monitors the escalating problem and may reveal patterns of aggression in the workplace, thereby allowing preventive strategies to be formulated. These may include education opportunities for the staff on communication and defusing techniques. If it is apparent that there is an increase in violent and aggressive situations, statistical evidence is useful when making a bid to management staff for more security staff, better protection or enhanced care facilities.

Mass Casualty Trauma Care

Some traumatic incidents, such as a transport crash or a bomb blast, will involve more than one or two people. When considering large numbers of traumatically injured people who need immediate medical care, the term 'major incident' is used. There is no one standard definition of a mass casualty event (formally known as a major incident); however, NHS England (2020) has stated:

a Mass Casualty Incident for health services as an incident (or series of incidents) causing casualties on a scale that is beyond the normal resources of the emergency and healthcare services ability to manage.

NHS England 2017, p. 7

Most definitions are deliberately nonspecific because what constitutes a mass casualty event for a small rural hospital may have minimal impact in a large urban hospital. Similarly, a large-scale disaster may affect only one hospital or may require the services of several hospitals within a region. The purpose of *emergency preparedness* (also known as emergency planning) for such situations within the NHS is to ensure that all the emergency services are able to work collaboratively and provide an effective response to any type of incident.

The persistent threat of global terrorism has resulted in the planning for dealing with and preparing for mass casualty incidents having had to be revised and revisited constantly over the past few decades (Park and Grier 2022) with each new incident, such the Grenfell Tower fire and terrorist attacks in Manchester and London, all in 2017. It is essential that every hospital has a major incident plan, including a chemical decontamination plan (NHS England 2018). The ED plays a major role in this, as it is required to provide the rapid initial response. However, most of the departments and services within a hospital also have a role to play in a major incident. Ward and critical care areas will need to discharge or transfer patients quickly to make bed space available for the major incident patients. All routine surgery and clinics should be immediately cancelled so that theatre space and personnel are available for emergency surgery. Extra intravenous fluids, blood products, medication and other equipment will be urgently needed, with porters or runners available to transport these vital supplies. Nonclinical staff will provide essential roles for registering and admitting patients, maintaining communication networks and providing support for patients being discharged and their relatives.

Types of mass casualty incidents include:
- transport (train, aeroplane, motor vehicle crashes)
- explosions (industrial or bomb blasts)
- industrial incidents (explosions, fire, chemical leaks)
- sporting/entertainment events where large numbers of people are gathered (e.g. Manchester bombing, 2017)
- environmental – natural (e.g. tsunami or earthquake) or collapse of a building or infrastructure
- chemical/biological spillages or deliberate releases
- radiation or nuclear incidents.

In the event of an incident, the police, fire service, ambulance service or local emergency planning officers may declare a major incident. In a large-scale incident where many casualties are predicted, more than one hospital will be involved in the response. The ED will be notified by the police or the local ambulance service, and informed of the type of incident that they are dealing with and the predicted number of patients. Usually, the nurse who receives the call will declare a hospital major incident through an emergency switchboard number. In order to prepare to receive the casualties, the department will be cleared as quickly as possible, restocking principal areas with extra equipment, such as decontamination equipment if dealing with a chemical incident, whilst calling in extra staff. Simultaneously, other areas and departments need to prepare to receive patients according to their local major incident plans.

The ED may be asked to provide an on-site mobile medical team (MMT). The MMT provided will depend on the local plan, and resources available at the hospital. Usually, there will be some ED nurses, an ED doctor, a surgeon and an anaesthetist. However, in some areas, there are dedicated prehospital care teams allied to a hospital (such as the Helicopter Emergency Medical Service in London) who will provide the MMT. It is vital that these staff

are adequately trained in their role (Department of Health [DH] 2015) and equipped with correct personal protective equipment as they will be required to support the ambulance service in difficult and potentially dangerous environments, such as a chemical or radiation spillage (NHS England 2022). If the major incident has a chemical, biological, radiological or nuclear (CBRN) involvement, then ideally no casualty should leave the scene of the incident until they have been thoroughly decontaminated by the ambulance and/or fire service. Inevitably, some casualties may 'slip through the net' and will require immediate decontamination on arrival to the hospital; therefore all ED personnel should be trained and practised in decontamination procedures (NHS England 2022).

Due to the volume of patients, it is important that careful attention is paid to adequate identification of all individuals. The police documentation team, which will be based in the hospital, should operate a 'casualty bureau', where all information regarding patients is collated. Members of the public can contact the bureau for further information regarding casualties. The hospital staff will have to keep this unit updated with details of patients. Many relatives will arrive at the hospital seeking information and the media will require regular press statements, as in all public interest events. It is important that this does not interrupt the care of the patients. The hospital will need to ensure that adequate facilities and support staff are in place to care for friends and relatives waiting to see the injured, whilst establishing separate communication networks for the media. Once all the casualties have been cared for and transferred to other areas for their definitive care, the ED must resume its customary work as soon as possible. However, the hospital will probably remain on major incident alert as the patients may require hours of surgery following injury and days in the critical care or ward areas. All of this will disrupt the normal flow of a hospital and the impact of this cannot be underestimated.

Major incidents are not just an ED problem. The whole hospital or healthcare trust will usually have a role to play. Trauma nurses *must* know their role in a major incident, regardless of the clinical setting in which they work (Reflection 26.4). Because of the relative infrequency of major incidents and the pattern of staff changes, it is recommended that hospitals carry out regular major incident exercises such as 'Off the shelf exercises' or simulated incidents, together with the ambulance and other emergency services, so as to ensure a rapid and effective response (Public Health England 2017).

Summary: Key Nursing Issues

- The trauma assessment framework 'C, A, B, C, D, E' is known as the primary survey: this helps to detect injuries and problems in the early stages of trauma care.
- Hypoxia and haemorrhage are common life-threatening problems for trauma patients.
- It is essential that nurses can identify abnormal observations, detect potential problems and access appropriate help promptly to avoid the patient deteriorating.
- Transferring or transporting trauma patients is a high-risk procedure that needs careful planning, preparation and the correct equipment.
- Trauma is a true multidisciplinary specialty where nurses work closely with medical staff, therapists, radiographers, etc., to ensure optimal care for the patient.

- Traumatic death is usually sudden and unexpected. This means that the nurse liaising with the patient's family should have clear, supportive communication skills.
- Trauma often has medico-legal implications and there are times when, by law, the patient's confidentiality has to be breached without their permission. The nurse must be absolutely certain of the facts before doing this.
- Major incident events resulting in large numbers of trauma patients need to be carefully planned for and practised.

Reflection and Learning – What Next?

- **Test** your knowledge by visiting the Evolve website 🌐 and answering the multiple-choice questions and critical thinking questions.
- **Consolidate** your learning by looking at some of the further reading suggestions, references and specialist websites.
- **Revisit** some of the additional material on the website.

- **Consider** what you have learnt and how this will help your professional development.
- **Reflect** on how you can apply this knowledge to the care of your patients.
- **Discuss** your learning with your assessor/supervisor, lecturer and colleagues.

References

Alshibani A, Banerjee J, Lecky F, Coats TJ, Conroy MS. New horizons in understanding appropriate prehospital identification and trauma triage for older adults. *Open Access Emerg Med*. 2021;13:117–135. doi:10.2147/OAEM.S297850.

Adulwahid MA, Booth A, Kuczawski M, Mason SM. The impact of Senior Doctor Assessment triage on emergency department measures: systematic review and meta-analysis of comparative studies. *Emerg Med J*. 2016;33:504–513.

American College of Surgeons (ACS). *Advanced Trauma Life Support Program for Physicians*. 10th ed. Chicago, IL: American College of Surgeons; 2018.

Bateman ME, Hammer R, Byrne A, et al. Death cafés for prevention of burnout in intensive care unit employees: study protocol for a randomized controlled trial (STOPTHEBURN). *Trials*. 2020;21:1019. https://doi.org/10.1186/s13063-020-04929-4.

Bloomer MJ, Ranse K, Adams L, Brooks L, Coventry A. Time and life is fragile": an integrative review of nurses' experiences after patient death in adult critical care. *Aust Crit Care*. 2022. https://doi.org/10.1016/j.aucc.2022.09.008.

Bickerton J, Dewan V, Allan T. Streaming A&E patients to walk in centre service. *Emerg Nurse*. 2005;13(3):20–23.

British Geriatrics Society. *Frailty: what's it all about?* British Geriatrics Society; 2018. bgs.org.uk.

Bryant EA, Tulebaev S, Castillo-Angeles M, et al. Frailty identification and care pathway: an interdisciplinary approach to care for older trauma patients. *J Am Coll Surg*. 2019;228(6):852–859. doi:10.1016/j.jamcollsurg.2019.02.052.e1.

Carberry M, Clement P, Headly E. How helpful are early warning scores? *Nurs Times*. 2014;110(1–3):12–14.

Cole E. *Trauma Care: Initial Assessment and Management of the Trauma Patient in the ED*. Oxford: Wiley–Blackwell; 2008.

Cole E, Crichton N. The culture of a trauma team in relation to human factors. *J Clin Nurs*. 2006;15:1257–1266.

Cole E, McGinley A. A structured approach to caring for the trauma patient. In: O'Shea R, ed. *Principles and Practice of Trauma Nursing*. Edinburgh: Elsevier; 2005:37–60.

Dattatri R, Jain VK, Karthikeyan P, et al. Anaesthetic considerations in polytrauma patients. *J Clin Orthop Trauma*. 2021;12:1. https://www.sciencedirect.com/science/article/pii/S0976566220304914.

Department of Health (DH). NHS England Emergency Preparedness, Resilience and Response Framework; 2015. https://www.england.nhs.uk/wp-content/uploads/2018/12/version1__Major_Incident_and_Mass_casualty_guidelines-Nov-2018.pdf.

Department of Transport. Reported Road Casualties in Great Britain: 2017 Annual Report; 2018. https://assets.publishing.service.gov.uk/government/uploads/system/uploads/attachment_data/file/744077/reported-road-casualties-annual-report-2017.pdf.

Falkenberg L, Zeckery C, Mommsen P, et al. Long-term outcome in 324 polytrauma patients: what factors are associated with posttraumatic stress disorder and depression symptoms. *Eur J Med Res*. 2017;22:14.

Findlay G, Martin IC, Carter S, et al. *Trauma: who cares? A Report on the National Confidential Enquiry Into Patient Outcome and Death (NCEPOD)*. London: NCEPOD; 2007:10–14.

Gabe B, Beck B. Trauma systems saves lives – is that enough? *Injury*. 2021;52(2):125 126.

GBD 2019 Diseases and Injuries Collaborators. Global burden of 369 diseases and injuries in 204 countries and territories, 1990–2019: a systematic analysis for the Global Burden of Disease Study 2019. *Lancet*. 2020;396:1204–1222.

Goldhill DR, McNarry AF. Physiological abnormalities in early warning scores are related to mortality in adult inpatients. *Br J Anaesth*. 2004;92(6):882–884.

Greaves I. Mechanism of injury. In: Greaves I, Porter KM, Ryan JM, eds. *Trauma Care Manual 2001*. London: Arnold; 2001:99–114.

Hackett J, Heavey E, Beresford B. 'It was like an airbag, it cushioned the blow': a multi-site qualitative study of bereaved parents' experiences of using cooling facilities. *Palliat Med*. 2022;36(2):365–374.

Hallet N, Dickens GL. De-escalation of aggressive behaviour in healthcare settings: concept analysis. *Int J Nurs Stud*. 2017;75:10–20.

Harris IA, Young JM, Rae H, et al. Predictors of post traumatic stress disorder following major trauma. *ANZ J Surg.* 2008;78(7):583–587.

Hatchimonji JS, Kaufman EJ, Babalola D, et al. Beyond pain and disability: the lasting effects of trauma on life after injury. *J Trauma Acute Care Surg.* 2022;93(3):332–339.

Hinderer K, von Rueden K, Friedmann E, et al. Burnout, compassion fatigue, compassion satisfaction and secondary traumatic stress in trauma nurses. *J Trauma Nurs.* 2014;21(4):160–169.

Ireland S, Gilchrist J, Maconochie I. Debriefing after failed paediatric resuscitation: a survey of current UK practice. *Emerg Med J.* 2008;25:328–330.

Jarman A, Chapman K, Vollam S, Stiger R, Williams M, Gustafson O. Investigating the impact of physical activity interventions on delirium outcomes in intensive care unit patients: a systematic review and meta-analysis. *J Intensive Care Soc.* 2023;24(1):85–95.

Kehoe A, Smith JE, Edwards A, et al. The changing faces of major trauma. *Emerg Med J.* 2015;32(12):911–915.

Kellezi B, Coupland Z, Morriss R, et al. The impact of psychological factors on recovery from injury: a multicentre cohort study. *Soc Psychiatry Psychiatr Epidemiol.* 2017;52(7):855–866.

Kubler-Ross E. *On Death and Dying.* London: Tavistock; 1984.

Leske JS, McAndrew NS, Brasel KJ, Feetham S. Family presence during resuscitation after trauma. *J Trauma Nurs.* 2017;24(2):85–96.

London Major Trauma System. Management of Older Major Trauma Patients. Third Edition. 2021. https://www.c4ts.qmul.ac.uk/downloads/pan-london-major-trauma-system-management-of-older-trauma.-third-editionapril-2021.pdf.

McCabe S, Maddineni S, Marini L, Rozeblit G. Vascular and interventional radiology in blunt abdominopelvic trauma – institutional practice and review of the literature. *J Trauma Treat.* 2016;5:324.

McCullough AL, Haycock DC, Forward DP, Moran CG. Early management of the severely injured major trauma patient. *Br J Anaesth.* 2014;113(2):234–241.

Meisner S. Trauma related deaths. In: Cole E, ed. *Trauma Care: Initial Assessment and Management of the Trauma Patient in the ED.* Oxford: Wiley–Blackwell; 2008.

Milne K, Penn-Barwell JG. Classification and management of acute wounds and open fractures. *Surgery.* 2023;41(2):93–99.

Ministry of Justice (MoJ). Guidance for registered medical practitioners on the Notification of Deaths Regulations. 2022. https://assets.publishing.service.gov.uk/government/uploads/system/uploads/attachment_data/file/1062499/registered-medical-practitioners-notification-deaths-regulations-25-march-2022.pdf.

Mohta M, Sethi AK, Tyagi A, Mohta A. Psychological care in trauma patients. *Injury.* 2003;34(1):17–25.

NHS Digital. Hospital admitted patient care activity 2020–21. 2022. https://digital.nhs.uk/data-and-information/publications/statistical/hospital-admitted-patient-care-activity/2020-21. Accessed 15 December 2022.

NHS England. *Emergency Preparedness, Resilience and Response.* Concept of Operations for Managing Mass Casualties; 2018. https://www.england.nhs.uk/wp-content/uploads/2018/03/concept-operations-management-mass-casualties.pdf.

NHS England. Hospital admissions for youths assaulted with sharp objects up almost 60%. 2019. https://www.england.nhs.uk/2019/02/teens-admitted-to-hospital/#:~:text=Cases%20involving%20all%20young%20people,with%20knives%20or%20sharp%20objects.

NHS England. *Clinical Guidelines for Major Incidents and Mass Casualty Events.* 2020. https://www.england.nhs.uk/wp-content/uploads/2018/12/B0128-clinical-guidelines-for-use-in-a-major-incident-v2-2020.pdf.

NHS England. *Emergency Preparedness, Resilience and Response (EPRR).* Hazardous materials (HAZMAT) and chemical, biological, radiological and nuclear (CBRN); 2022. https://www.england.nhs.uk/ourwork/eprr/hm/.

National Institute of Health and Care Excellence (NICE). *Major trauma: assessment and initial management.* NICE guideline [NG39]; 2016. https://www.nice.org.uk/guidance/ng39.

National Institute of Health and Care Excellence (NICE). Rehabilitation after traumatic injury should support people in resuming their lives. 2021. https://www.nice.org.uk/news/article/rehabilitation-after-traumatic-injury-should-support-people-in-resuming-their-lives.

Noble-Mathews PM. Pre-hospital care. In: O'Shea R, ed. *Principles and Practice of Trauma Nursing.* Edinburgh: Elsevier; 2005:61–70.

Nursing and Midwifery Council (NMC). The Code: Professional Standards of Practice and Behaviour for Nurses, Midwives and Nursing Associates. 2018. https://www.nmc.org.uk/globalassets/sitedocuments/nmc-publications/nmc-code.pdf.

Office for Health Improvement and Disparities. Guidance: Working definition of trauma-informed practice. 2022. https://www.gov.uk/government/publications/working-definition-of-trauma-informed-practice/working-definition-of-trauma-informed-practice.

Olive P, Hives L, Wilson N, et al. Psychological and psychosocial aspects of major trauma care in the United Kingdom: a scoping review of primary research. *Trauma.* 2022;25(4). doi:10.1177/14604086221104934.

Park CL, Grier GR. Provision of pre-hospital medical care for terrorist attacks. *Br J Anaesth.* 2022;128(2):e85–e89.

Peck GE, Heming Shipway DJ, Tsang K, Fertleman M. Cervical spinal immobilization in the elderly: a literature review. *Br J Neurosurg.* 2018;32:1–5.

Public Health England. 2017. https://www.england.nhs.uk/publication/off-the-shelf-exercises/.

Ramesh GH, Uma JC, Farhath S. Fluid resuscitation in trauma: what are the best strategies and fluids? *Int J Emerg Med.* 2019;12:38. https://doi.org/10.1186/s12245-019-0253-8.

Raymond A, Bazeer N, Barclay C, Krelle H, Idriss O, Tallack C, Kelly E. Our ageing population: how ageing affects health and care need in England. The Health Foundation; 2021. https://doi.org/10.37829/HF-2021-RC16.

Resuscitation Council UK. *The ABCDE Approach.* Resuscitation Council UK; 2021.

Rossaint R, Bouillon B, Cerney V et al. The European guideline on management of major bleeding and coagulopathy following trauma: fourth edition. *Crit Care.* 2016.12;20:100. doi: 10.1186/s13054-016-1265-x.

Royal College of Anaesthetists. Guidelines for the Provision of Anaesthesia Services (GPAS); 2021. https://rcoa.ac.uk/sites/default/files/documents/2021-03/GPAS-2021-16-TRAUMA.pdf.

Royal College of Physicians (RCP). *National Early Warning Score (NEWS) 2. Standardising the assessment of acute-illness severity in the NHS.* London: RCP; 2017. https://www.rcplondon.ac.uk/projects/outputs/national-early-warning-score-news-2.

Royal Society for the Protection of Accidents (RoSPA). *Make a real difference – become a RoSPA Fall Fighter.* Free Fall Prevention Course – RoSPA; 2022. https://www.rospa.com/home-safety/advice/falls-prevention/fall-fighter.

Shah A, Kerner V, Stanworth SJ, Agarwal S. Major haemorrhage: past, present and future. *Anaesthesia.* 2023;78:93–104.

Smith KA, High K, Collins SP. Self WH. A preprocedural checklist improves the safety of emergency department intubation of trauma patients. *Acad Emerg Med.* 2015;22:989–992.

Spahn DR, Bouillon B, Cerny V, et al. The European guideline on management of major bleeding and coagulopathy following trauma: fifth edition. *Crit Care.* 2019;23:98. https://doi.org/10.1186/s13054-019-2347-3.

Svoboda SJ, Owens BD, Gooden HA, et al. Irrigation with potable water versus normal saline in a contaminated musculoskeletal wound model. *J Trauma.* 2008;64(5):1357–1359.

The Royal College of Emergency Medicine. UK NHS Ambulance Services Pre-alert Guideline for the Deteriorating Adult patient. 2023. https://rcem.ac.uk/wp-content/uploads/2021/10/NHS_Ambulance_Services_pre_alert_criteria_guideline.pdf.

Tiel Groenestege-Kreb, van Maarseveen O, Leenen L, Howell SJ. Trauma team. *BJA.* 2014;113(2):258–265.

Trauma Audit Research Network (TARN). 2017. https://tarn.ac.uk.

Trauma Audit Research Network (TARN). 2022. http://www.tarn.ac.uk/Content.aspx?ca=16.

TCAR. Glossary. 2020. https://tcarprograms-uk.visionem.org/portal/glossary/.

van Maarseveen OEC, Ham WHW, Leenen LPH. The effect of an on-site trauma surgeon during resuscitations of severely injured patients. *BMC Emerg Med.* 2022;22:163.

Wibring K, Magnusson C, Axelsson C, et al. Towards definitions of time-sensitive conditions in prehospital care. *Scand J Trauma Resusc Emerg Med.* 2020;28:7. https://doi.org/10.1186/s13049-020-0706-3.

Williams B. The National Early Warning Score and the acutely confused patient. *Clin Med (Lond).* 2019;19(2):190–191. doi:10.7861/clinmedicine.19-2-190.

World Health Organisation (WHO). Injury-related disability and rehabilitation. 2008. https://www.who.int/violence_injury_prevention/disability/en/.

World Health Organisation (WHO). Why safe surgery is important. 2009. https://www.who.int/teams/integrated-health-services/patient-safety/research/safe-surgery.

World Health Organisation (WHO). Injuries and violence. 2021. https://www.who.int.

Department of Health. *Saving Lives, Valuing Donors – A Transplant Framework for England.* London: HMSO; 2003.

London Major Trauma System. Management of Elderly Major Trauma Patients 2017. 2017. http://www.c4ts.qmul.ac.uk/downloads/plmts-management-of-elderly-trauma-09022017.pdf.

Mackway-Jones K, Carley S. *Major Incident Medical Management and Support: The Practical Approach in the Hospital.* Oxford: Blackwell; 2005.

NCEPOD. *Trauma: Who Cares.* London: NCEPOD; 2007. https://www.ncepod.org.uk/2007report2/Downloads/SIP_summary.pdf.

National Institute of Health and Care Excellence (NICE). *Major trauma: assessment and initial management.* NICE guideline [NG39]; 2016. https://www.nice.org.uk/guidance/ng39.

Further Reading

Baxter J, Cranfield KR, Clark G, et al. Do lactate levels in emergency department predict outcome in adult trauma patients? A systematic review. *J Trauma Acute Care Surg.* 2016;81(3):555–566.

Cooper N. Acute care: recognising critical illness. 2004. http://student.bmj.com/issues/04/01/education/12.php.

Department of Health. *Comprehensive Critical Care – A Review of Adult Critical Care Services.* London: HMSO; 2000.

Useful Websites

The Brain Trauma Foundation, www.braintrauma.org
Support services and advice for head injured patients and their family, www.headway.org.uk
Support for spinal injured patients, www.spinal.co.uk
Support for patients and families following traumatic injuries, www.aftertrauma.org
Support for patients following a disfigurement, www.changingfaces.org.uk
Supporting Victims of Crime, www.victimsupport.org.uk
Youth Workers – supporting young people who are victims of violent/gang-related crime, www.stgilestrust.org.uk

27

Nursing the Unconscious Patient

CATHERYNE WATERHOUSE

Introduction

The unconscious patient presents a special challenge to the nurse. Medical management will vary according to the original cause of the patient's condition, but nursing care will be constant. The unconscious patient is completely dependent on the nurse to manage all their activities of living and to monitor their vital functions.

High-quality nursing care is crucial if the patient is to relearn to perceive self and others, to communicate, to control their body and environment and to become independent. The nurse must have a good understanding of the mechanisms that can contribute to unconsciousness, as well as a sound knowledge of the potential and actual physiological, psychological and social problems that these patients may face in the future.

Not all patients will make a complete recovery; some will die and others will be left with varying degrees of physical and cognitive disability. The nurse plays a pivotal role working with the multidisciplinary team to plan, implement and evaluate specific treatment regimens, whilst providing emotional support and reassurance to the patient and their relatives.

Defining Consciousness

Normal conscious behaviour is dependent upon the functioning of the higher cerebral hemispheres and an intact reticular activating system (RAS) (see later). Impaired, reduced or absent consciousness implies the presence of brain dysfunction and demands urgent medical attention. In order to appreciate the importance of altered states of consciousness, a basic understanding of the physiology of consciousness is required.

Hickey and Strayer (2019) define consciousness simply as 'a state of general awareness of oneself and the environment' and includes the ability to orientate towards new stimuli. The individual is awake, alert and aware of their personal identity and of the events occurring in their surroundings. Deep coma, the opposite of consciousness, is diagnosed when the patient is unrousable and unresponsive to external stimuli; there are varied states of altered consciousness in between the two extremes (Information 27.1). Even during normal sleep, an individual can be roused by external stimuli, in comparison to the person in a coma.

Anatomical and Physiological Basis for Consciousness

The reticular formation (RF) and the RAS (Fig. 27.1) are responsible for collating and transmitting motor and sensory activities and controlling sleep/waking cycles and consciousness.

The Reticular Formation (RF)

The RF is a network of neurons within the brain stem (Afifi and Bergman 2005, Moini and Piran 2020) that connect with the spinal cord, cerebellum, thalamus and hypothalamus. The RF is involved in the coordination of skeletal muscle activity, including voluntary movement, posture and balance, as well as automatic and reflex activities that link with the limbic system.

The Reticular Activating System (RAS)

The RAS is a physiological component of the RF and the neurons which radiate via the thalamus and hypothalamus to the cerebral cortex and ocular motor nuclei. It is concerned with the arousal of the brain in sleep and wakefulness. Two main parts have been identified: the mesencephalon and the thalamus.

The mesencephalic area is composed of grey matter and lies in the upper pons and midbrain of the brain stem. Stimulation produces a diffuse flow of nerve impulses which pass upwards through the thalamus and hypothalamus, radiating out across the cerebral cortex to provoke a general increase in cerebral activity and wakefulness (see Fig. 27.1). Signals from different areas in the thalamus initiate selective activity in the cortex protecting the higher centres from sensory overload. The reticular nucleus, which receives impulses from the RF, surrounds the front and sides of the thalamus. It is this nucleus that sends inhibiting messages back to the thalamic nuclei using several neurotransmitters including aminobutyric acid (GABA).

In order to function, the RAS must be stimulated by input signals from a wide range of sources. These are transmitted via the spinal reticular tracts and various collateral tracts from all the modalities of sensation, for example the specialised auditory and visual tracts. The RAS is also affected by signals from the cerebral cortex; that is, the RAS may first stimulate the cerebral cortex, and the cortical areas responding to reason and emotion may 'modify' the RAS, either positively or negatively, according to the 'decision' of the cerebral cortex.

Sleep is induced by a hormone called melatonin which is synthesised from serotonin in the pineal gland. When an individual is in a deep sleep, the RAS is in a dormant state. However, almost any type of sensory signal can immediately activate the RAS and waken the individual; for example, when daylight is detected by the retina of the eye, impulses are sent to the suprachiasmatic nucleus of the hypothalamus, activating sympathetic nerve fibres that will inhibit the secretion of melatonin in the pineal gland. This is called the 'arousal reaction' and is the mechanism by which sensory stimuli wake us from deep sleep (Martini et al. 2018). Lesions in this area can cause excessive sleepiness or even coma.

There are numerous pathways to both mesencephalic and thalamic areas, arising from the sensory, motor and cortical regions of the cerebral cortex that deal with a range of emotions. Whenever any of these areas becomes excited, impulses are transmitted into the RAS, thus increasing its activity. This is termed a 'positive feedback response'.

INFORMATION 27.1

Continuum of Levels of Consciousness

- *Full consciousness* – awake, alert, orientated, cognitive (mental) functioning intact
- *Confusion* – disorientated to time/place/person, short attention span, memory problems, may be agitated/restless/irritable
- *Lethargy* – orientated, slow speech, slow mental processes, slow motor activities
- *Obtundation* – rousable with stimulation, responds verbally with one or two words, follows simple commands, very drowsy
- *Stupor* – quiet, minimal movement, generally unresponsive except to vigorous stimuli, responds in normal way to painful stimuli
- *Coma* – unrousable, no verbal sounds, inappropriate or no response to stimuli
  It is difficult to classify levels of consciousness exactly, but this is a useful guide to help to describe various levels.

Adapted from Hickey JV, AL Strayer (2019). *The Clinical Practice of Neurological and Neurosurgical Nursing.* 8th ed. Wolter Kluwer.

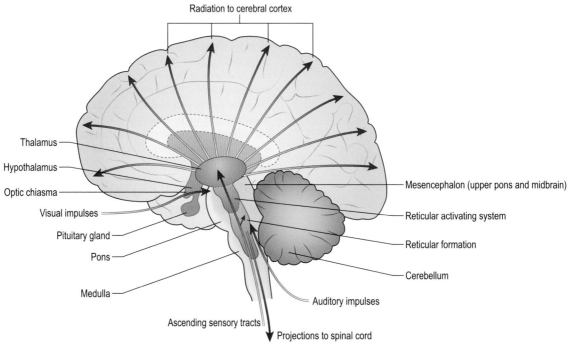

Figure 27.1 Midsagittal section of the brain, showing the reticular activating system and related structures.

The Feedback Theory

The cerebrum regulates incoming information by a positive feedback mechanism (Martini et al. 2018, Moini and Piran 2020). A second feedback cycle that stimulates proprioceptors in skeletal muscles is also shown in Fig. 27.2.

After a prolonged period of wakefulness, the synapses in the feedback loops become increasingly fatigued, reducing the level of stimulation and activity directed to the RAS and thereby inducing a state of lethargy, drowsiness and eventually sleep. Fig. 27.2 illustrates a number of activating pathways passing from the mesencephalon upwards.

The Content of Consciousness

The content of consciousness refers to the sum of cognitive and affective mental functions. It is dependent upon relatively intact functional areas within the cerebral hemispheres that interact with each other as well as with the RAS (Reflection 27.1).

Injury to, or disease of, the cerebral hemispheres may cause diffuse damage that can inhibit or block the signals from the

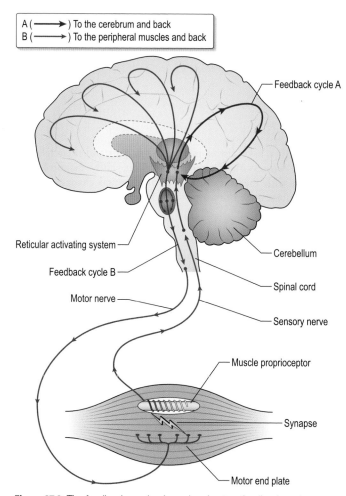

Figure 27.2 The feedback mechanism, showing two feedback cycles passing through the RAS. In cycle A, the RAS excites the cerebral cortex and the cortex in turn re-excites the RAS. This initiates a cycle that causes continued intense excitation of both regions. In cycle B, impulses are sent down the spinal cord to activate skeletal muscles. Activation of the muscle stimulates proprioceptors to transmit sensory impulses upward to re-excite the RAS. Consciousness results when the RAS, in turn, stimulates the cerebral cortex.

RAS, depressing the level of consciousness. The damaged cortex is unable to interpret the incoming sensory impulses and therefore cannot transmit them to other areas for appropriate action (Wijdicks 2021).

Localised damage to the cerebral hemispheres can affect consciousness to a lesser degree. For example, a patient who has aphasia caused by a stroke may appear awake and alert; however, their inability to understand or to use language may decrease their full awareness of self and their environment. Such localised defects are not generally regarded as a true altered state of consciousness, but this example highlights the difficulties in diagnosing conscious behaviour.

States of Impaired Consciousness

There is no international definition of levels of consciousness, but for assessment purposes, differing states of consciousness can be considered on a continuum between full consciousness and deep coma (Wijdicks 2021) (see Information 27.1). Consciousness cannot be measured directly but can be estimated by observing behaviour in response to stimuli. The Glasgow Coma Scale (GCS) (Teasdale 1974, 2014) is widely used as an assessment tool and helps to reduce subjectivity during assessment of conscious level.

Impaired states of consciousness can be categorised as acute or chronic. Acute states, for example drug or alcohol intoxication, are potentially reversible whereas chronic states tend to be irreversible as they are caused by invasive or destructive brain lesions. Deterioration or improvement will depend on several factors such as the mechanism, extent and site of injury; age; previous medical history; and length of time in coma. Common causes of altered level of consciousness are illustrated in Fig. 27.3.

Signs of deterioration in a patient's level of consciousness are usually the first indication of further impending brain damage. The nurse must be able to assess and observe the patient accurately so that appropriate interventions can be instituted if the level of consciousness deteriorates. Signs and symptoms may include:

- reduced level of awareness
- subtle changes in behaviour
- delirium and confusion
- persistent headache
- seizures
- coma.

Reduced Level of Awareness

Reduction in awareness reflects generalised brain dysfunction, as seen in systemic and metabolic disorders (see Fig. 27.3). These disorders interfere with the integrity of the RAS, affecting the patient's arousal response.

In the early stage, subtle changes may occur in the patient's behaviour. They may exhibit signs of hyperexcitability and irritability, alternating with drowsiness, progressing to confusion and increased levels of disorientation. Minor disturbance such as irritability can

REFLECTION 27.1

Causes of Altered Conscious Level

The clinical condition of unconsciousness is one of complex physiology. Review the contributory causes of altered consciousness shown in Fig. 27.3 and consider the underlying mechanism for each of them.

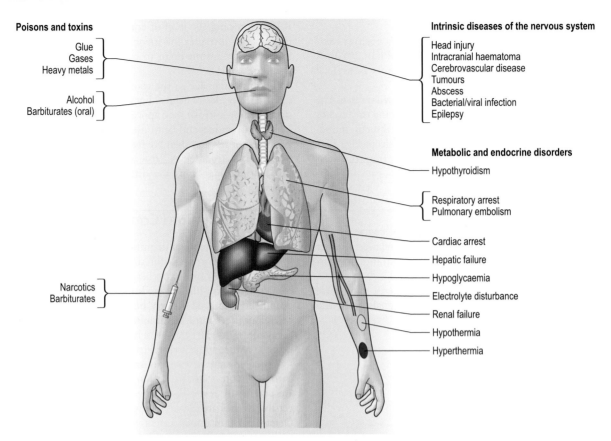

Poisons and toxins

Glue
Gases
Heavy metals

Alcohol
Barbiturates (oral)

Narcotics
Barbiturates

Intrinsic diseases of the nervous system

Head injury
Intracranial haematoma
Cerebrovascular disease
Tumours
Abscess
Bacterial/viral infection
Epilepsy

Metabolic and endocrine disorders

Hypothyroidism

Respiratory arrest
Pulmonary embolism

Cardiac arrest
Hepatic failure
Hypoglycaemia
Electrolyte disturbance
Renal failure
Hypothermia
Hyperthermia

Figure 27.3 Common causes of unconsciousness.

easily go undetected and comments from a relative such as 'she does not seem herself today' may represent a subtle change in behaviour that requires further investigation. It is important to pick up on these cues as they are often the first indication that the patient is developing behavioural, cognitive, motor or sensory changes even in people suffering mild brain dysfunction.

Any new or acute change from the patient's normal baseline behaviour must be reported and documented. The patient's nursing care plan will also need to be reevaluated and new goals for care set.

Cognitive changes, for example poor concentration or short-term memory problems, may only become apparent when a patient returns home. These can cause emotional distress for both the patient and family, particularly if they are disregarded and support is not provided. The primary care team plays a major role in supporting patients following an acquired brain injury, facilitating referral to specialist agencies (see www.headway.org.uk).

Delirium

Delirium, also known as an 'acute confusional state', is a fluctuating mental state characterised by confusion, disorientation, fear and irritability. The patient may be talkative, loud, aggressive, suspicious or extremely agitated. Delirium is common in critical care patients following a severe brain injury or stroke and those patients who have recently suffered a life-threatening illness or undergone a major surgical procedure. Similarly, delirium is experienced by patients at 'end of life' or elderly patients who may have difficulties with poor hearing or eyesight (Rahman 2020).

Delirium is very distressing for the patient and their relatives who may witness their altered behaviour. Early diagnosis and treatment with medication, and environmental changes such as reducing noise or sensory input may help to alleviate some of the symptoms.

Persistent Headache

Headaches can occur immediately following a mild, moderate or more severe brain injury and can be an indication of increasing intracranial pressure (ICP) within the head which could be life-threatening and demands urgent medical attention. Headaches can also be a recurring problem postinjury, lasting weeks and even months. These are also referred to as postconcussional syndrome, which include headaches, dizziness and difficulties with concentration; the symptoms are severely disabling for the patient and often prevent them from resuming their normal activities and returning to work.

Seizures

Seizures present because of sudden and erratic abnormal electrical disturbance in the brain and occur as a complication of injury to the brain, either traumatic or acquired, for example stroke or a neurological infection such as meningitis or encephalitis. Symptoms can vary from sudden loss of consciousness, convulsive limb movements, chewing or lip smacking or hallucinations where patients believe they see or hear something in the absence of any relevant sensory stimuli. Seizures can persist after the acute episode and patients can be diagnosed with epilepsy several months or years after the injury. There are many types of epilepsy and many different types of seizures requiring different treatment options, but most people learn to live and adapt their lifestyle to cope with their seizures (National Institute for Health and Care Excellence [NICE] 2022) (see Chapter 11).

Coma

Coma is a state of prolonged unconsciousness that can be caused by a variety of causes; the patient is unaware and unresponsive to their environment and cannot be roused by any stimulation even pain. Although coma is usually temporary and responds to treatment, it can vary in degrees and in some cases will develop into a permanent condition. Always assume that an unconscious patient is able to hear and understand what you say, particularly if you need to discuss sensitive issues with their relatives. Hearing can often be the last sense to be lost and the first one to come back before they are able to respond.

Chronic States of Impaired Consciousness

The chronic states of impaired consciousness tend to be irreversible as they are caused by invasive or destructive brain lesions. They are:

- dementia
- cerebrovascular accident (CVA)
- infection – cerebral abscess, encephalitis
- severe brain injury
- unresponsive wakefulness syndrome
- locked-in syndrome.

Dementia

This condition is caused by a generalised and progressive loss of cortical tissue in the brain. Mental functions progressively decline with global deterioration of memory, thought processes, motor performance, emotional responsiveness and social behaviour.

As the person deteriorates, speech and communication become difficult and behaviour may be increasingly inappropriate until control of basic and vital processes is completely disorganised. Alzheimer's disease is the most prevalent type of progressive dementia but there are numerous other causes.

Although dementia is an irreversible condition, new drug therapies are being developed with the aim of delaying the onset of the disease.

Cerebrovascular Accident (CVA)

CVA, also known as a stroke, refers to the sudden interruption in blood supply to the brain caused by a blockage within the lumen of the artery or a rupture of the artery resulting in the death of the brain tissue which it supplies. The symptoms of a stroke will depend on the area of the brain affected but invariably leaves the patient with some degree of weakness or paralysis and communication and swallowing difficulties. A severe stroke can cause loss of consciousness and difficulties maintaining their own respirations requiring support from a mechanical ventilator. Early medical interventions can significantly improve recovery including thrombolysis to dissolve the clot, thrombectomy where it may be possible to remove the clot or decompressive craniotomy to relieve the pressure within the brain.

Infection – Cerebral Abscess, Encephalitis, Meningitis

Infections of the central nervous system can be caused by several different pathogens. Bacteria can spread from other sources of infection such as the ear, sinuses or teeth or may be caused by a viral infection such as the herpes simplex virus. Clinical presentation often includes pyrexia, headache and neck stiffness. Analysis of the cerebral spinal fluid (CSF) following a lumber puncture aids early diagnosis and treatment.

Prolonged disorders of consciousness (PDOCs) include patients diagnosed as being in a coma, a minimally conscious state (MCS) or a vegetative state (VS), now referred to as the 'unresponsive wakefulness syndrome' (Pistarini and Maggioni 2021, Pundole and Crawford 2017).

PDOC is a complex neurological condition that may occur following a severe brain injury where the higher centres of the brain are severely damaged. Some patients may emerge from their coma, but only experience minimal awareness of their environment, whilst for others the condition is irreversible and permanent, continuing to survive for several years requiring full-time sensitive and ongoing specialist care often in a dedicated clinical setting (Wade et al. 2022). Invariably, diagnosis throws up numerous clinical and ethical dilemmas with guidance coming from the Royal College of Physicians (RCOP) (2020). Confirmation of diagnosis can take months and sometimes years augmented with functional neuroimaging (magnetic resonance imaging (MRI) and electroencephalography (EEG)). To enable clinicians to make a more accurate diagnosis, most neuro-rehabilitation units use a structured technique allowing them to assess sensory aspects of communication, movement, awareness and wakefulness, known as 'SMART' (sensory modality assessment and rehabilitation technique – www.smart-therapy.org.uk/) (Gill-Thwaites and Munday 2004).

There is ongoing debate, both in the UK and other countries, about the moral, ethical and legal issues surrounding the care and treatment of these individuals and the dilemma posed by some patients to 'the right to die' and withdrawal of treatment has received considerable professional, public and political attention over recent years (Kitzinger and Kitzinger 2015, RCOP 2020).

Locked-in Syndrome

This occurs when there is damage to the pons in the brain stem, resulting from cerebral vascular disease or trauma, paralysing voluntary muscles without interfering with consciousness and cognitive functions. The patient is unable to speak and is sometimes unable to breathe spontaneously, the latter requiring mechanical ventilation and respiratory support. However, the patient is able to control vertical eye movements and blinking and may be able to use these movements to develop a simple communication system. It is important to remember that the patient is cognitively aware, even if they appear to be mentally and physically inert (RCOP 2020).

Assessment of the Nervous System

The need to assess a patient's level of consciousness may arise at any time, in any ward, in any hospital. In 1974, Teasdale and Jennett developed the GCS, a framework used throughout the UK and worldwide as part of the neurological assessment and ongoing observation of the patient (see Fig. 27.4). It provides a standardised approach to observing and recording changes in the patient's level of consciousness, so that appropriate action can be taken (NICE 2023) (Evidence-Based Practice 27.1).

The Neurological Observation Chart

The Glasgow Coma Scale (GCS)

The GCS documents a baseline neurology that reflects the initial severity of the primary injury. Subsequent re-evaluation of their observations identifies early signs of deterioration (Teasdale 2014).

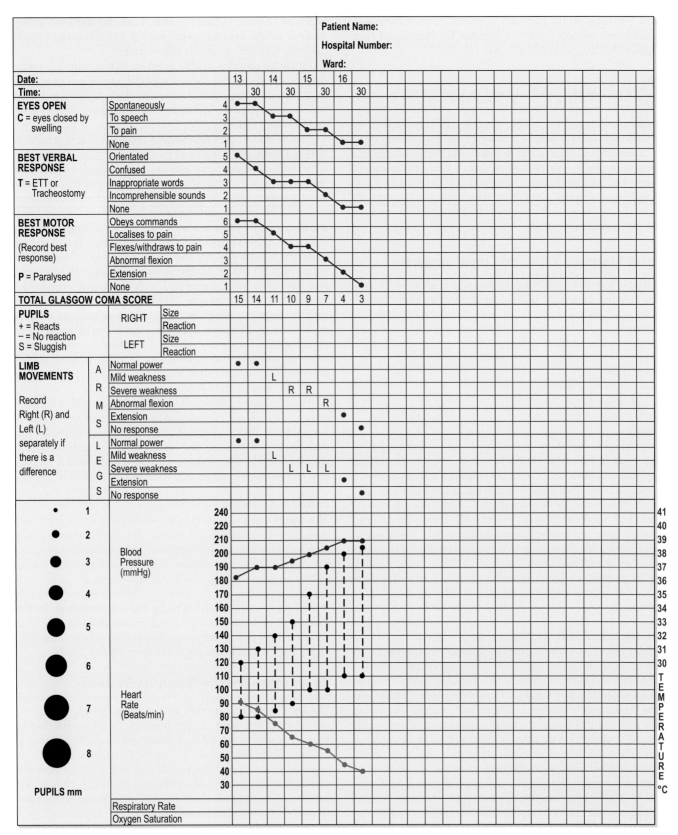

Figure 27.4 The neurological observation chart.

Figure 27.5 Applying a peripheral painful stimulus: fingertip stimulation.

When monitoring the patient's conscious level, the functional state of the brain is assessed as the nurse observes and describes three aspects of the patient's behaviour:
- eye opening
- verbal response
- motor response.

Each of these is independently assessed and documented (Fig. 27.4). The completed graph will display trends in neurological status, making it easier to evaluate whether the patient is improving or deteriorating. The frequency of recording will be based on the patient's clinical condition. The best response for each of the three behaviours is recorded as a numerical score. In the case of eye opening, the best response would score a 4, the best verbal response would score a 5 and the best motor responses would score a 6. The lowest response for each of the three parameters is a score of 1. Thus, the highest total score is 15 and the lowest is 3. However, to avoid ambiguity, it is important to communicate and explain exactly what the patient is doing, rather than relying on the scores which lack detail and substance.

A score of 15 indicates that the patient is alert, orientated and able to obey commands; a score of 8 or lower is generally considered to indicate that the patient is in a coma. However, it is important to consider each of the three responses (eye opening, verbal response and motor response) separately, taking into consideration any local interfering factors that prevent an accurate assessment such as communication difficulties (e.g. deafness) or paralysis if the patient is receiving muscle relaxants.

Eye Opening

This assesses the integrity of the RAS in the brain stem and is observed and recorded using the following categories.

Spontaneously = scores 4. The patient opens their eyes when first approached, which implies that the arousal mechanism is active.

To speech = scores 3. The nurse should speak to the patient by calling their name and asking them to open their eyes. It may be necessary to increase the level of the verbal stimulation to gain a reaction.

To pressure = scores 2. A gentle shake of the patient's shoulder may be sufficient to elicit a response. If the patient still fails to open their eyes, a painful stimulus must be used. Pressure is applied to the lateral inner aspect of the second or third finger using a pen or pencil, for a maximum of 15 seconds (Fig. 27.5). Nail bed pressure is contraindicated, as it will cause excessive bruising.

None = scores 1. If the painful stimulus does not elicit any response from the patient this indicates a deep depression of the arousal system, and the patient is recorded as having no eye opening.

Possible Assessment Problems

The patient who is in a deep coma with flaccid eye muscles will show no response to stimulation. However, if the eyelids are drawn back, the eyes may remain open. This is very different from spontaneous eye opening and should be recorded as 'none'.

Congenital deficits of the eye (see Chapter 15) must also be considered during the assessment. Inability to open the eyes due to bilateral orbital oedema, tarsorrhaphy (where upper and lower eyelids are sutured together) or ptosis (palsy of cranial nerve III) should be recorded as 'C' (closed) on the chart or 'not testable' due to local interfering factors (NT) (Teasdale 2014).

Opening of the eyes implies arousal, but it must be remembered that this does not necessarily mean that the patient is aware of their surroundings. This can be misleading and a source of false optimism for relatives.

Verbal Response

This assesses the area of the brain associated with receptive and expressive speech.

Orientated = scores 5. Patients are assessed as orientated in person, place and time if they can state their name, where they are and what the year and month are. Avoid asking them to state the day or the date as they are not easily remembered, especially after a period of time in hospital.

Confused = scores 4. The patient is able to produce phrases or sentences, but the conversation is rambling and inappropriate to the questions being asked.

Words = scores 3. The patient offers monosyllabic words, usually in response to physical stimulation. The words and phrases make little or no sense and may express obscenities.

Sounds = scores 2. The patient will moan or groan in response to painful stimulation. The verbal response may contain indistinct mumbling but no intelligible words.

None = scores 1. The patient is unable to produce any verbal response despite prolonged and repeated stimulation.

Possible Assessment Problems

Patients may be unable to understand the nurse's questions or commands because they do not understand the language or may have a hearing deficit. The patient's verbal response may be impaired as a result of a speech deficit such as a receptive or expressive dysphasia. If appropriate, written instructions and replies can be used to assess the patient's language ability. The verbal response may also be compromised by the presence of an endotracheal (ET) or tracheostomy tube. This is indicated on the patient's chart as 'NT'.

Motor Response

This assesses the patient's best motor response. Only the best response from the arms is recorded as leg responses to pain are less consistent and may be confused with a simple spinal reflex. The responses described here are shown in Fig. 27.6.

Obeys commands. Score = 6. The patient can follow instructions, for example 'put out your tongue', 'lift up your arms', 'show me your thumb'.

Localises to pain. Score = 5. If the patient does not obey commands, an external stimulus must be applied. In the absence of any facial, orbital or skull fractures, pressure is applied with the flat of the nurse's thumb over a branch of the fifth trigeminal cranial nerve, underlying the supraorbital ridge under the eyebrow (Fig. 27.7A). Pressure is gradually increased for a maximum of 10 seconds. Providing the patient has not sustained a cervical fracture, the 'trapezius pinch' (Fig. 27.7B) is a useful alternative which compresses the eleventh spinal accessory cranial nerve; the trapezius muscle (the large triangular muscle of the neck and thorax) is squeezed between the nurse's fingers and thumb. The response is recorded as 'localising to pain' if the patient moves their arm across the midline, to the level of the chin, in an attempt to locate and remove the source of the pain (Fig. 27.6C). During the course of the day, the patient may display a localising response to other sources of irritation, for example suctioning, nasogastric (NG) tube or urinary catheter, in which case, painful stimulus would not need to be applied.

Flexion to pain. Score = 4. Following the application of a central painful stimulus, either the trapezius squeeze or supraorbital ridge pressure, the patient responds by flexing their arm normally by bending their elbow and weakly withdrawing their hand; no attempt to localise towards the source of the pain is made.

Abnormal flexion. Score = 3. In response to a painful stimulus, the patient bends their elbow with adduction of the upper arms and abnormal posturing of the wrist and fingers, otherwise known as decorticate posturing. This indicates more severe dysfunction of the brain and is a poor prognostic sign.

Extension to pain. Score = 2. Following painful stimulation, the patient responds by rigid extension, that is, straightening the elbows and hyperpronation of the forearms, otherwise known as decerebrate posturing. The response usually includes spastic hand and wrist movements, with an inward rotation of the shoulders and forearms. The legs are generally straight, with the feet pointing outwards.

None. Score = 1. This response is only recorded when sufficient painful stimulus has been applied to provoke a response and no detectable movement has been observed.

Possible Assessment Problems

Variations in the motor response may occur during the assessment. Therefore, it is the best response that should be scored; for

Figure 27.6 Motor responses. (A) Obeys commands ('lift up your arms'). (B) Localising to pain. (C) Flexing to pain. (D) Abnormal flexion. (E) Extending to pain.

Figure 27.7 Applying a central painful stimulus. (A) Supraorbital ridge pressure. (B) Trapezius pinch.

example, if the patient localises to pain on the left side but flexes to pain on the right, the localising response is recorded. Asymmetrical responses are significant, indicating that a focal neurological deficit is present, but overall brain function is more accurately reflected by the level of best response on the better side (see limb movement, below).

When applying a painful stimulus, it is important to explain to the patient and their relatives what you are about to do and why you are doing it, otherwise they may feel that unnecessary distress is being inflicted.

For further information about the use of the neurological observation chart and GCS in practice, see Teasdale (2014), Braine and Cook (2017) and Reith et al. (2016).

Recording Other Measurements

A neurological assessment includes the recording of additional measurements as follows:
- vital signs:
  - blood pressure
  - pulse rate
  - respirations
  - temperature
- pupil size and reaction
- limb movements.

Vital Signs

Blood Pressure and Pulse. A rising blood pressure (elevated systolic pressure), widening of the pulse pressures and a slowing pulse (see Chapter 11), known as the 'Cushing's response', are very late signs of raised ICP and there may have been other signs such as subtle alterations in behaviour or fluctuating levels of consciousness which could have indicated a deterioration in neurological status.

Respiration. Factors that impair consciousness may also cause respiratory changes. The pattern and rate of respiration are directly affected by increasing brain injury that may produce an ataxic irregular or Cheyne–Stokes respiratory pattern, typified by periods of tachypnoea interspersed with periods of apnoea. It is important for the nurse to utilise the ABCDE approach to assessment, ensuring the patient has a clear airway, removing any obstructions (e.g. secretions or foreign bodies) and using airway adjuncts to maintain airway patency before assessing the rate, depth, rhythm and characteristics of breathing. Oxygen therapy should be commenced early, and the patient's oxygen saturation levels monitored to reduce the risk of hypoxia.

Temperature. A gradual elevation in temperature may indicate an early sign of infection in the lungs, urinary tract or wound. Rapid increases in body temperature are likely to be caused by damage to the hypothalamus (the body's temperature regulating centre). Each degree of rise in temperature increases the brain's metabolic rate and must be treated urgently to prevent further neurological deterioration.

Pupil Size and Reaction

Abnormal pupillary size and reaction can indicate brain dysfunction and/or raised ICP. It is important to note any changes, particularly if they occur in conjunction with other changes in the neurological observations. The size of both pupils is measured in millimetres and recorded using the guide included in the neurological observation chart. Reaction to light is recorded by a plus (+); no reaction is recorded by a minus (–). Pupil reactions should be assessed in dim surroundings, using a small bright flashlight. To elicit the direct-light

reflex, the nurse holds the patient's eyelids open, bringing the light in from the outer aspect of the eye and shining it directly into the eye. This should cause a brisk constriction of the pupil, and withdrawal of the light should produce brisk dilatation of the pupil. The size and reaction are observed and recorded on the chart. The shape of the pupils should also be assessed.

Abnormal Pupil Reactions

- A unilateral, unreactive pupil may be caused by an expanding mass, e.g. tumour, abscess and haematoma.
- Large dilated pupils may be an indication of drug toxicity, e.g. anticholinergic overdose.
- Fixed dilated pupils signify herniation of the brain stem and are associated with a poor prognosis.
- Bilateral pinpoint pupils can be difficult to assess as reacting but may be an indication of a brain stem haemorrhage or opioid toxicity.

Limb Movement

Disturbances of limb movement are an indication of localised (focal) brain damage and vary according to the site and extent of the damage; for example, the right arm and leg will be affected by a lesion in the left cerebral hemisphere due to the crossing over ('decussation') of most of the axons in the brain stem before they pass down the spinal cord. Diffuse brain damage will result in a greater disturbance of movement.

The nurse examines the arms and legs for movement and strength and compares the right and left sides. When differences exist, right and left are recorded independently. Responses can be elicited by asking the patient to grip the nurse's hand, to lift their arms forward or to bend their knees. To test strength in the legs, the nurse may ask the patient to push down against their hand. A painful stimulus is only applied if verbal requests fail to elicit a response.

Causes of Unconsciousness

Unconsciousness occurs when the RAS is damaged, or its function is depressed so that there is an interruption of the normal arousal mechanisms. This may be caused by a primary or secondary insult to the nervous system: primary insults are commonly caused by intrinsic disease to the brain; secondary involvement is most often caused by metabolic, endocrine or toxic conditions, where the critical insult is manifested elsewhere in the body. Table 27.1 identifies some of the signs and symptoms of changes in level of consciousness and possible causes. The major causes of unconsciousness are shown in Fig. 27.3.

Emergency Care of the Unconscious Patient

Whatever the cause of unconsciousness and wherever the event occurs, the patient's life depends on the knowledge and skills of those who find and care for them. The first aid and care that the patient receives until consciousness is regained will help to determine the outcome.

A Hospital Emergency

An individual can be rendered unconscious by any of the causes shown in Fig. 27.3. The measures a nurse should take on finding someone collapsed are as follows:
1. Press the emergency call button, shout or send someone for assistance.

TABLE 27.1   Clues to the Cause of Unconsciousness on General Physical Examination

Sign or Symptom	Possible Cause
Elevated temperature	Infection
	Heat stroke
Subnormal temperature	Dehydration
	Excessive intake of alcohol
	Barbiturate intoxication
	Hypothyroidism
	Exposure to the cold
Bleeding from the mouth	Epileptic seizure
	Trauma
Pulse irregularities	Hypoxia from inadequate cardiac output
Slow, regular respirations	Hypothyroidism
	Morphine or barbiturate intoxication
Cheyne–Stokes respiration	Bilateral cerebral dysfunction
	Late stages of increased intracranial pressure
	Severe cardiopulmonary disease
Ataxic, irregular (cluster) respirations	Lesions of the brain stem – signifies impending apnoea
Breath odour	Excessive intake of alcohol
	Hepatic dysfunction
	Renal dysfunction
	Ingested poisons
	Diabetes mellitus – ketoacidosis
Skin	
Jaundice	Hepatic dysfunction
Cyanosis	Cardiopulmonary problems
Rash	Infection, drug reaction, meningitis
Needle puncture marks	Substance use disorder
Hypertension	Raised intracranial pressure – tumours, abscess
	Intracranial haemorrhage – haematoma, stroke
Hypotension	Blood loss
	Septicaemia
	Myocardial infarction
	Pulmonary embolism

2. Following the ABC principles (see Chapter 2), call the arrest team and initiate cardiopulmonary resuscitation (CPR) if the individual is not breathing and the carotid pulse is absent.

3. If the person is breathing and a pulse is present, place them in a semiprone (recovery position, see Chapter 2) position. However, if spinal injury is suspected, maintain the patient's head, neck and spine in alignment until medical assistance attends. Stay with the person until assistance arrives and they can be moved to an appropriate place for further treatment and investigation.

Planned Admission

When an unconscious patient is to be admitted to hospital, prepare the bed area:

- Remove the top bedclothes and the head of the bed to facilitate easy transfer.
- Check that the oxygen supply and suction apparatus are functioning and that there is an adequate supply of relevant equipment.
- Ensure the following equipment is available for immediate use:
  - a resuscitation trolley containing the following:
    1. airway adjuncts – oropharyngeal (Guedel) airways (usually size 3 or 4 for an adult), I-Gel
    2. ambu bag with universal catheter mount
    3. suction equipment – including suction tubing and catheters
    4. laryngoscope and ET tubes (ETTs) sizes 6.5–10.00 mm
    5. lubricating jelly; strapping or tape (to secure the ETT); 5 mL syringe to inflate the ETT cuff
    6. emergency drug box
  - intravenous infusion stand
  - NG tube and associated equipment
  - neurological examination tray containing ophthalmoscope, reflex hammer, tuning fork, tongue depressor, sterile pin for assessment of sensation, cotton wool swabs to test corneal reflex
  - appropriate charts and admission forms.

Priorities of Nursing Management

The following checklist lists the priorities of nursing management in an emergency.

1. Maintenance of a clear airway.
   a. The patient's position – by positioning the patient correctly, it is possible to minimise the risk of the tongue falling back and obstructing the pharynx.
   b. Artificial airways – these include airway adjuncts inserted into the mouth, through the nose or into the trachea to optimise breathing and facilitate clearance of bronchial secretions.
   c. Suction – removes excess secretions and mucus from the trachea and lower airway when the patient's own cough is too weak to expectorate the secretions.
   d. Oxygen – is used to prevent hypoxia (low blood oxygen) and hypercapnia (high levels of carbon dioxide).
   e. NG tube – inserted via the nose into the stomach to provide enteral feeding until the patient is able to commence oral feeding. The National Patient Safety Agency (NHS Improvement 2016; National Nurses Nutrition Group [NNNG] 2016) has written guidance on the placement and safe management of the tube to reduce the risk of misplacement and aspiration.
2. Assessment of the central nervous system:
   a. GCS
   b. vital signs
   c. pupillary reactions
   d. limb movements.
3. Assessment of vital signs
   a. blood pressure
   b. pulse
   c. respiratory rate
   d. oxygen saturation
   e. urinary output (NEWS2 2017).

4. Maintenance of fluid balance.
   a. Intravenous infusion of fluids – maintains hydration until the patient is able to absorb enteral fluids or commence oral feeding. Crystalloid solutions of normal saline 0.9% are normally prescribed. Dextrose solutions are contra-indicated in patients following a head injury as dextrose increases ICP and leads to cerebral ischaemia. Mannitol or hypertonic saline (HTS) is an osmotic diuretic that reduces brain swelling associated with raised ICP, buying time for the underlying pathology to be treated or removed.
   b. Catheterisation of the urinary bladder, to facilitate accurate monitoring of hourly urine output.

Care of Relatives. A nurse who is not involved in the immediate care of the patient should be allocated to support the family/carers. It is a useful opportunity to gather the patient's biographical data and other information to help in planning the patient's care. A brief explanation of the management plan, supported with written information regarding hospital procedure or possible investigations, will help give some reassurance (Reflection 27.2).

Medical Management

An unconscious patient is a medical emergency, unless the unconscious state represents the terminal stages of a progressive disease process. Although life support measures take priority, such as provision of an adequate airway, control of haemorrhage and fluid or blood replacement, the cause of the unconscious state must be determined before the most appropriate treatment can be delivered.

The Medical History

The doctor or an experienced nurse will need to gain further information about the patient's medical history from the family or carers including the circumstances preceding and surrounding the onset of the unconscious state.

The Physical Examination

The general physical examination of the unconscious patient should include:
- Airway – look for chest movement, listen for breath sounds or abnormal noise, feel at the mouth/nose for exhaled air.
- Breathing – rate, depth, pattern of respiration, odour.
- Circulation – vital signs, skin colour, temperature.
- Disability – a neurological examination will include assessment of the cranial nerves, reflexes and motor and sensory function. A baseline assessment should be documented so that any future changes in the patient's condition can be observed. Analysis of capillary blood glucose levels will determine if the patient is hypoglycaemic and a metabolic cause for his level of consciousness.
- Exposure – other signs of trauma.

REFLECTION 27.2

Support of Families in Critical Care

Think about the relatives of a critically ill or highly dependent patient.
   What strategies might help to reduce their anxieties and enable them to be more involved with their relative's care?

Laboratory Tests

- Full blood count – measures haemoglobin levels, platelets and the number of red and white blood cells (neutrophils and lymphocytes).
- Blood glucose levels – to detect hypoglycaemia (low blood sugar levels) or hyperglycaemia (raised blood sugar levels).
- Urea and electrolyte levels – measures sodium, potassium and chloride levels in the blood that become deranged during periods of acute illness. If left untreated, abnormal levels can lead to confusion, cramps, irregular heart rhythm and ultimately death.
- Erythrocyte sedimentation rate (ESR) and C-reactive protein (CRP) are useful indicators for detecting acute and chronic inflammatory infection.
- Lactate – raised lactate levels is as strong indication of infection or sepsis.
- Blood gas analysis – measures partial pressure of carbon dioxide ($PaCO_2$) and oxygen (PaO_2) to assess the effectiveness of gaseous exchange in the lungs.
- Toxicology – detects the presence of drugs, alcohol, medication and other toxins or poisons.
- Urinalysis – for glucose, acetone, blood and infection.

Radiological Studies and Imaging

Once the patient has been resuscitated and their condition stabilised, radiological investigations can be requested:
- CT scan of head and cervical spine
- MRI scan to identify abnormalities in the soft tissue of the brain
- Plain X-rays if other injuries are apparent or suspected
- Cerebral angiography (CT angiography or invasive radiology) to identify any aneurysms or congenital malformations.

Further Investigations

Further investigations may be undertaken to aid diagnosis, for example
- Electroencephalogram (EEG) – records electrical activity within the brain, used in the diagnosis of epilepsy.
- Lumbar puncture (LP) – obtains cerebrospinal fluid and can be used diagnostically for signs of infection (meningitis, abscess.
- Electrocardiogram (ECG) – records the electrical activity of the heart and identifies a wide range of abnormalities.
- Positron emission tomography (PET scan) – uses a radioactive tracer to produce detailed images of the structure and functioning of specific organs and tissues (often used in research).
- Doppler studies – ultrasound uses reflected sound waves to evaluate blood flow through a vessel, e.g. in deep venous thrombosis (DVT), stroke.

Nursing Management of the Unconscious Patient

Breathing

Alterations in the rate, rhythm and pattern of respirations can be caused by a number of factors including electrolyte imbalance, trauma to the cervical spine, drugs, for example narcotics or sedatives, pulmonary disease such as pneumonia or atelectasis (see Chapter 3) or cardiac conditions (see Chapter 2). To prevent cerebral ischaemia and infarction caused by hypoxia, the nurse must perform regular respiratory assessment including rate, depth, type, colour of the patient as well as oxygen saturation (PO_2). The priority must be to maintain a clear airway:

- Remove any obvious potential obstruction to the airway, such as dentures or dental plates. Take note of the presence of loose teeth, caps or crowns, as these could become detached and obstruct the airway.
- Bleeding into the oropharynx from head or facial injuries, vomit and aspirate should be removed with a Yankauer suction probe (insertion of an NG tube will facilitate the emptying of the stomach reducing the risk of aspiration of gastric contents into the lungs).

Position of the Patient

Unconscious patients and those with head injuries, unless their condition contraindicates, should be nursed with the head of the bed tilted slightly upwards (10–30 degrees) to aid cerebral venous drainage and help reduce ICP (Hickey and Strayer 2019). Patients should be nursed in a semiprone or lateral recumbent position to prevent the tongue from obstructing the airway, reduce the risk of developing aspiration pneumonia from secretions and saliva and aid the prevention of pressure ulcers. Patients with actual or suspected spinal injury will be maintained in a position of spinal alignment supported with pillows.

Artificial Airways

The unconscious patient's cough reflex will be depressed or absent, affecting their ability to cough and protect and clear their own airway. The use of artificial airways and suctioning may be required.

Oropharyngeal Airway. The Guedel airway is easy to insert and is available in varying sizes. It prevents the tongue from obstructing the airway and allows the patient to breathe through the device into the pharynx. It also facilitates suctioning of secretions from the oropharynx and trachea. The oropharyngeal airway should be removed if it stimulates a gag or cough reflex which causes the patient to retch.

Nasopharyngeal Airway is often tolerated better by the patient; this is passed through the nose and does not exert a stimulus on the rear part of the tongue.

I-Gel, Supraglottic Airway. This is a thermoplastic device that is easily inserted into the airway that softens and moulds itself to form a high seal pressure around the pharyngeal and laryngeal structures. Prior to insertion the I-gel requires lubrication over the front, back and sides to enable it to slide in without causing trauma. In addition, it incorporates a gastric channel for insertion of a fine-bore NG tube to remove gastric aspirate and minimise the risk of aspiration.

Endotracheal Tube. An ETT is indicated if either the Guedel or nasopharyngeal airway proves inadequate or when mechanical ventilation is required. The tube is made of malleable plastic and has an inflatable cuff. The tube can be inserted orally or nasally into the trachea to the point just above the bifurcation of the bronchi. Breath sounds are determined immediately after insertion to make certain that the tube is properly positioned and is not obstructing one of the primary bronchi. An inflated cuff provides an airtight seal around the outside of the tube, preventing the aspiration of material from the mouth, nose and digestive tract into the lungs. If the patient continues to require airway support the ETT after 5–10 days, a tracheostomy will be considered because of the increased risk of erosion of the tracheal wall.

Tracheostomy Tube. A tracheostomy, a surgical opening in the anterior wall of the trachea, is usually indicated if intubation needs to be prolonged, or if there are difficulties in inserting an ETT. The tracheostomy tube bypasses the nose, pharynx and larynx, enabling air to flow directly into the lungs, thus reducing dead space and the effort required by the patient to breathe, and facilitates suctioning of bronchial secretions.

A variety of different types and sizes of tracheostomy tube are available. The tubes may be cuffed or uncuffed, fenestrated or unfenestrated to facilitate weaning and communication. Cuffed tubes are made with high-volume, low-pressure, soft cuffs to reduce the risk of pressure trauma to the trachea. The amount of air in the cuff should be measured at least 8-hourly, using a pressure gauge. Pressures should be maintained between 15 and 25 cmH$_2$O unless otherwise directed by medical staff.

Most tracheostomy tubes consist of three parts: an obturator inside the tube to keep it rigid during insertion, an outer cannula and an inner cannula. The advantage of a tube with an inner cannula is that this can be removed every 2–4 hours for cleaning, reducing the risk of airway obstruction with excess secretions. The procedure can be carried out without disturbing the outer tube, reducing the frequency of outer tube changes, thereby reducing the risk of trauma to the stoma and trachea.

The tracheal stoma must be cleaned using an aseptic nontouch technique. A sterile, nonadherent dressing should be applied around the stoma to collect secretions and minimise the risk of infection.

Suctioning

Tracheal or ET suctioning is performed to remove excessive secretions from the oropharynx, trachea and bronchi. In a patient with raised ICP, the procedure can provoke transient raised ICP and should be performed with care. The nurse's assessment of the patient's colour, respiratory rate and pattern will indicate how often this is required. Suction must be applied if one or more of the following occurs:

- signs of cyanosis
- increased and irregular respirations
- noisy, gurgling respirations
- reduced oxygen saturation (SpO$_2$).
  The following equipment is required:
- Suction device, collection jar with disposable liner, and disposable connecting tubing.
- Sterile suction catheters – catheter diameter should be less than half the internal diameter of the tube to allow airflow down the side of the catheter. Catheter size = (tube size - 2) × 2. For example, for a size 8 tracheostomy tube, it will be 8 - 2 = 6 × 2 = size 12 FG catheter.
- Sterile plastic gloves. The use of a closed suction catheter system and disposable suction equipment is recognised as good practice.

Procedure

Each hospital will have its own policy regarding suctioning, but the procedure described here is based on good practice and provides a general example (Klein et al. 2018).

1. Patients who are dependent on oxygen should continue with their therapy until immediately prior to insertion of the suction catheter and the supply must be replaced immediately afterwards.
2. Suction pressure is set below 16 kPa (120 mmHg) in adults.
3. Wash hands and pour the sterile normal saline into a sterile bowl, apply nonsterile examination gloves for your own protection.
4. Open the pack containing the sterile catheter and put a plastic sterile glove on the dominant hand.

5. Attach the catheter to the connecting tube, taking care not to contaminate the catheter.
6. Remove oxygen mask/nasal cannula from the patient.
7. Insert the catheter into the airway without applying suction and advance the catheter as far as it will easily pass, until resistance is met. This will usually cause the patient to cough.
8. Withdraw the catheter 1 cm and apply suction as the catheter is slowly withdrawn
9. Remove secretions within a time limit of 15 seconds.
10. Use the catheter once only and then wrap it around the gloved hand. Remove the glove with the catheter inside and discard both.
11. Rinse the suction tubing through with sterile water.
12. Give the patient at least 1 minute to recover before suctioning again. Give oxygen again, if prescribed.
13. If all the secretions have not been removed, repeat the procedure using a new sterile glove and sterile catheter.
14. If necessary, use a new catheter to suction the patient's mouth and nose at the end of the procedure. Nasal suction is contraindicated if the patient has sustained a frontal skull fracture or has nasal leakage of cerebrospinal fluid (CSF rhinorrhoea).
15. A saline nebuliser can deliver tiny droplets of moisture to the alveoli to optimise humidification and aid removal of secretions.

Humidification

Normally, the air drawn into the lungs is warmed, moistened and filtered through the nose and upper respiratory tract. To prevent irritation of the mucous membranes and production of dried tenacious secretions, patients with an ET or tracheostomy tube must receive effective humidification, preferably through a heated system, nebuliser or a heat and moisture exchanger (HME).

Oxygen

The amount of oxygen prescribed depends on the patient's clinical condition and the results from their arterial blood gases. A specimen of arterial blood is taken to ascertain the pH and partial pressures of oxygen (PaO_2) and carbon dioxide ($PaCO_2$). Severe deviations from normal are an indication for elective mechanical ventilation to ensure adequate oxygenation. Normal values are:

- pH, 7.36–7.44
- PaO_2, 11–15 kPa
- $PaCO_2$, 4.6–5.9 kPa.

There are various methods of administering oxygen and the doctor's prescription will include instructions about the rate of flow, duration of therapy and delivery system. The nurse must monitor the patients for complications (see Chapter 3).

Nursing and Physiotherapy

The prevention of respiratory complications is a priority in the nursing management of the unconscious patient, but infection may occur despite every precaution being taken. Effective respiratory management is dependent on good communication, skill and cooperation between the nurse, physiotherapist and medical team. Antibiotics can be effective if organisms are cultivated from the patient's secretions.

Communicating

The Patient

There is considerable anecdotal evidence of patients recalling, with startling accuracy, conversations they overheard whilst unconscious.

It is important that conversations not intended for the patient should not be held in close proximity, as unguarded or misinterpreted information can cause distress.

It is imperative that the nurse explains clearly and simply to the patient every aspect of their care, whether it is related to procedures being carried out or to the patient's progress (Reflection 27.3). The explanations and reassurances should be repeated whenever a procedure is carried out.

Pain is common following a traumatic brain injury. Pain may arise from muscular skeletal injuries, spasticity or headache. The recognition and diagnosis of pain in the unconscious patient are difficult and are further complicated by communication, cognitive and behavioural deficits. Most of the pain assessment scales, for example visual analogue or numerical rating scales, are unsuitable for the unconscious patient. It is important to be extra vigilant to the often-subtle signs of pain. Analgesia must be administered cautiously as oversedation can mask further signs of deterioration (pupil response, decreased respirations, decreased level of consciousness).

The Family and Others Significant to the Patient

Relatives and other visitors are likely to be distressed when they see the unconscious patient for the first time. A brief explanation of the immediate environment and the function of any equipment should be provided. Visitors should be encouraged to touch and speak softly to the patient. They should be given an opportunity to ask any questions and to speak with the doctor and nurse in charge of the patient's progress.

Rest and Sleep

Providing adequate rest and sleep for a patient in the acute clinical environment is one of the most difficult challenges confronting the nurse given the associated hospital environmental background noises. Patients whose level of consciousness fluctuates may experience periods of sleep and periods of wakefulness even though they may not be responsive to external stimuli.

It is easy to forget when we are providing 24-hour care that unconscious patients also need to have rest and sleep periods between nursing and other activities; nurses must consider this when planning their care. It can be detrimental to constantly stimulate the patient by undertaking frequent observations and procedures, and care should be coordinated with other members of the team who are attending to the patient (Hickey and Strayer 2019).

Acutely ill patients in intensive care will receive enteral feeding 24 hours/day to preserve gut integrity, increase immune function and reduce the risk of sepsis. As the patient's clinical condition improves or stabilises, intermittent or bolus NG feeding allows the patient to rest overnight (Reflection 27.4).

Diet and Hydration

The early commencement of fluid and nutritional support must be a high priority in the care of any unconscious patient. Failure

---

REFLECTION 27.3

Possible Barriers to Effective Communication

What do you understand by the term 'barriers to communication'?
List six potential barriers when caring for the unconscious patient and suggest strategies to enable you to cope with them.

to commence adequate fluid replacement and feeding can lead to dehydration and electrolyte imbalance, atrophy of skeletal muscle, increased risk of infection, immunosuppression and poor wound healing (BAPEN 2003).

Fluids

In the acute stage, fluids are usually administered intravenously, either peripherally or via a central line, titrated against the patient's fluid balance and serum electrolyte levels. Intravenous fluids are also given to:
- maintain hydration
- administer medications
- maintain normal electrolytes and correct imbalances.

It is essential that the correct fluids are administered at the prescribed rate to maintain fluid balance and meet metabolic needs. An infusion device is usually used to ensure accuracy.

The patient may also have an arterial line to facilitate frequent blood sampling. The line must be clearly labelled to distinguish it from other multiple venous lines or ports (see Chapter 19).

Nutrition

Provision of adequate nutrition is particularly important in the unconscious patient. Even brief periods of malnourishment will weaken the immune system with loss of energy and muscle mass.

Daily nutritional requirements are calculated on the basis of body weight, gender, height and age (http://www.bapen.org.uk). Unless the patient is nursed on a bed with an integral weighing scale, an estimated weight is often used.

Nasogastric Feeding. This is the most frequently used method of providing nutritional support, provided that the patient's alimentary tract is functional. The dietitian will assess the patient's nutritional requirements daily, titrating against clinical need. If the patient has a suspected base of skull fracture, CSF rhinorrhoea or severe facial/nasal fractures, an orogastric tube may be preferable.

The position of the tube must be checked according to local guidelines, which should reflect those of the NPSA (2016) (www.npsa.gov.uk).

Percutaneous Endoscopic Gastrostomy Feeding. Whenever possible, it is preferable to deliver food directly into the stomach to prevent the risk of translocation of bacteria from the unused gastrointestinal tract. Long-term feeding is better achieved by a percutaneous endoscopic gastrostomy (PEG) tube which has fewer associated complications than an NG tube and is more comfortable for the patient. Relatives/carers can be taught how to administer feeds through the tube if the patient is later cared for at home.

As the patient regains consciousness, they should be assessed by the speech and language therapist (SLT) to ensure that are they safe to swallow diet and fluids (see Chapter 22).

Parenteral Nutrition. Parenteral feeding is prescribed when the patient is unable to tolerate or fails to absorb enteral feeding. It is delivered either through a central venous line or a peripherally inserted central line (PICC line) (see Chapter 22). Patients who may benefit from parenteral nutrition include:
- patients with multiple traumas, particularly if there are gastrointestinal and/or facial injuries
- malnourished patients
- patients with sepsis or multisystem failure
- patients with inflammatory bowel disease which is extensive and life threatening
- patients in prolonged coma who are unable to tolerate enteral feeding.

For further information on enteral feeding and parenteral nutrition, see Chapter 22.

Elimination

The ability of the patient to control elimination is impaired due to their altered level of consciousness. Incontinence will lead to skin breakdown and loss of dignity. Initially, during the acute phase of admission, an indwelling catheter will enable an accurate measurement of urinary output. Local protocols should be followed regarding catheter care. Once the patient has stabilised, male patients may be able to manage with external penile collection devices such as a Uri-sheath. To optimise long-term care and patient comfort, a supra-pubic catheter may be recommended to reduce the incidence of urinary infection. The urine bypasses the urethra and flows into a catheter inserted directly into the bladder through the abdomen. To maintain the catheter, it should be turned within the stoma daily to prevent it adhering the bladder; the skin around the entry site should be cleaned twice a day.

The patient's bowel movements should be closely monitored, and a regular bowel regimen should be in place. Stool softeners and aperients may be administered in order to produce a regular stool. Diarrhoea should be quickly cleaned away and the skin inspected for signs of excoriation.

Personal Cleansing and Dressing

The unconscious patient is dependent upon the nurse to attend to all aspects of personal hygiene. A daily bed bath is necessary for most totally dependent patients, but care must be taken when turning the unconscious patient in bed as there is a danger that the airway may become compromised and the patient's chest movement may be impeded. To avoid this, turning should be planned and requires a minimum of two nurses to execute safely. If a mechanical hoist is available, the patient can be showered or bathed in a specifically designed bath. Many unconscious patients will require more than one bed bath a day to maintain their hygiene needs and personal comfort.

Hair washing may be difficult and if the use of a wet shampoo is impossible, a dry shampoo may be used. Nails should be kept short and clean; referral to a chiropodist may be necessary for some patients. Male patients will require a daily facial shave. If the patient has a moustache or beard, this should be trimmed as necessary.

Eye care must be performed on a frequent basis because unconscious patients do not blink, and the cornea will become dry. Without adequate eye care, this can quickly lead to corneal ulceration and permanent visual impairment. The eye and surrounding area should be cleaned with gauze and sterile normal saline, followed by the instillation of artificial tear drops at least four times a day. If the patient's eyelids do not close naturally, eye drops may need to be instilled more frequently. The eyes can be protected with a polyacrylamide hydrogel dressing or eye shield to prevent further damage to the cornea (Woodrow 2018). Electric fans directed towards the head and eyes can exacerbate corneal damage and must be avoided.

Oral hygiene should be maintained following thorough oral assessment to plan effective care (Woodrow 2018). The unconscious patient who has a Guedel airway or ETT in place may present with particular problems such as a dry mouth and difficult access to the oral cavity. A small toothbrush with a small amount of fluoride toothpaste and plain water should be used to clean the teeth, tongue and gums. Lubricants to prevent cracking of the lips and promote healing can also be useful. Dentures must be stored dry in a covered container labelled with the patient's name and hospital number and should be cleaned again and rinsed in cold water before reinsertion.

Maintaining a Safe Environment

The unconscious patient is physically vulnerable to a range of complications, such as pressure ulcers and infection, and nursing staff must always be alert to the need to maintain a safe environment.

Infection

The unconscious patient is particularly at risk of respiratory and urinary infection. All wounds and drains are also potential sites for infection. Gram-negative bacillary pneumonia causes 40%–60% of respiratory infections that are acquired in hospitals or institutionalised settings. Most people are resistant to this organism, which is constantly present in the environment, but certain factors contribute to the breaking down of physiological and immunological defences. The unconscious patient is exposed to many of these, particularly in the presence of invasive lines such as intravenous cannulae and urinary catheters. Antibiotic-resistant infections have become an increasing problem in hospital and primary care. Hospitals have their own local policies for screening of patients on their admission, this includes methicillin-resistant *Staphylococcus aureus* (MRSA), a potentially life-threatening organism and COVID-19 (Loveday et al. 2014) (see also Chapter 18).

The nurse needs to be aware of and conscientious about implementing trust policies in relation to standard infection control precautions (see Chapter 18). Handwashing is known to be the single most effective intervention to promote infection control in the clinical setting (Loveday et al. 2014, Royal College of Nursing [RCN] 2017).

Medication

The types of medication most commonly used in the unconscious patient include analgesics, anticonvulsants (see Seizure, later), antibiotics and laxatives. The hazards of administering medications are well documented, but the risks are increased in the unconscious patient for two reasons:

- The routes that are used carry a greater risk for the patient. The simpler and safer oral route is contraindicated. Other methods of administration have to be utilised, including intramuscular or intravenous injection instillation via a nasal or orogastric tube and occasionally the rectal route can be used.
- Patients cannot confirm their identity, so nurses must ensure that the right medication in the right dose is being given to the right patient via the right route at the right time (RCN 2020).

Motor and Sensory Loss or Impairment

The motor and sensory loss experienced by unconscious patients may be drug induced or part of an underlying disease process. Whatever the cause, the nursing intervention remains the same.

Motor Loss. See Mobility.

Sensory Loss. The sensory system is part of the body's defence system, and the unconscious patient is unable to process sensory information. It is imperative that the patient is not exposed to extremes of temperature, particularly in localised area of the skin, for example when heating or cooling devices are used.

Care must be taken when moving and positioning the patient as they will not be aware of any adverse friction or pressure. The patient may have a reduced or absent sensation of pain or, if experiencing pain, may be unable to communicate that feeling.

Seizure

The main role of the nurse when the unconscious patient, or indeed anyone, has a seizure is to ensure that the patient does not harm themselves. Depending on the type of seizure, the need for first aid may not be recognised, but always depends on the type and severity of the seizure (see www.epilepsy.org.uk).

- Do:
  - Stay calm.
  - Protect the patient from injury (especially the head).
  - Look for information/warning cards/jewellery.
  - Continually check the airway and remain with the patient until help arrives.
- Do not:
  - Restrain the patient in any way.
  - Try to move the patient (unless from immediate danger).
  - Give food or drink.
- Call an ambulance if:
  - This is the person's first seizure.
  - There is no sign of spontaneous recovery.
  - One seizure follows another.
  - A serious injury has occurred.

Status Epilepticus. (a prolonged seizure or a series of seizures without regaining consciousness) is always a medical emergency and demands urgent medical assistance. Further information about epilepsy can be found in Chapter 11.

Mobility

The nursing management of mobility and activity remains the same, whatever the cause of the unconsciousness. Lack of attention to mobility could lead to the development of:

- Contractures – permanent tightening of a muscle or tendon in response to increased muscle tone and involuntary movement preventing normal movement.
- Muscle atrophy/wasting – refers to a decrease in muscle mass following injury or disease to a nerve and occurs as a consequence of disuse due to immobility.
- Pressure ulcers – prevention is important for the comfort of the patient. Regular alteration of the patient's position and relief of pressure is paramount, particularly in the immobile, unconscious patient.
- Postural hypotension – a fall in blood pressure when the individual adopts an upright position after lying for long periods.
- Deep vein thrombosis (see Chapter 2).
- Hypostatic pneumonia (see Chapter 3).

Any one of these hazards will delay the patient's rehabilitation and cause additional pain and discomfort. Whilst the patient remains dependent, the nurse, working with the physiotherapists, is responsible for ensuring that the patient maintains a full range of movement. Correct positioning is important and the following should be considered:

- body alignment, especially if spinal injury is suspected
- use of aids such as pillows, foam pads or splints, to help to support weak or hemiplegic limbs
- avoidance of pressure, e.g. an arm trapped under the body, the pinna of the ear pressing on the pillow, bedclothes too tight
- changing the patient's position; this should be done frequently – at least every 2 hours is recommended
- avoidance of friction when moving the patient
- careful handling of joints and paralysed or weak limbs
- safety, e.g. if the patient is restless, padded bed rails may be required.

Safety/Restraint

Many patients experience disorientation, confusion or aggressive behaviour as they recover consciousness. This may be due to their underlying illness and pathology, medication, sensory deprivation or the unfamiliar environment. Healthcare teams face difficult decisions about identifying strategies to prevent the patient inadvertently dislodging tracheostomy tubes, invasive lines or dressings (Reflection 27.5). Diversional therapy, involving the patient's family and friends, or providing one-to-one nursing supervision may be useful. Balancing the best interests of the patient to ensure safety and promote their well-being can be difficult and presents unique challenges. When all other alternative therapies have failed, and only as a last resort, a short-term restraint measure, such as mittens, may be necessary. A risk assessment must be completed and continuously reevaluated to ensure the measures are discontinued at the earliest opportunity. No restraints should be applied without consultation with the patient, their family and the medical team involved with the patients' care (Nursing and Midwifery Council (NMC) (2022), Mental Capacity Act (2005) and Associated Code of Practice (2019). Deprivation of Liberty legislation (DOL's) was introduced in 2009 and in Scotland in 2000 (Adults With Incapacity (Scotland) Act), to safeguard and protect patients in hospital and care homes who lacked capacity to make their own decisions. Liberty Protection Safeguards (2023), aims to create a more streamlined framework to guide advanced decision making.

⊕See Evolve website Critical thinking question 27.1

Recovery From Coma

A multidisciplinary approach is essential to facilitate early mobilisation of the patient. Patients who have been nursed in bed for just a few days often experience dizziness and light-headedness due to postural hypotension when they sit up for the first time.

The physiotherapist will normally carry out an initial assessment, taking into consideration the patient's sensory or motor deficits, balance and trunk, head and neck control. Initially, the patient may be unsure and apprehensive about the prospect of getting out

REFLECTION 27.5

Managing Challenging Behaviour

Reflect on your experience and identify two issues about the ward environment or routine that may increase the risks to patients who are confused or disorientated or who may display challenging behaviour.
Consider how these patients are managed and any interventions that might help to reduce these risks.

of bed and will need constant reassurance. Once the patient is in a sitting position, the nurse should check the patient's vital signs and ask whether they are experiencing any untoward symptoms. If they are, an individualised mobility rehabilitation programme should be implemented at a slower rate. Specialist chairs are available that will provide additional support for highly dependent patients. It is more beneficial for patients to sit up for several short intervals rather than one long period (see Chapter 33).

Controlling Body Temperature

Body temperature is controlled by the heat-regulating centre in the hypothalamus, which acts like a thermostat, and must be maintained within a relatively constant range to sustain life, that is, 36–37.5°C. Pyrexia (an abnormally high temperature) is more commonly seen in the unconscious patient than hypothermia (an abnormally low temperature), although hypothermia may be the primary cause of unconsciousness.

Pyrexia may be caused by damage to the hypothalamus, an infective process or a metabolic disorder. For each degree of temperature above the normal range, the cerebral metabolism significantly increases, adversely increasing the brain's oxygen demands, which can have serious implications for the patient's eventual recovery and prognosis. In the acute stages the nurse must monitor the patient's temperature continuously with an electronic probe, sited over the patient's skin, inserted rectally or integrated into the patient's urinary bladder catheter. Normothermia is achieved using cooling blankets, electric fans and antipyretic medication, for example paracetamol.

Dying

Despite all intensive care measures, some patients will die. Active treatment may continue right up until the last moment, or it may be decided that any further active intervention would be futile. The emphasis would then move from curative to palliative care, ensuring that the patient is comfortable and pain free. If the patient is on a mechanical ventilator, they may fulfil the criteria required for assessing brain stem death.

Brain Stem Death

Patients who have sustained a catastrophic and irreversible brain injury may survive for a short period of time with life support interventions such as mechanical ventilation and drug therapies to maintain their cardiorespiratory functions.

When brain stem death is suspected, a range of neurological criteria are applied to diagnose and confirm irremediable structural brain stem death, in order that therapies can cease.

Brain stem death is clinically diagnosed by following a code of practice for the diagnosis and confirmation of death (AMRC 2008). Prior to performing the tests, the ventilated patient must fulfil a series of preconditions.

Preconditions. All reversible causes of coma have been eliminated, including:

- drug intoxication, e.g. as the result of an overdose, neuromuscular blocking agents or sedation to facilitate intubation
- primary hypothermia
- metabolic or endocrine imbalances such as uncontrolled diabetes.

Testing Brain Stem Function. The diagnosis of irreversible cessation of brain stem function is made by two doctors who have been registered with the General Medical Council for a minimum of 5 years and are competent to perform and interpret the results of the examination. If organ donation from the patient is being considered, neither doctor must be a member of the transplant team. There are six parts to the test:

1. The pupillary response to light is tested, using a bright torch; absence of response indicates loss of function. The examiner must be satisfied that a nonresponsive pupil is not due to the instillation of paralytic eye drops or damage to cranial nerve III.

2. The corneal reflex is tested by drawing a wisp of cotton wool across the exposed cornea. Absence of a blink response indicates loss of function, although the examiner should be satisfied that the presence of corneal oedema is not preventing the normal blink response.

3. Cranial nerve motor responses are tested by applying a painful stimulus at several sites (usually over the supraorbital ridge, compressing part of the trigeminal nerve). Again, no response indicates loss of function, although spinal reflexes can remain intact even in a brain-dead patient

4. The cough and gag reflexes are tested by agitating the ETT back and forth or by applying a suction catheter to the oropharynx and observing the patient's response. No response would indicate loss of the pharyngeal and laryngeal reflexes.

5. Absence of the oculovestibular reflex rules out the existence of normally functioning anatomical pathways within the brain stem and is a very sensitive test of brain stem function. It is tested by syringing 20 mL of ice-cold water into the patient's ears in turn and noting any eye movement in response. This is called 'cold caloric testing'. Before testing, the examiner should use an auroscope to look directly at the tympanic membrane to ensure that it is intact and that there is no obstruction preventing the water from making contact with the membrane.

6. Finally, the apnoea test is performed. Arterial blood gases are checked and $PaCO_2$ should be 5.33–6.00 kPa (40–45 mmHg). The patient is disconnected from the ventilator after providing a continuous flow of 100% intratracheal oxygen for 10 minutes. The patient's chest wall is observed closely for any respiratory movement and the $PaCO_2$ is allowed to rise above threshold level to stimulate breathing, usually to at least 6.65 kPa (50 mmHg).

The ventilator is then reconnected, and the entire process is repeated (either immediately or after a few hours) before the patient is declared brain-stem dead. It is at this time that the Specialist Nurse – Organ Donation (SNODs) will assess the patient as a potential organ donor and approach the families to discuss their wishes for end-of-life care including the opportunity to donate their organs and tissues, known as 'donation after brain stem death' (DBD). Patients who do meet the prerequisites for assessing brain stem death may still be able to donate their organs if the decision has been made to withdraw treatment due to futility and prolonging treatment is not in the best interests of the patient, known as 'donation after circulatory death' (DCD); these patients will be supported on the ventilator until a time when a planned withdrawal can take place with the family and transplant surgeons (British Medical Association [BMA] 2021).

For further information on brain stem death, see http://guidance.nice.org.uk/CG135, The Code of Practice for the Diagnosis and Confirmation of Death; on issues relating to organ donation and transplants, see www.uktransplant.org.uk and NHB Organ Transplantation and on DBD and DCD, see http://organdonationwales.org/Join-the-Organ-Donor-Register.

Physical and Psychological Care

The Patient. The principles of care for the dying unconscious patient are the same as those for all patients requiring palliative care (see Chapter 32). The unconscious patient must be treated with dignity and sensitivity even though they are unable to respond.

The Family. A sensitive and coherent strategy for caring for the relatives is needed. The nurse should know what information has been given to the relatives by other members of staff, including doctors. This will enable the nurse to reaffirm what has been said and avoid confusing the family members at a time when their ability to process information is drastically reduced (Reflection 27.6). They need to see and feel that the patient, even if unconscious and unresponsive, is still being treated as a person, through the humane, caring attitude of the nurse.

Some relatives may be helped by being encouraged to perform simple acts of care for the patient such as bathing them or combing their hair, reducing their feelings of passivity and helplessness.

Psychologically, this is a traumatic and emotionally distressing time for the patient's family, friends and/or those who have a significant relationship with the patient. They have perhaps spent the last few days (and in some cases, much longer than that) with the patient, in the unfamiliar technical surroundings. They may be relieved that an ending has been achieved or may find it difficult to accept the death, particularly if the patient has been artificially ventilated.

The support of a religious advisor may be appreciated, even if the patient or relatives have not previously held any religious beliefs. Bereavement counselling and support should be offered as well as practical information (preferably written) about registering the death and other formalities.

Inevitably, this chapter has focused on the care of unconscious people in hospital because, at the present time, only a small minority are cared for at home. Wherever the location of care, it is important for nurses to be sensitive to the fundamental needs of the unconscious patient and understand the emotional impact their condition has on their relatives, carers and friends. As noted at the outset of this chapter, caring for the unconscious person is a major challenge for the nurse and whatever the outcome, meticulous attention to nursing observations and care is vital (Reflection 27.7).

See Evolve website Critical thinking question 27.2

Summary: Key Nursing Issues

- Loss of consciousness may occur gradually or suddenly and be a temporary or a permanent state. Patients will be totally reliant on the nurse to maintain their safety and bodily functions.
- An individualised care plan should be written ensuring all activities of living are supported and provided for.
- Ensure a patent airway is maintained to prevent hypoxia.
- Assess respiratory function – rate, depth, oxygen saturation – and use airway adjuncts and apply oral/tracheal suction to remove secretions.
- Maintain hydration and nutrition with intravenous fluids and monitor blood chemistry levels. Commence enteral feeding via an NG feeding tube or PEG as soon as possible and assess swallow reflex before recommencing oral feeding.
- Elimination – measure urine output with a urinary catheter if accurate urine output is needed. Apply sheaths and pads and other appliances to manage urinary incontinence. Monitor bowel function and avoid constipation.
- Monitoring and observations – record vital signs, pulse, blood pressure, respirations, temperature.

- Monitor level of consciousness using the GCS and assess pupil reaction and limb movement.
- Maintain a safe environment by using bed rails and managing confused or challenging behaviour.
- Maintain personal hygiene with a bed bath at least daily and provide frequent eye and mouth care.
- Prevent pressure ulcers by risk assessment, use of pressure-relieving beds and equipment and adjusting the patient's position 2-hourly. Perform passive exercises and position limbs to reduce risk of contractures.
- Communicate with the patient as if he/she can hear and understand conversation and help the family to develop ways of communicating with the patient such as use of touch.
- Observe closely for signs of pain such as restlessness, vital signs, grimacing. Administer analgesia as prescribed.
- Maintain dignity and privacy by providing information for the patient and relatives in a confidential manner.
- Provide emotional support to the patient and family members.
- Promote sleep and rest and reduce stimulation, noise and external noxious stimuli where possible.

Reflection and Learning – What Next?

- **Test** your knowledge by visiting the Evolve website 🌐 and answering the multiple-choice questions and critical thinking questions.
- **Consolidate** your learning by looking at some of the further reading suggestions, references, and specialist websites.
- **Revisit** some of the additional material on the website.

- **Consider** what you have learnt and how this will help your professional development.
- **Reflect** on how you can apply this knowledge to the care of your patients.
- **Discuss** your learning with your mentor/supervisor, lecturer, and colleagues.

References

Adults With Incapacity (Scotland) Act. 2000. https://www.legislation.gov.uk/asp/2000/4/contents.

Afifi A, Bergman R. *Functional Neuroanatomy: Text and Atlas.* 2nd ed. McGraw Hill Professional; 2005.

AMRC. A Code of Practice for the Diagnosis and Confirmation of Brain Stem Death. Academy of Medical Royal Colleges; 2008.

BAPEN. *Malnutrition Universal Screening Tool (MUST).* Malnutrition Universal Screening Tool; 2003. bapen.org.uk.

Braine M, Cook N. The Glasgow Coma Scale and evidence informed practice: a critical review of where we are and where we need to be. *J Clin Nurs.* 2017;26(1):280–293.

British Medical Association (BMA). Organ donation. 2021. https://www.bma.org.uk/advice-and-support/ethics/end-of-life/organ-donation.

Gill-Thwaites H, Munday R. The Sensory Modality Assessment and Rehabilitation Technique (SMART): a valid and reliable assessment for vegetative state and minimally conscious state patients. *Brain INJ.* 2004;18(12):1255–1269.

Hickey JV, Strayer AL. *The Clinical Practice of Neurological and Neurosurgical Nursing.* 8th ed. Wolter Kluwer; 2019.

Kitzinger C, Kitzinger J. Withdrawing artificial nutrition and hydration from minimally conscious and vegetative patients: family perspectives. *J med Ethics.* 2015;41(2):157–160.

Loveday HP, Pratt RJ, Wilson JA, et al. National evidence based guidelines for preventing hospital acquired infections in NHS Hospitals in England. EPIC 3. *J Hosp Infect.* 2014;86S1:S1–S70.

Martini F, Nath J, Bartholomew E. *Fundamentals of Anatomy & Physiology.* 11th ed. Pearson; 2018.

Mental Capacity Act 2005 and Associated Code of Practice. http://www.justice.gov.uk/guidance/protecting-the-vulnerable/mentalcapacity-act/index.htm.

Mental Capacity (Amendment) Act. 2019. legislation.gov.uk.

Moini J, Piran J. *Functional and Clinical Neurology. A Guide for Professionals.* Elsevier. AP Academic Press; 2020.

National Institute for Health and Care Excellence (NICE). Epilepsies in children, young people and adults. NICE guideline [NG217]. 2022.

National Institute for Health and Care Excellence (NICE). *Head Injury: Assessment and Early Management Clinical Guideline.* London: NICE; 2023:CG176.

NEWS2. *National Early Warning Score.* Royal College of Physicians; 2017.

National Nurses Nutrition Group (NNNG). Good practice guideline-safe insertion of nasogastric NG feeding tubes in adults and ongoing care. 2016. www.nnng.org.uk.

NHS Improvement. Resource set. Initial placement checks for nasogastric and orogastric tubes. 2016. https://www.england.nhs.uk/wp-content/uploads/2016/07/Resource_set_-_Initial_placement_checks_for_NG_tubes_1.pdf.

Nursing and Midwifery Council (NMC). *The Code: Standards of Conduct, Performance and Ethics for Nurses and Midwives.* London: Nursing and Midwifery Council NMC; 2022.

Pistarini C, Maggioni G. Disorders of consciousness. *Clin Pathways Stroke Rehabilitation.* 2021;1:57–70.

Pundole A, Crawford S. *The Assessment of Language and the Emergence From Disorders of Consciousness. Neuropsychological Rehabilitation.* Routledge, Taylor & Francis Group; 2017.

Rahman S. *Essentials of Delirium: Everything You Really Need to Know for Working in Delirium Care*. London and Philadelphia: Jessica Kingsley Publishers; 2020.

Reith FC, Brennan P, Maas AI, Teasdale GM. Lack of standardisation in the use of the Glasgow Coma Scale. Results of international surveys. *J Neurotrauma*. 2016;33(1):89–94.

Royal College of Nursing. *Essential Practice for Infection Prevention and Control Guidance for Nursing Staff. Clinical Professional Resource*. London: Royal College of Nursing; 2017.

Royal College of Nursing. *Medicines Management: An Overview for Nursing. Clinical Professional Resource*. London: Royal College of Nursing; 2020.

Royal College of Physicians. *Prolonged Disorders of Consciousness Following Sudden Onset Brain Injury: National Clinical Guidance*. London: Royal College of Physicians; 2020.

Teasdale G. Forty years on: updating the Glasgow Coma Scale. *Nurs Times*. 2014;110(42):12–16.

Teasdale G, Jennett B. Assessment of coma and impaired consciousness. A practical scale. *Lancet*. 1974;304(7872):81–84.

Wade DT, Turner-Stokes L, Playford ED, Allanson J, Pickard J. Prolonged disorders of consciousness: a response to a "Critical Evaluation of the New UK Guidelines". *Clin Rehabil*. 2022;36(9):1141–1277.

Wijdicks EF. *Examining Neurocritical Patients*. 1st ed. Springer; 2021.

Woodrow P. *Intensive Care Nursing*. 4th ed. London: Routledge, Taylor & Francis Group; 2018.

Useful Websites

British Association of Neuroscience Nurses, www.bann.org.uk
British Brain and Spine Foundation, www.bbsf.org.uk
Epilepsy Action, www.epilepsy.org.uk
Headway – the brain injury association, www.headway.org.uk
Life NPH (Normal Pressure Hydrocephalus) Life NPH (Normal Pressure Hydrocephalus), www.allaboutnph.com
National Poisons Information Service National Poisons Information Service, www.npis.org
Organ/tissue donation and transplants, www.uktransplant.org.uk

28

Nursing the Critically Ill Patient

DEAN WHITING

CHAPTER OUTLINE

Introduction

The term 'critically ill' is used to describe people who have acute, life-threatening conditions but who may recover if they are given timely, appropriate, effective and often highly technical nursing and medical care. Critically ill patients come from diverse backgrounds and the conditions from which they suffer and the care and treatment they need are so varied that elements from every chapter in this book are relevant to their care. Patients who present in a critically ill state can be considered in three main categories:

- Those who have never had a significant illness and who have suffered a sudden, acute life-threatening event, e.g. extensive trauma, severe burns, near drowning, major childbirth complications or deliberate self-harm.
- Those who suffer from chronic illness, perhaps involving frequent previous hospital admissions, e.g. chronic obstructive pulmonary disease (COPD) or chronic pancreatitis, and who present as critically ill as a combination of their chronic illness with a life-threatening event.
- Those who have become critically ill because of surgery – in some cases, the life-threatening situation is not expected, while in others, postoperative critical care is a recognised necessity.

Critical care is an ever-evolving specialty that has grown in response to medical, surgical and technological advancements. The cost of providing critical care is high, and the range of cases is broad, including trauma, disease adverse events and surgery (Intensive Care Society [ICS] 2022). All critically ill patients require varying levels of organ support or intervention according to their clinical requirements, and critical care is categorised into three levels. This includes levels 2 and 3 for intensive care patients and level 1 for enhanced level care patients, as outlined in the ICS 2021 guidelines) (Information 28.1).

For over 15 years, the concept of critical care has expanded beyond traditional hospital departments, with the development of rapid response and critical care outreach teams (CCOTs) in most acute hospitals. The specialist teams are made up of specialist nurses, allied health practitioners (e.g. physiotherapists) and medical staff. These teams provide expert critical care input and skill sharing to the multidisciplinary team across all wards and departments outside of the dedicated critical care environment. The aim being to prevent unnecessary deaths and to avert admission by

Levels of Critical Care Support

Level 0 – ward care
- Patients whose needs can be met through normal ward care in an acute hospital.
- Patients who have recently been relocated from a higher level of care, but their needs can be met on an acute ward with additional advice and support from the critical care outreach team.
- Patients who can be managed on a ward but remain at risk of clinical deterioration.

Level 1 – enhanced care
- Patients requiring more detailed observations or interventions, including basic support for a single organ system and those 'stepping down' from higher levels of care.
- Patients requiring interventions to prevent further deterioration or rehabilitation needs which cannot be met on a normal ward.
- Patients who require ongoing interventions (other than routine follow-up) from critical care outreach teams to intervene in deterioration or to support escalation of care.
- Patients needing a greater degree of observation and monitoring that cannot be safely provided on a ward, judged on the basis of clinical circumstances and ward resources.

Level 2 – critical care
- Patients requiring increased levels of observations or interventions (beyond Level 1), including basic support for two or more organ systems and those 'stepping down' from higher levels of care.
- Patients requiring interventions to prevent further deterioration or to support ongoing rehabilitation needs, beyond that of Level 1.
- Patients needing two or more basic organ systems monitoring and support.
- Patients needing one organ system monitored and supported at an advanced level (other than advanced respiratory support).
- Patients needing long-term advanced respiratory support.
- Patients who require Level 1 care for organ support but who require enhanced nursing for other reasons, in particular maintaining patient safety if severely agitated.
- Patients needing extended postoperative care, outside that which can be provided in enhanced care units: extended postoperative observation is required either because of the nature of the procedure and/or the patient's condition and comorbidities.
- Patients with major uncorrected physiological abnormalities, whose care needs cannot be met elsewhere.
- Patients who require nursing and therapies input more frequently than available in Level 1 areas.

Level 3 – critical care
- Patients who need advanced respiratory monitoring and support alone.
- Patients who require monitoring and support for two or more organ systems at an advanced level.
- Patients with chronic impairment of one or more organ systems sufficient to restrict daily activities (comorbidity), and who require support for an acute reversible failure of another organ system.
- Patients who experience delirium and agitation in addition to requiring Level 2 care.
- Complex patients requiring support for multiple organ failure; this may not necessarily include advanced respiratory support.

From Intensive Care Society. Levels of Adult Critical Care. 2nd ed. 2021. https://ics.ac.uk/resource/levels-of-care.html

offering advice and reviewing patients at risk of deterioration or to ensure safe and timely transfer to critical care through early identification of patients requiring higher-intensity care (ICS 2022).

The National Early Warning Score system (NEWS 2) has been implemented in many hospitals to help identify patients at risk. These assessment tools use a range of clinical observations to generate an overall score to assess the patient and evaluate the risk of deterioration. The scoring system identifies patients at low, medium and high risk of deterioration and determines ongoing interventions such as increasing the frequency of observations or triggering a review by the medical team or by critical care outreach services (Royal College of Physicians 2017).

Critical care has also expanded into the community setting with the development of hospital at home services offering noninvasive ventilation (NIV) to patients with chronic diseases such as muscular dystrophy, motor neurone disease and high spinal injuries who require respiratory support and are managed at home with input from specialised home ventilation nurse practitioners.

The nursing of the critically ill patient is an extensive and specialised area of care that cannot be fully addressed in this chapter. The aim is to provide an overview and, where appropriate, provide links to other chapters and more specialised texts and journals.

The primary responsibility of the nurse in the critical care setting is to provide physical and psychological care for patients and help prevent complications. There are several different models of nursing that have been adapted to deal with all aspects of care for these patients, and due to the nature of their condition, a *systems approach* is the most logical method of reviewing the care requirements for individual patients. Tools such as daily goals sheets, a multidisciplinary tool to ensure that all aspects of the patient's care are considered, are helpful.

⊕ **See Evolve website Fig. 28.1**

Patient Safety

Patient safety is of paramount importance in critical care nursing and is high on the agenda of government and professional bodies. Broadly, it considers two separate dimensions including factors associated with the individual nurse and more broadly, the risk associated with error occurring in unsafe systems. Critical care practitioners have developed evidence-based 'care bundles' to optimise care. Care bundles are a group of interventions related to a disease process that, when executed together, result in a better outcome than when implemented independently (Institute for Healthcare Improvement 2018). The acquisition of healthcare-associated infections (HAIs) such as methicillin-resistant *Staphylococcus aureus* (MRSA) and *Clostridium difficile* receives a great deal of media attention and developing strategies to avoid harm is crucial. This includes measures to control antibiotic prescribing and compliance to isolating patients affected (National Institute for Health and Care Excellence [NICE] 2015).

MEETING THE PHYSICAL NEEDS OF THE CRITICALLY ILL PATIENT

Respiratory Needs and Care

Many disease processes may lead to the need for ventilatory support (Information 28.2). Mechanical ventilation is the artificial support of, or assistance with, breathing when adequate gaseous exchange and tissue perfusion can no longer be maintained (see Chapter 3, Nursing Patients With Respiratory Disorders). Ventilatory support can be administered 'invasively' through an endotracheal (ET) tube or tracheostomy or noninvasively through a mask or hood. Both methods can maintain vital respiratory function; the type of support required depends on the patient's underlying condition. Patients with type I or type II respiratory failure or acute pulmonary oedema are likely to have a good response to NIV, which may avoid intubation. High-flow nasal cannula (HFNC) is an innovative and effective treatment modality for treating respiratory failure from a range of causes. The therapy involves delivering heated humidified oxygen air mix at high flow (up to 60 L) that creates a positive pressure environment which 'washes out' gases in the nasopharynx assisting in carbon dioxide clearance. It is well tolerated by patients (Renda et al. 2018).

Ventilation Modes

Practitioners must have specialist training in the equipment and processes involved in the care of patients requiring ventilation in order to deliver optimal care and recognise complications. The ventilation modes and care outlined next give a brief overview. The patient's underlying medical condition, age and weight will determine the prescribed mode of ventilation.

Invasive Modes

- *Intermittent positive pressure ventilation (IPPV).* This delivers a preset tidal volume at a preset rate. It ignores the patient's own respiratory drive. Its use is restricted to heavily sedated or paralysed patients or those with central nervous system disturbance.
- *Synchronised intermittent mandatory ventilation (SIMV).* The positive pressure breaths are synchronised with the patient's own breathing and the patient is able to breathe spontaneously.
- *Biphasic positive airway pressure (BiPAP).* Used in invasive ventilation, this mode uses pressure control to deliver the tidal volume. It also allows spontaneous breathing and is often used in acute lung injury (ALI).
- *Assisted spontaneous breathing/pressure support (ASB/PS).* This senses when a patient takes a breath and gives them additional preset support. It can be used with SIMV or alone.
- *Positive end-expiratory pressure (PEEP).* PEEP increases functional residual capacity, i.e. the amount of air left in the lungs at the end of expiration. The pressure prevents small alveoli collapsing and allows a longer period of gas exchange. It is used as an adjunct to IPPV, SIMV and ASB/PS. High levels of PEEP can reduce venous return and reduce cardiac output.

The potential complications of mechanical ventilation are outlined in Information 28.3.

Noninvasive Modes

- *Continuous positive airway pressure (CPAP).* This is equivalent to PEEP but is delivered via mask or hood (see Fig. 28.1). Airway pressure is maintained above atmospheric pressure throughout the ventilatory cycle by pressurisation in the ventilatory circuit. This makes breathing easier for the patient and facilitates gas exchange.
- *NIV* supports the patient's breathing to a preset pressure level:
- *Inspired positive airway pressure (IPAP).* This is the pressure level the patient receives on inspiration. The patient initiates a breath, and this breath is then supported by the ventilator to the preset IPAP pressure.
- *Expired positive airway pressure (EPAP).* As the patient breathes out, the expired positive airway pressure prevents alveolar collapse.

This mode is frequently employed in type II respiratory failure or as a maximum treatment option if the patient is not suitable for invasive ventilation. NIV has become a popular choice for clinicians in recent years. It has the potential advantage over invasive methods of reducing the risk of infection and reducing length of stay (Duke 2018).

Close observations of the patient's face should be undertaken for pressure damage. Patients who are actively vomiting and those with gastrointestinal (GI) bleeds or facial trauma may not be suitable candidates for NIV. Clear explanations are required to ensure the patient understands the treatment. The patient is often anxious prior to treatment commencing due to feeling breathless, and

---

INFORMATION 28.2

Causes of Respiratory Failure

Acute Respiratory Failure Without Respiratory Distress

- Central airway obstruction
- Decreased level of consciousness
  - head injury
  - sepsis
  - drug overdose
- Neuromuscular pathway impairment – Guillain–Barré syndrome
  - myasthenia gravis
  - postoperative diaphragmatic paralysis
  - trauma
- Cardiovascular impairment – acute myocardial infarction
  - cardiogenic shock

Lung Parenchymal Disease

- Asthma
- Pneumonia
- ALI

Acute or Chronic Respiratory Failure

- Exacerbation of chronic obstructive airways disease (COAD)
- Chronic neuromuscular disease

INFORMATION 28.3

Potential Complications of Mechanical Ventilation

- Damage to the airways/lung parenchyma
- Barotrauma, tension pneumothorax, disconnection/occlusion of the ET tube
- Mechanical failure
- Subcutaneous emphysema
- Hypo/hyperventilation
- Pulmonary oedema/pleural effusions
- Nosocomial hospital-acquired infection (HAI), consolidation
- Low cardiac output
- Cardiovascular depression
- Arrhythmias
- Water retention
- GI haemorrhage, aspiration of stomach contents, paralytic ileus
- Impairment of the central nervous system, kidneys and liver function
- O_2 toxicity
- Altered body image
- Sleep deprivation
- Tracheal injury

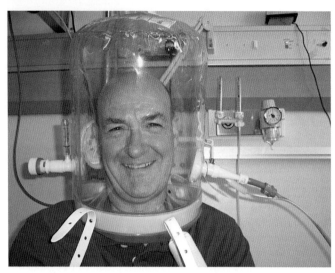

Figure 28.1 A continuous positive airway pressure hood.

the masks and hoods used can cause feelings of claustrophobia. The gradual implementation of treatment may be necessary to enable the patient to get used to the therapy.

Extracorporeal Membrane Oxygenation (ECMO)
In a small number of cases, patients who do not respond to standard ventilation may require ECMO. It is a supportive measure that uses an artificial lung (the membrane) to oxygenate the blood outside the body (extracorporeal). It is performed at specialist centres.

❖ Nursing Management and Health Promotion: Respiratory Care

Monitoring Respiratory Function and Maintaining Safe Ventilation
Monitoring and maintaining safe ventilation are crucial and once the patient is intubated and receiving ventilation support, constant and thorough observations are required as there are many associated complications (see Information 28.3).

Chest Auscultation. This should be performed at the start of a shift, as a baseline, and thereafter at the discretion of the nurse. It can offer a wealth of information about the patient's air entry – from an expiratory wheeze requiring treatment with a bronchodilator, to areas of reduced air entry due to secretion retention, consolidation or pulmonary oedema. Using a systematic approach, this can detect trouble early and assure appropriate intervention.

Ventilator-Associated Pneumonia. A ventilator-associated pneumonia (VAP) can be defined as a nosocomial airway infection that develops more than 48 hours after intubation. It is the most common HAI in critical care units, and it is associated with increased length of stay. There is good evidence that implementing a ventilator care bundle can demonstrate a significant reduction of VAP (Institute for Healthcare Improvement 2018).

Ventilator Care Bundle
The following components should be incorporated into the patient's daily care (Hellyer et al. 2016).
- Avoid the supine position; patients should be nursed in a semi-recumbent (30–45 degrees), head-up position, if practicable, to prevent oesophageal reflux and pulmonary aspiration, unless contraindicated.

- Sedation should be reviewed and if possible, stopped each day in order to assess the patient's readiness to wean and prevent oversedation. This daily screening reduces ventilator days and complications.
- ET and tracheostomy tubes with an additional port so that subglottic secretions can be cleared from the patient's oropharynx are available. Use of subglottic secretion drainage in ventilated patients reduces rates of VAP and intensive care unit (ICU) length of stay by preventing aspiration and lower airway colonisation from secretions that pool above the ET cuff.
- Regular ventilator circuit changes should be avoided so that soiled secretions do not migrate into the airways. Ventilator circuits should ideally be changed if visibly soiled or if faulty.

Humidification. As ET and tracheostomy tubes bypass the natural protective structures of the nasal passages, the oxygen used to ventilate the patient must be warmed to 32–36°C, humidified and filtered artificially without allowing condensate to backwash into the patient. Exposing the lungs and airways to cold gas has a number of potentially harmful effects: it can increase mucus viscosity, depress ciliary activity and obstruct the airways due to the build-up of the tenacious secretions. There are a number of humidification systems available. The heat moisture exchange filter (HMEF) is commonly used and is relatively cheap and disposable and often includes an additional microbiological filter. Temperature-controlled water humidifiers may be used if patients have tenacious secretions.

Ventilator and Endotracheal (ET) Tubes. The ventilator tubes must not be allowed to become kinked as this would reduce the desired respiratory effect. Patient comfort must be balanced with the safe and secure position of the ET tube in the patient's mouth. The ET tube must be secured to prevent movement which may compromise the patient's airway. This is achieved by tying the tube in place in the patient's mouth with cloth tape looped around the tube or by using commercially available tube attachment devices. These specifically designed holders better facilitate stabilisation and maximise comfort for the patient. In the case of a patient with a head injury, nonallergic adhesive tape should be used instead of a bandage to decrease the risk of raised intracranial pressure (ICP). Care should be given to pressure prevention and the position of the ET tube to prevent damage to the lip surface.

Ventilator tubes must not be allowed to drag as this in turn pulls on the ET tube, thereby applying pressure to the lips. Ventilators usually have an 'arm' which will support the weight of the tubes. To prevent water condensation in the tubing from entering the ET tube and the lungs, it is important that the tubes slope downwards from the patient towards the water traps. When turning the patient, care must always be taken to ensure that ET and ventilator tubes are guarded and supported.

Endotracheal Cuff Pressures. These need to be checked regularly using an ET cuff manometer. While cuff pressures of 30 mmHg are recommended, pressures of 17–23 mmHg have been shown to be adequate. For patients likely to require ventilatory support for a longer period, a tracheostomy is recommended; this will increase patient comfort, reduce sedation requirement and facilitate oral hygiene. Early tracheostomies can also reduce days on the ventilator and length of stay (Tanaka et al. 2022).

Ventilator Observations
Continual observation of the patient should include:
- the patient's colour to check if well perfused or cyanosed
- oxygen saturation (SaO_2; see Chapter 3)
- level of consciousness, i.e. if sedated or whether drowsy due to CO_2 retention

- chest movements, i.e. are both lungs being ventilated
- vital signs – changes in a patient's vital signs can indicate problems with ventilation; blood pressure, heart rate and rhythm, temperature and respiratory rate and pattern should all be closely monitored.

Observations of the ventilator should include:
- fraction of inspired oxygen (FiO_2)
- the prescribed ventilatory setting
- the expired minute volume
- the patient's tidal volume
- airway pressures and respirations (spontaneous and ventilator breaths).

End Tidal CO_2 ($ETCO_2$). Gives an indication of the amount of carbon dioxide in the exhaled air. A flat waveform would indicate a lack of ventilation and would be an indication of a misplaced or blocked tube.

All observations should be recorded regularly, typically hourly allowing for continual respiratory assessment and the early detection and treatment of any problems.

Arterial Blood Gases (ABGs). Judicious analysis of ABGs will most accurately reveal a patient's respiratory progress or deterioration and the adequacy of ventilatory support. Care must be taken not to oversample, to prevent iatrogenic anaemia.

Hyperoxia injures the lung and causes arterial vasoconstriction, alveolar-capillary 'leak' and fibrogenesis. Therefore a more targeted approach of maintaining oxygen saturations between 94% and 98% by titrating oxygen therapy will reduce the risk of complications. COPD patients will be prescribed a lower SaO_2 target (Singer et al. 2021).

Positioning

The position of the patient will depend on where the pulmonary abnormality is, and the patient should be positioned to maximise the matching of ventilation and perfusion. In a case of a left lower lobe collapse, it may be helpful to nurse the patient on the right side, thereby optimising the treatment to the affected area. Regularly turning patients will not only assist in the prevention of pressure ulcers but also facilitate pulmonary postural drainage. Nursing the patient in a semirecumbent position with a 30–45 degree head tilt reduces the risk of aspiration and VAP.

When a patient's oxygenation remains poor, despite high oxygen delivery and high PEEP levels (classically found in ALI), it may be decided to position the patient face down in the prone position. This manoeuvre increases lung compliance by recruiting under ventilated areas of the posterior lung bases and improves oxygenation (Hadaya and Benharash 2020).

Endotracheal Suction

ET suctioning is a procedure used to facilitate the clearance of secretions when a patient's normal cough mechanism is either inadequate or disrupted. This may occur where there is underlying respiratory or neurological disease or where the cough reflex is suppressed by sedation, muscle relaxants or anaesthetic agents during IPPV. Its purpose is the removal of pulmonary secretions, to avoid the problems associated with their retention, such as increased airway pressures, pneumothorax, cardiovascular instability, lobar consolidation, ventilation–perfusion mismatch, pneumonia, hypoxaemia and atelectasis. However, ET suction can produce complications and carries with it hidden risks (see Information 28.4). Maintaining a patent airway involves ET suctioning and, while it is essential to keep the airway clear of

---

INFORMATION 28.4

Potential Hazards of Endotracheal Suctioning

- Tracheal mucosal damage
- Hypoxaemia
- Atelectasis
- Arrhythmias
- Infections
- Excessive coughing
- Stress response
- Pain
- Aspiration of stomach contents

---

secretions, it is also important not to use oversuction and thereby cause unnecessary trauma, irritation and hypoxia.

Weaning

Weaning is the term used to describe the gradual transition from mechanical to spontaneous ventilation (self-ventilation). During the weaning phase, patients may alternate between these modes until they are able to cope continually on a reduced mode, ultimately achieving spontaneous breathing. It should be individually tailored and begun as soon as it is established that the patient is physically capable of maintaining respiration. The nurse has a key role to play in this. Patients who are likely to require ventilation over a longer period of time will be considered for a tracheostomy, which is more comfortable, and the patient will require less sedation (see Chapter 16, Nursing Patients With Disorders of the Ear, Nose and Throat). It is good practice to allow the patient to rest overnight by giving them increased ventilatory support, which will also allow the patient's $PaCO_2$ to return to normal. Each patient should be assessed for readiness to wean each day; an example of a sedation weaning tool can be found on the website.

Extubation

When spontaneous respiration is successfully maintained, the next step is the removal of the ET tube, a procedure known as extubation. Prior to this procedure, ABGs, oxygen saturation, tidal volumes, respiratory rate and pattern, vital signs, any evidence of tiring and the presence of a gag reflex together with a strong cough reflex must all be reviewed. Extubation should not be considered unless the patient can cough, swallow and protect the airway, and is sufficiently alert to cooperate. If possible, a planned extubation early in the day is ideal, with more staff on duty. Emergency equipment should be available in case rapid reintubation is necessary. More information and guidance on extubating patients can be found at Difficult Airway Society 2015 (Useful Websites).

Cardiovascular Care

In critical care settings, monitoring systems are essential to evaluate any potentially fatal physiological derangements and to allow timely treatment to correct any abnormalities. The cardiovascular system can be monitored by the measurement of volume, flow, pressure and resistance in different areas. Chapter 2 covers haemodynamic aspects of care and should be referred to in relation to this section. Patients admitted to critical care units undergo monitoring to glean information about tissue perfusion, blood volume, tissue oxygenation and vascular tone. It is the nurse's responsibility to carefully monitor these parameters and identify changes.

❖ Nursing Management and Health Promotion: Cardiovascular Care

Monitoring Heart Rate and Rhythm

The amount of information that can be gleaned from a three-lead electrocardiogram (ECG) and, more importantly, a 12-lead ECG must never be underestimated and a sound understanding of the heart's electrical activity facilitates this (see Chapter 2, Nursing Patients With Cardiovascular Disorders). Cardiac arrhythmias are commonplace in patients in critical care. Hypoxia, shock, electrolyte abnormalities, sepsis, vagal stimulation from ET suctioning, irritation from central venous or pulmonary artery catheters and medication are responsible for most cardiac arrhythmias; however, some will be the result of myocardial ischaemia in patients with underlying heart disease. Accordingly, where possible, the nurse needs to be aware of any cardiac impairment the patient may have. Monitoring should be continuous, to enable early detection and prompt treatment of underlying problems. For information about the conduction pathways of the heart, arrhythmias and their management, see Chapter 2.

Monitoring Arterial Blood Pressure

Critically ill patients generally have an arterial line inserted for the accurate measurement of arterial blood pressure and the provision of easy access to arterial blood for blood gas analysis. Common sites for the insertion of arterial lines are (in order of preference) radial artery, brachial artery, femoral artery and dorsalis pedis artery (see Chapter 18, Infection Prevention and Control, for care of patients with invasive lines). Together with the systolic and diastolic arterial pressure, the mean arterial pressure (MAP) is also recorded. This gives the measurement of perfusion pressure over much of the cardiac cycle. A MAP of 65–85 mmHg is generally the acceptable range. Below 50 mmHg is dangerous as it is inadequate to perfuse vital organs and tissues. Complications associated with arterial lines can and do arise (Information 28.5).

Monitoring Central Venous Pressure (CVP)

Central venous access is generally preferred over peripheral access, because it enables assessment of the patient's circulating blood volume as well as allowing the administration of intravenous medication such as inotropes, specific antibiotics/antifungals and certain electrolyte supplements that can only be infused centrally. Monitoring the CVP also allows for the assessment of the tone of the vascular system and the ability of the right side of the heart to accept and expel blood, itself influenced by left ventricle function (see Chapter 19, The Deteriorating Patient, Recognising and Managing Shock). The trend of readings, along with other clinical information, is more important than any one individual reading. Insertion of invasive lines is not without its complications. A care bundle should be implemented to manage the care, and the elements are outlined in Information 28.6. The principles of this care bundle are applicable to all invasive lines.

Monitoring Cardiac Output

There are several monitoring indices that can give greater insight into the patient's cardiac performance.

Pulmonary Artery Catheter

A pulmonary catheter enables the assessment of the functioning of the left ventricle and very often becomes part of the monitoring

---

INFORMATION 28.5

Complications Associated With Arterial Lines

- Infection/potential sepsis. Infection can occur during insertion or at the site. Strict adherence to asepsis and the use of occlusive dressing and chlorhexidine to clean the site will reduce this risk.
- Haemorrhage due to disconnection of the line. Check the Luer lock connections and ensure the line is not pulled when moving the patient.
- Air embolism. If air gets into the system, this could be 'flushed' into the patient. Care is required when setting up the transducer system.
- Vascular occlusion/thrombosis (distal circulation should be assessed regularly).
- Ischaemia of the distal limb.
- Poor reading. Lines should be re-zeroed each shift to calibrate the equipment to normal atmospheric pressure. The saline pressure bag should be maintained at 300 mmHg to maintain accuracy and the level of the transducer should be maintained at mid heart.
- Spasm of the artery. This can be caused by forceful flushing of the line or aspirating samples of blood too vigorously.
- Wrongful administration of medication. Arterial lines must be clearly identified to prevent them being confused with intravenous cannulae. Staff must be appropriately trained in their management to prevent this.

INFORMATION 28.6

Central Line Bundle

Insertion Bundle

- Hand hygiene and maximal barrier precautions
- Ensure the procedure is documented in the patient's notes
- Skin asepsis with 2% chlorhexidine
- Catheter site selection: the femoral site should be avoided where possible

Maintenance

- Assess patient daily to determine continued necessity for a central line
- Dressing should be intact, cleaning with chlorhexidine
- Needle-free access devices should be used

---

profile in situations causing either circulatory failure or acute respiratory failure. Its use is considered when information is required about fluid status, cardiovascular function or oxygen delivery. It provides information which guides the therapy of those patients on mechanical ventilation, circulatory assist devices or inotropic medication. The pulmonary artery wedge pressure (PAWP), or 'wedge', gives a more accurate indication of the fluid status of the patient. Elevated PAWP may be due to volume overload, left ventricular failure (LVF), mitral stenosis or regurgitation and cardiac tamponade. Abnormally low readings may be due to hypovolaemia (see Information 28.7).

Oesophageal Doppler Monitoring

Oesophageal Doppler monitoring is a minimally invasive monitoring device that measures the velocity of the blood flow by placing a probe in the oesophagus parallel with the descending aorta. It offers a reduced risk of morbidity and mortality in comparison to the pulmonary artery catheter. This form of monitoring is not suitable for all types of patients; it is most useful as a guide in deciding when, what and how much fluid replacement to give in cases of hypovolaemia.

Haemodynamic Cardiac Profile – Normal Readings

- Pulmonary artery pressure (PAP)
  - systolic: 15–25 mmHg
  - diastolic: 8–15 mmHg
- Pulmonary artery wedge pressure (PAWP): 6–12 mmHg
- Cardiac output (CO): 4–8 L/min
- Cardiac index (CI): 2.5–4.2 L/min per m2
- Systemic vascular resistance (SVR): 900–1600 dyn/s per cm5 (this measurement relates to the resistance to flow in the whole systemic circulation)
- Mixed venous oxygen saturations (SvO2): 65%–75%

INFORMATION 28.8

Inotropic Drugs Commonly Used in Intensive Care and Their Receptors

- Alpha: increase SVR, increase blood pressure (BP), affecting the coronary arterioles and vascular smooth muscle (noradrenaline)
- Beta 1: increase heart rate, increase contractility, affecting the SA node and myocardium (adrenaline, dopamine, dobutamine)
- Beta 2: increase contractility and decrease SVR, affecting the vascular and bronchial smooth muscle, AV node (adrenaline, dobutamine)
- Dopamine receptor (DA1): vasodilation affects kidney and heart (dopamine).

Pulse Contour Cardiac Output (PiCCO)

This method uses a standard central line with a temperature sensor on the distal lumen and a thermodilution sensor arterial catheter in the femoral artery. Injection of cold fluid into the CVP line is sensed by the arterial line. The method allows calculations of cardiac output, cardiac index and stroke volume; it also gives an indication of extravascular lung water. It has the advantage of being less invasive than a pulmonary artery catheter.

Inotropic Medication

Cardiac output monitoring is often used to determine inotropic therapy, as it clarifies whether there is a pressure problem (i.e. reduced blood pressure), a problem with the flow (i.e. decreased cardiac output) or a problem with oxygen delivery and consumption. Cardiac contractility can become impaired, either as a direct result of cardiogenic shock or secondary to hypovolaemic and septic shock. In such cases, inotropic medication such as noradrenaline, dopamine and dobutamine, which improve cardiac contractility, is used to support the patient until such time as definitive treatment is administered or the patient recovers. Administration is always via a central vein and the effects of inotropic therapy are monitored closely. Different combinations of inotropic medication may be advocated to achieve the desired effect. It is common practice to titrate inotropic therapy against MAP, generally aiming for a MAP of between 65 and 85 mmHg; inotropic medication is always reduced slowly by 1 mL at a time before discontinuation. These drugs are highly potent and it is essential that the nurses delivering them have appropriate training and understanding. A brief outline of the commonly used drugs and receptor effects can be found in Information 28.8.

Monitoring and Regulating Temperature

Despite a wide variety of heat-producing metabolic processes and the range of ambient temperatures to which the human body may be exposed, homeostatic mechanisms ensure that core body temperature is maintained with remarkable stability. However, critical illness can disturb temperature control, producing body temperatures at either end of the spectrum, that is, hypothermia (<35°C) or hyperthermia/hyperpyrexia (>38.5°C). High temperatures can have an adverse effect on ICP of patients with unstable head injuries and these patients may be actively cooled. Patients who have suffered cardiac arrest may benefit from therapeutic cooling for brain protection.

Prevention of Thromboembolism

Venous thromboembolism (VTE) is a potentially fatal risk factor in any hospitalised patient and it is significantly increased in critical care patients due to prolonged periods of inactivity, factors associated with the presenting disease process, sedation and paralysis to allow for ventilation. In addition to anticoagulation, compression hosiery and pneumatic compression devices are utilised to minimise risk of VTE events (NICE 2019). It is essential that the patient requirement for DVT prophylaxis is incorporated into the patient's daily assessment (Reflection 28.1).

REFLECTION 28.1

Case History: Mrs C

Mrs C is critically ill following a subarachnoid haemorrhage. She has no medical history of note. What is the most appropriate form of thromboprophylaxis for her?

Answer

Anticoagulants such as heparin will be contraindicated for her due to her recent bleed. She is in a high-risk group; therefore she would have antiembolism stockings and intermittent pneumatic compression applied.

For further reading, see NICE NG89: Venous thromboembolism in over 16s: reducing the risk of hospital-acquired deep vein thrombosis or pulmonary embolism (NICE 2019).

Sepsis

Sepsis is a condition of life-threatening organ dysfunction and hypoperfusion caused by dysregulated response to infection. Left untreated the patient may die. There continues to be a high mortality rate associated with sepsis (Bauer et al. 2020). There has been a great deal of focus on early recognition and treatment of the condition in recent years. Anyone presenting with a high temperature, tachypnoea or compromised circulation should be suspected of having sepsis. The 'Sepsis Six' bundle has been produced to guide staff in early recognition and treatment. The key actions are outlined and can be considered as giving 3 and taking 3 (Macik and Bridges 2018).

- 'Give 3':
  - Administer oxygen to maintain target oxygen saturations greater than 94% (or 88%–92% in people at risk of hypercapnic respiratory failure)
  - Give intravenous broad-spectrum antibiotics
  - Start intravenous fluid resuscitation
- 'Take 3':
  - Take blood cultures and consider other sampling
  - Check serial lactate level
  - Monitor hourly urine output

As well as organ dysfunction, different organisms can present with different features. Meningococcal septicaemia presents with a purple rash, which may lead to ischemia of the extremities requiring amputation. More information on meningococcal disease can be found on the Centers for Disease Control and Prevention website (see Useful Websites).

Immunocompromised patients, the young, elderly or patients with pre-existing comorbidities are more susceptible to sepsis.

Renal Care and Fluid Balance

With the kidney normally requiring 25% of the cardiac output, physiologically compromised patients are at high risk of developing acute kidney injury (AKI), a sudden and usually reversible failure of the kidneys to excrete the waste products of metabolism. This is a common problem in the critical care unit. AKI is characterised by a rapid decline in renal function over days or weeks, which results from the cessation of or decreased urine output and the accumulation of metabolites and electrolytes normally excreted by the kidney.

Causes are divided into prerenal, renal and postrenal. Systemic manifestations may accompany the development of renal insufficiency and these can include lowered haemoglobin level, fluid overload, breathlessness, arrhythmias due to electrolyte imbalance and confusion and itchy skin due to build-up of urea. The treatment of AKI is predominantly one of support until recovery occurs; the condition is nearly always recoverable.

❖ Nursing Management and Health Promotion: Renal Care

AKI is a common complication of critical illness. The primary goal of the critical care team must always be the prevention and detection of renal impairment. This involves knowledge of the causes of AKI and meticulous monitoring of the following.

Urine Output. In addition to the meticulous monitoring of all fluid intake, hourly urine output volumes must be recorded, together with an accurate 24-hour fluid balance of all fluid gains and losses. While a urine output of less than 0.5 mL/kg per hour (oliguria) over a 6-hour period is indicative of AKI, it is also acknowledged that AKI can occur in the absence of oliguria (non-oliguric AKI) when there is an elevated serum creatinine.

Urea and Electrolytes. Daily assays of urea and electrolytes will indicate the degree of renal insufficiency present. Urea, creatinine and some electrolyte levels rise with developing AKI, leading to varying degrees of metabolic acidosis. AKI is diagnosed when serum creatinine increases by greater than 26.5 μmol/L within 48 hours or to 1.5 times baseline within the previous 7 days. It should be noted, however, that elevated urea on its own may indicate merely that the patient is dehydrated. The nurse must know the normal plasma values for urea, creatinine and the more common electrolytes and the significance of any deviations, as some electrolyte abnormalities can produce life-threatening arrhythmias.

Fluid Therapy. Intravenous fluid therapy should be considered carefully in the management of the critically ill patient. This is particularly so in conditions such as sepsis, ALI or systemic inflammatory response syndrome (SIRS). In such situations, the permeability of capillary endothelial cells increases and the vessels become 'leaky', allowing large protein particles to pass into the interstitial space, thus reducing the capillary osmotic pressure. This facilitates the movement of water together with further protein molecules into the interstitial space, depleting intravascular volume and impairing

gaseous exchange. This results in peripheral oedema and, within the lungs, results in pulmonary oedema, causing hypoxaemia and consequently diminished oxygen delivery and consumption by peripheral tissues. Vascular volume must be restored. The three main groups of volume-expanding fluids are crystalloids, colloids and blood:

- Crystalloids are made up of nonionic solutes such as sodium chloride added to water; they do not contain oncotic particles and will therefore eventually move out of the vascular compartment (see Chapter 21). These fluids, unlike colloids, are cheap to produce and are not associated with immunologically mediated reactions.
- Colloids, which contain oncotic particles, generating oncotic pressure, are mainly confined to the intravascular space, at least when first administered.
- Blood and blood products also exert an oncotic pressure due to the large protein particles they contain and so are less likely to contribute to interstitial oedema. Haemoglobin targets for critical care patients are 7 g/dL for most patients. Patients with ischemic heart disease have a greater threshold of 9 g/dL.

Cardiovascular Status. Regular monitoring of the CVP, cardiac output and occasionally, pulmonary artery wedge pressure (PAWP) will indicate whether fluid input or inotropic support is required. The presence of peaked T waves on the ECG is suggestive of a rising plasma potassium level.

Nephrotoxic Medication. The use of nephrotoxics, for example gentamicin and nonsteroidal anti-inflammatory drugs (NSAIDs), should be avoided in those with impending renal failure or in those whose renal function is precarious.

Immediate Management of Diminishing Renal Function

- Optimise fluid balance either by giving a fluid challenge if vital signs indicate hypovolaemia or by using diuretic therapy if there are clinical signs of fluid overload. Furosemide, a potent loop diuretic, is the drug of choice.
- Correct electrolyte imbalances as necessary.
- Maintain haemoglobin within the target range.
- Ensure adequate nutritional input.
- Remove any known causative factors, e.g. nephrotoxic drugs.
- Exclude obstruction, e.g. make sure that the urinary catheter has not become blocked with sediment.
- Diuretic therapy. Diuretics will not alter the course of AKI; however, they may help maintain fluid balance.

Renal Replacement Therapy

A small number of patients in critical care will require renal replacement therapy (RRT) to manage their AKI. While not providing a 'cure', it enables the critically ill patient to be supported pending recovery from the underlying disease process or injury. There are no set criteria for when RRT should be commenced, however, it should be instituted before complications occur. Hyperkalaemia, severe fluid overload, gross uraemia and metabolic acidosis are all indications for treatment (Claure-Del Granado and Clark 2021).

Caring for patients with RRT is deemed part of the professional practice of experienced nurses working in critical care. They require a thorough knowledge of the reasons for its use, the equipment involved, the problems that can arise and how to respond to them.

Haemofiltration

Technology has advanced significantly since the 1970s when the process of RRT was first introduced.

Continuous venovenous haemofiltration (CVVH)/continuous venovenous haemodiafiltration (CVVHD) are the modes of choice in haemofiltration, as they allow the slow, steady removal of fluid volume. They also give the venous system time to compensate for fluid lost from the interstitial spaces. Most importantly, they avoid the rapid shift of solutes and electrolytes, thereby preventing the risk of cardiovascular instability. A further advantage of CVVH/CVVHD is that they do not require arterial access. Access for these modalities is via a double-lumen catheter, often referred to as a Quinton line, which is inserted into a main vein. In CVVH, the blood is pumped through an artificial kidney where fluid, solutes and electrolytes are moved across a semipermeable membrane by convection and ultrafiltration. A set amount of fluid is then added to the circuit to replace the removed fluid. Anticoagulation is necessary to prevent the blood clotting in the plastic circuit. The amount of fluid exchanged and replaced will be prescribed according to the urea and creatinine levels, fluid balance and stability of the patient. In CVVHD, there is an additional counter current running across the semipermeable membrane which increases the efficiency of the movement of urea and creatinine out of the patient's blood.

Nursing Responsibilities in RRT

- **Fluid balance.** Accurate measurement of input and output of fluid is essential, and RRT is reviewed daily by the critical care physicians. The nurse responsible for the patient should adjust filtration rates in accordance with the medical prescription.
- **Vital signs**. At the start of RRT, the patient's blood pressure may fall due to movement of fluid outside of the body and the temperature may also drop. It is generally believed that body temperature drops by 1°C with RRT in progress. To prevent this, the RRT machine warms replacement fluid. It should be noted that RRT may mask developing sepsis, as a recorded temperature of 37°C may equate to a patient temperature of nearer 38°C.
- **Urea, electrolytes and ABGs.** Regular assessment of urea, electrolytes and ABGs is necessary to assess acid–base balance. Electrolyte supplements are often required. Phosphate is normally elevated in AKI; however, it is removed very efficiently on RRT and may require supplementation. Replacement fluids have different concentrations of potassium and are prescribed to meet patient need.
- **Monitoring the activated clotting time (ACT).** The time it takes for a small sample of blood to clot is of particular importance if the patient is receiving heparin as anticoagulation therapy while on the haemofilter. Prostacyclin is an alternative agent which works by inhibiting platelet aggregation; it can be used for patients with a higher risk of bleeding or liver failure patients. It does, however, have strong side-effects, noticeably vasodilatation, causing facial flushing and significant hypotension. ACT is not required with prostacyclin. Citrate is also now commonly used as an anticoagulant; the mechanism of delivery means that it acts locally in the extracorporeal circuit, preventing the wider complications of systemic anticoagulation.
- **Preventing infection and maintaining asepsis** are vital. Patients on RRT are often immunocompromised and therefore are more susceptible to infection. Residual catheterisation may be performed every 2–3 days, preventing stasis of urine in the bladder, a potential source for infection. If urine volume is 250 mL or more, the catheter is normally left in situ, as this can be indicative of the return of renal function.
- **Maintenance of patient safety** is the nurse's responsibility. If venous access is via the femoral vein, the limb must be carefully observed to ensure optimal perfusion is maintained.

Furthermore, the prevention of air emboli, infection or haemorrhage, as a consequence of heparin use, should be borne in mind.

Neurological Care

Altered states of consciousness of critically ill patients fall into two distinct types of causes:

- intracranial pathology, such as intracranial haemorrhage, cerebral hypoxia, space occupying lesions such as tumours and abscesses
- systemic disease affecting the cerebral blood supply or oxygenation, such as sepsis, metabolic encephalopathy, hypoglycaemia, hepatic failure (hepatic encephalopathy), AKI, pancreatitis, respiratory failure or hypo/hyperthermia, exogenous agents, such as drugs and toxins, and drug withdrawal.

❖❖ Nursing Management and Health Promotion: Neurological Care

Neurological functioning is an important part of the overall clinical assessment and continuous care of those being nursed in critical care. The use of a standardised neurological assessment tool such as the Glasgow Coma Scale (GCS) is essential, enabling early detection of any deterioration and facilitating prompt treatment (see Chapter 11, Nursing Patients With Disorders of the Nervous System). In addition, patients with intracranial pathology may require invasive neurological monitoring of ICP and cerebral perfusion pressure (CPP). This is often indicated in patients who demonstrate a GCS of 8 or less and/or a grade 3 or 4 encephalopathy (Information 28.9). As with most clinical observations, it is the trend that is of greatest significance when monitoring ICP and CPP.

Monitoring Neurological Function

Glasgow Coma Scale (GCS). The GCS is the standard tool used in assessing neurological function. It is an objective way of measuring levels of consciousness (LOCs) and is discussed in Chapter 11, Nursing Patients With Disorders of the Nervous System, and Chapter 27, Nursing the Unconscious Patient.

Intracranial Pressure Monitoring (ICP). ICP is the pressure exerted by the intracranial contents against the skull. Normally, brain tissue constitutes 80%, cerebrospinal fluid (CSF) 10% and blood volume 10% of the intracranial contents. Severe head injuries remain the most common cause of raised ICP, but it may also occur in patients presenting with problems such as hepatic encephalitis due to fulminant hepatic failure. This is increasingly seen nowadays as the consequence of paracetamol overdose. The level at which treatment of raised ICP will be necessary depends on the patient's condition but is often set at around >20 mmHg. Medication of choice includes mannitol 20% given in conjunction

---

INFORMATION 28.9

Grades of Encephalopathy

- Altered mood, impaired concentration and psychomotor function, altered sleep rhythm
- Lethargy or apathy, disorientation to time inappropriate behaviour, obvious personality changes
- Semistupor, bizarre behaviour, gross disorientation
- Coma

Adapted from Vilstrup et al. (2014).

with albumin replacement; hypertonic saline (5%) is also effective in treating raised ICP. If ICP is unresponsive to these treatment modalities, barbiturate therapy such as thiopentone may be necessary, which lowers ICP by reducing metabolism to a minimum and lowering blood pressure by reducing venous and arterial tone, thus reducing cerebral perfusion; there is however no evidence this treatment improves outcome (Ragland and Lee 2016).

Cerebral Perfusion Pressure (CPP). The value of monitoring the ICP is that it allows the CPP to be calculated. This is done by subtracting the ICP measurement from the MAP of circulating blood within the cranial cavity (i.e. CPP = MAP – ICP). Generally, the aim is to maintain CPP above 70 mmHg, thus preventing underperfusion of the cerebral tissue.

Computed Tomography (CT) Scan. In relation to neurological functioning, CT scanning is usually performed to detect cerebral haematomas, oedema, infarctions, atrophy, hydrocephalus and tumours.

Cerebral Function Analyser Monitor (CFAM). This comprises a visual display unit which allows the continual monitoring and display of cerebral activity. It is used continuously at the bedside to assess whether the patient is appropriately sedated and is commonly used with patients receiving paralysing agents to detect whether or not they are having seizures.

Nursing Responsibilities and ICP

The maintenance of adequate ventilatory support is essential as hypercapnia and hypoxia will increase cerebral vasodilatation, causing an increase in ICP. Conversely, a low $PaCO_2$ below 3.5 kPa can cause cerebral ischaemia and a target range of 4.5–5.0 kPa is standard for most head-injured patients. Continual monitoring of the end-tidal CO_2 assists with this. To ensure adequate ventilatory support:

- Secure the ET tube with adhesive tape rather than a commercially available securing devices or ties around the neck to avoid restricting cerebral drainage.
- Ensure good head alignment, elevating the head of the bed to promote cerebral drainage.
- Keep all nursing procedures to a minimum and well spaced out. The nurse should consider ET suctioning. The procedure itself will cause a rise in ICP, however, retained secretions will also have a negative impact on ICP.
- Check pupil size and reaction hourly and following all nursing and medical procedures.
- Maintain an accurate fluid balance chart. Monitor and be aware of electrolyte levels, e.g. both hypo- and hypernatraemia can contribute to raised ICP.
- Prevent cerebral ischaemia and maintain CPP above 60 mmHg. Inotropes are often administered to achieve this.
- Provide adequate nutritional support. Patients with ICP problems are often in a hypercatabolic state.
- Assess the need and extent to which pressure area care is appropriate.
- Maintain the patient's temperature at normothermia. Administration of antipyretics such as paracetamol and active cooling may be necessary to achieve this. In some cases of severe cerebral insult, patients may require cooling to hypothermia.
- Seizures may occur after head injury due to direct brain irritation or secondary to hypoxia and hypotension (Kolls and Laskowitz 2018). Close observation for seizure activity and administration of anticonvulsants is necessary.

A therapeutic flowchart on the management of acute head injury can be found on the website.

See Evolve Critical thinking question 28.1

Sedation and Pain Management

❖ Nursing Management and Health Promotion: Sedation and Pain Management

Pain has been identified as a major problem for patients in the ICU. Pain is a subjective experience and the control of pain will require regular assessment and clear documentation. The challenge is to provide the most appropriate form of pain relief. Pain control is covered extensively in Chapter 20 and therefore this section will focus primarily on the assessment of sedation required.

Assessing the Need for Sedation and Analgesics

Most critically ill patients will, at some point during their stay, require sedation and/or analgesics. Sedation may be necessary to produce the respiratory depression required to facilitate adequate ventilation, to aid tolerance of the presence of the ET tube or to decrease anxiety in general. Views and practice have changed considerably over the years from the belief that patients should be heavily sedated and unaware of their surroundings to the current preferred state of lighter sedation while maintaining an optimal state of comfort. Sedation and analgesics can be administered continually or as a bolus, the prescribed regimen being tailored to the needs of each patient. The nurse must constantly assess the sedation level and a number of sedation scaling systems exist to assist with this (Information 28.10); this requires a sound knowledge of the issues surrounding sedation in the ICU, that is, sensory overload and sensory deprivation (see Meeting the Psychosocial, Cultural and Spiritual Needs of the Critically Ill Patient). Optimal sedation should enable the patient to be rousable on stimulation

---

INFORMATION 28.10

Richmond Agitation–Sedation Scale (RASS)

Score	Term	Description
+4	Combative	Overtly combative, violent, immediate danger to staff
+3	Very agitated	Pulls or removes tube(s) or catheter(s); aggressive
+2	Agitated	Frequent nonpurposeful movement, fights ventilator
+1	Restless	Anxious but movements not aggressive vigorous
0	Alert and calm	
−1	Drowsy	Not fully alert, but has sustained awakening (eye-opening/eye contact) to voice (>10 seconds)
−2	Light sedation	Briefly awakens with eye contact to voice (<10 seconds)
−3	Moderate sedation	Movement or eye opening to voice (but no eye contact)
−4	Deep sedation	No response to voice, but movement or eye opening to physical stimulation
−5	Unrousable	No response to voice or physical stimulation

INFORMATION 28.11

Possible Causes of Agitation

Internal – Associated With Illness or Physiology	External – Associated With Physical Environment	Caused by Treatment
Infection Sepsis Fever Encephalopathy Hypoxaemia Hypoglycaemia	Arterial hypotension Inflammation Brain injury Acute renal failure and uraemia Metabolic disturbance Sleep deprivation	Pain – surgical and less overt causes, e.g. ET tube, urinary catheter position Fear and disorientation Withdrawal from sedatives Anxiety and disorientation Alcohol and drug withdrawal Medication and side-effects

Reproduced with permission from Pinder S, Christensen M. Sedation breaks: are they good for the critically ill patient? A review. Nurs Crit Care. 2008;13(2):64–70.

but able to sleep/rest when undisturbed. Keeping the patient comfortable is a balance between under- and oversedation (further reading can be found in Neme et al. 2020).

Daily Sedation Breaks

Patients are assessed each morning by the nurse, and if appropriate the sedation is stopped and the patient allowed to wake. If the patient is cooperative the sedation remains off, but if the patient is distressed or agitated, it is recommenced at half the previous rate and titrated up until the optimal level is achieved. This intervention has been shown to reduce ventilator time and length of stay in critical care (Hellyer et al. 2016).

Agitation and Delirium

Agitation and delirium are common among critically ill patients and are multifactorial; the condition is also referred to as 'ICU psychosis'. Patients may experience anxiety, become paranoid and very disorientated to time and place, hallucinate and become agitated. It is physiological, treatment related and associated with the physical environment; the causes are summarised in Information 28.11. Pharmacological intervention can assist with management of these challenging situations; however identification and correction of underlying pathology are essential in management. The nurse has a key role to play in effectively communicating with and reorientating patients. Ensuring that communication aids such as glasses and hearing aids are worn and optimising the environment to ensure normal sleep patterns can be maintained are essential nursing interventions. Guidelines for the management of delirium are available to facilitate nursing care. Patient assessment for delirium can be done by using an assessment tool; Confusion Assessment Method for the ICU (CAM-ICU) is commonly used to assess patients. More information can be found at www.icudelirium.org.

🌐 See Evolve website Fig. 28.2

Pharmacological Interventions

Four main groups of drugs can be used to enhance patient comfort:

Sedatives. Propofol has anaesthetic properties and is commonly used to sedate patients who require short periods of mechanical ventilation. It is widely used as it provides a controllable level of sedation, which is easily maintained, and recovery is rapid, allowing weaning from the ventilator to progress. Midazolam has sedative, anxiolytic and amnesic properties and has a short half-life. However, it is largely hepatically metabolised and renally excreted and therefore could accumulate should these organs be impaired.

Analgesics. Alfentanil is a valuable analgesic in the ICU, especially when short-term supplementation is required. It is short-acting with a short half-life. Morphine provides safe analgesia but should be used with caution in those with liver and renal impairment.

Neuromuscular Blocking Agents. Commonly referred to as paralysing agents, neuromuscular blocking agents such as atracurium, are occasionally used in specific patient groups. They reduce O_2 consumption and stop respiratory drive in patients who have developed ALI, and lower ICP in head injury.

Antipsychotic Agents. ICU delirium is challenging to treat. Haloperidol or clonidine is usually the medication of choice but should not be given before first assessing the patient's vital signs, clinical condition and the underlying cause of their behaviour.

Nutritional and Gastrointestinal Care

The nurse plays a key role in the nutritional management of the critically ill patient. Critical care patients are at high risk of malnutrition, and the need for nutrition is well recognised. Where possible, such nutritional support should be via the enteral route and started as soon as possible after admission. This will maintain the patient's GI integrity, minimise translocation of organisms, decrease the incidence of infection and aid wound healing. The European Society for Clinical Nutrition and Metabolism guideline on clinical nutrition in the ICU is a useful tool in ensuring early establishment of enteral nutrition (Singer et al. 2019). Most patients in critical care can be fed enterally, the only absolute contraindication being true GI failure. Relative contraindications include bowel anastomosis distal to the feeding tube, pancreatitis or small bowel disease.

🌐 See Evolve website Fig. 28.4 for nasogastric protocol

❖ Nursing Management and Health Promotion: Nutritional and Gastrointestinal Care

Nasogastric (NG) Feeding

NHS Improvement (2016) outlines the steps required to check the correct position of the NG tube; this is done by checking of gastric pH using pH strips. If a pH of less than 5.5 is not obtained, a chest X-ray will be required to confirm the correct placement. Some patients may not absorb their feed due to factors such as opioids and immobility.

Naso-Jejunal Feeding

This involves the placement of a fine-bore tube into the jejunum and may be an alternative for patients who are not tolerating NG feeding. However, an endoscopy is required to achieve this. Some companies have manufactured tubes that can be passed without the requirement of an endoscope; however, the results are not fully consistent.

Parenteral Nutrition

For patients who cannot be fed through the enteral route, parenteral nutrition (PN) is the alternative. It consists of a lipid-based substance that requires administration via a large central vein. Because of the high risk of sepsis, PN should always be administered through a port on the central line that has not previously been used. Meticulous asepsis is required when changing the bags. Careful consideration of the patient's nutritional and electrolyte needs should be made; the dietician and pharmacist are helpful in assessing individual patient requirements. Critical care patients can undergo significant physiological stress and feeding can be a lifesaving intervention. Whilst the use of protocols shows positive results for ensuring early enteral nutrition, feeding regimens must be adapted to meet the patient's individual physiological needs.

Optimal Glucose Control

Critical care patients may have altered blood glucose levels due to acute disease processes, chronic diseases such as diabetes mellitus and administration of inotropic medications, steroids and PN. The 'International recommendations for glucose control in adult non diabetic critically ill patients' (Ichai and Preiser 2010) suggest avoidance of severe hyper- and hypoglycaemia in critically ill patients. They add that there is no universally accepted upper limit, although over 10 mmol/L should be avoided. The Institute for Healthcare Improvement (2008) recommends a target range of 3.5 and 8.5 mmol/L and large variations in glucose levels should be avoided. The brain needs a constant supply of glucose as it is unable to store it. Severe hypoglycaemia is considered at 2.2 mmol/L. In patients unable to express themselves, hypoglycaemia should be corrected even in the absence of clinical signs. The nurse has a key role in monitoring patients' blood glucose levels and administering insulin, usually according to a local protocol.

Maintaining GI Integrity

Maintaining normal bowel function in critical care patients is a real challenge, with patients at risk of both diarrhoea and constipation. The nurse plays a key role in monitoring bowel function.

Constipation

Opioids, immobility, surgery and spinal injury can cause constipation, and pain and abdominal obstruction can be consequences. Many critical care units have bowel management protocols which can reduce the risk with early implementation of aperients and suppositories when required; many units have a bowel protocol to ensure aperients are started early in the patient's stay to avoid complications and discomfort of constipation.

Diarrhoea

Enteral feeding, antibiotics and altered gut motility can cause patients to have diarrhoea, which is uncomfortable and embarrassing for patients as well as putting them at risk of dehydration and skin excoriation. Stool samples should be analysed to rule out any infective cause such as *C. difficile*. Skin can be protected by the use of bowel management systems which use a soft tube inserted into the rectum. Close monitoring of the patient's fluid and electrolyte balance along with reassurance is a key nursing requirement for these patients.

Stress Ulceration

This may develop due to damage to the mucosal layer of the GI tract, often during a period of ischaemic anoxia as part of a shocked state, and can cause haemorrhage (see Chapter 19, The Deteriorating Patient, Recognising and Managing Shock). In addition,

impaired production of gastric mucus, reduced epithelial renewal, disturbed acid–base balance, reflux of bile acids and the presence of uraemia all predispose the patient to gastric ulceration. Enteral feeding decreases the risk; however, in patients being supported by PN, prophylactic medication should be prescribed. However, this can lead to an increased susceptibility to VAP or drug toxicity (Buendgens et al. 2016).

Hygiene, Mobility and Wound Care

Critical care patients range from those who require assistance with all aspects of their care to the high-dependency patient who requires nursing input in the form of rehabilitation and mobilisation. Meticulous assessment skills and individualised nursing care are required to maintain optimal body tissue integrity and organ function.

❖ Nursing Management and Health Promotion: Hygiene, Mobility and Wound Care

Personal Hygiene

Assisting with the maintenance of personal hygiene not only promotes comfort and dignity, but also represents an opportunity for thorough assessment of the patient, including skin integrity, any potential sites of infection, for example cannula insertion site, and the peripheral circulation. The nurse should always maintain the dignity of the critically ill patient.

Oral Hygiene

Most seriously ill patients will encounter oral problems, some specific to the disease and others associated with the medication. There is, for example, an increased risk of mouth ulcers, dry, cracked oral mucosa or yeast growth in those with diabetes mellitus, acute or chronic breathing difficulties and thyroid dysfunction. Furthermore, with the use of certain antibiotics, diuretics or morphine and procedures such as intermittent suction, the potential for oral hygiene problems is heightened.

Eye Care

Critical care patients have reduced ability to use their protective blink reflex and poor eyelid closure. Artificial ventilation causes reduced tear production and decreases venous return leading to conjunctival chemosis. Microbial keratitis and corneal exposure are also risks in the ventilated and sedated patient. To prevent such complications, the Royal College of Ophthalmologists and ICS (2017) state that the eyes should be protected by ensuring eyelid closure, regularly assessed and any disease process referred to ophthalmology and any treatments, for example lubricants, administered when prescribed. The nurse should also ascertain whether the patient is wearing contact lenses upon admission and remove as appropriate.

Maintaining Skin Integrity and Promoting Wound Healing

A sound knowledge is necessary of the factors involved in successful wound healing and those that adversely affect its progress (see Chapter 23, Tissue Viability and Managing Chronic Wounds). The main types of wounds encountered in the ICU are surgical traumatic wounds and pressure ulcers (see Chapter 23).

Pressure Ulcers

Prevention is always better than cure and this is certainly the case when it comes to pressure ulcers. However, with the critically ill patient, the main priority is ultimately to maintain haemodynamic stability and optimise ventilation, and in some cases, this may be jeopardised by turning or rolling the patient. Therapeutic pressure relieving beds are regularly required for the maintenance of skin integrity. There is also a risk of tissue damage due to pressure from equipment, such as an ET tube pressing on the lip, a tightly taped three-way tap or tube pressing on the skin. Pressure ulcers may delay recovery, pose increased infection risks and entail much discomfort for the patient

Promoting and Maintaining Normal Tone, Power and Movement of the Musculoskeletal System

As well as regularly positioning the patient to optimise air entry and ventilation and maintain skin integrity, passive and active exercises should be carried out. In patients who have limited movement or who are unable to move at all, a regimen of passive movements can be implemented which will progress to active/assisted movements as the patient's condition improves. This can counteract effects of bed rest, for example VTE, contractures and foot drop. Physiotherapists play a vital role in assisting with mobilisation as the patient's condition gradually improves. Prolonged critical care stay is a debilitating process for the patient. Interventions that can help improve long-term functionality would be a useful addition to clinical care. Getting patients up to sit in a chair and trying to normalise their daily activity are an essential part of the recovery process.

Prevention of Healthcare-Associated Infection (HAI)

HAI currently attracts a great deal of media attention and its prevention is rightly high on the government's agenda. Critical care patients are at high risk of acquiring infection due to their immunocompromised state secondary to the disease process, and multiple tubes and invasive lines create access points for bacteria (Reflection 28.2). The nurse plays an essential role in its prevention. Excellent nursing care and the use of central line and VAP prevention bundles help in the prevention strategy and isolation of patients with MRSA and *C. difficile*. However, the single most important prevention strategy is handwashing. Nurses not only play a key role with their own practice but are also in a key position to remind other members of the multidisciplinary team to adhere to policy.

Meeting the Psychosocial, Cultural and Spiritual Needs of the Critically Ill Patient

❖ Nursing Management and Health Promotion: Meeting the Psychosocial, Cultural and Spiritual Needs of the Critically Ill Patient

It is important to support the patient psychologically and minimise the stress of the ICU environment. This can be achieved by:
- providing adequate information, reassurance and encouragement
- preventing sensory overload or sensory deprivation
- maintaining natural biorhythms/sleep patterns.

Providing Adequate Information, Reassurance and Encouragement

One of the most challenging aspects of critical care nursing is caring for the patient's psychological needs. The presence of ET

REFLECTION 28.2

Case Study: Mrs T

Mrs T is a 67-year-old woman who was admitted to critical care following a craniotomy and evacuation of subdural haematoma. On arrival from theatre, she was ventilated and had intravenous access and an arterial line. A central line was inserted to support Mrs T's blood pressure with the administration of inotropic medication. She had an indwelling urinary catheter and was commenced on antibiotic treatment.

Mrs T had a past medical history of chronic atrial fibrillation which was treated with warfarin. She also had gastric ulcer disease and was on long-term omeprazole, a protein pump inhibitor. Mrs T also had a hiatus hernia and it was technically very difficult to put down a nasogastric tube to allow enteral feeding to commence.

Mrs T was ventilated for 5 days and discharged on day 6.
What factors put Mrs T at risk of getting an infection?

Answer
- Mrs T had 5 days on a ventilator. Any ventilated patient is at risk of VAP. Neurological patients are also twice as likely to get VAP as general patients.
- Presence of invasive lines – central lines, intravenous cannulae, arterial lines and urinary catheters.
- Bacterial translocation. The passage of indigenous bacteria from the intestinal tract to other areas of the body which can cause sepsis and multiorgan failure in critical care patients. This risk can be reduced by early enteral feeding.
- Recent major surgery. Neurological surgery carries a risk of meningitis or, as with any operation, surgical site infection.
- Antimicrobial treatment. The widespread use of antibiotics also puts patients at risk of developing resistances. It also can alter the ecosystem in the patient's gut leading to overgrowth of some pathogens such as *C. difficile*. Mrs T is at increased risk of this infection due to being on a long-term PPI.
- Immunological competence. The majority of critical care patients develop a degree of immunological compromise due to their underlying conditions.
- Nutritional depletion. It is good practice in critical care to implement enteral nutrition early to reduce nutritional depletion, which is a significant factor in the body's ability to fight infection. In the case of Mrs T, this did not happen due to mechanical problems of siting a nasogastric tube.
- Staff: critical care has a large number of staff. The importance of handwashing cannot be stressed enough.

---

tubes, effect of medication such as sedatives and underlying medical conditions makes communication more difficult but good communication may enable patients to see monitoring equipment as helpful rather than frightening, even if they do not always remember being told about it.

Preventing Sensory Overload or Sensory Deprivation

Critical care is a strange, alien environment to patients, and they are prone to experiencing sensory deprivation. Ensuring that patients have their spectacles and hearing aids available is an important nursing role. As patients are recovering, access to mobile devices (when safe to do so), radios and televisions will help 'normalise' the environment.

Support for each patient is most likely to be optimised when nurses, visitors and the patient collaborate to achieve effective and sensitive communication. It is recognised that nurses who are known to the patient and those in whom they have confidence reduce levels of anxiety and panic.

Maintaining Natural Biorhythms/Sleep

Human beings have biological or circadian rhythms that are normally related to the sleep/wake cycle, including fluctuations in body temperature, blood pressure, heart rate and plasma levels of various hormones. In critical care, there is always a concern that activity and lighting may be constant because of the need for continuous observation and frequent treatment, leading to lack of sleep for patients and disturbance of their biological rhythms, and also contributing to the sensory–perceptual alterations and delirium known to affect a considerable proportion of critically ill people. Diminishing the amount of light, noise and disturbance as far as possible at night can help to minimise such potential problems. It is clear that nursing requires the application of sound knowledge, judgement and skill. Practice must be sensitive, relevant and responsive to the needs of the individual, and nowhere more so than when preventing sleep deprivation.

Cultural Needs and Spiritual Care

Spiritual health relates to having a sense of meaning, hope and purpose in life, not simply to having a religious faith. Cultural and personal values are relevant to purpose in life and should be considered in assessment and care. While it is important for nurses to consider a patient's cultural needs, they must be mindful not to stereotype or make assumptions based on how they perceive or understand the patient's culture. Culture and ethnicity are inextricably linked, and failure to consider culture can lead to a deficit in racially appropriate care.

Some critically ill patients may lose hope and 'give up', ceasing to fight for life, particularly when ill for days or weeks. This can contribute not only to their current physical and emotional experience but also to the outcome of the illness. Anything a nurse can do, either directly or with the help of the patient's family or friends, to help the patient draw on their usual resources and sources of support must be helpful.

Despite the clinical and technological advancements made within critical care, it is becoming ever clearer that systemic and structural inequalities, racism and racial bias exist with regards to the health of Black, Asian and Minority Ethnic (BAME) people and attention should be drawn to decolonising critical care for these patients. An example is awareness that some of the assessment tools, for example CAM-ICU and GCS, may be difficult to understand for non-English speakers and it is possible that nurses or other healthcare practitioners may inaccurately assess the level of consciousness, misdiagnose delirium or inappropriately deem the patient 'unable to assess'. The nurse should provide care that is free from implicit or explicit racism and free from prejudice by developing an understanding of cultural intelligence (Moorley et al. 2020).

The Role of Family and Friends

Family and friends play an important role in relieving social isolation, depersonalisation and disorientation for patients. Yet family and friends are unable to be of maximum help to patients unless they themselves are assured of any necessary help from the nurses in the form of access, information and emotional support. Nurses have a great influence on the extent to which family and friends can support the sick patient during intensive care, after transfer to a ward and then home. Families themselves need significant support when their relative is in critical care, and their anxiety can be relieved by clear explanations. Many critical care units have an open visiting policy, which is welcomed by families. Further reading on experiences of relatives and patients can be found on the Healthtalk website (see Useful Websites).

Due to the nature of critical illness, death rates are high in critical care. The nurse has an integral role in guiding families through difficult processes of end-of-life care.

Patient Diaries

Patient diaries are a simple yet valuable tool in assisting patients come to terms with their experience of critical illness and may reduce the risk of developing anxiety, posttraumatic stress disorder and depression. Nurses, members of the wider clinical team, family and friends are invited to regularly write in the diary for the patient. They 'fill the memory gaps' lost through periods of sedation and amnesia associated with medications and critical illness. They are written in everyday language and contain updates on the patient's condition, significant milestones, things that are happening at home and significant events that the patient may be missing. Patients generally find receiving the diary valuable, but this should be undertaken sensitively by a nurse who is able to explain and talk through the contents. Some units have guidelines on the use of patient diaries.

Organ Donation

Over the last 20 years, many people have been able to survive or have a significant improvement in their quality of life due to receiving heart, lung, kidney, liver or pancreas from a donor. While some organs, most frequently the kidney, can be 'living related' (donated by a close relative), the majority of organs are harvested from intensive care patients, most frequently after devastating brain trauma or haemorrhages. Patients who donate organs fall into two categories.

Donation after brain stem death (DBD): two senior doctors using a set of neurological criteria confirm the patient's death. These patients have an irreversible loss of capacity and consciousness. This diagnosis can only be made with patients on mechanical ventilation.

Donation after circulatory death (DCD): takes place after death which follows the planned withdrawal of life-sustaining treatments that have been considered to be of no overall benefit to a critically ill patient.

Organ donation is carefully regulated and managed in the UK nationally so organs can be matched to recipients. The patient's family plays an important role in the process and are included in the decision making with the Specialist Nurse – Organ Donation (SNOD) playing a key role in supporting the family. Many families get a degree of comfort that a tragic death of a loved one has helped others survive.

For more information on organ donation, visit NHS Blood and Transplant (see Useful Websites).

Summary: Key Nursing Issues

- Care of the critically ill patient is a diverse and ever-expanding field with advances in medicine and technology.

- Patient care is designed to support patients both mentally and physically through a life-changing and life-threatening experience and prevent further complications of infections or secondary complications.

- To be effective, nurses must have a sound knowledge and understanding of physiology and other sciences and how the body works in health as well as in illness.

- The practitioner has a responsibility to ensure that evidence-based care is used to prevent secondary complications to achieve the best possible care for patients and their families. One of the most effective ways of achieving this is by the implementation of care bundles where groups of interventions can be effective in improving patient outcome.

Reflection and Learning – What Next?

- **Test** your knowledge by visiting the Evolve website 🌐 and answering the multiple-choice questions and critical thinking questions.
- **Consolidate** your learning by looking at some of the further reading suggestions, references and specialist websites.
- **Revisit** some of the additional material on the website.

- **Consider** what you have learnt and how this will help your professional development.
- **Reflect** on how you can apply this knowledge to the care of your patients.
- **Discuss** your learning with your mentor/supervisor, lecturer and colleagues.

References

Bauer M, Gerlach H, Vogelmann T, Preissing F, Stiefel J, Adam D. Mortality in sepsis and septic shock in Europe, North America and Australia between 2009 and 2019 – results from a systematic review and meta-analysis. *Crit Care*. 2020;24(239). doi:10.1186/s13054-020-02950-2.

Buendgens L, Koch A, Tacke F. Prevention of stress-related ulcer bleeding at the intensive care unit: risks and benefits of stress ulcer prophylaxis. *World J Crit Care Med*. 2016;5(1):57–64.

Claure-Del Granado R, Clark WR. Continuous renal replacement therapy principles. *Semin Dial*. 2021;34(6):398–405. https://doi.org/10.1111/sdi.12967.

Duke G. Non-invasive ventilation. In: Bersten A, Soni N, Oh T, eds. *Oh's Intensive Care Manual*. 8th ed. Oxford: Butterworth-Heinemann; 2018:483–491.

Hadaya J, Benharash P. Prone positioning for acute respiratory distress syndrome (ARDS). *JAMA*. 2020;324(13):1361. doi:10.1001/jama.2020.14901.

Hellyer T, Ewan V, Wilson P, Simpson A. The Intensive Care Society recommended bundle of interventions for the prevention of ventilator-associated pneumonia. *J Intensive Care Soc*. 2016;17(3):238–243.

Ichai C, Preiser J-C. International recommendations for glucose control in adult non diabetic critically ill patients. *Crit Care*. 2010;14:R166.

Institute for Healthcare Improvement. Evidence-based care bundles; 2018. http://www.ihi.org/Topics/Bundles/Pages/default.aspx.

Intensive Care Society. *Levels of Adult Critical Care*. 2nd ed. 2021. https://ics.ac.uk/resource/levels-of-care.html.

Intensive Care Society. Guidelines for the provision of intensive care services; 2022. https://www.ficm.ac.uk/standardssafetyguidelinesstandards/guidelines-for-the-provision-of-intensive-care-services.

Kolls B, Laskowitz DT. Post traumatic seizures. In: Skolnick B, Alves W, eds. *Handbook of Neuroemergency Clinical Trials*. 2nd ed. New York: Academic Press, Elsevier; 2018:231–243.

Macik MB, Bridges E. Managing sepsis and septic shock: current guidelines. *Am J Nurs*. 2018;118(2):34–39.

Moorley C, Ferrante J, Dangerfield A. Decolonizing care of Black, Asian and minority ethnic patients in the critical care environment: a practical guide. *Nurs Crit Care*. 2020;25:324–326.

NHS Improvement. Patient Safety Alert: nasogastric tube misplacement: continuing risk of death and severe harm. NHS/PSA/RE/2016/006; 2016. https://improvement.nhs.uk/documents/194/Patient_Safety_Alert_Stage_2_-_NG_tube_resource_set.pdf.

National Institute for Health and Care Excellence (NICE). *Clostridium difficile* infection risk with broad spectrum antibiotics; 2015. https://www.nice.org.uk/advice/esmpb1/chapter/Key-points-from-the-evidence.

Pinder S, Christensen M. Sedation breaks: are they good for the critically ill patient? A review. *Nurs Crit Care*. 2008;13(2):64–70.

Ragland J, Lee K. Critical care management and monitoring of intracranial pressure. *J Neurocritical Care*. 2016;9(2):105–112.

Renda T, Corrado A, Iskandar G, et al. High-flow nasal oxygen therapy in intensive care and anaesthesia. *BJA*. 2018;120(1):18–27.

Royal College of Ophthalmologists and Intensive Care Society. Eye care in the intensive care unit. 2017. https://www.rcophth.ac.uk/wp-content/uploads/2021/01/Intensive-Care-Unit.pdf.

Royal College of Physicians. National Early Warning Score (NEWS) 2; 2017. https://www.rcplondon.ac.uk/projects/outputs/national-early-warning-score-news-2.

Sessler CN, Gosnell M, Grap MJ. The Richmond Agitation–Sedation Scale: validity and reliability in adult intensive care patients. *Am J Respir Crit Care Med*. 2002;166:1338–1344.

Singer M, Young P, Laffey J, et al. Dangers of hyperoxia. *Critical Care*. 2021;25(440). doi:10.1186/s13054-021-03815-y.

Singer P, Blaser A, Berger M, et al. ESPEN guideline on clinical nutrition in the intensive care unit. *Clin Nutrition*. 2019;38:48–79.

Tanaka A, Uchiyama A, Kitamura T, et al. Association between early tracheostomy and patient outcomes in critically ill patients on mechanical ventilation: a multicenter cohort study. *J Intensive Care*. 2022;10(1). doi:10.1186/s40560-022-00610-x.

Vilstrup H, Amodio P, Bajaj J, et al. Hepatic encephalopathy in chronic liver disease: 2014 Practice Guideline by the American Association for the Study of Liver Diseases and the European Association for the Study of the Liver. *Hepatology*. 2014;60(2):715–735.

Further Reading

Alobaidi R, Basu RK, Goldstein SL, Bagshaw SM. Sepsis-associated acute kidney injury. *Semin Nephrol*. 2015;35(1):2–11.

British Thoracic Society. BTS/ICS Guidelines for the ventilatory management of acute hypercapnic respiratory failure in adults. *Thorax*. 2016;71(suppl 2):ii1–ii35.

Department of Health (DH). *Comprehensive Critical Care. A Review of Adult Critical Care Services*. London: DH; 2000.

National Institute for Health and Care Excellence (NICE). Venous thromboembolism in over 16s: reducing the risk of hospital-acquired deep vein thrombosis or pulmonary embolism. NICE guideline [NG89]. 2019. https://www.nice.org.uk/guidance/ng89.

Neme D, Aweke Z, Micho H, Mola S, Jemal B, Regasa T. Evidence-based guideline for adult sedation, pain assessment, and analgesia in a low resource setting intensive care unit: review article. *Int J Gen Med*. 2020;13:1445–1452.

Wang F, Bo L, Tang L, et al. Subglottic secretion drainage for preventing ventilator-associated pneumonia: an updated meta-analysis of randomized controlled trials. *J Trauma Acute Care Surg*. 2012;72:1276–1285.

Useful Websites

Centers for Disease Control and Prevention – Meningococcal Disease. https://www.cdc.gov/meningococcal/index.html

Difficult Airway Society, www.das.uk.com/guidelines/das_intubation_guidelines

Healthtalk, https://healthtalk.org/introduction/intensive-care-patients-experiences/.

ICU Delirium, www.icudelirium.org/delirium.html

NHS Blood and Transplant – Organ Donation and Transplantation, www.odt.nhs.uk

29

Nursing the Patient With Burn Injury

BREEDA MCCAHILL

Introduction

Most people experience minor burns more than once in their lifetime but few have any concept of the devastation associated with severe burn injury. Extensive burn injury is catastrophic, both physically and psychologically, for the patient and their family. It is also one of the most challenging and arduous types of injury to treat. In order to help the patient and their family to achieve optimal outcomes, the responsibility of care must be distributed throughout the multidisciplinary team. However, the nurse, being the only professional in 24-hour attendance, will play an especially important role. Nurses also attend to many patients whose burns are not extensive, providing care in the community, in emergency departments (ED) and in general surgical wards. This chapter provides information which will help nurses care for patients with burn injuries in all settings.

Prevention of Burn Injuries

Burns are frequently described as being among the most serious of injuries because of the long-term problems which are often associated with them. Advances in treatment and improved facilities have led to a reduction in mortality rates (Kearney et al. 2018), but the resultant morbidity is such that prevention is the responsibility of all healthcare personnel.

Burn prevention programmes have led to substantial reductions in the incidence of burns in high-income countries. Studies emphasise that, in order to be effective, burn prevention programmes should involve assessment of the incidence of burn injuries, followed by the creation of targeted prevention campaigns based on these factors (Chana et al. 2022).

Assessment

This includes identifying the extent of the problem, its causative agents and any predisposing factors.

The Extent of the Problem

The exact prevalence of burn injury in the UK is difficult to determine as many people experience burns which do not require medical attention. However, it has been suggested that there are approximately 10,000 hospital burn admissions and 300 major burns in adults in England and Wales per year. In Scotland, there is an incidence of 500 hospital burn admissions per year, of which 25 are considered major burns (McCann et al. 2022).

Causative Agents

Scalds and flame burns are the most common type of burn injury. Contact burns (touching hot objects) also have a high incidence. Chemical and electrical burns occur less frequently.

Government statistics (Home Office 2021) identified the most common cause of death in domestic fires as careless handling of fire and hot substances, mainly smokers' materials. Nonfatal burn casualties result from the misuse of equipment or appliances, most commonly cooking appliances. Hot water in plumbing systems is also a considerable cause for concern in countries where there is no legislation governing the upper limit of plumbed water temperature. Although many authorities advocate a temperature of 50°C (which would take 2–3 minutes to cause a burn), because of altered sensation and reduced mobility in older people, this figure has been reduced to 44°C in residential accommodation for older people (Health & Safety Executive 2012).

Predisposing Factors

Epidemiological studies identify toddlers as being at greatest risk of burn injuries, with scalds accounting for most of these (Jordan et al. 2022). Adult high-risk groups include those with epilepsy (Ghoddusi et al. 2019) and those who smoke tobacco and drink alcohol in excess (Palmu et al. 2018). Older people have also been identified as being more susceptible to burn injury and as having a higher mortality rate following injury (Harats et al. 2019). Studies agree that males of all ages are at higher risk than females.

The common denominator of predisposition to burn injury appears to be a combination of reduced awareness of danger and decreased mobility.

Planning and Implementation

Planning for a burns prevention programme must be realistic. While it is impossible to modify certain risk factors, for example gender and age, having identified the groups most at risk, it should be possible to alter some of the related predisposing factors.

There are already numerous health education/promotion campaigns aimed at persuading the public not to smoke and to only drink alcohol in moderation. Unlike the promotion of commercial products, which is based on enhancing pleasure and promising immediate gratification, health promotion usually urges people to stop doing something which they find pleasurable in the hope of long-term benefit. Many of these campaigns are fear based; however, Kok et al. (2018) suggest that the evidence for this approach is poor. Blatant shock tactics are considered unacceptable and are likely to make people 'switch off'. It seems unlikely that those who do not comply would be influenced by the knowledge that smoking and drinking alcohol increase their risk of burn injuries. More subtle, but potentially potent, messages may be conveyed, for example, by incidental reference in popular television series.

Identification of the burn agent or energy source results from epidemiology studies. The agent may be a result of poor design of equipment, for example the hot water jug with a higher centre of gravity than a kettle, or a radiator which produces a high surface temperature. Once the problem has been recognised, design modification may be sufficient to eradicate the danger.

REFLECTION 29.1

Reducing Burn Injuries

Renuka and some friends returned home after a night out and, feeling hungry, decided to have some chips. Renuka put the chip pan on the stove, leaving the fat to heat whilst she checked her e-mail and put on some music. Some time later, smelling smoke, Renuka rushed back to the kitchen to find the pan in flames. In her panic, she tried to douse the flames by smothering them with a towel, which promptly caught fire. She then remembered to put the lid on the pan and turn off the stove. The noise alerted her friends, who phoned the emergency services for an ambulance and the fire service. Renuka was rushed to the nearest ED, where, on examination, she was found to have a total of 8%, mainly superficial, burns to her hands, forearms, chest and face.

Activity

- Reflect on the potential reasons why this burn injury occurred and why the chip pan was well alight before Will and his friends were aware of the fire.
- Visit the Fire Service website (https://www.fireservice.co.uk/safety/chip-pans/) and discuss with your mentor how you could use the Fire Service information to reduce burn injury caused by chip pan fires.

Product modification may be carried out voluntarily by manufacturers; however, legislation is often required. Since 1990, it has been against the law to sell new or re-upholstered soft furnishings which are padded with foam that is not combustion modified or which are covered with fabric that does not resist ignition tests for both smouldering cigarettes and match-like flames.

Previous legislation and regulations include the prohibition of the sale of highly flammable children's nightwear and the requirement that all new gas or electric fires and radiant oil-burning stoves are fitted with a fireguard that passes British Standards specifications.

With regard to the environment, probably the greatest single factor in reducing death and injury by fires in the home has been the introduction of smoke detectors/alarms. In North America, their installation into both new and established domestic properties is legally required. In the UK, legislation is more arbitrary and installation into established properties is voluntary; however, in 2022, the Scottish Government passed a new law whereby all homes, both new-builds and older properties, are now legally need to have interlinked smoke alarms. It must be recognised that the groups at highest risk of burns, that is, older or disabled people, may be less able than others to buy safer soft furnishings and heating appliances. Smoke detectors may be bought for as little as £5, but their fitting, although simple for the able-bodied, may be impossible for older or disabled individuals. Many UK fire services now offer free home safety visits, including free provision and installation of smoke detectors. Healthcare workers, therefore not only have a responsibility to disseminate information on the prevention of burn injuries, but also must work closely with other interested groups such as the Fire Service, The Royal Society for the Prevention of Accidents (see Useful websites) and both local and national government in order to lobby for more effective legislation and regulations (Reflection 29.1). Nurses working in the community have the opportunity to observe the environment and to give specific advice relating to burns prevention.

First Aid Treatment of Burns

Burn injuries result from the transfer of energy from a heat source to vulnerable tissues. The higher the temperature of the heat source and the longer it is in contact with the tissues, the greater will be the destruction.

The first priority of first aid treatment is to remove the individual from the source of heat. If the causative agent is electricity, it is important to switch off the supply, if possible, or to use non-conducting material to rescue the person.

Frequently, there is a continuing source of heat if the individual's clothing is on fire or saturated by a hot liquid. The most effective way to remove this continuing heat source is to throw cool liquid, which is neither flammable nor corrosive, over the affected material, thus dousing the flames or reducing the temperature of the scalding liquid. If no such cool liquid is immediately to hand, rapid removal of hot saturated clothing will arrest the heat transfer. Where clothing is on fire, it is important to stop the person running around as this will fan the flames. The person assisting should lay the victim on the ground and use heavy material such as a coat or blanket to smother the flames. If chemicals are the causative agent, prompt sluicing with copious amounts of water will dilute the strength of the agent and limit the penetration of the chemical into the skin, where it can continue to cause damage for many hours. Some common chemicals such as hydrofluoric acid which is used in both industrial and domestic settings are also treated with specific neutralising agents as advocated by Huang et al. (2021).

In the clinical situation, a useful means of identifying whether a chemical is acid or alkaline is to apply litmus paper, as this will give a pH reading.

After removal of the heat source from the skin, the next measure is to cool the superheated tissues. In their first aid clinical practice guideline, the British Burn Association (2018a) advises applying cool running tap water to the affected area for 20 minutes. They also suggest cooling is beneficial for up to 3 hours after injury, and should still be performed, even if there is a delay in accessing a method of cooling. For the face, however, cold soaks should be applied. The application of ice or chilled water below 8°C is contraindicated, as studies have found that this was associated with delayed healing (Wright et al. 2015). There is no doubt that continued cooling reduces pain from the burn wound, but if a large area of the body surface is involved, there is a risk of hypothermia.

Since patients with extensive burns have problems retaining body heat, the use of space blankets or other heat-retaining coverings is advised during transfer to hospital.

Many national and International burns first aid guideline also recommend polyvinyl chloride film, for example cling film as the temporary wound cover of choice while awaiting transfer to ED or Burns Services (McLure et al. 2021). The reasons for this are:
- It does not adhere to the wound surface and cause pain on removal.
- It conforms closely to the body contours and excludes air, thus reducing pain.
- The wound can be viewed without removal of the transparent film.

However, this kind of material should only be used after cooling of the burn wound is complete. It should not be layered and should never be wrapped around a limb to avoid a tourniquet effect should swelling occur. The use of ointments, lotions and powders should also be avoided in the immediate first aid period as they may change the appearance of the wound and thus impair the assessment of the burn depth.

To summarise, first aid treatment of burn injuries consists of:
- separating the individual from the source of injury
- cooling of the affected part with cold water for 20 minutes or application of cold water soaks to the face
- application of cling film; cold soaks may be used for wounds which are not extensive.

Assessing the Severity of Burn Injuries

The majority of patients with burn injuries do not require hospitalisation. The UK National Burn Care Referral Guidance (National Network for Burn Care 2012) identifies factors to be considered when deciding whether to refer patients to a burn service, rather than simply considering the size of the burn wound. The thresholds for adult patients for whom referral to or discussion with a burns service is advisable include those:
- whose burns exceed 3% of the body surface area
- with full-thickness burns
- with burns on functionally important areas such as face, hands, feet, perineum, joints or flexor surfaces
- with electrical or chemical burns
- with burns not healed within 2 weeks
- with associated injuries, e.g. smoke inhalation
- with any comorbidities that may affect treatment or healing of the burn.

For patients who do not fall into any of these categories, relief of pain and local treatment of the burn wound are generally all that is required. Both interventions will be described later.

Assessment of the severity of the burn injury involves estimation of the:
- extent of body surface area involved
- depth of tissue damage
- probability of associated respiratory tract injury.

Knowledge of the circumstances of the accident, for example whether electricity was involved, and information about the individual's general health and domestic situation will help in deciding whether the patient may, or may not, be managed by the primary healthcare team.

Extent of Burn

Whenever tissues are traumatised, the inflammatory response occurs, resulting in increased circulation to the area (hyperaemia) and increased movement of fluids from intravascular to interstitial compartments. If this occurs in a small area, that is, over less than 5% of the body surface, the effects are localised. However, when a larger percentage of the body surface is injured, there is a massive shift of fluids into the tissues with a corresponding reduction in circulating volume. It is generally accepted that children with burns involving more than 10%, and adults with burns of more than 15%, of body surface area will suffer from hypovolaemic shock unless there is prompt intravenous replacement of fluid (see Chapter 19, The Deteriorating Patient, Recognising and Managing Shock).

In order to estimate the percentage of body surface affected, the simplest and most easily remembered method is the long established 'rule of nines' introduced by Wallace in 1951 (Fig. 29.1). In this method, the head and upper limbs each equal 9%, while the anterior trunk, the posterior trunk and the lower limbs each equal 18%. The remaining 1% is usually applied to the perineum.

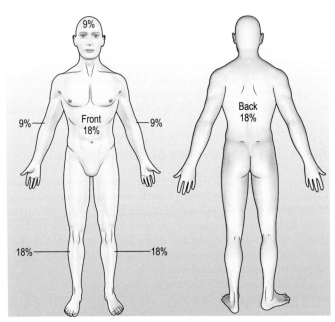

Figure 29.1 Wallace's rule of nines.

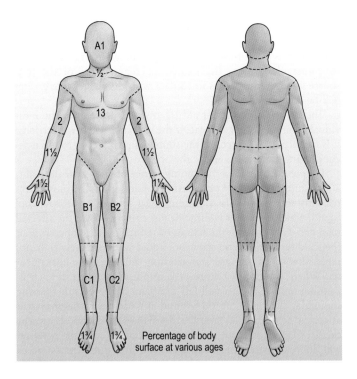

Percent of areas affected by growth

	0	1	5	10	15	Adult age
A = ½ head	9½	8½	6½	5½	4½	3½
B = ½ one thigh	2¾	3¼	4	4¼	4½	4¾
C = ½ one leg	2½	2½	2¾	3	3¼	3½

To estimate the total of the body surface area burned, the percentages assigned to the burned sections are added. The total is then an estimate of the burn size.

Figure 29.2 The Lund and Browder burn chart.

Another rapid approximation of the percentage can be made by using the palmar aspect of the patient's hand (with fingers together) as 1% of the body surface area.

The rule of nines should never be used for estimating burn percentage in young children as it does not allow for the different proportions of head and lower limbs in infants and toddlers. Under the age of 1 year the child's head equals 19% of the body surface area and the lower limbs are correspondingly smaller. A more accurate chart which allows for the changing proportions of different age groups and which shows percentages applicable to smaller, more specific areas of the body surface is the Lund and Browder (1944) burn chart (Fig. 29.2). This is generally in use in specialist units and is available in EDs throughout the UK.

Burn Depth

The depth of a burn influences the rate at which the wound will heal spontaneously. The longer the wound takes to heal, the greater the probability of infection and the worse the scarring and loss of function. There are a number of methods of classifying burn depth. In the UK, the most popular is to differentiate between partial-thickness and full-thickness skin destruction. Partial-thickness burns involve the epidermis and part of the dermis. Full-thickness burns destroy the epidermis and all of the dermis.

🌐 **See Evolve website Figs. 29.1 and 29.2**

Full-thickness burns may also involve deeper structures such as fat, muscle and bone. Partial-thickness burns are classified as 'superficial' or 'deep', depending on the amount of dermis involved. As a general rule, deep partial-thickness and full-thickness burns require skin grafting.

As may be seen from Fig. 29.3, the more superficial the injury, the greater the number of surviving epithelial sources from which cells migrate across the wound surface; thus, a more superficial burn heals more rapidly and causes less wound contraction. The effects of superficial partial-thickness burns and full-thickness burns are described below and in Table 29.1.

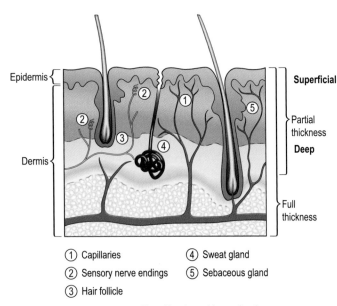

① Capillaries ④ Sweat gland
② Sensory nerve endings ⑤ Sebaceous gland
③ Hair follicle

Figure 29.3 Classification of burn depth.

Superficial Partial-Thickness Burns

These burns are very painful as the sensory nerve endings are stimulated by the injury or exposed to air. They are characterised by oedema, blister formation and serous exudate where the blisters

TABLE 29.1   Indications of Burn Depth

Depth	Signs and Symptoms	Related Anatomy/Physiology
Superficial partial-thickness burns	Very painful	Sensory nerve endings in the dermis are stimulated by the injury and/or exposed to air
	Oedema, blister formation, serous exudate where blisters have burst	As a result of the inflammatory response, the capillary walls are more permeable and fluid leaks into the interstitial spaces of the dermis, collecting below the nongerminating layers of the epidermis or exuding from the wound surface
	Wound surface warmer than unburned skin	Also due to the inflammatory response; arteriolar dilatation causes increased blood flow
	Wound appears bright pink and blanches with pressure	Due to increased blood flow; pressure greater than capillary blood pressure occludes the flow of blood
Full-thickness burns	Painless, no sensation	Sensory nerve endings in the dermis are destroyed
	Wound surface dry. No blistering	Cessation of blood flow through dermal capillaries
	No overt oedema	Necrosis of dermis renders it inelastic
	Wound surface cooler than unburned skin	Cessation of blood flow through dermal capillaries
	Wound colour may be white, brown, translucent showing thrombosed vessels, or bright red (does not blanch on pressure)	Cessation of blood flow through dermal capillaries. Brown or red appearance is caused by release of haem pigments from the destroyed erythrocytes (red blood cells)

burst. The blistering results from the increased permeability of the capillary walls, with fluid leaking into the interstitial spaces and from the wound surface. This fluid collects into blisters beneath the nongerminating layers of the epidermis. Heat radiates from the wound surface due to arteriolar dilatation and increased blood flow and as part of the inflammatory response. This also causes the typical bright pink appearance of the wound, which will blanch on pressure. On removal of the pressure, the hyperaemia is restored.

Full-Thickness Burns

These burns are insensate (without sensation), as the sensory nerve endings have been destroyed. There is normally no blister formation and the wound surface is dry. There is no overt oedema, the wound surface is cool to the touch and the colour may be white, brown or bright red with no blanching on pressure.

These characteristics are all due to the fact that there is no surviving circulation within the dermis. The brown or red colour is due to the release of haem pigments from destroyed erythrocytes. The area may appear translucent with thrombosed vessels being apparent. It is important to recognise that there is an inflammatory response in deeper tissues affected, but this is masked by overlying necrotic tissue. High temperatures (>60°C) cause coagulation of the tissue proteins and water is lost from the cells, interstitial spaces and blood vessels, resulting in a degree of contraction of the affected tissues. Destruction of the dermis renders the skin inelastic and the texture becomes firm and leathery. This is known as eschar.

Deep Partial-Thickness Burns

As the depth of destruction in this type of burn is between those of superficial partial-thickness and full-thickness burns, the presenting signs and symptoms are between the extremes in sensation, blistering, temperature and colour.

Problems in Assessment

The assessment of burn depth is an inexact science. Frequently, assessment of burn depth is dependent on the visual characteristics of the wound and sensation of the wound bed surface, the information regarding the circumstances of the accident, the agent

involved and the first aid measures carried out. Other more objective techniques including laser Doppler imaging and video microscopy have been used successfully in aiding assessment of burn depth (Ponticorvo et al. 2019), however these options are not readily available outside of specialist burn units.

Burn-Associated Respiratory Tract Injury

Inhibition of respiratory function may result from thermal injury to the skin of the trunk and neck. Hidden oedema formation below the leathery, inelastic eschar of circumferential full-thickness burns causes pressure on the deeper structures. In deep burns of the neck, this may cause compression of the trachea and, if there is involvement of the chest and upper abdomen, will inhibit expansion of the thoracic cavity. Decompression by escharotomy will be required (Reflection 29.2).

Inhalation of smoke and hot toxic gases is frequently associated with burn trauma. The main types of inhalation injury are:
- intoxication and hypoxaemia (reduced oxygen in arterial blood)
- thermal damage to the airways
- respiratory tract injury due to irritants.

Intoxication and Hypoxaemia

Intoxication and hypoxaemia most commonly result from inhalation of carbon monoxide (CO) and/or hydrogen cyanide produced by burning plastics.

CO, produced by the combustion of carbon and organic materials in a limited oxygen supply, has an affinity for haemoglobin many times that of oxygen. Therefore following inhalation of CO, there is displacement of oxygen from haemoglobin and the production of carboxyhaemoglobin (COHb) with resulting generalised hypoxia (reduced oxygen in the tissues). The symptoms of CO poisoning are related to the concentration of the inspired gas and to COHb levels and are recognised as mild headache, dizziness, confusion, irritability, nausea, vomiting and fainting. At higher levels, there will be convulsions, altered consciousness, respiratory failure and death. Diagnosis is suggested by the typical cherry pink appearance of the patient and confirmed by checking COHb levels. The formation of COHb can be reversed by the administration of high concentrations of oxygen.

Hydrogen cyanide is rapidly absorbed through the lungs and inhibits cell function, which results in metabolic acidosis. It causes loss of consciousness, neurotoxicity and convulsions.

Thermal Damage

The upper airway may be damaged by the inhalation of hot gases, hot vapours or combustible gas mixtures. Mucosal oedema will narrow the lumen of the airway. The diagnosis is suspected where there is a history of explosion, burns of the face, singed nasal hairs, erythema and ulceration of the oropharynx. Hoarseness and inspiratory stridor (harsh breathing sound due to turbulent airflow through narrowed airways) may present later. As signs of upper airway obstruction may take several hours to become apparent, constant supervision is required.

Hot, dry air seldom causes burns of the airway below the level of the epiglottis as the respiratory tract has an excellent heat exchange capability. Injury to the lower airway is most commonly caused by inhalation of toxic chemicals.

Inhalation of Irritant Chemicals

The combustion of various materials produces a wide spectrum of irritant chemicals, including chlorine, formaldehyde and phosgene. The extent of the resultant damage to the respiratory system is determined by the density of the smoke and the duration of exposure. Patients who are asleep or under the influence of drugs or alcohol at the time of the fire will tend to have a longer exposure time, as will those who have restricted mobility, for example older people or people with a disability.

When irritant chemicals bound to carbon particles settle on the respiratory endothelium, the following events occur:
- inflammatory response
- inflammation of the alveolar capillary membrane
- bronchospasm
- chemical denaturation (change in basic structure or nature) of proteins
- loss of surfactant production by type II alveolar cells.

Surfactant normally lowers the surface tension of the alveolar walls, thus preventing collapse, and also prevents the transudation of fluid from capillaries into the alveoli. Loss of surfactant production will therefore lead to atelectasis (see Chapter 3, Nursing Patients With Respiratory Disorders).

In summary, the pathophysiological results of the inhalation of irritant chemicals may include tracheobronchitis (inflammation of the trachea and bronchi), pulmonary oedema, atelectasis and airway obstruction. These are frequently compounded by infection.

In cases where the patient survives long enough for admission to hospital, the respiratory damage related to inhalation of smoke may take several hours or even days to become manifest. Suspicion should be aroused where:
- the fire occurred within an enclosed space, especially at night
- the history suggests exposure to smoke, especially if the patient required bodily rescue
- the patient's breath and clothing smell of smoke
- the conjunctivae are inflamed
- carbon particles are present in clothing, wounds, nose, mouth and sputum.

Other Injuries

The appearance of a patient with extensive burns may be so visually dramatic as to distract the assessor from checking for other, less obvious, injuries. Fractures, internal injuries and spinal cord damage may have been sustained, especially if the burn was a result of a road traffic accident, an explosion or high tension electricity, or if the patient jumped from a burning building.

The Patient With Extensive Burns

Early Problems and Nursing Care

The patient with extensive burns has multiple problems, the relative urgency of which will vary during the perhaps very prolonged period following injury. There is increasing awareness that extensive burn injury causes a systemic inflammatory response syndrome (SIRS) in which there is widespread disorganisation of the immune system, eventually resulting in multiple organ dysfunction syndrome (MODS) (Chapter 19, The Deteriorating Patient, Recognising and Managing Shock, and Chapter 28, Nursing the Critically Ill Patient) (Toliver-Kinsky et al. 2018).

During the first 36–48 hours, however, the most life-threatening problem, except where inhalation injury is present, will be burn shock. Shock is covered in Chapter 19, but a summary of events which have particular relevance to burns injury is given here (Table 29.2).

The initial physiological response to a burn injury results in plasma loss from the circulation. This is accompanied by:
- Gross oedema of the affected tissues.
- Hypovolaemia – as in all types of shock, this results in decreased circulation to the skin, muscle and internal organs. Cerebral and coronary perfusion, being of greatest priority, are temporarily maintained.
- Haemoconcentration – unlike the hypovolaemia which results from haemorrhage, the loss of plasma alone from the intravascular compartment causes an increase in the ratio of blood cells to plasma in the circulation, a raised packed cell volume (haematocrit). This increases the viscosity of the blood, further reducing the flow through the capillaries.

TABLE 29.2	Pathology and Related Signs and Symptoms of Burn Shock
Pathological Condition	**Clinical Signs and Symptoms**
Hypovolaemia	Thirst Rapid, weak pulse Hypotension Peripheral and splanchnic (relating to the viscera) vasoconstriction
Peripheral vasoconstriction	Pale skin and mucosa Extremities feel cold Patient complains of feeling cold
Reduced perfusion of kidneys	Oliguria, anuria Impairment of renal function Metabolic acidosis Renal failure may occur
Red cell haemolysis	Haemoglobinuria (haemoglobin in the urine) Renal failure may occur
Reduced perfusion of lungs	Rapid, shallow breathing Air hunger – gasping
Reduced perfusion of gastrointestinal tract	Reduced absorption and intestinal stasis Vomiting, loss of electrolytes and fluid Paralytic ileus, lack of bowel sounds Bacterial translocation through mucosa
Hypoxaemia/electrolyte imbalance	Restlessness, disorientation, confusion May lead to altered consciousness and death

In addition to suffering from burn shock, the patient may be emotionally shocked, in great pain and have extensive destruction of the skin and, possibly, deeper structures. There may be associated injuries, especially inhalation of smoke, and a preburn illness may be present.

Haemoglobinuria (haemoglobin in the urine) may develop in patients who have been badly burned, as thermal injury destroys red cells (intravascular haemolysis). The resultant free haemoglobin in the blood will damage the kidneys and can cause renal failure, especially if renal perfusion is poor due to hypovolaemia.

The Emergency Department

To those unfamiliar with burns, the patient with extensive burns may not appear to be critically ill. The loss of plasma from the circulation is less rapid than haemorrhage from ruptured vessels and the patient may appear quite well. Inexperienced staff should consult with their designated burns service to ensure that treatment is appropriate to the severity of the injury.

The International Society for Burn Injuries (2016) practice guidelines identify the following principles of primary assessment and management by medical personnel:

- **A** Airway maintenance and cervical spine control
- **B** Breathing and ventilation
- **C** Circulation; cardiac status, with control of haemorrhage if present
- **D** Disability, neurological status
- **E** Exposure with environmental control; evaluation of extent and depth of injury, including removal of jewellery and keeping the patient warm

These are followed by X-ray of the cervical spine, chest and pelvis to exclude associated injury.

After life-threatening conditions have been excluded or treated, the secondary survey should be commenced. This includes a patient history, description of the incident and complete examination.

Except in instances where nurses are specially educated, the role of nursing staff is to assist with the earlier procedures, to support the patient and their relatives and to keep meticulous records of fluid balance and of medications given.

🌐 **See Evolve website Critical thinking question 29.1.**

Transfer of the Patient With Extensive Burns

The patient should be prepared for transfer with the application of a temporary wound dressing, preferably cling film, and covered with a space blanket or layers of ordinary blankets. As described earlier, there is a high risk of hypothermia, especially during transfer. If there are airway problems, the patient must be accompanied by an experienced nurse, as well as by a member of the medical team Monitoring of vital signs and maintenance of the intravenous fluids are usually carried out by the nurse. The speed of travel is frequently rapid, which will make the task of monitoring and recording fluid balance and vital signs very difficult; nonetheless, these records are important and, along with the ED file, should be given to the staff of the burns unit on arrival.

Admission to a Regional Burns Unit

Reception of the Patient

When the patient arrives at the unit, they should be greeted sensitively and orientated as to place, as many regional burns units and national burn centres receive patients from a wide catchment area. Where possible, the patient should be reassured and given a simple explanation of what is being done at every stage of the admission procedure and thereafter, throughout their in-patient stay. The appearance and smell of the burn wounds may be very upsetting, not only for the patient but also for inexperienced staff. It is important for staff to appear calm and confident, thus helping to reassure the patient.

The receiving staff must use personal protective equipment (PPE), for example, waterproof gowns, plastic aprons or tabards and gloves. This is to protect staff against contact with wound exudate and fluids. These measures also prevent spread of infection within burn patients (Norbury et al. 2016).

The patient should be received into a single room warmed to a temperature of 28°C, as heat loss from the inflamed wounds, in addition to evaporative heat loss from the wound exudate, can be extensive.

Maintaining the Airway

If the patient has inhalation injury, endotracheal intubation and assisted ventilation may have been instituted in the ED or may be required at the time of admission to the unit. In any case, all nursing care and observations relative to this treatment must be carried out (see Chapter 3, Nursing Patients With Respiratory Disorders, and Chapter 28, Nursing the Critically Ill Patient).

Constant observation of respiratory rate and ease, and of the colour of unburned skin and mucosa, must be carried out and recorded. Humidified air or oxygen administered by face mask or nasal catheter may be required.

Weighing the Patient

If possible, an accurate body weight in kilograms should be obtained as this is one of the baseline measurements on which the volume of fluid replacement is calculated. Estimation of weight is sometimes carried out but, unless the person doing so is experienced in this, gross over- or undertransfusion may result. In many units the patient is weighed on a special bed or sling, still covered in the blankets and temporary dressings used for the transfer; these are then gently removed and the patient is covered with sterile sheeting, for example linen, foam or cling film. The original coverings are then weighed and their weight subtracted from the total in order to get a naked weight. It is important to record the weight immediately as the exact figure may easily be forgotten, especially if there is a great deal of activity in the room.

Wound Assessment

Medical staff will estimate the depth of the burn wounds and chart their position and extent. Colour photographs will usually also be taken for recording purposes. In addition to being useful baseline records of wound appearance and distribution, the photographs may, with the patient's permission, be used in evidence in any subsequent criminal or civil proceedings relating to the circumstances of the burn injury. Whilst the wounds are exposed, the nurse can take swabs for bacteriological examination from each wound site, for example right hand, left hand, chest and neck. This reduces the possibility of wound contamination and the discomfort and possible loss of dignity suffered by the patient during repeated removal of the wound coverings. The initial wound swabs usually show no bacteriological contamination but provide a useful baseline for further monitoring. The wounds are then covered with a temporary dressing. Specific care will be carried out once the patient's condition has been stabilised.

Bacteriology swabs from nose and throat are also obtained in order to identify commensals which may act as wound pathogens (Chapter 18, Infection Prevention and Control).

Analgesics

Intravenous analgesics, usually in the form of morphine, are administered by infusion pump, giving an initial dose and then at an hourly rate of 20–30 µg/kg. The intramuscular route is never used if the patient is in shock, as the medication will not be absorbed owing to the peripheral vasoconstriction.

Intravenous Fluid Replacement

Once an accurate body weight has been obtained and the percentage area of the burn estimated (Figs 29.1 and 29.2), medical staff will calculate the volume of intravenous therapy required by using these parameters within a fluid resuscitation formula. Gillenwater and Garner (2017) discuss that there are a number of different formulae available, however the Parkland Formula is most commonly used. Regulation of the rate of flow and recording of the volume transfused, as well as care of the intravenous cannula site, is the responsibility of the nurse. A volumetric intravenous pump provides accuracy for the infusion of volumes required in each period which may be very large.

Monitoring Urine Output

If this has not been carried out in the ED, an indwelling urinary catheter is inserted, the bladder emptied and the urine volume measured. A specimen is tested for specific gravity and tested using a urine testing strip. The appearance is noted. A urimeter, which allows hourly measuring and sampling whilst maintaining a closed system, is attached to the catheter. Gillenwater and Garner (2017) emphasise the importance of monitoring renal function and that this is most commonly performed through regular, hourly measurement of volume and composition of the urine. A volume of 0.5–1.0 mL/kg body weight hourly is generally accepted as indicating that intravenous fluid replacement is satisfactory, although urine concentration, measured by specific gravity or osmolality, must also be estimated in order to assess renal function.

The appearance of the urine is monitored for indications of haemoglobinuria, such as dark coloured urine and, if this is present, for indications that it is diminishing. It is important that the nurse inform the medical staff at the first indication of haemoglobinuria, as it is imperative that this is treated quickly.

Monitoring Vital Signs

Pulse. If the patient is shocked, the pulse will be rapid and weak. This, combined with generalised oedema, can make manual counting very difficult and mechanical aids are normally used.

Blood Pressure. Where all four limbs have been burned, it is not usual practice to record blood pressure. Indeed, even if one limb is unaffected it has been considered more important to ensure effective intravenous access and fluid replacement than to repeatedly constrict the vessels with a blood pressure cuff.

The routine measurement of central venous pressure or arterial pressure is not recommended in most UK burns units because of the risk of systemic infection associated with such invasive techniques, especially if the site of entry of the catheter is close to the burn wound.

Temperature. A good indicator of the state of peripheral perfusion is the difference between core and shell temperatures. In the normal person, under warm conditions, the temperature of a toe is 1–4°C lower than rectal temperature, but in the patient suffering hypovolaemic shock, the vasoconstriction is such that the difference may be as much as 15°C. Temperature monitoring is usually facilitated by the use of thermistor probes in preference to the repeated insertion of a rectal thermometer. In some units a specially designed probe is inserted into the external auditory meatus in preference to using the rectum. If thermistor probes are not available, it is possible to gauge the shell temperature by feeling the temperature of the peripheries, especially the toes or the tip of the nose.

In addition to monitoring the difference between a normal core temperature and changes in the shell temperature, measuring the core temperature will, of course, also indicate a trend towards hyperpyrexia or hypothermia.

Oral Intake

Because of the reduction in gastrointestinal tract perfusion which results from hypovolaemia, it is necessary to restrict the volume of oral fluids initially, even if the patient is very thirsty, until it has been established that there is no nausea or vomiting. If there is persistent vomiting, a nasogastric tube is passed and is either allowed to drain freely or aspirated hourly before small amounts of water are given.

Patient Behaviour

In addition to recording clinical measurements as described previously, it is useful for the nurse to keep a record of the patient's behaviour, noting for example restlessness, confusion, distress or apathy, as these, along with the measured recordings, will give a more complete picture of the patient's condition. If there is cause for concern,

Complications of Burn Injuries

In some patients with extensive burns, recovery from the initial injury may be complicated by severe episodes of conditions that include (see Chapter 19, The Deteriorating Patient, Recognising and Managing Shock, and Chapter 28, Nursing the Critically Ill Patient):

- severe sepsis
- acute/adult respiratory distress syndrome (ARDS)
- disseminated intravascular coagulation (DIC)
- gastrointestinal ulceration and haemorrhage
- systemic infection of the respiratory system or urinary tract, wound infection
- wound contraction and scar formation.

monitoring of neurological status is facilitated by use of the Glasgow Coma Scale (see Chapter 27, Nursing the Unconscious Patient).

The Postshock Phase

After the first 36–48 hours following injury, the fluid in the interstitial spaces is reabsorbed into the circulation and, although there is continuous fluid loss through exudate and evaporation from the wound surface, there is normally no longer a need for intravenous replacement of fluids. Unless complications arise (Information 29.1), the intermediate stage of management will have been reached.

Nursing management during the intermediate stage of burn injury recovery follows the basic principles of burn care whatever the extent of body surface involved. Thus, nursing priorities include:

- pain relief
- hydration and nutrition
- prevention of infection and local wound care
- psychosocial support for patients and relatives.

Hydration and Nutrition

Until wound closure is complete, there will be continuous loss of the water, protein and electrolytes which comprise the wound exudate (see Chapter 21, Maintaining Fluid, Electrolyte and Acid–Base Balance). In addition, nutritional requirements will be increased because of the elevation in the metabolic rate resulting from trauma, as well as the cellular requirements of wound healing. In patients whose burn area is less than 20% of the body surface, oral intake of a normal diet, perhaps supplemented with high-protein, high-calorie drinks, should be all that is required. However, dietary intake should be monitored to allow assessment by the dietitian and the patient should be weighed weekly. The patient should be encouraged to take fluids and the fluid balance should be monitored and charted.

In more extensive burns, metabolic requirements will be greatly increased, making enteral nutrition via a nasogastric tube necessary. There are a number of proprietary preparations of enteral feeds available and the dietitian will prescribe the type, volume and rate of administration for each individual. If there is a problem with using the nasogastric route, percutaneous endoscopic gastrostomy (PEG) may be performed. Parenteral nutrition is reserved for patients who are unable to achieve adequate nutrition by the preferred enteral route (Clark et al. 2017) (see Chapter 22, Nutrition and Health).

Prevention of Infection

Both nonspecific and specific mechanisms of the immune system are impaired in patients with extensive burns (see Chapter 7, Nursing Patients With Disorders of the Immune System, and Chapter 18, Infection Prevention and Control).

Because of the large areas of skin destruction and the presence of exudate and necrotic tissue, burn wounds rapidly become colonised with bacteria. It has been found that most of the bacteria are acquired from other contaminated patients or equipment in the ward or unit and therefore meticulous attention must be paid to the prevention of cross-infection (see Chapter 18). When possible, the patient should be nursed in a single room and standard infection control precautions implemented. Once the patient's wound becomes colonised with an organism, it will soon be found on their bedclothes, personal clothing and on the surface of dressings. PPE must be worn whenever the patient is attended to; this normally consists of plastic tabards or water-resistant gowns. Gloves should be worn during any direct contact with the patient and the immediate surroundings; clean rather than sterile gloves may be used for most procedures, apart from those requiring an aseptic technique. Adherence to good handwashing practice requires frequent emphasis (Coban 2012).

The bacteriological status of the wounds should be monitored regularly by obtaining wound swabs during dressing changes.

The Burn Wound

As for any wound, the aim of management is to provide the optimal environment for the natural healing processes to take place (see Chapter 23, Tissue Viability and Managing Chronic Wounds). However, most burn wounds involve larger areas of the body surface than is common in other types of wound and this presents many problems in wound management.

See Evolve website Critical thinking question 29.2

Most burn wounds exude copious amounts of fluid. This is evident in superficial partial-thickness wounds from the outset. In deeper wounds, the surface is initially dry and, depending on the depth of tissue destruction, it may take days before the eschar becomes saturated with fluid leaking from the damaged capillaries in the deeper tissues. Unless the superficial partial-thickness burn wound becomes infected, or is subjected to further trauma, it should reepithelialise in 7–10 days. As migration of the epithelial cells occurs, the exudate will gradually diminish. Singer and Boyce (2017) describe the major aim in burn wound care to be obtaining wound closure as soon as possible with the least amount of scarring, thus maximising functional and cosmetic outcome. In order to meet this goal, management must entail:

- meticulous cleansing and debridement of devitalised tissue in order to prevent infection
- facilitating reepithelialisation or granulation in preparation for any necessary wound grafting
- promoting patient comfort.

Pain Relief

It is generally agreed that patients with burns experience the greatest pain during therapeutic procedures (Scheffler et al. 2018). Pain-relieving strategies used in wound care include:

- the administration of morphine and other similar opioids timed to ensure optimal cover during the procedure

- patient-controlled analgesia by inhalation administration, e.g. Entonox (nitrous oxide and oxygen)
- relief of anxiety through explanation and, if necessary, complementary and alternative medicine (CAM) therapies (e.g. hypnosis) and other psychological coping strategies.

The degree of discomfort the patient experiences will be strongly related to the skill of the nurse to recognise and appreciate the individual's pain tolerance (see Chapter 20, Pain Management).

Wound Cleansing and Debridement

Burn wound cleansing can be very time consuming and, where wounds are extensive, will require a number of staff. In some units, patients with extensive burns will have dressings changed under general anaesthesia with the involvement of a full surgical team.

Depending on the size and site of the wound, other methods include irrigation via a syringe, showering or immersion in a special tub. What is important for both patient comfort and to limit heat loss, especially when the wounds are extensive or on the trunk, is to ensure that the solution used is warmed to body temperature.

Following cleansing, loose devitalised tissue is trimmed using sharp scissors. Specialists vary in their approach to the management of blisters: Ro et al. (2018) advise that blisters can be left intact and aspirated, whereas the British Burn Association (2018b) advocate deroofing blisters >6 mm to allow for a complete assessment of the burn wound surface and therefore accurate diagnosis of the burn wound depth (Evidence-Based Practice 29.1).

Promotion of reepithelialisation or granulation and the prevention of wound contamination are normally facilitated either by applying dressings or more infrequently by exposing the burn wound.

Dressing the Burn Wound

One of the main problems presented by the burn wound is the copious amount of exudate it produces. This strongly influences the choice of dressing material used. Many modern materials are designed to create the optimal environment for healing, that is, warmth and moisture, whilst removing excess exudate. This may be accomplished by highly absorbent materials, such as alginates, hydrocolloids or hydrophilic foams, or by materials that allow rapid transmission of water vapour (Kus and Ruiz 2020). These types of dressing can be used successfully in burns affecting a relatively small area, but a substantial margin must be in contact with unburned skin to prevent leakage of exudate. Thus, their use is often not feasible for large wounds.

EVIDENCE-BASED PRACTICE 29.1

Blister Management

Specialists vary in their approach to the management of blisters – the two following examples suggest very different management.

Activity

- Access and read the articles by British Burn Association (2018a, 2018b) and Ro et al. (2018).
- Search the literature to see if further research about blister management has been published and discuss your findings with your mentor.

For extensive burns in the initial stages of injury prior to surgery, conventional dressings that comprise of an inner layer of mesh, usually impregnated with paraffin and thick layers of cotton gauze, are usually used. Some burn units will also routinely apply silver-containing dressings at this stage. The materials may be retained with cotton conforming bandages, or on the trunk by stitching or stapling the gauze. The frequency of scheduled dressing changes depends on the depth and state of the wound and on the properties of any medication incorporated in the innermost layer. Superficial partial-thickness burns may have their dressings left undisturbed for 4–7 days, unless there are indications for investigating the wound, such as signs of infection. More frequent changes, daily, every second day or twice weekly, are required in deeper burns as the presence of necrotic tissue increases the likelihood of bacterial growth. In such cases, antibacterial agents are normally used. For many years, silver sulfadiazine cream, in the UK Flamazine, was a popular antibacterial application for burn wounds throughout the developed world. However, because of its tendency to change the appearance of the wound and to macerate nonviable tissue, making surgical excision difficult, other silver-containing wound products including Aquacel Ag and Acticoat (Aggarwala et al. 2021) are now regularly used in burn wound management. Silver sulfadiazine with cerium nitrate is also used in some UK burn units for treating extensive burns where the patient's medical condition does not allow for early excision and skin grafting to occur (Reese et al. 2022). The ideal wound cover is the patient's own skin in the form of an autograft which 'takes' to provide wound closure. Other types of skin graft, that is, from other humans, an allograft, or from animals, a xenograft, provide only temporary cover except in the case of identical twins. Sheets of epidermal cells (keratinocytes) may be cultured from the patient's own skin but it may take some weeks before sufficient material is available (Hickerson et al. 2019). However, there are now also many bioengineered skin substitutes widely available for the treatment of extensive burn wounds (Mason and Pham 2023).

Skin Grafting

The necrotic tissue has to separate from the wound bed before a wound bed surface, suitable for skin grafting, is produced.

Surgical removal of necrotic tissue is carried out usually within the first 4 days following injury. The tissue is either excised with a scalpel or shaved down to a viable (bleeding) surface with a skin grafting knife. This procedure can result in extensive blood loss, and multiple blood transfusions may be required. The freshly prepared wound bed is usually skin grafted immediately.

A skin graft 'takes' by the ingrowth of capillaries from the wound into the graft, a process that takes only a few days. This will be disrupted if there is any blood, serum or pus preventing contact between graft and wound. Other factors that can cause disruption of the graft include any shearing of the graft/wound interface and the presence of β-haemolytic *Streptococcus*, group A (*S. pyogenes*) bacteria which produce streptokinase, an activator of plasmin which is fibrinolytic. Nursing staff will be responsible for ensuring that there is no overt staining or blood on the postoperative dressing as this could indicate bleeding or a collection of fluid under the graft. If this occurs, the dressing will require to be removed for inspection of the area. An aseptic technique is employed and great care is required to prevent the graft shearing on its bed.

The skin graft donor area is a superficial wound and, as a result, can be very painful. For the first 48 hours or so, it produces large amounts of bloodstained exudate and is usually dressed with calcium alginate followed by a conventional dressing, which is managed in the same way as that covering a superficial partial-thickness burn. The speed of reepithelialisation depends on the depth of dermis removed along with the epidermis but is normally between 10 days and 2 weeks.

Ideally, the calcium alginate dressing is left intact until it falls off. Injudicious early investigation will cause further trauma, delay healing and lead to risk of infection.

The alginate dressing dries out as epithelialisation occurs but readily regains its gel consistency when soaked with normal saline.

Care of Special Areas

Face. The most common method of managing superficial and partial-thickness facial burns is that of exposure.

Approaches to the use of topical agents including antimicrobials, nonantimicrobials and skin substitutes differ between burns units (Hoogewerf et al. 2020), however it is important to cleanse the area regularly as if the exudate dries out and produces a thin scab, the face can feel mask like with decreased mobility around the eyes and mouth.

The face can become very oedematous, so the patient should be nursed upright with head elevated as soon as their condition allows.

Oedema of the Periorbital Region can cause closure of the eyelids. As this can be very frightening for the patient, the nurse should warn the patient that eyelid closure may occur but reassure that the swelling will lessen in a few days. Eye drops or ointment will be prescribed in order to reduce the possibility of conjunctivitis. The use of artificial tears will make the patient more comfortable.

Oedema of the Lips may cause eversion of the oral mucosa, which should not be allowed to dry out. The skin of the lips should be kept lubricated with yellow soft paraffin and care must be taken when oral hygiene is performed. The use of a soft toothbrush, by patient or nurse, will help to maintain normal mouth care and, if the patient is unable to eat, regular mouthwashes should be given. If oral intake is allowed, the patient may experience difficulty in drinking from a normal cup; a feeding cup with a spout is preferable to using a straw as the patient may find it difficult to exert just the right pressure to allow suction without collapsing the straw.

Oedema of the Ears may cause them to jut out at right angles to the head, making them more susceptible to further trauma. If the pinna produces exudate, this is liable to trickle into the external auditory meatus, where it will collect and dry out at the level of the ear drum, reducing the patient's ability to hear. This may not be detected until some time later, in which case it may prove very difficult to evacuate the plug. It is easy to avert this problem by inserting a small piece of gauze just at the opening of the meatus to absorb the exudate, changing it as necessary. The ears may be dressed lightly with a conventional dressing.

Nostrils (Anterior Nares) should be kept free of exudate build-up by regular cleansing with a dampened cotton bud. If exudate dries on the nasal hairs, the crust will occlude the nostrils and its removal will be very painful indeed. This problem may be prevented by the application of a light smear of soft yellow paraffin just inside the nostrils.

Beard Area. In male patients, hair becomes incorporated in the crust as it grows. This does not usually present problems until the scab is separating from the newly epithelialised facial skin; in the case of deep burns, the hair follicles will be destroyed and no hair growth will occur. Once the scab starts to lift, it may be rehydrated using a moisturising lotion or hydrogel; this causes swelling of the scab, which no longer fits the contours of the face, and softens it to allow painless removal.

Scab Removal. As the scab lifts on the rest of the face, loose areas should be trimmed with care. There may be a strong temptation on the part of both nurse and patient to remove as much as possible. However, it must be borne in mind that removing an adherent crust causes wound trauma and may increase the possibility of scar formation. Newly epithelialised skin needs to be moisturised regularly with a bland cream to stop it from drying out.

Hands. Burns involving the majority of the hand can cause excessive swelling to the hand. If this occurs, it can be managed by the application of polythene bags or gloves, with or without the addition of an antibacterial cream, in order to facilitate movement and thus prevent joint stiffness and allow the patient a degree of independence. Because the polythene does not allow evaporation of water, the wound environment is very moist and the nonburned skin will become macerated. As large volumes of exudate will collect, it is usual, before applying the bag, to apply several layers of gauze around the wrist to absorb some of the exudate. Initially, the bags should be changed on a frequent basis and the hand gently cleansed at each change. The use of polythene bags or gloves should however be discontinued as soon as swelling allows and conventional dressing should then be applied. Minor burns to the hand are treated with lighter dressings, which should not restrict mobility.

Limbs. In order to reduce oedema formation, burned limbs are elevated and exercised on a regular basis, unless freshly laid skin grafts preclude movement.

Joints. Wound contraction is an integral part of the healing process, but excessive contraction leads to dysfunction and deformity. As flexor surfaces are more liable to contract, joints must be correctly positioned, with compensatory hyperextension especially of the wrists and neck. Physiotherapy should be carried out regularly, with adequate analgesic cover, to maintain a full range of movement of all joints. However, splinting may be necessary to arrest or correct contracture formation.

Scar Formation

Scar formation is part of the maturation phase of the healing process. In wounds healing by secondary intention (see Chapter 23, Tissue Viability and Managing Chronic Wounds), the scar often appears red and is raised above the level of the surrounding skin (hypertrophic). Hypertrophic scarring is a well-known complication following burn injury and the resulting disfigurement causes great distress. The most common means of prevention is the application of external pressure, usually effected by the use of specially designed elasticated garments which can be made to fit any anatomical part. The garments should be worn, apart from bathing and skin care, for 24 hours a day; treatment should continue for at least 9 months and a pressure of at least 24 mmHg is necessary for the treatment to be effective. Patients are provided with several sets of garments, which are alternately washed and worn then replaced every 3 months.

Elastic garments are not very effective for applying pressure to concavities on the body surface, especially on the face around the nose and mouth. For treatment of these areas, a rigid, or semirigid, transparent face mask can be made. One technique that does not rely on pressure to reduce the hypertrophy and redness of scars is the use of silicone gel sheets (Anthonissen et al. 2016). These need to be retained in place with light bandages or adhesive tape and must be removed regularly for washing as they are reusable for a few applications.

Psychological Effects of Burn Injuries

The disfigurement and impaired function which result from wound contracture and scar formation are generally accepted as the major sequelae of burn injuries, causing great distress and psychological problems for the patient and their loved ones. This, however, describes the long-term view and does not take into account that, for the patient and their family, the psychological effects start at the time of injury. Many patients will be routinely reviewed by a clinical psychologist at this time and regularly thereafter.

The role of the nurse is to offer care that focuses on the individual, with the patient at the heart of all that is done and this is also applied to any issues that may arise from the psychological effects of burn injuries. The Nursing and Midwifery Council (2018) makes clear that the nurse must prioritise people, preserve their safety and practice effectively; they can do this by practising professionally and engendering trust.

Many patients voice their relief at being alive in the immediate period following the accident, but as the implications of their injury sink in, their emotions and behaviour may begin to go through a series of changes.

Smith et al. (2006) described three psychological phases experienced by patients hospitalised following burn injuries:

- acute
- subacute
- chronic.

The Acute Phase

During the early stages of treatment, the patient will be preoccupied by bodily feelings and by the care provided by nursing and medical staff. If the wounds are extensive and complications arise, the patient will be cared for in the intensive care unit (ICU), perhaps for long periods, which may result in various mental health problems (see Chapter 28, Nursing Critically Ill Patients). Nightmares associated with the accident are common at this stage, as are fears of dying. A constant presence, reassurance and reorientation may be necessary.

The Subacute Phase

When the patient reaches this stage, anxiety related to survival is replaced with fears for the future, both short and long term. In the short term, stress is related to anticipation of pain and many patients become depressed or are hostile towards the nursing staff. They may regress in their ability to cope with activities of living and demand care and attention. This is perhaps the most difficult phase for the unit staff to cope with. Pain control helps to reduce patient anxiety related to wound care, and physiotherapy and monitoring of pain should continue throughout the period of hospitalisation.

Longer-term anxieties include the fear of disfigurement (Reflection 29.3) and of losing function and former roles. Nursing staff can help the patient come to terms with their changed situation by being honest and supportive and allowing them to grieve. The first look in the mirror should not be accidental but a planned occasion with the patient making the choice whether to be alone or to be accompanied by nursing staff, a clinical psychologist or loved ones. Although the patient may have some idea of their changed appearance from watching the reactions of visitors, the true extent of disfigurement may only be seen on first looking in a mirror. If the hands are not injured, the patient may gauge contour and textural changes through touch, but the reality of their changed appearance will still be a great shock.

REFLECTION 29.3

Coping With Disfigurement

The disfigurement caused by burns injury causes psychological problems for patients and their family and friends. Disfigurement affecting the face and hands is obvious all the time, but scarring present on other body areas causes problems, such as with relationships or undressing in a communal changing room.

Activity

- Think about, or discuss with colleagues, how you might feel about obvious disfigurement. How would it change your life? For instance would you want to continue with your nursing course/career?
- Investigate the information, advice and services offered by the British Association of Skin Camouflage (BASC) (www.skin-camouflage.net/) and Changing Faces (www.changingfaces.org.uk/), for example, physical means to reduce the impact of disfigurement, the problems of discrimination at work and the relevant legislation.

Regression in physical ability may also be managed by behavioural modification, with the patient being set easily achievable tasks, such as pouring a drink from their own water jug and being encouraged to feel a sense of achievement on doing so. Many patients regress when there is a sudden, unexplained reduction in the amount of nursing care they receive. Explanation about their improving condition and patient involvement in identifying needs and planning the reduction of care can help to alleviate this problem.

The Chronic Phase

This phase is marked by the patient rediscovering former interests and pleasures. The patient may, for example, take more notice of the activity in the unit and of the other patients. When possible, mixing with the other patients should be encouraged. When disfigurement is highly visible, such as on the face and hands, the patient may not wish to mix with others and will require a great deal of support from staff as well as from family and friends.

Prior to discharge, patients frequently experience ambivalence about leaving the safe confines of the unit where they are known and accepted. The actual discharge may be graduated by the introduction of visits home and by giving the patient the opportunity to discuss the pleasures and problems encountered. Liaison with the primary healthcare team will ensure continuity of care, and involvement of social workers and occupational therapists in the community will provide financial and practical help in the resumption of home life.

After Discharge

It is possible that the patient will need to return to hospital for clinic appointments and, later on, for plastic reconstructive surgery to improve the appearance of the scars or to correct any functional problems the scars may be causing, a process which may involve many operations over a number of years. Many patients suffer long-term psychological problems including depression, anxiety and other post-traumatic stress symptoms.

No matter how high the standard of care provided, the patient who suffers extensive burns may never return fully to their former physical or emotional functioning – a fact which can only serve to emphasise the need for greater effort in the field of burn prevention.

Summary: Key Nursing Issues

- Burn prevention and health education are the most effective ways of decreasing burn mortality and morbidity.
- Accurate assessment of depth and extent of burn wound is necessary to initiate the most appropriate evidence-based treatment, thus giving the burn patient the best possible chance of survival as well as decreasing any long-term effects of scarring or contracture.
- Nursing patients with burn injury requires skill and can be challenging. A holistic approach is essential to achieve optimal

outcomes. This includes assessment, fluid replacement, pain relief, wound care (when many wound care products are not feasible for extensive burns), nutrition, prevention of complications, etc.
- The psychological effects of burn injury can often occur and can result in long-term psychological damage to the individual and the family. Nurses have a vital role in providing information and support.

Reflection and Learning – What Next?

- **Test** your knowledge by visiting the Evolve website 🌐 and answering the multiple-choice questions and critical thinking questions.
- **Consolidate** your learning by looking at some of the further reading suggestions, references and specialist websites.
- **Revisit** some of the additional material on the Evolve website.

- **Consider** what you have learnt and how this will help your professional development.
- **Reflect** on how you can apply this knowledge to the care of your patients.
- **Discuss** your learning with your mentor/supervisor, lecturer and colleagues.

References

Aggarwala S, Optom B, Harish V, et al. Treatment of partial thickness burns: a prospective, randomized controlled trial comparing four routinely used burns dressings in an ambulatory care setting. *J Burn Care Res.* 2021;42:934–943.

Anthonissen M, Daly D, Janssens J, et al. The effects of conservative treatments on burn scars: a systematic review. *Burns.* 2016;42:508–518.

British Burn Association. *First Aid Clinical Practice Guideline.* Prehospital Special Interest Group; 2018. Available at. https://www.britishburnassociation.org/wp-content/uploads/2017/06/BBA-First-Aid-Guideline-3.7.18.pdf.

British Burn Association. Clinical Practice Guideline for Management of Burn Blisters. 2018b. https://www.britishburnassociation.org/wp-content/uploads/2017/06/BBA-Burn-Blister-Management-Guideline-20.6.18.pdf.

Chana NK, Yarwood J, Smith J. Burn injuries in the older population and understanding the common causes to influence accident prevention. *Burns.* 2022;49(4):848–853. doi:10.1016/j.burns.2022.06.013.

Clark A, Imran J, Madni T, et al. Nutrition and metabolism in burn patients. *Burns Trauma.* 2017;5(11):1–12. doi:10.1186/s41038-017-0076-x.

Coban YK. Infection control in severely burned patients. *World J Crit Care Med.* 2012;4:4–101.

Ghoddusi JM, Mohammadi AA, Dastgerdi V. Burn: a predictable but preventable tragedy in epileptic patients. *World J Plast Surg.* 2019;8:254–258.

Gillenwater J, Garner MS. Acute fluid management of large burns: pathophysiology, monitoring, and resuscitation. *Clin Plast Surg.* 2017;44:495–503.

Harats M, Ofir H, Segalovich M, et al. Trends and risk factors for mortality in elderly burns patients: a retrospective review. *Burns.* 2019;45:1342–1349.

Health & Safety Executive. Managing the Risk From Hot Water and Surfaces in Health and Social Care. 2012. Available at: http://www.hse.gov.uk/pubns/hsis6.pdf.

Hickerson WL, Remmers AE, Recker DP. Twenty-five years' experience and beyond with cultured epidermal autografts for coverage of large burn wounds in adult and pediatric patients. *J Burn Care Res.* 2019;40:157–165.

Home Office. Detailed analysis of fires attended by fire and rescue services, England, April 2020 to March 2021. *Statistical Bulletin.* 2021;25. Available at https://www.gov.uk/government/statistics/detailed-analysis-of-fires-attended-by-fire-and-rescue-services-england-april-2020-to-march-2021.

Hoogewerf CJ, Hop MJ, Nieuwenhuis MK, et al. Topical treatment for facial burns. *Cochrane Database Syst Rev.* 2020;7:CD008058. doi:10.1002/14651858.CD008058.pub3.

Huang SW, Yeh FC, Ji YR, et al. Chitosan-based hydrogels to treat hydrofluoric acid burns and prevent infection. *Drug Deliv and Transl Res.* 2021;11:1532–1544.

International Society for Burn Injuries. ISBI practice guidelines for burn care. *Burns.* 2016;42:953–1021.

Jordan KC, Di Gennaro JL, von Saint André-von Arnim A, et al. Global trends in pediatric burn injuries and care capacity from the World Health Organization Global Burn Registry. *Front Pediatr.* 2022;10:954995.

Kearney L, Francis EC, Clover AJ. New technologies in global burn care – a review of recent advances. *Int J Burns Trauma.* 2018;8:77–87.

Kok G, Peters GJY, Kessels LT, et al. Ignoring theory and misinterpreting evidence: the false belief in fear appeals. *Health Psychol Rev.* 2018;12:111–125.

Kus KJB, Ruiz ES. Wound dressings – a practical review. *Curr Derm Rep.* 2020;9:298–308.

Lund CC, Browder NC. The estimation of areas of burns. *Surg Gynaecol Obstet.* 1944;79:352–358.

Mason S, Pham TN. Use of dermal regenerative templates for burns. *J Burn Care Res.* 2023;44:s19–s25.

McCann C, Watson A, Barnes D. Major burns: Part 1. Epidemiology, pathophysiology and initial management. *BJA Educ.* 2022;22:94–103.

Mclure M, Macneil F, Wood F M, et al. A rapid review of burns first aid guidelines: is there consistency across international guidelines? *Cureus.* 2021;13:15779.

National Network for Burn Care. National burn care referral guidance. 2012. https://www.britishburnassociation.org/wp-content/uploads/2018/02/National-Burn-Care-Referral-Guidance-2012.pdf.

Norbury W, Herndon D, Tanksley J, et al. Infection in burns. *Surg Infect.* 2016;17:250–255.

Nursing and Midwifery Council (NMC). The Code: Professional Standards of Practice and Behaviour for Nurses, Midwives and Nursing Associates. 2018. https://www.nmc.org.uk/globalassets/sitedocuments/nmc-publications/nmc-code.pdf.

Palmu R, Partonen T, Suominen K, et al. Alcohol use and smoking in burn patients at the Helsinki Burn Center. *Burns.* 2018;44:158–167.

Ponticorvo A, Rowland R, Baldado M, et al. Evaluating clinical observation versus Spatial Frequency Domain Imaging (SFDI), Laser Speckle Imaging (LSI) and thermal imaging for the assessment of burn depth. *Burns.* 2019;45:450–460.

Reese A, Keyloun J, Garg G, et al. Compounded cerium nitrate–silver sulfadiazine cream is safe and effective for the treatment of burn wounds: a burn center's 4-year experience. *J Burn Care Res*. 2022;43:716–721.

Ro HS, Shin JY, Sabbagh MD, et al. Effectiveness of aspiration or deroofing for blister management in patients with burns: a prospective randomized controlled trial. *Med (Baltimore)*. 2018;97:e0563.

Scheffler M, Koranyi S, Meissner W, et al. Efficacy of non-pharmacological interventions for procedural pain relief in adults undergoing burn wound care: a systematic review and meta-analysis of randomized controlled trials. *Burns*. 2018;44:1709–1720.

Singer AJ, Boyce ST. Burn wound healing and tissue engineering. *J Burn Care Res*. 2017;38:605–613.

Smith JS, Smith KR, Rainey SL. The psychology of burn care. *J Trauma Nurs*. 2006;13:105–106.

Toliver-Kinsky T, Kobayashi M, Suzuki F, et al.. 5th ed.The Systemic Inflammatory Response Syndrome. Total Burn Care19 Philadelphia: Saunders Elsevier; 2018:205–220.

Wallace AB. The exposure treatment of burns. *Lancet*. 1951;1:501–504.

Wright EH, Harris AL, Furniss D. Cooling of burns: Mechanisms and models. *Burns*. 2015;41:882–889.

Further Reading

Herndon D, ed. *Total Burn Care*. 5th ed. Philadelphia, PA: Saunders Elsevier; 2018.

Useful Websites

British Association of Skin Camouflage (BASC), www.skin-camouflage.net

Changing Faces, www.changingfaces.org.uk

Fire Service, www.fireservice.co.uk

The Royal Society for the Prevention of Accidents (RoSPA), www.rospa.com

30

Care and Rehabilitation of People With Long-Term Conditions

KATHARINE MARTYN

CHAPTER OUTLINE

Introduction

The prevalence of people living with one or more long-term conditions (LTCs) is increasing in all countries across the world and the World Health Organisation (WHO) 2023 considered LTCs to be the greatest challenge facing healthcare services in the 21st century. Related terms to LTC are noncommunicable diseases (NCDs) and chronic conditions. While there is an overlap between these terms, NCD is commonly used in an international context or associated with conditions such as cardiovascular, respiratory and diabetes that share common lifestyle risk factors. LTCs cover both physical and mental health including lifelong impairments, across all age ranges and patient demographics, often requiring both health and social care. The Kings Fund estimates that the care and management of LTCs account for 70% of the total health and social care budget and that this figure will continue to rise (Nuffield Trust 2021). Although previously the management of LTCs has been a low priority amongst doctors and policy-makers alike the NHS 5-year forward view (2014), NHS Long term plan (2019) and the Health and Care Act 2022 have increased the focus and driven a policy shift towards patient-centred, integrated planned care and management that recognizes the impact of LTC, to ensure people continue to live well and independently. When care for people with LTCs is managed effectively it is evident that this leads to better outcomes for the individual and a reduction in the need for admission into the hospital (Hiltunen et al. 2020). It is better for the individual and a more effective use of resources to reduce admission to hospital and develop effective care in the community.

Caring for patients with an LTC can present many challenges: the changing nature of LTC with advances in medicine and the emergence of 'new conditions' such as long COVID in the aftermath of the SARS-CoV-2 (COVID-19) pandemic, the need to balance the drive for optimal health against the patient's wishes, the constraints of evolving healthcare systems and the complexities of multidisciplinary and multiagency work to name a few. Nurses are required to constantly review their knowledge and skills as they collaborate with people as they manage their LTC, not only in the traditional sense of clinical skills and supportive care and advice but also to facilitate the patient's negotiation of an often complex health and social care system.

What Is a Long-Term Condition?

Capturing the complexity of LTCs is difficult and LTC can be poorly defined or diagnosed. The literature often refers to conditions such as diabetes or heart disease, but LTCs also include mental health and people with lifelong conditions, which can present with fluctuating health and social care needs. For example, following an acute SARS-CoV-2 infection, many people will suffer from a range of persistent nonspecific symptoms, and this condition, now coined long COVID-19 by recognised research institutes, is not easy to diagnose. Long COVID-19 can involve multiple organs and can affect many systems including, but not limited to, the respiratory, cardiovascular, neurological, gastrointestinal and musculoskeletal systems. The symptoms of long COVID include fatigue, dyspnea, cardiac abnormalities, cognitive impairment, sleep disturbances, symptoms of post-traumatic stress disorder, muscle pain, concentration problems and headache (Crook et al. 2021).

For many with lifelong conditions, there is limited need for continued support with many leading full and active lives, which is only disrupted during acute illness. Others require flexible support from social or health care to support exacerbations in their condition or changes in their situation, while some require packages of care encapsulating complex health and social care needs. These care packages can change due to ageing, a result of additional comorbidities or changing social support networks such as the death of a carer. The Equality Act (2010) and definitions provided by the WHO (2002) and Kings Fund (2013) speak of LTCs as 'conditions' that last for more than 12 months and for which there is no cure. However, adequately describing congenital and acquired conditions that are 'long-term' is challenging, as many people may not consider they have an LTC as framed through a biomedical lens. Although the terms 'long-term condition', 'lifelong condition', 'chronic disease' and 'chronic illness' and 'noncommunicable diseases' are often used interchangeably, the way these are applied reveals assumptions about enduring conditions and the individuals who experience them.

Multimorbidity

The proportion of patients in primary and secondary care settings with two or more medical conditions that fit the definitions of an LTC is rising, driven across all countries by changing demographics and aging populations (Ho et al. 2022). NICE (2016) suggests that the prevalence of multimorbidity is common in older adults and a retrospective study in England estimated that it affected 27.2% of a cohort of 403,985 people (Cassell et al. 2018) and in Scotland 23.2% of a population of 1,751,841 (Barnett et al. 2012). People with multimorbidity often have a high treatment burden attending multiple appointments, managing complex drug regimens and engaging with multiple professionals. The risk of polypharmacy and adverse drug reaction is also high due to treatment by multiple prescribers (NICE 2017). Nurses are increasingly engaged in the support and management of people with multimorbidity and this requires timely assessment and review using an interprofessional and integrated approach. Nurses in primary care acting as case managers have a pivotal role in ensuring that there is a holistic approach to the assessment and the use of screening tools such as the comprehensive geriatric assessment (CGA) and Screening Tool of Older Persons' potentially inappropriate Prescriptions/Screening Tool to Alert doctors to Right Treatment (STOPP/START) (O'Mahony 2023) for medication reviews avoiding unnecessary complications or admission into hospital (Nord et al. 2020).

Frailty

Our ageing population with those over 80 years set to exceed 3 million by 2043 (ONS 2018) adds to the complex health and social care picture. Whilst age alone does not determine health outcome, within this population, there are increasing numbers of people who become frail necessitating additional care and support (Reeves et al. 2018). Frailty is a distinctive health state defined by two models. The first, known as the phenotype model (Fried et al. 2001), describes a group of patient characteristics (unintentional weight loss, reduced muscle strength, reduced gait speed, self-reported exhaustion and low energy expenditure) which, if present, can predict poorer outcomes. Individuals who present with three or more of these characteristics are said to be frail. The second, the cumulative deficit model (Mitnitski et al. 2001), assumes that over time people accumulate deficits that can occur with aging, which combine to form the frailty index. In both models being frail is linked to poorer outcomes as body systems gradually lose their inbuilt reserves. People with LTC or disabilities may be frail; however, people who are just frail may not be consumers of healthcare services or known to the general practitioner until they are unable to manage independently or deteriorate because of a relatively minor infection or illness (Public Health England 2017). This makes the measuring of frailty prevalence in the UK uncertain. However recent estimates suggest that frailty affects as many as 8.1% of adults over the age of 50 in England (Sinclair et al. 2022). Frailty is identified using validated tools such as the gait Speed Test, PRISMA-7 and timed up and go test (Barry et al., 2014). NHS England systematically identifies people aged 65 or over who are living with moderate or severe frailty using the electronic frailty index (eFI) (NHS England 2024). The Rockwood frailty scale (Moorhouse and Rockwood 2012) is commonly used in the assessment process by medical and nursing teams, in both primary and secondary care settings.

Does It Matter What We Call It?

Terminology

Traditional definitions of long-term health conditions in healthcare practice have favoured a biomedical approach with a link to disease, illness and impairment. Therefore LTCs are often described as the result of protracted illness such as HIV or chronic obstructive pulmonary disease (COPD), and the disease impacts a person's functioning and lifestyle. This reductionist approach is increasingly limiting as it fails to account for the psychosocial consequences of living with an LTC. For example, during the COVID-19 pandemic, the impact of social isolation associated with lockdown and a reduction in service provision amplified the experiences of 'uncertainty' associated with living with an LTC limiting well-being and exacerbating frailty (Holland et al. 2021).

Models of Disability

Models of disability are often represented as opposing medical and social models. The medical model regards disability as a problem that is intrinsic to the person and caused directly by disease, a health condition, or trauma. Here, 'impairment' is not only used to describe disturbance in the body's structure and function. It is also seen as responsible for preventing the individual's participation in normal society and, therefore disabling them. This means that the management is diagnosis-related with a cure focus driven by medical interventions to restore an individual's ability to fully participate in society. Conversely, the social model assumes that disability exists where attitudinal or environmental barriers exclude people with impairments from full engagement in mainstream activities.

Disability is therefore a socially created problem that is distinct from and superimposed on impairment. From this standpoint, disability can be managed collectively by social action. Government legislation such as the Equality Act 2010 seeks to remove these barriers, providing greater opportunities to the individual. However, despite positive rhetoric around enablement and inclusion meaningful and sustainable societal change remains challenging.

There is a danger of seeing these models as absolutes, for example, in judging services simplistically as either focusing on medical intervention or not. The social model arose from the British disability movement and, in characterising disabled people as an oppressed group, has been central to its civil rights agenda, informing government policy and legislation, such as the Equality Act (2010). While the medical model might be criticised for defining people by their impairments and medicalising their lives, the social model arguably downplays the impact impairment has on daily personal experience and that many impairments have short- or long-term physical implications.

In contrast, the WHO's (2001) International Classification of Functioning, Disability and Health (ICF) was developed with the intent of synthesising the above models via a biopsychosocial approach. It acknowledges the importance of knowing the disease process while recognizing that the impact of the disease on the life of an individual will vary greatly and is independent of the specific disease identified. Its aims included establishing a common language to improve communication between service stakeholders and a framework that would allow international comparison. In so doing, it provides a conceptual basis for defining, measuring and formulating policy for health and disability. However, it has not been widely adopted in nursing practice and is primarily used by nurses working in the field of rehabilitation. However, when used it provides a common language and understanding between professionals enhancing effective collaborative working (Mizuma et al. 2020, Piexak et al. 2015, Sagahutu et al. 2020).

The ICF (WHO 2001) comprises two parts, each being made up of two components. Part One is concerned with functioning and disability, encompassing body structures and functions, activities and participation; Part Two addresses contextual environmental and personal factors. As shown (Fig. 30.1), these elements have an interactive and dynamic relationship. Research has indicated that it is now time to review and update the ICF in line with changing expectations and our increased understanding of participation and collaborative care (Sverker et al. 2020).

Factors Influencing Long-Term Conditions, Disability and Frailty

Lifestyle and Blame

An unhealthy lifestyle is increasingly associated with an increased risk of developing NCD and some LTCs, and guidance from the Chief Medical Officer (2020) clearly articulates the benefits of a healthy lifestyle in the prevention and management of many LTC with a focus on physical activity. A study on healthy lifestyle and life expectancy in people with multimorbidity has shown that engaging in a healthy lifestyle was associated with greater life expectancy (Chudasama et al. 2020). Also, public health guidance on type 2 diabetes and obesity focuses on healthier diets with a reduction in carbohydrates and processed food consumption. However, such guidance can lead to assumptions being made that on becoming unwell, individuals have failed to respond to preventive health education

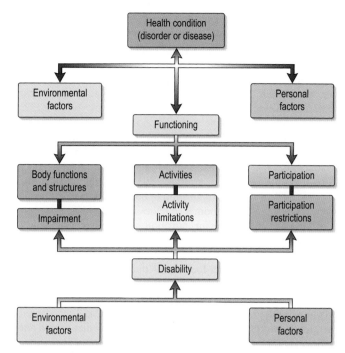

Figure 30.1 Interactions between the components of the International Classification of Functioning, Disability and Health. (Adapted with permission from World Health Organisation (WHO). *International Classification of Functioning, Disability and Health (ICF)*. Geneva: WHO; 2001.)

REFLECTION 30.1

The Impact of Language Used to Describe Disability

If you are able-bodied or able-minded, how do you feel about being described as an 'abled' or 'normie'? Think about how this makes you feel about terms you have used to describe disabled people.

REFLECTION 30.2

Health Behaviours and Individual Responsibility

Given the association between food advertising, social media and celebrity-led food programmes, cultural perceptions of food, availability, cost and access to healthier foods and concerns over weight and increase in incidence of obesity in the UK, can individuals be blamed for their behaviour? What other factors influence personal health choices?

---

campaigns. For example, for people who are obese assumptions can be made that the individual is simply eating too much, despite evidence to suggest that the issue is far more complex than that (Farrell et al. 2021). Beliefs concerning the origin of LTCs and disability appear, therefore, to reflect a combination of moral ideology and scientific principles (Reflection 30.1 and Reflection 30.2).

Food and Nutrition

Equitable access to healthy and nutritious food is of increasing concern across developed and developing countries alike. Changes to climate, political unrest and the 2020 COVID-19 pandemic have all heightened awareness of the fragility of global food supply chains while research increasingly clarifies the role of nutrition both in the prevention of NCD and in the management of LTCs (Douglas et al. 2020). All people with or without LTCs need a balanced diet that is based on at least five portions of fruit and vegetables, with an emphasis on plant based foods, less animal protein, fat or ultraprocessed foods that are low in fibre and high in salt and sugar. In achieving this using, a culturally appropriate Eat Well plate can provide guidance and support food conversations (NHS 2022). However, for many people with LTCs, disability and frailty the risk of malnutrition is high and this includes undernutrition, over nutrition (overweight and obesity) and micronutrient deficiency (Nathan 2021). UK national data indicate that malnutrition affects 11% of people visiting GP practices, 30% attending hospital outpatients, 29% of adults on admission to hospital and 35% of people recently admitted to care homes (Holdoway et al. 2017).

Addressing and enhancing nutrition support is challenging as malnutrition often occurs as a result of complex social, cultural, economic as well as health factors. Increasing awareness of peoples' struggle to afford healthier food across the life spectrum has led to an increase in food provision via food banks, emergency food parcels and other community groups. There are concerns however, that such provision while they can be a lifeline at times of heightened need, their role in addressing food insecurity or improving diet-related outcomes requires further development (Oldroyd et al. 2022).

Unemployment

Economic survival in preindustrial society largely depends on the capacity to engage in physical labour. Individuals restricted by the effects of protracted disease or impairment would thus have a limited function in their social group. This, together with likely dependency on others, could result in the perception that disabled people are of less value than their able-bodied counterparts.

One in five people of working age in the UK can be defined as disabled (DWP 2022), however, employment rates are lowest among disabled people, with only 53% in work, meaning there is a substantial employment rate gap in the UK between disabled and nondisabled people (82.0% in employment). There is a lot of variation in employment rates for different health conditions. For example, people whose main health condition is severe disfigurements, skin conditions and allergies are nearly three times more likely to be in employment compared with someone whose main health condition is severe or specific learning difficulties (72.5% compared with 25.6%). Disabled people whose main health condition is musculoskeletal are more likely to be in employment compared to those with a mental health condition.

In an industrialised society, technological developments and diversification of working practices should create opportunities for those with a wide range of disabilities to gain employment but the disability gap remains at 29% (Scope 2022)

Disability is considered a protected characteristic under the terms of the Equality Act 2010. The Act defines disability as an 'impairment that has a substantial and long-term adverse effect on one's ability to carry out normal day-to-day activities'. The Act seeks to protect those with disabilities from discrimination based on their disability and requires reasonable adjustments to be made to protect the individual from disadvantage. However, the onus is on individuals to demonstrate that they are disabled under the terms of the Act and assert their rights.

Work and the State Benefit System

There is a belief that individuals with a disability or LTC who claim state benefits are reluctant to work, however, research suggests that of the 5.3 million people with a nondisabling long-term health condition in the UK, 81.6% are in employment compared with 81.2% of the 28.4 million people with no long-term health conditions. This suggests that the existence of a health condition does not in itself affect the likelihood of people being in work, but whether it is perceived to limit a person's day-to-day activities.

The introduction of Personal Independence Payments (PIPs) creates additional bureaucracy and makes it increasingly difficult for individuals to access state support (Disability Rights UK 2017). Media representations of the benefits culture and fraudulent claims can leave people with LTCs feeling that they are perceived as 'spongers', yet entitlement to some payments assumes an all-or-nothing approach to fitness for work and limits the hours and the time recipients can engage in 'permitted work' without losing their entitlement. This traps individuals into remaining on benefits because it prevents them from testing their capabilities, gaining confidence and accumulating experience to assist in obtaining paid employment.

Stigma

According to Goffman's (1963) seminal text, the word 'stigma' was originally used with reference to visible signs inflicted to brand individuals (including slaves or criminals) unfit for participation in normal social interaction. These signs had moral and judgemental implications, such that the disgrace and shame of the stigma assumed more importance than its physical presence. The stigma attached to an LTC relates to deviation from the perceived norm and depends on the body part involved, visibility, controllability and diagnostic labelling. Dependency can also be stigmatising. Reliance on services, state benefits or other people means that individuals with LTCs are in a position of receiving without being able to contribute in return. To be labelled with an LTC is to be deemed exceptional and, in many cases, marginalised. People in this situation engage in constant efforts to make themselves acceptable and their stigmatising condition often dominates their social identity and relations with others (Reflection 30.3).

REFLECTION 30.3

Living With a Visible Long-Term Condition

D is 44 years old, is employed as a hotel receptionist and has had psoriasis for some years. He experiences periods of exacerbation and at present his scalp is covered in a thick, hardened layer of scales. When these areas are detached, his scalp surface weeps and becomes painful. Scales are also deposited on his clothing and in his immediate vicinity. D is conscious that people stare and look at his affected skin rather than making eye contact. When his children were small, one of them asked him not to attend a school play and eventually admitted it was due to being embarrassed by his appearance. D thinks that some people think his condition is contagious or caused by poor personal hygiene and believes this explains why bus passengers rarely occupy the space next to him until the vehicle becomes crowded.

D feels that he is managing his problems well. Since his job involves public contact, he has learned to project an outgoing and friendly image which he feels is stronger than the visual impression of the condition. Other people's behaviour still makes him uncomfortable and affects his confidence but he has learned to accept it as something he must live with.

Activity

Reflect on D's sense of stigmatisation. Consider the daily experience of someone with an obvious skin condition. Have you have ever felt embarrassed or uncomfortable when you encountered someone like this? How did you react?

People with less visible conditions such as epilepsy, autistic spectrum disorder, fibromyalgia and depression experience 'felt stigma', increasing the stress of managing their condition as denial and behavioural disengagement are frequently used as coping strategies (Bautista et al. 2015). The problem of constantly concealing part of oneself in order to pass as normal and avoid being found out is added to by difficulties in gauging which details to share with whom so that relationships can be maintained. Relatives also experience stigma by association and this affects their relationship with the individual and wider society. Cultural dimensions must also be considered in relation to stigma, particularly when supporting those with mental health conditions.

Others' behaviour towards people with long-term illness reinforces stigma when they generalise or make assumptions about impairments. For example, speak loudly to someone with a hearing impairment or communicate with others accompanying a disabled person rather than to the individual directly. This 'do they take sugar?' approach leaves people feeling less than adults. For example, C, an office administrator with cerebral palsy, described the public humiliation felt when waiting with a friend at a crowded supermarket checkout. The sales assistant confirmed the purchase with the friend before reluctantly taking C's money and then made a point of handing the friend the bagged items, change and receipt.

Healthcare workers often share society's view of disability. Reflecting this in their interactions with disabled people can compromise effective care (Kritsotakis et al. 2017). Perceiving disabled people to be dependent, managed or to be pitied gives rise to an approach that gives them a sense of being patronised, demeaned and disempowered. This adds to their feelings of inferiority and reduces confidence in the caregiver. Nurses working with people who have LTCs may experience a range of emotions when confronted with very real manifestations of human vulnerability. In response they may be distant in their approach but whilst distancing might provide short-term protection in shielding these emotions it accentuates the space between nurses and stigmatised people.

🌐 **See Evolve website Critical thinking question 30.1**

How Prevalent Are Long-Term Conditions?

The prevalence of LTCs is difficult to establish. This is due in part to their inherent interactive, dynamic, multidimensional and subjective natures. More people are now reporting a long-term health condition or disability in 2020 to 2021 than did so 8 years ago. The number of people reporting a long-term health condition increased by nearly 2 million (17.0%) between 2013/14 and 2020/21. Of these, nearly 1.4 million people (19.9% increase) stated that their condition limited their day-to-day activities (classifying them as disabled) with a further 0.43 million (15.2% increase) also stating that these activities were limited 'a lot' (classifying them as severely disabled) (DWP 2022). Of these 2 out of 50 were in receipt of care and almost 50% were of state pension age or older. Estimates in the UK are not definitive, given differences in definitions, sampling and data capture. There is no single register of people with LTCs and individuals do not have to be registered with local authorities to be defined as disabled or to receive services. Not all disabled people claim benefits, so capturing data only from recipients of these also provides a limited picture. With an ageing population and increasing multimorbidity, the true figure is likely to be much higher. Many patients with LTCs do not consider themselves to have a disability, despite meeting the criteria laid out in the Equality Act 2010, for example, patients with

mental health conditions and learning difficulties may not associate with being disabled, and therefore may also not be represented in official figures.

Consequences of Changing Morbidity and Mortality

Driven by improvements in public health, better housing, and food, and established vaccination programmes the continuing decline in mortality is reflected in an increased expectation of life for all age groups, a trend liable to continue. However, as life expectancy has increased so has the number of years living in poor health. This has implications for the number of people experiencing LTCs and disabilities because the prevalence of these rises with advancing age. Confirmation of this can be found in data from sources such as the UK Census or General Household Survey (GHS) self-reported limiting long-term illness (LLTI) or disability questionnaire (ONS 2022).

However, since 2019, the impact of the COVID-19 pandemic has highlighted how despite modern medicine and effective vaccination programmes we are vulnerable to new and emerging infectious diseases. SARS-CoV-2 (COVID-19) and subsequent variants have had an impact across all sectors of our society with those most disadvantaged, older, and with preexisting conditions suffering the most (Joy et al. 2020). In addition, the consequences of having had COVID-19 infection have led to an increase in people suffering from what is termed 'long COVID'. Long COVID is poorly understood but encapsulates a range of postviral syndromes and conditions that have a significant impact on a person's well-being. Estimates indicate that as many as 1.8 million people experience post-COVID-19 symptoms in the year following initial infection (NIHR 2021).

The National Picture

In 2019 over 18 million adults reported having a long-term illness (ONS 2020). The Department for Work and Pensions (DWP) calculates that more than 14.6 million people identify with having a disability (DWP 2022). There is no significant difference in the rates of self-reported long-term illness between men and women in the UK. Rates of long-term illnesses are closely correlated with increasing age, with over 6 million people over the age of 65 reporting they have one or more LTC (ONS 2020). Geographical comparison across the UK shows that England has the lowest rates, with Wales having the highest (ONS 2020). Social inequalities continue to impact the prevalence of LTCs with those with incomes of less than £10,00 per annum, three times more likely to have reported an LLTI than those with an income above £30,00 per annum; Black and minority ethnic elders reporting higher rates of LTC than White British elders. Hayanga et al. (2021) argued that some minoritised ethnic group people with multiple long term conditions (MLTCs) had poor disease management and called for better initiatives for managing health conditions and/or a need for enhanced strategies to reduce ethnic inequalities in healthcare.

Census questions have not considered types of LTCs and disabilities experienced or how these limit activities. Although the GHS samples only private households, it asks about the nature of health problems, coding replies according to the International Classification of Disease (ICD). Data from the 2011 survey show the prevalence of long-standing illness in children and adults to have risen from 21% to 35% between 1972 and 2011, while LLTIs increased from 15% to 21% (ONS 2021).

There is a striking similarity between the proportions of men and women experiencing various long-standing conditions. This

REFLECTION 30.4

Long-Term Conditions, Disability and Health

Reflect on what health means to people with long-term conditions or disabilities. Can they be 'healthy'?

could be partly due to women's longevity, but differences in lifetime behaviours and occupational factors could also be significant (Reflection 30.4).

While LTCs are widespread, only a proportion of those affected might be significantly impaired or disabled. It is, however, important to recognise that with improved management and treatment more people live longer lives with LTC, consequently, nurses must be equipped to recognise the impact of LTCs on independence and well-being and respond effectively across all health and social care settings.

Features of Living With Long-Term Conditions

As the prevalence of people living with one or more LTC increases, so understanding the uniqueness of the individual experience and how this impacts people, families, carers, health and social care workers is essential. Strauss et al. (1984) identified seven features of chronic illness and developed a framework to enable its impact to be understood more clearly and empathically (Fig. 30.2). This was furthered in the subsequent development of a trajectory model which aimed to give insight into experience over the course of an illness over time (Corbin and Strauss 1991; Fig. 30.3). These models are drawn on in the next section of this chapter.

Endurance

The time span of acute illness contrasts markedly with that of LTCs. Once treatment is initiated, acute illness is generally resolved within a short period and life is resumed as before, whereas the duration of LTCs is indefinite. This unwanted intrusion into an individual's life is often accompanied by the involvement of others who explore the most personal and private aspects of how you may live. The right to be private is overtaken by the need for support and care, and adjusting life to accommodate the working time frames of others can in itself add to the impact of the LTC. Building on Curtin and Lubkin's (1998) metaphor, this can be likened to a stranger arriving at someone's home unexpectedly and announcing that they are taking up permanent residence, regardless of whether there is a vacant spare room. In developing effective support care professionals should demonstrate knowledge and insight into the importance of understanding and respecting the continued development of self through the life course of an LTC, and develop positive, stable and consistent relationships with people with LTC (Hughes and Burch 2020). The use of diagnostic labels can be of benefit to some patients as they can provide relief and validate individuals' feelings that 'something isn't right' (Locker 2008), however, for some patient's diagnostic labelling becomes a limiting and stigmatising title. People with long-term mental health conditions, for example, often speak of feeling stigmatised, even when they feel they are managing well with minimal support (Brouwers 2020). How different LTCs are perceived by the individual also reflects society's view, for example, with a diagnosis

Salient features of chronic illness

- Chronic illnesses are long-term by nature
- Chronic illnesses are uncertain
- Chronic illnesses require proportionately great efforts at palliation
- Chronic illnesses are multiple diseases
- Chronic illnesses are disproportionately intrusive
- Chronic illnesses require a wide variety of ancillary services
- Chronic illnesses are expensive

Individual experience

Key problems

Chronic illnesses cause multiple key problems for daily living, including;
- Prevention and management of medical crises
- Control of symptoms
- Carrying out prescribed regimens and management of related problems
- Prevention of, or living with, social isolation
- Adjustment to changes in the course of the disease
- Attempts at normalising interaction with others and style of life
- Funding – finding money to survive partial/complete loss of employment or pay for treatment
- Confronting psychological, marital and familial problems

Basic strategies

- Individuals and families need to develop basic strategies (standard methods or techniques) to manage key problems

Organisational and family arrangements

- Basic strategies require the assistance of others acting as *agents* (family, friends, acquaintances or strangers who act in a rescuing or protective capacity)
- Agents' arrangements must coordinate efforts, understandings and agreements, relying on trust, interactional skill and financial, medical and familial resources

Consequences

- The way organisational and family arrangements are carried out influences how problems are managed, with consequences for individuals and their families

Figure 30.2 Strauss et al.'s (1984) features of chronic illness and framework for understanding individual experience.

of cancer individuals may find that support is readily available from family, friends and health professionals. For others such as those with psychosis accessing support can be more challenging, whilst those with lifelong conditions such as autism or Tourette's syndrome may feel that that support is limited as they do not 'fit' with any particular health or social care professional domain.

Adulthood is a dynamic period usually associated with autonomy and control. It is a time of life in which people expect to nurture others, rather than to be nurtured. The limitations imposed by LTCs and need for ongoing care conflict with these expectations and can be damaging to the individual's self-esteem. Accepting

Chronic illness trajectory: stages of chronic illness

- Pre-trajectory – before the onset of symptoms and formal diagnosis. Genetic or lifestyle factors for the development of a long-term condition are in place
- Onset – symptoms appear, the diagnosis is made and the individual starts to learn how to manage its implications
- Stable – the individual manages life activities within limitations and symptoms are controlled, with care taking place in the home
- Unstable – symptoms cannot be controlled or the condition reactivates, life is disrupted and the individual experiences difficulty managing activities. Care takes place at home
- Acute – severe, unrelieved symptoms or complications require acute intervention, hospitalisation and temporary reduction or suspension of life activities
- Crisis – a life-threatening episode requiring urgent intervention, with life activities suspended until resolution is achieved
- Comeback – the individual's efforts result in gradual return to relative stability and an acceptable way of life
- Downward – gradual or rapid deterioration, increasing disability and difficulty in managing symptoms
- Dying – the terminal stage where body processes begin to shut down, the individual relinquishes life activities and prepares for death

Figure 30.3 Stages of chronic illness, as featured in the trajectory model. (After Corbin JM, Strauss A. A nursing model for chronic illness management based upon the trajectory framework. *Sch Inq Nurs Pract.* 1991;5:155-174 and Henly SJ, Wyman JF, Findorff MJ. Health and illness over time: the trajectory perspective in nursing science. *Nurs Res.* 2011;60(3 Suppl):S5-14.)

help can be difficult enough; however, people with LTC or disabilities can be offered unnecessary assistance based on presumed need and their preferences overlooked. For example, a person described wheeling herself manually through a town centre on her way to meet a friend and suddenly finding herself moving at speed towards a department store. A helpful member of the public had thought this was her destination, decided that it would be easier for her to be pushed, ignored her requests to stop and took her response as a personal rejection: 'I was disoriented and motion sick. But what really got me was they acted like I was ungrateful and being too independent! My chair is part of me – it's the same as pulling their legs out from under them and dragging them off without permission.' Unsurprisingly, some users prefer not to have grab handles on their chairs.

Living with an LTC impinges on home, work-related and social activities. Experience leads individuals to develop a repertoire of strategies for managing their conditions around these. For instance, when attending events where food and drink are available, some people with diabetes mellitus are guided by their condition, rather than purely by desire. If they do not wish to bring this to wider attention, they might avoid alcoholic drinks on the pretext of wanting to 'keep a clear head'. Conversely, others might learn to alter their insulin injections to allow for indulging in food and drink that they prefer. Creative nonadherence (Taylor 2021) to treatment or 'intelligent cheating' is common in LTCs. It can result in errors, but careful adaptation reflects individuals' assertion of control and successful renegotiation of life situations in their own context. Strategies used can require the ongoing assistance of relatives, friends, acquaintances or strangers who might

function in various ways to assist in maintaining treatment programmes or protect the individual from harmful effects of the disorder. For example, someone with epilepsy might need help from workmates, such that harmful objects are moved should an unexpected seizure occur.

The enduring nature of LTCs also results in repeated interaction between individuals and service providers, perhaps over a period of months or years. This leads to individuals becoming familiar with organisations and staff with whom they come into contact, having implications for the development of complex relationships between them. Familiarity helps staff in monitoring self-management and detecting subtle changes in health but can make maintaining social boundaries difficult. Frequent attendance with problems that are vague or irresolvable can also mark patients as unpopular. The current emphasis on self-management advocated by health systems, and charitable organisations seeks to empower and liberate individuals to take control (Patients Association 2022). However, whilst this is welcomed by many, for some this focus may further exacerbate how difficult and challenging they are finding their LTC. This is particularly true of those experiencing socioeconomic deprivation who subsequently suffer further mental distress and poor health (Woodward et al. 2023) Depending on the dominant approach in a particular setting, either asserting oneself or passivity can be regarded as resistance to adopting the patient role and result in individuals acquiring a reputation for being 'demanding' or 'difficult'.

Uncertainty

Living with LTC(s) from an older person's perspective can be like living in a world with diminishing horizons as they navigate insecurity, uncertainty, unpredictable health, indeterminate prognosis and constant change (Åberg et al. 2020). At any age, there is sometimes a lengthy and complicated journey to diagnosis or recognition of the impact of their symptoms, with repeated visits to physicians and outpatient clinics and for some people, it is sometimes hard to convince health workers of the legitimacy of their condition.

Biographical disruption (a term used to describe the way individuals with chronic illness are faced with losing life as lived previously, sense of self in relation to this and their vision of the future) leads to grieving for previously taken-for-granted opportunities and ambitions (Reflection 30.5). The restriction, discomfort and possible dependence (actual or imposed by carers) that accompany LTCs may force the individual to forgo their desire for independence and autonomy

Fear of dependence, which in itself causes uncertainty, is a fundamental human concern in cultures valuing self-reliance and physical and economic independence. Following diagnosis, this problem is shared to an extent by health workers who must decide how much to share regarding the likely course of conditions and difficulties of treatment. Although it is seen as important to provide sufficient information to enable patients to exert maximum control over their situation, staff might question this in situations where only limited solutions can be offered (Rees 2023).

The Impact of Fluctuation

Fluctuations in symptoms, and the energy to manage them, make it impossible to forecast the occurrence of 'good days' and 'bad days' and this is compounded because a 'good day' can turn abruptly into a 'bad day' and vice versa. Uncertainty is also present because many LTCs are episodic, involving recurrent unpredictable exacerbations, followed by periods of remission or control.

Living With Biographical Disruption

J is 30 years old, works as a cook in an independent school and lives on the premises. Her social life revolves around sporting activities, an interest shared with her boyfriend. J was diagnosed as having multiple sclerosis (MS) 2 years ago when she was admitted to hospital following a fall. She had begun to find coordination difficult and became known for dropping and spilling things but thought this was due to overwork.

J's approach to MS was to get on with living. Within a short period, however, her balance deteriorated, walking became difficult and she tired easily. Having valued her physical fitness, she experienced frustration at her loss of ability, felt as though her body had betrayed her and was increasingly tearful. She had always been independent and wanted this to continue. Her boyfriend tried to support her but this was hard at times. His friends advised him not to remain in the relationship purely because of his concern for J, and his feelings for her were sometimes confused.

Meanwhile, J was preoccupied by questions about her future. How long would she be able to continue work? Would alternative employment be possible? Giving up her job would mean losing her home. Her parents wanted her to live with them but J worried her mother would be overprotective. However, her boyfriend was her greatest concern. J loved him and hoped that their relationship would last. She wanted to have children and already felt time was running out. J felt it impossible to discuss this, fearing that this could press her boyfriend to make an immediate decision and that she may lose him altogether. Her conclusion was that with MS she could no longer be sure of anything.

Activity

J has clear concerns about what is happening and what this could mean for her future. Reflect on J's experience and the aspects of living she feels anxious about, visit the MS Society's website and explore the pages for people aged 18–40 (http://www.mssociety.org.uk/pieces/index.html). Why might learning more about MS enable J to manage her situation?

Since the onset and duration of exacerbations cannot be anticipated, individuals and their carers must be vigilant for them and ready to respond at any time. This means that individuals and their families can find it difficult to maintain continuity or plan their activities ahead and, as a result, cannot participate fully in community life. Friends might, for instance, eventually hesitate to extend invitations when people have repeatedly refused or withdrawn from events. Regret, resentment and social isolation can follow as activities are curtailed (Biordi and Nicolson 2009). For example, somebody with type 1 diabetes is constantly vigilant as to their blood glucose levels and must ensure they eat at regular intervals. Whilst technology and the use of glucose sensors and insulin pumps have reduced the need for continued 'finger pricking', the need to constantly be aware of their condition to avoid hypoglycaemic or hyperglycaemic events remains.

Fluctuation in LTCs also influences the way in which individuals perceive themselves and are perceived by others. Crucially, the invisibility of some conditions can cause others to question the reality of their experience and even doubt that it exists. For example, long COVID-19 does not easily fit into the dominant evidence-based practice and the biomedical model of health. Like other postviral syndromes such as myalgia encephalomyelitis (ME), chronic fatigue syndrome (CFS) or fibromyalgia, objective indicators of the disease process can be absent. Despite patient narratives, patients' accounts of their health are frequently disbelieved, and their narratives are not taken seriously leading to stigma and epistemic injustice, which introduces a lack of trust in the therapeutic relationship (Ireson et al. 2022). This means that the consequences of living with an LTC are disregarded. Individuals are believed to be directly affected only when it becomes noticeable, so variation in ability, during a particular day or period of exacerbation, is misunderstood. Nurses lacking knowledge of LTCs can be quick to make judgements as to why people could perform activities yesterday but not today or cannot be certain of their capability for tomorrow. This can have harmful consequences. For instance, staff caused an immobile man with Parkinson's disease considerable distress when they implied he was lazy because they had seen him walking previously. He was actually unable to move due to the unpredictable 'on–off effect' associated with his response to long-term medication.

Beneficial Effects of Uncertainty

Paradoxically, uncertainty in LTCs can be presented as an opportunity to reappraise life's possibilities (Kimbell et al. 2016). Whether of sudden life-changing onset or signalling that changes will occur, diagnosis can prompt individuals to reflect on the way life had been lived and to search for new meaning in exploring events, reprioritising and seeking new challenges. As one person explained: 'If anyone asks, I tell them I wouldn't do away with having had my stroke now. Yes, I'd do away with its problems, but I've learned who my real friends are, that I don't want to spend all my waking hours in the office, and discovered I can do things I'd never thought of as "me" before too – like disability sport and joining a service users' group.' Uncertainty can also motivate concordance with treatment since this provides a tool for maintaining some stability.

Transition

During an individual's life course, there are many transitions as they move from childhood to adulthood. For some these transitions are more frequent between periods of wellness and illness, whilst for others, they mark the passage of time, the impact of ageing and the shift between active treatment, palliative and end of life care. An individual diagnosed with an LTC in young adulthood may have many years of health and independence before other health conditions impact their abilities to remain independent. Transition can also be a feature of how care is experienced as traditional models of caring practice led by nurses is replaced with a multidisciplinary team and integrated care teams, and the shift towards community-focused acute services such as virtual hospitals. How we support people during periods of transition can have a lasting impact on their health and well-being in the future and each must be planned and managed sensitively to ensure every person reaches their full potential (NICE 2016).

Palliative Emphasis

As the prospect of cure is remote in LTCs, measures to improve or maintain quality of life assume primary importance. More emphasis is placed on palliation, that is, alleviating pain, discomfort and nausea, providing symptomatic relief and addressing problems created by restricted activity. Palliation is of greater significance than in acute illness because people with LTCs must live with both the conditions' features and the cumulative side-effects of the treatment.

Decisions as to which palliative measures are suggested depend on their availability, acceptance by individuals and the medical profession, evidence base, perceived benefit and financial constraints.

Integrating effective palliative care into long-term care is challenging, in part due to diverse views (within health professionals and patients) as to what palliative care is, and when to introduce this to patients and their carers (Cloutier et al. 2021). Improvements in quality of life following palliation are difficult to measure objectively and this has implications for the allocation of resources, as discussed later.

Individuals have considerable personal resilience and many try to resolve problems before seeking help or as an adjunct to it. This is commonly seen when the treatment itself or its side-effects become intolerable. Complementary therapies are used commonly by people who feel that orthodox treatments have nothing further to offer but, in LTCs, this also represents an assumption of control where it otherwise seems to have been lost. This is also evident in patients who use recreational drugs, such as cannabis, to alleviate symptoms of either disease or treatment. Patient control is important because stress both results from the experience of living with LTCs and exacerbates symptoms, being associated with relapse. Mental distress can also lead to the development of anxiety-related and depressive disorders. Stress management is aided by therapies that pay explicit attention to the mind–body relationship, and approaches that mobilise individuals' inner resources, such as mindfulness-based interventions (Hodge et al. 2015), are also practiced alongside conventional treatment. However, recent research suggests that the effectiveness of practising mindfulness to reduce stress in palliative care patients is minimal (Latorraca et al. 2017).

Comorbidity

The systematic and degenerative effects of many LTCs mean that the failure of one organ or system leads eventually to the involvement of others. In addition, the impact of polypharmacy and ageing populations adds to a complex picture of comorbidities. For example, people living with HIV have an increased risk of NCDs compared with non-HIV-positive people (d'Arminio Monforte et al. 2020). Complications associated with type 2 diabetes might result in nerve impairment and an increased risk of peripheral neuropathies. Impaired sensation in the extremities can in turn predispose the patient to an increased risk of falls, poor recovery from injury and greater susceptibility to infection. Amputation of an affected limb leads to further alteration of physical, psychological and social functioning. Efforts to adjust are also complicated by the multiplication of symptoms and resulting impairment. For example, chronic pain both inhibits movement and correlates with atrophy in the brain's prefrontal cortex, which impairs decision-making.

Since contemporary medical services are organised by area of specialisation, people may require referral to a multitude of specialties, such as a surgeon, medical physician, specialist psychiatrist for substance misuse, as well as a range of specialist nurses, and other health professionals. Defining specialists' boundaries and intraservice communication is not always straightforward, so individuals have difficulty identifying from whom to seek advice for different aspects of their condition and whose recommendations should take precedence at any one time.

To be confronted with the inevitability of deterioration is a substantial psychological challenge to individuals and their carer. Those fearing the prospect of total disability might regard any development of their condition, or the onset of a new condition, with anxiety and anger, directing these emotions toward others. Carers may experience the brunt of these emotions as they deal with changing and increasing support needs, new service interventions and a drain on their emotional and physical reserves.

Healthcare professionals can be perceived as being incapable of resolving certain issues or, in the case of problems arising from treatment. This has obvious implications for the quality of nurse–patient relationships, which to be genuinely therapeutic must be characterised by mutual trust and cooperation (Reflection 30.6).

Intrusiveness

A significant aspect of living with LTCs is the daily requirement of monitoring and managing their features (Roddis et al. 2016). Such work is unrewarding, unrelenting and inescapable. As someone with CFS explained: 'For one wonderful moment when you wake up you forget. But there it is. Again. Any novelty around pills and things has gone and there's no time off.' Becoming accustomed to

---

REFLECTION 30.6

Different Approaches to Managing a Long-Term Condition

Until recently, L, a 68-year-old man who has COPD (chronic obstructive pulmonary disease), was making progress in managing his condition but he had recently been under pressure at work and become depressed. He had hoped to retire at 66 but due to changing financial circumstances has had to continue working. He has missed recent appointments with the practice nurse, and was reluctant to admit this or to disclose his feelings to his GP but was reassured to be received positively and told that commonly prescribed medication for his depression should help. The GP added, this to his drug regimen; however, L was distressed to find he now had sexual dysfunction. In addition he was struggling to maintain his weight and was feeling increasingly tired and lethargic. These developments deepened L's sense of hopelessness; he felt a failure, and related stress exacerbated his dyspnoea.

L began to fear what might happen next and his trust in the healthcare team was badly shaken. This was underlined when, during his next GP visit, the issues seemed to be put down to his mental ill-health and the importance of its continued treatment was emphasised. The consultation was short and L was shaken as he had not thought he had mental ill-health, he had just felt stressed in the workplace. It seemed to L as though he was expected to comply with what was deemed to be in his best interests without any discussion or acknowledgement that, from his perspective, the side-effects of treatment were making his situation much worse.

Despite having lost motivation to attend, L decided to keep his forthcoming appointment with the practice nurse at the COPD clinic. This was because, while other healthcare team members seemed to be 'always on at him' about condition management, her previous approach to his smoking cessation had involved listening without judgement to difficulties he was having, identifying his personal barriers and considering pros and cons around genuinely realistic solutions. L reasoned that it would be easier to explain to her that this experience was more than he could tolerate and to ask about other treatment options.

Activities

Reflecting on L's circumstances:

- Why should people be aware of both the benefits and drawbacks of treatment?
- What could happen to an individual's long-term condition management if they are unable to share their views with the healthcare team?
- Identify why L perceived his relationship with the nurse positively. You could think about organisational issues such as availability and continuity, together with attributes such as knowledge of long-term conditions, being open to patients' insights, skilled interaction, developing rapport and demonstrating empathy.

this is challenging because it involves a fundamental shift from the former self and life towards recognition and acceptance of a new normal (Chew et al. 2014).

Loss, Grief and Adaptation

Grief experienced in LTCs resembles that in bereavement. It can be associated with loss of a body part, image, function, social status or role and can occur suddenly when an LTC is acquired or over time as it progresses. People can also experience loss of identity because it reflects their previous, nonimpaired self and they feel they have become less of a person than they were. Awareness of models of grief or response towards threat to self-integrity (e.g. Kubler-Ross 1969, Morse 1997, respectively) guides nurses in supporting individuals to work towards adaptation to unwanted change. However, many of the traditional models focus on the intrapsychic process and patterns of grieving without full exploration of the embodied experience with physical symptoms seen as a reflection of the mind. Brinkmann (2017) argued that grief does not simply impact the body but is enacted by the embodied grieved person. In the grief experienced by people who have LTCs the process is painful, and unpredictable and fluctuates in their struggle to manage the powerful reactions created. Attending to embodied activities can provide meaning and bring about a sense of recovery as people adjust to their new and often different life.

For some, grief remains unresolved and can be more disabling than the condition itself. Here, it is essential for nurses to recognise the meaning of what has been lost and understand that addressing this is key to renewing self-identity (Telford et al. 2006). Again, this means considering biopsychosocial issues beyond diagnostic labels and accounting for other health problems present. Adaptation is complicated, particularly because 'good' adaptation is judged by others and not by the person experiencing the grief. The emotional burden experienced by the individual can be increased by shame and guilt at failing to recover or adjust as quickly as expected. Health workers need to recognise this and avoid comparing individuals with others who have adapted successfully despite being 'worse off'. Creating artificial hierarchies of suffering and invalidating someone's experience is unhelpful. Although it is not truly possible to walk in another's shoes, trying to understand the person's own perspective is paramount. Individuals can feel responsible for not doing better, in the light of images of disabled people as 'brave' with an innate capacity to tolerate adversity or assumptions that they must simply adjust to the obvious. Pressure can be added where media portrayals of triumph over tragedy create models of behaviour that individuals feel they must live up to.

Impact on Home Life and Relationships

LTCs often impose changes to normal domestic routines to allow for physical limitations and the sustained requirements of treatment programmes. Structural alteration of housing might also be required to install equipment and reassign room space for access to facilities. These adaptations, together with the intrusion into living spaces by nurses and health professionals, and alterations in appearance and behaviour associated with the condition, will impact on other members of the household. Families' daily activities are often centred on supporting individuals and it might not be possible for them to pursue interests they once enjoyed together. Providing ongoing care changes relationships and compels those who have assumed an unexpected caring role to make fundamental changes to their lifestyle. The strategies used to manage conditions can have implications for everyone taking part. For example, the schedule of dialysis for people with chronic kidney injury requires

them to have fixed periods of treatment across a week limiting the opportunity for them to be flexible in their other activities. It can disrupt well-established routines and individuals and carers are faced with developing a lifestyle structured by the demands of the presenting condition, within which spontaneity has no place.

Adopting the roles of carer and cared for also impacts established relationships and it cannot be assumed that even in loving relationships the changing role is easy. For example, it can be difficult for a disabled person to blend the role of partner with that of someone now needing support to manage incontinence from the other in a relationship. The inevitable triad between the cared for, carer and partner and the dynamic relationship between them all are eloquently captured by McKinney (2018) in her critical autoethnography of the experience.

Despite increased recognition of the needs and rights of carers within the legislation, carers continue to experience considerable difficulty in navigating through convoluted support systems administered by local and central government. Dealing with this is stressful and demands resources which, by nature of their activities, carers simply do not have.

Financial and Employment Issues

LTCs also have economic implications. Even if the person is not totally incapacitated, continued employment might be impossible because of the demands that disorders and their treatment make on time, strength and stamina. Difficulty in adhering to work schedules and nonattendance during exacerbations can give the impression that individuals are unreliable. Employers' inclusion of related absences in cumulative records of sick leave, raising issues of work capability, while offering incentives to reward low absenteeism disadvantage disabled people. Individuals might also be assigned less demanding roles and be overlooked for training or promotion because they are perceived to have limited potential, so are not deserving of the investment (Taylor 2021). Gaining employment is problematic in itself; employers may see the prospect of incapacity and variable function as risk and hidden costs, including lost production and redeployment of other workers.

It is understandable that, despite there being advantages in disclosing health status to an employer, people with LTCs are often reluctant to do so. It can lead to an individual's competence being doubted, reduces self-esteem and gives rise to guilt and fear of letting others down. This can result in individuals working harder than others to prove their worth when the effort needed to manage their conditions means that their energy margins are already stretched (Holland and Collins 2018). Employers do not always recognise the implications of this or of the 'reasonable adjustments' required by the Equality Act 2010.

Effect on Social Activities

LTCs affect the ability to participate in social activities. The impact of this depends in part on the strategies people use to deal with the features of their disorder. For example, a patient requiring diuretics in the morning for heart failure may need to urinate frequently throughout the day. Individuals may respond by not taking their medication in the morning, staying at home or planning outings carefully with short journeys and using known venues with accessible toilets.

Complex Service Use

The Department of Health and Social Care (DHSC) is responsible for supporting and advising ministers helping them shape and implement policy that delivers the government's objectives. The

DHSC is responsible for setting direction and anticipating the future and to lead debate ensuring it protects and improves global and domestic health. In 2022, the Health and Social Care Act in England continues to drive forward the agenda to ensure that people with LTC needs have planned and coordinated care, which is patient-centred and makes good use of available resources.

An abundance of statutory, voluntary and independent agencies are concerned with supporting people with LTCs in the UK. The NHS, the Department of Work and Pensions (DWP) and local authority social services are principal sources of statutory support. Provision can be fragmented due to the number of medical specialties and personnel involved, ineffective interagency coordination, differing access criteria and service targets. Transfers between care settings or the UK's administrative areas can add to this. For example, where an individual's relocation means that they cross regional or country boundaries and move into an area administered by another agency, it is likely that they will have to make a new application for services or equipment that they received previously. There is a risk of refusal if their needs are deemed inconsistent with priorities in the new locality, which can have a detrimental effect on independence and quality of life.

Integrated care systems (ICSs) in England replaced clinical commissioning groups in 2022, as partnerships of organisations come together to plan and deliver joined-up health and care services and to improve the lives of people who live and work in their area. These partnerships involve the NHS, local councils, community and voluntary organisations, local residents, people who use services, their carers and representatives and other community partners with a role in supporting the health and well-being of the population. In doing so ICSs aim to

- support people to stay well and independent, act sooner to help those with preventable conditions such as type 2 diabetes
- support those with long-term physical and mental health conditions
- care for those with multiple needs and
- effectively use collective resources to provide care as soon as possible.

Similar divisions occur in the devolved nations of Wales and Northern Ireland, and in Scotland, with health and social care partnerships.

Barriers to Seeking Support

Definitions used by formal agencies to categorise individuals and allocate resources lack compatibility with disabled people's experience. For example, assessment to determine eligibility for benefits and services might fail to acknowledge that LTCs fluctuate. If assessed during a period of relative wellness, the type and level of support required at other times might not be apparent. Some benefit claim forms acknowledge this but completing them can be dispiriting because their lengthy 'I need help with …' approach throws what individuals cannot do into sharp focus. This also discourages claims from those who are able to perform activities to some degree but with considerable difficulty, for example, being able to prepare a simple main meal independently even though problems with manual dexterity, pain, fatigue and managing spillages mean this takes several hours. The situation is compounded by having to reapply for benefits when only time-limited awards are made, despite the well-established existence of an LTC.

People might avoid seeking support because they perceive the organisation of services to be complex and arbitrary or fear that this could trigger state interference in their lives, whereas

appealing against the refusal of awards requires energy which individuals might not have. Ineffective communication presents an obstacle when those entitled to benefits lack information or have difficulty interpreting the information given. In addition, some people might be reluctant to seek or accept help because to do so would conflict with cultural values regarding responsibility and self-sufficiency.

Strategies adopted to manage an individual's problems also require the coordinated effort of everyone involved. The establishment and maintenance of arrangements rely on trust, skilled interaction, sufficient resources and realistic negotiation of the roles, responsibilities and expectations of all concerned. This does not apply only to formal care. Someone whose mobility is severely limited, for instance, due to long-standing arthritis, might have an array of relatives and friends to do shopping, pick up drug prescriptions, change light bulbs or batteries and walk their dog. The continued success of this depends on each person involved having a clear appreciation of what is required, as well as an understanding of their own contribution to the individual's chain of support.

Nursing Management

Location and Management of Care

Nurses encounter adults with LTCs in a range of community and institutional settings, including the person's own home, care homes and hospitals providing acute, rehabilitative, intermediate or continuing care. Statutory and other agencies have responded to the shift towards user-focused community care. This is supported by the aspirations of the Health and Care Act 2022 by attempting to meet rising demand, while accounting for the shortcomings of long-term institutionalisation. In addition, it is widely recognised that for many people with LTCs admission to hospital is not always necessary and that using intensive home-based care preventively or aiding them to return home more quickly and improve quality of life. The development of Community Health Services is key to improving out-of-hospital care, and includes services in people's own homes, care homes, intermediate care facilities and clinics. To achieve this, nurses working as community matrons or case managers need to work collaboratively with other primary, acute, mental health and social care providers (Stanhope and Lancaster 2016). Home-based care is viewed as resource effective, while also being preferable for and preferred by individuals.

Integrated Care

ICSs established across England in July 2022 consist of partnerships of organisations that come together to plan and deliver joined-up health and care services. Similar strategies are evident in the devolved countries of Scotland, Wales, and Northern Ireland.

In achieving these goals it is important that NHS, local government and their voluntary, community and social enterprises plan and deliver services. The House of Care model provides a framework that considers the expertise of the person with the LTC, and their communities alongside health and care professionals committed to partnership working. This whole system approach requires commissioners of services to be clear about what they want to provide, which populations of people require a customised House of Care approach, the model of care delivery (where, when and whom) and how this will be achieved including a financial model that can support what needs to be done. Carers and Community nursing services are essential to this providing a platform for promoting health and working effectively together.

Telecare, Virtual Wards and Hospital at Home

The direct and indirect costs of LTCs are high. Long-term medication to control or palliate symptoms has significant financial and ethical implications. Rationing of healthcare has become more explicit in the face of growing demand and the increased availability of treatment options, coupled with pressure to reduce expenditure (Robertson 2016). Limited resources mean that decisions are concerned with identifying the potential benefit to individuals and justifying whether such expenditure on a single patient is warranted or making population-based cost: benefit calculations, for example, per quality adjusted life year (QALY). The latter approach has, however, been criticised for discriminating against people with LTCs and older individuals whose life expectancy is by definition limited, and where quality of life measures 'perfect health' rather than what it means to individuals against the background of their specific life circumstances. NICE uses these indicators when identifying treatment options for individuals with long-term illnesses (Reflection 30.7).

During COVID 19 strategies implemented in the novel coronavirus pandemic enabled continued medical care while maintaining social distancing and allowed those at greater risk of morbidity and mortality to get medical assessments without leaving their home. Telehealth and telecare initiatives support this home-based approach and while not new, the improvements in technology make it widely available, low cost and more acceptable for patients and healthcare teams. However, technical issues such as internet access, Wi-Fi signal and bandwidth connectivity impact on its use, with many professionals and patients preferring more traditional phone consultations (Bokolo 2020). Moreover there is a lack of a fully developed legal framework to regulate the use of innovative IT solutions such as telemedicine in healthcare (Maret et al. 2020). The use of wearable devices has also increased and their feasibility in monitoring physiological measurements such as blood pressure and blood glucose, movement identification and fall risk, and mental well-being could help to improve outcomes for older adults in their own homes or in other residential health and care settings (Lu et al. 2020).

The concept of the virtual ward and Hospital at Home ensures that people have contact with appropriate health professionals and timely interventions to support acute illness events without leaving their homes (Kanyimo 2022). Community virtual wards (CVWs) are led by consultants supported by advanced practitioners and built around an experienced team of health professionals, coordinated by dedicated case managers, and are based on a conceptual model of risk. CVWs target support and interventions for older people in the community that are likely to experience adverse health outcomes. Specific pathways currently address the needs associated with frailty and respiratory infections. This model improves health-related quality of life, reduces unplanned hospital admissions, reduces the length of stay (LOS)

after Emergency Department (ED) presentation and statistically significantly reduces ED presentations. Delivery of acute interventions and remote monitoring is key to the concept of a virtual ward, and can involve sending data from devices such as pulse oximetry or blood glucose monitors to a central server, where they are compared against patient norms and clinicians are alerted if needed. Importantly, ongoing data capture also enables the effects of treatment and lifestyle changes to be monitored over time.

Reablement teams provide intensive time-limited intervention to assist people in regaining skills and independence on return home from hospital or residential care. Implemented since the early 2000s reablement interventions and activities are developed collaboratively with clients to focus on activities of living (AL) that enable people to continue to live safely and independently. These can also be supported with telecare to include safety monitoring, medication reminders, providing access to information, asking individuals questions to check and improve their knowledge of self-management (NHS England 2018).

Supporting Transition of Care

Moving into a care home can be perceived negatively as a last resort but can come as a relief when, for instance, someone is unable to maintain their desired lifestyle, an inflexible care package is in place or services no longer meet their needs. As one man with motor neurone disease (MND) stated: 'things just got too much, my home wasn't really mine. I'd lost count of the number of care workers who'd been in my underwear drawer or gone upstairs without asking and don't want to count any more.' Nurses have an important role in supporting individuals and their carers in considering options, adjusting to new environments, grieving for their past life and constructing a future such that they feel 'at home' in every sense and consider theirs a place for living. The quality of daily life in care homes depends on four key factors: the acceptance and adaptation of the resident to their new living situation, resulting in behaviours that preserve independence; connectedness with peer residents; a reciprocal relationship with staff; and improved familial relationships. The resident may no longer feel a burden to carers and be able to regain some independence and re-establish traditional familial roles.

A homelike environment is crucial to the new resident regaining control and adapting to their new lifestyle. The freedom of one's own room and bathroom, the opportunity for flexible unregimented living as well as meaningful activities and opportunities within and outside the care home are important to establish this care home as a place that provides support but is also a home. The attitude and competence of carers directly influence the resident's experiences within the assisted living/nursing home/residential care. Staff continuity, a feeling of attachment with care givers, staff understanding of the resident's life story, trust and a sense of safety are all identified as fostering a positive care home experience for the resident (Bradshaw et al. 2012).

Service contact with people who have LTCs can occur intermittently and recurrently in relation to establishing diagnoses, managing exacerbation or when conditions necessitate rehabilitation, stabilisation or palliation. It is also important to remember that it might result from the development of unrelated health problems: so, for example, nurses working in an ambulatory care unit will need to adapt their approach to care for someone with an acquired brain injury who has been admitted for laparoscopic surgery. Likewise, practice nurses will need to consider how cervical cytology screening can be made accessible for disabled women who are unable to adopt the customary position on the bed.

REFLECTION 30.7

Ethical Issues and Resource Allocation

Where resources are limited, it could be argued that efforts should be directed towards patients for whom improvement can be assured, rather than those who have long-term conditions or are disabled.

Activities

Using ethical principles to underpin your thinking, reflect on why patients with long-term conditions should be given equal or priority consideration.

Care management in the form of integrated care pathways (ICPs) has particular relevance in LTCs because these present a structured means of planning and delivering coordinated, patient-oriented care as part of a sequential journey, instead of as a series of separate episodes.

What Is Rehabilitation?

Definitions of rehabilitation vary, in line with its perceived purpose, but it is best described as an ongoing process that begins as soon as individuals are clinically stable, is independent of the location of care, reflects a transferable underpinning philosophy and involves shifting degrees and forms of support. This means that rehabilitation takes place wherever the patient is (and not on the ward next door, the unit downstairs or in the hospital across town).

Rehabilitation is frequently associated with 'restoration' but, this does not necessarily equate with returning someone to their former life. Rather, it implies enabling individuals to acquire the knowledge and skills needed for optimal biopsychosocial functioning, so that they can manage their impairments and reconstruct their lives. This requires an approach that embraces autonomy, independence, empowerment, problem-solving and learning because taking a purely functional view can fail to address the qualitative aspects of living with impairment. Rehabilitation was traditionally focused on physical health but it can also apply to mental health and the concept of recovery as a process, as opposed to an outcome model, can provide a framework for considering rehabilitation in that context (Jatta et al. 2022).

The Rehabilitative Process

The principles of rehabilitation apply to the care of people with long-term congenital or acquired conditions, though the emphasis given to it will depend on the individual's health and the presence of any other life-threatening or acute illness.

Davis and Madden's (2006) continuum of rehabilitation (Fig. 30.4) demonstrates that goals and interventions evolve according to the stroke survivor's needs and degree of impairment.

Thus during the initial stage when individuals are unconscious, rehabilitative care might involve providing stimulation, coming to know about them as people and supporting relatives/friends. Once individuals are fully responsive, have regained physical function and enter the second stage, interventions could include continual assessment of functional and cognitive ability, managing challenging behaviour, re-establishing daily activities, offering choice and involving relatives/friends in care. A more active rehabilitative programme assumes prominence in the third stage, with care in specialist settings concentrating on the individual's level of participation and quality of life. Interventions entail empowerment though shared goal planning, facilitating movement towards maximum potential in daily living, providing a coordinated rehabilitation programme and psychologically supporting all concerned. Having achieved this, the fourth stage focuses on maintaining quality of life and enabling individuals to live with their impairments, or LTC, through community and third-sector support, or through outpatient care, reassessment and problem-solving.

Team-Working

Effective rehabilitation requires input from several disciplines, and team-working is generally accepted as central to this. Contributory characteristics include clear communication, acceptance of collective responsibility, purpose and action, understanding each other's roles and overlap, a common goal and flexibility (WHO 2011). In

Stage 4

Where the individual has reached their full potential and is either at home or in alternative accommodation

Goal: to focus on enabling them to live with impairments and maintaining quality of life

Interventions include: follow-up appointments with the rehabilitation team, reassessment and revised or further interventions, provision of respite care, attendance of day facilities

Stage 3

A more active rehabilitation programme is needed, perhaps with transfer to a dedicated unit

Goal: to focus on the individual's level of participation and quality of life

Interventions include: enabling achievement of potential in daily activities, empowerment through involvement and informed choice, ensuring cross-disciplinary continuity, providing individuals and their families with psychological support and a supportive, structured environment

Stage 2

The individual has recovered consciousness, is fully responsive and regaining some physical function

Goal: depends on individual need. Can include to maintain a safe, comfortable environment or focus on functional or cognitive abilities

Interventions include: managing challenging behaviour, assessing ability (functional and cognitive), establishing alternative means of communication, establishing daily activities (e.g. using toilet facilities instead of a commode), providing choices, giving support to and involving relatives

Stage 1

The initial critical stage taking place at first contact (e.g. in an Accident and Emergency Unit) when the individual is unconscious

Goal: to preserve life

Interventions include: preventing complications, providing stimulation, supporting relatives

Figure 30.4 Continuum of rehabilitation. (After Davis S, Madden S. Rehabilitation at a macro and micro level. In: Davis S, ed. *Rehabilitation: The Use of Theories and Models in Practice*. Edinburgh: Churchill Livingstone; 2006:3-22.)

addition using a patient-centred approach that includes the individuals and their carers ensures goals and outcomes are agreed. The terms used to describe teams reflect their ways of working, for example, whether they are multi-, inter- or transdisciplinary.

Interdisciplinary working implies a greater commitment to collaboration and shared decision-making, authority and responsibility. This is achieved through the collaborative setting of person-oriented goals, using integrated pathways and records, transcending professional or role boundaries, and leadership based on skill, as opposed to professional grouping. Obstacles to this can be attitudinal, for example, perceived loss of professional autonomy or status, and organisational, such as uniprofessional education, different working patterns and lines of accountability (Weller et al. 2014).

The Nursing Role

While the contribution of health professionals is crucial during diagnosis, rehabilitation and exacerbation, individuals and their carers are responsible for managing conditions on a daily basis. The nursing role is, therefore, far from restricted to the delivery of direct care and increasingly nurses will be working as part of an integrated care team, led by themselves or others. In Ireland, the Integrated Care Programme for Older Persons (ICPOP) 2021, provides a useful framework for delivering effective healthcare that leverages existing health and social care provision based on collaboration between older people, carers and health professionals, including nurses. Importantly in effective healthcare delivery, effective and positive communication is essential and nurses are well placed to ensure that the needs and wishes of the individual are understood and that care delivery is coordinated without unnecessary repetition. People with LTCs often complain about how different professionals ask the same questions, and as a result, care feels disjointed and unplanned. An integrated approach has been shown to improve the patient experience and satisfaction with care delivery (Duhoux et al. 2022).

When working in a collaborative manner to support optimal self-management, the nurse must also be prepared to adopt a flexible approach. During some phases of long-term illness it may be necessary to act directly for patients and carers, while, at other times, support will focus on facilitating review by other health professionals, the performance of self-care activities, imparting knowledge, teaching practical skills or giving emotional support to aid adaptive behaviour. Nurses need to be committed to forming and maintaining collaborative, empowering relationships (Goedhart et al. 2017). Individuals can be disabled where nurses are accustomed to acting as 'doer' such as when using a wheelchair to move a patient's location, without giving them the opportunity to walk with support due to the time it may take. This can occur due to perceived time pressures and risk reduction that are influenced by professional, organisational and systemic factors, which either enhance or inhibit relational quality, shared decision-making, mutual commitment and nurses' confidence and capacity to enable individuals to be independent.

Empowerment

The notion of empowerment has particular value for people living with LTCs because they are likely to have lost control and confidence in their own abilities. Empowerment is an enabling process that enhances personal control and facilitates the process of recreating self. Although self-management groups provide a means of empowerment, they also reflect preparedness to assert the value of experiential knowledge and to question that of medicine. This opposes traditional roles and leads professionals to control information and dismiss patients' efforts to theorise about or explain their conditions.

Conversely, patients can feel coerced into partnership, experiencing tension at being expected to both drive their care and 'do as they are told' in accepting this. Rehabilitation is a difficult process to enter into and requires individuals to be receptive and committed to intensive, new learning at a time when they are dealing with the physical impact of disability and related psychosocial issues.

Nurses need to recognise that not all individuals are motivated to participate actively in their rehabilitation and that support and patience are needed to enable them to work towards their potential at their own pace (Kings Fund 2012).

The complexity of LTCs and their impact on lifestyle and functioning have already been emphasised. It is all too easy for nurses to make assumptions about the problems experienced by individuals on the basis of medical diagnosis alone. There are additional implications arising from classifying people as 'the long-term ill' or 'the disabled'. Overuse of these labels can give the impression of homogeneous groups for whom care can be planned unilaterally. It also opposes the idea that individuals with LTCs should be regarded as team members in shaping the rehabilitation process.

Nursing Roles in Rehabilitation

Rehabilitation nursing is recognised as a specialty but roles are not clearly defined and nurses do not always feel their contribution is recognised by other team members. McPherson (2006) argues that skills claimed in areas such as team-working, communication, assessment, facilitating independence in AL, health promotion, working with person-centred goals, empowerment and acting as advocate for individuals and their families apply equally to roles of others working in the field. They maintain a 24-hour presence is not reason enough to assert nurses' unique role but this does provide opportunities for them to 'close the circle in the rehabilitation process' by encouraging people to incorporate new skills and therapeutic activity into daily life (therapy 'carry-on'), leading, educating, coordinating and sharing their ongoing observations with team members whose decision-making might otherwise be based on snapshot evaluation.

In addition, nurses integrate the management of pain, continence, nutrition, tissue viability and the need for balanced rest and stimulation into the individual's overall rehabilitation programme. The important thing is not so much what nurses do but the way care is provided. Rehabilitation is not effective because it provides life-saving interventions but by focusing on enabling individuals to achieve their own goals by identifying how barriers can be overcome (Kings Fund 2012). This also involves 'being with' the person and sharing their journey through the development of a supportive, empathic relationship.

Prescribing and Deprescribing

People living with LTCs are often prescribed many medications and although poorly defined a prescription of five or more drugs is termed polypharmacy. Polypharmacy contributes to the health concerns experienced as additional medications are prescribed to compensate for the side-effects of treatments or medications already prescribed. Older people are at increased risk of drug-related complications including drug therapy problems related to interactions, drug toxicity, falls with injury, delirium and nonadherence. Polypharmacy is associated with increased hospitalisations, increased care in the community and higher costs to individuals and healthcare systems. Nurses have a key role in ensuring there are processes in place for timely medication review that require an interdisciplinary approach that avoids episodic care. Using a systematic approach can facilitate good interprofessional working and collaboration, as the responsibility to ensure appropriate prescribing is nested with all prescribers. One such approach is supported by the use of tools to minimise potentially inappropriate prescribing, such as STOPP/START (O'Mahony et al. 2023). Although time-consuming, the inclusion of tools to support medication review with appropriate deprescribing using a patient-centred approach is warranted (Oboh and Qadir 2017).

Using Frameworks and Models to Guide Practice

As discussed earlier, although a variety of characteristics are shared by people with LTCs, there is considerable diversity in their response. A nursing approach that recognises explicitly the uniqueness of individuals and enables the totality of their situation to be understood must therefore be adopted.

Various conceptual models have been devised to articulate beliefs about nursing's essential components and underpinning theory. In representing the reality of practice, concepts of person, environment, health and nursing are central to them. These models offer a foundation for the development of nursing as a discipline and, if adopted by a nursing team, promote consistency and continuity of nursing action. The selection of a particular model for practice depends largely on the extent to which it reflects the patient/client focus, nursing team's own values and perceived goals related to interventions.

While a number of models have relevance for nursing people with LTCs, those identified subsequently might have particular interest for those working in this area. Discussion of the models is necessarily brief in this chapter and readers are encouraged to refer to the referenced sources to gain a better understanding.

Recovery Model

The recovery-orientated approaches in mental health focus on fostering personal growth, encouraging active participation based on a coaching style approach to enable the individual to live their 'best life possible' (Roberts and Wolfson 2004). Increasingly models of care are influenced by the concept of recovery. The guiding principles of recovery are based on hope and the belief that an individual can have a meaningful life despite persistent symptoms. As such recovery is considered a conceptual framework that focuses on development and support of self-management strategies (Jacob 2015).

The recovery model whilst originating within the context of mental illness is relevant to the care and management of many people with LTCs. The aim of the recovery model is to get people to a point where they can live healthy, productive lives, in a sustainable way through building resilience to cope with challenges, validating personal experiences, cultivating strategies for coping and improving quality of life. Arguably such an approach is well suited to those living with an LTC. It empowers people to clarify their values, establish goals and complete action plans that provide them with the direction needed to pursue their vision of a valued life. Used as a philosophical approach alongside more traditional frameworks within nursing practice enhances collaborative and co-constructed models of working.

Orem's Self-Care Model

The self-care deficit nursing theory (SCDNT, Orem 2001) is likely to appeal to nurses who consider its emphasis on client autonomy and motivation to be consistent with the aim of helping individuals to accept responsibility for themselves. This might seem appropriate, given the role people with LTCs play in managing their condition. Its concern with independent action is, however, more complex than face value suggests. The concept of self-care must be seen in the context of the model's other components, so that underlying theory can be understood and the whole operationalised.

Self-care is the contribution people make to their own continued existence and involves practising activities to maintain health and well-being. Nurses assist patients and their associates to achieve self-care, taking individual ability and need into account. Following negotiation with all concerned, care is organised in terms of one of three nursing systems. These are wholly compensatory, partly compensatory or supportive–educative, that is, the nurse may perform activities for the individual, assist the individual in carrying out shared activities or help them to develop the ability to act on their own behalf. The decision to use a nursing system or a combination of systems is not static but changes in response to patient need over time.

Orem's model can be used in a variety of settings. The importance of partnership with patients and carers is acknowledged and their involvement in planning nursing interventions considered essential. Attention is given to the notion that people are active in learning to live with the effects of LTCs and exploits their motivation to do so. The variation in nursing activity necessary to address the range of problems likely to be experienced during the course of such disorders is also accounted for.

Roy's Adaptation Model

Roy's adaptation model (Roy and Andrews 2008) might be thought suitable in LTCs because it views human behaviour as being influenced by an interrelated set of biological, psychological and social systems, each of which is directed towards achieving a state of relative balance. This will, as far as possible, promote regularity of function and aid the individual to adapt positively to environmental stimuli (or stressors).

Roy identifies three types of stimuli to which individuals are exposed: focal, contextual and residual. A focal stimulus is something that has an immediate effect on the person, a contextual stimulus is a contributory circumstance and a residual stimulus arises from beliefs or attitudes relating to past experiences. Maladaptation occurs where the effect of any stimulus exceeds someone's capacity to make a positive response. This results in a threat to continued health and well-being. Roy's model accepts that individuals possess a unique capacity to deal with stimuli, such that people react differently when faced with the same events. The ability to adapt thus varies from person to person.

Nursing intervention is needed when an individual's usual methods of coping with stressors prove ineffective. The nursing role centres on promoting adaptation in maintaining health and during periods of illness, and is concerned with manipulating stimuli, enabling people to respond positively.

This model also has value for care in LTCs in a variety of settings. Its focus is congruent with the belief that individuals manage and adapt to the same events differently, considers it desirable for them to develop the ability to live with the effects of their conditions and engages them collaboratively in their care. Nurses are encouraged to consider factors that influence the individual's context, not merely the immediate problems confronting them. In this way it is possible for nurses to appreciate the effects of a condition over time and how the individual feels about this. The model assists nurses in identifying successful past coping mechanisms and elements likely to impede future adaptation, so that intervention may be planned with realisable goals. Care can therefore be tailored in relation to individual resources.

The Roper–Logan–Tierney (RLT) Model

The RLT model for nursing (Holland et al. 2008, Roper et al. 2000) has been widely adopted in the UK and thus is one with which many nurses are familiar, and can be readily applied to all healthcare settings.

In addition, it is based on ideas drawn directly from practice, and the AL terminology is one that is familiar to other health and social care workers. As such, although the RLT model can be poorly used as a 'checklist', when used in its entirety it is effective when planning integrated care. With the development of integrated services that may be led by other health professionals, having a common language, such as AL, in the assessment of care needs, alongside a recovery approach to goal identification can inform and support the development of a coordinated and sustained plan. Roper et al.'s portrayal of an uncomplicated view of nursing is a deliberate attempt to provide a flexible framework that can be applied across settings. In this model, the focus of nursing intervention is on assisting individuals in the prevention, resolution and management of problems and ultimately to regain independence in AL independently or with support.

The RLT model applies readily to LTCs because it is grounded on a model for living, demonstrating that health status and lifestyle are closely related. An awareness of this helps nurses to perceive their role in terms of health promotion and maintenance, as well as dealing with acute condition-oriented problems. In the assessment and planning process, problems can be defined as actual or potential with nursing goals described using the Specific, Measurable, Achievable, Relevant, and Time-Bound (SMART) framework. The model's purpose of equipping practitioners with a means to plan and deliver individualised care in relation to both nurse-initiated and multiprofessional activity facilitates collaboration. Fig. 30.5 outlines the model's five components. These will be considered in turn and applied to the care of people with LTCs.

Activities of Living (AL)

Living can be described as a fusion of the 12 AL (see Fig. 30.5), which individuals experience and carry out differently. Although the AL are the core of the RLT model and present a framework for assessment, there is a danger that some nurses use it simply as a 12-point checklist and the model's other dimensions may be overlooked as a result. For example, identifying an old woman who has osteoporosis and is admitted to hospital following a fall as simply 'having problems mobilising' would not necessarily take into account issues such as her social circumstances, her values and beliefs about her diagnosis or the systemic effects of her condition. The effectiveness of her existing long-term pain management, coping strategies psychological impact have not been looked into. Factors such as living in a first-floor flat, whilst being fiercely independent and rejecting additional support, leaves this patient more vulnerable.

The performance of any AL requires the coordination of a complex pattern of behaviour. The ability to communicate, for example, relies on skills including the reception and interpretation of information and the formulation and transmission of appropriate verbal and nonverbal responses. This is influenced by many variables, such as the efficiency of physiological and psychological functions. Thus there is considerable scope for error and it is likely that people with LTCs will experience a wide range of associated problems. For instance, some individuals may not understand or express ideas verbally following a stroke, while others find no difficulty in this area but are unable to articulate words clearly (see Chapter 11, Nursing Patients With Disorders of the Nervous System). In either case, individuals will be limited in their ability to make their thoughts and feelings known and this will cause frustration for all concerned.

Speech deterioration also takes place in, for example, Parkinson's where communication can be further inhibited by memory impairment and loss of facial expression. The latter provides the listener with poor feedback and results in the absence of important nonverbal cues. As mentioned, alteration in the person's

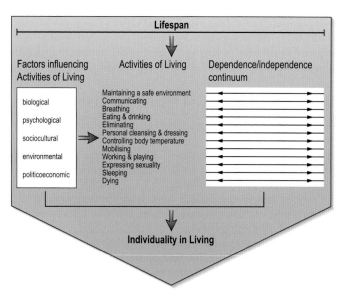

Figure 30.5 The Activity of Living (AL) model. (From Holland K, Jenkins J, Solomon J, Whittam S. *Applying the Roper–Logan–Tierney Model in Practice*. 2nd ed. Edinburgh: Churchill Livingstone; 2008 with permission.)

physical appearance can also present a barrier to communication, in that people might avoid casual social contact with them or make assumptions about their mental state.

It is common for people with LTCs to find that disruption in the performance of one AL leads to difficulty in the performance of others. For instance, someone who has long-term mental health issues and COPD who experiences shortness of breath might also find their capacity to communicate, eat and drink, reach the toilet, attend to personal hygiene, walk, work, socialise and sleep compromised.

Lifespan

This component of the model represents the passage through life from conception to death. The progression along the lifespan is marked by continual change, as the individual moves through a series of developmental stages, each of which is associated with the expression of different levels of physical, cognitive and social function. As mentioned previously, adulthood is generally characterised by self-reliance centring on occupational and family interests but there is, of course, considerable diversity in individual lifestyle and behaviour during this life stage. Chronological age alone does not give the nurse enough information to appreciate the likely impact of LTCs. Rather, the nurse will need to gain an understanding of which developmental tasks someone has already achieved, those they aspire to and the value placed on each by the individual and those close to them.

Obtaining this kind of information reveals the existence of actual or potential problems requiring nursing intervention. For example, a woman who has multiple sclerosis (MS) and wishes to become pregnant may have to confront issues such as sexual dysfunction, the impact of discontinuing disease-modifying or other medication and whether her functional impairment would present difficulties in meeting the needs of a newborn. Once the nurse recognises this as causing emotional distress, it can be accounted for in the care planning process; for example, the woman's need for accurate, evidence-based information may be met by referral to a specialist nurse and a suggestion that she obtain peer support from the MS Society.

The Dependence/Independence Continuum

This component acts as a reminder that individuals are not always able to perform each AL unaided (Holland et al. 2008). Some people have yet to acquire the necessary skills or do not have the means to develop them, whilst illness or trauma causes others to lose abilities they once had.

No single measure reflects the capacity for independent function in all AL, since it can be argued that few people, if any, are truly self-sufficient. In addition, the concepts of dependence and independence have meaning only when considered in relation to each other. For these reasons, any form of assessment will have a subjective bias which is determined by the nurse's interpretation of an individual's abilities in comparison with clinical, developmental and social norms. This means, for example, that assumptions about the inevitability of universal deterioration in advancing age need to be questioned.

The interactive nature of the AL and the fact that difficulty in carrying out one can affect adversely the performance of others have implications for the maintenance of independent action in LTCs. In recognition of this, it is essential that attention is paid to each of them when assessing a patient's dependence/independence status. For example, altered mobility associated with systemic lupus erythematosus (SLE or lupus) can also interfere with shopping for and preparing meals, while sports activity and keyboard skills might be made difficult by reduced physical dexterity or fatigue.

Factors Influencing the Activities of Living

Understandings the factors that influence the individual way that AL are performed, regardless of the point reached in the lifespan or the level of dependence held is central to effective management of LTCs. The five influential factors identified in the RLT model assist nurses in taking a holistic view of an individual's situation:

- biological
- psychological – incorporating intellectual and emotional factors
- sociocultural – incorporating spiritual, religious and ethical factors
- environmental
- politico-economic – incorporating legal factors.

These factors, acting singly or in combination, influence each AL to some degree. Consideration of these factors during assessment provides the basis for a deeper understanding of the cause of an individual's difficulties, as well as indicating likely outcomes. This has particular relevance for people with LTCs, given the timescales involved, the multiple effects of such disorders, the pattern of relapses that may be a characteristic of their condition and the impact of pharmacy and comorbidities. For example, knowledge of normal anatomical structure and physiological function enables the nurse to appreciate the effects of spinal cord injury (SCI) on physiological parameters but not in how they will address their changing life. The biological focus is useful both in guiding immediate action to alleviate existing problems and in devising care to prevent the onset of anticipated complications, such as autonomic dysreflexia, constipation and pressure ulcers. However an exploration of psychological and sociocultural and environmental status will reveal someone's capacity to acquire further information, resources and motivation to develop the skills necessary for self-management.

The social and cultural determinants associated with everyday living including role function may be significant in how a person adapts to having an LTC. A man who develops Guillain–Barré syndrome (GBS), for instance, may perceive that his role as provider and protector of the family group is threatened when he is no longer earning and requires help to perform basic living activities.

Increasingly we are concerned with how environmental factors such as noise, climate and atmospheric pollution can affect the performance of AL. For example, people with asthma or COPD experience worsening of their symptoms during periods of poor air quality and disturbed sleep if their home is adjacent to a busy motorway. The structure and layout of buildings in which activities are performed are also of significance here. Someone with poor physical health who lives in a top-floor flat without a lift might not be able to negotiate the stairs easily. This would further limit their activities and worsen their health in broad terms. Access to GP surgeries can be difficult if they are sited at some distance from public transport or on uneven terrain and the interior of older facilities might not be optimally disabled-friendly. This may discourage users from attending and result in inadequate monitoring of self-management and lack of attention to some features of their conditions. Admission to hospital can present an additional source of anxiety because the disruption to social networks and support, distance between home and the facilities and the need to share bathroom and sleeping accommodation can interfere with an individual's routine or draw attention to what others might consider to be idiosyncratic behaviour.

Increasingly health and social care struggles to meet the needs of a diverse and ageing population. Despite new innovations such as telemedicine and virtual wards, building and sustaining an effective health workforce is challenging. Concerns over staffing levels, external pressures to address healthcare waiting lists and challenges to resourcing have additional implications for individual lifestyles. For example, if seating of a suitable height cannot be obtained for someone who has difficulty standing, it will not be possible for them to remain independent in personal hygiene. Similarly, someone who is obese can experience considerable difficulty in maintaining independence when using a temporary chair, or a bed that is too small, that does not meet their needs, forces the adoption of an uncomfortable posture increasing risk of skin damage and limits their mobility.

Applying the Roper–Logan–Tierney Model Using the Nursing Process

Assessment

Initial assessment is important in LTCs because it presents a structured method of data collection, which will create a total picture of the person and, thus provide a baseline against which change can be measured. In some cases, for example, in the immediate aftermath of trauma or a stroke, priority will necessarily be given to managing threat to life or pain and distress, with more comprehensive details of daily activities gathered over time. It must be emphasised, however, that circumstances are seldom static in LTCs, so continued planned assessment and review is essential and should be considered at any stage of the nurse–patient relationship.

Assessment based on a person-centred approach, which values the input of the individual and where relevant their carers, supports engagement in the process. In specialist units and ICPs, the format taken is based on an interdisciplinary approach, with a single member of the healthcare team taking the lead while drawing on the expertise of both the individual and other health professions. Using a systematic approach that starts with comprehensive history-taking identifies the issues to be considered before focussing on the presenting symptoms and the priorities of the individual, alongside that of the health professional (Bickley et al. 2017).

Several issues require attention during the assessment of people with LTCs, regardless of the setting, some of which relate directly to traumatic or disease processes and include the type and duration of the presenting condition. Adopting a person-centred approach when applying the selected assessment framework and integrating tools such as the Malnutrition Universal Screening Tool (MUST) for nutrition, or mini mental health assessment for low mood can help to identify current concerns while collecting information about successful and less successful strategies previously used, and any new features or ongoing treatment needed. This will help nurses understand how individuals, and when appropriate their carers, incorporate interventions into daily life and the degree of efficacy achieved. The collation of objective and subjective data is crucial here. For example, spasticity (uncoordinated, involuntary muscle contractions associated with painful spasms, stiffness and changed movement) is an observable phenomenon in MS and this can prompt nurses to explore how it affects individuals, whereas invisible problems, such as fatigue or pain, might not be evident unless patients explain their impact. Symptoms such as fatigue are subjective and experiential in nature, and may be poorly recognised or described. Nurses need to be prepared to assess how this presents for individuals (e.g. 'so debilitated', 'completely wiped out') to enable exacerbating factors to be identified. In addition understanding people's beliefs and understanding around sexuality, death or dying will require a sensitive approach that enables open discussion about how their health status is currently affecting them and their concerns for the future.

🌐 **See Evolve website Critical thinking question 30.2**

The RLT model prompts nurses to consider the individual's abilities as well as impairments in carrying out the AL, through reference to the dependence/independence continuum. Any equipment used to assist independence can be identified and carer involvement, resource use and support services can be explored. Independence needs to be judged in terms of whether activities can be completed safely and if individuals can use them when unsupervised or unaided. It is not that an activity is undertaken 'perfectly' but that it meets the needs of the individual. In this way, for instance, someone with significant physical impairment due to SCI can be assessed as having task independence because they are in a position to instruct others in the correct management of their care. This part of the assessment can also help to determine whether people have a realistic idea of their situation.

Although much of the assessment data can be obtained from patients, other sources of information must be included. The views of formal and informal carers should be used to build up a more detailed impression of behaviour and events. This can be captured in the use of 'This is me' documentation developed by the Alzheimer's Society (2022) for people with dementia, which can be very useful for many other situations where communication is difficult. For example, when someone with MND or dementia is admitted for respite care, a community nurse might share an observation that during recent months there has been a marked deterioration in the relationship between the patient and their partner, although the couple strenuously denies that this has taken place. This could then be explored with reference to the features and progression of the condition, and demands on the carer, so that key problems are identified and accounted for in the plan for care (Reflection 30.8).

Diagnosis

The diagnosis section of the nursing process alludes to the ability to systematically interpret the information identified within the assessment process, and the subsequent clinical decision to inform planned interventions. This can produce either single or multiple diagnoses for a patient. In LTCs it is likely that the patient would experience multiple comorbidities and it is important that these are

REFLECTION 30.8

Recognising the Importance of Individual Experience

Living with long-term conditions is influenced by a range of interacting physical, psychosocial, politico-economic and spiritual factors. It is also clear that people share some experiences of long-term conditions but have individual approaches to living with and managing them.

Activities

- Reflecting on your experience, think about two people with long-term conditions whom you know or have met in your practice. Identify examples of physical, psychosocial, politico-economic and spiritual factors affecting each of their lives.
- Which similarities and differences do you see?
- Consider how coming to know the individual could enhance their care.

looked at both individually and as a combined entity. For example, a medical diagnosis of stroke provides information about the patient's pathology. The complementary nursing diagnoses of impairment in verbal communication, risk for falls, interrupted family processes and powerlessness provide a more holistic understanding of the impact of that stroke on this patient and their family – they also direct nursing interventions to obtain patient-specific outcomes.

Some aspects of this assessment may involve dealing with consequences of active treatment. Increasingly nurses are monitoring the impact of long-term medication for a primary illness and the prescription of medication and treatment for the side-effects or consequences of the first-line treatment option. In COPD, patients are often treated with doses of corticosteroids. These can be changed depending on severity of acute illness, often with patients maintained on a low therapeutic/prophylactic dose. The side-effects of corticosteroids are multiple, but one major factor would be vulnerability to other infections.

Planning

Care is planned to address the actual and potential problems identified during assessment. The priority given to each depends on the individual's situation, though, again, life-threatening, or distressing problems assume precedence over those with a less immediate impact. Aside from this, priority setting in LTCs should always be negotiated with the individual, and their main carer, and include the appropriate health professionals. An open discussion is useful in clarifying the meaning of each problem to the individual, determining how problems are related to each other, discussing options for addressing them and creating a shared awareness of difficulties. This helps to foster collaborative relationships and enhances the commitment of all concerned.

The aim of the care plan is to assist the patient in preventing, solving, alleviating or managing problems as far as is possible by using best practice. Goals are set for each problem and appropriate strategies devised to attain them. In LTCs, it is particularly important that goal-setting reflects the individual's capacity for achievement, is meaningful and is consistent with personal values and priorities. Both short- and long-term goals can be specified. However, given the instability of many LTCs, it might be inappropriate to select broad objectives for eventual achievement, such as acceptance of the condition and total self-management. It is preferable to simplify these by dividing them into a series of short-term goals, so that progress can be achieved and motivation maintained. This provides patients with a stimulus and sense of purpose (Holland et al. 2008). Goals must also be expressed in understandable, measurable terms so that their attainment is obvious to patient and carer. Regular goal planning meetings with individuals, their carers and other interdisciplinary team members to identify needs, set SMART goals and review progress are essential for supporting people to live well with LTC.

The way in which AL are addressed during assessment, whether related problems are identified and how care is planned depends on nurse's knowledge, skills and behaviours including social and cultural values. For instance, although promoting sexual health is generally agreed to be part of their role, nurses do not necessarily address this proactively and prefer to wait for patients to voice related concerns. Consideration of gender preferences, including those who have transitioned, is an important aspect of personal identity during assessment and planning of nursing interventions. LGBTQ+ older adults are more likely than non-LGBTQ+ peers to have chronic conditions, and rely on support networks that may not be legally recognised (family of choice) (Hiedemann and Brodoff 2013, Orel 2017). However, given its intimate nature, people, and healthcare professionals, might be reluctant to explore this, or disregard preferences by focusing on cis-gender normative approaches to healthcare. This means that sexual expression risks being neglected, whether this concerns the sexual act, relationships, care givers or how individuals dress and present themselves.

This is particularly important in LTCs because associated changes in appearance, body image or function have significant effects on sexual health. For example, impaired mobility can prevent attention to personal hygiene and preferred management of body hair, limit clothing choices, restrict body positioning, cause pain and dominate one's appearance as a disabled person. Incontinence causes embarrassment and sensory alteration affects stimulation and perceived pleasure from physical contact. In addition, the use of catheters or other less invasive continence aids may be experienced as challenging. Chronic pain is associated with depression which decreases libido, as does some antidepressant medication (see Reflection 30.6). Specific conditions also influence sexual expression directly or indirectly due to the impact of polypharmacy. Gynaecological, breast and male reproductive cancers have an obvious relationship with this activity. Acquired brain injury can be followed by changes in libido, erectile dysfunction and inability to orgasm. Changes in male fertility might occur here and in SCI, where ejaculatory failure, retrograde ejaculation, raised testicular temperature and chronic infection are implicated (Bickley et al. 2017). Not all nurses are able to give advice on sexual healthcare, but they should provide support by having an awareness of potential problems, being sensitive, being willing to present patients with an 'open door' to discuss them when ready and by planning for specialist referrals.

Care plans should describe prescribed interventions and patient participation in detail, communicating clearly what can be expected from everyone involved. This offers a means of ensuring continuity of care and can help to prevent confusion, such as when individuals are learning to develop a routine for renal dialysis in a domestic setting. It also articulates nursing's contribution to interdisciplinary planning, for instance with reference to care pathways. Where collaborative plans are used, it is important to identify which team member is best placed to support progression towards each goal and to ensure that everyone concerned is committed to the agreed process and outcome (Booth and Jester 2007).

🌐 **See Evolve website Critical thinking question 30.3**

Implementation

The actions proposed in the care plan are realised in this phase of the nursing process. It is tempting to believe that most nurses will experience little difficulty in this area because they are familiar with the idea of 'doing'. However, as care delivery changes, with a greater focus on integration and collaboration, so nurses' roles change as the emphasis from 'doing' to managing and coordinating becomes paramount, and increased depth of knowledge, and new skills are required.

The delivery of care in relation to the AL should be consistent with the way in which individuals with LTCs usually behave, whether they normally require assistance and how independence and autonomy are maintained. As in Orem's (2001) model, this may require the nurse to act for the patient, to supplement and develop the person's self-care capability or in promoting health to aid learning. Determining the emphasis to be placed on each of these approaches in a given situation requires nurses to be responsive to the individual's experience of their condition in the light of issues considered in the first part of this chapter, while being aware of the possibilities of nursing roles.

Implementation also involves supporting patients to optimise their strengths in developing their own knowledge and applying skills learned during therapy sessions. Peer support and learning from others who have moved further in the rehabilitative process can be invaluable here, however, practices need to be adapted to fit individual impairments and preferences. For example, many people with LTCs have limited movement. Universal risk assessment will identify those most liable to develop pressure ulcers but tissue viability is of greater concern to people with paralysis and sensory deficit, such as following SCI. Here, instinctive movements to ensure circulation and prevent pressure damage cease, while the lower body's skin quality and muscle bulk decline. This means that individuals need to learn the serious consequences of pressure ulcers and take responsibility for avoiding them by incorporating careful movement and transfers, turning and skin inspection into daily life. Psychological factors will also influence patients' level of engagement and, thus determine when intervention would be most appropriate. The development of a therapeutic relationship with individuals and their carers is a sound basis from which to work. Individuals can discern quickly whether nurses have a genuine interest in their well-being and are more likely to be responsive to them. For instance, a simple act of communication shaped McCrum's (2008) feelings of being cared for after a stroke, while a nurse focusing on their own religious beliefs and preferences alienates the patient following his SCI.

It is important for nurses to gain patients' trust and to recognise that, under normal circumstances, they and their carers have – or will have – responsibility for managing their condition and daily life. In both hospital and community settings, nurses must enable people to retain control of their situation rather than expecting them to conform to alien norms and expectations.

In LTCs, nursing intervention is far from restricted to the delivery of physical care, although the value of this should not be underestimated. Assisting another person in carrying out any activity, such as washing and dressing, requires more than the ability to reproduce simple practical actions. The promotion of health and self-care capability requires an understanding of an individual's developmental level as well as of effective teaching techniques. This involves the use of refined communication skills, as does the role of coach, counsellor and supporter to both patients and carers.

The wishes of the individual and ability or desire of family members to engage and participate in long-term care vary. Initiating early discussions and engagement in the assessment process, goal planning and care delivery can give an indication of this and provide opportunities for the nurse to provide information, support and training for the role. Assumptions should not be made that people will be able to participate or support their family member, or that lack of engagement means lack of care. Carers can feel pressured to participate or guilty at not being able to, even though they have the right to refuse engagement or to continue caring, they may find sharing this with nurses is difficult. It is important to try to understand people's decisions and avoid making judgements. Family members might care very much for an individual but just not as others expect. Culture influences the way people view illness, disability, gender roles, religious adherence and the performance of daily activities. Their involvement also depends on existing family dynamics, structure, physical location and culture. An extended family might provide several carers whose availability makes role sharing feasible. While family members who are geographically distant may wish to engage in decision making and remote support via phone or online contact but only be able to offer some direct assistance during times of hospitalisation, transition and relapse.

Nurses may need to support families to manage their expectations. Some carers may have unrealistically high expectations of an individual's independence or, conversely, hinder their progress by being overprotective and performing activities for them. Nurses need to be prepared to advocate on behalf of patients who may find it hard to share concerns with their families or express their needs. They should, however, recognise when personal characteristics and poor relationships can make caring inappropriate.

When helping an individual to adapt to living with an LTC, nurses should present explanations honestly and positively, to foster realistic hope for the future. Nonverbal communication, especially touch, can be a helpful way to strengthen a caring relationship, providing this is culturally, age and gender appropriate.

Extending traditional nursing skills in relation to touch, or signposting to others for interventions such as massage has significant benefits for people in this situation. The provision of massage, for example, can be of value in assisting individuals to deal with stress, enhance self-worth, contribute to palliation and facilitate sympathetic reconnection with a body that has 'let them down'. As with all complementary therapies, nurses should ensure that the care provided is safe, in patients' best interests, that they are trained and competent to practise, have involved interdisciplinary members in decision-making and obtain informed consent (Nursing and Midwifery Council 2018).

Evaluation

The effectiveness of nursing interventions is judged by evaluating whether goals have been achieved. This phase of the nursing process lends meaning to those that precede it. The extent to which goals have been achieved should be measured objectively where possible. It is also possible to identify movement on the dependence/independence continuum in response to interventions, teaching programmes or how patients manage symptoms.

The evaluation of some aspects of care is, however, largely dependent on subjective data. For instance, it is difficult to measure to what extent an individual has adapted to the idea of having an LTC. Evaluation in this area could be guided instead by how the individual is speaking about their LTC and the care planned, and their engagement with nurses and other health professionals and by interpreting behavioural cues; for instance, by observing whether they are active in information-seeking and practising new skills, appear depressed or avoid discussion of the condition and its related problems. It is essential to combine observation with listening to what the person says about their experience. The use of tools such as symptom diaries and pain scales can be helpful in mapping patient experience and identifying trends. Measuring functional outcomes without acknowledging their context provides an inadequate indicator of progress. An individual might, for example, be able to get up, shower and dress but take until 10:30 to do so. This might be judged as successful in some respects but not in others. The person can perform the named activities independently but when 'bodily housekeeping' becomes a job, engagement with other activities or paid employment is not possible, forcing reliance on benefits and/or social care. For the individual this level of independence is important, and maintaining positivity and hope, so that individuals continue a forward trajectory is important.

The achievement of any goal relies on wide-ranging situational variables. It is therefore sometimes difficult to identify whether strategies have been successful. The contribution of human, material and environmental factors can all influence outcomes. Non-achievement should not be viewed as 'failure', as this has negative connotations and is liable to demotivate but should be considered a stimulus for reassessment and an opportunity to revise better targeted problem statements and to set new goals. Nurses must think creatively when identifying why goals were not achieved and in searching for solutions (Reflection 30.9).

The importance of the nurse's own self-evaluation must not be forgotten. As noted earlier, nurses sometimes find it difficult to work within the boundaries of their occupational role where

---

REFLECTION 30.9

Case History: the Importance of Understanding the Individual's Perspective of Their Rehabilitative Experience

Team members working with 81-year-old B aimed to reduce his risk of falling post-traumatic injury. Care included advising him to consider safety a priority by focusing consciously on balancing during activity, wearing orthoses (braces, splints or in-shoe devices used to support and correct limb function), using a Zimmer frame and avoiding simultaneous movement and talking.

On evaluation, staff found it hard to understand why B felt that the goal of being able to manage this confidently had not been achieved; after all, he had fallen less frequently since the plan had been implemented and was observed to be moving more steadily.

In later discussion with a nurse, B agreed that this was true when walking on even surfaces in a hospital setting but it had raised awareness that he would not be able to manage independently at home, keep his garden tidy or attend village social events easily. He was fearful of being discharged when he was not ready but at the same time did not want to stay in hospital any longer than he needed. This had upset him, and he was feeling angry as he felt that his needs had not be considered but that nobody was interested in his feelings, and that he was simply expected to do his exercises and feel grateful for the care and support he was receiving.

The nurse reassuringly explained that what was meaningful to B was important for his rehabilitation. The team reviewed B's specific circumstances and the timescale for the goal was revised. It was also suggested that he considered what changes he thought he could make, including changes to his home or with the support he needed. B remained unhappy about the prospect of making changes to his home but agreed to speak with occupational therapy to see what they could advise. He also agreed to a home visit.

Activity

Reflecting on assessment and planning processes, how might the problem noted at the evaluation stage of B's care have been avoided?

relationships develop with individuals and their families over time. They can find it difficult to accept the inevitability of the patient's decline and to have a meaningful role where medicine deems that nothing more can be done. As a result, the emotional labour in sustaining long-term care can be high. It is possible that they will identify with the patient, particularly if they occupy the same stage of the lifespan. Some nurses will be unable to form close protracted relationships due to differences in personality, culture and attitude. Individual nurses must recognise that they cannot be all things to all people. Exposure to another's traumatic experience is a source of vicarious stress and the cumulative impact of working with LTCs adds dimensions to this. Nursing teams should be supportive of their members in enabling them to share feelings of vulnerability or emotional distress without fear of disapproval, to develop strategies for managing their own experience of sharing difficult journeys while working in restrictive service environments and to offer genuine opportunities for clinical supervision and reflection.

Summary: Key Nursing Issues

- LTCs are congenital or acquired, associated with a protracted disease processes or the consequence of trauma, might be controlled or palliated but not cured, and impact profoundly on all aspects of people's lives.
- Related impairments can result in disability, stigmatisation and, in turn, marginalisation. Society's perceptions of disabled people as dependent, incapable or objects of pity and curiosity are shared to some extent by health workers.
- Developments in screening, diagnostic methods, treatment and care delivery, together with an ageing population and policy drivers, mean that, regardless of the setting in which they work, most nurses will encounter people with LTCs.
- Living with an LTC is characterised by accommodating its lifelong presence in daily activities, identifying the need for and obtaining appropriate support and dealing with uncertainty.
- Managing impairments and controlling a condition's features and the side-effects of treatment are complicated by deterioration over time, unpredictable relapses and multiple pathology.
- Effective, evidence-based care requires not only a full understanding of specific conditions but, also, grounding in human and physical sciences, so that individual experiences and priorities can be understood.
- Nursing roles in LTCs are collaborative and enabling in nature, involving the expression of technological, rehabilitative, caring and interpersonal skills which are transferable across settings.
- Despite many conditions requiring complex and varied service use, individuals and their carers are responsible for their day-to-day management.
- Integrating principles of inclusivity and individuality into approaches to all patients as a matter of course means that differences will be anticipated, and positive responses made naturally, instead of dealing with differences reactively and leaving disabled people's needs unmet.
- Self-management of LTCs differs from traditional approaches to care and requires nurses to be provided with knowledge and skills to deliver person-focused interventions, promote self-care of conditions and their psychosocial implications and enable patients to exercise control in decision making.

Reflection and Learning – What Next?

- **Test** your knowledge by visiting the Evolve website 🌐 and answering the multiple choice questions and critical thinking questions.
- **Consolidate** your learning by looking at some of the further reading suggestions, references and specialist websites.
- **Revisit** some of the additional material on the Evolve website.
- **Consider** what you have learnt and how this will help your professional development.
- **Reflect** on how you can apply this knowledge to the care of your patients.
- **Discuss** your learning with your supervisor/assessor, lecturer and colleagues.

References

Åberg C, Gillsjö C, Hallgren J, Berglund M. "It is like living in a diminishing world": older persons' experiences of living with long-term health problems - prior to the STRENGTH intervention". *Int J Qual Stud Health Well-being*. 2020;15(1):1747251.

Alzheimer's Society 'This is me'. https://www.alzheimers.org.uk/get-support/publications-factsheets/this-is-me

Anthony Jnr, B. Use of telemedicine and virtual care for remote treatment in response to COVID-19 pandemic. *J Med Syst*. 2020;44(7):132.

Barnett K, Mercer SW, Norbury M, et al. Epidemiology of multimorbidity and implications for health care, research, and medical education: a cross-sectional study. *Lancet*. 2012;380(9836):37–43.

Barry E, Galvin R, Keogh C, Horgan F, Fahey T. Is the Timed Up and Go test a useful predictor of risk of falls in community dwelling older adults: a systematic review and meta-analysis. *BMC Geriatr*. 2014;14:14.

Bautista E, Shapovalov D, Shoraka A. Factors associated with increased felt stigma among many individuals with epilepsy. *Seizure*. 2015;30:106–112.

Bickley LS, Szilagyi PG, Bates B. *Bates' Guide to Physical Examination and History Taking*. 12th ed. Philadelphia, PA: Wolters Kluwer; 2017.

Biordi DL, Nicolson NR. Social isolation. In: Larsen PD, Lubkin IM, eds. *Chronic Illness: Impact and Interventions*. 7th ed. Sudbury: Jones and Bartlett; 2009:85–116.

Booth S, Jester R. The rehabilitation process. In: Jester R, ed. *Advancing Practice in Rehabilitation Nursing*. Oxford: Blackwell; 2007:1–13.

Bradshaw SA, Playford ED, Riazi A. Living well in care homes: a systematic review of qualitative studies. *Age Ageing*. 2012;41:429–440.

Brinkmann S. The body in grief. *Mortality*. 2017;24(3):290–303.

Brouwers EPM. Social stigma is an underestimated contributing factor to unemployment in people with mental illness or mental health issues: Position paper and future directions. *BMC Psychol*. 2020;8(1):36.

Cassell A, et al. The epidemiology of multimorbidity in primary care: a retrospective cohort study. *Br J Gen Pract*. 2018. http://bjgp.org/content/early/2018/03/12/bjgp18X695465.

Chew B-H, Shariff-Ghazali S, Fernandez A. Psychological aspects of diabetes care: effecting behavioral change in patients. *World J Diabetes*. 2014;5:796–808.

Chief Medical Officer 2020 available at Health matters: physical activity - prevention and management of long-term conditions - GOV.UK (www.gov.uk).

Chudasama YV, Khunti K, Gillies CL, Dhalwani NN, Davies MJ, Yates T, Zaccardi F. Healthy lifestyle and life expectancy in people with multimorbidity in the UK Biobank: A longitudinal cohort study. *PLoS Med*. 2020 Sep 22;17(9):e1003332.

Cloutier D, Stajduhar KI, Roberts D, Dujela C, Roland K. 'Bare-bones' to 'silver linings': lessons on integrating a palliative approach to care in long-term care in Western Canada. *BMC Health Serv Res*. 2021;21(1):1–610.

Corbin JM, Strauss A. A nursing model for chronic illness management based upon the trajectory framework. *Sch Inq Nurs Pract*. 1991;5:155–174.

Crook H, Raza S, Nowell J, Young M, Edison P. Long covid - Mechanisms, risk factors, and management. *BMJ (Online)*. 2021;374:n1648.

Curtin M, Lubkin IM. What is chronicity?. In: Lubkin IM, Larsen PD, eds. *Chronic Illness: Impact and Interventions*. 4th ed. Sudbury: Jones and Bartlett; 1998:3–25.

d'Arminio Monforte A, Bonnet F, Bucher H, Pourcher V, Pantazis N, Pelchen-Matthews A, Touloumi G, Wolf E. What do the changing patterns of comorbidity burden in people living with HIV mean for long-term management? Perspectives from European HIV cohorts. *HIV Med*. 2020;21(2):3-1.

Davis S, Madden S. Rehabilitation at a macro and micro level. In: Davis S, ed. *Rehabilitation: The Use of Theories and Models in Practice*. Edinburgh: Churchill Livingstone; 2006:3–22.

Department for Work and Pensions (DWP).The employment of disabled people 2021 updated Feb 2022. https://www.gov.uk/government/statistics/the-employment-of-disabled-people-2021/the-employment-of-disabled-people-2021. Accessed January 2024.

Disability Rights UK (2017). Disability Rights UK response to the Work and Pensions Committee inquiry on Personal Independence Payment (PIP). https://www.disabilityrightsuk.org/disability-rights-uk-response-work-and-pensions-committee-inquiry-personal-independence-payment-pip.

Douglas F, MacIver E, Yuill C. A qualitative investigation of lived experiences of long-term health condition management with people who are food insecure. *BMC Public Health*. 2020;20(1):1309.

Duhoux A, Dufour É, Sasseville M, Laroche D, Contandriopoulos D. Rethinking Primary Care Delivery Models: Can Integrated Primary Care Teams Improve Care Experience? *Int J Integr Care*. 2022;22(2):8.

Equality Act 2010. https://www.legislation.gov.uk/ukpga/2010/15/contents.

Farrell E, Hollmann E, Roux CW, Bustillo M, Nadglowski J, McGillicuddy D. The lived experience of patients with obesity: A systematic review and qualitative synthesis. *Obes Rev*. 2021;22(12):e13334.

Fried LP, Tangen CM, Walston J, et al. Frailty in older adults: evidence for a phenotype. *J Gerontol A Biol Sci Med Sci*. 2001;56(3):M146–M157.

Goedhart NS, van Oostveen CJ, Vermeulen H. The effect of structural empowerment of nurses on quality outcomes in hospitals: a scoping review. *J Nurs Manag*. 2017;25:194–206.

Goffman E. *Stigma*. Harmondsworth: Penguin; 1963.

Hayanga B, Stafford M, Bécares L. Ethnic inequalities in healthcare use and care quality among people with multiple long-term health conditions living in the united kingdom: A systematic review and narrative synthesis. *Int J Environ Res Public Health*. 2021;18(23):12599.

Health and Care Act 2022. https://www.legislation.gov.uk/ukpga/2022/31/contents/enacted.

Hiedemann B, Brodoff L. Increased risks of needing long-term care among older adults living with same-sex partners. *Am J Public Health*. 2013;103(8):e27–e33.

Hiltunen A, Hörhammer I, Silander K, Kaikuluoma J, Linna M. Integrating health service delivery for geriatric patients after hospital admission—A register study on the outcomes and costs. *Health Serv Manage Res*. 2020;33(1):24–32.

Ho IS, Azcoaga-Lorenzo A, Akbari A, et al. Variation in the estimated prevalence of multimorbidity: systematic review and meta-analysis of 193 international studies. *BMJ Open*. 2022 Apr 29;12(4):e057017.

Hodge E, Bui E, Goetter E, et al. Change in decentering mediates improvement in anxiety in mindfulness-based stress reduction for generalized anxiety disorder. *Cognit Ther Res*. 2015;39:228–235.

Holdoway A, Anderson L, McGregor I, et al. *A guide to managing adult malnutrition in the community*. second edition; 2017. https://www.malnutritionpathway.co.uk/library/managing_malnutrition.pdf.

Holland K, Jenkins J, Solomon J, et al. *Applying the Roper–Logan–Tierney Model in Practice*. 2nd ed. Edinburgh: Churchill Livingstone; 2008.

Holland P, Collins A. 'Whenever I can I push myself to go to work': a qualitative study of experiences of sickness presenteeism among workers with rheumatoid arthritis. *Disabil Rehabil*. 2018;40:404–413.

Holland C, Garner I, Simpson J, et al. Impacts of COVID-19 lockdowns on frailty and wellbeing in older people and those living with long-term conditions. *Adv Clin Exp Med*. 2021;30(11):1111–1114.

Hughes S, Burch S. 'I'm not just a number on a sheet, I'm a person': Domiciliary care, self and getting older. *Health Soc Care Community*. 2020;28(3):903–912.

ICPOP, 2021 Integrated Care Programme for Older Persons. https://www.icpop.org/integrated-care-programme.

Ireson J, Taylor A, Richardson E, Greenfield B, Jones G. Exploring invisibility and epistemic injustice in Long Covid—A citizen science qualitative analysis of patient stories from an online Covid community. *Health Expect*. 2022;25(4):1753–1765.

Jacob KS. Recovery Model of Mental illness: a complementary approach to psychiatric care. *Indian J Psychol Med*. 2015;37:117. doi:10.4103/0253-7176.155605.

Jatta S, Ian B, Robert M. Inequalities in recovery or methodological artefact? A comparison of models across physical and mental health functioning. *SSM Popul Health*. 2022;17:101067.

Joy M, Richard Hobbs FD, Bernal JL, et al. Excess mortality in the first COVID pandemic peak: Cross-sectional analyses of the impact of age, sex, ethnicity, household size, and long-term conditions in people of known SARS-CoV-2 status in England. *Br J Gen Pract*. 2020;70(701):E890–E898.

Kanyimo E. Using virtual wards and long-term conditions management network to improve practice and performance. *BMJ Open Qual*. 2022;11(4):e001952.

Kimbell B, Murray SA, Macpherson S, Boyd K. Embracing inherent uncertainty in advanced illness. *BMJ*. 2016;354. doi:10.1136/bmj.i3802.

Kings Fund. *Leadership and Engagement for Improvement in the NHS: Together We Can*. London: Kings Fund; 2012.

Kings Fund. Roberts S, Dixon A. Delivering better services for people with long-term conditions. Building the house of care. 2013. https://www.kingsfund.org.uk/insight-and-analysis/reports/better-services-people-long-term-conditions.

Kritsotakis G, Galanis P, Papastefanakis E, et al. Attitudes towards people with physical or intellectual disabilities among nursing, social work and medical students. *J Clin Nurs*. 2017;26:4951–4963.

Kubler-Ross E. *On Death and Dying*. New York: Macmillan; 1969.

Latorraca C, Natimbianco A, Pachito D, et al. Mindfulness for palliative care patients: systematic review. *Int J Clin Pract*. 2017;71(12). doi:10.1111/ijcp.13034.

Locker D. Living with chronic illness. In: Scambler G, ed. *Sociology as Applied to Medicine*. 6th ed. Oxford: Saunders Elsevier; 2008:83–96.

Lu L, Zhang J, Xie Y, Gao F, Xu S, Wu X, Ye Z. Wearable Health Devices in Health Care: Narrative Systematic Review. *JMIR Mhealth Uhealth*. 2020;8(11):e18907.

Maret D, Peters OA, Vaysse F, Vigarios E. Integration of telemedicine into the public health response to COVID-19 must include dentists. *Int Endod J*. 2020.

McCrum R. *My Year Off: Rediscovering Life After a Stroke*. London: Picador; 2008.

McKinney EL. Two's company, three's a crowd: disabled people, their carers and their partners. *Disability Society*. 2018;33(2):272–284.

McPherson K. Rehabilitation nursing: final frontier? *Int J Nurs Stud*. 2006;43:787–789.

Mitnitski AB, Mogilner AJ, Rockwood K. Accumulation of deficits as a proxy measure of aging. *Scientific World J*. 2001(1):323–336.

Mizuma K, Amitani M, Mizuma M, et al. Clarifying differences in viewpoints between multiple healthcare professionals during discharge planning assessments when discharging patients from a long-term care hospital to home. *Eval Program Plann*. 2000;82:101848–101849.

Morse J. Responding to threats to integrity of self. *ANS Adv Nurs Sci*. 1997;19:21–36.

Moorhouse P, Rockwood K. Frailty and its quantitative clinical evaluation. *R Coll Physicians Edinb*. 2012;42:333–340.

Nathan A. Malnutrition: Impact on long-term conditions. *InnovAiT*. 2021;14(4):263–265. doi:10.1177/1755738020919143.

NHS England. *The Eatwell Guide*; 2022. https://www.nhs.uk/live-well/eat-well/food-guidelines-and-food-labels/the-eatwell-guide.

NHS England. Living well, ageing well and tackling premature mortality. 2024. https://www.england.nhs.uk/ourwork/clinical-policy/.

NHS England. *Five Year Forward View*. London: NHSE; 2014. https://www.england.nhs.uk/publication/nhs-five-year-forward-view/.

NHS England. *Technology Enabled Care Services*. London: NHSE; 2018.

NHS England Long Term Plan, London 2019 https://www.longtermplan.nhs.uk/wp-content/uploads/2019/08/nhs-long-term-plan-version-1.2.pdf.

National Institute for Health and Care Excellence (NICE). *Multimorbidity: clinical assessment and management Nice Guidelines* [NG56]. 2016. https://www.nice.org.uk/guidance/ng56.

NICE. Multimorbidity and polypharmaacy key therapeutic topic [KTT18]. 2017. https://www.nice.org.uk/advice/ktt18.

NIHR 2021 Researching Long Covid Available at Researching long COVID | NIHR Living with Covid19 (nihr.ac.uk).

Nord M, Östgren CJ, Marcusson J, Johansson M. Staff experiences of a new tool for comprehensive geriatric assessment in primary care (PASTEL): a focus group study: Primary care staff experiences of geriatric assessment. *Scand J Prim Health Care*. 2020;38(2):132–145.

Nursing and Midwifery Council (NMC) (2018). The Code: Professional Standards of Practice and Behaviour for Nurses, Midwives and Nursing Associates. https://www.nmc.org.uk/globalassets/sitedocuments/nmc-publications/nmc-code.pdf.

Oboh L, Qadir MS. Deprescribing and managing polypharmacy in frail older people: a patient-centred approach in the real world. *Eur J Hosp Pharm Sci Prac*. 2017;24(1):58–62.

Oldroyd L, Eskandari F, Pratt C, Lake AA. The nutritional quality of food parcels provided by food banks and the effectiveness of food banks at reducing food insecurity in developed countries: a mixed-method systematic review. *J Hum Nutr Diet*. 2022;35(6):1202–1229.

O'Mahony, D, Cherubini A, Guiteras AR et al. STOPP/START criteria for potentially inappropriate prescribing in older people: version 3. *Eur Geriatr Med*. 2023;14:625–632.

Office for National Statistics (ONS). National population projections 2018. https://www.ons.gov.uk/peoplepopulationandcommunity/populationandmigration/populationprojections/bulletins/nationalpopulationprojections/2018based#changing-age-structure.

Office for National Statistics (ONS). *Proportion of People With Long term Conditions*. London; 2020.

ONS. People with long-term conditions, UK: January to December 2019. 2021. https://www.ons.gov.uk/peoplepopulationandcommunity/healthandsocialcare/conditionsanddiseases/adhocs/11478peoplewithlongtermhealthconditionsukjanuarytodecember2019.

Office for National Statistics (ONS). *Available at People with long-term health conditions*. UK: January to December 2019 - Office for National Statistics; 2022.

Orel NA. Families and support systems of LGBT elders. *Annu Rev Gerontol Geriatr*. 2017;37(1):89–109.

Orem DE. *Nursing: Concepts of Practice*. 6th ed. St Louis, MO: Mosby; 2001.

Patients Association. 2022 Available at Self-management | The Patients Association (patients-association.org.uk).

Piexak D, Cezar-Vaz M, Bonow C, Costa Santos S. How nurses are using the International Classification of Functioning, Disability and Health: an integrative review. *Aquichan*. 2015;15:351–367.

Powell A. *Commons Briefing Paper CBP 7540*. London: House of Commons; 2018.

Public Health England. *Health Profile for England: 2017*. London: PHE; 2017. https://www.gov.uk/government/publications/health-profile-for-england.

Rees M. Patient autonomy and withholding information. *Bioeth*. 2023;37(3):256–264.

Reeves D, Pye S, Ashcroft D M, Clegg A, Kontopantelis E, Blakeman T, et al. The challenge of ageing populations and patient frailty: can primary care adapt? *BMJ*. 2018;362:k3349. doi:10.1136/bmj.k3349.

Roberts G, Wolfson P. The rediscovery of recovery: open to all. *Adv Psychiatr Treat*. 2004;10(1):37–48.

Robertson R. *NHS Rationing Under the Radar*. London: Kings Fund; 2016.

Roddis J, Holloway I, Bond C, Galvin K. Living with a long-term condition: understanding well-being for individuals with thrombophilia or asthma. *Int J Qual Stud Health Well-being*. 2016;11. doi:10.3402/qhw.v11.31530.

Roper N, Logan W, Tierney AJ. *The Roper, Logan and Tierney Model of Nursing*. Edinburgh: Churchill Livingstone; 2000.

Roy C, Andrews HA. *The Roy Adaptation Model*. NJ: Prentice Hall: Englewood Cliffs; 2008:3.

Sagahutu JB, Kagwiza J, Cilliers F, Jelsma J. The impact of a training programme incorporating the conceptual framework of the International Classification of Functioning (ICF) on behaviour regarding interprofessional practice in Rwandan health professionals: A cluster randomized control trial. *PLoS One*. 2020;15(2):e0226247.

Scope. Disability facts and figures. https://www.scope.org.uk/media/disability-facts-figures/Sinclair, D.R., Maharani, A., Chandola, T. et al. Frailty among older adults and its distribution in England. *J Frailty Aging*. 2022;11:163–168. doi:10.14283/jfa.2021.55.

Stanhope M, Lancaster J. *Public Health Nursing: Population-Centered Health Care in the Community*. St Louis, MO: Elsevier; 2016.

Strauss AL, Corbin J, Fagerhaugh S. *Chronic Illness and the Quality of Life*. St Louis, MI: Mosby; 1984.

Sverker A, Thyberg I, Valtersson E, Björk M, Hjalmarsson S, Östlund G. Time to update the ICF by including socioemotional qualities of participation? The development of a "patient ladder of participation" based on interview data of people with early rheumatoid arthritis (the Swedish TIRA study). *Disabil Rehabil*. 2020;42(9):1212–1219.

Taylor SE. *Health Psychology*. 11th ed. New York: McGraw–Hill; 2021.

Telford K, Kralik D, Koch T. Acceptance and denial: implications for people adapting to chronic illness: literature review. *J Adv Nurs*. 2006;55(4):457–464.

The Nuffield Trust Supporting patients to manage their long-term condition(s) 2021. Available from Supporting patients to manage their long-term condition(s) | The Nuffield Trust

Weller J, Boyd M, Cumin D. Teams, tribes and patient safety: overcoming barriers to effective teamwork in healthcare. *Postgrad Med J*. 2014;90:149–154.

Woodward A, Davies N, Walters K, et al. Self-management of multiple long-term conditions: A systematic review of the barriers and facilitators amongst people experiencing socioeconomic deprivation. *PLoS One.* 2023;18(2):e0282036 -e0282036.

World Health Organisation (WHO). *International Classification of Functioning, Disability and Health (ICF).* Geneva: WHO; 2001.

World Health Organisation (WHO). *Innovative Care for Chronic Conditions – Building Blocks for Action.* Geneva: WHO; 2002.

World Health Organisation (WHO). *WHO Multi-Professional Patient Safety Curriculum Guide.* Geneva: WHO; 2011.

World Health Organisation (WHO). *WHO. World health statistics 2022: monitoring health for the SDGs, sustainable development goals.* Geneva: WHO; 2022.

World Health Organization (WHO). United Nations agencies launch first report on the decade of healthy ageing, 2021-2030. 2023. https://www.who.int/news/item/22-11-2023-united-nations-agencies-launch-first-report-on-the-decade-of-healthy-ageing--2021-2030.

Further Reading

Evandrou M, Falkingham J, Feng Z, Vlachantoni A. Ethnic inequalities in limiting health and self-reported health in later life revisited. *J Epidemiol Community Health.* 2016;0:1–10. doi:10.1136/jech-2015-206074.

31

Nursing the Patient With Cancer

SUSANNE CRUICKSHANK

CHAPTER OUTLINE

COVID-19

COVID-19's effect on cancer patients is a key concern to the cancer community resulting in delayed or decreased diagnosis, tests and treatment. The pandemic has had a significant impact on various aspects of healthcare, including cancer care, with many numbers of missed diagnoses as well as delayed treatments as a result of health systems that remain under pressure and patients who may have been and may still be unwilling to seek care. In the UK, during the first wave of the pandemic, regardless of continued reassurances from government that urgent care services were still available some people with potential cancer symptoms did not contact their doctor, as many felt fear of contracting COVID-19 and avoided placing extra strain on the NHS.

This resulted in suspected cancer referrals falling significantly when compared with the same period in 2019, in the UK and in other countries. Along with interruptions in cancer screening programmes (such as mammograms, colonoscopies and smears) and delays in scans and diagnostics, a spike has been seen in late cancer presentations and diagnoses; this makes some previously curable tumours more difficult to treat, along with this it brings further excess deaths.

Cruickshank S. COVID-19: The impact on people affected by cancers, oncology nurses and the wider health community. *Enferm Clin.* 2021:31:201-202.

Introduction

Cancer remains one of the top priorities in healthcare alongside heart disease, stroke and diabetes. It can profoundly affect every aspect of a person's life: physical, psychological, social or spiritual. The management of cancer is changing rapidly with many advances in technology, new treatments and new knowledge, improving survival outcomes. Nurses are at the forefront of care for cancer patients and their families.

Despite improvements in survival that have been significant for some cancer groups, the term 'cancer' still creates feelings of fear, uncertainty and thoughts about pain and death (Reflection 31.1). This is fuelled by groups of cancers that continue, despite new treatments, to have poorer outcomes, that is lung and pancreatic. In addition, government policy on prevention can appear controversial and contradictory. This creates misinformation and inconsistency surrounding knowledge of the disease. However, new trials in the UK looking at lung cancer screening are hoping to improve outcomes for people.

Cancer is not only a serious health concern but also a social problem, costing much in human and financial terms. One in three people in the UK risk developing cancer in their lifetime. One in four deaths was attributable to cancer in 2020 (Cancer Research UK). The incidence of different cancers and the death rate associated with them can vary both within the UK and globally. (See Sung et al. 2021 on behalf of GLOBOCAN, and Useful Websites and Further Reading: Cancer Research UK, World Health Organisation 2022)

Oncology as a Specialty

The UK political and healthcare agenda has recognised cancer as a high priority area for decades. The first important documentation to drive organisational change in cancer services across the country was initiated by the publication of the Calman–Hine/Calman report (Department of Health 1995). The Calman report focused on the patient and their family, care being delivered in specific designated cancer centres and cancer units in partnership with each other. The report recommended a seamless service integrating primary, secondary and tertiary care, with real commitment to psychosocial as well as medical needs. It also provided the opportunity to think about cancer control, early screening and detection programmes.

Subsequent policy documents have influenced the progression of cancer services and, following devolution, England, Wales and Scotland have set out their own policy directions for health (Department of Health 2007 and Scottish Government 2008). NHS England (2016) launched their new cancer strategy in 2016 and NHS Long Term Plan (2019a). The specific cancer part focuses on earlier diagnosis, faster diagnosis, prevention, personalised care and improving quality of life outcomes while recognising many patients may have other conditions.

The ambitions will be delivered in a way that improves quality of life outcomes, improves patient experience outcomes, reduces variation and reduces inequalities.

Nursing plays a central role in achieving these outcomes; the student nurse and nurses at all levels need to understand the multidisciplinary nature of cancer management within and outside the hospital, appreciating the roles of all those providing patient care. The Royal College of Nursing (RCN 2022) has developed a career and education framework for cancer nursing. It has been written to provide clarity about the cancer-specific nursing outcomes, and minimum standards, of theoretical and practice requirements necessary to provide excellent safe, effective and timely cancer care by nurses. It acknowledges that cancer is every nurse's business; those working towards qualification (preregistration) support staff and nurses in nonspecialist and specialist areas. This has informed the ACCEND programme (Aspirant Cancer Career and Education Development programme) (Health Education England 2022). The ACCEND programme aims to provide transformational reform for the career pathways and associated education, training, learning and development opportunities for the workforce providing care to people affected by cancer (see Useful Websites ACCEND for education and development).

The Fundamental Process of Cancer

The formation of cancer is a very complex process which involves the disruption of the regulation of growth of normal cells in the body. The process is called carcinogenesis. Any organ within the body has the potential to become cancerous however, some cancers are more common and some of these are directly linked to exposure to a known carcinogen.

In recent decades, molecular biology has made great progress in unravelling the steps involved in this process of cell transformation and is improving our ability to understand, classify, diagnose and treat cancer. A critical component in understanding the cancer process and rationale for treatment is a knowledge of the structure and function of cells, the role of deoxyribonucleic acid (DNA) and the cell cycle. (See Ashalford et al. 2019, Further Reading and Useful Websites, e.g. Cancerquest.)

To maintain functional cells through cell division the normal regulatory function of the cell will employ chemical signals to drive and halt growth; this is controlled by genetic components of the cell. The chemical signals are protein components of growth factors, receptors, and messenger and regulatory proteins. The chemical signals act within individual cells and are also utilised when communicating with neighbouring cells in regulating growth. Damage to the genetic components of the cells can result in loss of function and ability to regulate growth. As the scientific evidence for the chemical signals is complex this text will concentrate on the key genetic components involved.

During scientific research on viruses and how they propagate and reproduce within their host, scientists discovered extremely important genes involved in regulation of cell growth. These genes were called proto-oncogenes and had the ability to promote cell growth (switch on). When one of these genes becomes damaged and permanently switched on it is referred to as an oncogene. The ability of the cell to inhibit (switch off) growth is regulated by a tumour suppressor gene, the activity of which was revealed when investigating the childhood hereditary cancer retinoblastoma. When this gene is damaged the function is lost and the cell can no longer switch growth off. Another gene implicated in the replication repair process is called the mismatched repair gene. This gene repairs damaged DNA after replication. When this gene is damaged the cell accumulates lots of mismatched DNA which in turn promotes cell growth. The last essential gene controls the process of apoptosis (programmed cell death) – when the cell has divided a certain number of times it commits cell death. Therefore damage in this gene results in an inability to programme the cell to die. Such damage may occur from either error in DNA replication during mitosis or exposure to environmental agents. In the transformation to a cancerous growth, there is a progressive series of mutations of genes regulating cell division and differentiation.

Cancers develop when the cell can no longer regulate its own growth, resulting in the cells being able to divide rapidly. To survive within the host the forming tumour seeks out a new blood supply to maintain its growth which results in small fragments of tumour splitting off and travelling to distant sites to form secondary tumours (metastases); the cancer is said to have metastasised.

Tumours grow by repeated cell divisions; their rate of growth is often defined in terms of doubling time. Tumours vary greatly in their doubling time but, contrary to popular belief, their growth is not as rapid as that of normal tissues. For a tumour growth to exceed 1 or 2 mm, it requires a blood supply for survival; therefore the formation of a capillary network from the surrounding host tissue is initiated by proteins or angiogenic factors, for example, fibroblast growth factor (FGF) and tumour necrosis factor (TNF).

Tumour Pathology

A tumour may be benign or malignant. 'Cancer' is a general term used to describe all malignant neoplasms, that is a new growth of tissue, or tumour.

Usually benign tumours are:
- well differentiated – still closely resemble the host tissue
- slow growing
- enclosed in a capsule
- noninvasive – do not invade locally or metastasise.

Once removed, benign tumours rarely recur. However, a benign tumour can cause problems or even death in certain sites. For example, a benign brain tumour can cause pressure on the brain (see Chapter 11, Nursing Patients With Disorders of the Nervous

System) and some benign tumours cause problems in other ways, such as bleeding or secreting excess hormones.

Malignant tumours are characterised by the presence of malignant cells. Each cancer is distinguished by the nature, site or clinical course of the tumour. There are particular characteristics associated with tumour growth:

- The degree of cell differentiation – ranging from well differentiated (looks like the tissue around it) to totally undifferentiated (few cells appear like the surrounding tissue).
- The growth rate – can be highly variable, may be uncoordinated; some are slow growing having no enclosing capsule.
- The invasive nature – can spread locally by infiltration and by metastatic spread to other sites in the body.

Malignant tumours destroy vital structures but, it is when they metastasise that results in premature death without effective treatment. It is, however, important to remember that survival outcomes continue to improve for people with a primary tumour and a secondary one, meaning they will be 'living with a cancer diagnoses for many years'.

Understanding the molecular biology of cancer is very important if one is to identify and obtain a definitive cancer diagnosis, identify the best treatments and predict prognosis. Increasing knowledge about newer biological factors such as HER2/neu receptors, HER2 and CDK 4/6 inhibitors, antiangiogenic agents and proliferative index (rate of cell division in the tumour) has altered the way adjuvant treatments are prescribed and these indicators are increasingly used to predict prognosis. The HER-2/neu receptor belongs to the epidermal growth factor receptor family, which is one of the receptors critical in controlling the pathway for epithelial cell growth and differentiation, and possibly angiogenesis (Nagy et al. 2021). Overexpression of the HER-2/neu protein is observed in up to 25% of breast cancers. ER2-overexpressing tumours treated with anti-HER2 (trastuzumab and pertuzumab) therapy have improved disease-free and overall survival in both the adjuvant and metastatic disease (Arnaud et al. 2021).

Identification of the steps involved in carcinogenesis has led directly to the discovery of molecular tumour markers (Table 31.1). Among the cancers for which molecular diagnostics has had an impact is chronic myeloid leukaemia (CML). The marker of this disease is the Philadelphia chromosome, which is detectable in 95% of cases. This additional information enhances the ability to accurately diagnose and determine prognosis.

Tumours may be classified not only by their biological behaviour but also traditionally by their tissue of origin. Most tumours retain sufficient characteristics of the normal differentiated cell to allow recognition of the type of tissue from which they were derived, which is the basis for the classification of tumours by tissue type (Table 31.2).

The Physical Effects of Cancer

The manifestations of cancer depend directly or indirectly on the location, size and type of tumour involved and the site of any metastases present. The most common sites of metastatic deposits are the lungs, bones, brain and liver.

Direct Tumour Effects include the following:

- Obstruction of duct and tracts, e.g. the oesophagus, causing dysphagia.
- Compression of major blood vessels such as the superior vena cava (Wells 2016), causing ischaemia, oedema of the head, neck and right arm, and dyspnoea.
- Compression of neighbouring tissues and organs, e.g. brain metastases may cause pressure and local oedema, which can compromise brain function and level of consciousness.
- Pressure on regional nerves, causing pain and/or paralysis, e.g. metastases in the vertebrae may cause spinal cord compression (SCC) and result in pain or loss of sensation and paralysis and is considered an oncological emergency (Lawton et al. 2019).
- Invasion of small local blood vessels, causing chronic bleeding and anaemia; when major vessels such as the carotid artery erode, a haemorrhage may be sudden and fatal.
- Uncontrollable growth causing necrosis or ulceration which may be internal or external – often termed 'a fungating tumour.'
- Infiltration by the cancer cells into the bone marrow compromising haemopoiesis (blood cell production) and leading to increased susceptibility to infection.
- Metabolic alterations – there are many tumour-specific metabolic imbalances such as those affecting the kidneys, liver and pancreas. Hypercalcaemia is the most common oncological emergency and is associated with cancer of the breast, bone, lung and kidney. It is caused by local bone metastases directly stimulating osteoclast activity (causing breakdown of bone structure) and the release of humoral hypercalcaemia factors. (See Further Reading, e.g. Pugh et al. 2015, UK Acute Oncology Society Website.)

TABLE 31.1 Examples of Molecular Genetic Markers Used in Cancer Diagnosis and Prognosis

Cancer	Genetic Marker	Principal Application
Chronic myeloid leukaemia	Philadelphia chromosome t(9;22)(q34;q11) [BCR/ABL]	Primary diagnosis, detection of residual disease after treatment
Non-Hodgkin's lymphoma Follicular Burkitt's	t(14;18)(q32;q21) [BCL2/IGH] t(8;14)(q24;q32)	Primary diagnosis, detection of residual disease after treatment As above
Neuroblastoma	MYCN amplification	Prognosis
Breast cancer	HER2-neu/ERB2 amplification	Prognosis
Familial Cancers		
Breast	BRCA1, BRCA2	Diagnosis of hereditary predisposition
Colon	APC, MSH2, MLH1	As above
Wilms' tumour	TP53 mutation	As above
Retinoblastoma	RB mutation	As above

TABLE 31.2 Classification by Tissue Type of Malignant Tumours

Tissue of Origin	Malignant Tumour
Epithelial	**'Carcinoma'**
Squamous: surface epithelium, cell lining covering body cavities, organs and tracts	Squamous cell carcinoma, e.g. lung, skin, stomach
Glandular: glands or ducts in the epithelium	Adenocarcinoma, e.g. breast, lung, colon
Transitional cells: bladder lining	Transitional cell carcinoma, e.g. bladder
Basal cells: skin layer	Basal cell carcinoma (BCC), 'rodent ulcer'
Liver	Hepatocellular carcinoma
Biliary tree	Cholangiocarcinoma
Placenta	Choriocarcinoma
Testicular epithelium	Seminoma, teratoma, embryonal carcinoma
Endothelial cells	Angiosarcoma
Mesothelial: covering the surface of serous membranes	Mesothelioma, e.g. pleura, peritoneum
Connective Tissue	**'Sarcoma'**
Bone	Osteosarcoma
Cartilage	Chondrosarcoma
Fatty tissue	Liposarcoma
Fibrous tissue	Fibrosarcoma
Lymphoid tissue	Lymphomas
Bone marrow	Leukaemias, e.g. ALL, CML
Muscle	**'Myosarcoma'**
Smooth muscle	Leiomyosarcoma
Striated muscle	Rhabdomyosarcoma
Cardiac muscle	Cardiac sarcomas
Neural	
Meninges	Meningeal sarcoma
Glia	Glioblastoma multiforme
Neurones	Neuroblastoma, medulloblastoma
Germ Cells	
Testes or ovary	Teratoma, germ cell

ALL, Acute lymphoblastic leukaemia; *CML,* chronic myeloid leukaemia.

Indirect Tumour Effects. A group of rare degenerative disorders broadly termed as 'paraneoplastic syndromes' may be the presenting features before diagnosis in 10%–15% of patients (Gonzalez 2022). Early detection is important as these symptoms can often be ameliorated.

Cancer Recurrence

The exact manner in which a cancer moves from being a carcinoma in situ to one which is capable of invasion and spread to other organs or tissues is not clear; however, it is thought to be partly due to physiological changes occurring in tumour cell membranes which reduce their adhesion to other cells. Tumours also produce proteolytic (protein-dissolving) enzymes, which may assist in the invasion of normal tissue. Malignant cells also seem to lose contact inhibition, failing to recognise their boundaries and to cease growth on meeting a different tissue type. For example, tumours of glandular lung tissue may continue invasion through the pleura to the chest wall. The risk of cancer recurrence is always present when a diagnosis has been given. Two-thirds of patients develop metastases and most deaths from cancer are due to metastases that are resistant to conventional therapies (Gallicchio et al. 2022). (See Useful Websites, e.g. Cancerquest; tumour biology and surveillance research programme, National Cancer Institute.)

Metastatic invasion (spread) may occur in one of four ways (Fig. 31.1):
- via the lymphatic system
- via the bloodstream (arteriovenous)
- via serous cavities
- via the cerebrospinal fluid (CSF).

Lymphatic Spread. Tumour cells may invade the lymphatic vessels and grow in clumps and cords, establishing themselves en route in local lymph nodes. This is termed 'regional spread'.

Arteriovenous Spread. Tumour cells enter blood vessels near the primary tumour or are shed into the blood via the thoracic lymph duct. They then become enmeshed in the next capillary network they encounter. For example, a gastrointestinal tumour will typically spread via the hepatic portal vein, initially to the liver.

Serous Cavity Spread. Serous membranes such as the pleura or the peritoneum may be invaded by tumours, either locally from the primary tumour or from nearby metastases. This can cause excess serous fluid to be produced and the formation of malignant pleural effusions or ascites. This process is commonly known as 'seeding'.

CSF Spread. Tumour cells may spread directly in the CSF. Some brain tumours metastasise along the spinal cord in this way.

Survival is referred to in 5-, 10- and 15-year intervals and, while more cancer patients are surviving, the term 'cure' is used with caution. It is important for healthcare professionals to clarify their meaning for patients, as the uncertainty surrounding cancer and cancer recurrence creates distress for the patient and their family. McHale et al. (2020) and Cruickshank et al. (2017; 2020) are undertaking a programme of research to test interventions to relieve this distress in clinical practice, delivered by specialist cancer nurses.

The Psychosocial Impact of Cancer

There are psychosocial implications for patients and families from diagnosis, through treatment, the development of recurrence and end of life. It is now widely accepted that quality of life in cancer patients is an important consideration and may be improved by psychological interventions at specific stages (Brown et al. 2021). These important areas are explored further in this chapter.

Epidemiology of Cancer

Epidemiological studies provide data about possible causes of different forms of cancer and inform the strategies for cancer prevention and screening. The most commonly diagnosed cancers in the UK are breast, lung, colorectal and prostate; together these four

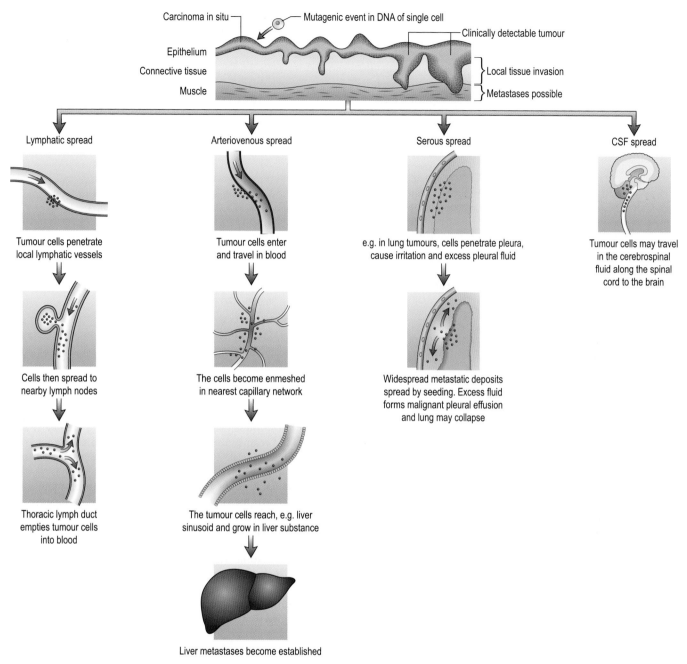

Carcinoma in situ — ┌── Mutagenic event in DNA of single cell

Clinically detectable tumour

Epithelium

Connective tissue

Muscle

Local tissue invasion

Metastases possible

Lymphatic spread

Tumour cells penetrate
local lymphatic vessels

Cells then spread to
nearby lymph nodes

Thoracic lymph duct
empties tumour cells
into blood

Arteriovenous spread

Tumour cells enter
and travel in blood

The cells become enmeshed
in nearest capillary network

The tumour cells reach, e.g. liver
sinusoid and grow in liver substance

Liver metastases become established

Serous spread

e.g. in lung tumours, cells penetrate pleura,
cause irritation and excess pleural fluid

Widespread metastatic deposits
spread by seeding. Excess fluid
forms malignant pleural effusion
and lung may collapse

CSF spread

Tumour cells may travel
in the cerebrospinal
fluid along the spinal
cord to the brain

Figure 31.1 The cancer process. *CSF,* Cerebrospinal fluid.

cancers make up over 50% of all new cancers each year (Cancer Research UK 2023a). The 20 most commonly diagnosed cancers are shown in Fig. 31.2.

Cancer is associated with increasing age. Around 75% of people diagnosed with cancer are aged 60 years and over (Cancer Research UK 2023a). Cancer is very rare in children; approximately 1% of cancers are diagnosed in children, teenagers and young adults (Cancer Research UK 2023b). (See Further Reading, e.g. Olsen and Smith 2018, and Useful Websites: TYAC and Children with Cancer UK.)

The incidence of cancer in the UK is one of the highest in the northern hemisphere. Predominantly, cancer is a disease of well-resourced countries but it is clear that patterns of cancer are set to increase in developing countries over the next decade (Sung et al. 2021). The greater incidence in the northern hemisphere may be

partly attributed to the availability of screening, diagnostic and reporting procedures, improved overall life expectancy and diet. Geographical variations across the world in the incidence of cancer provide clues to the lifestyles of different populations.

In Mozambique, a high incidence of liver cancer is thought to be associated with aflatoxin from mould found on stored peanuts. Since the introduction of more appropriate storage practices, the incidence of liver cancer has been falling. The Japanese have a low incidence of breast cancer in comparison with the UK and United States but a higher incidence of stomach cancer.

Epidemiological investigation of genetic predisposition to cancer is growing rapidly as developments in molecular biology make it possible to study genetic markers in large populations. The completion of the Human Genome Project is accelerating the discovery of such markers (see website for archive information).

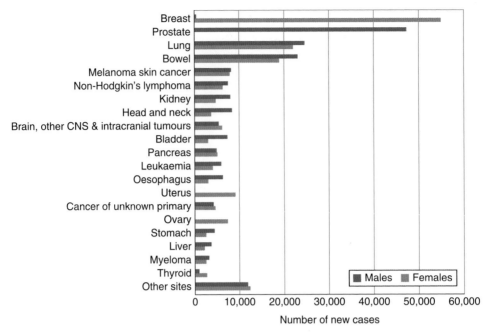

Figure 31.2 The 20 most commonly diagnosed cancers (excluding nonmelanoma skin cancer), UK, 2018. (From Cancer Research UK, https://www.cancerresearchuk.org/health-professional/cancer-statistics/incidence/common-cancers)

Aetiology of Cancer

The cause of cancer is the combined interaction of genetic and environmental factors and it is difficult to separate the two completely. Although all cancers have a genetic origin at the cellular level, this does not mean that all cancer is inherited. Genetic changes or mutations may be either *somatic* (acquired) or *germline* (inherited).

- *Germline mutations* are those present in the gamete (oocyte or spermatozoon) of a parent that can be passed to the offspring. The mutation is present in every cell of the body.
- *Somatic mutation* is when an individual body cell, post conception, acquires a gene alteration. If not repaired, the mutation is passed on to all future cells through mitosis. These clonal changes are unique to the cells in that particular tissue and are not inherited.

Many questions remain to be answered regarding the exact mechanisms involved in the cellular mutations that lead to cancer. However, epidemiological studies have identified certain causative factors, termed 'carcinogens'.

Carcinogens are factors that both initiate and promote changes in the cell which lead to cancer. Both are required to cause the cancer:

- *Initiation* – a mutagenic event occurs in the DNA of a single cell.
- *Promotion* – repeated exposure to carcinogenic agents may or may not cause this initiated cell to proliferate to form a tumour.

Carcinogenic factors and substances can be either intrinsic or extrinsic.

Intrinsic Factors

Heredity. Inherited cancers constitute 5%–10% of all cancers. Several genes have now been identified that are responsible for predisposing individuals to develop certain cancers. Cancers that occur with increased frequency in families are components of various hereditary cancer syndromes, for example, hereditary nonpolyposis colon cancer (HNPCC).

Cancer susceptibility genes such as *BRCA1* and *BRCA2* have been identified in breast and ovarian cancer. Women who inherit a mutation in these genes may face a 50%–85% lifetime risk of developing breast cancer including an increased risk for ovarian cancer (Dullens et al. 2020). Testing for these particular genes is now available (see NHS website).

Hormones. Certain hormones are thought to promote some tumours. Early menarche, late menopause and nulliparity are associated with an increased lifetime risk of breast cancer. The Million Women Study (2003) was a landmark study that followed up women over 20 years to understand their risk of breast cancer. They found that the use of combined oestrogen plus progesterone hormone replacement therapy (HRT) also increases the risk of breast cancer. High testosterone levels have also been related to increased risk of prostate cancer (Michaud et al. 2015).

Immunity. Individuals with impaired immunity are more susceptible to cancer; for example, people with HIV disease have a higher incidence of anal cancer than the normal population (Colón-López et al. 2018; Kiplagat et al. 2022). It is the prolonged immunosuppression that may predispose these patients to cancer rather than the infectious agent per se.

Pre-Existing Disease. Any tissue subjected to constant irritation or to a disease process has an increased susceptibility to malignant change.

Age. The increased incidence of cancer with age is thought to be attributable to:

- prolonged exposure to carcinogens
- decreased resistance to carcinogens
- hormonal changes that occur with age.

Extrinsic Factors

At least 70% of cancers occur in epithelial cells which are constantly exposed to external, ingested or inhaled substances. Extrinsic factors related to lifestyle and the environment are important in the process of carcinogenesis. These factors include physical agents, chemical agents, viruses and diet.

Physical Agents

Radiation. Radiation is known to cause cellular mutations and cancer. Survivors of the atomic bomb explosions in Hiroshima and Nagasaki in Japan experienced a high incidence of leukaemia and skin cancer. Early research showed an increase in the incidence of leukaemia among the children of fathers working in the nuclear industry, possibly due to germ cell mutations (Gardner et al. 1990). The nuclear industry is tightly controlled but despite this catastrophic events such as Chernobyl 1986 and Fukushima in 2011, still occur. In recent times conflicts such as the one in Ukraine around their nuclear reactor poses a risk.

There is also increasing focus on the use of ionising radiation for medical diagnostic purposes which has increased over the last three decades. Moderate to high doses of radiation are well established causes of cancer, especially for exposure at young ages. However, cancer risk from low-dose medical imaging is unclear (Ali et al. 2020).

Ultraviolet Light (UVL). There is overwhelming evidence that repeated exposure to solar UVL is the primary cause of basal and squamous cell carcinoma (see Chapter 14, Nursing Patients With Skin Disorders). Data establishing a direct causal relationship with sunlight are more complex but suggest a promotional role of sunlight in the cause of melanoma. Light-skinned or freckled individuals who are unable to manufacture sufficient protective melanin are particularly at risk (see Chapter 14).

Chemical Agents

Tobacco. Ninety per cent of all lung cancers can be attributed to tobacco smoking. The temporal relationship between smoking and lung cancer was defined in the 1950s by studies undertaken by Doll and Hill (1954). Cigarette smoking has now clearly been identified as a major cause of cancers of the mouth, pharynx, larynx, bladder and pancreas, whilst contributing to many others. Risk is more dependent on duration of smoking than on consumption. Smoking 20 cigarettes a day for 40 years is eight times more hazardous than smoking 40 cigarettes a day for 20 years. People who stop smoking even well into middle age avoid most of their subsequent risk of lung cancer, and stopping before middle age avoids more than 90% of the risk attributable to tobacco (Islami et al. 2015). It is also evident that nonsmokers are at risk from exposure to other people's smoke: one-quarter of lung cancer cases in nonsmokers are estimated to be due to passive smoking (International Agency for Research on Cancer (IARC) 2023). The introduction of e-cigarettes into Europe in 2006 has helped many smokers quit; they are believed to be 95% less harmful than using tobacco, and are supported in their use by Public Health England (McNeill et al. 2015). However, opinions are changing about the safety of these long term and among young people (Feeney et al. 2022).

Alcohol. The International Agency for Research on Cancer (IARC) (2023) review on human carcinogens reported that consumption of alcoholic beverages is causally associated with cancers of the oral cavity, pharynx, larynx, oesophagus, liver, colorectum and female breast, even for low and moderate alcohol intakes. The risk of cancer increases in a dose-dependent manner.

Other Chemicals. Carcinogenic chemicals present occupational hazards. Some of these, but by no means all, are now subject to control through regulation or ban. These controlled substances, and associated cancer sites, include:

- asbestos (lung, mesothelium and larynx)
- vinyl chloride (liver)
- certain chemical dyes (bladder)
- arsenic (lung and skin)
- some hardwood dusts (nasopharynx).

Viruses

Although cancer is not contagious, some cancers are associated with viral infections. For example, the Epstein–Barr virus (EBV) causes a systemic infection that may precede Burkitt's lymphoma, a malignant disease common in parts of Africa. Patients with chronic hepatitis B are more susceptible than others to liver cancer. The human papilloma virus (HPV), which may be sexually transmitted, is associated with cervical cancer, and a vaccine against some types of HPV has created opportunities to prevent some cases of cervical cancer.

Diet

Epidemiological studies that isolate diet as a causal factor in the development of cancer are extremely problematic to undertake. Nevertheless, dietary factors have been implicated as a major cause of the high incidence of cancer in the West. Countries where the average diet is high in fat and protein appear to have a high incidence of breast cancer, and low-fibre diets are thought to contribute to bowel cancer.

Cancer Prevention and Screening

Prevention of cancer is a major focus of research and education. The goal of primary prevention is to reduce the risk of the healthy population developing cancer. Secondary prevention aims to detect early-stage, curable cancer. Primary prevention is therefore the most effective and economic method of controlling cancer (Papadimitriou et al. 2021).

Nurses have a responsibility to incorporate health promotion, health education and disease prevention in their role as well as the care of those who are ill. This wider role is reflected in their pre- and postregistration education and the Nursing and Midwifery Council Code (2018). Community health practitioners work in primary care offering a range of health promotion programmes, as well as screening for ill health. Antenatal care, well-woman or well-man clinics, sexual health and family planning centres and other health screening clinics all provide opportunities for teachable moments about cancer prevention. Within hospitals, clinical nurse specialists incorporate cancer awareness and secondary prevention in their roles, with many involved in local and national initiatives such as cancer site-specific awareness weeks and health promotion in schools.

Primary Prevention

Primary cancer prevention includes activities such as:
- identifying risk factors in individuals or groups
- counselling high-risk individuals to promote behaviour modification
- genetic screening
- implementation of new cancer prevention programmes, e.g. smoking cessation, healthy eating and early diagnosis campaigns.

Media reporting of cancer risk development requires cautious interpretation and should be put into perspective by reference to the original studies on which it is based. It is important to remember that substances that are carcinogenic in animals are by no means always so in humans. Moreover, everyday exposure to some substances implicated is so minimal as to make risk insignificant. Some media scares do little to promote health; fear of cancer is one of the most common reasons why people avoid screening or fail to present with symptoms. Other reasons may include the influence of culture, family and friends.

Health Promotion Programmes

Health promotion/education programmes have some measure of success. The 'detect cancer early' campaign was first launched by the Scottish Government in 2012 and much of the focus remains on detecting cancer earlier when there is a better chance of cure. NHS England (2019b) has refreshed their strategy, which has a strong focus on prevention by supporting patients to adopt improved healthy behaviours. This will both help people to live longer, have healthier lives, and reduce the demand for and delays in treatment and care.

Through working partnerships with the community and the food industry, strategies to promote healthy eating include a national 'Five a Day' programme, improving accessibility to affordable fresh fruit and vegetables, and advocating five portions of these daily (see Chapter 22) (Reflection 31.2).

Attitudes

Psychologists developed the Health Belief Model (Strecher and Rosenstock 1997) to predict an individual's preventive health behaviour and account for some of the factors that determine attitudes to health and illness. The Health Belief Model states that an individual feels vulnerable to a disease if they believe they are susceptible to developing it and believe the disease to be serious. Preventive action will be taken only after the individual has balanced the benefits of that action against its physical, psychological and financial costs (Soerjomataram and Bray 2021).

Despite being taught about the risks of smoking, teenage smokers may consider themselves to be young and healthy and therefore not 'at risk'. Young people in general are motivated by short-term rather than long-term rewards. Smoking in some subcultures and families is associated with attributes such as maturity or rebelliousness, which the young person and their peer group may value. Later, the physical addiction to nicotine becomes a coping mechanism for life's stresses and social deprivation. For some people, the avoidance of lung cancer is not worth the cost of surrendering the immediate gratification and social status offered by smoking.

REFLECTION 31.2

Lifestyle and Cancer: Reducing the Risk

Access the European Code Against Cancer and Cancer Research UK websites and consider their advice on reducing cancer risk.

Activities

- Reflect on how you could modify your own lifestyle to reduce cancer risk.
- Discuss with your assessor/supervisor how you could use the European Code Against Cancer when talking with patients about reducing cancer risk.

Resources

European Code Against Cancer, https://cancer-code-europe.iarc.fr/index.php/en/.
Cancer Research UK, https://find.cancerresearchuk.org/?xss-q=prevention.

Clearly, consideration of the wider causes of individual behaviour would lead those involved in health promotion to an awareness of the social and political action necessary. The causes of social deprivation need to be considered alongside individual behaviour. Preventive services must be readily accessible, based on the expressed needs of the community and client centred.

The concepts of health and ill health are open to wide interpretation. An essential aspect of communication is that everyone understands and attaches the same meaning to language used. If adherence to healthcare programmes is to be achieved, nurses need to understand an individual's personal health beliefs and how information is interpreted.

COMMUNITIES OF CARE

People who are homeless or vulnerably housed are subject to disproportionately high risks of physical and mental illness, they are further disadvantaged by difficulties in access to services. People experiencing homelessness can face many barriers to accessing healthcare services including cancer services. These barriers often mean that they do not access primary care. Their health conditions are not well managed and their care is often crisis-led. People who are experiencing homelessness are more likely to use the emergency department and to have emergency admissions to hospital.

Homeless people find themselves at the junction of two very difficult challenges, battling homelessness as well as a life-threatening disease. The obstacles they face in accessing cancer services are many and complex, requiring dedicated efforts from nurses and other health and care professionals to bridge the gap and offer them the care and support they urgently need.

The National Institute for Health and Care Excellence (NICE) has produced draft guidelines, these include recommendations on ways to improve access to and engagement with health and social care services for people experiencing homelessness. It also offers advice on how care providers and practitioners across disciplines and agencies can collaborate to support and improve outcomes for those who experience homelessness (see Overview | Integrated health and social care for people experiencing homelessness | Guidance | NICE).

Secondary Prevention: Screening

The prognosis and outcome of patients with cancer are improved considerably if the tumour is detected at an early stage. Complete cure can only be assured if precancerous tissue can be identified and treated, as in the case of cervical intraepithelial neoplasia (CIN).

Cancer Screening Difficulties

The development of an accurate and cost-effective method of screening at-risk sections of the population is problematic for several reasons. The test must have both a high degree of sensitivity, reducing the risk of false-negative results, and specificity, reducing the psychological trauma and expense of treating false-positive results.

It must be possible to identify an at-risk group; otherwise the cost of screening becomes prohibitive. Finally, and most problematically, it must be determined whether detecting the cancer type at an early stage will prolong life (Yaffe et al. 2019).

The general cancer screening programmes currently offered (in the UK) are:
- breast cancer screening
- cervical cancer screening

- colorectal cancer screening
- lung cancer screening.

Additionally, there is the Prostate Cancer Risk Management programme (Public Health England 2016). (See Useful Websites, NHS Cancer Screening Programmes.)

Breast Cancer Screening

Despite recent debates about the quality of over 40 years of trials, it is generally agreed that there is a clear benefit and reduction in mortality from breast cancer from screening women over the age of 50 years by mammography every 2 years (IARC 2015) and programmes continue. In the UK mammography is routinely offered every 3 years to women aged between 50 and 70 years. However, the age range for routine invitation for screening is to be extended to include women aged 47 to 73. Accepted screening techniques include mammography and clinical breast examination. The value of screening women of 40 years or younger remains controversial however, an American guideline update by Oeffinger et al. (2015) provides an overview of the evidence in this area and a recommendation in the United States to screen all women every 2 years from age 40 is being considered (Tanne 2023). The denser breast tissue of premenopausal women makes mammograms difficult to interpret in this age group. In future, genetic screening and new technologies such as digital mammography may be of benefit.

Cervical Cancer Screening

Cervical cancer is one of the most common female cancers in under-resourced economies. Since the introduction of the Papanicolaou ('Pap') smear test in the mid-1960s, there has been a steady decline in mortality rates in the UK. Women in the UK are first offered screening at age 25 years (age 18 years in Scotland). This continues every 3 years until they reach the age of 49 years. Thereafter the test is offered at 5-year intervals until women reach the age of 64. Women aged 65 or over are only offered a smear test if they have not had a smear since they reached 50 or have had an abnormal smear in any of the previous three smears. However, some GPs may offer early screening as part of their consultation with women regarding sexual health.

Uptake of the service by groups at highest risk, that is women over the age of 40, of lower socioeconomic status and in minority ethnic groups, could be better. Barriers to cervical screening include lack of sensitivity and trust in health professionals, possible feelings of guilt and embarrassment, judgemental attitudes and a lack of privacy and supportive care in clinics (Crawford et al. 2016). It is important for staff working in screening services to have well-developed interpersonal and communication skills to alleviate any fears or anxieties. In addition, clinic schedules should allow time to provide support.

The World Health Organization (WHO) has recommended a self-care strategy to encourage women to access a cervical kit and self-sample. Self-sampling involves an individual obtaining a kit and collecting one's own vaginal sample. A Cochrane review by Staley et al. (2021) assessed the effectiveness of interventions aimed at women, to increase the uptake, including informed uptake, of cervical screening. They concluded evidence to support methods of intervention is low with the exception of invitational letters.

Colorectal Cancer Screening

The natural history of colon cancer, with the relatively long time from biological onset to the development of cancer, makes it a good candidate for screening. A national bowel screening programme based on faecal occult blood (FOB), using a home screening kit, was rolled out in 2006 (England) and 2007 (Scotland). The service became available throughout the UK in 2009.

Screening is routinely offered every 2 years to people aged 60–69 years (in England) and 50–74 years (in Scotland). However, people aged over 70 years in England can request a screening kit (see NHS Cancer Screening Programme). People with an unclear result will have the FOB test repeated. Where an abnormal result occurs, the person is offered an appointment with a specialist nurse to discuss colonoscopy (see Chapter 4). Campaigns by individuals such as Dame Deborah James who set up Bowelbabe (https://www.bowelbabe.org/) have been initiated to promote a greater awareness of the early warning signs of colon cancer (see Chapter 4).

Lung Cancer Screening

Despite the devastating impact of lung cancer, screening programmes are only just due to start in the UK. Screening for lung cancer using low-dose computed tomography (LDCT) has been established as an effective screening modality that reduces lung cancer mortality (Toumazis et al., 2020). In 2022, the UK Cancer Screening Committee recommended that people at high risk of lung cancer are invited to screening. This is called targeted lung cancer screening.

When it starts everyone aged between 55 and 74 who either smoke or used to smoke will be invited for an LDCT scan of the lungs. How often people will be invited is still to be decided.

Screening Options for Other Cancers

Screening programmes for the following cancers are always being reviewed, including:

- prostate cancer
- ovarian cancer.

Prostate Cancer. There is at present no consensus regarding the most appropriate screening method. There are three main screening modalities: digital rectal examination (DRE), serum prostate-specific antigen (PSA) and transrectal ultrasonography (TRUS). There are wide ranges in the estimates of sensitivity and specificity. Interest in PSA (a blood test) emerged in the late 1980s. However, PSA may be elevated in men with noncancerous conditions. There is currently no evidence that prostatic screening improves clinical outcomes; in fact, there are issues of uncertainty surrounding the appropriateness and type of treatment for men with early-stage prostatic cancer, since it has a long asymptomatic latency period.

A Prostate Cancer Risk Management programme is available to improve men's understanding of the benefits and limitations of PSA testing based on best available evidence (Public Health England 2016).

Ovarian Cancer. This cancer is sometimes referred to as the 'silent killer' because it often presents late and has the highest mortality rate of all malignant gynaecological cancers. Transvaginal ultrasound and detection of a raised cancer antigen (CA125) in the blood provide two possible techniques for the screening of ovarian cancer. However, as with PSA, CA125 may be elevated in nonmalignant conditions. A UK collaborative trial of ovarian cancer screening (UKCTOCS) (Jacobs et al. 2016) found that although the mortality reduction was not significant in the primary analysis, there was encouraging evidence of a mortality reduction in years 7–14. However, it was not able to draw firm conclusions on the efficacy and cost-effectiveness of ovarian cancer screening. Women known to have a high familial risk of developing ovarian cancer are offered annual screening as part of a national familial ovarian cancer screening study.

Medical Intervention and the Nurse's Role

Diagnosis and Staging

Patients present with cancer at different stages of the disease and may be asymptomatic or symptomatic.

The staging of a cancer is the process whereby the extent of the disease is established; this involves a variety of tests (see the appropriate chapter for the staging of a particular tumour site). The diagnosis and staging can be long, complex, and distressing for the patient and their family, raising many issues of uncertainty. However, accurate staging of the extent of the disease is vital for the following reasons:

- Different forms of treatment are known to be effective for specific tumours and at specific disease stages. For example, thoracic surgery for a patient with disseminated small-cell lung carcinoma (SCLC) and metastases in the ribs would be inappropriate given the metastatic spread of the disease. Staging avoids human and financial cost of using inappropriate treatment. Another example is a test that can identify HER2 +ve breast cancer. One in five breast cancers test positive for a protein called human epidermal growth factor (HER2), a protein that promotes the growth of cancer cells. Choosing treatments that target HER2 is important to improve survival outcomes.
- It provides a better estimation of prognosis.
- It allows clinicians to determine a patient's eligibility to enter a clinical trial of a new treatment.

The Tumour, Node (Lymph) and Metastasis (TNM) System

The most common internationally used method of defining disease stage is the TNM system (Union for International Cancer Control 2023), in which:

- T denotes the size or extent of local invasion of the primary tumour
- N refers to the spread to local lymph nodes
- M refers to the presence of metastases.

Agreed staging criteria exist for each cancer, such as those staging systems used for lung cancer (Information 31.1) (see Chapter 3, Nursing Patients With Respiratory Disorders), gynaecological, testicular cancers and so on (see Chapter 8, Nursing Patients With Disorders of the Breast and Reproductive Systems). Reflection 31.3 illustrates the staging system through the experience of a young man with testicular cancer.

Some types of cancer – usually those that are disseminated at presentation – cannot be effectively staged with the TNM system and have necessitated the development of other systems.

Patients may be restaged at various times following a diagnosis of cancer in order to measure their response to treatment, or the extent of disease recurrence/progression and/or when new symptoms arise that are unknown.

🌐 **See Evolve website Critical thinking question 31.1**

Psychological Impact of Diagnosis and Staging

Primary Diagnosis

It is common for patients to be aware that they have cancer before they are told formally of their diagnosis. This awareness

---

INFORMATION 31.1

Summary of the TNM Staging System for Lung Cancer

T (Primary Tumour)

TX	Positive cytology only
Tis	Carcinoma in situ
T1	Tumour ≤3 cm in diameter. No proximal invasion
T2	Tumour >3 cm in diameter, within 2 cm from carina or invading the visceral pleura or partial atelectasis
T3	Tumour of any size extending into the chest wall, diaphragm, pericardium, mediastinal pleura or within 2 cm of carina, total atelectasis
T4	Tumour of any size with invasion of mediastinal organs or vertebral body, malignant pleural effusion

N (Lymph Nodes)

N0	Nodes negative
N1	Positive nodes in ipsilateral hilar nodes
N2	Positive ipsilateral, mediastinal and subcarinal nodes
N3	Positive contralateral mediastinal or hilar nodes, scalene or supraclavicular nodes

M (Distant Metastases)

M0	No metastases
M1	Metastases present

The disease is then staged using the above information, as follows:

Stage IA	T1	N0	M0
Stage IB	T2	N0	M0
Stage IIA	T1	N1	M0
Stage IIB	T2	N1	M0
	T3	N0	M0
Stage IIIA	T1–3	N2	M0
Stage IIIB	T4	Any N	M0
Stage IV	Any T	Any N	M1

Adapted from Wittekind C, Compton CC, Greene FL, Sobin LH. TNM residual tumor classification revisited. *Cancer.* 2002;94(9):2511–2516.

---

derives from their experience of symptoms, tests and, in some cases, surgery and from the nonverbal communication of staff or relatives. Full disclosure of diagnosis is very important to allow patients to make informed decisions about their treatment and care. It is no longer appropriate to withhold information to an individual.

Reflection 31.4 provides an opportunity for you to reflect on patient experiences of being given a diagnosis of cancer.

Even if they suspect their diagnosis, patients often use different ways, such as denial and anger, as a coping mechanism. These are early emotional reactions experienced by people facing any actual or potential life crisis or loss, as described by Kübler-Ross in her seminal text (1973).

Disease Recurrence

The discovery that the disease has recurred after a symptom-free period may provoke further psychological distress. Fear of cancer recurrence (FCR) is defined as 'fear, worry, or concern about cancer returning or progressing' (De Vries et al. 2014, p. 3267). The period of waiting for test results, whether at initial diagnosis

REFLECTION 31.3

Staging Dan's Testicular Cancer

Staging System Generally Used in the UK

Stage I	Tumour confined to testes
Stage II	Pelvic and abdominal lymph node involvement
Stage III	Mediastinal and/or supraclavicular lymph node involvement
Stage IV	Distant metastases, e.g. lung

Dan, a 22-year-old student, discovered a testicular swelling but chose to ignore it initially because he misinterpreted it as a sports injury and he was busy with exams. As time passed he felt embarrassed and frightened. Nine months later he presented to the student health centre because he was becoming breathless far more readily than usual and suffered a constant backache. These symptoms were due to lung metastases and referred pain caused by metastases in the para-aortic lymph nodes.

Dan was admitted to a surgical ward, where a biopsy under anaesthesia was performed. A frozen section taken for histology showed a testicular teratoma. A left orchidectomy was then performed.

Following postoperative recovery, Dan was transferred to an oncology ward for staging. Dan lived too far away to travel to the department each day; otherwise the necessary tests could have been performed while he was an outpatient. Dan wanted to know why staging was needed and the specialist nurse explained the purpose of staging and outlined the tests that would be necessary. The tests were carried out and their results were as follows:

- chest X-ray: showed multiple lung metastases
- thoracic computed tomography (CT) scan: confirmed lung metastases
- abdominal CT scan: showed a large para-aortic lymph node and no liver metastases
- blood samples for full blood count, urea, creatinine and electrolytes, liver function and tumour markers (alpha-fetoprotein (AFP) and human chorionic gonadotrophin (hCG)).

These tests showed that Dan had stage IV testicular teratoma (see staging system above). Dan asked the specialist nurse to explain the results and treatment options to him and his parents, who were extremely concerned.

Even extensive disease is curable with cisplatin-based chemotherapy. Accordingly, this was the treatment course chosen following further discussion with Dan.

Note. Creatinine clearance measures the rate at which the kidneys are able to clear creatinine (a byproduct of metabolism) from the blood. It is calculated from the serum creatinine using an equation that includes age, gender and lean body weight to establish baseline measurements for subsequent assessment of any nephrotoxicity (damage to kidney tissue or function) induced by platinum compounds.

Activities

- Consider how you would react if you discovered a lump in a testis or a breast. Would you seek medical advice quickly, assume it to be completely innocent and forget it, or would you think it could be cancer but wait and hope the lump goes away?
- Discuss the role of the specialist nurse in supporting patients during the staging phase of a cancer with your supervisor/assessor.

REFLECTION 31.4

Supporting Patients and Families at Diagnosis

Listen to some patients talking about their diagnosis of lung cancer at Healthtalk.org (see Resource).

Activities

- Write a few notes about how you felt listening to the patients talking about their diagnosis.
- How can you as a nurse support this period for patients and their families?

Resource

Healthtalk.org. People's experiences – lung cancer. 2016. www.healthtalk. org/peoples-experiences/cancer/lung-cancer/topics.

It is important to know why each test is being performed and what it will entail for the patient. Enabling people to make decisions about their cancer is known as 'Health literacy' and is 'the personal characteristics and social resources needed for individuals and communities to access, understand, appraise and use information and services to make decisions about health' (NHS England 2023). Cancer literacy poses a unique set of challenges compared to other conditions because there are several time critical decisions to be made by the patient and clinicians. Cancer treatment can be complex and include many health professionals, tests, treatment and the need to manage side-effects (Sørensen et al. 2020). The nurse, acting as patient advocate, should ensure they are able to offer additional support and revisit this information again with the patient if necessary (NMC 2018). The patient may have fears they wish to express and/or clarification about their understanding of the decisions they need to make. An opportunity to discuss these openly is important. The nurse is well placed to do this.

Aims of Treatment

Cancer treatments can be broadly described as:
- curative – given with the intention of eradicating the disease
- palliative – given with the intention of controlling the disease and distressing symptoms.

Adjuvant treatments, such as a drug, that assist or increase the action of other drugs or therapies are often used in cancer treatment, for example, systemic anticancer treatment (SACT) used after removal of the tumour by surgery. The aim is to improve the chance of cure and the risk of a cancer recurrence.

Treatments, such as radiotherapy, used to reduce the tumour size before other treatment (e.g. surgery) are termed *neoadjuvant*. The aim is to improve the outcome of surgery and to reduce the risk of metastatic spread.

The transition from cure to palliative therapy may occur gradually over time but should always be discussed openly with the patient. Treatments for cancer vary considerably and can include surgery, radiotherapy, chemotherapy, biological and hormonal agents, immunotherapy or all of these treatments.

Response to Treatment

Response to treatment can be described as:
- complete – the tumour has disappeared
- partial – the tumour has decreased by at least 50%

or when a recurrence is suspected, can cause anxiety to both the person and their family.

Psychological Support

The nurse has an important role providing both practical information prior to and following each test, and emotional support.

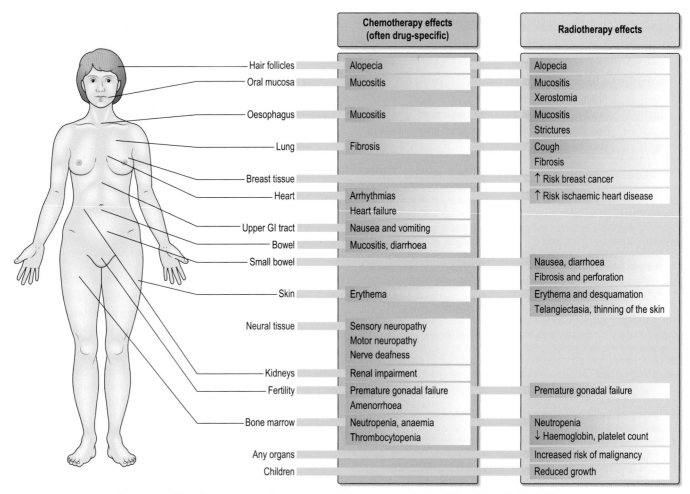

Figure 31.3 Side-effects of chemotherapy and radiotherapy – acute *(in pink)* and late *(in blue)*. (Reproduced with permission from Boon NA, Colledge NR, Walker BR. *Davidson's Principles and Practice of Medicine.* 20th ed. Edinburgh: Churchill Livingstone; 2006.)

- minimal or stable – there is very little change in tumour volume
- progressive – 25% increase in tumour volume.

Unfortunately, cancer treatments can have side-effects which may seriously reduce quality of life. Fig. 31.3 outlines side-effects associated with both chemotherapy and radiotherapy, and further coverage is provided in the appropriate sections later. Thus the decision to treat a patient must be carefully balanced between the costs and benefits of treatment for the patient and should ideally be taken jointly by the healthcare team and the patient.

Treatment Modalities

The principal forms of cancer treatment are:
- surgery
- radiotherapy
- chemotherapy – both cytotoxic chemotherapy and biological response modifiers (BRMs)
- immunotherapy.

Surgery

Surgery remains the most successful method of achieving long-term cure for patients with various types of localised tumour. Surgical removal of tumours of the skin (nonmelanoma), thyroid gland, uterus, colon and rectum (early stage) are associated with

an excellent chance of cure. Tumours that have disseminated at presentation are usually inoperable.

Surgery can also be used as an adjuvant treatment, for example, in the resection of diseased bone after radical chemotherapy for osteosarcoma, or as palliative surgery, for example, a stent insertion or bypass of the common bile duct can be performed to relieve jaundice in cancer of the head of the pancreas, leading to an improved quality of life.

Psychological Support

Surgical techniques, pre- and postoperative nursing care and the psychological problems associated with undergoing surgery are discussed in Chapter 25 The Care of a Person Undergoing Surgery. Important issues for nurses to consider around surgery are the possibility of the patient receiving the diagnosis during the perioperative period, alterations to body image and slower recovery time if treated with chemotherapy or radiotherapy prior to surgery. Reflection 31.5 provides an opportunity for you to reflect upon a patient's experiences having breast surgery.

Radiotherapy

Radiotherapy is the use of ionising radiation to destroy cancer cells. Approximately 70% of all patients with cancer receive radiotherapy. Note that radioactive substances may also be used

REFLECTION 31.5

A Patient's View of Care Prior to and Following Breast Cancer Surgery

These extracts are taken from a paper written by Niven and Scott (2003) in which they consider the appropriate use of nurse resource and the importance of 'hearing the patient's voice'. While now 20 years old, the account is very powerful because the patient was a nurse and coauthor of the paper.

Being 'prepped' consisted of having my breast, axilla and back painted. The sensation was pleasant; the last pleasant sensation there would be for a breast that had, in its time, been appreciated by baby and lover alike. There was no avoiding the issue, this was what I was going to lose. The nurse and I didn't talk. She didn't fill the moment with idle chit chat or pseudo empathy, which I would have found offensive and would have demanded social responses from me that I would have struggled to make. The nurse treated the task and thus me and my soon to be no more breast, with respect. While sharing none of the horrors of pubic shaving, this pre-operative preparation was an activity that called for high calibre nursing skills. I was very grateful for the way it was managed; it preserved my dignity, did not exacerbate an intrinsically distressing situation and gave me a sense of, literally 'being in good hands'. ....

On return from theatre it was trained staff who washed me, made me comfortable, gave me iced water to drink while checking heart rate, blood pressure, oxygen saturation, drain and wound. The sense of being completely cared for when I was in that post anaesthesia dependency state was wonderfully comforting and reassuring. For a short while I was completely in their hands and their competence was very obvious. Each task done well reinforced the sense of that competence. So it was as important that the water from the face cloth didn't run down my front as that the drain wasn't pulled or the wound exposed, forcing me to look at it rather than letting me choose my moment. These demonstrations of hands on competence created a climate of confidence in the nurses' expertise.

(Niven and Scott 2003, pp. 202–203)

Activities

- Consider the extract above, especially the patient's response to the supportive and competent care provided by the trained staff.
- Access and read the full paper.
- Reflect on the patient's account of her first postoperative shower (Niven and Scott 2003, p. 203) – a seemingly 'basic' activity delegated to a nursing assistant, which the patient regarded as a key nursing activity.
- Discuss with your supervisor/assessor the patient's observations on the lost opportunities for a trained nurse to monitor the wound and assess the patient's psychological state, such as her readiness to look at the wound.

References

Niven CA, Scott PA. The need for accurate perception and informed judgement in determining the appropriate use of nursing resource: hearing the patient's voice. *Nurs Philos.* 2003;4:201-210.

for some nonmalignant conditions, such as hyperthyroidism (see Chapter 5).

Radiation physics and biology are complex topics which are subject to intense research and development.

There are two kinds of radiation:

- particle radiation, e.g. alpha particles, beta particles, electrons, protons, neutrons which have a mass, limiting their depth of penetration

- ionising electromagnetic radiation, e.g. gamma (γ) rays and X-rays – these are similar to light, radio or microwaves, but have a very much higher energy level and are deeply penetrating.

Alpha particles are of low energy; they can be absorbed by a sheet of paper and are too weak to kill cancer cells. Electrons are of higher energy and can penetrate anything up to the density of wood. In radiotherapy, electrons are used to treat superficial areas located a few centimetres beneath the skin, for example, a 'booster' treatment to the site where the tumour was in breast cancer is known to prevent local recurrence. Gamma rays are short, very powerful waves that require lead or concrete to absorb them. They are emitted from the nuclei of radioactive elements, for example, caesium and cobalt, and are able to penetrate deeply into the body tissues.

The most common form of radiotherapy now is the X-ray. These rays are artificially generated when a stream of electrons bombard tungsten metal targets, releasing energy in the form of X-rays.

Radioactivity

Understanding ionising radiation requires a basic understanding of subatomic, atomic and molecular structure. All matter is made up of atoms, which consist of a central nucleus containing positively charged protons and uncharged neutrons, orbited by negatively charged electrons, equivalent in number to the protons. The negatively charged electrons (–) orbit the nucleus, being held in place by the attractive force of the positively charged protons (+); hence a stable state is maintained.

However, as the number of protons increases, an excess number of neutrons are required in order to hold the nucleus together. This imbalance causes the spontaneous disintegration of the nucleus with an associated emission of charged particles and radiation energy.

Some elements exist in a variety of states, depending on the number of neutrons in the nucleus. These are termed the isotopes of an element. Two isotopes of iodine (I), for example, are ^{127}I and ^{131}I. The latter is a radioisotope (also known as radionuclide), that is, it is unstable, because the nuclei of its atoms have a disproportionate number of neutrons. Radioisotopes may be naturally occurring, such as radium-226 (^{226}Ra), which is now seldom used in radiotherapy, or artificially manufactured by bombarding elements with neutrons in a nuclear reactor, for example, cobalt-60 (^{60}Co).

The Effects of Radiation

Radiation kills cancer cells by:

- a direct hit – when the radiation damages DNA directly; or
- an indirect hit – when the radiation produces free radicals in water adjacent to the DNA, which then damage the DNA.

Radiosensitivity of a given tumour is closely related to cell proliferation activity. As malignant cells are constantly dividing, they are all radiosensitive, although to varying degrees. Unfortunately, rapidly dividing healthy cells, such as those of the skin, the epithelium of the gastrointestinal and urinary tracts, the gonads and the bone marrow, are also vulnerable to radiation damage; this accounts for the unwanted side-effects of radiotherapy. Fig. 31.4 illustrates the difference between the radiation responses of tumour cells and normal cells.

In theory, all tumour cells could be eradicated by radiotherapy. However, the often narrow difference between the dose required to produce lethal damage to the tumour and that which causes irreversible damage to normal tissue (therapeutic ratio), makes it

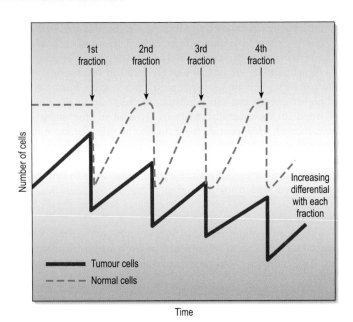

Figure 31.4 The difference between normal and tumour cell kill and recovery in radiotherapy. Normal cells have the capacity to recover to their previous population level more rapidly than malignant cells. Therefore successive treatments given after normal cell population recovery but before malignant cell population recovery will result in minimal damage to normal tissue but successive reductions in tumour size.

difficult to achieve optimal dosing without causing unacceptable side-effects.

Radiotherapy is prescribed as an 'absorbed dose'. The unit used is the Gray (Gy), where 1 Gy = 1 joule as absorbed by 1 kg of body tissue. The dose prescribed will vary, depending on several factors such as the volume and site of the area to be treated, sensitivity of the surrounding normal tissue, radiosensitivity of the particular tumour and also treatment intent, that is curative or palliative.

Sources of Radiation

Radiotherapy is given in a variety of ways, according to tumour type and stage and, occasionally, the patient's condition. Teletherapy (from the Greek téle – 'far'), sometimes called 'external beam therapy', is the most common method of treatment. Brachytherapy (from the Greek brachys – 'short') is administered via radioactive sources placed within a body cavity or tumour bed. Cyber knife, stereotactic radiosurgery and stereotactic body radiation therapy (SBRT) have enabled precision radiotherapy to be introduced, which can concentrate radiotherapy to the tumour and minimise doses to the surrounding tissues, thus reducing side-effects.

External Beam Radiotherapy. External beam radiotherapy is administered by machines which are categorised according to the level of energy of radiation produced and depth of penetration (kilovoltage, orthovoltage, megavoltage, cobalt machine). The linear accelerator or 'LINAC' is the predominant equipment in use throughout the world. The process of radiotherapy is complex and involves an understanding of the principles of medical physics, radiobiology, radiation safety, dosimetry, radiation treatment planning, simulation and interaction of radiation with other treatment modalities. Treatment involves the calculation of an overall dose of radiation sufficient to achieve the aim of the treatment plan, which will either be curative (known as 'radical' treatment) or palliative. The overall dose is then usually divided into a number of smaller doses, called 'fractions'. The purpose of delivering

the overall dose in a number of fractions is to allow healthy cells to recover during treatment.

The patient's initial visit to the department involves a planning session (simulation) which, if complex, may necessitate more than one visit. Absolute accuracy in devising the unique plan for each patient is vital, the aim being adequate dosage to the tumour and minimum exposure of healthy tissues and organs. Localisation of the tumour is made using an X-ray simulator, which mimics the treatment machine, and information from CT or magnetic resonance imaging (MRI) scans. This information is then used by the planning computer staff to determine a beam configuration that conforms precisely to the target organ or site. Patient immobilisation is important, particularly for patients with head and neck tumours. A close-fitting individualised Perspex shell is made in the mould room, which is worn throughout treatment. Some individuals may find this claustrophobic.

In most centres, the treatment field, or reference points, is marked out on the patient's skin using small permanent tattoos.

Proton Beam Therapy (PBT). Proton beam therapy provides radiation by delivering a beam of proton particles, rather than X-rays.

Brachytherapy. Brachytherapy is a type of radiation treatment where a sealed radioactive source is placed, inside, on or near the tumour to minimise side-effects. There are two main types of brachytherapy: low-dose rate (LDR) and high-dose rate (HDR).

LDR brachytherapy. Small radioactive seeds are implanted near or in the tumour. Often used for localised prostate cancer tumours

HDR brachytherapy. Similar principles to LDR but the radiative source is removed from the patient at the end of each treatment session. Delivers more intensive short-lived dose for example in high-risk localised gynaecological cancers.

Other Treatments. include:

SIRT (Radio-Embolisation) is 'Selective Internal Radiotherapy,' also called 'Radio-Embolisation' (RE). It is a method of treating malignant liver tumours, whether those tumours originate from the liver itself, or have spread to the liver from elsewhere in the body (e.g. bowel cancer).

IORT (Intraoperative Radiotherapy) is the application of therapeutic levels of radiation to a target area, such as a tumour, while the area is exposed during surgery. The treatment can be applied using low energy (0 kV) X-rays, or with electrons (intraoperative electron radiotherapy [IOERT]). These techniques are most commonly used in the treatment of breast cancer, but can be used for other tumours, for example, cancer of the cervix.

Radiotherapy Treatment Intent

This may be:

- curative
- adjuvant or neoadjuvant
- palliative.

The goal of radiotherapy in early-stage cancer is curative. Certain tumours such as skin cancer, Hodgkin's lymphoma, cervical cancer, cancer of the larynx and seminoma (germ cell tumour, testicular in origin) are particularly radiosensitive. Treatment can take up to 30 days and is associated with side-effects, but prognosis is very good long-term.

Adjuvant Radiotherapy. Radiotherapy is commonly used as an adjuvant treatment which forms part of the treatment plan. It is given either pre- or postoperatively, and increasingly alongside other systemic anticancer therapy especially for cancer of the breast, prostate, colon and rectal cancer. Chemotherapeutic agents such as cisplatin, 5-fluorouracil (5-FU), doxorubicin or mitomycin C are sometimes given alongside radiotherapy in cancers of the cervix, anus, head, neck and lung to achieve a greater cell kill.

Palliative Radiotherapy. Cancers at a more advanced stage where cure or eradication is not possible constitute 50% of all radiotherapy treatments given. It involves a shorter course of treatment at much lower doses than either radical or adjuvant therapy. Its aim is to maximise symptom relief and quality of life and minimise side-effects. Examples include haemoptysis in lung cancer or rectal bleeding in rectal cancer and SCC which presents as an emergency whereby the use of radiotherapy may alleviate symptoms and further distress for the patient.

SBRT is increasingly the approach used in palliative settings where side-effects can be minimised while providing maximum accuracy when treating the tumour.

Total Body Irradiation radiotherapy to the whole body is referred to as total body irradiation (TBI) and is often required to treat conditions such as leukaemia. This treatment must be followed by a haemopoietic stem cell transplantation (HSCT; bone marrow transplant [BMT]) to restore bone marrow function (see Chapter 13, Nursing Patients With Blood Disorders).

Hemibody (half body) radiation provides effective palliation for patients with extensive bone metastases, as are common, for example, in prostate or breast cancer.

The decision making and planning surrounding any course of radiotherapy involves a team approach. Informed consent is essential as is patient and carer education.

Radiation Protection

There is much fear and misconception amongst both professionals and the public about the dangers of radiation exposure. Indeed, radiation is potentially extremely hazardous, and exposure to high doses can cause several side-effects, together with cell mutations that may lead to carcinogenesis, or to congenital abnormalities if pregnant women are exposed.

Every institution dealing with radiation is legally obliged to appoint a radiation protection officer, to follow stringent guidelines for radiation monitoring and to provide education for staff and patient protection. If these are adhered to, radiation damage risk is negligible. Staff most at risk are those working constantly with unsealed sources. Staff working in areas of potential radiation exposure should wear personal dosimeters or film badges to monitor their individual exposure (see Further Reading, e.g. Health and Safety Executive UK 2023).

Side-Effects of Radiotherapy (see Fig. 31.3)

Side-effects occur when normal tissue is irradiated. Manifestation of side-effects varies greatly from patient to patient, depending on the location and amount of tissue being irradiated, the dose and its fractionation, and the patient's physical and psychological state. Treatment techniques are constantly being developed to improve accuracy of delivery and minimise side-effects. Patients may suffer from systemic side-effects such as fatigue, lethargy, nausea, anorexia and headaches but in general, radiotherapy affects only those tissues being irradiated. For example, a patient receiving treatment for bladder carcinoma will experience localised bladder irritation while radiotherapy to the brain will cause loss of hair on the head.

Side-effects may be 'early' (acute), occurring within days of commencing treatment, continuing for a period of weeks following treatment completion. Long-term or 'late' side-effects usually present 18 months to 2 years after treatment. Acute problems manifest in areas of rapid cell growth and division and are usually reversible. The nursing management of the most common side-effects forms a major part of the nursing role in the radiotherapy department (Table 31.3). Skincare is particularly important during and after a course of radiotherapy (see Further Reading, e.g. The Society and College of Radiographers 2020).

Late side-effects occur as, due to DNA damage, slowly dividing cells fail to replicate. Problems are most often a consequence of damaged vasculature and are usually permanent. Examples include fibrosis of the lung, chronic bowel inflammation and lymphoedema. Monitoring of late side-effects is undertaken during follow-up outpatient clinics.

Psychological and Supportive Care

Patients receiving radiotherapy are often perceived as self-caring. Their problems and needs are often hidden as treatment is mostly on an outpatient basis with the added stress of daily travel to and from the department. It is important to remember that radiotherapy treatment is not always an isolated event but usually precedes or follows other forms of cancer treatment. Although it brings its own problems and side-effects, its impact needs to be considered in the context of the patient's overall experience. That experience may be affected by existing psychosocial, physical and functional needs related to other existing disease or to financial or social constraints.

Myths and Fears

Few therapeutic modalities in medicine induce more misunderstanding, confusion and misapprehension than radiotherapy. For many patients, the news that they are to receive radiotherapy comes soon after knowledge of their cancer diagnosis when they are already coping with multiple stressors and feelings of loss. Myths and fears compound these stresses (see also Reflection 31.6).

❖❖ Nursing Management and Health Promotion: Radiotherapy

Nurses can do much to alleviate the patient's fears and anxieties, helping to make the experience of radiotherapy more tolerable. Supportive care relies on the understanding of the impact of cancer and its treatment viewed from the perspective of the patient.

REFLECTION 31.6

Starting Treatment at the Radiotherapy Unit

Look at the radiotherapy services in Glasgow:
https://www.beatson.scot.nhs.uk/about-us/video-tours/
This will allow you to see what radiotherapy machines look like.

Activities

- Find out where your nearest radiotherapy unit is and whether there is a virtual tour for staff and patients to view.
- Consider the benefits of this form of visual information for patients and their families.
- Reflect on how a patient might feel arriving at the department for their first treatment. Compare your impressions with those of another student.

TABLE 31.3	Nursing Management of the Side-Effects of Radiotherapy		
Irradiated Body Part/Organ	**Radiation Effect**	**Nurse Intervention**	**Rationale**
General	Fatigue	Forewarn patients of fatigue during and after radiotherapy. Provide appropriate information about pattern of symptoms	To foster independence, encouraging energy-saving activities but not inactivity. Exercise can help
		Assess and promote self-care strategies. Refer to appropriate healthcare professional as necessary	To prevent feelings of social isolation, low mood and to decrease anxiety
		Assess baseline fatigue levels prior to treatment starting	To monitor changes over time and need for further intervention
		Check for physical, biochemical and psychological causes of fatigue	Electrolyte imbalances/anaemia may be corrected. Appropriate psychological support can be given
		Encourage patients to maintain a daily record of fatigue levels and the relationship to activities	Enhances the ability to control activities or plan ahead, goal-setting and prioritising
Skin (See Further Reading Radiographer's guidelines)			
Particularly areas where the skin is thin, moist, e.g. skin folds, axilla, groin, breast and perineum. Light skin is especially sensitive	Three-stage reaction: 1. Erythema: redness, heat, itchiness	No metal-containing skin preparations	Metal may intensify radiation reactions
		Gentle washing with warm water and gentle drying, no rubbing	Friction causes irritation. Ink marks must not be washed off
		Application of simple moisturiser	Soothing and minimises friction, keeps skin supple
		If itchy, an antihistamine cream may be prescribed. Apply 1% hydrocortisone	To alleviate discomfort and itch
		Avoid exposure to the sun and extremes of heat and cold	UV light may intensify any reaction
		Encourage nonconstrictive clothing in lightweight, natural fabrics: no tight or elastic clothing	Reduces sweating and friction
	2. Dry desquamation: dryness, scaliness, tight feeling, pain on movement	1% hydrocortisone or lanolin cream (centres vary in their recommendations)	Soothing emollient and/or anti-inflammatory
		Expose skin to fresh air or cool fan	Cooling has a short-term analgesic effect
		For moderate to severe reaction, or if skin folds involved, consider application of a nonadhesive tape, ensuring it is removed with baby oil	Preventive measure and promotes wound healing as it is permeable. Removing with oil ensures the skin is not damaged
	3. Moist desquamation: blisters, loss of surface epithelium, pain, susceptibility to infection Occasionally progresses to necrosis	A break in treatment may be required Analgesics Observation for signs of infection	To prevent further skin breakdown and discomfort Infection exacerbates skin damage and may become systemic
		Use of hydrogel/hydrocolloid/alginate dressings Dressing plan: assessment, dressings, evaluation using wound care principles	To promote wound healing To record any changes, evaluating the effectiveness of the intervention applied
Scalp	Alopecia (in treatment field only). Loss of any body hair occurs from weeks 2–3	Reassure the patient that hair will usually grow back in 2–3 months, although it may be of a different texture and colour	Hair loss poses a very stressful threat to body image, especially for women
		Organise provision of a wig Wearing of scarf/turban at night	Prevents distress of hair on pillow
Brain	Cerebral oedema (within week 1 of treatment) (see Chapter 11)	Administer prescribed corticosteroids Observe and report alterations in mental status Ensure patient safety	Anti-inflammatory Enables prompt medical intervention

TABLE 31.3	Nursing Management of the Side-Effects of Radiotherapy—cont'd		
Irradiated Body Part/Organ	Radiation Effect	Nurse Intervention	Rationale
Mouth (see Useful Websites, e.g. Multinational Association of Supportive Care in Cancer)	1. Mucositis due to damaged, sloughed oral mucosa	Comprehensive dental review prior to treatment	To identify potential infection risks and carry out any necessary dental work, giving time for wound healing
	Opportunistic infection may ensue, e.g. candidiasis ('thrush')	Regular use of an oral assessment tool	To monitor any changes, evaluating interventions
		Teaching and encouraging frequent routine systematic oral hygiene, initiated prior to treatment if possible	To reduce the amount and severity of mucositis and encourage compliance. Also to minimise the risk of infection
		Use of a soft toothbrush, fluoride toothpaste and regular 0.9% sodium chloride mouthwashes	To minimise damage to the oral mucosa and prevent build-up of plaque
		Use of antibacterial/antifungal preparations, e.g. chlorhexidine, nystatin	To prevent or treat infection
		Regular analgesics: topical, e.g. benzydamine, and systemic including opiates	Oral pain is excruciating and always to the forefront of consciousness
		Use of cellulose film-forming agents to line the mucosa	Forms a thin protective film which relieves pain and discomfort
		Observe for signs of dehydration and inadequate nutrition, liaising with the dietitian (see Useful Websites, e.g. National Cancer Institute)	Prompt parenteral hydration and dietary supplements or enteral feeding may be commenced
	2. Xerostomia (dry mouth) due to altered salivary gland function. May be permanent. Causes difficulty in chewing, swallowing and talking	Frequent mouth rinses with 0.9% sodium chloride and sodium bicarbonate	Comforting, aids swallowing, buffering of oral environment
		Frequent sips of water	
		Use of artificial saliva	Lubrication of mucosa
		Moist soft diet	Easier to tolerate
		Avoidance of spices, alcohol, smoking, extremes of temperature	These are mucosal irritants
	3. Taste changes due to xerostomia and damaged taste buds	Assist patients to experiment with other foods	To maintain nutritional intake
	4. Dental decay due to xerostomia and radiation gingivitis	Pretreatment dental referral	Any caries will be exacerbated by radiation and form foci for infection
		Avoidance of high-sugar-content foods and fluids	Sugar alters natural slightly alkaline pH of oral environment and demineralises teeth
Neck area	1. Pharyngitis, laryngitis, causing pain, hoarseness, loss of voice, dry cough and occasionally respiratory stridor	Discourage smoking	Mucosal irritant
		Encourage patient to rest voice	
		Observe respiratory status and colour	Medical intervention: corticosteroids or even a tracheostomy may be necessary
		A cough suppressant	Prevents mucosal irritation caused by coughing
		Topical analgesics prior to food, e.g. aspirin gargles, anaesthetic throat spray; systemic analgesics	Promotes comfort and aids swallowing
	2. Oesophagitis (upper one-third) causing dysphagia	Maintain nutrition. Soft diet, referring to the dietitian for supplements	These patients are often already malnourished
		Avoid irritant foods, strong alcohol and smoking	
Thorax	1. Oesophagitis (lower two-thirds) causing 'heartburn'	As above; also administer antacids prior to food. Some antacids also contain topical anaesthetics	Lines oesophagus and prevents pain and trauma of swallowing and from gastric acid reflux
	2. Pneumonitis due to inflammation. May cause dyspnoea, productive cough and haemoptysis	Discourage smoking	Irritant
		Observe for signs of infection: pyrexia, cough, purulent sputum	Enables prompt commencement of antibiotics
		Oxygen as prescribed	
		Assessment and management of breathlessness	Patient comfort and integrated approach to managing this distressing symptom
	3. Dyspepsia, nausea and vomiting (less severe than with abdominal radiation)	(see below)	

Continued

TABLE 31.3	Nursing Management of the Side-Effects of Radiotherapy—cont'd		
Irradiated Body Part/Organ	**Radiation Effect**	**Nurse Intervention**	**Rationale**
Abdomen and pelvis	1. Nausea and vomiting due to inflammation of gastrointestinal epithelium; also a generalised radiation reaction	Encourage a small meal 3 hours before treatment and light snacks after	Some patients are unable to eat after treatment due to nausea
		Regular and appropriate antiemetics	Regular administration required to prevent and relieve nausea
		Distraction/relaxation techniques	There may be a contributing psychological factor in nausea
		Monitor fluid and food intake	To avoid fluid balance problems and malnutrition
	2. Diarrhoea, possibly accompanied by rectal bleeding	Maximise privacy	
		Administer antimotility medication as prescribed	
		Low-residue, bland diet, low fat	Better tolerated by damaged mucosa
		Observe for dehydration (see Chapter 21)	Avoid dehydration
		Maintain high fluid intake	
		Observe perianal skin: gently apply barrier cream after washing if necessary	To prevent skin excoriation
	3. Cystitis due to inflammation of bladder epithelium. Predisposition to urinary tract infection (UTI)	Encourage high fluid intake (3 L daily)	Prevents stasis of urine and sloughed epithelium
		Encourage and/or assist with personal hygiene	Helps prevent ascending urinary tract infection
		Regular collection of urine specimens for microbiology	Enables prompt antibiotic treatment of UTI
	4. Altered sexual function (depends on treatment site and dosage)	Psychological support and counselling	Loss of any degree of sexual function is very threatening to most people's self-image; opportunity to talk this through is vital
		Include partner in discussion if patient wishes	To gain understanding and support and minimise body image problems
		Assess the need for psychosexual counselling	To maintain a healthy relationship and sexuality
	Men:		
	Erectile dysfunction (usually temporary)	Psychological support	To explore possible options to help with erectile difficulties
	Sterility (usually permanent) Decreased libido	Offer sperm banking if appropriate	To enable sperm to be used for artificial insemination
		Monitor hormone levels Testosterone replacement therapy Patient/couple education and psychological support	To improve libido and promote healthy sexuality
	Women:		
	Sterility (if ovaries are irradiated). May be temporary or permanent	Advise continued contraception during and for several months after treatment. Hormonal contraception is contraindicated with some cancers, e.g. breast	Fertility is not always immediately affected and any pregnancy may not be viable
	Dyspareunia due to vaginal fibrosis and dryness	Advise use of vaginal lubricant	To promote comfort and ease of penetration
		Use of barrier contraceptives, e.g. condom during intercourse	There may be a burning sensation associated with semen and this will help to decrease irritation
		Education and use of vaginal dilators during (if tolerated) and for up to 2 years after treatment	To prevent vaginal stenosis and postcoital bleeding
	Loss of libido	Patient/couple education and psychological support, sensitively explaining that this is usually temporary	To maintain healthy sexual relationships
	Premature menopause (if ovaries irradiated)	Inform of possibility and potential menopausal symptoms	To help women manage menopausal symptoms
		Discuss possible strategies in managing the hot flushes, preventing osteoporosis, and so forth	
		Hormone replacement therapy should be discussed if appropriate	

A thorough needs assessment is fundamental to enable effective interventions to support the patient and their family throughout treatment. Bonevski et al. (2000) was one of the first studies to allow patients to identify needs they may have experienced in the last month because of having cancer. It considered needs associated with psychological, health system and information, physical and daily living, patient care and support, sexuality and financial issues. The authors found real benefits for both patients and clinicians in using this tool to assess the magnitude of needs that occur in clinical oncology settings. Their assessment tool has been used widely across the work (Cochrane et al. 2021). There are a number of needs assessment tools that can be used, but, in the UK, many nurses use the Macmillan Concerns Checklist as part of a recovery package. The recovery package (Macmillan Cancer Support 2018) is a series of key interventions which, when delivered together, can improve outcomes for people living with and beyond cancer.

Information is seen as crucial for successful interactions between patients and healthcare professionals, relieving anxiety and promoting a sense of control (Faller et al. 2016). Nurses are responsible, therefore, for becoming accurately informed themselves – about radiotherapy in general, and about each patient's individual treatment plan and likely side-effects.

Good practice is that written information should be accompanied by verbal explanation wherever possible. There is now a comprehensive range of patient information materials from a wide range of support agencies such as Macmillan Cancer Support and Tenovus (see Useful Websites), alongside telephone information helplines. Individual cancer alliances, hospitals and networks are also involved in the development of local information, ensuring patients receive accurate information at the appropriate time across all care settings. The internet has many sites providing high-quality information, but caution must be taken that they are trusted sites otherwise they can cause more harm than good. Over the past few years, there has been a rapid development of apps to provide information and support tools. (See Further Reading – McGrady et al. 2023).

Studies have also shown that many patients want as much information as possible to enable them to prepare for treatment, decrease their fears and anxieties and increase their understanding of treatment. Information requested includes:
- how treatment works
- the effectiveness of treatment
- likely side-effects
- preventive and self-care strategies
- impact of treatment on their lives and their families (Farrington and Townsend 2014).

Nurses have an increasingly important role in radiotherapy care, with both nurses and therapy radiographers developing advanced practitioner roles through which innovative approaches to care are more and more evident. Advanced practice is characterised by the following principles: autonomous practice, critical thinking, high levels of decision making and problem solving, values-based care and improving practice (Carvalho et al. 2022; RCN 2018). Employment of both nurse specialists and therapy radiographers to provide information and counselling services, practitioner-led review and follow-up clinics, telephone follow-up and nursing interventions for side-effects can make a positive contribution to patient care (Brown et al. 2021; Humphris et al. 2019). (See Useful Websites, e.g. Health Education England Aspirant cancer career and education development programme.)

Systemic Anticancer Treatment: Chemotherapy

Chemotherapy literally means 'treatment with chemicals' and therefore can refer to any form of medication therapy, but especially drugs used to treat cancer and antimicrobial drugs. However, in common usage the term refers to cytotoxic drugs. Cytotoxic (toxic to cells) chemotherapy involves the use of medication to disrupt the cell cycle and thus ultimately kill malignant cells.

Cytotoxic drugs, like radiation, are toxic to both healthy and malignant dividing cells and interfere with cell reproduction (see Fig. 31.3). There are many different cytotoxic agents, each with a different mode of action and function at different phases in the cell cycle (see Useful Websites, e.g. British National Formulary, and Further Reading, e.g. Tortora and Derrickson 2017).

Cytotoxic drugs are usually classified according to their chemical structure, cell cycle activity and primary mode of action. The classic categories include:
- alkylating agents
- antimetabolites
- antitumour antibiotics
- vinca alkaloids (plant alkaloids)
- taxanes
- miscellaneous compounds.

The action of some of these is described in Information 31.2. (See Further Reading, e.g. Lister et al. 2020).

Modes of Cytotoxic Chemotherapy Treatment

Cytotoxic chemotherapy differs from radiotherapy in that it is a systemic rather than a localised treatment modality. It can be used to treat any cancer that has a risk of metastasising. Despite newer drugs being introduced, many of the chemotherapy drugs used in current practice date back to the 1940s, 50s and 60s. Complete responses are seen in up to 20% of adults with Hodgkin's lymphoma, and 70% of childhood leukaemias. Chemotherapy is used mainly as an adjuvant treatment in solid tumours to prevent future recurrence.

Adjuvant and Palliative Chemotherapy. For the most part, chemotherapy is used:
- as the sole, or most important, treatment
- as a means of reducing the size of the tumour to aid the success of subsequent surgery or radiotherapy, i.e. 'debulking' of tumours, such as those of the head, neck and bladder
- following radiotherapy or surgery to eradicate remaining tumour cells or any micrometastases; this is common in breast, colorectal and ovarian cancer
- to treat a recurrence
- for palliation of symptoms – some tumours are partially chemoresponsive, so that treatment may relieve symptoms and improve the quality of, and possibly lengthen life
- within a trial for investigation of the usefulness of a new medicine.

Combination Chemotherapy. This is the use of a variety of agents. The purpose is to use a combination of drugs with different modes of action to reduce the risk of drug resistance. This interaction is more effective than using the drugs separately. It also allows drugs with different toxicities to be given at a maximum dose without causing unacceptable or irreversible toxicity.

Administration of Chemotherapy

Chemotherapy is scheduled at regular intervals, sometimes called 'pulses' or 'cycles'. The purpose is to prevent the cancer cells recovering and repairing. The specific regimen or protocol of drugs to be used is then calculated based on the patient's body surface area (BSA). The goal is to provide a concentration of the drugs that is

INFORMATION 31.2

Classification of Cytotoxic Agents

Alkylating Agents

Alkylating agents are highly reactive and are cell cycle phase nonspecific (CCPNS). Their primary mode of action is to join together or cross-link the two strands of DNA, preventing them from separating and therefore replicating. Cyclophosphamide is an example of a cytotoxic which acts in this way. Another group of alkylating agents are platinum-based compounds, for example, cisplatin and carboplatin, which cause interstrand and intrastrand linkages.

Antimetabolites

These are cell cycle phase specific (CCPS), exerting their effect in the S phase. They are structural analogues of normal intracellular metabolites essential for cell function and replication and so are used to disrupt cellular metabolism. Methotrexate, for example, inhibits the enzyme necessary for the conversion of folic acid to folinic acid. Folinic acid is necessary for the formation of purines and pyrimidines, components of DNA. Folinic acid rescue, in the form of folinic acid replacement, is necessary 12–24 hours after the administration of methotrexate to prevent the death of too many healthy cells. Other antimetabolites include 5-fluorouracil (5-FU) and cytosine arabinoside.

Plant Alkaloids

Many plants and plant extracts continue to be screened to identify new cytotoxic agents. To date these include the vinca alkaloids, taxanes and topoisomerase inhibitors. Mitotic inhibitors include vincristine, vindesine and vinblastine, which are CCPS acting in the mitosis phase. They bind to microtubule proteins, blocking spindle formation and preventing cell separation.

The taxanes (docetaxel and paclitaxel), on the other hand, promote assembly of the microtubule which results in a very stable microtubule that is non-functional.

Topoisomerase inhibitors (etoposide, teniposide, irinotecan and topotecan) interfere with DNA replication by binding to DNA and the topoisomerase enzymes.

Antitumour Antibiotics

Some classes of antibiotic have been found to be cytotoxic. In general, they are CCPNS and interfere with DNA function, although several other mechanisms of action may occur, such as alteration of the cell membrane or inhibition of certain enzymes. The most widely used is doxorubicin because it has a broad spectrum of activity; others include mitoxantrone and bleomycin.

Cytotoxic agents are constantly being researched and developed. There are several which do not fit into the above categories and whose action may not be fully understood.

INFORMATION 31.3

Safe Administration of Chemotherapy

Cytotoxic agents can be dangerous if they are not handled appropriately. They are considered hazardous drugs and the Health and Safety Executive are responsible to ensure measures are in place in hospitals to ensure the patients and the staff are safe (Cruickshank and Turner 2016, HSE 2023).

Extravasation

Some cytotoxic agents, for example, doxorubicin and vincristine, are termed 'vesicants' and can cause severe burns and tissue damage if they leak from the vein into the subcutaneous tissue (Fig. 31.5). If extravasation is suspected, the infusion should be stopped and an experienced clinician informed immediately. There are various antidotes available, but more scientific research is required. (Each hospital has a local policy; see guidelines by Fidalgo et al. 2012.)

Staff Protection

There has been concern for many years regarding the potential exposure and subsequent effects in healthcare workers. The scientific evidence indicates that staff handling these medications do so with extreme caution. The Royal College of Nursing, the UK Oncology Nursing Society (UKONS) and the British Oncology Pharmacy Association (BOPA) worked together to produce up-to-date guidance about maintaining safe practice for healthcare workers, which is available online through a flickbook (see British Journal of Nursing (BJN) 2016).

Handling Body Fluids

Many cytotoxic agents are excreted unchanged in urine and faeces, and both should be treated as hazardous for at least 48 hours and up to 7 days. It is therefore important to wear gloves when handling the body fluids of patients receiving chemotherapy, and to teach patients and their families to take appropriate precautions (see BJN 2016).

References

British Journal of Nursing. Be compliant, protect each other and stay safe: avoiding accidental exposure to cytotoxic drugs. *Br J Nurs.* 2016;24(16 Suppl):S1-S54.

Fidalgo JAP, Fabregat G, Cervantes A, et al; on behalf of the ESMO Guidelines Working Group. Management of chemotherapy extravasation: ESMO–EONS clinical practice guidelines. Ann Oncol. 2012;23(Suppl 7):vii167–vii173.

Health and Safety Executive Radiation Guidance 2023. https://www.hse.gov.uk/radiation/

UKONS (2018). Acute Oncology Initial Management Guidelines. https://ukons.org/news-events/acute-oncology-initial-managment-guidelines-latest-version/.

---

sufficient to achieve a therapeutic cytotoxic effect without causing too much toxicity to normal cells. Numerous routes are used in the administration including:

- oral
- subcutaneous
- intramuscular
- intravenous
- directly into blood vessels supplying the cavity containing the tumour or into the tumour itself; such routes include intrahepatic, intra-arterial, intrapleural, intraperitoneal and intrathecal.

Intravenous administration may be delivered as a 'bolus', a short infusion or as a continuous infusion. Continuous infusions may be delivered using a medication delivery pump via a vascular access device (VAD) such as a skin-tunnelled catheter (STC), a totally implanted port (TIP) or a peripherally inserted central catheter (PICC) (see Lister et al. 2020).

Side-Effects of Chemotherapy

Chemotherapy causes several side-effects affecting a patient both physically and psychologically. It is nurses who deliver most of the chemotherapy in outpatient departments and the community, thus there is a consensus that this requires special chemotherapy education to fulfil this role (RCN 2022) (Information 31.3).

Each cytotoxic agent causes different side-effects, varying in intensity with dosage and method of administration (see Useful Websites e.g. British National Formulary, Reflection 31.7). Nursing management of the potential side-effects requires an in-depth knowledge of the common and uncommon toxicity profiles of each

Figure 31.5 Extravasation. Skin necrosis due to extravasation of anthracycline chemotherapy (e.g. doxorubicin). (Reproduced with permission from Boon NA, Colledge NR, Walker BR. *Davidson's Principles and Practice of Medicine.* 20th ed. Edinburgh: Churchill Livingstone; 2006.)

REFLECTION 31.7

Anticipating the Side-Effects of Chemotherapy

Listen to a patient who is receiving combination chemotherapy at Healthtalk.org (see Resources).

Activities

- Write a few notes about how you felt listening to the patient's experience of side-effects such as nausea/vomiting, or hair loss.
- Next time you are helping to care for a patient who is having chemotherapy, find out the usual doses and the emetogenic (ability to cause nausea and vomiting) potential of each of their drugs. Are there other side-effects and how are they managed?

Resources

British National Formulary, www.bnf.org.uk.
Healthtalk.org. 2023. People's experiences – lung cancer. www.healthtalk.org/peoples-experiences/cancer/lung-cancer/topics.
Manufacturers instruction guidelines.
Roila F, Molassiotis A, Herrstedt J, et al; on behalf of the participants of the MASCC/ESMO Consensus Conference, Copenhagen 2015. Consensus guidelines for the prevention of chemotherapy and radiotherapy-induced nausea and vomiting: ESMO Clinical Practice Guidelines. Ann Oncol. 2016;27(Suppl 5):v119-v133. Your hospital pharmacy cytotoxic manual.

agent given in the regimen. In the UK, all nurses require specific training. UKONS (2019) introduced a passport to ensure a consistent approach to learning for nurses and evidence of competence.

Physical and emotional responses to chemotherapy vary greatly between patients and it is important that nurses consider both when assessing the patient (Pedersen et al. 2013). A toxicity assessment tool is widely used in outpatient chemotherapy units to provide a consistent approach to care and encourage patients to participate in this care. The following is a brief summary of some of the potential physical side-effects of chemotherapy (see Useful Websites, e.g. British National Formulary, Multinational Association of Supportive Care in Cancer, National Cancer Institute).

Myelosuppression is the most common dose-limiting toxicity of chemotherapy but also potentially the most lethal. To understand the potential damage that chemotherapy may cause to the bone marrow, it is helpful to review normal blood cell development (see Further Reading, Tortora and Derrickson 2017). The suppression of the production of blood constituents by the bone marrow occurs to varying degrees after almost all types of cytotoxic chemotherapy. Cell cycle phase-specific (CCPS) agents (e.g. antimetabolites, natural products) tend to cause a rapid decline to a low point (nadir) in the marrow cells, usually 7–10 days after drug administration, although with some drugs the nadir may be reached earlier. Cell-cycle phase-nonspecific (CCPNS) drugs (doxorubicin, cisplatin) have nadirs around 10–14 days, while with others the nadir is 26–30+ days. Such factors need to be considered in the planning of treatment regimens. Since the prime function of neutrophils is phagocytosis, neutropenia eliminates one of the body's prime defences against bacterial infection (see Chapter 13). The longer the nadir period, the greater the opportunities to develop infections. Thrombocytopenia is usually delayed but, if active bleeding occurs, transfusions of platelets may be given. In view of the significant problems associated with bone marrow suppression, therapeutic use of haemopoietic growth factors such as granulocytic colony-stimulating factor (GCSF) is normal practice (Gawade et al. 2020). Studies have shown that these factors can significantly reduce or prevent myelosuppression induced by chemotherapy (Aras et al. 2020).

See Evolve website Critical thinking question 31.2

Stomatitis/Mucositis induced by chemotherapy is strongly associated with myelosuppression. Some cytotoxic agents have a direct effect on the oral mucosa, causing thinning and ulceration within 4–7 days of administration. Patients may experience mild redness and swelling along the mucocutaneous junction of the lip, mouth dryness and a burning sensation in the lips. Nausea, vomiting and a reduced food and fluid intake compound this effect, making the mucosa an ineffective barrier to opportunistic infection. Within 10–16 days, myelosuppression causes the already compromised mucosa to be even more susceptible to infection and haemorrhage. Regular thorough assessment and care of the oral mucosa is a vital part of a supportive care strategy (Multinational Association of Supportive Care in Cancer [MASCC] 2023). A meaningful and validated assessment tool should be used at least daily and more often if mucositis is severe. It will contain questions about eating, swallowing, pain and so on.

Oral care interventions should aim to provide adequate pain relief, prevent or treat infection and promote healing (see Further Reading, e.g. Multinational Association of Supportive Care in Cancer, Mucositis study group).

Nausea and Vomiting. Chemotherapy drugs can be characterised as having mild, moderate or severe emetogenic potential and therefore antiemetic medication should be prescribed accordingly. There are three types of nausea/vomiting that patients may experience:
- anticipatory
- acute
- delayed.

Antiemetics such as the 5-HT$_3$ antagonists (e.g. ondansetron, granisetron) have vastly improved the management of chemotherapy-related nausea and vomiting. MASCC and The European Society for Medical Oncology (ESMO) produced useful guidance in 2016 about how and when the different medications should be used (Roila et al. 2016). These medications have their own side-effect profile, including constipation (ondansetron) and headaches (granisetron). Corticosteroids such as dexamethasone potentiate the effect of these antiemetics and are most effective in delayed vomiting. Again, they have their own toxicity profile, such as indigestion, hyperactivity and mood disturbance, and may mask signs of infection in myelosuppressed patients. Relaxation, meditation and sedatives such as lorazepam have also been found to be helpful for some patients, especially with anticipatory nausea/vomiting.

Alopecia is caused by chemotherapy agents such as doxorubicin, taxanes and topoisomerase inhibitors, and may range from slight thinning to complete hair loss. It is important to note that not all chemotherapy causes hair loss and nurses must be careful they provide specific information related to the specific drug to prevent unnecessary distress. The severity of hair loss is directly related to the specific drug, dose and regimen. It usually occurs approximately 2 weeks after therapy has started and is temporary, with hair regrowth occurring about 6 weeks after the completion of treatment. Hair loss includes complete loss of eyebrows, eyelashes, body and facial hair. Patients should be offered the choice of a wig prior to any hair loss to enable close matching to their own hair. Promoting a positive self-image by offering advice to minimise hair loss, the use of fashion accessories and offering the opportunity to speak with other patients is important, as the psychological impact of alopecia should not be underestimated (Versluis et al. 2022).

Scalp cooling techniques have been developed with varying degrees of success (Fischer-Cartlidge et al. 2018). Earlier scalp cooling techniques involved wetting the scalp and applying ice packs, but more sophisticated refrigeration systems are now available which offer a more uniform cooling at a constant rate (Fischer-Cartlidge et al. 2018). Observations from clinical practice suggest that scalp cooling can slow down the rate of hair loss when used with single-agent drugs with a short half-life at low dosages, for example, doxorubicin, cyclophosphamide, docetaxel.

Sexual Dysfunction may occur due to vascular changes and hormonal imbalance. Amenorrhoea and menopausal symptoms may be induced due to ovarian failure and follicle destruction. Women under 35 years of age have a greater chance of resumption of the menses on completion of treatment; however, this may not occur for 6–12 months. In men, erectile dysfunction can occur.

Infertility may occur, depending on the agent, its dosage, the patient's age and gender, and other as yet unknown factors. Infertility may be temporary or permanent. Alkylating agents such as cyclophosphamide, chlorambucil and the nitrosourea compounds are certain to induce infertility. Patients should be informed about this side-effect. However, barrier methods of contraception are encouraged, as the exposure of a fetus to cytotoxic agents may result in congenital abnormalities or loss of the pregnancy.

In certain circumstances, some patients may receive counselling for sperm banking or oocyte harvesting. These options raise emotional and ethical dilemmas which may compound patients' existing stress concerning their diagnosis and treatment. Opportunities to discuss menopausal consequences of cancer treatment must be included pretreatment to allow women opportunities to reflect on the impact on their fertility long term (Cruickshank and Hume 2014; Fenlon et al. 2018).

Other Side-Effects. It is not possible to address all the potential side-effects of chemotherapy in this chapter (see Further Reading, e.g. MASCC 2018 and Useful Websites, e.g. British National Formulary). However, apart from the more common ones previously mentioned, it is important to remember the long-term effects, which include cardiotoxicity, pulmonary fibrosis, myalgia, neuropathy and renal toxicity. In addition, much nursing research has focused attention on fatigue and the need to develop positive interventions such as energy conservation (see Further Reading, Curiglano et al. 2020).

Biological Response Modifiers

Biological response modifiers (BRMs), often referred to as the fourth treatment modality, involve the therapeutic use of substances known to occur naturally in the body. Most of these are involved in some way in the immune response (see Chapter 7, Nursing Patients With Disorders of the Lymphatic and Immune Systems), controlling cell-mediated and humoral responses; hence some of these developments are termed 'immunotherapies'. Immunotherapy is a rapidly growing area of treatment (Peterson and Steele-Moses 2016).

As the landscape of cancer treatment changes and new therapies become available, nurses will need to be aware of how new treatments will affect patients and their practice.

Cytokines

Cytokines are substances released from an activated immune system. Interferon α_{2a}, for example, is an activator of natural killer cells and protects host cells against viruses. It has been found to maintain remission in hairy cell leukaemia and is being used with some success in certain patients with renal cancer and AIDS-related Kaposi's sarcoma. Side-effects include flu-like symptoms and mood disturbances, which may be very unpleasant. Other similar substances include TNF and interleukin 2 (IL-2).

Monoclonal Antibodies

During the 1980s, significant strides were made in the field of antibody therapy, which promotes specific targeting of cells through an antigen–antibody response. Tumour cells have antigens on their surface, and monoclonal antibodies to these antigens can now be manufactured commercially. Examples of monoclonal antibodies used in the clinical setting are rituximab and trastuzumab. Rituximab is directed against the CD20 antigen expressed in over 90% of B cell lymphomas and chronic lymphocytic leukaemia (CLL). Trastuzumab is directed against the human epidermal growth factor HER2-neu (c-erb2) proto-oncogene. In clinical studies, HER2 protein overexpression and gene amplification have been associated with a higher frequency of tumour recurrence and a reduction in overall survival time. Trastuzumab is presently used alongside other chemotherapy agents for the treatment of women with both primary and metastatic breast cancer whose tumours overexpress the HER2-neu protein (see Chapter 8).

Cancer Vaccines

Based on the antibody–antigen response mechanism, several vaccines have been developed for use in melanoma and trialled with encouraging responses. There are two vaccine programmes offered in England to protect against some types of the human papillomavirus (HPV). One is for children who are 12–13 years of age, and one is for gay, bisexual and other men who have sex with men (MSM) up to 45 years of age. The vaccine is effective at stopping people getting the high-risk types of HPV that cause cancer such as cervical, anal, genital, mouth and throat (head and neck).

Biological therapies have very different toxicity profiles from those of chemotherapy and include infusion syndrome, flu-like symptoms such as fever, chills, headache, malaise, arthralgia and fatigue. These symptoms require additional knowledge by the nurse as the timing of appropriate interventions such as premedications is important to safely administer these drugs and, side-effects can occur many weeks after the treatment is received (see Further Reading, e.g. McGowan 2015).

Psychological Support During Chemotherapy and BRM

There is increasing recognition, supported by research, that chemotherapy can lead to psychological distress and thus affect an individual's quality of life (Smith 2015). In a study, nurses reported that patients were often anxious, distressed or frightened and emphasised that patients required individualised, clear information about their disease and treatment. Psychological, social and financial support for themselves and their families were also seen to be important. Nurses perceived that patients required more psychological support at the beginning and at the end of treatment, which may be difficult times for patients. The importance of talking and providing information was seen as an essential intervention for meeting patients' psychological needs (Milant et al. 2016).

Nurses working in cancer settings delivering SACT have their own patient caseload where care priorities include assessment of treatment toxicities, cannulation, administration of bolus and intravenous chemotherapy, and coordinating the chemotherapy/BRM regimens in collaboration with the oncologist. Some nurses are now prescribers and can prescribe the SACT. The continuity of care engendered by this approach allows a trusting supportive relationship to be built between nurse and patient.

Some areas in the UK offer home chemotherapy. Specialised nurses, who may be hospital or community based, deliver chemotherapy to patients in the comfort of their own homes.

Hormonal Agents

Hormonal agents are used to treat specific cancers. They are specifically used with tumours that grow when exposed to hormones. There are several ways oestrogen and testosterone will be blocked. One method may be surgical removal of the ovaries (oophorectomy) or testes (orchidectomy) to reduce the growth stimulus to tumours of the breast or prostate provided by oestrogen and testosterone, respectively. Alternatively, this may be achieved using medication such as tamoxifen. Tamoxifen blocks the action of oestrogen by binding to oestrogen receptor sites on the tumour cells. The introduction of aromatase inhibitors such as anastrozole, letrozole and exemestane is expanding the treatment options available for postmenopausal women. They act on the cancer cells differently from tamoxifen, by preventing rather than blocking the effect of oestrogen.

Corticosteroid hormones, such as prednisolone and dexamethasone, are also widely used, the former in conjunction with cytotoxic medication as primary treatment, usually for lymphomas, and the latter for its anti-inflammatory action in symptom control and the control of emesis.

Clinical Trials

Despite an enormous amount of worldwide investment in research, cancer remains overall an incurable disease. However, it must be acknowledged that globally cancer survival is improving among some cancers (Allemani et al. 2018).

Most cancer centres are involved in multiple research trials, and through the clinical networks it has been possible to recruit patients from smaller units. Nurses should be familiar with the clinical trials available in their area to understand the implications, support patients' decisions and provide nursing care.

New treatment methods for cancer are tested on fully informed and consenting patients by means of a series of trials termed phase I, II and III trials. During phase I, the maximum tolerable dose is established, and information is obtained about the drug's toxicity profile; phase II trials discover which type of cancer is most responsive; and finally, phase III trials discover the extent to which the treatment improves survival. In phase III trials, patients from the target group are randomly selected to receive either the new treatment or the best established one. Phase IV trials continue once the drug has approval for clinical use to monitor, report and collate adverse and other reactions not reported in earlier phases. Survival rates are then compared.

New approaches to using radiotherapy, chemotherapy and biological agents are constantly being tested in this way (Further Reading Cancer Research UK 2023).

Complementary Therapies

The uncertainty that surrounds cancer and the impact it has on daily life has seen an increasing interest in complementary and alternative medicine (CAM) therapies. Based on the connection between body and mind, these therapies focus on a more 'holistic' approach to health in which the individual is encouraged to take control of their own life, both mentally and physically. Such therapies include homeopathy, acupuncture, therapeutic touch, massage, aromatherapy, relaxation techniques, yoga, hypnotherapy, nutrition, self-help groups and stress management.

The evidence is often scant for any effect of a complementary method on patient-relevant endpoints such as relief of disease symptoms, reduction of treatment side-effects or prolonged survival. However, many patients use dietary, massage, nutrients, etc. to help them cope with the treatment. It is important to check with the patient what they are taking and discuss with the pharmacist. It is important that health professionals respect an individual's beliefs and choices, recognising the potential benefits of a combined approach to cancer treatment. To avoid potential harm, only certified practitioners with knowledge of interactions or contraindications should deliver complementary therapies.

The Cancer Nurse

Cancer and its treatment have a unique impact on an individual's life. Although the physical problems experienced by cancer patients may be similar to those of patients with many nonmalignant conditions, the combination of these problems with the chronic nature of cancer, the highly toxic effects of treatment and the profound psychological impact of the disease mean that cancer nurses require specialised knowledge and skills. Cancer nursing as a specialty has been in existence for many years in the UK and is continually developing. Key skills in cancer nursing are those that help the cancer patient and their carers to adapt to the reality of living with cancer while maximising quality of life. The introduction of advanced nurse practitioners into cancer services complements the work of the clinical nurse specialists. See Barnwell (2015) and Health Education England ACCEND programme for an example of the role.

Hospital–Community Liaison

Cancer is a chronic illness characterised by remissions, exacerbations and progressive physical changes. More patients with cancer are living longer. Health professionals caring for cancer patients should view care as a continuous process, whether it takes place in the hospital or in the community setting. Supporting the patient through the cancer journey requires the skills of all members of the multiprofessional team in conjunction with the patient and family. Shared care protocols came about in response to the recognition of unfulfilled needs of patients receiving active treatments at home, for example, immunotherapy or continuous chemotherapy infusions. Such protocols promote the philosophy of continuity of care between hospital and community. Effective communication and discharge planning are essential to optimal care. Without proper coordination and integration of services, the cancer patient's 'journey' through the healthcare system can be a bewildering and demoralising experience. Reflection 31.8 presents the need for good discharge planning and liaison between hospital and community nurses.

Cancer patients spend most of their lives at home, interrupted by short hospital admissions. As a result, much of the psychological and physical adjustment to cancer takes place at home. Community initiatives and services are set up to support patients, their families and other carers from diagnosis to terminal illness and end-of-life care, helping patients in decision making and achieving optimal independence and quality of life.

Cancer Care in the Community

Community nursing staff are involved in cancer care during five phases:

- prevention programmes
- diagnosis
- treatment-related support
- rehabilitation following initial cancer treatment
- palliative care and end-of-life care.

Practice nurses, community nurses, liaison nurses, health visitors and GPs are generally involved in prevention schemes. District nurses coordinate and carry out a needs assessment for patients throughout their time in the community. Although work began in 2000 to introduce community cancer care nurses with specialist oncology knowledge and skills into practices (Gorman et al. 2000), this has never really evolved into standard practice. Towards the later stages of the disease, symptoms may become more problematic and place more strain on carers; at this stage, Macmillan Cancer Support, Marie Curie or community palliative care nurses who have close links with the hospice and hospital-based palliative care teams may become involved. These nurses have specialist skills in managing complex symptoms, providing psychosocial support and planning care in conjunction with the district nurse and other members of the primary care team.

The Role of the District Nurse

The role of community staff is changing rapidly as the demographics of patients alters, more older people, comorbidities and complex care (Griffiths 2017). Another major role of the district nurse involves coordination of the primary care team and integration of statutory and nonstatutory services. Because of the nature of cancer, the need for these services is considerable. The statutory services available include all those necessary for the care of long-term illness in the community (see Chapter 32, Nursing Patients Who Need Palliative Care).

Nonstatutory Services in the Community

Nonstatutory services for cancer patients are particularly comprehensive in their provision and include the following.

Support and Self-Help Groups. Such groups can reduce the isolation of the cancer experience. The sharing of feelings and experiences provides emotional support, fosters hope and encourages a sense of self-worth and purpose. Many local groups exist for patients and/or their carers.

Support and Information Centres. Empowerment of individuals, thereby allowing them to help themselves, is the basis of the recovery programme developed by Macmillan Cancer Support in conjunction with health professionals in the UK. Information, emotional support, relaxation and stress management are provided in thoughtfully designed environments for those affected by cancer, including carers, partners, relatives and friends. Programmes have been developed to provide opportunities for people to live and cope with a cancer diagnosis. Maggie's Cancer Caring Centres and Macmillan Information Centres are just two examples. Many other UK cancer support centres provide similar assistance and access to CAM therapists.

Counselling Services. Counselling may be necessary to assist the patient and their family to adapt emotionally to cancer and can help to relieve anxiety and depression. The Cancer Counselling Trust provides this service by telephone and in person.

Financial Aid. The financial burden of cancer is now well documented. The Macmillan Cancer Support fund can provide financial aid to meet the cost of aids, appliances, heating, bedding, holidays and other special needs but is means tested. Other charities may also provide financial assistance. The government provides a benefit to people who are within 6 months of dying.

Nursing Services. Marie Curie Cancer Care charity provides nursing staff, including a night nursing service, to allow carers some respite or sleep.

Nursing Frameworks for Cancer Care

No one framework or model of nursing can be suitable for every cancer patient or care setting. Integrated care pathways (ICPs) are an example of a framework that aims to integrate evidence-based practice through a documented plan of anticipated care for a group of patients with a particular diagnosis or set of symptoms. Each professional involved in the patient's care has a clearly defined role and the plan of care leads the patient towards a required goal.

Family Coping

A cancer diagnosis can have a devastating effect on the patient's family and loved ones in the following ways:

- Cancer can disrupt patterns of familial and other interpersonal interaction. Reactions vary from overprotection and excessive vigilance to distancing behaviour and even the complete breakdown of relationships. Many patients, especially in the early stages of the disease, may feel that they have to be the strong one emotionally, supporting and holding the family together. A study by Petren et al. (2021) looked at relational turning points in spousal relationships. Their findings highlighted the stress and strain, changes in relationship and changes in family role experienced throughout the treatment trajectory, not just at diagnosis.
- Cancer disrupts planning for the future. The uncertainty involved disrupts family plans and dreams for holidays, retirement, parenthood and so forth. Roles within the family change, particularly if the patient is a breadwinner or parent. Such change is stressful and can undermine the patient's sense of self-worth and purpose. Loss of income and increased expenditure due to the illness can create financial hardship, isolation and feelings of low esteem.

Nursing Interventions. After assessment of family dynamics and needs, the following nursing interventions may help to alleviate some of these problems:

- Providing regular information about the patient's status and plans for care, preferably facilitating open communication between the patient and their family, which is associated with lower anxiety levels (Johnston et al. 2019). Shared information helps to promote a positive attitude and improves adaptation and communication within the hospital setting and at home.
- Encouraging relatives to express their feelings of fear, loss, guilt and exhaustion (Cruickshank et al. 2017; 2020).
- Encouraging realistic, mutual goal-setting, e.g. the timing and planning of holidays.
- Encouraging family members to adapt the patient's role within the family to maintain a sense of belonging and worth, e.g. by exchanging physical tasks for clerical ones.

- Referring families promptly to the social work department for financial assistance and, if necessary, rehousing.
- Recognising signs of exhaustion in carers, giving them 'permission' to take time off and arranging respite care or hospital/hospice admission for the patient if necessary.
- Encouraging continued social involvement, suggesting appropriate activities if necessary.
- Suggesting referral to a psychologist or Relate counsellor if family relationships appear to be breaking down.

Diet and Exercise

Cancer patients lose weight because of metabolic changes caused by the tumour; this is referred to as cancer cachexia syndrome (Petermann-Rocha et al. 2021). The associated weight loss can have a negative impact on a patient's body image and sexuality; it represents a major source of concern for both patient and family, often acting as a barometer of the patient's condition.

Causes of malnutrition and weight loss in cancer patients include the following:

- Reduced food intake due to:
  - Anorexia: due to multiple causes, e.g. release of cytokines such as TNF and IL-1 is thought to delay gastric emptying, thus delaying digestion, suppressing the appetite and causing satiety (Shaw and Eldridge 2015).
  - Taste changes: may occur in any cancer patient; they are most common following radiotherapy to the head or neck due to destruction of salivary tissue. These changes involve a lowered threshold for bitter tastes, and therefore aversion to meat; raised threshold for sweet tastes, and hence many foods taste bland and 'cardboard-like'; alteration of the taste of tea and coffee.
  - Early satiety: metabolic abnormalities directly related to tumour burden may result in early satiety, a premature feeling of fullness, usually progressing over the day.
  - Other symptoms: such as pain, nausea, vomiting and drowsiness.
  - Physical difficulties: due to oral prostheses or badly fitting dentures; also to the tumour and treatment, e.g. oesophageal obstruction, chemotherapy-induced mucositis.
  - Anxiety and depression.
- Malabsorption due to:
  - Resection of tumours of the gastrointestinal tract, leading to decreased enzyme production and increased transit time.
  - Impairment of nutrient absorption resulting from chemotherapy and abdominal radiotherapy.
- Excess expenditure of nutrients, due to:
  - In many patients, raised basal metabolic rate (BMR), partly due to the demands of the tumour.
  - Loss of body protein due to vomiting, diarrhoea, haemorrhage, oedema, from stomas, fistulas and in exudates from ulcerations.

Exercise. Irrespective of stage of cancer, or treatment, there is increasing evidence of the benefits of maintaining levels of exercise among people affected with cancer (Macmillan Cancer Support 2018, Malek et al. 2017, Further Reading – WHO Guidelines on physical activity and sedentary behaviour 2020).

Prehabilitation. (prehab) is a term used regularly to describe the process that seeks to prepare people for cancer treatments by optimising their health by prescribing exercise, nutrition and psychological interventions (Giles and Cummins 2019).

Nursing Interventions. Actions that the nurse can take to help the patient overcome or manage difficulties with eating and drinking include the following:

- Using a screening tool such as Malnutrition Universal Screening Tool (MUST) to assess the patient's current nutritional status and potential for further deterioration (British Association for Parenteral and Enteral Nutrition (BAPEN) 2003; 2023). Weekly weighing is adequate; more frequent weighing may cause the patient to become anxious and demoralised.
- Identifying the major factors that contribute to the nutritional deficit.
- Referring 'at-risk' patients to a dietitian.
- Referring to a speech and language therapist (SLT) those patients with an identified swallowing or aspiration problem.
- Referring to an occupational therapist (OT) to assist with functional or practical difficulties.
- Referring to a social worker for a care package to assist with shopping and meal preparation.
- Enlisting the help of relatives and friends to offer the patient's favourite foods whilst respecting autonomy. However, it is important to explain that there are very real reasons for the patient's reluctance to eat. Provision of dietary information, recipes and self-care measures may be helpful.
- Offering frequent, small, high-calorie attractive meals and snacks throughout the day; negotiating with the catering department for flexibility in portion size and for a supply of nutrient-rich foods to be kept at unit/ward level.
- Encouraging patients to take fluids in the form of high-energy drinks; discouraging drinking at mealtimes, to avoid early satiety.
- Decreasing satiety by the avoidance of high-fat foods which delay gastric emptying; the use of drugs, e.g. metoclopramide, may promote gastric emptying.
- Reassuring the patient that taste changes are to be expected and may disappear in time; offering taste-enhancing herbs, spices, marinades (unless mucositis is a problem) and alternatives to tea and coffee.
- Supporting the patient if there is further weight loss despite sufficient calorie intake, due to abnormal metabolism.
- Using gentle exercise, relaxation to stimulate the appetite.
- Controlling other symptoms. Antiemetics and analgesics (topical and systemic) should be administered 30 minutes before meals.
- Encouraging regular oral care, such as mouthwashes, before and after meals.
- Eliminating nauseating environmental stimuli at mealtimes, such as bedpans, odours and disturbing procedures.
- If intake is consistently inadequate and/or weight loss continues, commencing other forms of feeding: enteral feeding by nasogastric tube if absorption is adequate; parenteral if not (see Chapter 22, Nutrition and Health).

Expressing Sexuality

Following treatment for cancer, up to 50% of patients who were sexually active before the illness report some reduction in sexual interest or activity. Healthcare professionals may fail to take the initiative in addressing their patients' sexual problems within the context of treatment for chronic and life-threatening illness. Although some nurses find it difficult to discuss sexuality and intimacy with patients, patients are experiencing a number of late effects that benefit from open discussions (Martin et al. 2022; Schover et al. 2014).

Sexuality involves more than sexual intercourse. It includes self-image in relation to gender, role behaviour within a partnership and many forms of love and affection between partners. Fertility affects both males and females and support is needed to cancer patient and partner to deal with the psychological impact of this (White and Butcher 2016). A cancer patient's sexuality may be altered for many reasons, including:

- The physical effects of the tumour, e.g. lesions of the spinal cord, may interfere with the nerve pathways necessary for sexual sensation or motor function.
- Symptoms caused by the tumour, e.g. pain, immobility, nocturia, dysuria, vaginal or rectal bleeding and fatigue, can all contribute to a decrease in desire for sexual intimacy.
- The physical effects of treatment, e.g. hormone manipulation may alter sexual function; surgery may alter the anatomy, for example, prostate surgery may cause pelvic nerve damage resulting in erectile dysfunction; pelvic irradiation may reduce vaginal lubrication causing painful intercourse (dyspareunia).
- Body image problems, e.g. following mastectomy or stoma formation; less obvious changes may also contribute, e.g. varying degrees of weight loss or hair loss.
- Anxiety and depression related to the cancer diagnosis resulting in low self-esteem.

Nursing Interventions. The nurse can provide support for the cancer patient experiencing problems with the expression of sexuality in the following ways:

- Initiating discussion to give the patient 'permission' to voice their concerns. Once the discussion is initiated, the patient will indicate whether they wish to pursue the topic.
- Anticipating problems before treatment: explaining how long problems will last and that they are to be expected; describing measures that can be used to relieve them (see Table 31.3, for examples of interventions for patients receiving radiotherapy).
- Opening discussion with nonthreatening subjects such as contraceptive advice or the alterations in partnership roles due to illness. This will aid progression to potentially more personal issues.
- Ensuring that anxiety and depression are treated and body image problems addressed. Severe body image problems may require psychological therapy.
- Involving partners in discussion and physical care as appropriate.
- Facilitating the privacy of couples in hospices and hospitals.
- Referral to a psychosexual practitioner who specialises in working with cancer patients.

Communicating

From the cancer patient's perspective, patient-focused communication can be the most important aspect of treatment, in part because of its capacity to exacerbate or allay the fear that often accompanies cancer (Fallowfield and Jenkins 2004). Communication encompasses three areas of activity, which may be described as:

- cognitive – the giving and receiving of information
- emotional – the feeling and expression of psychological responses
- spiritual – the expression and feeling of thoughts relating to existential issues beyond the self.

Although this division can help in identifying specific nursing activities, the three areas are interrelated. Providing information in a sensitive, caring manner affords emotional support, and many people do not consciously make the distinction between the emotional and spiritual dimensions.

Cognitive Activity

The patient's need for information in relation to diagnosis and treatment has been examined in earlier sections of this chapter. To this discussion the following observations may be added:

- Knowledge is power: power that enables independence, choice, autonomous decision making and realistic goal-setting for patients and their families. Information promotes the patient's sense of control over their life.
- Studies of patients' perceived needs rank information and support as a key component for coping with cancer (Armes et al. 2009).
- Lack of information can deepen a depressive reaction to a cancer diagnosis.
- Patients have traditionally expected their needs for information to be met by doctors, and their needs for support to be met by nurses. However, in practice, particularly with the evolution of specialist nurses, this is changing. Patients will choose the person they wish to obtain information from depending on their needs.
- Nurses, by their behaviour and nonverbal communication, may indicate they are too busy to answer questions at that particular time. They may also feel they lack the information the patient is seeking, or fear that information-giving may lead to an emotional unburdening by the patient, for which they may lack the personal resources necessary to cope.
- Patients and their families need information on the cause of the cancer, the possible course of the disease, treatment options, the role of the healthcare team, available services and sources of further information.
- Patients vary greatly in their desire for, and receptivity to, information.

Nursing Interventions. The following advice may assist the nurse to meet the patient's communication needs:

- Be equipped with the information that the patient needs. Be assertive in obtaining this information from other members of the healthcare team so that consistent information is given to the patient.
- Be present at as many interactions between the patient and the doctor as possible. Afterwards reinforce messages and ensure that the patient has understood.
- Find out what the patient already knows and has been told, and what they want to know. In general, follow the patient's agenda.
- Bear in mind that when receiving information most people remember only three specific points; the first three points made are those most likely to be remembered.
- Avoid jargon: 'your white cell count will fall', for example, may mean nothing to most patients. Information about how they will feel and what they will experience is most important to most patients.
- Be prepared for the patient to forget or deny receiving the information given.
- Reinforce verbal information with written information. Many cancer charities produce excellent literature, as do many hospitals. This information is written at a level (usually age 9 years) to facilitate understanding.
- Be prepared for information-giving to lead to emotional issues. Allow time for this or promise to return at an arranged time – and do so.
- Give the patient and their relatives the same information. Give each the opportunity to receive this information both together and separately, so that personal anxieties can be expressed privately and within the family group.

Emotional Activity

Enabling patients and their families to cope with the emotional impact of cancer demands effective listening skills and is an essential component of counselling (Reflection 31.9).

The following considerations should be borne in mind by the nurse in addressing the cancer patient's emotional needs:

- During any stage of the disease, the cancer patient is suffering the effects of various actual or potential losses. These may include loss of a body part or function, loss of self-image, loss of work or leisure activities, loss of family or social role, loss of control over life, loss of goals and dreams for the future and, ultimately, loss of life itself. Loss is the predominant factor in all sadness and depression.
- There are many uncertainties involved in cancer; uncertainty leads to anxiety.
- While the majority of cancer patients adjust emotionally and cope reasonably well with loss and uncertainty, there is psychological distress and even psychiatric illness among this client group.

REFLECTION 31.9

Communication Skills in the Care of Lara

This is an example of how one nurse offered her support to a young woman with acute leukaemia and her family.

While waiting for confirmation of the diagnosis, I did a lot of listening. I listened to the expression of shock, fear and guilt. I did not negate their concerns or try to offer false assurances.

It was clear that one of the most useful things I could do for this distraught family, who were in a strange and overwhelming place, was to assist them, little by little, in gaining control over their experiences. This involved helping them to anticipate and be prepared for what was to come, for how it might feel or look physically or emotionally. It also involved helping them to continue in their usual roles as much as possible, and engaging them in the decisions affecting Lara's care.

Although she knew that she had less than a 50% chance of survival, Lara concentrated on the here and now: the pain associated with frequent intravenous therapies, bone marrow and lumbar punctures; the embarrassment of hair loss; the isolation from her friends; and the nausea and vomiting associated with her chemotherapy. I followed her lead by responding to her immediate concerns.

I used a variety of approaches in working with her, depending on what kind of day she was having. Sometimes we would just joke around; other times we would talk about more serious issues – not just her illness but her personal life, as well as my own.

I was always open with her, accepted her feelings, and never made light of them. I did not assure her that 'it would get better soon' or that 'I knew how she must be feeling' because I truly did not know whether she would get better or how she actually felt.

Lara was just plain miserable. All I could do was to listen, acknowledge how awful it must be, and honestly say that she must feel like crying. Permission to cry was all she needed to let the tears flow. One day, she looked me directly in the eyes and said, 'I'm so sick, am I going to die?' Although it was a matter of seconds before I answered, it seemed like hours as my mind groped for the right words. I did not avert my gaze and answered from my heart: 'I'm afraid, Lara, you are so sick that you could die.'

Activities

- Reflect on how the nurse followed the agenda set by Lara and responded to the situation as it developed, rather than imposing a preconceived structure for communication.
- Discuss with some fellow students how you would feel if a patient asked 'I'm so sick, am I going to die?'

- A great deal of this emotional turmoil, anxiety and depression passes undetected and unrelieved (Fallowfield and Jenkins 2004). Early research focused on prediction and early detection of affective disorders, through screening and improving communication skills of health professionals as well as therapeutic interventions (Maguire 1995) and was the catalyst for attention given to a person's psychological and emotional consequences of cancer. These researchers also helped establish the role of clinical nurse specialist and the importance of providing psychosocial support.
- Emotional distress may result in somatic symptoms such as confusion, immobility, insomnia and pain. Oxlad et al. (2008) described these physical manifestations as being similar to chronic disease and therefore a clear history must be taken of the patient's symptoms. Long-term distress may exacerbate disease progression.
- Patients' reactions to cancer vary greatly, depending on personality, past experience and learned coping strategies.
  Nursing Interventions. The following strategies can be employed to give patients support as they adjust emotionally to their illness and treatment:
- Give the patient 'openings' to state what is on their mind, e.g. by concluding an information-giving session by asking them how they feel about the information, or by remarking upon a worried or sad expression.
- Do not be afraid of saying the wrong thing.
- Learn and apply interviewing techniques used in counselling, e.g. reflecting a patient's question or statement. This gives the patient the chance to realise what has been said and to expand on it, and the nurse time to reflect on what is meant. Constant reflection of questions, however, will irritate patients. Once the patient's main concerns have been established, it may be time to give direct answers.
- Resist giving 'pat' answers and false reassurances. Many of the dilemmas faced by cancer patients have no ready solution. Do not be afraid to admit that answers cannot be given to all the patient's questions about the future. Try, however, to leave the patient with some hope, help the patient to identify something positive in their situation on which to focus.
- Assist the patient to identify realistic goals in order to foster hope. These goals should originate from the patient but often need an objective person to identify them. Examples may be the goal of getting through treatment and remaining positive about the future, of living until a daughter's wedding or returning to work part-time.
- A certain degree of worry and sadness is to be expected. Be alert to signs of disabling anxiety (somatic stress symptoms, lack of concentration, feelings of panic) or depression (a 'flat' mood, an exaggerated feeling of guilt and self-blame, suicidal ideation). If these are noted, refer the patient to a psychologist or psychiatrist. Anxiolytic and antidepressant medication and various forms of psychological therapy may be required before other forms of counselling therapy can be effective.
- FCR is a natural response to a cancer diagnosis, experienced on a continuum from none to severe. It is also one of the most frequent unmet needs reported in the immediate post-treatment phase (Armes et al. 2009; Cruickshank and Hume 2014). When severe it can lead to distress, difficulty coping and poorer physical health, leading many to seek help from health professionals such as doctors and specialist breast cancer nurses (De Vries et al. 2014, Thewes et al. 2016, Yang et al. 2017).

- Patients may react to their disease with denial, anger, bargaining, depression and acceptance (Kübler-Ross 1973). Counselling cannot force the patient to move from one stage to another, but it does allow them to express feelings and perhaps make progress. The nurse should give patients permission to express their feelings in any safe way they choose and should not feel a sense of failure when a patient becomes emotionally distraught. The expression of emotions is therapeutic and is an important part of psychological adaptation.
- Supporting patients and their families through the cancer experience is very demanding emotionally. It is important for nurses to recognise the resultant stress in themselves and their colleagues and to seek and offer active support (see later).

Spiritual Activity

A full consideration of the cancer patient's quality of life must recognise the spiritual dimension of the experience, which might be described, in the most basic terms, as the search for meaning and purpose. Because spirituality involves the contemplation of things that affect us but lie beyond our control, cancer has the capacity to precipitate a spiritual crisis (see Further Reading, e.g. Quinn and Connelly 2023).

Stress in Cancer Nursing

In 1988, Speck stated that the most important ethical choice made by cancer nurses is whether or not to engage in '*an intense, personalised involvement*' with their patients in response to human need. The emotional work of cancer nurses is complex. Working with cancer patients can be very rewarding but occupational stress can occur when faced daily with stories of sadness and distress.

A systematic review by Gomez-Urquiza et al. (2015) found that oncology nurses present with high levels of emotional exhaustion and personal accomplishment. It is believed a large proportion of these nurses are at risk of burnout. Age, work experience, workload and communications skills can influence burnout.

The constructive expression of emotions is as important as stress control. Establishing an environment of trust and mutual respect where it is safe to admit to colleagues feelings of inadequacy, grief and guilt, and even personal fears about cancer and death, is beneficial in relieving stress. A report by Macmillan Cancer Support that looked at the workforce in primary care (UK) identified pressure and low morale among nurses, allied health professionals and GPs, which can lead to stressful working environments. Providing support to staff to ensure their own well-being is maintained is very important for patient care. Such support should also be provided on an organised basis in the form of support groups and counselling services, as formal support groups are often catalysts for social support, problem solving and task sharing (Reflection 31.10). Reflective practice, clinical supervision and mentorship are also important concepts that enable and empower individuals within their nursing practice (Caley et al. 2017).

New Directions for Cancer Care

Seminal work by Slevin et al. (1990) pointed out that those who do not have cancer, whether they are members of the public or professionals, have very little concept of the experience of cancer or of how the cancer patient perceives quality of life, their future and the decisions that must be made. Cancer is a chronic illness, and more patients are surviving and living with their disease than previously. These patients have needs and expectations – physical, psychosocial

REFLECTION 31.10

Stress in Cancer Nursing

Caring for cancer patients and their families is intensely rewarding but the emotional involvement required can have negative consequences for the nurse.

Activities

- Think about a patient with cancer that you have cared for on placement. Reflect on the positive aspects of your professional relationship with the person – for the patient and for your professional development.
- How were you affected by caring for this person? Discuss your thoughts with a fellow student or your supervisor/assessor.
- Find out what support services are available in your area for nurses and other health professionals who care for cancer patients.

and spiritual. While they may survive, they may not necessarily thrive. In this situation, cancer rehabilitation is paramount to support patients in effectively managing their illness on a day-to-day basis.

There has been an increase in strategies aimed at self-care management, with individuals, families and communities playing a larger role in determining and meeting their own health needs. The internet has empowered patients by providing access to information about their disease and treatment and opening up communication links with fellow patients. Advances in molecular biology may lead to the identification of high-risk groups and better targeted prevention and screening as well as treatment. New challenges lie ahead for nurses in all fields for role development, research and education to support patients and their families through the cancer experience. The Royal College of Nursing (2022) career and education framework for cancer nursing, and its translation into the ACCEND programme is a step forward in providing guidance to the future nursing workforce when facing the challenges ahead.

Summary: Key Nursing Issues

- Cancer is a major healthcare condition. One in three people in the UK risk developing cancer in their lifetime.
- The term 'cancer' evokes a variety of emotions for people and families including shock, disbelief and a fear of pain and death. Many people with cancer are surviving longer but this is not the case for all types of cancer. Although cancer management and treatment involve a large team of health and social care professionals and the voluntary sector, nurses are at the forefront of prevention and early detection, delivery of cancer treatments and providing supportive care.
- Nurses need to understand the biology of cancer – how it develops and why it spreads – and recognise the features associated with common cancers.
- Patients need accurate information about their cancer and treatments. Nurses have an important role in providing general

information but for more specialist information it is important to seek help from a cancer nurse or palliative care specialist.
- Cancer affects not only the patient but also their family, partners and friends.
- Cancer can be extremely debilitating. Nurses must listen to the patient and act on their symptoms. Distinguishing between cancer symptoms and those of treatment is very important.
- The psychological impact of a cancer diagnosis and subsequent treatment can be very difficult for patients. Nurses are often witness to this. Nurses are not the sole providers of care and support and they must be mindful that there are many other professionals, such as psychologists, social workers, GPs and voluntary cancer services, who can also support patients. Nurses are often in a position to help patients to access these services.

Reflection and Learning – What Next?

- **Test** your knowledge by visiting the Evolve website 🌐 and answering the multiple choice questions and critical thinking questions.
- **Consolidate** your learning by looking at some of the further reading suggestions, references and specialist websites.
- **Revisit** some of the additional material on the Evolve website.

- **Consider** what you have learnt and how this will help your professional development.
- **Reflect** on how you can apply this knowledge to the care of your patients.
- **Discuss** your learning with your assessor/supervisor, lecturer and colleagues.

References

Ali YF, Cucinotta FA, Ning-Ang L, Guangming Z. (2020) Cancer risk of low dose ionizing radiation Frontiers in Physics https://doi.org/10.3389/fphy.2020.00234.

Allemani C, Matsuda T, Di Carlo V the CONCORD Working Group. Global surveillance of trends in cancer survival 2000–14 (CONCORD-3): analysis of individual records for 37 513 025 patients diagnosed with one of 18 cancers from 322 population-based registries in 71 countries. *Lancet*. 2018;391(10125):1023–1075.

Aras E, Bayrakter-Ekincioglu A, Killickap S. Risk assessment of febrile neutropenia and evaluation of G-CSF use in patients with cancer: a real-life study. *Support Care Cancer*. 2020;28:691–699. https://doi.org/10.1007/s00520-019-04879-x.

Armes J, Crowe M, Colbourne L, et al. Patients' supportive care needs beyond the end of cancer treatment: a prospective, longitudinal survey. *J Clin Oncol*. 2009;27:6172–6179.

Arnaud A, Grenier J, Boustany R, Kirscher S, Mege A, de Rauglaudre G, Vazquez L, Debourdeau P. Role of supportive care in improving the quality of life and reducing unscheduled hospital care in patients with metastatic breast cancer. *Support Care Cancer*. 2021 Jul 29: 3735–3742.

Ashalford, Raynsford, Taylor. Pathophysiology & Pharmacology in Nursing (Transforming Nursing Series) ed 2 2019 (ed 3, due October 2023).

Barnwell A. Advanced nursing practice in colorectal and stoma care. *Gastrointest Nurs*. 2015;13(1):42–49.

Bonevski B, Sanson-Fisher R, Girgis A, et al. Evaluation of an instrument to assess the needs of patients with cancer. Supportive Care Review Group. *Cancer*. 2000;88(1):217–225.

British Association for Parenteral and Enteral Nutrition (BAPEN). *Malnutrition Advisory Group*. The malnutrition universal screening tool (MUST); 2003. http://www.bapen.org.uk/pdfs/must/must_full.pdf.

British Association for Parenteral and Enteral Nutrition (BAPEN) (2023) updated resources. https://www.bapen.org.uk/

Brown T, Cruickshank S, Noblet M. Specialist breast care nurses for support of women with breast cancer. *Cochrane Database Syst Rev*. 2021(2): Art. No.: CD005634.

Caley L, Pittordou V, Adams C, Gee C, Pitkahoo V, Matthews J, Cruse S, Muls A. Reflective practice applied in a clinical oncology research setting. *Br J Nurs*. 2017 Sep 7;26(16):S4–S17.

Cancer Research UK (2023a) Cancer incidence for common cancers in adults – UK statistics. https://www.cancerresearchuk.org/health-professional/cancer-statistics/incidence [accessed 22nd June 2023]

Cancer Research UK (2023b) Cancer incidence in children and young people – UK statistics. https://www.cancerresearchuk.org/children-and-young-people [accessed 22nd June 2023]

Cardis E, Hatch M. The Chernobyl accident — an epidemiological perspective. *Clin Oncol*. 2011;23(4):251–260. https://doi.org/10.1016/j.clon.2011.01.510.

Carvalho, et al. Advanced nursing practice: a review of scopes of practice in cancer care. *Br J Nurs*. 2022;31(21):1104–1110.

Clero, et al. Lessons learned from Chernobyl and Fukushima on thyroid cancer screening and recommendations in case of a future nuclear accident. *Environ Int*. 2021(146). https://doi.org/10.1016/j.envint.2020.106230.

Cochrane A, et al. Unmet supportive care needs associated with quality of life for people with lung cancer: a systematic review of the evidence 2007-2020. *Eur J Cancer Care (Engl)*. 2021;31(1):e13525.

Colón-López V, Shiels MS, Machin M, et al. Anal Cancer Risk Among People with HIV Infection in the United States. *J Clin Oncol*. 2018 Jan 1;36(1):68–75.

Crawford A, Benard V, King J, Thomas CC. Understanding barriers to cervical cancer screening in women with access to care: Behavioral Risk Factor Surveillance System 2014. *Prev Chronic Dis*. 2016;13:160225.

Cruickshank S, Hume A. The experience of providing support about menopausal symptoms to women with breast cancer. *Eur J Oncol Nurs*. 2014;18(1):110–117.

Cruickshank S, Steel E, Fenlon D, et al. A feasibility study of the Mini-AFTER telephone intervention for the management of fear of recurrence in breast cancer survivors: a mixed-methods study protocol. *Pilot and Feasibility Studies*. 2017;4:22. https://pilotfeasibilitystudies.biomedcentral.com/articles/10.1186/s40814-017-0161-8.

Cruickshank, et al. Specialist breast cancer nurses' views on implementing a fear of cancer recurrence intervention in practice: a mixed methods study. *Support Care Cancer*. 2020;28:201–210. https://doi.org/10.1007/s00520-019-04762-9.

Cruickshank S, Turner J. British Journal of Nursing (2016). Be Compliant, protect each other and stay safe: avoiding accidental exposure to cytotoxic drugs. *Br J Nurs*. 2016;suppl 2:S1–S56.

Cruickshank S. COVID-19: The impact on people affected by cancers, oncology nurses and the wider health community. *Enfermería Clínica*. 2021;31:201–202.

Department of Health. 1995. A policy framework for commissioning cancer services: a report by the Expert Advisory Group on Cancer to the Chief Medical Officers of England and Wales. http://tinyurl.com/y5rx6mlw.

Department of Health. 2007. Cancer Reform Strategy. http://tinyurl.com/y4twfhvh.

De Vries J, Oudsten D, Jacobs PMEP, Roukema JA. How breast cancer survivors cope with fear of recurrence: a focus group study. *Support Care Cancer*. 2014;22(3):705–712.

Doll R, Hill AB. The mortality of doctors in relation to their smoking habits. A preliminary report. *Br Med J*. 1954;1:1451–1455.

Dullens B et al. (2020) Cancer Surveillance in Healthy Carriers of Germline Pathogenic variants in BRCA1/2: A review of secondary prevention guidelines (20) https://doi.org/10.1155/2020/9873954

Faller H, Koch U, Braller E, et al. Satisfaction with information and unmet information needs in men and women with cancer. *J Cancer Surviv*. 2016;10(1):62–70.

Fallowfield L, Jenkins V. Communicating sad, bad, and difficult news in medicine. *Lancet*. 2004;363:312–319.

Farrington N, Townsend K. Enhancing nurse-patient communication: a critical reflection. *Br J Nurs*. 2014;23(14):771–775.

Feeney S, Rossetti V, Terrien J. E-Cigarettes—a review of the evidence—harm versus harm reduction. *Tobacco Use Insights*. 2022;15. https://doi.org/10.1177/1179173X221087524.

Fenlon, et al. MENOS4 trial: a multicentre randomized controlled trial (RCT) of a breast care nurse delivered cognitive behavioural therapy (CBT) intervention to reduce the impact of hot flushes in women with breast cancer: Study Protocol BMC Women's. *Health (N Y)*. 2018;18:63. https://doi.org/10.1186/s12905-018-0550-z.

Fidalgo JAP, Fabregat G, Cervantes A, et al; on behalf of the ESMO Guidelines Working Group. Management of chemotherapy extravasation: ESMO–EONS clinical practice guidelines. *Ann Oncol*. 2012;23(Suppl 7):vii167–vii173.

Fischer-Cartlidge E, et al. Scalp Cooling Implementation of a program at a multisite organization. *Clin J Oncol Nurs*. 2018;22(5):534–541.

Gallicchio L, et al. Estimation of the number of individuals living with metastatic cancer in the United States. *J Natl Cancer Inst*. 2022;114(11):1476–1483.

Gardner MJ, Snee MP, Hall AJ, et al. Results of case control study of leukaemia and lymphoma in young people near Sellafield nuclear plant in West Cumbria. *Br Med J*. 1990;300:423–429.

Gawade, et al. Patterns of granulocyte colony-stimulating factor prophylaxis in patients with cancer receiving myelosuppressive chemotherapy. *Support Care Cancer*. 2020;28:4413–4424.

Giles C, Cummins S. Prehabilitation before cancer treatment. A great idea in theory, somewhat trickier in practice. *BMJ*. 2019;366:l5120. https://doi.org/10.1136/bmj.l5120.

Gomez-Urquiza JL, Aneas-Lopez AB, De La Fuente-Solana EI, et al. Prevalence, risk factors, and levels of burnout among oncology nurses: a systematic review. *Oncol Nurs Forum*. 2015;43(3):E104–E120.

Gonzalez S. Paraneoplastic syndromes review: The great forgotten ones. *Crit Rev Oncol Hematol*. 2022:174. https://doi.org/10.1016/j.critrevonc.2022.103676.

Gorman DR, Mackinnon H, Storrie M, et al. The general practice perspective on cancer services in Lothian. *Fam Pract*. 2000;17(4):323.

Griffiths J. Person-centred communication for emotional support in district nursing: SAGE and THYME model. *Br J Community Nurs*. 2017;22(12):593–597.

Health and Safety Executive Radiation Guidance (2023). https://www.hse.gov.uk/radiation/.

Health Education England 2022 Aspirant Cancer Career and Education Development Programme (ACCEND). https://www.hee.nhs.uk/our-work/cancer-diagnostics/aspirant-cancer-career-education-development-programme/accend-framework.

Humphris G et al. (2019) Emotional talk of patients with breast cancer during review appointments with therapeutic radiographers: effects on fears of cancer recurrence 27: 2143-2151.

International Agency for Research on Cancer (IARC). Breast cancer screening update – viewpoint of the IARC Working Group. *N Engl J Med*. 2015;372(24):2353–2358.

International Agency for Research on Cancer (IARC) Working Group on the Evaluation of Carcinogenic Risks to Humans. 2023. Personal habits and indoor combustions. IARC Monograph Volume 100 E. https://monographs.iarc.who.int/

Islami F, Torre LA, Jemal A. Global trends of lung cancer mortality and smoking prevalence. *Transl Lung Cancer Res*. 2015;4(4):327–338.

Jacobs IJ, Menon U, Ryan A. Collaborative trial of ovarian cancer screening (UKCTOCS): a randomised controlled trial. *Lancet*. 2016;387(10022):945–956.

Johnston L, Young J, Campbell C. The implementation and impact of Holistic Needs Assessments for people affected by cancer: A systematic review and thematic synthesis of the literature. *Eur J Cancer Care (Engl)*. 2019;28(3):e13087.

Kiplagat J, Tran DN, Barber T, Njuguna B, Vedanthan R, Triant VA, Pastakia SD. How health systems can adapt to a population ageing with HIV and comorbid disease. *Lancet HIV*. 2022 Apr;9(4):e281–e292.

Kübler-Ross E. *Death, the Final Stage of Growth*. New York: Prentice Hall; 1973.

Lawton AJ, et al. Assessment and management of patients with metastatic spinal cord compression: a multidisciplinary review. *J Clin Oncol*. 2019;37(1):61–71.

Macmillan Cancer Support. 2018. The recovery package. https://be.macmillan.org.uk/be/s-689-recovery-package.aspx

Maguire P. Psychosocial interventions to reduce affective disorders in cancer patients: research priorities. *Psychooncology*. 1995;4:113–119.

Malek L, Wan BA, Chow E, Merrick J. Cancer and exercise: facts and myths. *J Pain Manag*. 2017;10(2):129–130.

Martin R et al. 2022. Female sexual function in bladder cancer: a review of the evidence. https://doi.org/10.1002/bco2.186

McHale CT, Cruickshank S, Torrens C, et al. A controlled pilot trial of a nurse-led intervention (Mini-AFTERc) to manage fear of cancer recurrence in patients affected by breast cancer. *Pilot Feasibility Stud*. 2020;6:60.

McNeill A, Brose LS, Calder R, et al. 2015. E-cigarettes: an evidence update. A report commissioned by Public Health England. https://tinyurl.com/ycgdxu3n.

Michaud JE, Billups KL, Partin AW. Testosterone and prostate cancer: an evidence-based review of pathogenesis and oncologic risk. *Ther Adv Urol*. 2015 Dec;7(6):378–387.

Milant A, Metsala E, Hannula L. Reducing the psychological distress in patients undergoing chemotherapy. *Br J Nurs*. 2016;25(4 Suppl):S25–S30.

Million Women Study Collaborators. Breast cancer and hormone replacement therapy in the Million Women Study. *Lancet*. 2003;362(9):419–427.

Multinational Association of Supportive Care in Cancer (MASCC) Mucositis study group. https://mascc.org/resources/mascc-guidelines/

Multinational Association of Supportive Care in Cancer (MASCC). 2018. Oral Care Study Group resources. https://mascc.memberclicks.net/oral-care.

Nagy Á, Munkácsy G, Győrffy B. Pancancer survival analysis of cancer hallmark genes. *Sci Rep*. 2021;11:6047.

NHS England. 2016. Achieving World Class Cancer-Outcomes: Taking the Strategy Forward. https://www.england.nhs.uk/wp-content/uploads/2016/05/cancer-strategy.pdf.

NHS England. Long Term Plan 2019a. https://www.longtermplan.nhs.uk/online-version/

NHS England. Cancer Plan 2019b. https://www.england.nhs.uk/cancer/strategy/

NHS England. Enabling people to make informed decisions. https://www.england.nhs.uk/personalisedcare/health-literacy/ [accessed 8.7.2023]

Niven CA, Scott PA. The need for accurate perception and informed judgement in determining the appropriate use of nursing resource: hearing the patient's voice. *Nurs Philos*. 2003;4:201–210.

Nursing and Midwifery Council (NMC). 2018. The Code: Professional Standards of Practice and Behaviour for Nurses, Midwives and Nursing Associates. https://www.nmc.org.uk/globalassets/sitedocuments/nmc-publications/nmc-code.pdf.

Oeffinger KC, Fontham ETH, Etzioni R, et al. Breast cancer screening for women of average risk: 2015 guideline update from the America Cancer Society. *JAMA*. 2015;314(15):1599–1614.

Oxlad M, Wade TD, Hallsworth LB, Koczwara B. 'I'm living with a chronic illness, not … dying with cancer': a qualitative study of Australian women's self-identified concerns and needs following primary treatment for breast cancer. *Eur J Cancer Care (Engl)*. 2008;17(2):157–166.

Papadimitriou N, Markozannes G, Kanellopoulou A, et al. An umbrella review of the evidence associating diet and cancer risk at 11 anatomical sites. *Nat Commun*. 2021;12:4579. https://doi.org/10.1038/s41467-021-24861-8.

Pedersen B, Koktved DP, Nielson LL. Living with side effects from cancer treatment – a challenge to target information. *Scand J Caring Sci*. 2013;27:715–723.

Peterson JJ, Steele-Moses SK. Update on new therapies with immune checkpoint inhibitors. *Clin J Oncol Nurs*. 2016;20(4):405–410.

Petermann-Rocha F, et al. Frailty, sarcopenia, cachexia and malnutrition as comorbid conditions and their associations with mortality: a prospective study from UK Biobank. *J Public Health*. 2021;44(2):c172–c180.

Petren RE, et al. Relational turning points in spousal relationships during the journey with cancer. *Medsurg Nurs*. 2021;30(3):187–196.

Public Health England. 2016. Prostate cancer risk management programme. https://www.gov.uk/guidance/prostate-cancer-risk-management-programme-overview.

Roila F, Molassiotis A, Herrstedt Jon behalf of the participants of the MASCC/ESMO Consensus Conference, Copenhagen 2015. Consensus guidelines for the prevention of chemotherapy and radiotherapy-induced nausea and vomiting: ESMO Clinical Practice Guidelines. *Ann Oncol*. 2016;27(Suppl 5):v119–v133.

Royal College of Nursing (RCN). 2018. Advanced level nursing practice: Introduction. https://www.rcn.org.uk/professional-development/publications/pub-006894.

Royal College of Nursing (RCN). 2022. Career and education framework for cancer nursing. https://www.rcn.org.uk/Professional-Development/publications/career-pathway-and-education-framework-for-cancer-nursing-uk-pub-010-076

Schover LR, der Kaai M, Dorst E, et al. Sexual dysfunction and infertility as late effects of cancer treatment. *EJC Suppl*. 2014;12(1):41–53.

Scottish Government. 2008. Better cancer care. http://www.scotland.gov.uk/Publications/2008/10/24140351/0.

Scottish Government. 2012. Detect cancer early. https://www.gov.scot/Topics/Health/Services/Cancer/Detect-Cancer-Early.

Shaw C, Eldridge L. Nutritional considerations for the palliative care patient. *Int J Palliat Nurs*. 2015;21(1):7–15.

Slevin ML, Stubbs L, Plant H, et al. Choices in cancer treatment: comparing the views of patients with cancer with those of doctors, nurses and the general public. *Br Med J*. 1990;300:1458–1460.

Smith HR. Depression in cancer patients: pathogenesis, implications and treatment (Review). *Oncol Lett*. 2015;9(4):1509–1514.

Soerjomataram I, Bray F. Planning for tomorrow: global cancer incidence and the role of prevention 2020–2070. *Nat Rev Clin Oncol*. 2021;18:663–672.

Sørensen K, Makaroff LE, Myers L, et al. The call for a strategic framework to improve cancer literacy in Europe. *Arch Public Health*. 2020;78:60.

Staley H, et al. Interventions targeted at women to encourage the uptake of cervical screening. *Cochrane Database Syst Rev*. 2021(9): Art. No.: CD002834. doi:10.1002/14651858.CD002834.pub3.

Strecher VJ, Rosenstock I. The health belief model. In: Glanz K, Lewis F, Rimer B, eds.. San Francisco: Jossey-Bass; 1997. *Health Behaviour and Health Education*. 2:41–59.

Sung et al. Global Cancer Statistics 2020: GLOBOCAN Estimates of Incidence and Mortality Worldwide for 36 Cancers in 185 Countries 2021. https://doi.org/10.3322/caac.21660

Tanne JH. Breast Cancer: US recommends women start screening at 40. *BMJ*. 2023;381. https://doi.org/10.1136/bmj.p1077.

Thewes B, Lebel S, Leclair S, Butow P. A qualitative exploration of fear of cancer recurrence (FCR) amongst Australian and Canadian breast cancer survivors. *Support Care Cancer*. 2016;24(5):2269–2276.

Toumazis I, et al. Risk-Based lung cancer screening: a systematic review. *Lung Cancer*. 2020;147:154–186.

Tschudin V, ed. *Nursing the Patient With Cancer*. 2nd ed. Hemel Hempstead: Prentice Hall; 1996.

UK Oncology Nursing Society UKONS Systemic anti-cancer therapy (SACT) competency passport. 2019. https://www.ukons.org/site/assets/files/1138/ukons_sact_electronic_passport_version_4.pdf.

Acute Oncology Initial Management Guidelines. https://www.ukons. org/site/assets/files/1134/acute_oncology_initial_management_guidelines.pdf.

Union for International Cancer Control. TMN Classifications of Malignant Tumours https://www.uicc.org/what-we-do/sharing-knowledge/tnm [accessed 15.7.2023]

Versluis A, et al. Dear hair loss – illness perceptions of female patients with chemotherapy-induced alopecia. *Support Care Cancer*. 2022; 30:3955–3963.

Wells FC. Case study of an oncological emergency: Superior Vena Cava Syndrome (SVCS). *Can Oncol Nurs J*. 2016;26(1):77–82.

White ID, Butcher J. Special issue: Working with the sexual consequences of cancer and its treatment. *Sex Relation Ther*. 2016;31(4): 411–413.

World Health Organisation, WHO recommendations on self-care interventions Human papillomavirus (HPV) self-sampling as part of cervical cancer screening and treatment, 2022 updatE file:///C:/Users/user/Downloads/WHO-SRH-23.1-eng.pdf

Yaffe MJ. PhD, CM and others, Breast Cancer Screening: Beyond Mortality. *J Breast Imaging*. 2019;1(3):161–165.

Yang Y, et al. The relationship between cancer patient's fear of recurrence and chemotherapy: A systematic review and meta-analysis. *J Psychosom Res*. 2017;98:55–63.

Further Reading

Boulanger J, Ducharme A, Dufour A, et al. Management of the extravasation of anti-neoplastic agents. *Support Care Cancer*. 2015;23: 1459–1471. https://doi.org/10.1007/s00520-015-2635-7.

Calzone KA, Masny A. Genetics and oncology nursing. *Semin Oncol Nurs*. 2004;20(3):178–185.

Cancer Research UK (2023) What clinical trials are? Find a clinical trial | Cancer Research UK.

Curiglano, et al. Management of cardiac disease in cancer patients throughout oncological treatment: ESMO consensus recommendations. *Ann Oncol*. 2020;31(2):171–190.

Health and Safety Executive. 2015. Occupational exposure to ionising radiation. http://www.hse.gov.uk/statistics/ionising-radiation/cidi.pdf.

McGowan D. Safe handling and administration of MABS: the guidance. *Br J Nurs*. 2015;24(Suppl 16a):S14–S20.

McGrady, et al. 2023 Systematic evaluation of the behavior change techniques and quality of commercially available cancer self-management apps. *JCO Oncol Pract*. 2023;19(2):e228–e237.

Olsen PR, Smith S. *Nursing Adolescents and Young Adults With Cancer, Developing Knowledge, Competence and Best Practice*. London: Springer; 2018.

Pugh A, et al. Acute oncology: a developing subspecialty. *Br J Nurs*. 2015;24(16):S18–S25.

Quinn B, Connolly M. Spirituality in palliative care. *BMC Palliat Care*. 2023;22:1.

Royal College of Nursing (RCN). 2016. Standards for infusion therapy. https://www.rcn.org.uk/professional-development/publications/pub-005704.

Lister Hofland, Grafton. *The Royal Marsden Manual of Clinical Nursing Procedures*. 10th ed. London: Wiley Blackwell; 2020.

Tortora GJ, Derrickson B. *Principles of Anatomy and Physiology*. ed 15 New York: John Wiley & Sons, Inc; 2017.

The Society and College of Radiographers (2020) Radiation Dermatitis Guidelines for Radiotherapy Healthcare Professionals. https://www.sor.org/getmedia/53bd52ff-679e-48de-82a0-dc8dae570896/2020_version_4_final_practice_guideline_radiotherapy_skin_care_llv1.pdf [accessed 8.7.2023].

World Health Organisation (2020) Physical activity and sedentary behaviour. https://apps.who.int/iris/bitstream/handle/10665/337001/9789240014886-eng.pdf.

Useful Websites

About the Human Genome, https://web.ornl.gov/sci/techresources/Human_Genome/index.shtml

ACCEND Aspirant Cancer Career and Education Development, https://www.e-lfh.org.uk/programmes/aspirant-cancer-career-and-education-development-programme-accend/

British National Formulary, www.bnf.org.uk

Cancer Care Map, https://www.cancercaremap.org/

Cancerquest for further biology, https://www.cancerquest.org/

Cancer Research UK, https://www.cancerresearchuk.org/

Children with Cancer UK, https://www.childrenwithcancer.org.uk/

European Code Against Cancer, https://cancer-code-europe.iarc.fr/index.php/en/

Healthtalk.org, www.healthtalk.org/peoples-experiences/cancer/

Macmillan Cancer Support, www.macmillan.org.uk

Maggie's Centres, https://www.maggies.org

Marie Curie Cancer Care, https://www.mariecurie.org.uk/

Multinational Association of Supportive Care in Cancer, https://www.mascc.org

National Cancer Institute (NCI)

(US government with information about types of treatment and side-effects), https://www.cancer.gov/cancertopics

National Extravasation Information Service (NEIS), www.extravasation.org.uk/home.html

NHS Cancer Screening Programmes, www.cancerscreening.nhs.uk

South East Scotland Cancer Network, https://www.nhsresearchscotland.org.uk/research-areas/cancer

Teenager and Young People with Cancer (TYAC), https://www.tyac.org.uk/

Tenovus, https://www.tenovuscancercare.org.uk/

World Health Organization, https://www.who.int/health-topics/cancer

32

Nursing Patients Who Need Palliative Care

JANE MARQUESEN, ELAINE CROSBY-JONES

CHAPTER OUTLINE

Introduction

Caring effectively for people with a progressive, life-limiting illness presents a number of challenges for the multiprofessional team. Nurses have an important role to play in assessing care needs and managing the impact of an incurable illness on the patient and their family. Nursing knowledge and skills are vital contributions to the delivery of high-quality palliative care that enables patients to experience a good quality of life and a peaceful, dignified death, and their family to cope with bereavement.

The first part of this chapter defines palliative care and explores the fundamental principles of this approach. Consideration is given to how palliative care is provided within different settings and the range of services and teams which may be involved. The middle section has two parts: first it focuses on how the principles of palliative care may be applied in clinical practice, including communication with patients and families, and secondly on the evidence-based strategies for the management of common, distressing symptoms. The chapter concludes by exploring issues specific to the final phase of the patient's illness and considering how these may be addressed by effective end-of-life care.

What Is Palliative Care?

The most widely accepted definition of palliative care was first provided by the World Health Organisation (WHO) in 1990. The most recent version (WHO 2020) states:

> *Palliative care is an approach that improves the quality of life of patients (adults and children) and their families who are facing problems associated with life-threatening illness. It prevents and relieves suffering through the early identification, correct assessment and treatment of pain and other problems, whether physical, psychosocial or spiritual.*

This clearly portrays palliative care as an active approach to assessing and managing care needs, far from the perspective that 'nothing more can be done' for the patient when their illness cannot be cured. The aim is to support the patient in living as comfortable and fulfilling a life as possible as their illness progresses towards death. It is important for healthcare professionals to recognise that dying is more than a physical experience and that suffering has psychological, social and spiritual dimensions which can also envelop those closest to the patient. This requires consideration not just of the physical disease process, but also the effects on the patient as an individual and their family and those important to them when planning and delivering care. The palliative care approach is therefore person centred, holistic and multi-dimensional (Reflection 32.1).

Historically, a number of terms have been associated with palliative care. These include 'care of the dying', 'hospice care', 'supportive care', 'terminal care' and 'end-of-life care'. These terms are often used

Figure 32.1 The scope of palliative care.

(Fig. 32.1). This includes all stages of the disease trajectory including whilst the patient is receiving treatments which, although cure is not possible, may prolong their life or help control symptoms. Supportive care is integral to the palliative approach in helping the patient and family cope with the impact of the disease and the uncertainties and losses of the dying process. Terminal care or, more appropriately, end-of-life care refers to the last stage of the patient's illness which is generally considered the last 6–12 months of life, where there is increasing disability and dependence and death is anticipated in the near future. End-of-life care is delivered in the last days of the patient's life and will be considered in more depth later in this chapter.

The Development of Palliative Care

In the UK, the palliative care approach was pioneered by Dame Cecily Saunders, attributed as founding the modern hospice movement with the opening of St Christopher's Hospice, London, in 1967. This was a milestone in the history of palliative care, from which has evolved the person-centred, holistic approach underpinned by research and evidence-based practice that is now recognised worldwide (St Christopher's Hospice 2023).

In 1987, 20 years after the opening of St Christopher's Hospice, palliative care was awarded the status of a medical specialty by the Royal College of Physicians in recognition of the growing body of knowledge and expertise in care of the dying generated within the hospice setting. In the mid-70s a nurse specialist role was established in palliative care as the 'Macmillan Nurse' (Seymour et al. 2002). Since then, there have been further significant advances in clinical practice, research and education for healthcare professionals. As a result, there is now a substantial evidence base underpinning palliative care and greater expectations from both professionals and the public that suffering can be alleviated and a 'good death' achieved.

This is reflected in the wide range of guidelines, protocols and standards available to guide clinical practice and the delivery of care, including those from government advisory bodies and regulatory organisations such as the National Institute for Health and Care Excellence (NICE), Health Improvement Scotland (HIS), the Care Quality Commission (CQC) and Health Education England (in England) and the Care Inspectorate in Scotland.

As the majority of care for the dying is delivered within hospitals, the community and care homes (both residential and nursing), palliative care is a core responsibility of all health and social care professionals in these settings. Yet, increasing societal awareness and expectations of palliative care contrast sharply with reports of inequitable access, variation and deficiencies in care provision and the unmet needs of dying patients (CQC 2016).

This has prompted development in two main areas:

- the expansion of hospice and specialist palliative care services
- introduction of frameworks to support professionals in delivering palliative care within mainstream services in both hospital and community settings.

interchangeably and thus are open to misinterpretation. Reigada et al. (2020) highlights the importance of the use of language and its influence on the messages being transferred to patients and caregivers which impact their access and understanding of palliative care.

A number of factors may have contributed to the varied terminology used to describe palliative care. Improved health and social care alongside advances in medical technologies have caused an epidemiological shift in the main causes of death within the developed world. From the late 19th century onwards, mortality rates from infectious diseases, childhood illnesses and maternal deaths have gradually declined. As a result, the average life expectancy has significantly increased and has now reached the highest level on record for both men and women (excluding 2020–2021 COVID-19 pandemic mortality rates) (Office for National Statistics 2021). This has led to a steady rise in the incidence of life-limiting illnesses with more prolonged disease trajectories such as cancer, chronic respiratory and cardiovascular disease, for which more sophisticated diagnostic and treatment options have improved prognosis and length of survival. This means that an increasing number of people are living longer with progressive and ultimately fatal conditions. Meier et al. (2016) provide a comprehensive and thought-provoking review of what constitutes a good death or successful dying. They point out that the concept of a good death has shifted from an event that is simply free from pain and suffering towards a more all-encompassing view which takes into account death from a sociological and philosophical perspective examining whether a person's preferences around dying or death were met or not. This is now commonly referred to as 'living whilst dying' and 'the dying process', which can extend over weeks, months, even years. To support such preferences, community support is essential. Sallnow et al. (2016) reviewed the impact of a community approach to palliative care concluding that issues such as carer support, community capacity, well-being and social isolation were key factors associated with supporting end-of-life care.

Following the WHO definition, the palliative approach is applicable from the time a life-limiting illness is diagnosed, throughout the patient's illness and into bereavement support for the family

The Expansion of Hospices and Specialist Palliative Care Services

Hospices were the first specialist palliative care services, and there are currently over 200 hospices across the UK serving over 300,000 people and their families for end-of-life care services and support yearly (Hospice UK 2023). Patients may be admitted for a variety of reasons, including assessment, rehabilitation and symptom management, respite stays to give families and carers a short break and care at end of life.

From the 1990s onwards, the specialty of palliative care expanded with the development of services within the hospital and community. These include specialist hospital palliative care teams, day hospices and community palliative care teams. Provision for end-of-life care is currently delivered by a patchwork of providers and funded by a mixture of public, private and charitable sources (Hospice UK 2021). Charities such as Macmillan Cancer Support had in the past provided the financial backing to initiate a number of specialist posts for cancer care. Today, specialist palliative care nurses often work independently as part of a larger multidisciplinary team and are considered a reference point for clinical advice and guidance. The role of the specialist palliative care nurse includes planning care from admission to discharge as well as family support and dealing with the breadth of physical, psychosocial and spiritual concerns commonly seen in the context of palliative and end-of-life care for malignant and nonmalignant diagnosis (Connolly et al. 2021).

The core dimensions of specialist palliative care services are:

- Multiprofessional teams of health and social care professionals with advanced knowledge and skills in palliative care, having completed postqualification accredited education and substantial clinical experience. They include palliative medicine consultants and clinical nurse specialists, together with a range of expertise provided by physiotherapists, occupational therapists, dietitians, pharmacists and social workers.
- The provision of specialist interventions and direct care for patients and families with moderate to high complexity of palliative care needs.
- The provision of advice and support for other professionals within general hospital and community care settings in applying the principles of palliative care in clinical practice.
- Advancing the specialty of palliative care through research, audit, education and practice development initiatives (Scottish Government 2015).

Specialist palliative care services are not always involved in the care of all patients with a life-limiting illness but operate on an advisory and referral basis where the generalist nurse might need advise or there are more complex assessed needs. Other health and social care professionals, such as GPs and district nurses in the community and ward teams in hospitals, can request advice regarding how to address the needs of patients and families under their care. They can also refer patients and families with more complex needs for specialist assessment and direct intervention, for example in managing difficult pain and other symptoms, and psychological and spiritual distress. In this way, the expertise of the specialist team is shared through interprofessional working to address palliative care needs, although the referring team retains overall clinical control and responsibility for the patient (Reflection 32.2).

Supporting General Palliative Care Within Community and Hospital Settings

Current healthcare strategy emphasises the need to ensure access and delivery of a high standard of palliative care for all patients

---

REFLECTION 32.2

Availability of Specialist Palliative Care Services

Specialist palliative care services vary from area to area. For example, the provision of services in a city may be quite different from those provided in a sparsely populated rural area.

Activities

- What specialist palliative care services are available in your area?
- What are the criteria for referring patients to these specialist palliative care services?
- Reflect on the range of services offered and the benefits to patients and their families.

Resource

Hospice UK. Homepage. https://www.hospiceuk.org/.

---

with a life-limiting illness within all care settings (National Palliative and End of Life Care Partnership 2021, Scottish Government 2015). Traditionally, hospices have provided care predominantly for people with cancer. Over 50% of those admitted to hospice services have a cancer diagnosis. Although community services provided by hospices such as: hospice at home, counselling and pre and post bereavement services provide access to hospice services to people with cancer as well as nonmalignant diagnosis to provide better provision of palliative care to all (Scobie and Hutchings 2023).

It has already been highlighted that the incidence of both malignant and nonmalignant life-limiting illnesses is rising, with a corresponding increase in demand for palliative care. Since the COVID-19 pandemic, where inpatient hospice services has declined, the need for palliative care in community locations has been highlighted (Hospice UK 2021). In addition, greater awareness of inequality of access to effective care across settings and for some patient groups (mental health, learning disabilities, homelessness, prisons and those who identify as lesbian, gay, bisexual, transgender, queer or questioning, intersex or asexual [LGBTQ+]) has made strengthening the delivery of palliative care within mainstream hospital and community services a priority. Developments towards this include the Ambitions for End of Life Care and Equality for Hospice and End of Life Care [Hospice UK 2021, National Palliative and End of Life Care Partnership 2021].

The Palliative Care Approach in Practice

This part of the chapter considers the palliative care approach in clinical practice. A model of palliative care is presented which can be used as a guide to apply the principles of palliative care when caring for patients and families.

The Principles of Palliative Care– A Model for Practice

The model for practice is presented as a guide for the clinical nurse in the 21st century (Fig. 33.2). Using this model means challenging assumptions and looking for creative and workable solutions to problems, critically reading literature and appraising research and, in partnership with the multiprofessional team, implementing reflective, evidence-based practice.

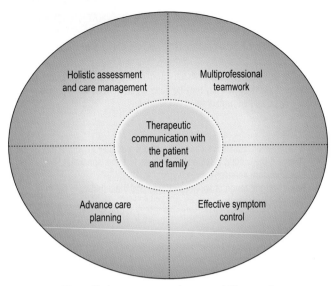

Figure 32.2 The palliative care approach – a model for practice.

Each dimension of the model is presented and discussed. It is important to recognise that these dimensions are interrelated and interdependent.

Fundamental to person-centred palliative care is therapeutic communication with the patient and family and those important to the patient; therefore, this forms the core of the model. Holistic assessment and care management relate to the overarching aim of palliative care and the patient experiencing a quality of life and a dignified death. Ongoing holistic assessment of a person with recognition of the wide range of physical, psychological, social and spiritual issues which may arise from a life-limiting illness and the individual responses of the patient and family to their situation. Multiprofessional teamwork emphasises that the knowledge and skills of different health and social care professionals are vital contributions to the provision of holistic palliative care. Effective symptom control maximises independence and comfort and thus allows both the patient and family to focus on goals and activities which are important to them. The dimension of advance care planning identifies palliative care as a proactive approach to care as well as responsive to the current needs of the patient. Planning ahead for anticipated changes in condition allows the patient's wishes to be considered regarding their future care and treatment, a quality of life to be maintained and the distress of unnecessary hospital admissions avoided.

Therapeutic Communication

Effective communication with the patient and family is central to the delivery of palliative care. Knowing how the illness affects the person, what they think and how they feel about their situation provides the basis for care appropriate to their individual needs and goals. If a key aim of palliative care is that the patient experiences a quality of life, then professionals need to understand exactly what that means for them. Quality of life is a subjective experience and therefore we need to consider what is important to the patient and what gives their life meaning. How do they perceive the illness affects them, their family and their quality of life?

Eliciting this information requires effective and sensitive communication between professionals and patients. This can be termed therapeutic communication, which differs from the social communications integral to everyday life in relation to context, purpose and the communication skills used by the professional.

The purpose of therapeutic communication is primarily supportive to the patient and family in the context of care provision and provides the medium by which professionals can gain an accurate understanding of care needs. Therapeutic communication also allows information needs to be identified and addressed, at a level appropriate to the individual patient and family to ensure their understanding. The provision of information has been shown to reduce distress and enhance compliance with treatment and the ability to cope with the practicalities of living with and dying from a life-limiting illness. Professionals have a responsibility to be aware of how well they communicate with patients and families, and this can be supported by critical reflection on practice. This responsibility extends to then developing the necessary knowledge, skills and confidence in the use of strategies that support effective interaction with the patients and families under their care. However, in summarising research in this area, communication skills training requires more attention to ensure it is effective in developing the right skills, which has been most acutely highlighted with communication barriers experienced by those who identify with LGBTQ+ groups (Brighton et al. 2017, Cloyes et al. 2018). A full discussion regarding the skills and strategies for therapeutic communication is beyond the scope of this chapter; however, some key points are considered here.

Therapeutic interaction with patients and/or families may take the form of an assessment interview, a one-to-one discussion or interaction with patient and family together. Preparation is important in ensuring that the nurse has as much information as is available regarding the patient's condition, history and circumstances. Patients often feel they have to repeat information over and over again to different professionals and this can be frustrating and extremely tiring for those already fatigued because of their illness. The patient's case notes should be read, as they may contain a great deal of the required information regarding diagnosis, previous treatment, current issues and problems. Members of the multiprofessional team may be able to provide further details, including those in other care settings: for example, the district nurse may be able to provide useful information for hospital staff regarding the care needs of the patient at home and any family issues. It is wise to remember, however, that the nature of a life-limiting illness means that issues and problems change over time and that how they are perceived by the team caring for the patient may be different from those causing the greatest concern for the patient. This means the nurse should work from an informed basis but check and expand their understanding of the patient's situation and, importantly, related perceptions and concerns.

The ideal situation for therapeutic communication is one in which privacy is provided without interruption. The patient's physical comfort should be attended to. The purpose should be made explicit and the patient's consent obtained to proceed. Patients and families need to feel secure that confidentiality will be maintained. It is often believed that patients realise they are being cared for by a multiprofessional team and that they therefore implicitly agree that information given to one professional may be openly shared with others. This should not be assumed. It is useful to remind patients and families that information which is relevant to their care is shared within the multiprofessional team and to emphasise that they do not have to talk about areas they prefer to keep private. The ethics of confidentiality are beyond the scope of this chapter (see Griffith and Tengnah 2023, Nursing and Midwifery Council [NMC] 2018 and Further Reading.

Attention to nonverbal behaviours such as maintaining appropriate eye contact, sitting rather than standing beside the patient and adopting an open posture, slightly leaning forward rather than sitting back with crossed arms and legs, can display warmth and respect. The use of paralinguistic responses can encourage the patient to continue to talk and shows the nurse is paying attention. Active listening is a key skill and incorporates close attention to not just what the patient is saying verbally but also their facial expression, tone of voice and behaviour, which can convey the meaning and emotion behind their words.

The flow of discussion should be paced according to the patient, who is encouraged to talk about their main problems and concerns. Open questions such as 'Can you tell me how this affects your day-to-day life…?' give the patient the opportunity to provide rich and detailed information from their perspective. In contrast, closed or focused questions such as 'How many times a day does this happen?' provide more specific information, particularly when clarification is needed or when the patient is too tired or breathless for a lengthy discussion.

From skilful use of questioning, it should be possible to appraise the patient's understanding of their illness and expectations regarding care. Patients are individuals in how they cope with a life-limiting illness. This includes what they understand about their illness from the information provided by professionals, how they interpret changes in their condition and their social circumstances and their psychological coping style. This can also influence what they wish to discuss and when, and their choice to do so should be respected. Asking an open question such as 'Can you tell me what you understand about…?' allows the patient to exert some control over what is discussed and how they respond. If the patient becomes tired or upset at any time, the nurse must enquire if they wish to stop. The patient may wish to conclude the interview or, where the expression of the emotions is appropriate and needed by the patient, they may simply wish some time. In this situation, the importance of sensitivity and the nurse's presence should not be underestimated. An upset or distressed patient should not be abandoned. If, however, they require some private time alone or with their family, then reassurance should be given that the nurse will return at an agreed time in the very near future or sooner, should they request.

There may be occasions where the nurse does not have the information required to answer a question or address a concern. Honesty is the best policy, alongside acknowledgement that the question or concern is important to the person. Reassurance can be given that the nurse will direct their question or concern to an appropriate member of the multiprofession team. Dying patients and their families do not expect every professional to have all the answers; however, dishonesty or failing to acknowledge their concerns can undermine their trust and confidence in and openness with the multiprofessional team (Dixon et al. 2015, National Audit of Care at End of Life [NACEL] 2023).

When speaking to families, it is important to note that where the patient has capacity, their permission and wishes should be ascertained regarding disclosure of information. Family members can offer useful information regarding care needs and may be the greatest source of support for the patient, including supporting their wish to be cared for at home. Family dynamics do vary, however, and therefore an understanding of roles and relationships ensures that the patient's wishes can be respected whilst addressing the concerns of the family, reinforcing the principle that family support is an integral part of palliative care (Leadership for the Alliance of the Care of Dying People [LACDP] 2014).

In concluding the interaction, summarising key points that have been discussed is a useful strategy. This lets the patient and/or family see that the nurse has listened and understood what they have said and provides the opportunity for them to add more detail or correct any misunderstandings. The summary should include agreeing on any required actions or changes to the plan of care and allows the nurse to ensure their understanding of any information given. Screening for any other issues gives patients and/or families the opportunity to raise any concerns which they have not yet mentioned. Following such interactions, the nurse will clearly and succinctly document relevant information and communicate any immediate issues to the appropriate multiprofessional team member. The sharing of information in order to maintain continuity of care requires robust electronic documentation systems that enable the multiprofessional teams to have the most current and accessible information (National Palliative and End of Life Care Partnership 2021). In this way, care is patient centred and consistent whilst avoiding the need for patients to repeatedly provide the same information to different team members.

Holistic Assessment and Care Management

Holistic assessment is a key activity in palliative care and directs the use of appropriate strategies for care needs associated with the physical, psychological, spiritual and social impact of the illness on the patient and family. A number of approaches may be used; these include quantitative measures such as rating scales to measure the severity of a symptom, for example pain assessment tools (see Chapter 20, Pain Management), and more qualitative approaches such as history taking. Whatever approach is used, it is imperative that it is multidimensional so that the assessment captures a full and comprehensive picture of the palliative care needs of the patient and family. Some key assessment questions that can be adapted for a holistic assessment include:

- Can you describe what … is like?
- How bad is it – at worst/at best?
- How often does … happen?
- What makes … better/worse?
- What do you think is causing …?
- How does … make you feel?
- What does … mean to you?
- How does …. affect your day-to-day life?

A plan of care can then be devised which reflects the principles of palliative care. Attention to detail is important, as is continuous review because of the complex and progressive nature of the dying process.

Multiprofessional Teamwork

From review of the principles of palliative care, it can be identified that no one profession can meet all the care needs of the patient and family. A holistic approach requires the skills and expertise of different professionals. Nurses play a central role within the multiprofessional team which includes facilitating communication and coordinating the input of other team members in patient care. This may include a range of professionals including the physiotherapist, occupational therapist, chaplain, social worker and dietitian.

Effective multiprofessional teamwork is, however, more than just a group of professionals involved in the care of the same patient and family. A number of authors have outlined the challenges for the multiprofessional team in palliative care (Klarare et al. 2013, O'Connor and Fisher 2011, Warner et al. 2021). These include ensuring a shared understanding of goals and objectives and that a blurring of traditional role boundaries can occur when all professionals share a holistic perspective. Effective communication and coordination of activity across a wide team are essential to avoid the risk of fragmented care and key needs not being identified and properly addressed.

Advance Care Planning

A thorough understanding of the pathophysiology of the patient's illness offers direction for anticipating likely disease progression and associated issues. Effective palliative care requires consideration of what problems may arise and, where possible, the instigation of measures to prevent them or facilitate their timely management. This includes ensuring adequate medications are available, including on a prn 'as required' basis should the patient's symptoms worsen. Unnecessary hospital admissions can potentially be avoided by providing ready access to equipment and increased social support should the patient's condition deteriorate and ensuring that out-of-hours services have essential access to information. Incorporating advance care planning discussion for patients with life-limiting diagnosis does not improve the patient's care experience but enhances the therapeutic relationship and can be influential in reducing over treatment (Fleuren et al. 2020).

Ascertaining the wishes of the patient regarding future care and treatment is an important part of care planning, and nurses play a key role in acting as the patient's advocate and supporting an informed choice. This may include decisions concerning resuscitation which can present a number of ethical and practice issues for nurses. Guidance on the decision making, ethical issues and how to approach the conversation for resuscitation is provided by the Resuscitation Council UK (2023a).

Currently in the UK, it is a criminal offence to assist or encourage suicide; healthcare professionals, including nurses, are often asked by patients and their relatives for advice in this area. The NMC provides limited advice for nurses with regards to this, instead referring nurses to act lawfully at all times and emphasising that they must practice within their code of professional conduct (NMC 2018). The Royal College of Nursing (RCN) (2016), however, has provided helpful advice on how to respond to people who seek advice assisted suicide. They highlight the need to explore the reasons why people express the wish to die, advising that it is helpful to ask questions to understand the emotional and practical concerns, showing empathy and understanding of their situation and to offer helpful interventions to improve their quality of life. Appropriate referral to experienced palliative care practitioners would be recommended. It needs to be clear that as a nurse, you would not be able to act unlawfully and as such you cannot do anything to assist them to shorten their life. The patient's preferences regarding place of care during their illness and at the end of life should also be explored using therapeutic communication. Patient's wishes may change over time and therefore decisions should be sensitively revisited as appropriate when circumstances change. The use of an advance care planning document such as ReSPECT (Resuscitation Council UK 2023b) to communicate and respect patient choice alongside clinical judgement across care settings has been advocated in England and Wales (see also Gold Standards Framework, ACP, 2023).

Effective Symptom Control

The key components of symptom control in palliative care are well described (see Cherny 2021 and Further Reading). In summary, the multiprofessional team must work with the patient to:
- make a thorough assessment of each symptom

- discuss causes and treament options
- plan symptom management in light of the patient's expectations and priorities
- evaluate regularly with changing condition and progressive disease.

When administering medications for symptom control, the most appropriate route for the patient must be considered. If, for example, the patient is regularly nauseated or is vomiting, then they are unlikely to fully absorb oral medications and, likewise, if drowsy at the end of life, may be unable to swallow. In such situations, parenteral administration is appropriate, usually via continuous subcutaneous (SC) administration by syringe pump. This avoids the need for repeated injections and is less invasive than the intravenous route. Patient choice must also be considered: for example, some patients with stable pain may prefer an adhesive transdermal analgesic that is changed every 3 days to taking oral analgesics regularly by mouth.

The effective control of some common distressing symptoms is discussed next.

❖ Nursing Management and Health Promotion: Common Distressing Symptoms

Many health authorities provide evidence-based clinical practice guidelines for the management of symptoms in palliative care. These often provide helpful advice that is contextualised to the particular area. This part of the chapter focuses on the management of four common distressing symptoms: pain, nausea and vomiting, constipation and breathlessness. See Cherny 2021 and Further Reading for information about other symptoms, such as cough, hiccup, delirium, etc.

Pain

Pain is one of the most feared symptoms of a terminal illness and is estimated to occur in between 35% and 95% of patients with cancer depending on the stage and type of cancer. The incidences of pain are less evident in research for nonmalignant palliative diseases but the presence and fear of pain when dying from chronic diseases are well documented (Klint et al. 2019). Despite the complexity of this symptom, a vast amount of knowledge is available regarding strategies for effective management. However, pain that is not identified will not be treated, and pain will not be treated vigorously enough if its severity is underestimated.

It has now been accepted that the patient's self-report is the most reliable indicator of pain. However, there are challenges to this in practice. Self-report of pain may not be an option in the confused or nonverbal patient. Observation of behaviour and proxy reporting from carers then become the main method of assessing the pain of these individuals (Schofield 2018).

In addition, there are personality, attitudinal and cultural reasons why people do not reveal their pains. These range from struggling to acknowledge an increase in pain as they perceive this may signify progression of their disease and they may be unwilling to admit that the best efforts of the multiprofessional team have been to no avail.

Patients who are dying commonly have more than one pain. The nurse committed to helping the patient must therefore systematically assess and document the following information about each pain the patient is experiencing:
- location
- severity

- radiation – does the pain move or travel from its original site?
- type – is the pain described as dull/gnawing/shooting/burning/spasmodic?
- when *the pain* started
- aggravating factors
- alleviating factors.

The severity of pain can be assessed using visual or numerical analogue scales, for example by asking the patient to score their pain on a scale of 1–10 where 0 equals no pain and 10 equals the most severe pain possible. Some patients may prefer rating their pain as none/mild/moderate/severe or simply using their own terms. It is important to find a way of rating pain severity that is clearly understood by both the patient and the multiprofessional team. From this shared understanding of how bad the pain feels, management strategies can be targeted most effectively and patient distress minimised. Professionals must remember that in a palliative context, the patient may have been experiencing pain for some time. The physiological indicators common to those with acute pain, for example tachycardia and raised blood pressure, may therefore be absent.

It is also important to ask the patient about their pain now and when at its worst. This can detect the presence of 'incident pain' which is pain that only happens at certain times or is triggered by specific events; for example, the patient may rate their hip pain as 0 out of 10 when sitting at rest but 9 out of 10 when trying to walk or bend. This has obvious implications for the patient's quality of life and maintaining their independence for as long as possible.

How the patient describes the character of their pain helps determine the type of pain they are experiencing. Pain that is described as shooting or burning may denote nerve or neuropathic pain whilst aching and gnawing pain over a joint may indicate bone pain from secondary cancer or severe arthritis. The type of pain is a key factor in selecting the most appropriate choice of analgesics and interventions.

The nurse should discuss the findings from the assessment with medical staff and other relevant members of the multiprofessional team, such as the physiotherapist. It is essential that this be done in an informed manner by giving a detailed description of the pain as outlined earlier. It is poor practice when requesting medical attendance or input from other professionals for the nurse just to give the blank statement that the patient is in pain.

An accurate diagnosis of new pain is usually derived from observation, discussion and physical examination by the doctor. A full assessment is essential, as new pain may require laboratory or radiological investigations and other treatments, as well as analgesics.

Analgesic medications, given regularly to prevent the recurrence of pain, are central to effective pain management in palliative care. It is essential that an adequate, regular dose is calculated and administered, enabling the patient to be as comfortable as possible without being drowsy.

Principles have been established by the WHO to guide healthcare professionals in the effective management of pain. In addition, guidelines such as the Scottish Intercollegiate Guidelines Network (SIGN) (2022) publication *Control of Pain in Adults With Cancer* are readily available online, along with the NICE guidelines for palliative care for adults requiring strong opioid for pain relief (NICE 2016). Registered nurses must have a working knowledge of these principles and guidelines to promote good multiprofessional understanding and patient confidence.

WHO Key Principles of Pain Control and the Analgesic Ladder

The key principles of the WHO approach are that analgesics be given by the mouth, by the clock and by the ladder.

By the Mouth

This convenient and easy route of administration should be the method of choice for as long as possible. When the patient can no longer tolerate oral medicines, the SC route is most frequently used for SC injections or by setting up a syringe pump.

By the Clock

Persistent severe pain must be prevented; it is inhumane to simply wait for pain to return and escalate before administering the next dose, and regular analgesia may be necessary to achieve stable pain control. This requires professionals to be knowledgeable about the duration of action of different analgesic preparations. For example, normal-release morphine solution is effective for 4 hours; therefore, it can be safely administered regularly every 4 hours. Other controlled-release preparations, such as MST Continus, last 12 hours and so should be administered every 12 hours to provide stable levels of background analgesia. In an inpatient setting, care must be taken that the patient receives their analgesics at an appropriate time and does not have to wait for drug rounds for the analgesics they need to control their pain.

By the Ladder

The analgesic ladder developed by the WHO in 1996 details a three-step approach to using mild to strong analgesics to control pain (see Useful Websites, e.g. WHO guidelines for the pharmacological and radiotherapeutic management of cancer pain in adults and adolescents). This was developed for cancer pain but is now commonly applied to those with noncancer life-limiting illness. The ladder combines primary analgesics and adjuvant therapies.

The WHO (2018) recommends that the strength of analgesia required should be matched with the severity of the pain and from this they developed the analgesic ladder. Commonly used analgesics are outlined in Information 32.1.

INFORMATION 32.1

Analgesic Medications Commonly Used for Cancer Pain

Step 3

Opioids for Moderate to Severe Pain
Morphine normal release – as an oral solution, e.g. Oramorph, or tablets, e.g. Sevredol
Morphine controlled release, e.g. MST Continus or MXL
Morphine by SC injection
Oxycodone normal release as an oral solution or capsule, e.g. Oxynorm
Oxycodone controlled release, e.g. Oxycontin
Oxycodone by SC injection

Step 2

Opioids for Mild to Moderate Pain
Codeine often combined with paracetamol, e.g. co-codamol 30/500

Step 1

Nonopioids for Mild Pain
Paracetamol or nonsteroidal anti-inflammatory drugs (NSAIDs)

If the patient's management starts on *step 1* of the ladder (mild pain), paracetamol may be given until the ceiling of 4 g in 24 hours has been reached, that is, the upper dose limit of this drug. If it does not control the pain, then a drug on *step 2* (mild to moderate pain) will be prescribed. Co-codamol 30/500, a combination of paracetamol and the step 2 opioid codeine, is commonly used. It is referred to as co-codamol 30/500 as each tablet contains codeine 30 mg and paracetamol 500 mg. It will be given up to the ceiling of two tablets 6-hourly. When that is ineffective in controlling the patient's pain, the step 2 opioid is stopped and a drug on *step 3* (moderate to severe pain) will be prescribed. It is essential to note that paracetamol may be continued simultaneously with a step 3 opioid as the analgesic action is different from opioids and the combination can therefore be synergistic in relieving pain. The decision to use a step 3 opioid should be based on patient need and the severity of pain and not their prognosis. The outdated practice of saving morphine for the last few weeks of life is misinformed.

An immediate-release oral preparation of morphine, such as Oramorph liquid or Sevredol tablets, will be prescribed with the intention of establishing a regimen that will relieve the pain without causing oversedation. This process is known as titration. A common starting dose of immediate-release morphine is 5–10 mg, except in older, frail or cachexic patients, when 2.5 mg might be the starting dose. It will be prescribed to be taken 4-hourly round the clock, for example at 06.00, 10.00, 14.00, 18.00, 22.00 and, if awake, at 02.00 h.

Should the patient be in pain between doses, a breakthrough dose equivalent to the standard 4-hourly dose will be given. If a breakthrough dose is given, the timing of the next regular dose must not be altered. For example, if a patient has Oramorph at 06.00 h and requires a breakthrough dose at 09.00 h, the dose due at 10.00 h will still be given on time. Once a stable dose of analgesic has been reached for 24–48 hours, the dose of normal-release medication can be converted into a sustained-release preparation. For example, the patient receives 10 mg of normal-release morphine every 4 hours, therefore over a 24-hour period, they receive 6 doses × 10 mg = 60 mg in total. This can be converted to an equivalent dose of MST Continus 30 mg every 12 hours. Guidance for transferring patients from oral morphine to SC morphine sulphate and other step 3 opiates is available from SIGN (2022). It is essential that nurses are aware that patients may have more than one pain and that different analgesics may well be required for effective pain relief (Reflection 32.3).

Some common side-effects might be expected when a patient commences on step 3 opioids. Transitory effects may be slight sleepiness and nausea; these usually pass in a few days. More troublesome are constipation and a dry mouth. Constipation *must* be treated prophylactically; a laxative such as Docusate Sodium or a macrogol (polyethylene glycols) such as Movicol must be prescribed at the same time as the opioid.

Occasionally, unacceptable side-effects may occur. 'Opioid toxicity' is a term used to denote a range of side-effects which can be distressing and, if untreated, life-threatening. Early signs are subtle and include vivid dreams, seeing shadows moving at the periphery of their visual field and mild confusion. This can progress to worsening confusion, agitation, muscle twitches and hallucinations and ultimately lead to respiratory depression, sedation and even death. Opiate toxicity may arise where the dose of opioid has been rapidly escalated or, alternatively, where dehydration or renal failure occurs and opioid metabolites normally excreted via the kidneys accumulate in the bloodstream. Such side-effects must be reported to the medical team as soon as detected. The dose of opioid will be reduced and intravenous fluids may be required to

help excretion of metabolites. Opioid toxicity from morphine and other intolerable side-effects including intractable constipation might cause the physician to prescribe a second-line opioid such as oxycodone, fentanyl or alfentanyl. This is referred to as opioid switching or rotation and should be done under the guidance of specialist palliative care services (Schuster et al. 2018).

Adjuvant medications are frequently given along with analgesics in the effective management of pain and may be given in conjunction with a primary analgesic on any step of the ladder (Table 32.1). Some pains do not respond well to the primary

---

REFLECTION 32.3

Michelle: Assessment and Management of Pain

Michelle is a 39-year-old mother of two (Jack, aged 9, and Sophie, who is 7 years of age). Her mother (Kate) is caring for the children and visits Michelle every day. Michelle is a company director and is separated from her husband. She has advanced breast cancer with metastases to bone, liver and brain. Whilst you are helping Michelle to wash one morning, she complains of pain. On further questioning, she describes three pains.

- First, she rubs the upper right quadrant of her abdomen and states that a feeling of extreme pressure builds up from deep inside her body. It has been getting steadily worse over the last few weeks, especially if she tries to lie on her right side.
- Second, Michelle describes the tight band of headache that is frequently worse on waking in the morning.
- Third, Michelle grimaces as the skin over her right femur is washed. When encouraged, she points with her finger to a specific area of pain in the bone that is causing discomfort.

The first pain is visceral pain caused by the liver being enlarged with metastases and a stretched liver capsule. Michelle has been prescribed diamorphine by continuous SC infusion and the adjuvant medication dexamethasone for this pain. Before admission, Michelle was trying to take MST Continus 60 mg 12-hourly for this pain; however, nausea and vomiting affected concordance. Cyclizine, an antiemetic, has been added to the diamorphine by SC infusion to alleviate the nausea/vomiting whilst assessment as to cause is undertaken.

The second pain around Michelle's head is likely to be caused by pressure from the oedema due to cerebral metastases. The dose of dexamethasone already prescribed for her liver pain has been increased to reduce the oedema. In addition, paracetamol 4 g in 24 hours will now be prescribed to help relieve this headache. The doctor has discussed with Michelle the role of palliative radiotherapy in treating this problem. Pain from extensive bone metastases was a considerable problem almost 1 year previously although successfully managed with hemibody radiotherapy.

It is likely that the third pain in Michelle's femur is due to bone metastases. The paracetamol being commenced for her headaches may also help to relieve bone pain. In addition, nonsteroidal anti-inflammatory drugs (NSAIDs), which can bring considerable relief, should be considered.

Michelle reports that she feels less able to cope with her pain when she is tired and feels low in mood, particularly when she cannot do the things she previously enjoyed, including as part of caring for her children.

Activities

- Reflect on the complex nature of Michelle's different pains and discuss with your assessor/supervisor the importance of a thorough pain assessment for patients who need palliative care.
- Consider how analgesics (primary and adjuvant), adjuvant drugs and nonpharmacological treatment all have a role in relieving Michelle's pain.
- Consider the guidance on transferring patients from oral to SC analgesia (Scottish Intercollegiate Guidelines Network (SIGN). Our guidelines. 2022. sign.ac.uk).

TABLE 32.1	Adjuvant Analgesics Commonly Used for Cancer Pain	
Medication	**Example**	**Indications**
Nonsteroidal anti-inflammatory drugs (NSAIDs)	Naproxen Diclofenac	Bone pain, inflammatory pain, soft tissue infiltration
Corticosteroids	Dexamethasone Prednisolone (less commonly used due to increased fluid retention)	Raised intracranial pressure Neuropathic pain from nerve compression or destruction Soft tissue pressure or infiltration Hepatomegaly (enlarged liver)
Tricyclic antidepressants	Amitriptyline	Neuropathic pain from nerve compression or destruction Paraneoplastic neuropathies
Anticonvulsants	Gabapentin Pregabalin	Neuropathic pain from nerve compression or destruction Paraneoplastic neuropathies
Bisphosphonates	Zoledronic acid Pamidronate	Bone pain

analgesics codeine, morphine and the medications that are collectively known as opioids. Bone pain and neuropathic pain present particular challenges and commonly require adjuvant analgesics (Cherny and Fallon 2015).

Approximately 80%–90% of pain due to cancer can be relieved with oral analgesics and adjuvant medications following the WHO guidelines (Cherny and Fallon 2015). The remaining percentage of pain can be challenging to manage and may require input from specialist palliative care or pain services. For detailed information on complex pain problems, see SIGN (2022), Cherny (2021) and NICE (2016).

There are now new pain assessments, interventions and new delivery methods that were unavailable in 1996 when the WHO ladder was revised. WHO, however, now recognises that despite the mainstay of cancer pain therapy remaining analgesic medications, radiotherapeutic, anaesthetic, neurosurgical, psychological, physiotherapeutic, spiritual and social interventions all play a role (WHO 2019). WHO, however, acknowledges that the analgesic ladder remains a useful tool (WHO 2019)

Fear of Addiction

One barrier to effective pain control in palliative care is the fear that patients, families and some healthcare professionals have of addiction to opioids. This fear is unfounded when the patient has physical pain. The confusion frequently arises when the patient on opioids requires increasing doses to relieve the physical pain arising from progressive disease.

An understanding of the terms 'addiction', 'tolerance' and 'dependence' is useful to reassure the patient and family. Addiction, that is, psychological dependence and craving, is usually seen in individuals who are taking morphine in the absence of physical pain. In contrast, tolerance is an involuntary physiological

response when, having taken the opioids for some time, the patient requires larger doses to benefit from the same analgesic effect. Physical dependence is another physiological response which patients may experience when an opioid is stopped suddenly, such as flu-like symptoms which can be avoided by gradual dose reduction. Tolerance and physical dependence are not the same as addiction and it is important to note that the requirement for increasing doses is most commonly due to disease progression and not pharmacological tolerance (NICE 2016).

Nausea and Vomiting

Nausea and vomiting are common and distressing symptoms in palliative care. The pathophysiology of nausea and vomiting is complex and incompletely understood. There is no antiemetic ladder to guide the multiprofessional team, but a useful guide suggests that where possible, antiemetics should be administered orally, unless active vomiting precludes this (Collis and Mather 2015).

An understanding of the pathophysiology of nausea and vomiting is important to allow the nurse to participate actively in planning care and to explain care to patients and their families.

In order for vomiting to occur, there must be detectors to identify the need to vomit, a coordinating centre and effectors which make the vomiting take place. The main receptors involved in controlling the experience of nausea and need to vomit are located in the:

- gastrointestinal tract
- chemoreceptor trigger zone (CTZ), a specialised area of the brain on the floor of the fourth ventricle
- inner/middle ear
- higher brain centres.

Fig. 32.3 illustrates the location of these receptor sites.

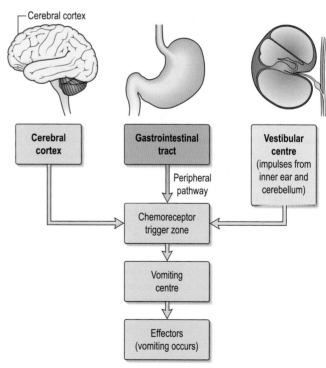

Figure 32.3 The vomiting reflex. (Adapted from Bruce L, Finlay T, eds. *Nursing in Gastroenterology*. Edinburgh: Churchill Livingstone; 1997 with permission.)

Messages from each of these receptor sites are transmitted to the vomiting centre in the medulla (part of the brain stem), which coordinates vomiting. Transmission from the gastrointestinal tract to the vomiting centre is via the vagus nerve. As this nerve innervates other tissues, vomiting may be stimulated by disease or trauma to other organs, for example the pharynx, liver or bladder. Direct stimulation of the vomiting centre by pressure, trauma or disease may also cause vomiting.

In advanced cancer, the vomiting centre can be activated in a number of ways:
- Vagal stimulation caused, e.g. by gastric or bowel distension, liver capsule stretch, mediastinal disease or genitourinary problems.
- Stimulation from the CTZ caused by chemical abnormalities in the blood, e.g. uraemia, hypercalcaemia (excessive calcium level in the blood), drugs or bacterial toxins.
- Stimulation from the inner/middle ear due to infection, movement or local tumour.
- Stimulation from higher central nervous system centres by anxiety, fear or revulsion.
- Direct stimulation from raised intracranial pressure.

Many neurotransmitter receptors have been identified as playing a part in vomiting pathways and understanding of this is developing. What is important in terms of patient care is to appreciate that particular antiemetics are thought to block messages about the need to vomit at specific points along the vomiting pathways. It is this action which produces improvement or control of nausea and vomiting. Some of the commonly used antiemetics in palliative care act centrally at the vomiting centre, vestibular centre and/or the CTZ. Some antiemetics act peripherally in the gastrointestinal tract and some act at both levels. Specific antiemetics must therefore be selected for specific causes of nausea and vomiting. Further information regarding antiemetic medication and prescribing may be found in the British National Formulary (BNF) (see also Lench 2019 and Useful Websites, e.g. palliativedrugs.com). A table outlining the commonly used antiemetic drugs is also provided on the companion website.

Careful assessment is crucial. Working with the patient, the team puts together a detailed picture of these symptoms. The importance of the clinical picture in assessing and managing nausea and vomiting has been recognised (Collis and Mather 2015). The challenge for the multiprofessional team in caring for a patient who is vomiting is to tailor symptom management to the patient's problems, expectations, priorities and wishes. A comprehensive physical examination of the patient is another important source of information. Blood tests may be requested to measure serum urea, calcium and other electrolyte levels, which in some cases may be contributing to nausea/vomiting or be deranged as a result of this.

The multiprofessional team may also consider nonpharmacological measures. The potential benefits of nonpharmacological interventions such as transcutaneous electrical nerve stimulation (TENS), acupuncture and guided mental imagery are acknowledged in the literature, but more research is required. Nursing measures are important, such as encouraging fluid intake, avoiding exposure to strong smells, ensuring good oral hygiene and providing small portions of food.

🌐 **See Evolve website Critical thinking question 32.1**

Constipation

Constipation affects approximately 40% of palliative care patients (McIlfatrick et al. 2019). It may lead on to other serious problems such as faecal impaction, overflow diarrhoea, urinary dysfunction, vomiting and even confusion (Sykes et al. 2007). Careful assessment, management and documentation of this symptom may make the difference between the patient staying at home and hospital admission. The nurse's role in this is crucial. McIlfatrick et al. (2019) provide a good reference point for the assessment, prevention and treatment of constipation in palliative care. Many factors may work together to cause constipation. Sometimes, constipation is disease related. For example, for the patient with cancer, the site of the tumour or the presence of hypercalcaemia may be contributing causes. Eating very small helpings of food with little fibre, drinking considerably less than before and restricted mobility may all contribute to the development of constipation. If the patient is nauseated or experiencing vomiting, then they may be reluctant to eat and drink. When opioids are added to this scenario, constipation becomes a certainty. Opioids have a number of effects on the bowel. They reduce peristalsis, inhibit fluid secretion, increase sphincter tone and diminish sensitivity to rectal distension (Larkin et al. 2008). In this way, the patient can quickly become constipated, struggling to expel small, dry, hard stools.

Anticipation and assessment of this symptom form the basis for effective management. In other words, the nurse does not wait until the patient complains of constipation, but is constantly alert to this possibility, reviewing the situation each day. As part of the holistic assessment of the patient, the nurse needs to take a careful and sensitive history, including:
- previous bowel habits
- the most recent stool (when it was passed, what it was like, any problems experienced)
- intake of diet and fluids
- compliance with laxative regimen
- other medications taken
- accessibility and acceptability of toilet arrangements.

Where constipation is suspected, abdominal and digital rectal examinations are indicated. Depending on local policy and practising within The Code (NMC 2018), a competent registered nurse may perform a digital examination of the rectum. A plain X-ray of the abdomen may be useful in assessing the extent of constipation.

The management of constipation requires more than prescribing and administering laxatives. It involves attention to the relief of pain and other symptoms, to fluids and diet and to adapting toilet facilities to ensure accessibility, comfort and privacy.

An understanding of laxatives is vital, especially for nurse prescribers. Oral and rectal laxatives may be classified as shown in Information 32.2.

A combination of a stimulant and faecal softener, for example Docusate Sodium, gives the most favourable results, at an acceptable dose and with a minimum of unwanted side-effects. The dose should be titrated against patient response. Recently, macrogols such as Movicol have grown in popularity.

As the majority of patients prefer oral to rectal measures, the nurse should endeavour to keep the use of enemas and suppositories to a minimum. All rectal measures act to a greater or lesser extent by stimulating the anocolonic reflex. When rectal treatment is given, the prescriber should review the oral laxative

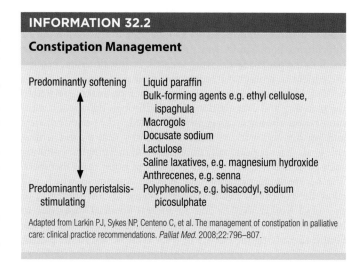

prescription and increase the dose as appropriate. The European consensus group on constipation provides a comprehensive guide (Larkin et al. 2008) but many specialist palliative care teams will have devised a multiprofessional protocol for the use of oral and rectal laxatives, but a case history of a patient with constipation (Ziyad) is also provided on the companion website, which you might want to use for discussion with your assessor/supervisor.

Breathlessness

Breathlessness is a common and distressing symptom of many life-limiting illnesses, including advanced cancer, chronic obstructive pulmonary disease (COPD) and heart failure. Ascertaining the subjective experience for the patient is a vital part of the holistic assessment, as measurable signs such as increased respiratory rate and oxygen saturation are inadequate for fully understanding the total experience of breathlessness for the patient. Patients commonly report feeling such as having to 'fight for air' and that an acute episode can be like choking or suffocating as if 'they are not going to get another breath'. Anxiety and fatigue are therefore commonly associated with breathlessness.

A thorough assessment of the patient is important to exclude reversible causes of breathlessness, such as infection or pulmonary embolus (Chin and Booth 2016). For many patients, their breathlessness is part of a progressive disease process and ongoing management includes both medication and nonpharmacological strategies including breathing control techniques, fan therapy, relaxation and anxiety management, which help to maintain steady breathing during exertion and avoid precipitating an acute attack. Pacing and prioritising activities help patients to manage their energy and achieve daily tasks which are important to them with as little energy expenditure as possible. The occupational therapist and physiotherapist can play key roles in helping the patient to control their breathing and to remain as independent as possible using these strategies. Nurse-led clinics are available in some areas and offer support to patients in coping with the distress associated with breathlessness as well as practical advice regarding the strategies described earlier. Chin and Booth (2016) state that non-pharmacological interventions should be delivered by a multidisciplinary team, with an interest in breathlessness, and that this support should be accessible by patients in all care settings. It is important not to forget that supportive measures such as ensuring a well-ventilated room, the use of a fan and not rushing the

patient can reduce the labour of breathing whilst providing small, easily taken meals can help maintain energy levels.

Medication plays an increasing role in managing breathlessness as the illness progresses. Opioids such as morphine and oxycodone are commonly used via oral and parenteral routes and have been shown to be effective in relieving the sensation of breathlessness (Scottish Palliative Care Guidelines 2022). An immediate-release morphine liquid may be given as a trial dose and according to response can be titrated. Patients usually require lower doses than when given for pain and the interval between doses may be longer. A starting dose may be 2 mg of immediate-release morphine taken on a 4–6-hourly basis, with 2-hourly prn or as required basis may be given to titrate the therapeutic dose (Scottish Palliative Care Guidelines 2022). This can be taken before exertion and in situations where breathlessness can be anticipated. Where the patient is continually breathless at rest, a regular normal-release preparation or a sustained preparation such as MST Continus can be taken, or when the oral route is not viable this can be administered via continuous SC infusion by syringe pump. The patient must be monitored for opiate side-effects such as drowsiness, nausea and constipation and unfounded fears of addiction or hastening disease progression elicited and addressed.

Anxiolytics are another group of commonly used medications for breathlessness and work by relieving feelings of anxiety. There are short-acting preparations, such as the benzodiazepines, for example lorazepam which is administered buccally or sublingually and so rapidly absorbed to relieve intermittent episodes of acute panic and anxiety. Midazolam is a short-acting parenteral benzodiazepine which can be given by SC injection or added to an infusion by syringe pump. Other preparations such as diazepam are longer acting and so useful for continuous or background anxiety, and diazepam can be administered rectally (PR).

When the patient is breathless due to a lack of oxygen, the administration of oxygen can help. In advanced illness, patients may be breathless without lacking oxygen and therefore this is unlikely to help (Scottish Palliative Care Guidelines 2022). Careful assessment of need is required as inappropriate use is unlikely to help, can cause dry, uncomfortable oral or nasal mucosa and ties the patient to nasal cannulae or oxygen mask and tubing. In addition, there can be health and safety issues which must be considered, including the inflammability of oxygen which may be a particular concern in the home setting, where relatives may smoke (see also Johnson and Currow [2021]).

⬤ See Evolve website Critical thinking question 32.2

❖ Nursing Management and Health Promotion: Care of the Dying Patient and Their Family

This section of the chapter will focus on the end-of-life phase of the patient's illness including care in the last days of life and the provision of bereavement support for families and carers.

Caring for a patient who is facing their own mortality and supporting their family and carers through this difficult time can be challenging for health and social care professionals. This time requires careful consideration and skilled communication to enable the patient and family to come to terms with the reality of expected death. Making the adjustment from thinking of oneself as a relatively healthy person who will die someday in the future to thinking of oneself as an ill person who is dying right now is a very big step. Theorists have described the potential emotions and behaviours of people in this situation. Many variables influence the responses of the dying patient and the family, the most notable being personal characteristics, level of social support, past experience of illness and death, age, culture, religious belief and the characteristics specific to the illness. Several theories of the bereavement process have been proposed. Bayliss (2008) and Greenstreet (2004) review a number of seminal theories you may be familiar with and also some of the more contemporary perspectives.

Loss is an abiding feature in the life of a person who is dying – loss of future, loss of role, loss of independence. This period in the palliative care patient's life has been compared to bereavement. Many patients perceive that those who are dying are shunned by health professionals because they cannot be cured. The nurse caring for the dying person needs to be aware of this and must demonstrate the importance of the individual by displaying interest and respect, for example by consulting the patient about their wishes, needs and priorities and thereby helping to maintain self-esteem.

A useful starting point for understanding an individual's response to a life-threatening illness is to consider the question: 'What does this illness mean to this person?'

Suffering

Pain and suffering are terms that are sometimes used as if they had the same meaning; this demonstrates a deep misunderstanding of the experience of human suffering. Physical pain can usually be controlled or reduced, whereas suffering is a much more complex phenomenon, encompassing emotions and psychosocial concerns that, in some instances, may elude control.

Patients and families may suffer because of unresolved issues from the past. There may be guilt, remorse, loss of hope and fear of the future. People who are dying have lost control over their future, may have suffered multiple losses in relation to their previous lifestyle and are often witnessing their decline into total dependence on others. In addition, they may be suffering through observing the effect their imminent demise is having on their family and may be worried about how their survivors will cope. Family members may suffer by watching their loved one's decline and feeling unable to help. Previous experience of poor symptom control in a dying relative or friend may be the cause of considerable anxiety for both patient and family in anticipating the future.

Coping styles have attracted much interest in the literature. There is no doubt that some people cope much more effectively than others in stressful situations. Some, but not all, individuals are flexible in being able to change their lifestyle to their new circumstances, to seek information, to be involved in decision-making, to maintain hope and to preserve their self-worth.

Many factors are involved. These are as diverse as personality, the manner in which the bad news of the diagnosis was broken and the social support available. A previous coping style is not always useful in relation to facing a life-threatening illness. This can be very distressing for patients and families as they struggle with new and fearful situations. For example, a person who tends to cope with stressful life events by being very busy, active and organisational, who needs to feel 'in control' of what's going on around them, may struggle with the constraints imposed by their illness and treatment and lack of control over their day-to-day life. The physical effects of their illness including fatigue and reduced functional ability may preclude the busyness by which they usually avoid dwelling on more emotive issues whilst dependence on others may seem intolerable. How the person sees themselves may change markedly from employee, provider for the family, parent

and this can reduce self-worth. Responses such as emotional withdrawal or strong emotions such as anger due to frustration can be difficult for both family and professionals to deal with and can result in the patient feeling very isolated. In this situation, helping the patient to remain as in control of their situation as possible is needed, including their involvement in decision-making related to the planning and organisation of care. Through therapeutic communication, the nurse can gently acknowledge the person's distress and loss but also work with them to identify realistic and achievable goals that are personally important and meaningful. Fulfilling such goals may require the involvement of other team members. The occupational therapist may provide equipment which will allow the patient to retain a greater degree of independence, or the social worker may be able to address financial issues due to inability to work which relieves the pressure of providing for the family. Identifying the essence of what is important to the patient and how this can be achieved in another way can have a profound effect on the patient's quality of life. For example, a father who highly values playing football with his son as important to their father–son relationship and who can no longer participate due to the physical effects of the illness may find satisfaction and worth in this role by spending time with his son in another way, such as doing his homework with him – something he could never do before his illness because he was working.

Changing coping styles within the time limitations of a life-limiting illness is not generally an option. What is recommended is to adapt existing strategies and provide extra, positive coping strategies to enable individuals to achieve some relief from their suffering.

The assessment of psychological needs, coping styles and how the person is adapting to their situation is integral to holistic assessment. Therapeutic communication forms the basis of this, alongside observation of behaviour and social interactions with others, including family and friends. Whenever the patient is consistently anxious or distressed or when the usual approach to pain management does not appear to be having the desired effect, the nurse caring for the dying patient and their family must consider whether all avenues have been explored to alleviate suffering. Where measures by the multiprofessional team caring for the patient and family appear not to be fully addressing suffering and psychological distress, referral for more specialist input is required. This may be, for example, to specialist palliative care services, a psychologist, social worker or chaplain. Within the multiprofessional team, it is the nurse that usually spends more time with the patient and family than any other professional group and plays a key role in coordinating the input of other team members. The nurse should therefore be alert to the need for further referral for the patient and family and aware of what resources and services are available in their area should such a situation arise.

Realising the enormity of suffering that may be experienced by both patient and family can be daunting when providing palliative care; however, help and support can and should be offered. By building up a supportive relationship with the patient and the family and through therapeutic communication, the nurse may gain some insight into what would be useful for the individual.

Regular communication with the family is a good method of giving support. Family members should never feel they have to constantly search for someone to talk to about the patient or that the nurse or doctor is always too busy. A conscious effort must be made to show respect for family members which can include knowing and using their names and displaying warm body language towards them. Regularly approaching the family and listening to their concerns are important, and exploring who they have within the family circle to give support can help them identify practical solutions to easing the stresses of their caring role. Practical solutions within clinical areas may include providing privacy for the patient and family to talk and so maintain the interpersonal contact between patient and family essential for maintaining family bonds and ties.

Mind and body are inextricably linked. The stresses caused by suffering may evoke physiological effects on the body, such as muscle tension which can exacerbate pain, anxiety which interferes with sleep and nausea which reduces appetite. Many palliative patients seek to use complementary and alternative medicine (CAM) therapies, and whilst these may be of benefit to patients and make them feel better, the evidence base to support these therapies is weak and thus they are not universally available. Relaxation, massage, music therapy and other distractions may help to relieve the stresses of dying.

It is important to remember that a life-limiting illness can affect the very meaning individuals attach to their life and raise a number of spiritual concerns. Spirituality and religion are commonly considered to be the same. A person's religion may be integral to their spirituality; however, 'spirituality' is a much wider term which includes the meaning patients attribute to their illness and the dying process. Thought-provoking accounts of this aspect of care are given in a number of texts (see Further Reading, e.g. Goodhead and Hartley 2017).

Whenever the patient is consistently anxious or distressed or when the usual approach to pain management does not appear to be having the desired effect, the nurse caring for the dying patient and their family must reconsider whether there is a requirement for specialised support from a chaplain, counsellor or clinical psychologist.

End-of-Life Care

When it is recognised that the patient has entered the last phase of their illness, there is a shift in the priorities and the organisation of care. The focus moves from achieving a quality of life and supporting the patient in prioritising comfort and controlling symptoms whilst their illness is progressing to ensuring a peaceful death and supporting the family in coping with their impending loss.

Recognising that the patient has entered the terminal phase of their illness allows the multiprofessional team to plan end-of-life care. This includes consideration of the patient's expressed wishes regarding care and where they wish to die. It is important to recognise, however, that the patient's wishes can change over time as their circumstances change. Perspectives change between thinking of dying as something that will happen in the future and when later faced with the reality of this in the immediate future. Sensitive revisiting of such issues may therefore be required, as appropriate to the patient's condition and their ability to participate in such discussions.

Over recent years, defining criteria for diagnosing that the patient is in the terminal, dying phase has received considerable attention (Boyd and Murray 2010, Highet et al. 2014). This follows recognition that the trajectories of different illnesses can vary markedly. The typical cancer trajectory, for example, is a steady decline where the patient becomes progressively weaker, usually over a period of months, with a period of rapid escalation in the last few weeks of life. This makes the terminal phase of the illness

recognisable as the patient becomes progressively weaker and more dependent, is bed bound, eats and drinks less and sleeps for longer periods. In contrast, patients with organ failure including heart failure and chronic respiratory disease most commonly experience this deteriorating condition over 2 to 3 years; however, this is also punctuated with increasingly frequent acute exacerbations. The outcome of these exacerbations becomes more unpredictable as the illness progressively fails to respond to treatments, and death can occur suddenly during an acute exacerbation or may occur following a period of general decline.

A third trajectory, most commonly experienced by people with dementia and general ageing, is the longest trajectory of palliative care and is that of progressive decline which may last over a few years. Patients can be very frail and dependent for some time and this can result in professionals failing to recognise that the illness has now reached the stage where the patient is in the terminal phase and imminently dying. Patients are at risk of pneumonia and other such conditions which may act as a terminal event that precipitates their death.

This emphasises that, to provide palliative care, nurses must therefore have a sound understanding of the pathophysiology of the patient's illness and the likely disease trajectory. The decision that the patient is in the terminal phase and at the end of life should be made in a multiprofessional team context. Commonly used criteria include:

- The patient is bed bound and semicomatose/comatose.
- The patient is unable to take oral tablets and fluids/only sips of fluids.
- Reversible causes of deterioration in the patient's condition have been excluded.

Essential features of end-of-life care include stopping inappropriate interventions such as blood tests and antibiotics. The patient's medications should be reviewed to ensure that any unnecessary medications are withdrawn and the patient only receives those that will help to make them more comfortable. Essential medications directed at controlling symptoms and ensuring comfort, such as analgesics and antiemetics which the patient was previously taking by mouth, may require to be given parenterally via continuous SC infusion by syringe pump. Anxiolytic medications such as the benzodiazepines, for example lorazepam and midazolam, are frequently prescribed in palliative care to help the patient sleep at night and to relieve anxiety, terminal agitation or distress (Krakeauer 2021).

It must be noted, however, that the patient's symptoms can change at the end of life and prn medications must always be available in case of any breakthrough symptoms. Appropriate anticipatory prescribing means that if medication is required, there is no delay due to waiting for prescriptions to be written. This is also necessary to consider for patients who may never have experienced any symptoms before, as symptoms may occur during this phase. The following medications may be prescribed for intermittent SC injection:

- analgesia – usually morphine or oxycodone as first line
- a broad-spectrum antiemetic, e.g. levomepromazine
- an anxiolytic in case of terminal anxiety and distress, e.g. midazolam
- an antisecretory medication, e.g. hyoscine butylbromide or glycopyrronium, in case respiratory secretions become problematic.

A common symptom in the last days of life is increased or retained small amounts of secretions that accumulate in the oropharynx or bronchial tree, which the patient close to death cannot clear by coughing or swallowing due to overwhelming fatigue and often unconsciousness. This causes a gurgling noise when the patient breathes in and out which is commonly termed 'the death rattle'. This noise can be distressing for families to hear, therefore explanation and reassurance are essential. It is often compared to snoring; the person snoring is not aware or distressed by the snoring but the noise can be difficult for others to hear it occurring. Unless secretions are purulent and copious, suctioning usually has limited effect and the administration of antisecretory medications is required. Careful positioning can also help, with the patient's head to the side supported by pillows and avoiding semirecumbent or supine positions.

In addition to supporting care for the patient, attention to the psychological and spiritual care of the patient and family is important. Care at this time includes supporting the family in spending as much time with the patient as is wished and sensitively answering any questions they may have. This may include explaining what is happening and the physical changes they see as the patient is dying.

Attention to and respect for religious and cultural beliefs are an essential dimension of palliative care throughout the patient's illness. In relation to end-of-life care and following the patient's death, there may be customs and traditions important to the patient and family which must be followed. A useful resource is *Spiritual Care: A Multi-Faith Resource for Healthcare Staff*, which can be accessed from NHS Education for Scotland (see Useful Websites).

The Gold Standards Framework (Clifford et al. 2016, Thomas et al. 2022) outlines good practice in relation to the provision of palliative care in community settings, including the patient's own home, nursing homes and community hospitals. The aim is to support local processes of care delivery by GPs and primary care teams. There are seven standards for the provision of palliative care, referred to as the seven Cs:

- communication
- coordination of care
- control of symptoms
- continuity including 'out of hours'
- continued learning for the multiprofessional team
- carer support
- care in the dying phase.

Implementation of the Gold Standards Framework or equivalent has been identified as a requirement by both the Scottish Government and Department of Health in their respective strategies for palliative care: Strategic Framework for Action on Palliative and End of Life Care 2016–2021 (Scottish Government 2015) and the End of Life Care Strategy (Department of Health 2008). Reflection 32.4 provides an opportunity to reflect on end-of-life care.

The Liverpool Care Pathway (LCP) was developed as an evidence-based care pathway to inform the provision of end-of-life care for patients who were in nonspecialist settings such as acute hospitals. In 2013 the LCP came under intense media scrutiny largely due to inappropriate use in some care settings, with some reports of its use contributing to the hastening of death. Each of the four nations' governments in the UK decided to withdraw its use and it was phased out in 2014.

To address the void in guidance for practitioners providing palliative care, the Scottish Government outlined a principles-based approach (Scottish Government 2019) and the Leadership Alliance for the Care of Dying People: One Chance to Get it Right (LACDP 2014) developed the five Priorities for Care of the Dying Person.

REFLECTION 32.4

End-of-Life Care

Access the information available on the Gold Standards Framework and the Supportive and Palliative Care Indicators Tool websites. Reflect on the principles of palliative care (Reflection 32.1) and consider the following.

Activities

- How do you think these tools could support nursing practice?
- What may be the benefits to (a) patients, (b) families and (c) the multiprofessional team in using these tools to support palliative care?

Resources

Gold Standards Framework. Welcome to Gold Standards Framework. https://www.goldstandardsframework.org.uk/.
Supportive and Palliative Care Indicators Tool (SPICT), https://www.spict.org.uk/.

The Needs of the Professional

It is important to recognise one's limitations and feelings towards mortality when caring for people who are approaching death. A number of research studies, including that of Ekedahl and Wengstrom (2007), have identified that nurses also experience existential concerns and other stressors in caring for people who are dying. Often, it is useful to reflect with a colleague or clinical supervisor how one feels regarding this type of caregiving. This is not a sign of weakness or inability. To the contrary, acknowledgement of one's own feelings may help develop an empathic understanding of what the patient and family are experiencing at this time and positive strategies for coping with the emotional cost of caring. Failure to do so can result in nurses distancing themselves as a protective mechanism which can interfere with therapeutic communication and leave patients and families feeling isolated. The multiprofessional team may also suffer (Davis 2005) and a culture of mutual support must be developed by those caring for the dying.

Bereavement Support

Bereavement support for the family begins before the patient dies, in supporting family members in adjusting to the impending death of the patient. Care around the time of death plays a crucial role in facilitating adjustment to loss and a future without the patient. This includes allowing the family time to be with the patient, to say goodbye and to ventilate their grief where wished.

Many people go through the bereavement process with no professional support, finding that informal support from family and friends is sufficient. For a minority of individuals, professional help is, however, required. Recognised risk factors for a complicated bereavement include sudden, unexpected death, traumatic death, an ambivalent relationship with the deceased and previous mental health, drug or alcohol issues.

As the nurse working in the hospital setting who has cared for the patient until death, your involvement with family members may end here; however, in other settings, such as the community or hospice settings, your involvement may also extend to bereavement care of the family. Relatives of those you have cared for in practice may also ask you where they can receive support. It is therefore helpful to be ready to answer these questions promptly and accurately. The nurse should also be able to identify those at risk of a complicated bereavement and ensure they know where to access support where required.

Sources of Bereavement Support

There are a number of agencies available to provide professional bereavement services; however, they are individual to regions and countries (in the UK). Examples include hospital-based services, chaplaincy or psychologist/psychiatric services, local hospices, Cruse Bereavement Care and Macmillan Cancer Support as well as GP surgeries and hospital palliative care teams. Some of these may also provide information for grieving children and adolescents (Together for Short Lives 2023).

Increasingly, information is being provided online, making it easy for those with computer skills and internet access to gain information and support. However, these are open to interpretation and some may include chat rooms. A selection of reliable sources is provided on the companion website.

The advantages of online help include its availability 24 hours a day, so the individual may access this source as and when is convenient to them. Each site offers practical advice as well as some offering discussion boards. Discussion boards may help the bereaved identify with others who are experiencing similar feelings regardless of whether they participate in posting messages or not.

However, there are disadvantages. People who prefer to talk to someone about their feelings may not find this method helpful but they may be able to access sources where they may talk over the phone or in a local group/individual setting. Not everyone has computer/internet access or the reasonable level of navigation skill required.

Health Promotion in Palliative Care

For many, including the general public, applying the term 'health promotion' to care of dying patients may seem inappropriate. Yet it should be apparent from reading this chapter that health promotion is a key aspect of palliative nursing care. This includes providing information, equipment and support for patients and families to enable them to retain as much independence as possible and to focus on a quality of life throughout their illness. Specific examples include addressing patient concerns regarding addiction when taking morphine, ensuring they know that normal-release morphine preparations should be taken every 4 hours and how to avoid opiate-induced constipation by concurrent use of laxatives, facilitating compliance, reducing anxiety and alleviating pain. Effective management of pain contributes to avoiding suffering and distress which can lead to depression and enhances the person's ability to be physically active, so reducing the risks of immobility such as pressure ulcers (see Chapter 23, Tissue Viability and Managing Chronic Wounds). Advance care planning and therapeutic communication can support the patient in accepting the reality of their situation and making decisions that are important to them with regard to treatment and place of care/death, avoiding later distress from unfinished business. Supporting the family in coping with loss and preparing for the patient's death, including identifying and utilising positive coping mechanisms, can facilitate successful adjustment to their bereavement and thus is also a key dimension of health promotion.

Recently, the need to address public awareness and attitudes towards death and dying has been recognised. Changing societal perspectives are described by Kellehear (2007) and the requirement to consider these in service planning is outlined within national strategy (National Palliative and End of Life Care Partnership 2021, Scottish Government 2015).

Summary: Key Nursing Issues

- This chapter has introduced you to the philosophy of palliative care which includes the assessment and management of the symptoms of advanced illness as well as the provision of compassionate care for the patient and family, ensuring their psychological and spiritual needs are met.
- The principles of palliative care were introduced which outlines the need for therapeutic communication with the patient and their family, holistic assessment and care management,

effective symptom control, good multiprofessional team working and advance care planning.
- Adoption of this model for practice may help the nurse to apply the philosophy of palliative care within any care setting.
- Palliative care undeniably requires a multiprofessional approach; however, nurses fulfil key responsibilities as palliative care is an integral aspect of their role.
- When cure is not possible, prioritising symptom control and patient comfort is considered to be the very essence of nursing.

Reflection and Learning – What Next?

- **Test** your knowledge by visiting the Evolve website 🌐 and answering the multiple-choice questions and critical thinking questions.
- **Consolidate** your learning by looking at some of the further reading suggestions, references and specialist websites.
- **Revisit** some of the additional material on the Evolve website.

- **Consider** what you have learnt and how this will help your professional development.
- **Reflect** on how you can apply this knowledge to the care of your patients.
- **Discuss** your learning with your assessor/supervisor, lecturer and colleagues.

References

Bayliss J. Rethinking loss and grief. In: Nyatanga B, ed. *Why Is It so Difficult to Die?* 2nd ed. London: Quay Books; 2008:241–254.
Boyd K, Murray SA. Recognising and managing key transitions in end of life care. *BMJ.* 2010;341:c4863.

Brighton LJ, Koffman J, Hawkins A, et al. A systematic review of end-of-life care communication skills training for generalist palliative care providers: research quality and reporting guidance. *J Pain Symptom Manage.* 2017;54(3):417–425.
Care Quality Commission (CQC). A different ending. 2016 May: https://www.cqc.org.uk/publications/themed-work/different-ending-end-life-care-review.

Cherny NI. Chronic cancer pain syndromes. In: Cherny NI, Fallon M, Kaasa S et al, eds. *Oxford Textbook of Palliative Medicine*. 6th ed. Oxford: Oxford University Press; 2021:345–363.

Cherny NI, Fallon M. Cancer induced bone pain. In: Cherny NI, Fallon M, Kaasa S et al, eds. *Oxford Textbook of Palliative Medicine*. 5th ed. Oxford: Oxford University Press; 2015:841–859.

Chin C, Booth S. Managing breathlessness: a palliative care approach. *Postgrad Med J*. 2016;92(1089):393–400.

Clifford C, Thomas K, Armstrong-Wilson J. Going for Gold: the Gold Standards Framework programme and accreditation in primary care. *End of Life J*. 2016;6:e000028.

Cloyes K, Hull W, Davis A. Palliative and end of life care for lesbian, gay, bisexual and transgender (LGBT) cancer patients and their caregivers. *Semin Oncol Nurs*. 2018;34(1 February):60–71.

Collis E, Mather H. Nausea and vomiting in palliative care. *BMJ*. 2015;351.

Connolly M, Ryder M, Frazer K, et al. Evaluating the specialist palliative care clinical nurse specialist role in an acute hospital setting: a mixed methods sequential explanatory study. *BMC Palliat Care*. 2021;20:134. https://doi.org/10.1186/s12904-021-00834-y.

Davis H. The emotional load of caring: care for those for whom there is no cure. In: Nyatanga B, Astely-Peper M, eds. *Hidden Aspects of Palliative Care*. London: Quay Books; 2005:143–158.

Department of Health: End of Life Care Strategy – promoting high quality care for all adults at the end of life. 2008.

Dixon J, King D, Matosevic T, et al. *Equity in the Provision of Palliative Care in the UK: A Review of the Evidence*. Personal Social Services Research Unit, London School of Economics and Political Science; 2015. https://www.mariecurie.org.uk/globalassets/media/documents/policy/campaigns/equity-palliative-care-uk-report-full-lse.pdf.

Ekedahl M, Wengstrom Y. Nurses in cancer care – stress when encountering existential issues. *Eur J Oncol Nurs*. 2007;11(3):228–237.

Fleuren N, Depla MFIA, Janssen DJA, Huisman M, Hertogh CMPM. Underlying goals of advance are planning (ACP): a qualitative analysis of the literature. *BMC Palliative Care*. 2020;19:27. https://doi.org/10.1186/s12904-020-0535-1.

Gold Standards Framework. Advance care planning. 2018. https://www.goldstandardsframework.org.uk/advance-care-planning.

Greenstreet W. Palliative care nursing. Why nurses need to understand the principles of bereavement theory. *Br J Nurs*. 2004;13(10):590–593.

Griffith R, Tengnah C. *Law and Professional Issues in Nursing*. 5th ed. Exeter Learning Matters; 2020.

Highet G, Crawford D, Murray SA, Boyd K. Development and evaluation of the Supportive and Palliative Care Indicators Tool (SPICT): a mixed-methods study. (Development and evaluation of SPICT). *BMJ Support Palliat Care*. 2014;4(3):285–290. doi:10.1136/bmjspcare-2013-000488.

Hospice UK. 2021. Equality in Hospice and End of Life Care, Challenges and Change. Available at: https://hukstage-new-bucket.s3.eu-west-2.amazonaws.com/s3fs-public/2021-10/Equality%20in%20hospice%20and%20end%20of%20life%20care%20-%20May%202021_0.pdf.

Hospice UK. 2023. Homepage. https://www.hospiceuk.org/.

Johnson MJ, Currow DC. Breathlessness and other respiratory symptoms in palliative care. In: Cherny NI, Fallon M, Kaasa S et al, eds. *Oxford Textbook of Palliative Medicine*. 6th ed. Oxford: Oxford University Press; 2021:589–603.

Kellehear A. *A Social History of Dying*. Cambridge: Cambridge University Press; 2007.

Klarare A, Hagelin CL, Fürst CJ, Fossum B. Team interactions in specialized palliative care teams: a qualitative study. *J Palliat Med*. 2013; 16(9):1062–1069.

Klint A, Bondesson E, Rasmussen B, Fürst C, Schelin M. Dying with unrelieved pain—prescription of opioids is not enough. *J Pain Symptom Manage*. 2019;58(5):784–791.

Krakeauer EL. Medical and ethical considerations in palliative care sedation. In: Cherny NI, Fallon M, Kaasa S et al, eds. *Oxford Textbook of Palliative Medicine*. 6th ed. Oxford: Oxford University Press; 2021:1180–1188.

Larkin PJ, Sykes NP, Centeno C, et al. The management of constipation in palliative care: clinical practice recommendations. *Palliat Med*. 2008;22:796–807. https://doi.org/10.1177/0269216308096908.

Leadership for the Alliance of the Care of Dying People (LACDP). 2014. One chance to get it right; improving people's experience of care in the last few days and hours of life. https://assets.publishing.service.gov.uk/government/uploads/system/uploads/attachment_data/file/323188/One_chance_to_get_it_right.pdf.

Lench C. Nausea and vomiting in palliative care. *Clin Med*. 2019;19(4):299–301.

McIlfatrick S, Muldrew D, Beck E, et al. Examining constipation assessment and management of patients with advanced cancer receiving specialist palliative care: a multi-site retrospective case note review of clinical practice. *BMC Palliative Care*. 2019;18 Article number: 57.

Meier EA, Gallegos JV, Thomas LP, et al. Defining a good death (successful dying): literature review and a call for research and public dialogue. *Am J Geriatr Psychiatry*. 2016;24(4):261–271.

National Audit of Care at End of Life. Fourth Round of the Audit 2022/2023. Report England and Wales. 2023. https://s3.eu-west-2.amazonaws.com/nhsbn-static/NACEL/2023/NACEL%202022%20Summary%20Report%20-%20Final.pdf.

National Institute for Health and Care Excellence (NICE). *Palliative Care for Adults: Strong Opioids for Pain Relief. NICE Clinical Guidance*. National Institute for Health and Care Excellence; 2016.

National Palliative and End of Life Care Partnership. Ambitions for Palliative and End of Life Care: A National Framework for Local Action: 2021–2026. May 2021. ambitions-for-palliative-and-end-of-life-care-2nd-edition.pdf.

Nursing and Midwifery Council (NMC). *The Code: Professional Standards of Practice and Behaviour for Nurses, Midwives and Nursing Associates*. Read The Code online – The Nursing and Midwifery Council; 2018. nmc.org.uk.

O'Connor M, Fisher C. Exploring the dynamics of interdisciplinary palliative care teams in providing psychosocial care: 'Everybody thinks that everybody can do it and they can't'. *J Palliat Med*. 2011;14(2):191–196.

Office for National Statistics. National Life Tables—Life Expectancy in the UK: 2018–2020. *Census*. 2021. ons.gov.uk.

Reigada C, Arantzamendi M, Centeno C. Palliative care in its own discourse: a focused ethnography of professional messaging in palliative care. *BMC Palliat Care*. 2020;19:88. https://doi.org/10.1186/s12904-020-00582-5.

Resuscitation Council UK. *For Health Professionals and Healthcare Organisations*. Resuscitation Council UK; 2023a. https://www.resus.org.uk/.

Resuscitation Council UK. *ReSPECT for Healthcare Professionals*. Resuscitation Council UK; 2023b. https://www.resus.org.uk/respect/respect-healthcare-professionals.

Royal College of Nursing. *When Someone Asks for Your Assistance to Die. RCN Guidance on Responding to a Request to Hasten Death*. 2nd ed. London: RCN; 2016. Available at: https://www.rcn.org.uk/professional-development/publications/PUB-005822.

St Christopher's Hospice. More than just a hospice. 2023. stchristophers.org.uk.

Sallnow L, Richardson H, Murray SA. The impact of a new public health approach to end-of-life care: a systematic review. *Palliat Med*. 2016;30(11):200–211. doi:10.1177/0269216315599869.

Schofield P. The assessment of pain in older people: UK national guidelines. *Age Ageing*. 2018;47:i1–i22. doi:10.1093/ageing/afx192.

Schuster M, Bayer O, Heid F, Laufenberg-Feldmann R. Opioid rotation in cancer pain treatment. *Dtsch Arztebl Int*. 2018;115(9):135–142.

Scobie S, Hutchings R. End of life care explained: what it is, how it is provided and what are the challenges. *Nuffield Trust*; 2023. Available at: https://www.nuffieldtrust.org.uk/resource/end-of-life-care-explained-what-is-it-how-is-it-provided-and-what-are-the-challenges.

Scottish Government. Caring for people in the last days and hours of life – national statement. 2014. https://www.gov.scot/Publications/2014/12/9301.

Scottish Government. Strategic framework for action on palliative and end of life care 2016–2021. 2015. http://www.gov.scot/Resource/0049/00491388.pdf.

Scottish Intercollegiate Guidelines Network (SIGN). *Control of Pain in Adults With Cancer*. Edinburgh: SIGN; 2022. https://www.palliativecareguidelines.scot.nhs.uk.

Scottish Palliative Care Guidelines. 2022. Available at: https://rightdecisions.scot.nhs.uk/scottish-palliative-care-guidelines/?UID=80514845720236111189 10.

Seymour JE, Clark D, Hughes P, et al. Clinical nurse specialists in palliative care: (3). Issues for the Macmillan Nurse role. *Palliat Med.* 2002;16:386–394.

Shaw KL, Clifford C, Thomas K, Meehan H. Improving end-of-life care: a critical review of the Gold Standards Framework in primary care. *Palliat Med.* 2010;24(3):317–329.

Sykes N, Ripamonti C, Bruera E, et al. Constipation, diarrhoea and intestinal obstruction. In: Fallon M, Hanks G, eds. *ABC of Palliative Care*. Oxford: Blackwell Publishing; 2007:29–35.

Thomas K, Armstrong-Wilson J, Clifford C. The Gold Standards Framework Hospital programme: implementation and progress. *Int J Palliat Nurs.* 2022;28(4):172–177.

Together for Short Lives. 2023. Together for Short Lives: Children's Charities – Children Hospices. https://www.togetherforshortlives.org.uk/.

Warner R, Hoinville L, Pottle E, Taylor C, Green JSA. Refocusing cancer multidisciplinary team meetings in the United Kingdom: comparing urology with other specialties. *Ann R Coll Surg Engl.* 2021;103(1). https://doi.org/10.1308/rcsann.2020.0212.

World Health Organisation. *WHO guidelines for the pharmacological and radiotherapeutic management of cancer pain in adults and adolescents*. WHO; 2019. https://www.who.int/publications/i/item/9789241550390.

World Health Organisation. *Palliative Care*. Geneva: WHO; 2022. Cancer, https://www.who.int/news-room/fact-sheets/detail/palliative-care.

Further Reading

Cherny N, Fallon M, Kaasam S et al, eds. *The Oxford Textbook of Palliative Medicine*. 6th ed. New York: Oxford University Press; 2021.

Gold Standards Framework. *Overview of the work of the National GSF Centre in End of Life Care*. Welcome to Gold Standards Framework; 2017. https://www.goldstandardsframework.org.uk/.

Goodhead A, Hartley N. *Spirituality in Hospice Care*. London: Kingsley; 2017.

Griffith R, Tengnah C. *Law and Professional Issues in Nursing*. 6th ed. Exeter: Learning Matters; 2023.

Leadership for the Alliance of the Care of Dying People (LACDP). One Chance to Get It Right. https://assets.publishing.service.gov.uk/government/uploads/system/uploads/attachment_data/file/323188/One_chance_to_get_it_right.pdf.

National Palliative and End of Life Care Partnership. Ambitions for Palliative and End of Life Care: A National Framework for Local Action 2021–2026. 2021. ambitions-for-palliative-and-end-of-life-care-2nd-edition.pdf (england.nhs.uk).

Nicol J, Nyatnga B. *Palliative and End of Life Care in Nursing (Transforming Nursing Practice Series)*. London: Sage; 2017.

Nyatanga B. *Why Is It so Difficult to Die?* London: Quay Books; 2008.

ReSPECT. The ReSPECT process creates personalised recommendations for a person's clinical care and treatment in a future emergency in which they are unable to make or express choices. www.respectprocess.org.uk.

Royal College of Nursing. End of life care. Clinical. Royal College of Nursing. rcn.org.uk.

Walshe C, Preston N, Johnston B. *Palliative Care Nursing. Principles and Evidence Base for Practice*. 3rd ed. London: Open University Press; 2017.

World Health Organisation (WHO). *Cancer Pain Relief. Cancer Pain Management Guidelines*. Geneva, Switzerland: World Health Organisation; 2023. who.int.

Worthington R. *Ethics and Palliative Care: A Case Based Manual*. Oxon: Radcliffe Publishing; 2005.

Useful Websites

British National Formulary (BNF), https://bnf.nice.org.uk/.

Cruse Bereavement Care, Home – Cruse Bereavement Support

Education for Scotland Spiritual Care: A Multi-Faith Resource for Healthcare Staff 2021 https://www.nes.scot.nhs.uk/media/ay4je0io/multi-faith-resource-for-healthcare-staff.pdf

Gold Standards Framework, www.goldstandardsframework.org.uk

GOV.UK, Bereavement website, What to do when someone dies: step by step, www.gov.uk

Hospice UK, Homepage

International Association of Palliative and Hospice Care, https://www.hospiceuk.org/

Macmillan Cancer Support (incorporating Cancer BACUP), https://www.macmillan.org.uk/

Marie Curie, https://www.mariecurie.org.uk/

National Institute for Health and Care Excellence (NICE), www.nice.org.uk, www.palliativedrugs.com (provides a formulary of medications used for palliative care and a discussion forum used by experts in palliative care from around the world. Access is free, although registration is required)

Scottish Intercollegiate Guidelines Network, www.sign.ac.uk

Scottish Partnership for Palliative Care, www.palliativecarescotland.org.uk

Sue Ryder Care, www.suerydercare.org

World Health Organisation (WHO) (2018), WHO guidelines for the pharmacological and radiotherapeutic management of cancer pain in adults and adolescents, https://apps.who.int/iris/handle/10665/279700

World Health Organisation (WHO), Palliative care, https://www.who.int/news-room/fact-sheets/detail/palliative-care

33

Nursing Care for Older People

JITKA VSETECKOVA, CHERYL HOLMAN

Introduction

The reduction of mortality rates and fertility rates over time has shaped the age structure of UK society. It is a 21st century phenomenon that more people reach old age and live longer; consequently, there is a larger proportion of older people in the population overall. This trend is expected to continue, and the Government Office for Science (GOS) (2019) predicts that 70% *of population growth between 2014 and 2039 will be in the 60+ age group. Although the process of population ageing is more advanced in wealthy countries, there has been a rapid increase in the number of older people across the world including developing regions and it is predicted by 2050, the number of people aged 65 years or over worldwide is projected to be more than twice the number of children under age 5 and about the same as the number of children under age 12.*

(United Nations Department of Economic and Social Affairs 2022).

Clearly, each older person's needs are different according to their individual circumstances and personalities, but it is helpful to have a critical understanding of some of the significant social trends that impact on people's health in later life. In economically developed countries, most people are living well in old age and for many people, it is a time when they have access to financial and time resources (Hill et al. 2022). Factors such as social class, gender and ethnicity can impact on a person's potential in early as well as later life (Heaslip et al. 2022) and manifest in social determinants of health such as housing conditions, income through pensions and access to independent living. Another sociological perspective is that old age is shaped by the beliefs and practices of individuals and communities (Rajan-Rankin 2018). This can be seen in cultural differences in expectations of work and retirement, family size and divorce and how care for vulnerable people is organised in communities. A blend of social factors, cultural beliefs and personal circumstances are likely to influence people's capacity to embrace opportunities in old age (Heaslip et al. 2022), perceive their own health and negotiate some of the challenges of old age.

Increase in longevity is an indicator of a society's success. Opportunities in old age have altered and expectations of older people are changing. The large numbers of people born between the mid-1940s and mid-1960s, known as Baby Boomers (Martin et al. 2021), are different from their parents' generation and are likely to have fewer children and more open attitudes towards divorce and dynamic family lives and relationships. This cohort of older people hopes for leisure in a long retirement and may achieve it due to financial stability through home ownership (Genoe et al. 2019).

Significance of an Ageing Population

Biggs (2014) suggests that a deep reflection on the meaning of a long life is required by ageing societies to ensure new and positive ways to achieve an integrated population. He challenges assumptions that caring for older people is perceived as a burden by younger generations and proposes re-examining intergenerational relationships. Importantly for healthcare providers, he supports a long-term commitment to the promotion of health and the prevention of illness in later life. Key issues related to a health in later life are: staying well and keeping fit and managing long-term conditions (Carrier 2022).

There is a suggestion that healthy ageing is closely linked to an active lifestyle and this is not just about being physically active but also participating socially and emotionally in life (São José et al. 2017). There is a developing body of research which indicates physical exercise, diet, technology and types of social engagement might help older people maximise their health and wellbeing, whether they are living in the community on their own or in assisted living or a long-term facility (Borgstrom et al. 2022). The approach used by these researchers is exemplary in that it brings together knowledge from a wide range of disciplines, involves older people themselves and adopts a holistic perspective, but may inadvertently contribute to an assumption that there is an ideal way to age (São José et al. 2017). Healthcare practitioners need to be aware of evidence that underpins health and health promotion in old age but also be prepared to care for individuals who do not fit a blueprint of a healthy lifestyle.

Although patterns of illness continually change, the increase in longevity for so many people has given rise to an increase in noncommunicable diseases common to old age. It is suggested that in England, more than 40% of those over 65 report having chronic diseases and 15% more say they have two chronic diseases (OECD/European Observatory on Health Systems and Policies 2019). The common chronic illnesses are coronary heart disease, diabetes, cancer, hypertension, musculoskeletal conditions and mental health problems (NHS 2019). The care for people with long-term conditions is complex and frequently challenges the resources of health services. Having a long-term condition impacts on a person's quality of life which is further exacerbated by comorbidities (Carrier 2022). Kingston et al. (2018) explain comorbidities as the coexistence of two or more diseases in the same person and that the coexisting diseases may have occurred by chance or be connected to each other. People with physical chronic health problems often concurrently experience mental health problems such as depression, anxiety and, especially, dementia. Approximately 944,000 people have dementia in England, and this figure is predicted to double in the next 30 years (Dementia Statistics Hub 2018).

A sole focus on individual ageing can hide the social inequalities in later life. The chances of having a decent old age are not only dependent on physical and mental health but also vary according to where you live, your access to resources such as heating and financial income from a pension (Centre for Ageing Better 2022) and the disadvantage of poverty and discrimination accumulate in old age. Age UK (2021), citing figures from the Department of Work and Pensions (2021), reports that poverty levels amongst pensioners in the UK have increased from 1.5 million (14%) in 2013–2014 to 2.1 million 18% in 2021. A person's potential to make the most of old age is shaped by access to wealth and some groups such as those living in rented accommodation and people from Black and Asian communities are more likely to be vulnerable to inequalities in accessing health assets (Age UK 2019). Lack of resource in old age has serious implications for health and wellbeing. Every year, older people die due to their homes being too cold, and estimates show that, on any night in England, around 400 older people aged 55 and above may be sleeping rough, and at least 10 times that number will be spending the night in short- and long-term homelessness accommodation (Centre for Policy on Ageing 2017).

A consequence of an ageing society is that most of its citizens die in old age. In England and Wales in 2022, the most common age of death was 87 for men and 89 for women (Office for National Statistics [ONS] 2022). The death rate increased during the COVID-19 pandemic, and it was the leading cause of death in 2021 (ONS 2022) followed by diseases that are usually the common causes of death in old age such as dementia and Alzheimer's disease and ischaemic heart diseases (ONS 2022). Death in old age is frequently preceded by physical and psychological deterioration known as frailty. Physical frailty is linked to very old age, loss of independence and health and increasing a person's risk of illness and death (Sieber 2017). Older people themselves tend to articulate the way they live in frailty in a more holistic and subjective way, referring to the value of relationships and responding to the ups and downs of life (Nicholson et al. 2017). It is important that frailty is not solely understood in terms of health and social care needs so that having a meaningful and self-determined life is important throughout the whole life course.

It is the job, increasingly, of nurses and other members of the multidisciplinary team to work with individual older people who have health and social care needs. It is important that healthcare workers such as nurses, doctors, social workers and therapists work together to coordinate appropriate care of a high standard.

What Happens When We Age?

Research into the physical aspects of ageing has shifted focus from investigations into the diseases that are common in old age to discoveries about old age itself. Insights into ageing at a cellular, tissue and systems level mean that scientists are starting to be able to understand how the ageing process correlates with disease processes (Campisi et al. 2019). Given that old age is a significant risk factor for many long-term conditions, it is predicted this branch of research will increase the impact that health advice will have on the lives of older people.

That biological ageing takes place is beyond dispute (Campisi et al. 2019), despite the efforts of people to deny this or to hide the effects of the ageing process. The changes of ageing not only depend on an individual's makeup and external environment but also how they perceive and experience ageing changes. Attitudes toward old age and how societies are organised to meet the needs of its older and vulnerable citizens also affect health outcomes in later life (Biggs 2014). Older people have diverse experiences and individual personalities; it is important nurses recognise any personal bias they may have and avoid stereotypes (Reflection 33.1).

The next section describes possible physical and psychological changes that may take place in later life, but it should be remembered that these are only a guide to what may occur, rather than a template of what will happen.

Changes in Blood Pressure Control

In later life, the blood vessels are less adaptable because of structural alteration; this can lead to changes in blood pressure. The heart and blood vessels become less responsive to epinephrine and norepinephrine, which means that the homeostatic mechanisms for maintaining blood pressure become less efficient (Moini 2019). One tangible outcome of this is a tendency towards postural hypotension, whereby a sudden change in position from sitting to standing is less well tolerated and blood pressure remains low, sometimes leading to dizziness, loss of balance and falls (Gilani et al. 2021).

In normal ageing, there is an increased thickness of the deep layers of the arteries and a decrease in vascular elasticity. This in turn leads to an increased stiffness of the vascular walls and can develop into hypertension (Moini 2019). Hypertension is when a person's blood pressure is repeatedly high (over 140 mmHg for the systolic blood pressure and over 90 mmHg for diastolic blood pressure) and is common in old age, especially for women (Moini 2019). High blood pressure is usually treated because it causes a person to be at a higher risk of other conditions common to older people, such as coronary heart disease and stroke (Nilsson 2017).

Changes in Exercise Tolerance

Along with changes in the cardiovascular system, there are changes in the respiratory system such that it becomes less efficient at extracting oxygen from the blood (De Favari Signini et al. 2022). This is not usually a problem but it may lead to exercise intolerance. The older person may well be able to go about their normal level of activity as these systems have considerable reserve capacity but will, for instance, be less able to run to catch a bus than they were when they were younger. If a person responds to these changes by maintaining physical fitness and being actively engaged in life, described as active ageing, it may have a positive impact on their overall health and wellbeing (Hijas-Gomez et al. 2020).

Changes in Muscles, Bones and Teeth

Healthy bones and muscles are important in old age. Reduction in muscle mass, muscle strength and physical function is called sarcopenia (Petermann-Rocha et al. 2022) and is linked to poor health outcomes and death. Its development is caused by multiple factors such as hormone changes, lifestyle choices and a person's genetic make-up. The loss of bone mass starts earlier in women than men and is particularly marked in the postmenopausal years, whether a person goes on to develop osteoporosis depends on their bone health in earlier life and the rate of degeneration in later life (Choi et al. 2021). Osteoporosis is common, especially in women, and increases the risk of fractures as the bone becomes more fragile (Choi et al. 2021). Although there are changes to the mouth and teeth in later life, most oral conditions are preventable and treatable. It is important that older people are offered advice and care to prevent dental caries and preserve healthy gums and teeth. This is important for wellbeing and impacts on long-term health (Patel et al. 2021).

Changes in Resistance to Infection

The changes in the immune system that occur with age are complex. The impairment and dysregulation of the body's innate and acquired ability to develop cellular defence in later life is known as immunosenescence (Vetrano et al. 2021). With respect to acquired immunity, there are important changes in the development of T cells which hinder the response to old and newly encountered infective agents. A significant aspect of cellular level ageing results in a chronic low-grade inflammation which reduces the effectiveness of vaccination and is thought to be the trigger for a range of age-related diseases such as type 2 diabetes and Alzheimer's disease (Haynes 2020). If a person becomes frail (having reduced muscle tone, experiencing chronic fatigue and reduced levels of activity), the incidence of infections such as influenza and pneumonia increases and there is additional impact on the effectiveness of vaccination (Vetrano et al. 2021). In turn, although there is little research, it is assumed that multiple infections of these types impact a person's physical and cognitive function.

The interplay between factors such as the changes in immune response in ageing, frailty and opportunity of cross-infection in communal living means people living in care homes are particularly vulnerable to infections such as COVID-19 (Shepherd et al. 2022) and its complications (Haynes 2020). There is a need for research to evaluate the development of systematic rapid responses to infection outbreaks in communities such as care homes which can inform protocols for effective practice (Shepherd et al. 2022).

Changes in Sensory Perception

Most people adapt successfully to the changes to the nervous system in later life and the impact of ageing on the way people perceive and make sense of their surroundings (Moini 2019). There is an inevitable decline in vision as we age, and one in five people aged 75+ are living with sight loss and one in two people aged 90+ (Age UK 2019). The most common causes of sight loss are age-related macular degeneration (AMD) and cataracts (RNIB 2021). AMD distorts central vision over time due to deterioration of the macular which is the tiny part of the retina at the back of the eye and cataracts blur vision as the lens of the eye becomes opaque (Moini 2019).

In the ear, the bones that transmit sound waves from the outer to the inner ear tend to become fused together, thereby reducing their ability to transmit sound, leading to reduced hearing – presbycusis (Moini 2019). This does not mean that all older people are blind and deaf, but this reduction in hearing and vision has to be taken into account when considering their care and support. For example, managing a resident's hearing loss in a care home can prevent loneliness and improve their quality of life (Age UK 2019).

Similarly, it is clear that older people can suffer from pain. Dong et al. (2020) suggest that older people are more likely to experience chronic pain and that it is often more complex and less likely to be reversible. It is important that older people are encouraged to describe their pain so that it can be assessed and managed effectively.

Changes in Thought Processes

Older people are no less intelligent, no less able to remember and recall and no more stubborn than their younger counterparts. There are complex age-related changes in the brain, including a decrease in size of some areas of the brain, and there is a progressive loss of neural tissue but due to the plasticity of the brain neurones, the brain adapts and reshapes to overcome losses (Moini 2019). There is some change in short-term memory with ageing (McCrae 2018), but this does not usually interfere with leading a normal life. Some older people do suffer from age-associated memory impairment (Livingstone et al. 2020) however, it is unclear whether or not this is a precursor to dementia. Intelligence, measured using standard IQ tests, does not decline with age. There is some change in intelligence, with a decline in fluid intelligence (e.g. problem-solving) and an increase in crystallised intelligence (the application of learning to new problems), but these changes do not have a significant impact on daily living (McCrae 2018).

Changes in Emotional Life

There are theories that relate to psychological and sociological changes in later life. The classic study of Erikson et al. (1986) identified stages of ageing during which the ageing person either manages or fails to come to terms with their life in order to develop as a person. The ultimate stage during later life leads to the older person being at peace with life and reconciled to what they have, or have not, done and experienced. The activity theory of ageing and the disengagement theory of ageing (Guyette 2018) acknowledge psychosocial changes with ageing: the former that as people age they give up certain activities and take up others, and the latter, that as people age, they give up activities and gradually withdraw from life and from society. Broadly speaking, these types of theories try to explain how people sustain themselves and grow whilst negotiating losses and challenges that may be incurred through ageing. Sometimes, this relates to social or culturally determined losses such as retirement or the family position of grandparents, whilst other challenges are brought on by individual circumstances such as illness and physical dependence (Reflection 33.2).

⊕ **See Evolve website Critical thinking question 33.1**

Working With Older People

Nurses increasingly work with older people whether or not they specialise in this area and it is important they are treated with appropriate dignity and respect (National Institute for Health and Care Excellence [NICE] 2019). Some nurses choose to work exclusively with older people in hospitals and the community. However, with the increasing proportion of older people in our

society, unless the choice is made to specialise in working with children or in maternity care, nurses will meet older people in general medical and surgical wards, in the community and in many specialist areas. The largest group of users of health and social care services are people aged over 65 years. Health and social care is provided for older people in many different settings by a range of professionals which makes the drive for joined up working very important (NICE 2019).

The organisation of care is complex and it is important that service users and their carers are at the centre of the planning process so that care meets the needs of the individuals (Bunn et al. 2017). For example, if an older person living in a residential care home has a fall, they might have support from their family and the staff who work there. They may have an assessment by a general practitioner or district nurse and be referred to a falls clinic provided by a local hospital or community services. In addition, the person might access privately funded services such as chiropody or optometry as well as needing advice about making adjustments to their living conditions from social services. The role of the nurse working with older people in this type of situation is not only about the provision of care; it also involves working closely with older people and their families and carers and liaison with other members of the multidisciplinary team to coproduce care packages (Bunn et al. 2017).

The nurses' skills in communication, leadership and education are key to the organisation and delivery of care that maximises an older person's potential for health and wellbeing (Reflection 33.3).

The Development of Key Policies and Concerns

At the start of the 21st century, The Health Advisory Service (HAS 2000) produced a pivotal report entitled *Not Because They Are Old*, which made specific reference to the care for older people in acute wards in general hospitals. The report can be described as 'pivotal' because it gave rise to critical determinants of the quality of care in key areas for older people's services and attempted to set standards in rooting out age discrimination, person-centred care, intermediate care helping older people maintain their independence, general hospital care, stroke care, falls, mental health in older people and the promotion of health and active life in old age.

The reports influenced education and the quality of care for older people, however, in 2013, an investigation carried out in a healthcare trust in England (Francis 2013) still found an unacceptable standard of nursing care across a wide range of disciplines, including the care for older people. Francis (2013) surmised that the situation had arisen due to a lack of response by leaders when concerns were raised, not listening to patients and an organisational focus on the wrong priorities. The Francis Report made recommendations about patient safety, quality of care and leadership and

REFLECTION 33.2
Changes in Later Life and Nursing Assessment

Read the section 'What happens when we age?' in this chapter.

Activities
- List the specific considerations for assessing an older person based on your knowledge of what happens when we age.
- For each subheading, write a nursing action that should be carried out when assessing an older person. State your reasons for identifying the nursing actions based on the changes that occur in later life.

REFLECTION 33.3
Networks of Care for Older People

Think about an older person for whom you have helped provide care.

Activities
- List all the healthcare professionals who were involved in their care. Now list all nonprofessionals who were involved in their care.
- Look at your lists and decide in each case whether the nurse's role was to liaise, coordinate or educate.

suggested there was a need to change the culture of care across the whole care system. Following the report, the legal responsibilities of health and social care services for preventing substandard care and abuse were set out in the Health and Care Act 2022 (Bottery et al. 2022). This marked a change in attitudes towards quality of care which had significance for all nurses caring for older people.

Interwoven with policy aimed at the provision of healthcare are the arrangements and funding for social care which is the practical support for people with ongoing needs due to illness or healthcare issues. This can be provided in residential or care homes or people's own homes. Successive governments have failed to adequately address the responsibilities and funding for social care resulting in a lack of choice in the provision, varied access to quality social care and families and individuals often being left with an unexpected financial burden (DHSC Reforming Adult social care in England 2023). The COVID-19 pandemic had a devastating impact on those being care for in residential accommodation (Shepherd et al. 2022) but the extra funding required to deliver support during the COVID-19 has prompted policy development to provide oversight of adult social care (Bottery et al. 2022). It remains to be seen whether the reconstructed aims to provide better quality social care and to give individuals and families more affordable choices in its provision will be realized.

In the current health and economic climate, we are more and more aware of the needs to self-manage and become partners in our healthcare as we age. This highlights a need for evidence-based public health interventions that use accessible language to bring evidence-based recommendations to the ageing populations. The World Health Organisation (WHO) has embraced this positive concept of ageing, defining active ageing as 'the process of optimising opportunities for health, participation, and security in order to enhance quality of life as people age' (WHO 2020). Further to the WHO (2017) Global Strategy and Action Plan, the United Nations (UN) General Assembly declared 2021–2030 the UN Decade of Healthy Ageing (WHO 2020).

Translating research evidence around ageing and healthy lifestyle is not something that has been massively happening in the past but there are some interventions that emerged and support well ageing populations to understand better what ageing naturally brings about and offers easy to do steps, accompanied by 'bitesize' pieces of knowledge and information that supports the ageing populations in following the steps that lead to healthy ageing and more effective self-management.

An example could be the Ageing Well Public Talks Series (AWPTS) developed and delivered via The Open University in partnership with older people, public, voluntary and private sector partnerships. The AWPTS are structured around Five Pillars for Ageing Well (Nutrition, Hydration, Physical, Social and Cognitive Stimulation). Being mindful of the 'Five Pillars for Ageing Well' helps to support the wellbeing of ageing populations in the form of an educational intervention that brings about facilitated learning. The AWPTS is unique in its use of Participatory Public Engagement as the main vehicle for codesign, coproduction, codelivery and impact. The AWPTS brings and translates the available scientific evidence to the public and invites members of the public to share their own experience. This empowers and enables participants to make lifestyle choices that support them living longer and healthier lives.

This then further supports self-management and becoming partner in one's own healthcare. The timing seems to be perfect for such an intervention that takes all known barriers into account to engage wide and diverse audiences, especially when inviting

representatives from diverse populations to shape the direction, coproduction and delivery of the programme of talks.

The AWPTS and related portfolio of work (see Useful Websites section) have been viewed by over 75,000 people since its inception in 2019 and achieved an excellent momentum because of the motivation of all involved in its coproduction, codelivery and also because of the significant and palpable need for this intervention across communities and across borders. The AWPTS and the related portfolio of work:

- Create bridges between communities to allow for a mutual flow of information/knowledge exchange.
- Engage diverse communities in discussions about their health and wellbeing and thus empower the communities to self-manage and become partners in their own healthcare.
- Cofacilitate a step change in user behaviour and support existing health and social care services provision.
- Contribute to the government's (local and central) NHS agendas for prevention of ageing decline and hospital admissions through self-management.
- Connect sustainable, already existing work and support programmes offered by various organisations and networks that already exist in four nations (England, Wales, Northern Ireland and Scotland) and internationally (China, Nepal, Canada, United States, Brazil, Czech Republic, France, Greece, Ireland, Switzerland and Hungary) by working closely with wide and diverse communities in several areas of the country via a continuously widening network of partners.

AWPTS are regularly evaluated and widely support codesign, coproduction and cofacilitation/codelivery in a participatory fashion by the ageing populations, clinicians, practitioners and other third sector stakeholders who support ageing populations in their professional roles. The feedback highlights the impact of the AWPTS on their personal lives, increased confidence and skills to self-manage and/or professional practice, developing their skills and increasing their knowledge and ability to engage with communities of older people supporting thus their self-management. Interventions such as AWPTS make a difference to the lives of ageing populations, professionals, practitioners, volunteers and carers (formal and informal) and others across our health and social care economies in a way that has a potential to either prevent and or support effective self-management when living with a long-term condition(s).

Long-Term Conditions

The effects of living with a long-term condition have been identified as having significant and far-reaching impact on a person's life (Carrier 2022). Ten million UK citizens live with a long-term condition which compromises psychosocial and physical health and wellbeing. Living with long-term conditions often from early years or early adulthood throughout life practically means the as the population ages (ONS 2021, United Nations 2019), more people will enter older age carrying the consequences of decades of chronic illness or long-term conditions. Ageing with a lifelong nonpreventable long-term condition may have minimal to medium impact on life expectancy but significantly reduces healthy life expectancy or disability free life expectancy (ONS 2021, Toye et al. 2019) and creates personal as well as economic burden. The common long-term conditions of old age include cancer, heart disease, diabetes, stroke and dementia. A person may require care when their health degenerates due to a single long-term condition, but in old age, it is more likely the consequence of comorbidity also called multimorbidity; this can be when the person has two (or more) nonrelated conditions or when one long-term condition leads to another (McKee et al. 2021). This has emerged as one of the greatest challenges facing health services (Pearson-Stuttard et al. 2019). Many people with physical long-term conditions have significant mental health problems which impacts on their quality of life (Pearson-Stuttard et al. 2019). This is a key driver for the integration of physical and mental health, primary and secondary care and health and social care. Health and social care should reflect the priorities of the service users and foster growing essential skills in caring for the growing population of adults, particularly older adults, with multiple long-term conditions (Tinetti et al. 2019). Having two or more chronic conditions in middle age is associated with an increased risk of dementia later in life (Hassen et al. 2022) and this in turn increases the need for healthcare professionals to acquire varied and complex skills (Sherlaw-Johnson et al. 2018). It is suggested that working in close partnership with patients and their carers is central to improving their access to services and the quality of care delivered. Sherlaw-Johnson et al. (2018) further suggest that primary care hubs that are dedicated to the care of older people with complex health needs can have a positive impact on quality of care, and on the experiences of both patients and staff.

Equity, Dignity and Care for Older People

It is important that care offered to older people is equitable to the care given to younger people. This means that decisions about access to treatment and care should not be based on age and that it is not appropriate to restrict specific services to certain populations based on age criteria (Government Equalities Office and Equality and Human Rights Commission 2015, Sundgren et al. 2020). Diverse needs in relation to culture, ethnicity, religion, gender, sexuality and disability should be considered and respected in an older client group as in any other. People from all walks of life should be treated with dignity, confirming a person's feeling of self-worth and protecting them from humiliation (Clancy et al. 2021). It is especially important that the provision of health and social care preserves and promotes dignity when an individual has a stigmatised identity, whether it is providing health promotion for a homeless person (Kneck et al. 2021) or end-of-life care for an older person in prison (Novisky et al. 2022).

In delivering individualised and equitable care strategies, it is important to generate knowledge that addresses issues that affect particular groups, for example the cultural significance of food and nurture especially for those from Black and Asian communities (Nair et al. 2022) and that staff working in residential care need appropriate skills and attitudes to be able to provide sensitive care for people who are lesbian, gay, bisexual and transgendered (Bristow et al. 2023). In Evidence-Based Practice 33.1, the key themes of these studies are identified.

Equitable care means that the care services predominantly offered to older people should be of a similar quality to other services. Care for all older people should promote a person's self-respect and usually involves giving respect (Social Care Institute for Excellence 2020b). At the simplest level, this might mean older people's care environments have proper facilities that are clean, well maintained and of sufficient quality to provide privacy. At the more complex level, it means developing a culture of care that respects the personal needs of individuals and generates an evidence base for understanding what is important for specific groups. It is argued that in order to deliver this type of care, nurses need to hold the right values and work in a culture that encourages

compassion both for the service user and the care givers (Maddox et al. 2022).

Person- and Relationship-Centred Care

In person-centred care, nurses and carers get to know the patient, client or resident in an intimate way and this is achieved through a real connection with the other person and their family (Ebrahimi et al. 2021). By taking this approach, communication and care interactions are more likely to prioritise the older person's needs rather than those of the care organisation. It can be argued that by prioritising the individual in person-centred care, there is a missed opportunity to focus on the relationships that mediate care (De Witt and Fortune 2017). This may diminish the importance of the interpersonal processes, the needs of carers and the social systems to the delivery of high-quality and compassionate care. A relationship-centred care framework acknowledges the needs of those delivering care and shifts the focus to the organisation of care rather than just the individuals providing it (Ryan 2021). The reciprocity of the caring relationship is captured in Nolan et al.'s (2001) Senses Framework, where care delivery is of an optimal standard, when the culture of an organisation provides a certain atmosphere or feeling that promotes a sense of security, continuity, belonging, purpose, fulfilment and significance. Importantly, these senses should be felt not only by the older people being cared for but also the staff working with them. Ryan (2021) argues that although there may be subtle differences in these approaches, over time, key themes have emerged from these approaches that evidence person- and relationship-centred care is practiced by nurses:

- *Building therapeutic relationships:* where a continuous, close working relationship underpins the delivery of care.
- *Maintaining identity:* stresses the importance of finding out about the person being cared for and ensuring their uniqueness and individuality is encouraged.
- *Sharing power:* where the person being cared for is enabled to make decisions for themselves and so that their care is consistent with their values and wishes.
- *Engaging with people in a holistic manner:* Recognising care goes beyond physical care and includes psychological, social and spiritual dimensions to the whole person.
- *Relationships as significant:* Understanding that the person being cared for may exist in a range of social networks including family and friends and that the people and the organisation delivering care are also a meaningful part of these relationships.
- Ryan (2021) concludes that there is a range of evidence available to support nurses and the multidisciplinary team in the delivery of person- and relationship-centred care in a range of contexts.

Consent and Older Adults

In poor health, in a state of confusion or when dying, older people may become frail and vulnerable. This does not mean that their rights can be overridden, even in the apparent pursuit of the older person's best interests; action taken must not cause an affront to dignity. According to the Mental Health Capacity Act 2005, wherever possible, the consent of a person to treatment or even a seemingly innocuous nursing intervention is required; treatment, including life-saving treatment, cannot be forced on an older person without consent. Clearly, patient and staff safety is a paramount consideration, but restraint has such harmful consequences (Duxbury et al. 2019) that it should only be applied in conditions that put the person at risk of harm (NHS England 2017). Frail older people who have cognitive impairment and are physically dependent on staff for the fundamental aspects of care are more likely to be subjected to physical restraint (Pu et al. 2020) so it is important nurses and carers understand their responsibilities for recognising abusive care and safeguarding the rights of vulnerable older people.

Communication and Older People

Communication with older people, especially those who have sight and hearing impairment, can be made more effective by the following (Davis et al. 2021, Jack et al. 2019):

- Make time to listen to the older person's ideas, concerns and point of view.
- If you want the person to talk, especially about sensitive issues, ensure privacy and give them your full attention.
- If the person has a communication difficulty, make sure your face can be seen and do not cover your mouth when speaking.
- If the older person wears a hearing aid and/or glasses, make sure they are accessible and in working order.
- Remember, anxiety, pain or confusion is likely to interfere with the ability to communicate. You will need to adapt your communication to the individual's needs. You may need to administer analgesics to control the pain before giving information or have a family member present to help the person cope with their anxiety.
- Be aware of cultural differences; e.g. in some cultures, it is a sign of respect to make eye contact, in others it is a sign of disrespect.
- If the older person does not understand you, choose different words and avoid jargon where possible.
- Visual cues may be helpful, especially if you are trying to explain a complex issue. Charts and pictures can be helpful and interpreters may be necessary for deaf people or people who do not speak English.
- Be mindful of the environment; e.g. consistent lighting can be helpful for individuals with visual impairment and reduce background noise if the person has a hearing impairment.

Perhaps the most important form of communication between nurses and older people in their care is the indirect communication made via the relationships they form. Ryan (2021) suggests that older people prefer nurses to try to make a meaningful connection with them and to involve them in their care.

Providing this sort of caring relationship can be very challenging when there are competing demands on the practical and emotional resources available in particular care environments (Davis et al. 2021). Making time to listen to older people and find out about their life history, their family lives and their hopes and concerns is skilled work and a very important role for the nurse working with older people. It is important that staff are supported so they can develop the skills and resources to be able to do this (Reflection 33.4).

REFLECTION 33.4

The Importance of Relationships When Caring for Older People

Think about a time you were involved in the care of an older person.

Activities
- Do you feel you got to know them well?
- What questions could you have asked to find out more about their background or family circumstances?
- Are there any topic areas you would avoid asking about?

Depression and Older People

Depression is a very common mental health problem in later life (McCrae 2018). It is difficult to get an accurate picture of how many older people suffer with depression due to underdiagnosis but it is a significant problem that affects people's quality of life. Depression increases an older person's risk of suicide and older people are more likely than younger people to complete suicide (Walker et al. 2018). The incidence of depression increases considerably for older people entering institutional settings (Wang et al. 2021). Depression is said to occur when a person's mood is lowered, there is a decrease in their enjoyment of their usual activities and there is a reduction in their levels of energy. They may be bothered by a persistent sense of hopelessness or feeling down (NICE 2022). It is important that nurses and carers understand depression in old age, so that older people have proper assessment and access to appropriate care. A key issue is to recognise that whilst anxiety and confusion may be conditions that are experienced separately, they are linked to depression and require thorough investigation (Walker et al. 2018).

There are significant risk factors linked to depression in old age. These include long-term conditions, social isolation, residential care and being a carer (McCrae 2018). Frailty is also relevant but it is a two-way connection: frailty may be a risk factor for depression or depression could lead to frailty (Soysal et al. 2017). There are also factors that protect older people from depression, such as a high degree of self-esteem, the presence of a confidante and access to high-quality support (Worrall et al. 2020). Older people are vulnerable to depression when the risk factors overwhelm their protective resources.

There are a range of treatments and therapeutic approaches. Appropriately prescribed medications and psychologically based therapies such as psychodynamic, systemic, cognitive behavioural or interpersonal therapy may be helpful for depressed older people (NICE 2022). Less formal interventions such as activity-based programmes, for example music therapy, may also be helpful (Aalbers et al. 2017). A criticism of mental healthcare for older people is that there is an overreliance on medications as a treatment and lack of referral for psychologically based interventions (McCrae 2018). Worse still, there is sometimes a complete focus on the physical needs of older people at the expense of their emotional wellbeing. Noonan (2018) suggests that nurses should be aware of the risk factors of suicide. These include one or more of the following: older age, being male, gestures of self-harm or attempts at suicide, an apparent wish to die or evidence of planning suicide, drug or alcohol use disorder (Walker et al. 2018) and chronic condition causing chronic pain (Conejero et al. 2018). Severe depression can lead to suicide and a referral to specialist services should be made if an older person appears to be at risk.

Delirium, Mild Cognitive Impairment and Dementia

Delirium is an acute disorder which affects a person's attention and thought processes and is frequently missed by healthcare professionals (Wilke et al. 2023). The effects are that the person is hyperactive, becoming restless and agitated or hypoactive, staring in to space and being drowsy and withdrawn or there are intermittent periods of hypoactivity and hyperactivity (Wilke et al. 2023). It is important that nurses recognise the difference between delirium, which is sometimes called acute confusion, and dementia. Delirium usually develops over a short period of time, hours or days,

and is generally caused by a complex network of factors including inflammation, disorders of electrolyte balance or hypoxia (Tahir et al. 2020). Frequently, the conditions underlying delirium are reversible. In contrast, dementia is caused by specific illness that results in progressive confusion, for example Alzheimer's disease. Dementia is unlikely to be significantly reversed and it is gradual in onset (McCrae 2018).

Whilst a person is in a state of delirium, they may not understand their surroundings and become anxious. It is important for the nurse to protect them from harm by being aware of their physical environment and provide psychologically supportive care (Dixon 2018). The principles of care for a person with delirium include finding out the cause of the delirium and treating it, promoting their physical health, ensuring their safety and including family carers in decision making (Dixon 2018).

Sometimes, an older person notices a chronic memory decline but does not meet the diagnostic criteria of dementia or delirium. This intermediate state, between normal ageing and dementia, is termed mild cognitive impairment (MCI) (Livingstone et al. 2020). There two types of MCI; one refers to the loss of memory (amnestic MCI) and the other affects other cognitive functions such as a decline in language use or the ability to judge distances and space (Bermejo-Pareja et al. 2020). A person who experiences delirium or MCI has a greater risk of having dementia.

Dementia is caused by disease processes such as Alzheimer's or vascular degeneration in the brain. Dementia is a severe and devastating disorder. There are approximately 850,000 people with dementia in the UK, and the number is expected to reach over a million by 2025 (Office for Health Improvements and Disparities [OHID] 2022a). The UK government reports improvements in healthcare and the wellbeing of people living with dementia and their carers as part of the Prime Minister's Challenge: Implementation Plan on Dementia 2020 (DHSC 2019), and although no treatments are available for the most common dementias, research is beginning to uncover the complexity of the disease and suggest modifiable lifestyle (Livingstone et al. 2020). Professionals may be able to impact population levels of dementia by encouraging people to be more physically active, eat healthily and maintain a healthy weight, drink less alcohol, stop smoking and be socially active and control diabetes and high blood pressure (OHID 2022a). For individuals the emphasis is living well with dementia in communities which support people with dementia and their families to live a good life at home or residential care (OHID 2022a).

There are a range of types of dementia which have specific trajectories; initially, symptoms usually include impaired memory, disorientation, poor concentration, emotional changes and a withdrawal from social activities (Alzheimer's Association 2022). It is important for people in confusional states to undergo psychiatric assessment. Early diagnosis of dementia allows people to access appropriate services as well as advice and help with memory loss and appropriate medication (Social Care Institute for Excellence 2020a). Over time, dementia can result in severe disability and loss of function (Røsvik et al. 2020). Care practices should preserve the person's dignity and sense of self-worth by treating them as an individual and encouraging them to be independent. The Alzheimer's Society provides good information about issues such as helping the person with dementia to eat, drink, dress and wash. For example, laying out clothes on the bed for the person with dementia will remind them of dressing activities and provide the optimal opportunity for choice and independence (www.alzheimers.org.uk) (Reflection 33.5).

REFLECTION 33.5

Providing Good Care for People With Dementia

Think about other ways to promote and stimulate the person's memory so they have more choice and independence.

Activities

- What types of tools have you used to assess a person's cognitive state?
- What do you know about memory clinics and patients who are referred to them?
- List ways you can improve your care for people with dementia.
- Go to the Alzheimer's Society website and look at the examples of good practice they give. How did yours compare?
- Are there any gaps in your knowledge about caring for people with dementia?
- You can become a Dementia Friend by getting training from the Alzheimer's Society.

REFLECTION 33.6

Advice and Support for Older People and Their Carers

Consider how confident you are in your role as information provider. Advice and support for older people with dementia and their carers are provided by the charity Dementia UK (http://www.dementiauk.org) and more generally for carers by the charity Carers UK (http://www.carersuk.org). Both charities have a helpline.

Activities

- Identify ways you can improve your role as information provider.
- What sort of questions do you think carers and relatives ask the helpline?
- How can you help carers and relatives find out information?

INFORMATION 33.1

Principles of Practice in the Prevention of Falls

- There should be a person-centred approach.
- There should be a multidisciplinary approach to care.
- Organisational issues such as education, training and audit should be integral to falls prevention strategies.
- Individuals contacting healthcare professionals should be assessed for risk routinely.
- Assessment of older people's risk of falling should be multifactorial.
- In hospital, any issues assessed to be risk factors should be treated, improved or managed during the patient's stay.
- Interventions should be multifactorial.
- Exercise and strength training are recommended.
- Home hazard and safety intervention should be in place on discharging older people at risk.
- Assessment of medications should be integral to falls prevention strategies.

Reference

National Institute for Health and Care Excellence (NICE). Falls in older people. Quality standard [QS86]. 2017. https://www.nice.org.uk/guidance/qs86.

quality standard for the assessment and prevention of falls in older people (NICE 2017a) and makes recommendations for practice (Information 33.1).

Central to best practice is an assessment of multiple factors, including the person's individual circumstances and environment. The purpose of the assessment is to identify risk factors with the view to developing a strategy to reduce the risk (NICE 2017a). It is not possible for risk to be completely eliminated but it is important to identify potential hazards and educate the person at risk. Age, gender, underlying medical conditions, side effects of medication, poor mobility, mental health and cognition and vision are known to place people at higher risk of falls (WHO 2021). It is important that practitioners and professionals have the knowledge and skills to support their patients depending on their needs (OHID 2022b).

Falls are an ongoing and traumatising problem for older adults and the available evidence suggests that rather than a single intervention to prevent falls, a multifactorial approach that includes effective self-management is deemed the most effective (Wilkinson et al. 2018). Healthcare professionals have an important role in working with older adults and carers and would ideally assess their patient's risk of falls by routinely screening if the patients have fallen in the last year, observing their gait and balance and referring to appropriate agencies for interventions to reduce risk of falls (Wilkinson et al. 2018).

Strength and Balance Training

Exercise as part of a multifactorial approach can improve muscle strength and balance may improve confidence and stability (Sherrington et al. 2020). Falls commonly occur in the bedroom and involve the process of transferring from bed to chair. Some exercise classes specifically target this activity, whereas others are more general and include walking and low-impact weight-bearing exercise. Sustained exercise in later life is helpful for general wellbeing and preventing falls. Regular exercise programmes that are tailored to the individual and monitored by appropriately trained healthcare professionals are recommended (Sherrington et al. 2020).

Nurses are likely to come across people living with dementia and it is important they have the skills and knowledge to adapt their care appropriately (Keuning-Plantinga et al. 2021). The areas for knowledge and skills development for all nurses and carers include dementia awareness, for example, having a positive attitude and understanding the diagnosis process, providing compassionate care and understanding the perspective of the person living with dementia (Skills for Health 2018). The progression of dementia takes a long time and it is important that nurses and carers are sensitive to the changes and losses involved. Care plans need frequent review, and appropriate referral and communication with relevant members of the multidisciplinary team are necessary to ensure continuity. Underpinning this are the needs and wishes of the person with dementia and their family. It is a key role of the nurse to provide practical and emotional support to relatives and informal carers (Reflection 33.6), give information, coordinate resources and assess the needs of relatives and carers of older people.

Preventing Falls in Older People

An important concern for older people is the risk of having a fall. Falls in old age are common and costly and the risk of falls causes anxiety and impacts on a person's everyday life and independence (Wilkinson et al. 2018). The NICE has produced a

Home Hazard Assessment and Prevention

Additional aspects of the multifactorial approach include adjusting the environment to avoid trips and accidents. Areas of high risk such as bathrooms and bedrooms can be adapted to ensure there is enough space and clutter is removed (Wilkinson et al. 2018). Aids to provide physical support, such as hand rails, can be fitted. Preventative measures such as removal of loose-fitting carpets and thorough cleaning after spillage can be effective. Good practice in care homes and hospitals includes accurate record keeping of incidents and accidents, heightened supervision at busy times and ensuring older people have had sensory and cognitive assessment (Wilkinson et al. 2018). Appropriate skills training in falls prevention and especially in relation to people with mental health needs is important to improve practice (OHID 2022b).

Medications and Falls

It is important to review older people's medications regularly. This is especially relevant as the combination of drugs and specific medications such as sedatives and those prescribed for mobility problems can increase the risk of falling if not properly monitored. It is good practice to keep the dose and the number of medications prescribed to a minimum where possible (Nazarko 2022). It is also important that older people understand their medications to maximise their effectiveness. They should be given a full explanation of what the medication is for, the possible unwanted side-effects and how to get help if they do experience side-effects. For example, if a person is prescribed diuretics, they may suffer dizziness and loss of balance when getting up (postural hypotension). It is good practice to ensure people are aware of the potential for this happening so they can adjust their behaviour by getting up slowly and feel less anxious should it occur (Nazarko 2022). Prescribing medicines for frail older people is different from prescribing for fit younger people (Lau et al. 2020). It is important to take steps to avoid the negative effects of polypharmacy by ensuring any prescribed medication is necessary via regular and systematic review (see Information 33.2).

Nutrition and Older People

Over a million older people in the UK are estimated to be malnourished or at risk of malnourishment (Malnutrition Task Force 2017). Older people and especially those living in residential care are more likely to suffer from more problems with nutrition than younger people (Nazarko 2018). Malnourishment impacts on an older person's health and wellbeing by increasing their risk of pressure sores, infection and admission to hospital; it also delays recovery from illness and surgery (Malcomson and Mathers 2018). The reasons why older people suffer from poor nutrition are varied. The Malnutrition Task Force (2017) categorises risk factors as medical and disease related, especially having a long-term condition such as depression or dementia; physical factors such as reduced mobility, poor dentition and sensory loss; and social factors, for example loneliness and low income. Although there is considerable awareness of these factors, the incidence of malnutrition in older people continues to increase. Malcomson and Mathers (2018) further argue that the societal perspective matters enormously and brings about an urgent imperative to discover, and to implement, accessible, affordable, cost-effective lifestyle interventions which enable all to age well, stay physically, cognitively and socially active to maintain independence and minimise the end-of-life pronounced frailty and multimorbidity due to undernutrition or malnutrition.

Nurses have a considerable responsibility in hospital, at home and in care homes when it comes to nutritional status of older people,

---

INFORMATION 33.2

Principles of a Medication Review for a Person With Multiple Medical Conditions

1. The aims of treatment from the patient's point of view should be established. The patient should be asked: 'What matters to you?'
2. In partnership with the patient, the reviewer(s) should list all the patient's medications, including herbal and traditional remedies, and make sure the patient knows what their medication is for. It should be established which drug therapies are essential.
3. Any unnecessary medications should be identified and alternative approaches explored with the patient.
4. It should be established whether the therapeutic aims of the drug therapies are being achieved and whether the medications are being taken as per prescription.
5. It should be established whether the patient is at risk of or experiencing an adverse drug reaction (ADR).
6. The cost-effectiveness of the drug therapy should be considered.
7. The outcomes of the review should be discussed with the patient and the drug therapy should be tailored to the patient's preferences to ensure maximum effectiveness.

Adapted from Scottish Government Polypharmacy Model of Care Group (2018).

---

especially when it comes to disease-related malnutrition (DRM) (Hiesmayr et al. 2019). Hiesmayr et al. (2019) suggest that political action is needed in the current economic and healthcare climate to raise awareness and increase formal education for healthcare practitioners and stakeholders on all aspects related to DRM. Support responsibilities within hospitals, induce routine and benchmarking data collection and adequate reimbursement schemes are crucial to tackle efficiently poor nutrition. Nurses should be able to screen for nutritional problems and pass this information to the doctor or the dietitian as appropriate. Principles of nutritional screening include gathering nutritional measurements such as height, weight and body mass index and noting any unplanned weight loss and the effects of acute illness. Screening tools can ensure the assessment is systematic and evidence based (Hiesmayr et al. 2019). Assessment should investigate whether the older person is dehydrated by asking them about their fluid intake and observing them for signs of dehydration such as dry or discoloured skin, concentrated urine and change in urine output. Nurses and carers should also be aware of medications such as diuretics that affect fluid and electrolyte balance (NICE 2017b) and have a basic knowledge of nutrition to be able to identify basic food groups in order to advise on adequate nutritional intake. Nurses also need to be aware of people with conditions such as dysphagia (difficulty swallowing), which require a more specialised assessment (NICE 2017b).

It is important to ensure that mealtimes are a time when people can eat their meals without unnecessary interruptions and that people with special needs receive adequate support and practical help. Reber et al. (2019) report that in patients with risk of malnutrition, nutrition intake was improved with enriched meals or oral nutritional supplements; food intake was monitored and was associated with better outcomes and reduced healthcare costs. Further to that, careful planning around the support of people with problems that may impact on their ability to eat, such as confusion or difficulties with fine movements of the hand, needs to be incorporated into the organisation of care (Hiesmayr et al. 2019).

Staff need to understand the importance of good nutrition and be able to use relevant equipment, aids and any dietary supplements

(NICE 2017b). They should consult with relatives and involve the older person in order to find out their individual preferences. The Alzheimer's Society offers further guidance about practical care at mealtimes. Hiesmayr et al. (2019) further highlight the human right for proper nutrition care, that was acknowledged in the Cartagena declaration (Cardenas et al. 2019). The declaration includes 13 principles, such as empowerment, dignity, ethical principles, justice and equity, and urges the United Nations and the Human Rights Council to recognise the Right to Nutrition Care as a human right in line with the 'Sustainable Development Goals'.

Continence and Older People

People can suffer from incontinence at any age but, as with many physical problems, there is an association between incontinence and ageing (Ostaszkiewicz et al. 2020). When referring to incontinence, it is usually urinary incontinence that is being implied, but frail older people or those with dementia may also experience faecal incontinence (NHS England 2018). Urinary incontinence is associated with older age and the at-risk groups include women, especially those who have had children, are going through the menopause or who have had a hysterectomy, or men who have had prostate surgery. Incontinence can lead to multiple problems that span the psychological, the social and the physical. People should be treated sensitively and with respect as urinary incontinence can be profoundly embarrassing and it may cause anxiety and depression (NHS England 2018). Urinary incontinence can arise for several reasons and is classified as follows (National Institute on Aging 2022):

- Urge incontinence when there is detrusor muscle dysfunction leading to an inability to suppress spontaneous contractions of the bladder leading to sudden voiding of urine.
- Stress incontinence when there is urine leakage due to incompetence of the pelvic floor muscles and, while this is common in women following childbirth, it can arise in men following pelvic surgery.
- Outflow obstruction arises when there is something blocking the outflow of urine from the bladder; for example, it may arise in constipation, prostatic hyperplasia or as a result of a tumour. This leads to urine overflowing periodically under the pressure in the bladder.
- Total incontinence – when no urine is stored in the bladder, which causes frequent leakage or constant passing of urine.
  It is possible to have more than one type of incontinence.

When a person is incontinent, it is important to collect data about when and how often the incontinence occurs as well as any associated symptom. This requires sensitivity but should include specific questions to obtain the relevant information. It is important to ask specific questions to identify certain types of incontinence. For example, answering 'yes' to the question 'Do you get so desperate to pass water that you find it hard to hold on?' may indicate that the person has urge incontinence. Answering 'yes' to the question 'Do you leak urine if you cough, laugh or exert yourself?' is likely to indicate stress incontinence. A thorough assessment is important to establish the right approach to care and treatment (National Institute on Aging 2022). The person with the continence problem can be asked to keep a diary to establish patterns of incontinence, and investigations into other underlying problems such as confusion or diabetes may be necessary.

Active treatment is dependent on the type of incontinence and may involve bladder control training, medication, education or behavioural changes (National Institute on Aging 2022). For people with dementia and those living in residential care, the attitude and practices of those delivering care can be crucial to care that

promotes the privacy and dignity and more research is needed to promote personalised care and independence (National Institute of Health and Care Research [NIHR] 2022).

End-of-Life Care

End-of-life care usually refers to the support and care given to a person during the time when they are living with the practical and emotional concerns about dying although their death is not obviously imminent. Terminal care usually means the care provided immediately preceding a person's death – perhaps in the last few days of life (Handley et al. 2022). End-of-life care is significant for older people because it can be supportive and validate a person's life. The delivery of relationship-centred care is central to end-of-life care in residential care. The palliative care expertise in care homes was disrupted by the COVID-19 pandemic, and Bradshaw et al. (2023) recommend further integration of care homes in health and social care services along with workforce development and especially support for care home managers.

Honest and sensitive communication is a key skill in providing end-of-life care. For instance, it is important to establish what the older person would prefer to happen should their condition deteriorate or should they suffer a cardiac arrest (Nursing and Midwifery Council [NMC] 2018). When a nurse or carer talks about these issues with the older person, they should try to explain the possible limits of the medical intervention and clarify the older person's expectations (Boyd et al. 2022). If the nurse does not feel able to talk about dying in this way, it is essential to refer to a more experienced nurse or another member of the multidisciplinary team so that the older person is helped to express their hopes and fears.

Older people often experience a complex array of losses towards the end of their lives. There are many frameworks that explain the experience of grief following a loss. One that is familiar to nurses is described by Kubler-Ross and Kessler (2005). They suggest that when a person is faced with significant loss such as death or losses related to increased dependence, they have to grieve. They describe five stages of grief: denial, anger, bargaining, depression and acceptance. Nurses and carers have a role in supporting older people to work through the feelings that can be stirred up as part of the grieving process. For example, when circumstances necessitate moving to continuing care, it is important for nurses and carers to help the older person identify, express and acknowledge their feelings in order to make the appropriate transition.

Nurses and carers can be supportive by developing a therapeutic relationship with the person and using the communication skills outlined earlier in this chapter. They should also be alert to recognise when symptoms persist and intensify as this can indicate that the person may be experiencing depression. In this case an appropriate referral should be made for specialist help from mental health services (McCrae 2018).

A palliative care approach is helpful in making sure the person can maintain optimal levels of quality of life whilst being comfortable and free of distressing symptoms (Handley et al. 2022). Practical support for older people at the end of their lives should prioritise pain relief, aid coping with chronic fatigue and assist with any problems related to eating and drinking. Palliative approaches are often appropriate over long periods of time and should be integral to the organisation of care for older people with long-term conditions, especially dementia which adds another level of complexity (Handley et al. 2022). Community and care home staff should have the relevant training and support to ensure that high levels of communication and clinical care are delivered appropriately.

Summary: Key Nursing Issues

- Old age is a varied and interesting aspect of life, and nursing older people is important and rewarding. Making time to listen to older people and find out about their life history, their family lives and their hopes and concerns is the most skilled and most important role of the nurse working with older people.
- Older people are no different from other people nurses come into contact with in the course of their work; like any patient, the older person requires sensitivity, tact and professionalism.
- Dignified care should promote a person's self-respect and usually involves giving respect. At the simplest level, this can mean proper toilet facilities and curtains to provide privacy. At the more complex level, it means developing a culture of care that respects the personal needs of individuals.
- The physical and psychological changes of ageing depend not only on an individual's makeup and external environment but also on how they perceive and experience ageing. Most people experience some physical, psychological and social changes in later life.
- Changes in blood pressure control, exercise tolerance, muscles, bones and teeth, reaction to temperature, sensory perception and resistance to infection are common but by no means inevitable.
- The effects of long-term conditions have a significant impact on an older person's life. The common long-term conditions of old age include cancer, heart disease, diabetes, stroke and Alzheimer's disease.
- Older people generally suffer from more problems with nutrition than younger people, and older people in hospital suffer greatly from nutritional problems. Undernutrition leads to weight loss and vulnerability to secondary problems of infection, skin breakdown and poor recovery from illness and from surgical procedures.
- Relationship-centred care is central to quality care for older people. It acknowledges the needs of those delivering care and shifts the focus to the organisation of care rather than just the individuals providing it. The organisation should promote a sense of security, continuity, belonging, purpose, fulfilment and significance, which should not only be felt by the older people being cared for, but also the staff working with them.

Reflection and Learning – What Next?

- **Test** your knowledge by visiting the Evolve website 🌐 and answering the multiple-choice questions and critical thinking questions.
- **Consolidate** your learning by looking at some of the further reading suggestions, references and specialist websites.
- **Revisit** some of the additional material on the Evolve website.
- **Consider** what you have learnt and how this will help your professional development.
- **Reflect** on how you can apply this knowledge to the care of your patients.
- **Discuss** your learning with your supervisor/assessor, lecturer and colleagues.

References

Aalbers S, Fusar-Poli L, Freeman RE, et al. Music therapy for depression. *Cochrane Database Syst Rev*. 2017(11):CD004517. https://www.cochrane.org/CD004517/DEPRESSN_music-therapy-depression.

Age UK. *Later Life in the United Kingdom*. Age UK publication; 2019. https://www.ageuk.org.uk/search/?q=Later+Life+in+the+United+Kingdom+2019.

Age UK. *Poverty in Later Life*. Age UK; June 2021. https://www.ageuk.org.uk/globalassets/age-uk/documents/policy-positions/money-matters/poverty_in_later_life_briefing_june_2021.pdf.

Alzheimer's Association. Alzheimer's disease facts and figures. *Alzheimers Dement*. 2022;18(4):700–789. https://doi.org/10.1002/alz.12638.

Bermejo-Pareja F, Contador I, del Ser T, et al. Predementia constructs: mild cognitive impairment or mild neurocognitive disorder? A narrative review. *Int J Geriatr Psychiatry*. 2020;36(5):743–755. https://doi.org/10.1002/gps.5474.

Biggs S. Adapting to an ageing society the need for cultural change. *Policy Q*. 2014;10(3):12–16.

Borgstrom E, Gopinath M, Vseteckova J. Learning in the Fourth Age: the role of physical activity interventions for people living in long term facilities. *Int J Educ Ageing*. 2022;5(2):25–38.

Bottery S, Jeffries D. The Kings Fund. *Ideas that Change Health and Care. Social Care 360*. The Kings Fund; 2022. https://www.kingsfund.org.uk/publications/social-care-360.

Boyd KJ, Clark C, Stevens E. Communication. In: Pryde N, ed. *Enhanced Palliative Care: A Handbook for Paramedics, Nurses and Doctors*. Class Professional Publishing; 2022.

Bradshaw A, Ostler S, Goodman C, et al. Provision of palliative and end-of-life care in UK care homes during the COVID-19 pandemic: a mixed methods observational study with implications for policy. *Front Public Health*. 2023;14(11):1058736. https://doi.org/10.3389/fpubh.2023.1058736.

Bristow K, Timmins L, Braybrook D, et al. LGBT+ partner bereavement and appraisal of the Acceptance-Disclosure Model of LGBT+ bereavement: a qualitative interview study. *Palliat Med*. 2023;37(2):221–234. https://journals.sagepub.com/doi/10.1177/02692163221138620.

Bunn F, Burn A, Robinson L, et al. Healthcare organisation and delivery for people with dementia and comorbidity: a qualitative study exploring the views of patients, carers and professionals. *BMJ Open*. 2017;7:e013067. doi:10.1136/bmjopen-2016-013067.

Campisi J, Kapahi P, Lithgow G, Melov S, Newman JC, Verdin E. From discoveries in ageing research to therapeutics for healthy ageing. *Nature*. 2019;571:183–192. https://doi.org/10.1038/s41586-019-1365-2.

Cardenas D, Bermudez C, Barazzoni R. The Cartagena Declaration: a call for global commitment to fight for the right to nutritional care. *Clin Nutr*. 2019;38:2458–2459. doi:10.1016/j.clnu.2019.07.015.

Carrier J. *Managing Long-Term Conditions and Chronic Illness in Primary Care: A Guide to Good Practice*. 3rd ed. Routledge; 2022.

Centre for Ageing Better. The state of ageing. 2022. ageing-better.org.uk.

Centre for Policy on Ageing. Rapid review. Diversity in older age – older homelessness. 2017.http://www.cpa.org.uk/information/reviews/CPA-Rapid-Review-Diversity-in-Older-Age-Older-Homeless-People.pdf

Choi KH, Lee JH, Lee DG. Sex-related differences in bone metabolism in osteoporosis observational study. *Med (Baltimore)*. 2021;100(21):e26153. https://doi.org/10.1097/md.0000000000026153.

Clancy A, Simonsen N, Lind J, Liveng A, Johannessen A. The meaning of dignity for older adults: a meta-synthesis. *Nurs Ethics*. 2021;28(6):876–894. https://doi.org/10.1177/0969733020928134.

Conejero I, Olie E, Courtet P, Calati R. Suicide in older adults: current perspectives. *Clin Interv Aging*. 2018;13:691–699. doi:10.2147/CIA.S130670. https://pubmed.ncbi.nlm.nih.gov/29719381/.

Davis L, Botting N, Cruice M, Dipper L. A systematic review of language and communication intervention research delivered in groups to older adults living in care homes. *Int J Lang Commun Disord*. 2021;57(1):182–225. https://doi.org/10.1111/1460-6984.12679.

De Favari Signini É, Castro A, Rehder-Santos P, et al. Integrative perspective of the healthy aging process considering the metabolome, cardiac autonomic modulation and cardiorespiratory fitness evaluated in age groups. *Sci Rep*. 2022;12:21314. https://doi.org/10.1038/s41598-022-25747-5.

De Witt L, Fortune D. Relationship-centered dementia care: insights from a community-based culture change coalition. *Dementia*. 2017;18(3). https://doi.org/10.1177/1471301217708814.

Dementia Statistics Hub. Alzheimer Research UK. 2018. https://dementiastatistics.org/statistics/dementia-maps/

Department of Health and Social Care (DHSC). Dementia 2020 Challenge: 2018 Review Phase 1. February 2019. https://ssets.publishing.service.gov.uk/government/uploads/system/uploads/attachment_data/file/780777/dementia-2020-challenge-2018-review.pdf.

Department of Health and Social Care (DHSC). Reforming adult social care in England. 2023. https://www.nao.org.uk/wp-content/uploads/2023/11/Summary-reforming-adult-social-care-in-England-summary.pdf.

Dixon M. Assessment and management of older patients with delirium in acute settings. *Nurs Older People*. 2018;30(4):35–42.

Dong H, Larsson B, Dragioti E, Bernfort L, Levin L, Gerdle B. Factors associated with life satisfaction in older adults with chronic pain (PainS65+). *J Pain Res*. 2020;13:475–489.

Duxbury J, Baker J, Downe S, et al. Minimising the use of physical restraint in acute mental health services: the outcome of a restraint reduction programme ('REsTRAIN YOURSELF'). *Int J Nurs Stud*. 2019;95:40–48.

Ebrahimi Z, Patel H, Wijk H, Ekman I, Olaya-Contreras P. A systematic review on implementation of person-centered care interventions for older people in out-of-hospital settings. *Geriatr Nurs (Minneap)*. 2021;42:213–224. https://doi.org/10.1016/j.gerinurse.2020.08.004.

Erikson EH, Erikson JM, Kivnick HQ. *Vital Involvement in Old Age: The Experience of Old Age in Our Time*. New York: Norton; 1986.

Francis R. *Report of the Mid Staffordshire NHS Foundation Trust Public Inquiry. Executive Summary*. London: TSO; 2013.

Genoe MR, Liechty T, Marston HR. Leisure innovation and the transition to retirement. *Leisure Sci*. 2019;44(4):440–458. https://doi.org/10.1080/01490400.2019.1597791.

Gilani A, Juraschek SP, Belanger MJ, Vowles JE, Wannamethee SG. Postural hypotension. *BMJ*. 2021;373:n922. https://doi.org/10.1136/bmj.n922.

Government Equalities Office and Equality and Human Rights Commission. Equality Act 2015. https://www.gov.uk/guidance/equality-act-2010-guidance.

Government Office for Science (GOS). *Future of an Ageing Population*. London: Government Office for Science; 2019. https://assets.publishing.service.gov.uk/government/uploads/system/uploads/attachment_data/file/816493/future-of-an-ageing-population.pdf.

Guyette F. Successful aging: social theory, scripture, church teaching. *J Relig Spiritual Aging*. 2018;30(3):199–211. https://doi.org/10.1080/15528030.2018.1428921.

Handley M, Parker D, Bunn F, Goodman C. A qualitative comparison of care home staff and palliative care specialists' experiences of providing end of life care to people living and dying with dementia in care homes in two countries: a focus group study. *Palliat Med*. 2022;36(1):114–123. doi:10.1177/02692163211043374.

Hassen C, Fayosse A, Landré B, et al. Association between age at onset of multimorbidity and incidence of dementia: 30 year follow-up in Whitehall II Prospective Cohort Study. *BMJ*. 2022;376:e068005. doi:10.1136/bmj-2021-068005.

Haynes L. Aging of the Immune System: Research Challenges to Enhance the Health Span of Older Adults Frontiers in Aging. 2020;1. https://doi.org/10.3389/fragi.2020.602108.

Health Advisory Service (HAS). *Not Because They Are Old*. London: HAS; 2000.

Heaslip V, Thompson R, Tauringana M, Holland S, Glendening N. Health inequity in the UK: exploring health inequality and inequity. *Pract Nurs*. 2022;33(2):72–76.

Hiesmayr M, Tarantino S, Moick S, et al. Hospital malnutrition, a call for political action: a public health and nutrition day perspective. *J Clin Med*. 2019;8(12):2048. doi:10.3390/jcm8122048.

Hijas-Gomez AI, Ayala A, Rodríguez-García MP, et al. The WHO active ageing pillars and its association with survival: Findings from a population-based study in Spain. *Arch Gerontol Geriatr*. 2020;90:104114. ISSN 0167-4943. https://doi.org/10.1016/j.archger.2020.104114.

Hill PL, Pfund GN. Purposeful retirement expectations and their associations with retirement planning. *Aging Ment Health*. 2022;26(9):1882–1888. https://doi.org/10.1080/13607863.2021.1963948.

Jack K, Ridley C, Turner S. Effective communication with older people. *Nurs Older People*. 2019;31(4):40–48. doi:10.7748/nop.2019.e1126.

Keuning-Plantinga A, Roodbol P, van Munster BC, Finnema1 EJ. Experiences of informal caregivers of people with dementia with nursing care in acute hospitals: a descriptive mixed-methods study. *J Adv Nurs*. 2021;77:4887–4899. https://doi.org/10.1111/jan.15042.

Kingston A, Robinson L, Booth H, Knapp M, Jagger C. Projections of multi-morbidity in the older population in England to 2035: estimates from the Population Ageing and Care Simulation (PACSim) model. *Age Ageing*. 2018;47(3):374–380. https://doi.org/10.1093/ageing/afx201.

Kneck A, Mattson E, Salzmann-Erikson M, Klarare A. "Stripped of dignity" – women in homelessness and their perspectives of healthcare services: a qualitative study. *Int J Nurs Stud*. 2021;120:103947. https://doi.org/10.1016/j.ijnurstu.2021.103974.

Kubler-Ross E, Kessler D. *On Grief and Grieving. Finding the Meaning of Grief Through the Five Stages of Loss*. London: Simon and Schuster; 2005.

Lau S, Lun P, Ang W, et al. Barriers to effective prescribing in older adults: applying the theoretical domains framework in the ambulatory setting – a scoping review. *BMC Geriatr*. 2020;20:459. https://doi.org/10.1186/s12877-020-01766-7.

Livingstone G, Huntley J, Sommerlad A, et al. Dementia prevention, intervention, and care: 2020 report of the Lancet Commission. *Lancet*. 2020;396(10248):413–446. https://doi.org/10.1016/S0140-6736(20)30367-6.

Maddox L, Barreto M. The team needs to feel cared for: staff perceptions of compassionate care, aids and barriers in adolescent mental health wards. *BMC Nurs*. 2022;21(206). https://doi.org/10.1186/s12912-022-00994-z.

Malcomson FC, Mathers JC. Nutrition and ageing. *Subcell Biochem*. 2018;90:373–424. doi:10.1007/978-981-13-2835-0_13. PMID: 30779016.

Malnutrition Task Force. *State of the Nation: Older People and Malnutrition in the UK Today*. London: Malnutrition Task Force; 2017.

Martin G, Roberts S. Exploring legacies of the baby boomers in the twenty-first century. *Sociol Rev*. 2021;69:4. https://doi.org/10.1177/00380261211006326.

McCrae N. Functional mental health disorders ion older people. In: Norman I, Ryrie I, eds. *The Art and Science of Mental Health. Principles and Practice*. 4th ed. McGraw-Hill; 2018.

McKee M, Dunnell K, Anderson M, et al. The changing health needs of the UK population. *Lancet*. 2021;397:1979–1991. doi:10.1016/S0140-6736(21)00229-4.

Moini J. *Anatomy and Physiology for Health Professionals*. 3rd ed. Jones and Bartlett Learning; 2019.

Nair P, Borrado-Martin Y, Anantapong K, et al. Experiences of carers and people with dementia from ethnic minority groups managing eating and drinking at home in the United Kingdom. *Nutrients*. 2022;14(12):2395–2417. https://doi.org/10.3390/nu14122395.

National Institute on Aging (NIA). *Urinary incontinence in older adults*; 2022. https://www.nia.nih.gov/health/urinary-incontinence-older-adults.

National Institute for Health and Care Excellence (NICE). *Falls in older people*. Quality standard [QS86]; 2017. https://www.nice.org.uk/guidance/qs86.

National Institute for Health and Care Excellence (NICE). *Nutrition support for adults: oral nutrition support, enteral tube feeding and parenteral nutrition*. Clinical guideline [CG32]; 2017. nice.org.uk/guidance/cg32.

National Institute for Health and Care Excellence (NICE). Quality statement 1: Empathy, dignity and respect. 2019. https://www.nice.org.uk/guidance/qs15/chapter/quality-statement-1-empathy-dignity-and-respect.

National Institute for Health and Clinical Excellence (NICE). *Depression in adults: recognition and management.* Clinical guideline [CG90]; 2022. https://www.nice.org.uk/guidance/ng222/resources/depression-in-adults-treatment-and-management-pdf-66143832307909.

National Institute of Health and Care Research (NIHR). *Continence, dementia, and care that preserves dignity*; 2022. https://evidence.nihr.ac.uk/themedreview/continence-dementia-and-care-that-preserves-dignity/.

Nazarko L. Fit for life: improving nutrition in care home residents. *Nurs Resident Care.* 2018;20(6):250–255.

Nazarko L. Falls 3: medication can harm as well as heal: how it can increase the risk of falls. *Br J Care Assist.* 2022;16(11):516–525. https://doi-org.ezproxy.herts.ac.uk/10.12968/bjha.2022.16.11.516.

NHS (2019). NHS Long Term Plan. Version 1.2. NHS England. https://www.longtermplan.nhs.uk/

NHS England. Safeguarding Adults. 2017. https://www.england.nhs.uk/wp-content/uploads/2017/02/adult-pocket-guide.pdf.

NHS England. Excellence in continence care, practical guidance for commissioners, and leaders in health and social care. 2018. https://www.england.nhs.uk/wp-content/uploads/2018/07/excellence-in-continence-care.pdf.

Nicholson C, Gordon AL, Tinker A. Changing the way "we" view and talk about frailty.... *Age Ageing.* 2017;46(3):349–351.

Nilsson PM. Blood pressure strategies and goals in elderly patients with hypertension. *Exp Gerontol.* 2017;87:151–152. https://doi.org/10.1016/j.exger.2016.04.018.

Nolan M, Davies S, Grant G. Quality of life, quality of care. In: Nolan M, Davies S, Grant G, eds. *Working With Older People and Their Families: Key Issues in Policy and Practice.* Buckingham: Open University Press; 2001.

Noonan IPS. Assessing and managing the risk of self-harm and suicide. In: Norman I, Ryrie I, eds. *The Art and Science of Mental Health. Principles and Practice.* 4th ed. McGraw-Hill; 2018.

Novisky MA, Chelsey SN, Prost S. Older Adult's perspectives on death and dying in prison. *J Crim Justice.* 2022;83(2022):101930. https://doi.org/10.1016/j.jcrimjus.2022.101930.

Nursing and Midwifery Council (NMC). The Code: Professional Standards of Practice and Behaviour for Nurses, Midwives and Nursing Associates. 2018. https://www.nmc.org.uk/globalassets/sitedocuments/nmc-publications/nmc-code.pdf.

OECD/European Observatory on Health Systems and Policies. *United Kingdom: Country Health Profile 2019, State of Health in the EU.* Brussels: OECD Publishing, Paris/European Observatory on Health Systems and Policies; 2019.

Office for Health Improvements and Disparities (OHID). Dementia: applying all our health. 2022a. https://www.gov.uk/government/publications/dementia-applying-all-our-health/dementia-applying-all-our-health.

Office for Health Improvements and Disparities (OHID). Falls: applying all our health. 2022b. https://www.gov.uk/government/publications/falls-applying-all-our-health/falls-applying-all-our-health.

Office for National Statistics (ONS). Deaths registered in England and Wales: 2021. 2022. https://www.ons.gov.uk/peoplepopulationandcommunity/birthsdeathsandmarriages/deaths/bulletins/deathsregistrationsummarytables/2021.

Ostaszkiewicz J, Dickson-Swift V, Hutchinson A, et al. A concept analysis of dignity-protective continence care for care dependent older people in long-term care settings. *BMC Geriat.* 2020;20:266. https://doi.org/10.1186/s12877-020-01673-x.

Patel J, Wallace J, Doshi M, et al. Oral health for healthy ageing. *Lancet Healthy Longe.* 2021;2(8):E521–E527. https://doi.org/10.1016/S2666-7568(21)00142-2.

Pearson-Stuttard J, Ezzati M, Gregg EW. Multimorbidity—a defining challenge for health systems. *Lancet Public Health.* 2019;4:e599–e600.

Petermann-Rocha F, Balntzi V, Gray SR, et al. Global prevalence of sarcopenia and severe sarcopenia: a systematic review and meta-analysis. *J Cachexia Sarcopenia Muscle.* 2022;13(1):86–99. https://doi.org/10.1002/jcsm.12783.

Pu L, Moyle W. Restraint use in residents with dementia living in residential aged care facilities: a scoping review. *J Clin Nurs.* 2020;31:13–14. https://doi.org/10.1111/jocn.15487.

Rajan-Rankin S. Race, embodiment and later life: re-animating aging bodies of color. *J Aging Stud.* 2018;45:32–38. https://doi.org/10.1016/j.jaging.2018.01.005.

Reber E, Norman K, Endrich O, Schuetz P, Frei A, Stanga Z. Economic Challenges in nutritional management. *J Clin Med.* 2019;8:1005. doi:10.3390/jcm8071005.

Røsvik J, Rokstad AMM. What are the needs of people with dementia in acute hospital settings, and what interventions are made to meet these needs? A systematic integrative review of the literature. *BMC Health Serv Res.* 2020;20:723. https://doi.org/10.1186/s12913-020-05618-3.

RNIB. Key information and statistics on sight loss in the UK. 2021. https://www.rnib.org.uk/professionals/health-social-care-education-professionals/knowledge-and-research-hub/key-information-and-statistics-on-sight-loss-in-the-uk/.

Ryan T. Facilitators of person and relationship-centred care in nursing. *Nurs Open.* 2021;9:892–899. https://doi.org/10.1002/nop2.1083.

São José JM, Timonen V, Amado CAF, Santos SP. A critique of the active ageing index. *J Aging Stud.* 2017;40:49–56.

Scottish Government Polypharmacy Model of Care Group. *Polypharmacy Guidance: Realistic Prescribing.* 3rd ed. Edinburgh: Scottish Government; 2018. https://www.therapeutics.scot.nhs.uk/wp-content/uploads/2018/04/Polypharmacy-Guidance-2018.pdf.

Shepherd V, Islam I, Wood F, et al. Development of a core outcome set for the evaluation of interventions to prevent COVID-19 in care homes (COS-COVID-PCARE Study). *BMC Geriatr.* 2022;22:710. https://doi.org/10.1186/s12877-022-03395-8.

Sherlaw-Johnson C, Crump H, Arora S, Holder H, Davies A, Meaker R. Patient-Centred Care for Older People With Complex Needs. Evaluation of a New Care Model in Outer East London. *Nuffield Trust.* 2018. https://www.nuffieldtrust.org.uk/sites/default/files/2018-04/1524661229_bhr-2-complex-care-web.pdf.

Sherrington C, Fairhall N, Wallbank G, et al. Exercise for preventing falls in older people living in the community: an abridged Cochrane systematic review. *Br J Sports Med.* 2020;54:15. https://doi.org/10.1136/bjsports-2019-101512.

Sieber CC. Frailty – from concept to clinical practice. *Exp Gerontol.* 2017;87:160–167. https://doi.org/10.1016/j.exger.2016.05.004.

Skills for Health. *Dementia Training Standards Framework.* Skills for Health, Skills for Care, Health Education England; 2018. https://www.skillsforhealth.org.uk/info-hub/dementia-2015-updated-2018/.

Social Care Institute for Excellence. Dementia. Why early diagnosis of dementia is important. 2020a. https://www.scie.org.uk/dementia/symptoms/diagnosis/early-diagnosis.asp.

Social Care Institute for Excellence (SCIE). Dignity in care. 2020b. https://www.scie.org.uk/dignity/care.

Soysal P, Veronese N, Thompson T, et al. Relationship between depression and frailty in older adults: a systematic review and meta-analysis. *Ageing Res Rev.* 2017;36:78–87.

Sundgren S, Stolt M, Riitta S. Ethical issues related to the use of gerontechnology in older people care: a scoping review. *Nurs Ethics.* 2020;27(1):88–103.

Tahir TA, Khan R, Saxena A, Delirium Hasnain M. Psychiatric aspects of general medicine. *Med (Baltimore).* 2020;48(12):779–783. https://doi.org/10.1016/j.mpmed.2020.09.003.

Tinetti ME, Green AR, Ouellet J, Rich MW, Boyd C. Caring for patients with multiple chronic conditions. *Ann Intern Med.* 2019 Feb 5;170(3):199–200. doi:10.7326/M18-3269 Erratum in: Ann Intern Med. 2019 Mar 5;170(5):356.

Toye F, Seers K, Barker K. Living life precariously with rheumatoid arthritis – a mega-ethnography of nine qualitative evidence syntheses. *BMC Rheumatol.* 2019;3:5. https://doi.org/10.1186/s41927-018-0049-0.

United Nations. World Population Ageing 2019. 2019. https://www.un.org/en/development/desa/population/publications/pdf/ageing/WorldPopulationAgeing2019-Highlights.pdf.

United Nations Department of Economic and Social Affairs, Population Division. World Population Prospects 2022: Summary of Results. UN DESA/POP/2022/TR/No. 3. 2022. https://www.un.org/development/desa/pd/sites/www.un.org.development.desa.pd/files/wpp2022_summary_of_results.pdf.

Vetrano DL, Triolo F, Maggi S, et al. Fostering healthy aging: the interdependency of infections, immunity and frailty. *Ageing Res Rev*. 2021;69:p101351. https://doi.org/10.1016/j.arr.2021.101351.

Walker H, Fleming M, Gillespie M. The person with depression. In: Norman I, Ryrie I, eds. *The Art and Science of Mental Health Nursing: Principles and Practice*. 4th ed. McGraw Hill; 2018.

Wang F, Liu S, Zhang Q, Ng CH, Cui X, Zhang D, Xiang YT. Prevalence of depression in older nursing home residents in high and low altitude regions: a comparative study. *Front Psychiatry*. 2021;12:669234. doi:10.3389/fpsyt.2021.669234.

World Health Organization. Global strategy and action plan on ageing and health. 2017. https://apps.who.int/iris/bitstream/handle/10665/329960/9789241513500-eng.pdf.

World Health Organization. UN Decade of Healthy Ageing: baseline report. 2020. https://apps.who.int/iris/bitstream/handle/10665/338677/9789240017900-eng.pdf.

World Health Organization. Falls. 2021. https://www.who.int/news-room/fact-sheets/detail/falls.

Wilke S, Steiger E, Bärwolff TL, Kleine JF, Müller-Werdan U, Rosada A. Delirium in older hospitalized patients—a prospective analysis of the detailed course of delirium in geriatric inpatients. *PLoS One*. 2023;18(3):e0279763. https://doi.org/10.1371/journal.pone.0279763.

Wilkinson A, Meikle N, Law P, et al. How older adults and their informal carers prevent falls: an integrative review of the literature. *Int J Nurs Stud*. 2018;82:13–19. https://doi.org/10.1016/j.ijnurstu.2018.03.002.

Worrall C, Jongenelis MI, McEvoy PM, Jackson B, Newton RU, Pettigrew S. An exploratory study of the relative effects of various protective factors on depressive symptoms among older people. *Front Public Health*. 2020;8. https://doi.org/10.3389/fpubh.2020.579304.

Further Reading

Mental Capacity Act. 2005. http://www.legislation.gov.uk/ukpga/2005/9/pdfs/ukpga_20050009_en.pdf.

Norman I, Ryrie I, eds. *The Art and Science of Mental Health. Principles and Practice*. 4th ed. McGraw-Hill; 2018.

Pryde N, ed. *Enhanced Palliative Care: A Handbook for Paramedics, Nurses and Doctors*. Class Professional Publishing; 2022.

Shaw B, Menzies L, Bernardes E, Baars S, Nye P, Ethnicity Allen R. *Gender and Social Mobility*. Social Mobility Commission; 2016. https://assets.publishing.service.gov.uk/government/uploads/system/uploads/attachment_data/file/579988/Ethnicity_gender_and_social_mobility.pdf.

The King's Fund. Health and Care Act 2022. 2022. https://www.kingsfund.org.uk/topics/health-and-care-act-2022.

Useful Websites

Hour Glass, https://wearehourglass.org/
Age UK, www.ageuk.org.uk
Alzheimer's Society, www.alzheimers.org.uk
British Society for Research on Ageing, www.bsra.org.uk
Cancer Research UK, www.cancerresearchuk.org
Carers UK, www.carersuk.org
Dementia UK, www.dementiauk.org
My Home Life, www.myhomelife.org.uk
Ageing Well Public Talk Series, https://wels.open.ac.uk/research/projects/ageing-well-public-talks

Glossary

6 Cs The 6 Cs – care, compassion, courage, communication, commitment and competence – are a central plank of Compassion in Practice.

Abortion/miscarriage The legal definition of 'abortion' refers to the premature delivery of a non-viable fetus, spontaneously or by induction. In the UK, a fetus is considered viable from the 24th week of pregnancy. The term 'miscarriage' is recommended when the pregnancy loss is spontaneous and is generally more acceptable to women who lose a wanted pregnancy.

Acidaemia A high level of acid (hydrogen ions) in the blood which results in a below normal blood pH, less than 7.35 (greater than 44 nmol/L H+).

Acidosis The processes that lead to excess acid in the body.

Acute coronary syndrome A continuum of manifestations of coronary heart disease (CHD). It includes unstable angina and acute myocardial infarction which have as common underlying pathology the abrupt, total or subtotal occlusion of a coronary artery.

Acute pain Often described as being short-lived, that is, less than 6 weeks, and commonly nociceptive pain associated with surgery, trauma or acute disease.

Adaptive specific immunity The specific immune responses comprising the humoral (antibody-mediated) immune response, initiated by B lymphocytes, and the cell-mediated response, initiated by T lymphocytes.

Ageing The normal structural and physiological changes that occur with time. The process of growing old.

Age-related macular degeneration (AMD) Degenerative changes in the macular region of the retina that may lead to central vision loss. AMD may be described as 'dry' or 'wet'.

Albuminuria The presence of albumin in the urine.

Alkalaemia Low level of acid (hydrogen ions) in the blood and an above-normal pH.

Alkalosis The processes that result in low levels of acid (excess of alkali) in the body.

Allergen A usually innocuous substance capable of stimulating an allergic reaction.

Alzheimer's disease A neurodegenerative brain disorder characterised by progressive dementia. The onset is subtle and includes progressive memory loss (particularly short-term or recent), failing intellectual ability, confusion, restlessness, speech problems, motor retardation, depression and personality changes.

Ambulatory surgery (day surgery) Surgery undertaken on the day of admission. If recovery is problem free, the patient is discharged that day to the care of the primary care team. Procedures include cataract surgery, minor gynaecological and orthopaedic procedures and endoscopic examinations.

Amnesia Loss of memory.

Anaemia Decreased oxygen-carrying capacity of the blood, due to a reduced number of erythrocytes and/or the amount of haemoglobin within the erythrocytes.

Anaesthesia Loss of sensation.

Analgesics Drugs such as paracetamol or morphine that relieve pain.

Anaphylaxis Sudden life-threatening allergic reaction. An exaggerated type I hypersensitivity response to an antigen, such as peanuts or a penicillin.

Aneurysm A localised dilatation of a blood vessel. It usually occurs in an artery such as the aorta, carotid artery, cerebral arteries and popliteal artery.

Angina pectoris Part of the spectrum of acute coronary syndrome. Discomfort or pain felt in a variety of sites including the chest, throat and arms, resulting from a transient, reversible episode of inadequate coronary circulation.

Antibodies (immunoglobulins) Globular proteins able to recognise and bind to a specific antigen, usually a microorganism.

Antigen Foreign cell/substance that induces a specific immune response in the host.

Anuria Complete cessation of urine production by the kidneys.

Aphthous ulcers, aphthae Shallow, painful ulcers usually affecting the oral mucosa.

Apyrexia Without fever.

Arrhythmia A term used to imply an abnormality in either electrical impulse formation or electrical impulse conduction within the heart, e.g. atrial fibrillation.

Ascites (hydroperitoneum) An accumulation of fluid in the peritoneal cavity.

Aseptic no touch technique (ANTT) A set of principles and practices used in healthcare settings to prevent the transmission of infections during medical procedures. Also known as aseptic technique.

Asthma An obstructive pulmonary disease characterised by chronic inflammation of the airways with bronchial wall hyperactivity leading to bronchospasm and airway narrowing.

Ataxia Uncoordinated voluntary movement.

Atelectasis Alveolar collapse.

Atheroma Plaques of fatty material in the lining of arteries. Eventually the build-up reduces the lumen of the artery which results in ischaemia. A thrombus may develop if a plaque ruptures, which leads to further blockage of the artery.

Atherosclerosis Coexisting atheroma and arteriosclerosis.

Autoantibodies Abnormal antibodies that bind to self-antigens of normal body cells.

Autoimmune disorders Those that occur when the normal tolerance to 'self' breaks down and autoantibodies against self-antigens are formed.

Autologous Describes a situation in which the person's own cells are used for a graft, such as blood transfusion, skin or bone marrow.

AVPU Acronym from 'Alert, Voice, Pain, Unresponsive'. A system by which a healthcare professional can measure and record a patient's level of consciousness.

Biological response modifiers (BRMs) (immunotherapies) Substances that occur naturally in the body and can be used therapeutically. Most are involved in some way in the immune response. It may be possible to manipulate the immune system such that it recognises tumour cells as antigens and causes the body to reject them. Examples include cytokines and monoclonal antibodies.

Biopsy The procedure of obtaining a sample of tissue for examination from a specified area.

Body image The image held in the person's mind of their body.

Bradykinesia Slowness of movement.

Breast Screening Programme The NHS Breast Screening Programme is a national screening programme that aims to detect breast cancer early in women. The programme offers mammograms to women aged 50 to 70 years every three years. In some areas, the programme has been extended to include women aged 47 to 73 years.

Breast ultrasound A scan using high-frequency sound waves to image the breast tissue.

Breathlessness See Dyspnoea.

Burn assessment Involves factors including extent (size), depth, location, complexity and the possibility of respiratory involvement. Patient-related factors such as age are also considered.

Burn injury Tissue damage caused by moist and dry heat, flame, electricity, friction, chemicals (acids and alkalis) and radiation (sunlight and ionising radiation).

Burn sequelae (long term) Include psychosocial problems, wound contracture and scarring, and loss of function.

Burns prevention Involves assessment of the incidence of burn injuries, the causative agents and any predisposing factors, followed by planning, implementation and evaluation of appropriate interventions.

Cancer Cancer initiation is a very complex process involving the disruption of the regulation of growth of normal cells in the body. 'Cancer' is a general term describing any malignant tumour, the growth of which is purposeless, parasitic and at the expense of the host. It has a tendency to destroy tissue locally, attack adjacent tissue and spread to distant sites (metastasise).

Candidiasis (thrush) Fungal infection caused by *Candida*, usually *Candida albicans*. Affected areas include the mouth and gastrointestinal tract, respiratory tract, nails, skin or genitourinary tract (balanitis, vulvovaginitis). Risk factors include debilitation, e.g. by cancer, or immunosuppression, and long-term or extensive treatment with antibiotics and other drugs, such as corticosteroids. Candidiasis is also associated with immunodeficiency conditions including HIV disease.

Cardiac arrest Failure of the heart to pump sufficient blood to maintain cerebral function. The main mechanisms of cardiac arrest are:
pulseless ventricular tachycardia and ventricular fibrillation (VF)
ventricular asystole
pulseless electrical activity (PEA).

Cardiac output The volume of blood ejected from the ventricles in 1 minute.

Cardiogenic shock That caused by myocardial dysfunction, such as following an extensive myocardial infarction.

Cardiovascular disease (CVD) Diseases of the heart and blood vessels. The main diseases are CHD and stroke, but CVD also includes congenital heart disease and peripheral vascular disease.

Carer A person who accepts the responsibility for caring for another (child, person with an illness or disability, or an older person). Usually describes unpaid family, friends and neighbours in the UK, and not paid helpers such as care workers or nurses.

Cast (1) Exudate or other matter that has been moulded to the shape of a structure in which it has collected. (2) Splinting device comprising layers of bandages impregnated with plaster of Paris, fibreglass or resin; used to immobilise and hold bone fragments in reduction and to support and stabilise weak joints.

Cataract Opacity of the crystalline lens. Usually age related, but may be congenital, iatrogenic or due to inflammation, trauma or metabolic causes.

Cell-mediated immunity The adaptive specific immune response initiated by T lymphocytes important for dealing with intracellular organisms, such as viruses. Also causes graft rejection.

Central venous pressure (CVP) The blood pressure within the right atrium and vena cava. It provides information about blood volume or venous system capacity. It can also give an indication of vascular tone and pulmonary vascular resistance, as well as of the effectiveness of the right heart pump.

Chemotherapy Chemicals of various types, administered to delay or arrest growth of cancer cells.

Chlamydiae Microorganisms belonging to the genus *Chlamydia*. Subgroups of *Chlamydia trachomatis* lead to reproductive tract infections in adults which are sexually acquired. Men may be asymptomatic, but can have urethritis or epididymitis. Most chlamydial infections are symptomless in women; however, untreated women may develop pelvic inflammatory disease with damage to the uterine tubes with risk of ectopic pregnancy or infertility.

Chronic obstructive pulmonary disease (COPD) Chronic airflow limitation. There is increased airway resistance with impaired airflow, e.g. pulmonary emphysema, chronic bronchitis. Some authorities include asthma.

Chronic pain (persistent pain) Pain unresolved after 3 months. Subdivided into chronic non-malignant pain (nociceptive and/or neuropathic pain) and malignant (life-threatening) pain.

Cirrhosis 'Hardening' of an organ with degenerative changes and fibrosis. For example, liver cirrhosis is caused by viruses, other microorganisms, toxins including alcohol and nutritional deficiencies.

Climacteric The normal changes that occur leading up to the menopause (cessation of menstruation). The changes of the climacteric are usually gradual and may occur over several years.

Colloid A non-crystalline substance. It is diffusible but insoluble in water, thus it does not pass through a semi-permeable membrane.

Coma See Deep coma.

Compartment syndrome Occurs when tissue pressure within a compartment increases to the point that circulation and function of tissues are compromised. This results in tissue death (necrosis) and permanent loss of function, which can occur within 6–8 hours.

Computed tomography (CT) A computer-constructed imaging technique of a thin slice through the body, derived from X-ray absorption data collected during a circular scanning motion.

Concordance The making of decisions about treatment and management in negotiation and partnership with the patient. It is very different from compliance where the patient is expected to agree to treatment decisions made by a healthcare professional.

Consciousness A 'state of general awareness of oneself and the environment' and includes the ability to orientate towards new stimuli. The individual is awake, alert and aware of their personal identity and of the events occurring in their surroundings.

Consent Informed consent to treatment, surgery and any intervention that requires physical contact is a legal requirement. Depending on the intervention, consent may be verbal, written or implied, i.e. by non-verbal communication.

Constipation The infrequent and difficult passing of hard stools.

Continence Having voluntary control over voiding urine and passing faeces.

Coping In a neutral sense, the term 'coping' refers to the way in which the individual responds to a stressful situation or to the perception of threat, by attempting consciously and unconsciously to maintain equilibrium.

Core body temperature See Deep body (core) temperature.

Coronary heart disease (CHD) Includes angina pectoris and myocardial infarction; caused by a deficient supply of oxygenated blood to the myocardium.

Corticosteroids Three types of hormones produced by the adrenal cortex: glucocorticoids, mineralocorticoids, sex hormones. Also applied to synthetic steroids such as prednisolone.

COVID-19 Short for "coronavirus disease 2019," is an infectious disease caused by the severe acute respiratory syndrome coronavirus 2 (SARS-CoV-2). First identified in December 2019 and has since spread globally, leading to the ongoing COVID-19 pandemic.

Creatinine A substance produced during the metabolism of creatine phosphate in muscle tissue. It is normally removed from the blood by the kidneys and excreted in the urine. Measurements of creatinine in blood and urine are used to assess renal function.

Critical care support See Levels of critical care support.

Crystalloid A clear solution containing molecules small enough to pass through semi-permeable membranes, i.e. between the blood and the interstitial fluid.

Cyanosis Bluish discoloration of the skin, mucous membranes, or nail beds due to low oxygen levels in the blood, can be more challenging to detect in individuals with darker skin tones. In people with darker skin tones, other signs of cyanosis may be more noticeable, such as a bluish tint in the lips, gums or tongue or a dusky appearance of the skin.

Debridement Removal of dead or devitalised tissue. This can be achieved in various ways including autolysis with dressings, or sharp or surgical debridement.

Deep body (core) temperature The temperature (close to 37°C) of the organs of the central cavities of the body, i.e. cranium, thorax and abdomen.

Deep coma Deep coma is the opposite of consciousness, it is defined as being unrousable and unresponsive to external stimuli; there are varied states of altered consciousness in between the two extremes.

Defaecation The passage of faeces which may be involuntary or voluntary.

Dehiscence Breakdown of a surgical wound, most commonly due to infection or undue strain on wound edges.

Delirium An acute confusional state. A fluctuating mental state with disturbance of awareness and thought processes characterised by confusion, disorientation, fear, irritability and disturbed or agitated behaviour.

Dementia A progressive irreversible brain disorder leading to memory disturbance, impaired cognition, disorientation and personality changes. The many causes include Alzheimer's disease and vascular degeneration.

Dentition The natural teeth present in the dental arches of a person. The 20 primary teeth and later the 32 permanent teeth of the secondary dentition.

Detrusor The smooth muscle of the walls of the bladder, which contracts to empty the bladder.

Diabetes mellitus A metabolic disorder characterised by chronic hyperglycaemia with disturbances of carbohydrate, protein and fat metabolism which results from defects in insulin secretion, insulin action or both.

Diabetic ketoacidosis (DKA) Uncontrolled lipolysis in the absence of insulin, gluconeogenesis, ketogenesis and glycogenolysis combine to raise the blood glucose level still further, increase osmotic diuresis, and exacerbate fluid imbalance and metabolic acidosis.

Dialysis Renal replacement therapy. A process involving diffusion, osmosis and filtration in which solutes (waste, electrolytes) and excess fluid are removed across a selectively permeable membrane in patients with renal failure.

Diarrhoea Loose, frequent watery stools.

Diffusion The passive (requiring no energy) movement of solutes from an area of higher concentration to an area of lower concentration, which results in an equal concentration in both areas.

Dignity A complex concept with many definitions. Dignified care is that which promotes the person's self-respect and usually involves respect. See Person-centred care.

Disability The medical model regards disability as a problem which is intrinsic to the person and caused directly by disease, a health condition or trauma. In this model, 'impairment' is not only used to describe disturbance in the body's structure and function. It is also seen as responsible for preventing the individual's participation in normal society and, therefore, disabling them. Conversely, the social model is based on the assumption that disability exists where attitudinal or environmental barriers exclude people with impairments from full engagement in mainstream activities. This defines it as a socially created problem which is distinct from and superimposed on impairment.

Donor area/site The area used to take a skin graft to treat a burn injury.

Dyspareunia Difficult or painful sexual intercourse for a woman.

Dyspepsia Indigestion. A feeling of fullness after eating and discomfort in the epigastrium. Causes include peptic ulcer, chronic cholecystitis and gallstones.

Dysphagia Difficulty swallowing. Causes include oesophageal stricture or tumour, stroke, motor neurone disease.

Dysphasia Loss of ability to understand/produce language.

Dyspnoea Difficulty in or laboured breathing. May be due to respiratory conditions, anaemia or cardiovascular conditions.

Dysuria Pain or discomfort on micturition. Often due to bacterial infection (urethritis, cystitis, prostatitis) but may be associated with bladder tumours or calculi, or changes to urethral mucosa during the climacteric.

Elective surgery Planned surgery rather than an emergency procedure.

Embolism Obstruction of a blood vessel by a mass of undissolved material. Usually caused by a thrombus (clot), but other causes include malignant cells, fat, amniotic fluid, gases, bacteria and parasites.

Emollient An agent that moisturises and lubricates the skin. Used as soap substitute/bath additive or 'leave on' preparations.

Encopresis The involuntary or voluntary passage of a normal consistency stool in a socially unacceptable place.

End of life care (terminal care/phase) Care delivered in the last days of life. The focus moves from achieving a quality of life and supporting the patient in 'living whilst dying' whilst their illness is progressing, to ensuring a peaceful death and supporting the family in coping with their impending loss. Readers should be aware that the terminology is sometimes used differently.

Enteral feeding The delivery of nutrients directly into the stomach or small intestine via a tube.

Enuresis Any involuntary loss of urine; it may be primary or secondary. Nocturnal enuresis is urinary incontinence occurring during sleep, in the absence of organic disease or infection.

Epilepsies A group of conditions resulting from intermittent, uncontrolled discharge of neurones within the CNS. Manifests seizures which can range from a major motor convulsion to a brief period of lack of awareness and can occur in any individual at any time.

Epistaxis Bleeding from the nose. Causes include nasal trauma, infection or tumour, hypertension, coagulation problems and sudden changes in atmospheric pressure.

Erectile dysfunction (ED) The inability to achieve and maintain an erection sufficient for sexual intercourse.

Erythema Skin redness due to vascular congestion or perfusion.

Escharotomy Incision(s) into eschar for decompression. Used in full-thickness burn injury occurring circumferentially around a limb, to prevent compression of the deeper structures, especially the blood vessels, or when full-thickness burn injury of the chest/upper abdomen inhibits respiratory movement.

Expert Patient Programme (EPP) The UK Government's EPP initiative stems from recognition that traditional cure-oriented services have not dealt comprehensively with problems faced by people with long-term conditions and that partnership enhances self efficacy. EPPs are led by lay people rather than healthcare professionals. EPPs aim to increase people's confidence, resourcefulness and control, thereby improving quality of life and reducing service use.

External fixation Used to keep bone fragments in position by skeletal pins inserted into the bone on either side of the fracture and held in alignment by a scaffold or a ring fixator.

Exudate Wound fluid which ranges from a watery consistency to being thick and tenacious. It is serous fluid which is beneficial for moist wound healing and bringing growth factors to the wound. However, enzymes in exudate can cause wound and skin breakdown if not controlled.

Falls prevention A person-centred, multidisciplinary approach to care. Education, training and audit are integral to falls prevention strategies. People in contact with health professionals should be assessed for risk routinely. Assessment of risk of falling and interventions should be multifactorial.

Fever High deep/core body temperature due to an upward reset in the hypothalamic set-point temperature.

First aid The immediate management of a person following sudden illness or injury before the arrival of a qualified health professional. The aims are to preserve life, prevent deterioration and promote recovery.

Fluid replacement Various ways of replacing fluid lost from the body – oral, enteral, subcutaneous, rectal, parenteral.

Fracture A break in the continuity of a bone resulting from direct or indirect trauma, repetitive stress applied to a bone or disease affecting bone.

Frailty Weakness and/or infirmity occurring not only as the result of medical condition(s) but also as a result of the difficult losses sometimes experienced in later life.

Frequency Voiding of urine more often than is acceptable to the person. Usually it is more often than before and in smaller volumes.

Full-thickness burn injury Destroys the epidermis and all of the dermis; may also involve deeper structures such as fat, muscle and bone.

Gastritis Acute or chronic inflammation of the stomach lining.

Gingivitis Inflammation of the gingivae (gums).

Glasgow Coma Scale (GCS) A reliable rating scale of conscious level for trauma and neurological patients that assesses their best motor, verbal and eye opening response. The best response for each of the three aspects is recorded as a numerical score: best eye opening is 4, best verbal is 5 and the best motor is 6. The lowest response for each of the three parameters is a score of 1. Thus the highest total score is 15 and the lowest is 3.

Glomerular filtration rate (GFR) The volume of plasma filtered by the kidneys in one minute. In health it is typically around 120 mL/min.

Glucagon A catabolic pancreatic hormone secreted in response to falling blood glucose. It causes glycogenolysis and the release of glucose from the liver and increased fat and protein breakdown in order to provide an alternative source of glucose via lipolysis and gluconeogenesis.

Gonorrhoea Caused by the bacterium *Neisseria gonorrhoeae*, it is a sexually acquired infection in adults. Newborns may be infected during a vaginal delivery leading to gonococcal conjunctivitis. Gonococcal vulvovaginitis in prepubertal girls may point to sexual abuse. Most women with uncomplicated gonorrhoea are asymptomatic, whereas men have dysuria and purulent urethral discharge.

Grading A classification of cancers based on histopathological characteristics.

Granulation New red, moist tissue in a wound. Comprises new capillaries held in a matrix of collagen and other cells found in a healing wound.

Haematemesis Vomiting of blood. It is bright red in recent bleeding, darker in colour or resembling 'coffee grounds' due to the action of gastric acid in earlier bleeding. Bleeding usually originates from the upper gastrointestinal tract due to gastritis, peptic ulceration, oesophageal varices, tumour, drug-induced erosions or blood coagulation disorders. Blood swallowed following oral trauma, dental procedures or epistaxis may be vomited.

Haematopoiesis Formation of blood cells from pluripotent stem cells present in the red marrow.

Haematopoietic growth factors Substances controlling haematopoiesis. They include hormones, cytokines and growth factors including erythropoietin, colony-stimulating factors (CSFs), thrombopoietin and interleukins.

Haematopoietic stem cell transplantation (HSCT) The transplantation of healthy haematopoietic progenitor cells to re-establish healthy bone marrow function in someone whose bone marrow has been destroyed or depleted by disease or its treatment.

Haematuria Blood present in the urine. It may be macroscopic, when it may be bright red, dark red or smoky in appearance; or microscopic when it is detected by dipstick urine tests or microscopy. Causes include urinary tract infection, glomerulonephritis, cancer, kidney trauma, urinary calculi, anticoagulant drugs or blood coagulation disorders.

Haemofiltration A form of renal replacement therapy in which the patient's blood is passed through a filter allowing separation of an ultrafiltrate containing fluid and solutes. This is discarded and replaced with an isotonic solution. It is usually continuous as in continuous venovenous haemofiltration (CVVH).

Haemophilias A group of inherited disorders in which an essential coagulation factor is either partly or completely missing. A person with haemophilia bleeds for longer than normal. Haemophilia is a recessive X-linked condition (sex-linked inheritance) which nearly always affects males, while females carry the defective gene. However, it is possible for a female to have haemophilia or a bleeding tendency.

Haemoptysis Coughing up of blood or blood-stained sputum/mucus from the respiratory tract. The amount ranges from blood-streaked sputum up to a life-threatening haemorrhage. The blood may be bright red, pink and frothy or described as rusty looking. Causes include pneumonia, lung abscess, tuberculosis, chronic bronchitis, lung cancer, pulmonary infarction, left ventricular failure, anticoagulant drugs and blood coagulation disorders.

Hand hygiene Considered to be the most important step in preventing healthcare-associated infection (HCAI). Recognising the times when hand hygiene is required is crucially important. These are: before touching a patient, before invasive procedures including aseptic tasks, after body fluid exposure risk, after touching a patient and touching patient surroundings. An effective hand hygiene technique is important in ensuring adequate hand hygiene standards. This includes ensuring thorough cleansing and drying of all areas of the hands and avoiding recontamination when closing taps and disposing of paper towels.

Healthcare-associated infection (HCAI) Previously known as hospital-acquired infection (HAI) or nosocomial infection. Refers to infection acquired during receipt of some form of health care.

Healthy diet One that provides the appropriate amounts of all nutrients in the correct proportions to meet body requirements.

Hearing loss (deafness) May be total or partial and can affect all age groups. It may be conductive (e.g. cerumen) or sensorineural (e.g. damage to the organ of Corti or the cochlear part of the VIIIth cranial nerve).

Heart failure A clinical syndrome that results from an inability of the heart to provide an adequate cardiac output for the body's metabolic requirements. It may be acute or chronic. Heart failure may involve either ventricle or both together.

Highly active antiretroviral therapy (HAART) Combination of three or more different types of antiretroviral drugs active against HIV at different stages of replication.

Histamine H₂-receptor antagonists Drugs such as ranitidine that reduce gastric acid production by blocking the histamine H_2 receptors. Used in gastro-oesophageal reflux disease and peptic ulceration.

Homeostasis The autoregulatory mechanisms whereby functions such as blood pH, glucose, body temperature and so on are maintained within set parameters.

Hormone Chemical messenger secreted by endocrine glands, neurones and other structures. Usually travelling in the bloodstream, hormones maintain homeostasis by acting on and coordinating activity within target organs or tissues.

Hormone therapy The use of drugs to replace, manipulate or block the production and function of circulating hormones.

Hospice care Care provided for people with life-limiting illnesses and their families, including end of life care. Care may be offered at home, as day-care and in hospice premises.

Human immunodeficiency virus (HIV) The virus causing AIDS.

Human papilloma virus (HPV) HPV is a group of more than 150 related viruses. Each HPV virus is given a number which is called its HPV type. HPV is named for the warts some HPV types can cause. Some other HPV types can lead to cancer. Men and women can get cancer of mouth/ throat, and anus/rectum caused by HPV infections. Men can also get penile HPV cancer. In women the infection can also cause cervical, vaginal, and vulvar cancers.

Humoral (antibody-mediated) immunity Adaptive specific immune response initiated by B lymphocytes. The humoral response deals mainly with extracellular organisms through the production of antibodies (immunoglobulins).

Hypercalcaemia Excessive level of calcium in the blood.

Hypercapnia Increased carbon dioxide tension in arterial blood.

Hyperchloraemia Excessive level of chlorides in the blood.

Hyperglycaemia Increased level of glucose in the blood.

Hyperkalaemia Excessive level of potassium in the blood.

Hypermagnesaemia Excessive level of magnesium in the blood.

Hypernatraemia Excessive level of sodium in the blood.

Hyperphosphataemia Excessive level of phosphates in the blood.

Hyperpyrexia Core body temperature above 40–42°C due to an altered set-point.

Hypersensitivity and allergic reactions Abnormal and excessive immune responses following contact with an antigen (allergen). Effects range from local tissue damage to life-threatening anaphylaxis.

Hypertension An abnormally high arterial blood pressure involving systolic and/or diastolic readings.

Hyperthermia An abnormally high body deep/core temperature caused by loss of thermoregulatory control.

Hypertonic solutions Those with a higher osmotic pressure relative to another solution such as serum.

Hypertrophic scar Scar that appears red and is raised above the level of the surrounding skin. A complication of burn injury.

Hypervolaemia Increased volume of circulating blood.

Hypocalcaemia Decreased level of calcium in the blood.

Hypochloraemia Decreased level of chlorides in the blood.

Hypoglycaemia Decreased level of glucose in the blood.

Hypokalaemia Decreased level of potassium in the blood.

Hypomagnesaemia Decreased level of magnesium in the blood.

Hyponatraemia Decreased level of sodium in the blood.

Hypophosphataemia Decreased level of phosphates in the blood.

Hypothermia A state in which the deep/core body temperature is lower than the thermoregulatory set-point. Usually considered to be below 35°C.

Hypotonic solutions Those with a lower osmotic pressure relative to another solution such as serum.

Hypovolaemia Reduced volume of circulating blood.

Hypoxaemia Reduced oxygen content in arterial blood, evidenced by decreased PaO_2.

Hypoxia Reduced oxygen in the tissues.

Immunity An innate or acquired state of immune responsiveness to an antigen.

Immunodeficiency Defective immune responses, leading to increased susceptibility to infection, autoimmune diseases and cancer.

Immunoglobulins See Antibodies.

Immunosuppressants Drugs that suppress the immune responses, e.g. ciclosporin, tacrolimus.

Immunotherapy See Biological response modifiers.

Impaired glucose tolerance (IGT) and Impaired fasting glycaemia (IFG) Stages in the natural history of diabetes rather than a class of diabetes.

Infection prevention Measures required routinely in order to minimise the risk of infection to patients, their relatives/carers and staff. These include standard precautions (e.g. hand hygiene, personal protective equipment, environmental cleaning), decontamination of reusable medical devices, transmission-based precautions, aseptic and clean techniques, use of evidence-based practice guidelines, antimicrobial stewardship and outbreak management.

Infertility A couple is said to be subfertile if they have been having unprotected sexual intercourse for 12 months without conception occurring. It may be primary or secondary where there has been a previous pregnancy, irrespective of the outcome.

Inflammation A non-specific defence mechanism initiated by tissue injury. The injury may be caused by trauma, microorganisms, extremes of temperature and pH, ultraviolet (UV) radiation, or ionising radiation. A phase in wound healing.

Insomnia Sleeplessness. An inability to initiate sleep or to stay asleep or waking in the early hours. Sleep is of poor quality and the person does not feel refreshed.

Insomnia treatments Include pharmacological solutions, alternative approaches, e.g. developing good sleep habits ('sleep hygiene'), complementary and alternative medicine therapies (CAM) and cognitive-behavioural therapies.

Insulin An anabolic pancreatic hormone secreted in response to a rising blood glucose level. Insulin has numerous effects on the metabolism of carbohydrate, fat and protein.

Internal fixation An operative fracture reduction whereby metal pins, plates, screws or nails are used to hold the bony fragments in position.

Intracranial pressure (ICP) Pressure exerted inside the skull by the brain, cerebrospinal fluid and blood volume contained within the cranium.

Intracranial pressure monitoring Invasive technique involving direct measurement of ICP. A typical system comprises a fibreoptic transducer-tipped catheter, which can be placed in the lateral ventricle, subdural or extradural space.

Ischaemia Lack of oxygenated (arterial) blood to an area of tissue, causing tissue destruction. Can be a result of a compromised vascular system due either to atherosclerosis or to localised pressure, both of which cause arterial occlusion.

Isotonic Having equal tension. Any solution which has the same osmotic pressure as the fluid with which it is being compared.

Jaundice Yellow discoloration of the skin, sclerae and mucosae. It is due to an increase in the level of bilirubin in the blood. It may be accompanied by pruritus.

Joint arthroplasty (joint replacement) The surgical insertion of inert prostheses of similar shape into joints, such as hip, knee and shoulder. May be total, as in replacing the head of femur and acetabulum, or partial.

Laxatives (aperients) Drugs used to prevent or relieve constipation. Administered orally or rectally (suppositories or enema).

Leg ulcer A leg ulcer is the loss of skin below the knee on the leg or foot, which takes more than two weeks to heal.

Lesion An area of skin with changes to texture, elevation or colour which is bordered by normal skin.

Leukaemia A group of blood disorders in which there is abnormal and excessive proliferation of malignant leucocytes. Typically divided into acute and chronic types, and further subdivided into myeloid or lymphoid types depending on the type of leucocytes affected.

Levels of critical care support Level 0 – Patients whose needs can be met through normal ward care in an acute hospital. Level 1 – Patients at risk of their condition deteriorating, or those recently relocated from a higher level of care, whose needs can be met on an acute ward with additional advice and support from the critical care team. Level 2 – Patients requiring more detailed observation or intervention including support for a single failing organ system or postoperative care and those 'stepping down' from a higher level of care. Level 3 – Patients requiring advanced respiratory support alone or basic respiratory support together with support of at least two organ systems. This level includes all complex patients requiring support for multiorgan failure.

Life-limiting illness A progressive and ultimately fatal condition. Includes inherited diseases such as muscular dystrophy as well as cancer, chronic respiratory and cardiovascular disease, stroke and dementia.

Locked in syndrome Damage to the pons in the brain stem, resulting from cerebral vascular disease or trauma, paralyses voluntary muscles without interfering with consciousness and cognitive functions. The patient is unable to speak and is sometimes unable to breathe spontaneously. However, they are able to control vertical eye movements and blinking and may be able to use these movements to develop a simple communication system.

Lund and Browder's charts Used to calculate more accurately a burn area. They allow for the changing proportions of different age groups and show which percentages are applicable to smaller, more specific areas of the body surface.

Lymphoma A group of malignant disorders characterised by a proliferation of lymphoid cells originating in the lymph nodes or lymphoid tissue. Traditionally divided into two groups: Hodgkin's lymphoma (HL) and non-Hodgkin lymphoma (NHL).

Magnetic resonance imaging (MRI) A non-invasive imaging technique that uses a powerful magnetic field combined with radiofrequency pulses to excite hydrogen nuclei in the body. When the hydrogen nuclei settle, the signal from the body is measured and reconstructed, using computer software, into two-dimensional or three-dimensional images.

Major incident preparedness (emergency planning) The emergency preparedness for major incidents within the NHS to ensure that all the emergency services are able to work collaboratively and provide an effective response to any type of incident.

Mammogram Breast X-ray that involves compression of the breast tissue both laterally and medial-obliquely before the X-ray is taken.

Mastectomy Surgical removal of the breast.

Mechanical ventilation Artificial support of, or assistance with, breathing when adequate gaseous exchange and tissue perfusion can no longer be maintained. Respiratory support may be invasive through an endotracheal tube or tracheostomy or non-invasive through a mask or hood.

Melaena Black stools with tar-like consistency with a distinctive odour. They contain digested blood and are evidence of upper gastrointestinal bleeding, such as from oesophageal varices, peptic ulceration, stomach cancer, or small bowel disease.

Menopause The cessation of menstruation, a single event occurring during the climacteric.

Menstrual (uterine) cycle The endometrial changes caused by the ovarian hormones. They correspond to the hormonal events of the ovarian cycle and can be divided into three phases: proliferative phase (follicular or pre-ovulatory), secretory phase (luteal or post-ovulatory) and menstrual phase.

Mouth care See Oral hygiene.

Multidisciplinary team (MDT) A team of healthcare professionals assigned to plan, treat, care and meet the needs of the individual with a particular condition or need, such as a woman with breast cancer when the team would usually include surgeons, pathologists, radiologists, specialist nurses, radiographers, and others.

Multiple organ dysfunction syndrome (MODS) A syndrome in critically ill patients in which more than one organ system (e.g. renal, coagulation, respiratory and gastrointestinal) fails to function normally and may progress to multiple organ failure. It requires appropriate organ support such as mechanical ventilation and haemofiltration.

Myeloma (multiple myeloma) An uncommon malignant disorder characterised by abnormal and unregulated proliferation of plasma cells which develop from mature B lymphocytes.

Myocardial infarction (MI) Part of the spectrum of acute coronary syndrome. There is death (necrosis) of part of the myocardium (heart muscle) from deprivation of oxygenated blood following occlusion of a coronary artery.

Nasal obstruction Results from a number of causes, e.g. infection, polyps. The most common symptoms are obstructed breathing and increased nasal discharge.

Negative feedback A homeostatic mechanism whereby increased levels, for example, of a specific hormone in the blood 'turn off' or cancel the stimulus causing hormone secretion. Once hormone levels are below the normal range, the stimulus is 'turned on' and again causes the hormone to be secreted.

Neurogenic shock A type of distributive shock, which is due to altered vascular resistance.

Neurological assessment Includes the Glasgow Coma Scale, vital signs – blood pressure, pulse rate, respirations, temperature, and also pupil size and reaction and limb movements.

Neuropathic pain Describes pain that persists beyond the original cause, such as a nerve injury or infective cause.

Neutropaenia A decrease in the number of circulating neutrophils to below 1.0×10^9/L.

NEWS 2 (National Early Warning 2) A tool used in healthcare settings, particularly in hospitals, to quickly assess and track the severity of illness in patients. It is based on a scoring system that takes into account various physiological parameters, such as respiratory rate, oxygen saturation, temperature, systolic blood pressure, heart rate, and level of consciousness.

Nociceptive pain Somatic or visceral pain that results from stimulation of nociceptors following tissue damage or inflammation, e.g. surgery, infection or trauma.

Nocturia Waking up to void urine at night.

Non-rapid eye movement (NREM) sleep Four sleep stages associated with differing electrical activity of the brain.

Non-specific immunity Natural non-specific immunity includes intact skin/mucosae, specialised epithelial surfaces, body secretions containing antibacterial substances such as lysozyme and immunoglobulins and the microorganisms of the normal flora. The inflammatory process and phagocytosis are also included. Additionally, natural killer (NK) cells detect and destroy damaged or malignant cells and virus-infected cells, and undertake non-specific immunosurveillance.

Nutritional science The science of the macronutrients and micronutrients needed to maintain health.

Obesity The condition of excessive accumulation of fat in the body, leading to an increase in weight beyond that considered desirable.

Oedema Abnormal collection of fluid in the tissues, such as around the ankles. Fluid may also collect in the pericardial or pleural cavities or in the abdominal cavity.

Oliguria Reduced urine output.

Oral assessment Thorough examination to assess the condition of the oral cavity, preferably using a valid and reliable tool for the care setting.

Oral cancers Cancers affecting the lips, floor of the mouth and tongue, the palate and the salivary glands.

Oral candidiasis See Candidiasis.

Oral hygiene Measures required to ensure the mouth is clean and healthy, including a thorough oral assessment, sufficient fluid intake (especially oral fluids), teeth and oral surface cleaning and regular dental examination.

Orodental disease Includes both conditions of the teeth (plaque, calculus, caries) and periodontal conditions affecting the supporting structures of the teeth (gingivitis, periodontitis).

Orofacial trauma Soft tissue injuries range from simple lacerations, knife wounds and bites to multiple injuries resulting in tissue loss. Bone injuries include fracture of the mandible and fracture of the maxillae, malar (zygomatic) and nasal bones (middle third fracture). Causes include violence, road traffic accidents, work accidents, sport, falls and burns.

Osmolality The concentration of a solution expressed as osmoles of solute per kilogram of solvent.

Osmolarity The concentration of a solution expressed as osmoles of solute per litre of solvent.

Osmosis Passive movement of fluid from an area of lower concentration (of solutes) to an area of higher concentration, in an attempt to dilute the 'stronger' solution and achieve an equal balance on both sides of the membrane.

Osteoarthritis (OA) Slow deterioration of the articular cartilage in a synovial joint. OA may be primary or secondary; the former is more common in older people, especially females.

Oxygen therapy A potent drug used to relieve breathlessness and manage hypoxaemia.

Pain management (palliative care) Analgesic medications, given regularly to prevent the recurrence of pain, are central to effective pain management in palliative care. An adequate, regular dose is calculated and administered, enabling the patient to be as comfortable as possible without being drowsy.

Pain threshold The least experience of pain that a person can recognise.

Pain tolerance This the most pain that a person is prepared to abide.

Palliative care The active holistic care of a patient with advanced progressive illness. Management of pain and other symptoms and provision of psychological, social and spiritual support. The aim of palliative care is to achieve the best quality of life for patients and their families. End of life care includes palliative care.

Paraesthesia Abnormal sensation, e.g. tingling or 'pins and needles'.

Parenteral nutrition Nutrients in solution infused directly into the venous system.

Partial-thickness burn injury Injury involving the epidermis and part of the dermis. Classified as 'superficial' or 'deep', depending on the amount of dermis involved.

Perioperative care Care throughout the surgical experience from pre-admission, pre-operative period, anaesthesia and surgery, recovery to postoperative period.

Peripheral vascular disease (PVD) Pathological processes affecting both the peripheral arterial and venous circulations.

Personal protective equipment (PPE) The disposable, single-use clothing and equipment, e.g. disposable gloves, aprons/gowns, goggles/visors and masks/respirators, available to healthcare workers, and at times visitors, to protect them from exposure to microorganisms no matter in which setting they are working.

Pneumonia Lower respiratory tract infection. Characterised by inflammation of the lung parenchyma, usually resulting from bacterial and viral infection, but may be fungal or parasitic.

Positron emission tomography (PET) scan Imaging technique that produces three-dimensional images illustrating metabolic activity in particular areas of the body. It employs cyclotron-produced isotopes of extremely short half-life that emit positrons which are introduced into the patient. As positrons react with electrons in the body gamma rays are emitted, which are detected by a specialist gamma camera.

PrEP Pre-exposure prophylaxis. When people at very high risk for HIV take HIV medicines daily to lower their chances of getting infected. PrEP can stop HIV from taking hold and spreading throughout the body. It is highly effective for preventing HIV if used as prescribed.

Pressure ulcer Pressure ulcers are also known as pressure sores or bedsores. They are injuries to the skin and underlying tissue, primarily caused by prolonged pressure on the skin, sheer or friction.

Primary and secondary surveys Assessment and management of the trauma patient includes the initial assessment (primary survey) which has five components ('A, B, C, D, E'):

Airway with cervical spine control

Breathing and ventilation

Circulation and haemorrhage control

Disability and dysfunction

Exposure and environmental control

The secondary survey only commences when the primary survey is complete and the patient's condition is stabilised. The secondary survey may not take place in the ED, as the critically injured patient is likely to require surgical intervention to stabilise their condition. If the patient's condition does permit, then the secondary survey involves a full head-to-toe examination and gives the nurse the opportunity to complete a thorough assessment, including documenting wounds (location, surface area and depth), skin integrity, tetanus status, allergies.

Protein pump inhibitors (PPIs) Drugs such as lansoprazole that inhibit gastric acid production by blocking the 'proton pump' in the parietal cells of the stomach. Used with antibacterials to eliminate *Helicobacter pylori*, for gastro-oesophageal reflux disease, peptic ulceration.

Proteinuria Protein in the urine.

Pruritus Intense itching. Generalised pruritus may be associated with jaundice, cancer, renal failure or Hodgkin's lymphoma. Localised pruritus affecting the vulva or perianal area may be due to a number of causes, e.g. vaginal candidiasis.

Public health nutrition The promotion of good nutritional health and the prevention of diet-related illness in groups of people, rather than the nutritional care of individuals.

Pyrexia Deep/core body temperature above normal.

Radiotherapy The use of ionising radiation to kill dividing cells in a therapeutic approach.

Rapid/premature ejaculation (PE) Persistent or recurrent ejaculation with minimal stimulation that causes marked interpersonal distress.

Rash A skin eruption. A collection of numerous lesions, with some coalescing.

Reconstructive breast surgery A surgical method using implants or autologous tissue flaps to re-create the breast once a mastectomy has been performed.

Re-feeding syndrome The term 're-feeding syndrome' is applied to the problems arising from sudden feeding in a very malnourished patient. This is caused by a rapid shift of electrolytes, glucose and water from extracellular to intracellular compartments, causing deficits in the extracellular fluid.

Rehabilitation Definitions vary, in line with the perceived purpose, but it is best described as an ongoing process which begins as soon as individuals are clinically stable, is independent of the location of care, reflects a transferable underpinning philosophy and involves shifting degrees and forms of support.

Respiratory failure Results from a situation where the lungs fail to oxygenate the blood sufficiently or excrete waste carbon dioxide.

Reticular activating system (RAS) A diffuse functional area of the reticular formation. It has connections with other brain areas including the thalamus, hypothalamus, cerebral cortex and ocular motor nuclei. Involved in levels of consciousness, cortical arousal and sleep/wake cycles.

Reticular formation (RF) A network of neurones within the brain stem that connect with the spinal cord, cerebellum, thalamus and hypothalamus. Involved in the coordination of skeletal muscle activity, including voluntary movement, posture and balance, as well as automatic and reflex activities that link with the limbic system.

Retinopathy Disease of the retina. Associated with hypertension, diabetes mellitus, abnormal retinal vessels and sun damage.

Rheumatoid arthritis (RA) A systemic autoimmune disease of connective tissue. There is joint inflammation due to inflammatory changes in the synovial membrane. The synovium becomes thicker, very vascular and there may be joint effusion. As proliferative tissue spreads as a 'pannus' over the articular cartilage, the cartilage is slowly eroded. Systemic inflammatory effects include pericarditis, alveolitis, pleuritis, eye involvement and bowel vasculitis, as well as general malaise, fever and anaemia.

Rigidity Increased resistance to passive movement; it is not velocity dependent.

Scabies A parasitic skin disease caused by the itch mite (*Sarcoptes scabiei*). Highly contagious, scabies spreads in situations where there is frequent intimate personal contact.

Screening Secondary preventive measure to identify potential or incipient disease at an early stage when it may be more easily treated.

Sepsis State of being infected with pus-forming (pyogenic) microorganisms.

Sepsis Six The Sepsis Six is an initial resuscitation bundle designed to offer basic intervention within the first hour of initial identification of sepsis.

Seroconversion Conversion from a negative blood test where specific antibodies are not present to a positive test in which specific antibodies present in the serum confirm that a response to an antigen has taken place.

Shock A state in which there is inadequate flow of oxygenated blood to the tissues, which results in cell hypoxia and inadequate tissue perfusion.

Sickle cell disease An inherited haemoglobinopathy.

Sinusitis Inflammation of one or more paranasal sinuses.

Skin graft A sheet of skin containing dermis and epidermis applied to a raw surface such as burn injury.

Spasticity Increased muscle tone; there is velocity-dependent increase in tonic stretch reflexes.

Staging (of cancer) This is a way of describing the size of a cancer and how far it has grown. When a diagnosis of cancer is made, tests are carried out to determine how big the cancer is and if it has spread into surrounding tissues as well as to other parts of the body. There are a number of staging systems in use.

Standard precautions The measures applied at all times when performing healthcare activities in order to minimise the risk of spreading microorganisms to patients, healthcare staff and others, including hand hygiene, dealing with blood and body fluid spillages, PPE, prevention of exposure to infection. Applied routinely in all situations, whether or not an infection has been identified.

Stoma An opening, such as a colostomy.

Stomatitis Inflammation of the mouth.

Stress Can be considered as a disturbed homeostasis that can result in physiological and psychological imbalances. The impact of stress occurs only when the cumulative effects of stressors surpass the individual's ability easily to return to equilibrium.

Stress management The methods used to manage stress include deep breathing, improving diet and regular exercise.

Stroke (cerebrovascular accident) Sudden loss of blood supply to an area of the brain causing a neurological defect lasting more than 24 hours.

Stroke volume The volume of blood ejected from the heart by each ventricular contraction.

Superficial burn injury A type of partial-thickness burn injury in which there is limited dermal involvement.

Swallowing (deglutition) A process initiated voluntarily but completed through involuntary reflex action. It has three stages: the voluntary oral stage, pharyngeal stage (reflex) and oesophageal.

Symptom management in palliative care Effective symptom management requires a thorough assessment of each symptom, e.g. pain, nausea and vomiting, breathlessness, cough, hiccup and constipation, before discussing causes and options with the patient. Management is planned in consideration of the patient's expectations and priorities and evaluated regularly.

Terminal care Care in the last stage of a patient's illness, where there is increasing disability and dependence and death is anticipated in the near future. See End of life care.

Testicular cancer Cancers of the testes are divided into two groups: germ cell tumours (the majority) or stromal tumours. The two basic groups are further subdivided. Testicular cancer is a relatively rare cancer, but is the most common cancer in males aged 15–44 years and is one of the most curable solid tumours.

Thalassaemia An inherited haemoglobinopathy.

Thermogenesis Production of body heat, either chemically by the release of noradrenaline (non-shivering thermogenesis [NST]) or physically by skeletal muscle contraction (shivering thermogenesis).

Thrombocytopenia Decrease in the number of platelets (thrombocytes) in the blood.

Thrombosis The formation of a thrombus (clot) in the heart, artery or vein.

Tinnitus Usually a subjective sensation of sound in the ear. It is often accompanied by vertigo and/or deafness.

Tonsillectomy Surgical removal of the palatine tonsils.

Tracheostomy An opening through the skin and structures of the neck into the trachea.

Traction A pulling force applied to a part or parts of the body; counter-traction, a pulling force in the opposite direction, is also applied. Counter-traction is usually supplied by the patient's body weight. Traction may be skeletal or skin traction, balanced/sliding or fixed.

Trans man A trans man (sometimes trans man or transman) is a man who was assigned female at birth. The label transgender man is not always interchangeable with that of transsexual man, however the two labels are often used in this way. Transgender is an umbrella term that includes different types of gender-variant people (including transsexual people).

Transmission-based precautions (TBP) Incorporating isolation procedures, previously often known as 'barrier nursing'. Should be applied in addition to standard precautions when highly transmissible or antimicrobial-resistant microorganisms are present in a patient. The procedures are commonly categorised by the organism's main route of transmission, the most common being contact, droplet and airborne.

Trans woman A trans woman (sometimes trans woman or transwoman) is a woman who was assigned male at birth. The label transgender woman is not always interchangeable with that of transsexual woman, however the two labels are often used in this way. Transgender is an umbrella term that includes different types of gender-variant people (including transsexual people).

Trauma nursing Includes several roles: initial care in the emergency department, care of relatives, involvement in organ and tissue donation, health promotion/injury prevention and rehabilitation.

Tremor Rhythmic, involuntary movement – may occur at rest or on movement.

Trichomoniasis Inflammation of the vagina (vaginitis) or urethritis in males caused by the motile protozoan *Trichomonas vaginalis* (TV). Usually sexually acquired.

Tuberculosis (TB) A chronic granulomatous infection caused by the bacterium *Mycobacterium tuberculosis*. Mainly affects the lungs (pulmonary TB) but may affect the kidneys, uterine tubes, bones and joints, gastrointestinal tract and lymph nodes, or cause meningitis.

Uraemia (azotaemia) Increased levels of waste products including urea and other nitrogenous substances in the blood. It leads to electrolyte and acid–base imbalance. Caused by severely impaired renal function or renal failure.

Urgency The sensation of an immediate need to pass urine, it may have a motor or sensory cause.

Urinary catheterisation The passage of a tube through the urethra or suprapubically through the abdominal wall into the bladder to drain urine. Also required for certain investigations, e.g. cystometry, and to administer intravesical medication.

Vegetative state (VS) Describes a condition that may occur following a severe brain injury, where there is extensive damage to the cerebral cortex. Although the patient has sleep/waking cycles, the higher centres of the brain are destroyed. The brain stem is functioning but the cerebral cortex is not and patients can survive for several years requiring full-time nursing care.

Venous disease Includes venous insufficiency, venous ulcers, venous thromboembolism (VTE) (deep vein thrombosis, pulmonary embolism), and varicose veins.

Ventilator acquired pneumonia (VAP) Pneumonia diagnosed more than 48 hours following the insertion of an endotracheal tube and the commencement of mechanical ventilation.

Vertigo A disturbance of equilibrium in the absence of an external cause which creates a sensation of rotating motion of oneself or one's surroundings. Often described as a whirling sensation, but rocking and swaying sensations are also reported. May be accompanied by pallor, nausea and vomiting.

Visual impairment (VI) Some degree of low vision, sight impairment or total blindness. Important causes worldwide include cataract, trachoma caused by *Chlamydia trachomatis*, onchocerciasis (river blindness – caused by *Onchocerca volvulus*, a parasitic microfilarial worm), xerophthalmia (vitamin A deficiency), glaucoma, macular degeneration, diabetic and other retinopathies and trauma.

Wallace's rule of nines A simple method of assessing the percentage of body surface area affected by a burn injury, using standard body maps. In adults, the head and upper limbs each equal 9%, while the anterior trunk, the posterior trunk and the lower limbs each equal 18%. The remaining 1% is usually applied to the perineum.

Weaning The gradual transition from mechanical ventilatory support to spontaneous ventilation (self-ventilation).

Wound assessment The state of the wound and surrounding skin is assessed using a range of wound criteria. Wound assessment charts will usually collect information around key parameters which suggest if the wound is healing, deteriorating or static. Key parameters include: cause and location of the wound, size of wound, pain, condition of surrounding skin, volume of exudate, odour and type and amount of tissue, e.g. necrotic tissue, slough, granulation, epithelialisation.

Wound dressing Product applied to surgical or medical wounds, e.g. pressure ulcers. Dressings should be permeable to water vapour and gases but not to bacteria or liquids, thus retaining serous exudate. Vitally they do not adhere to the wound surface, thereby reducing damage to new tissue during dressing change.

Wound healing A complex series of events comprising haemostasis, inflammation, proliferation and maturation. The events depend on many patient and environmental factors and can easily be disrupted by inappropriate care.

Index

Page numbers followed by '*f*' indicate figures, '*t*' indicate tables, and '*b*' indicate boxes.